ESSENTIAL ADOLESCENT MEDICINE

NOTICE

Medicine is an ever-changing science. As new research and clinical experience broaden our knowledge, changes in treatment and drug therapy are required. The authors and the publisher of this work have checked with sources believed to be reliable in their efforts to provide information that is complete and generally in accord with the standards accepted at the time of publication. However, in view of the possibility of human error or changes in medical sciences, neither the editors nor the publisher nor any other party who has been involved in the preparation or publication of this work warrants that the information contained herein is in every respect accurate or complete, and they disclaim all responsibility for any errors or omissions or for the results obtained from use of the information contained in this work. Readers are encouraged to confirm the information contained herein with other sources. For example and in particular, readers are advised to check the product information sheet included in the package of each drug they plan to administer to be certain that the information contained in this work is accurate and that changes have not been made in the recommended dose or in the contraindications for administration. This recommendation is of particular importance in connection with new or infrequently used drugs.

ESSENTIAL ADOLESCENT MEDICINE

Donald E. Greydanus, MD, FSAM, FAAP, FIAP(H)

Professor, Pediatrics & Human Development
Michigan State University College of Human Medicine
Pediatrics Program Director
Michigan State University/Kalamazoo Center for Medical Studies
Kalamazoo, Michigan

Dilip R. Patel, MD, FSAM, FAAP, FAACPDM, FACSM

Professor, Pediatrics & Human Development
Michigan State University College of Human Medicine
Michigan State University/Kalamazoo Center for Medical Studies
Kalamazoo, Michigan

Helen D. Pratt, PhD

Licensed Clinical Psychologist
Professor, Pediatrics & Human Development
Michigan State University College of Human Medicine
Director, Behavioral & Developmental Pediatrics
Pediatrics Program
Michigan State University/Kalamazoo Center for Medical Studies
Kalamazoo, Michigan

McGraw-Hill
Medical Publishing Division

NEW YORK / CHICAGO / SAN FRANCISCO / LISBON / LONDON
MADRID / MEXICO CITY / MILAN / NEW DELHI / SAN JUAN
SEOUL / SINGAPORE / SYDNEY / TORONTO

Essential Adolescent Medicine

Copyright © 2006 by The McGraw-Hill Companies, Inc. All rights reserved.
Printed in the United States of America. Except as permitted under the United
States Copyright Act of 1976, no part of this publication may be reproduced or
distributed in any form or by any means, or stored in a data base or retrieval system without the prior written permission of the publisher.

1 2 3 4 5 6 7 8 9 0 DOC/DOC 0 9 8 7 6 5

ISBN 0-07-143843-2

This book was set in Times Roman by International Typesetting and
Composition.
The editors were James F. Shanahan and Robert Pancotti.
The production supervisor was Sherri Souffrance.
Project management was provided by International Typesetting and
Composition.
The indexer was Susan G. Hunter.
RR Donnelley was printer and binder.

This book is printed on acid-free paper.

Library of Congress Cataloging-in-Publication Data

Essential adolescent medicine / editors, Donald E. Greydanus, Dilip R. Patel, Helen D. Pratt.
   p. ; cm.
  Includes bibliographical references and index.
  ISBN 0-07-143843-2 (alk. paper)
  1. Adolescent medicine. I. Greydanus, Donald E. II. Patel, Dilip R. III. Pratt, Helen D.
  [DNLM: 1. Adolescent Medicine. 2. Adolescent Development. 3. Adolescent
  Psychology. 4. Health Behavior—Adolescent. WS 460 E78 2005]
  RJ550.E875 2005
  616′.00835—dc22
                                2005041602

This magnum opus *is dedicated to Margaret Elizabeth Greydanus and Adele Dellenbaugh Hofmann, with much love and admiration for two remarkable women who are for all seasons and for all times. This "fourth" is for you.*

Requiescat in Pace cum Deo.

CONTENTS

CONTRIBUTORS

JOYCE A. ADAMS, MD
Clinical Professor of Pediatrics
School of Medicine
University of California, San Diego
San Diego, California

KAREN H. ALBRITTON, MD
Director, Adolescent & Young Adult Oncology
Assistant Professor, Center for Sarcoma & Bone Oncology
Dana Farber Cancer Institute and Harvard University
Boston, Massachusetts

LEAH K. ANDREWS, MBCHB, FRANZCP
Senior Lecturer, Psychiatry
School of Medicine
University of Auckland
Auckland, New Zealand

ROBERTA K. BEACH, MD, MPH
Professor Emeritus of Pediatrics and Adolescent Medicine
University of Colorado School of Medicine
Denver, Colorado

DAVID L. BENNETT, MBBS, FRACP
Head, Department of Adolescent Medicine
Director, New South Wales Centre for the Advancement of
    Adolescent Health
Clinical Associate Professor, Department of Paediatrics &
    Child Health
The University of Sydney
The Children's Hospital at Westmead
Westmead, New South Wales, Australia

SWATI Y. BHAVE, MD, DCH, FCPS, FIAP, FAAP
Consulting Pediatrician, Indraprastha Apollo Hospital
New Delhi, India
Former Professor of Pediatrics, BJ Medical College
Pune, India
Former Associate Professor and Consulting Paediatrician
Bombay Hospital & Medical Research Centre
Mumbai, India
Director, "Expressions India"
Mumbai Branch, India

W. ARCHIE BLEYER, MD
Director Emeritus, Community Clinical Oncology Program
Professor and Chair Emeritus of Pediatrics
Chair, Children's Cancer Group
Adolescent and Young Adult Committee
The University of Texas M.D. Anderson Cancer Center
Houston, Texas

MARGARET J. BLYTHE, MD
Professor of Pediatrics
Director of Adolescent Clinical Services
Indiana University School of Medicine
Indianapolis, Indiana

CARTER D. BROOKS, MD
Professor, Pediatrics & Human Development
Michigan State University College
    of Human Medicine
Pediatrics Program
Michigan State University/Kalamazoo Center for
    Medical Studies
Kalamazoo, Michigan

JON B. BRUSS, MD, MSPH, MBA
Vice President and Chief Medical Officer
PediaMed Pharmaceuticals, Inc.
Florence, Kentucky

MOZHDEH B. BRUSS, PHD, MPH, RD
Assistant Professor, Family and Consumer Sciences
Western Michigan University
Kalamazoo, Michigan

PETER CHOWN, BSCPSYCH, MAPS
Psychologist and Consultant
New South Wales Centre for the Advancement of
    Adolescent Health
New South Wales, Australia

GLENN CRAIG DAVIS, MD
Dean, College of Human Medicine
Michigan State University
East Lansing, Michigan

DAVID S. DICKENS, MD
Clinical Assistant Professor of Pediatrics &
    Human Development
Michigan State University College of Human Medicine
Associate Director of Clinical Services
Division of Pediatric Hematology/Oncology & Blood and
    Bone Marrow Transplantation
DeVos Children's Hospital
Grand Rapids, Michigan

MARTIN B. DRAZNIN, MD
Professor, Pediatrics & Human Development
Michigan State University College of Human Medicine
Director, Pediatric Endocrine Division
Pediatrics Program
Michigan State University/Kalamazoo Center for
    Medical Studies
Kalamazoo, Michigan

ARTHUR N. FEINBERG, MD
Professor, Pediatrics & Human Development
Michigan State University College of Human Medicine
Pediatric Clinic Director
Michigan State University/Kalamazoo Center for
    Medical Studies
Kalamazoo, Michigan

LISA A. FEINBERG, MD
Clinical Associate, Department of Pediatric Gastroenterology
Cleveland Clinic Foundation
Cleveland, Ohio

DAVID R. FREYER, DO
Associate Professor of Pediatrics & Human Development
Michigan State University College of
    Human Medicine
Director of Clinical Research Programs
Division of Pediatric Hematology/Oncology & Blood and
    Bone Marrow Transplantation
DeVos Children's Hospital
Grand Rapids, Michigan

RENUKA GERA, MD
Professor and Associate Chair, Department of
    Pediatrics/Human Development
Division of Pediatric and Adolescent
    Hematology/Oncology
Principal Investigator, Children's Oncology Group
Michigan State University
East Lansing, Michigan

NEVILLE H. GOLDEN, MD
Professor of Clinical Pediatrics
Albert Einstein College of Medicine
Director, Eating Disorders Center
Division of Adolescent Medicine
Schneider Children's Hospital
North Shore Long Island Jewish Health System
New Hyde Park, New York

TATIANA PAVLOVA GREENFIELD, MD, PhD
Fellow, Section of Adolescent Medicine
Department of Pediatrics
Indiana University School of Medicine
Indianapolis, Indiana

DONALD E. GREYDANUS, MD, FSAM, FAAP, FIAP(H)
Professor, Pediatrics & Human Development
Michigan State University College of Human Medicine
Pediatrics Program Director
Michigan State University/Kalamazoo Center for
    Medical Studies
Kalamazoo, Michigan

DOUGLAS N. HOMNICK, MD, MPH
Professor, Pediatrics & Human Development
Michigan State University College of Human Medicine
Director, Pediatric Pulmonary Division
Pediatrics Program
Michigan State University/Kalamazoo Center for
    Medical Studies
Kalamazoo, Michigan

RENÉE R. JENKINS, MD
Professor and Chair, Department of Pediatrics &
    Child Health
Howard University College of Medicine
Washington, D.C.

JENNIFER JOHNSON, MD, MS
Emeritus Professor of Pediatrics
University of California, Irvine
Irvine, California

MELISSA KANG, MBBS, MCh
Lecturer, Department of General Practice
The University of Sydney at Westmead Hospital
Consultant, New South Wales Centre for the Advancement
    of Adolescent Health
New South Wales, Australia

DAVID W. KAPLAN, MD
Division of Adolescent Medicine
University of Colorado
Children's Hospital Denver
Denver, Colorado

PARITOSH KAUL, MD
Assistant Professor of Pediatrics
Section of Adolescent Medicine
University of Colorado School of Medicine
Westside Teen Clinic
Denver Health
Denver, Colorado

CHARLES F. KOOPMANN, JR., MD
Professor and Associate Chair, Otolaryngology-Head &
    Neck Surgery
Professor, Department of Pediatrics
University of Michigan School of Medicine
UMMC-Pediatric Otolaryngology
University of Michigan Health System
Ann Arbor, Michigan

DANIEL P. KROWCHUK, MD
Professor, Pediatrics and Dermatology
Department of Pediatrics
Wake Forest University School of Medicine
Director of Adolescent Medicine and Co-Director of
    Pediatric Dermatology
Brenner Children's Hospital
Winston-Salem, North Carolina

ROSHNI KULKARNI, MD
Professor, Pediatrics & Human Development
Director, Division of Pediatric and Adolescent
    Hematology/Oncology
Pediatric Director, MSU Comprehensive Center for
    Bleeding & Clotting Disorders
Michigan State University College of Human Medicine
East Lansing, Michigan

BENNETT L. LEVENTHAL, MD
Professor of Psychiatry
Director, Center for Child Mental Health &
    Developmental Neuroscience
University of Illinois College of Medicine
Chicago, Illinois

EUGENE F. LUCKSTEAD, SR., MD
Professor, Pediatrics and Cardiology
Department of Pediatrics
Texas Tech Medical School–Amarillo
Amarillo, Texas

ANNE LYREN, MD
Associate Director, Rainbow Center for Pediatric Ethics
Assistant Professor of Pediatrics
Rainbow Babies & Children's Hospital
Cleveland, Ohio

MARY D. MOORE, MD
Director, Pediatric Rheumatology
Pediatrics Program
Michigan State University/Kalamazoo Center for
    Medical Studies
Kalamazoo, Michigan

H. NOUBANI, MD
Pediatric Cardiology
Department of Pediatrics
Texas Tech Medical School–Amarillo
Amarillo, Texas

DILIP R. PATEL, MD, FSAM, FAAP, FAACPDM, FACSM
Professor, Pediatrics & Human Development
Michigan State University College of Human Medicine
Michigan State University/Kalamazoo Center for
    Medical Studies
Kalamazoo, Michigan

VENUS PAXTON, MD
Department of Psychiatry
University of Chicago
Chicago, Illinois

MAIJA PETERSONS, PHD, RD
Professor, Family & Consumer Sciences
Western Michigan University
Kalamazoo, Michigan

HELEN D. PRATT, PHD
Licensed Clinical Psychologist
Professor, Pediatrics & Human Development
Michigan State University College of Human Medicine
Director, Behavioral & Developmental Pediatrics
Pediatrics Program
Michigan State University/Kalamazoo Center for
    Medical Studies
Kalamazoo, Michigan

TINA R. RAINE, MD, MPH
Associate Professor
Department of Obstetrics, Gynecology, and
  Reproductive Sciences
University of California, San Francisco
San Francisco General Hospital
San Francisco, California

MARY ELLEN RIMSZA, MD
Professor, School of Health Management and Policy
W. P. Carey School of Business
Arizona State University, Tempe
Professor of Pediatrics
Mayo Graduate School of Medicine, Scottsdale
Professor of Clinical Pediatrics
University of Arizona College of Medicine
Tucson, Arizona

ELLEN S. ROME, MD, MPH
Head, Section of Adolescent Medicine
The Cleveland Clinic Children's Hospital
Associate Professor of Pediatrics
The Cleveland Clinic Lerner College of Medicine at
  Case Western Reserve
Cleveland, Ohio

JOHN D. ROWLETT, MD
Assistant Professor of Pediatrics
Medical College of Georgia
Augusta, Georgia
Director of Pediatrics
Georgia Emergency Associates
St. Joseph/Candler Hospital
Savannah, Georgia

JOHN N. SCHUEN, MD
Assistant Clinical Professor of Pediatrics
Michigan State University College of Human Medicine
Chief, Division of Pediatric Pulmonary &
  Sleep Medicine
Director, Pediatric Sleep Laboratory
DeVos Children's Hospital at Spectrum Health
Grand Rapids, Michigan

AJOVI B. SCOTT-EMUAKPOR, MD, PhD
Professor, Department of Pediatrics/Human Development
Director, Pediatric & Adolescent Sickle Cell Program
Division of Pediatric and Adolescent
  Hematology/Oncology
Michigan State University
East Lansing, Michigan

AMIT SEN, MBBS, MD, MRCPSYCH (UK), CCST
Senior Consultant Child & Adolescent Psychiatry
Sitaram Bhartia Institute of Science & Research
Head of Mental Health Program
Salaam Balak Trust
New Delhi, India

ERIC J. SIGEL, MD
Associate Professor of Pediatrics
University of Colorado Denver Health Science Center
Children's Hospital Denver
Denver, Colorado

TOMAS JOSE SILBER, MD
Director, Adolescent Medicine Fellowship
Director, Office of Ethics
Children's National Medical Center
Professor of Pediatrics, George Washington University
Washington, D.C.

RUSSELL W. STEELE, MD
Professor and Vice Chairman
Department of Pediatrics
Louisiana State University Health Sciences Center
Division of Infectious Diseases
Children's Hospital
New Orleans, Louisiana

MICHAEL STEPHENS, MD
Assistant Professor of Pediatrics
Medical College of Wisconsin
Children's Hospital of Wisconsin
Milwaukee, Wisconsin

HELGA V. TORIELLO, MS, PhD
Professor, Pediatrics & Human Development
Michigan State University
Genetics Services
Spectrum Health
Grand Rapids, Michigan

ALFONSO D. TORRES, MD
Director, Pediatric Nephrology
Pediatrics Program
Michigan State University/Kalamazoo Center for
  Medical Studies
Kalamazoo, Michigan

DAVID H. VAN DYKE, MD
Professor of Neurology and Pediatrics
Michigan State University
East Lansing, Michigan

JULIAN H. WAN, MD
Associate Clinical Professor, Pediatric Urology
University of Michigan School of Medicine
Ann Arbor, Michigan

STEVEN WERLIN, MD
Professor of Pediatrics
Medical College of Wisconsin
Children's Hospital of Wisconsin
Milwaukee, Wisconsin

JOHN SCOTT WERRY, MD
Professor Emeritus of Psychiatry
University of Auckland School of Medicine
Auckland, New Zealand

PATIENCE HAYDOCK WHITE, MD
Professor of Pediatrics and Medicine
George Washington University School of
    Medicine and Health Sciences
Research Director, Adolescent Employment
    Readiness Center
Children's National Medical Center
Washington, D.C.

FOREWORD

Adolescent medicine as a subspecialty of pediatrics has only recently been defined. Starting in the late 1700s and continuing to the present, there has been interest in the physical and psychologic growth and development of adolescents and in their unique medical and psychosocial needs. The first formal unit for adolescent medicine was developed in 1951 at the Boston's Children's Hospital by Dr. J. Roswell Gallagher. The Society for Adolescent Medicine was established in 1968 and research presentations were begun in that forum in 1973.

As we start the twenty-first century, we find that many of the unique characteristics of adolescents are being defined by our greater understanding of both biology and behavior and of the interface between biology and behavior. Our increased understanding of hormonal assays, neurotransmitters, and brain functioning, as well as increased sophistication in evaluating the cognitive and intellectual capacities of adolescents allow us to appreciate both the complexity and the predictability of adolescent growth and behavior.

Despite this increasing sophistication, there is ever-increasing morbidity related to adolescent biologic changes, adolescent behavioral changes, and a vastly changing unstable world. As the adolescent matures, there is less predictability in many adolescents' families, schools, and communities. Thus, we see the emergence of medical and behavioral conditions resulting from violence, dysfunctional families, premature sexual behavior, and substance abuse. Many "adult" morbidities, including hypertension, obesity, arteriosclerotic disease, and gastrointestinal conditions, are now being identified in adolescence and childhood. The antecedents of adolescent medical and behavioral morbidity may even start as early as the prenatal period. Thus, to comprehend fully the impact of morbidity in adolescence, the practitioner must understand the science of adolescent biology and behavior and the psychosocial ecology of the family, the schools, and the community.

Essential Adolescent Medicine introduces readers to the practice of adolescent medicine with a thorough discussion of growth and development, office care of the adolescent, and contemporary subjects such as end-of-life care. Medical conditions are reviewed thoroughly, including sleep disorders and disorders of genetics, areas about which scientific information has emerged quickly. A separate section on sexual and gynecologic health is a contemporary review of current information. The editors dedicate a separate section to eating disorders because of the morbidity related to both the restriction of food and the overuse of food in our society. Sports medicine also takes an important place in this edition, as it is growing in importance. The mental health section covers many of the most vexing conditions of adolescents.

We welcome this text as an important update about the most challenging adolescent patients for whom we care. Despite many opportunities for the world to be a more pessimistic place than it was previously, those of us who work with adolescents remain optimistic as these patients continue to adapt to a rapidly changing world.

Elizabeth R. McAnarney, MD
Professor and Chair
Department of Pediatrics
University of Rochester Medical Center
Rochester, New York

PREFACE

All of us pass through different phases like childhood, adolescence, adulthood, parenthood, others. In each phase, we experience certain difficult periods and come out with wonderful discoveries. With some insight into our lives, we can definitely say that "Teen years" or "Adolescence" is one of the most challenging periods![1]

The term *adolescence* was first used in the fifteenth century and is derived from the Latin word *adolescere*, meaning "to grow into maturity." Adolescence is the critical process in which the human being leaves the dependency of childhood and enters a period of dramatic changes, which leads to adulthood. Physiologic, psychologic, and sociologic issues occur during this complex developmental time that acts as a unique bridge, accepting the successes and failures of childhood and setting in the changes necessary for an autonomous adulthood. The peak rates of growth and development during adolescence are exceeded only by those of fetal life and early infancy.

Worry about the adolescent has been a universal theme of human society, probably since *Homo sapiens* emerged more than 50,000 years ago.[2] In the eighth century B.C., Hesiod lamented a universal concern about teenagers:

I see no hope for the future of our people if they are dependent on the frivolous youth of today, for certainly all youth are reckless beyond words....

When I was a boy, we were exceedingly wise and impatient of restraint.[3]

Interest by American clinicians in the issues of adolescents started with the work of G. Stanley Hall (1844–1924), the first person in the United States to earn a PhD in psychology. Hall wrote the first classic text on adolescence and coined the term *Sturm und Drang* (storm and tempest) to describe the process of adolescence as turbulent.[4]

Some of Hall's conclusions were based on work performed in the physiology lab of H. P. Bowditch,[5] the scientist whose monumental work on growth in 1877 led to the classic work of J. M. Tanner[6] published in 1955 and 1962.

The first American medical clinic for adolescents was established in 1918 at Stanford University. The concept of a clinic for adolescents was later augmented by the work of Dr. J. R. Gallagher, who established an adolescent clinic in 1951 in Boston.[7] Gallagher also published the first textbook on medical care of teenagers.[8] This classic book had three editions, in 1960, 1966, and 1976. Gallagher's view that the opinions of adolescents should be valued more than those of the parents remains controversial in today's milieu. Gallagher is honored by today's adolescent medicine clinicians as the "father of adolescent medicine" in American medicine of the twentieth century. In the preface to the first edition of his book, Gallagher noted:

Adolescents are different, and it is clearly desirable to think about them in different terms than one does of a little child or an adult. So, too, is the doctor's relationship to these patients different; no longer is it the parent who tells all the story, and now the patient requires very considerable evidence of his doctor's interest in him. How to talk to these young people (or better how to get them to talk to you!), how to deal with them effectively, how to utilize for their own good their tendency to accept advice from and to imitate and to talk freely to other adults than their parents—these we have considered to be important topics.[8]

The official recognition of adolescents as worthy of inclusion in the health care provided by pediatricians was by the American Academy of Pediatrics in 1972; the Academy noted that pediatricians should care for those up to age 21. Promotion of the study of adolescence was fostered effectively in the last quarter of the twentieth century by the Society for Adolescent Medicine (SAM). SAM was established in 1968 and has influenced the education and research of adolescent medicine for many educators, clinicians, and researchers who have sought continually to improve the lives of adolescents in the United States and throughout the world.[9] It was Adele D. Hofmann who picked up the mantle of J. Roswell Gallagher and produced a classic text of adolescent medicine in 1983.[10] This text, like Gallagher's work, went on to three editions (1983, 1989, and 1997) and stimulated other texts of adolescent medicine in the 1990s and early in the twenty-first century.

Essential Adolescent Medicine considers intrinsic concepts of adolescent medicine as outlined in the six parts of the book. Part I presents an introduction to adolescent medicine, with discussions on growth and development, caring for teens in the office, legal and ethical aspects, cultural diversity, transition to adulthood, and end-of-life concepts. Part II presents an overview of much of the *medicine* of adolescent medicine. This part of the book deals with the key organ systems of the body, including concepts of pulmonology, cardiology, gastroenterology, neurology, endocrinology, nephrology, and others. Part III examines sexuality and gynecology, Part IV reviews eating disorders, and Part V considers concepts of sports medicine. Finally, Part VI presents an overview of mental health and the adolescent: substance abuse disorders, disruptive behavioral disorders, mood disorders, anxiety disorders, attention-deficit/hyperactivity disorders, and schizophrenia.

Much has been learned since the days of Hesiod regarding behavior and biology in adolescents. The editors of this text hope that this work will be useful to the many clinicians who care comprehensively for adolescents and their families. A wide variety of experts in the field of adolescent medicine have been gathered and I thank them all for working with us on this exciting project. I thank my co-editors, Dilip R. Patel, MD, and Helen D. Pratt, PhD, for their wonderful assistance in the development of this *magnum opus* and for their continued colleagueship and friendship. I am also grateful to the medical publishing division of McGraw-Hill for allowing us to produce this book. I especially thank James F. Shanahan and Robert Pancotti at McGraw-Hill for wonderful encouragement and superb technical assistance in the development of *Essential Adolescent Medicine*.

Events in twentieth century America resulted in diverse opinions about the process of adolescence and the role of youth; the twenty-first century continues to struggle with these different opinions. However, we can change history's lament about the impossible adolescent and teach society about the positive effects that each generation of adolescents will have for the future. We clinicians, privileged to care for adolescents, can be of immense positive influence in this regard.

I am full of hope, and even while I speak in some distress.

My hope is that tomorrow's child will speak of great progress![11]

Donald E. Greydanus, MD, FSAM, FAAP, FIAP(H)

References

1   Nair MKC: *Adolescence and Family Life Education.* Standard Press: Bangalore, India, 2002.

2   Magner LN: *A History of the Life Sciences,* 3d ed. New York: Marcel Dekker, 2002, 502 pp.

3   Greydanus DE: Adolescent sexuality: An overview and perspective. *Pediatric Ann* 11:714–726, 1982.

4   Stanley HG: *Adolescence: Its Psychology and its Relationship to Physiology, Anthropology, Sociology, Sex, Crime, Religion, and Education.* New York: Appleton, 1904.

5   Bowditch HP: *Growth of Children.* Boston, MA: AJ Wright State Printer, 1877.

6   Tanner JM: *Growth at Adolescence.* Oxford: Blackwell Scientific Publications, 1955; 1962.

7   Gallagher JR: The origins, development, and goals of adolescent medicine. *J Adolesc Health Care* 3:57–63, 1982.

8   Gallagher JR: *Medical Care of the Adolescent.* New York: Appleton-Century-Crofts, 1960.

9   Brown RC, Cromer BA, Brookman RR, Moore E: The Society for Adolescent Medicine: The first thirty years. *J Adolesc Health* 23:133–174, 1998.

10 Hofmann AD: *Adolescent Medicine.* Menlo Park, CA: Addison-Wesley, 1983, 448 pp.

11 WHO, UNCF: A Healthy Start in Life. *Report on the Global Consultation on Child and Adolescent Health and Development. March 12–13, 2002.* Stockholm, Sweden. WHO: Geneva, Switzerland, 2002.

ESSENTIAL ADOLESCENT MEDICINE

INTRODUCTION TO ADOLESCENT HEALTH

1

ADOLESCENT GROWTH AND DEVELOPMENT

Eric J. Sigel

INTRODUCTION

Adolescence is an exciting and dynamic time, both from a biologic as well as a developmental and psychologic perspective. Understanding adolescent growth and development provides the foundation for understanding healthy teenagers as well as identifying aberrations that allow the practitioner to intervene accordingly. First, normal pubertal physiology and growth will be addressed, providing the reader a framework to understand the biology of puberty. Second, developmental milestones will be defined, which will allow the reader to identify normal development and understand some of the risk morbidities that occurs during this time.

Adolescence conjures myriad definitions interpreted differently by society, media, and biology. For the sake of addressing adolescent growth, the definition of an adolescent implies the time when a still unknown process initiates the transformation from latency to full adult physical maturity, beginning as early as 7 or 8 years, and culminating between 16 and 18 years. Adolescent psychologic development may begin as early as when initial physical changes occur, but is classically described as occurring between the ages 12 and 21, extending beyond pubertal completion. Some social scientists now define adulthood beginning at age 26, which would then expand the range of adolescence lasting until 25.

Recent Issues in Assessing Initiation of Puberty

Debate exists in assessing whether puberty has truly decreased in onset over time. Two major studies have been completed and written about recently, the PROS[1] (Pediatric Research in Office Settings) study first published in 1997, and the NHANES III[2] (National Health and Nutrition Examination Survey) data, collected during 1988–1994 and written about extensively in the last several years.[3] Data for both were robust, though each had limitations. Discussion about results has been intense. Authors using the same NHANES data arrived at different conclusions regarding the age of onset of menses, depending on the statistical method used. A commentary by Herman-Giddens, et al.[4] provides an excellent discussion about the issues raised. Interpreting results from different studies does indicate that girls are in fact reaching menarche at an earlier age and puberty overall seems to be occurring earlier in both boys and girls.

Intellectual and practical challenges exist for the clinician as well. Detection of, and what constitutes the initiation of puberty has been debated. It is recognized that the disinhibition of the hypothalamic-pituitary-gonadal axis and subsequent physical changes of the breast bud and testicle is the hallmark of the initiation of puberty. However, adrenarche, under the stimulation of adrenal androgens separate from gonadal production, often appears early, specifically in Black girls. Clinicians certainly use pubic hair staging in pubertal assessment, but it is unclear how this sign should be used in the evaluation of precocious puberty. Additional challenges include how and when clinicians should actually assess the initiation of puberty. The PROS study used visual sexual maturity rating (SMR) or Tanner stages, instead of direct palpation of breast buds (Fig. 1-1). With increased adiposity, it can be difficult to distinguish breast tissue from fat. One study[2] that used NHANES data, concluded that the median age to reach genital stage 2 in White boys is 10.03 years while median age for thelarche, or breast stage 2 for White girls is 10.38 years, which suggests that puberty may begin earlier in boys than girls (Figs. 1-1 to 1-3). This fact contradicts what is standardly accepted. Additional research from Biro,[v] in a paper published in 1995, has suggested to create an extra SMR stage (genital 2A and 2B) that is

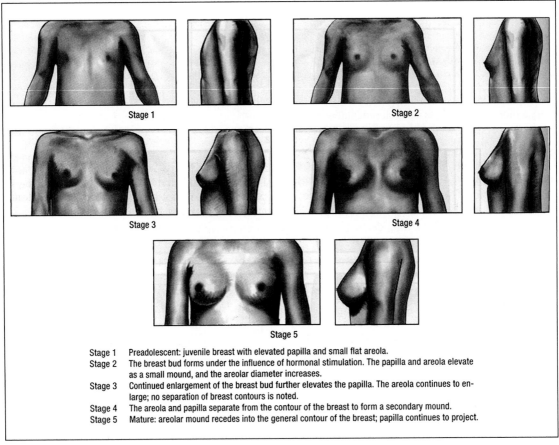

Stage 1

Stage 2

Stage 3

Stage 4

Stage 5

Stage 1   Preadolescent: juvenile breast with elevated papilla and small flat areola.
Stage 2   The breast bud forms under the influence of hormonal stimulation. The papilla and areola elevate as a small mound, and the areolar diameter increases.
Stage 3   Continued enlargement of the breast bud further elevates the papilla. The areola continues to enlarge; no separation of breast contours is noted.
Stage 4   The areola and papilla separate from the contour of the breast to form a secondary mound.
Stage 5   Mature: areolar mound recedes into the general contour of the breast; papilla continues to project.

FIGURE 1-1

MATURATIONAL STAGES OF FEMALE BREAST DEVELOPMENT.
Source: Used with permission from: Hofmann AD, Greydanus DE. Adolescent medicine, 3d ed., Stamford, CT: Appleton & Lange, 1997,16.

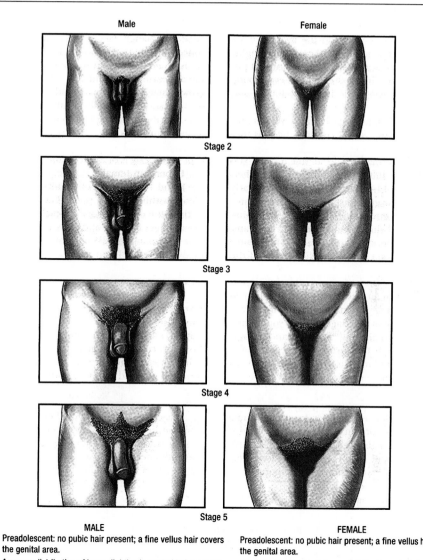

Male   Female

Stage 2

Stage 3

Stage 4

Stage 5

MALE

Stage 1	Preadolescent: no pubic hair present; a fine vellus hair covers the genital area.
Stage 2	A sparse distribution of long, slightly pigmented hair appears at the base of the penis.
Stage 3	The pubic hair pigmentation increases; the hairs begin to curl and to spread laterally in a scanty distribution.
Stage 4	The pubic hairs continue to curl and become coarse in texture. An adult type of distribution is attained, but the number of hairs remains fewer.
Stage 5	Mature: the pubic hair attains an adult distribution with spread to the surface of the medial thigh. Pubic hair will grow along linea alba in 80% of males.

FEMALE

Preadolescent: no pubic hair present; a fine vellus hair covers the genital area.

A sparse distribution of long, slightly pigmented straight hair appears bilaterally along medial border of the labia majora.

The pubic hair pigmentation increases; the hairs begin to curl and to spread sparsely over the mons pubis.

The pubic hairs continue to curl and become coarse in texture. The number of hairs continues to increase.

Mature: pubic hair attains an adult feminine triangular pattern, with spread to the surface of the medial thigh.

FIGURE 1-2

MATURATIONAL STAGES OF MALE AND FEMALE PUBIC HAIR DEVELOPMENT.
Source: Used with permission from: Hofmann AD, Greydanus DE. Adolescent medicine, 3d ed., Stamford, CT: Appleton & Lange, 1997,16.

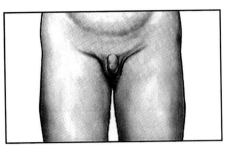

Stage 1

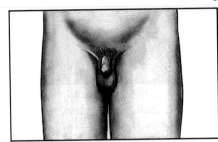

Stage 2

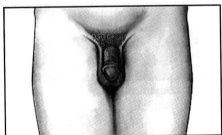

Stage 3

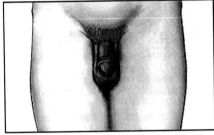

Stage 4

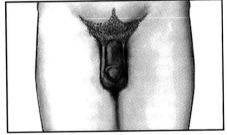

Stage 5

Stage 1   Preadolescent: testes, scrotum, and penis identical to early childhood.
Stage 2   Enlargement of testes as result of canalization of seminiferous tubules. The scrotum enlarges, de-
           veloping a reddish hue and altering its skin texture. The penis enlarges slightly.
Stage 3   The testes and scrotum continue to grow. The length of the penis increases.
Stage 4   The testes and scrotum continue to grow; the scrotal skin darkens. The penis grows in width, and
           the glans penis develops.
Stage 5   Mature: adult size and shape of testes, scrotum, and penis.

FIGURE 1-3

MATURATIONAL STAGES OF MALE GENITAL DEVELOPMENT.
Source: Used with permission from: Hofmann AD, Greydanus DE. Adolescent medicine, 3d ed., Stamford, CT: Appleton & Lange, 1997,16.

shown to have clinical relevance but would require direct palpation and sizing of the testicle, which has not generally been put in practice.

PHYSIOLOGY OF PUBERTY

Intense research has focused on discovering the elusive initial signal that marks the beginning of puberty. Leptin[6] has received attention as the signaling agent that initiates puberty, but further study has not borne this out. Leptin levels do begin to rise 2–3 years earlier than the rise in pubertal hormones,[7] but the increase may be a direct reflection of adiposity. Increasing adiposity[8] and obesity itself has been associated with the initiation of puberty. Girls with higher BMI (Body Mass Index) show evidence of earlier maturation compared to girls with normal BMI, though more research needs to be done to definitively associate degree of adiposity with initiation of puberty. Adrenal adrenarche also has been studied as a possible precursor or signaling agent, but is also as yet unproven.

Regardless of where the green light to start puberty comes from, the initial endocrine change that represents the hallmark of pubertal initiation is the appearance of gonadotropin releasing hormone (GnRH). The hypothalamic-pituitary-gonadal axis has been suppressed to this point. The presence of GnRH, released from the hypothalamus begins to stimulate the pituitary gland. Follicle stimulating hormone (FSH) and luteinizing hormone (LH) are released from the pituitary, initiating the stimulation of gonadal steroids. Gonadal steroids—testosterone and estradiol—are then released by the testis and ovaries that begins a cascade effect, which leads a healthy individual through the process of puberty.

Once circumstances are right, GnRH begins to increase in amplitude during sleep. GnRH is released in pulsatile form into the pituitary portal plexus, binding to surface receptors on the anterior pituitary, resulting in release of gonadotropins. Initially, GnRH stimulation occurs only at night, with resultant pulsation and increase in amplitude of FSH/LH. Over time, daytime pulsations begin as well. LH pulse

depends on GnRH pulsation throughout puberty, while FSH pulsation becomes independent of GnRH as gonadal activity increases. A negative feedback loop—FSH/LH on the hypothalamus and gonadal steroids on both the hypothalamus and pituitary—exist that allows puberty to occur slowly over time. Contributing to the feedback loop are peptides, secreted by the gonads. Inhibin and follistatin decrease FSH biosynthesis and its secretion at the pituitary level, while activin increases biosynthesis of FSH.[9] Inhibin levels rise during puberty.[10]

The first hormonal changes begin to occur between ages 6 and 8. Hormonal adrenarche may begin at this time, with release of androgenic hormones from the adrenal gland. Main contributors include dehydroepiandrosterone (DHEA), DHEA-sulphate (DHEAS), and androstenedione. This appears to be independent of hypothalamic/pituitary stimulation as gonadal hormones remain at prepubertal levels. Some evidence indicates a slow increase of adrenal androgens from as early as 3 years old.[11] Increase in gonadal androgens appears approximately 2 years after the rise of adrenal androgens. Adrenal androgens can be converted to active testosterone and estradiol in extra glandular tissue. DHEA and DHEAS continue to rise throughout puberty, reaching a peak between ages 20 and 30. Some feel that the presence of androgens is what leads to reversing the inhibition on the hypothalamus.

Female Physiology

On average, girls begin puberty about one or two years earlier than boys, with the average initiation of puberty happening around age 10. In the ovaries, LH stimulates the theca interna cells to synthesize estrogen precursors and FSH stimulates the production of the enzyme aromatase, which converts androgen precursors to estrogen. Estradiol is the major estrogen, 90% of which is secreted by the ovary. The remaining fraction of estradiol comes from the extraglandular conversion of testosterone and androstenedione.

As estrogens are produced, they begin to have end-organ effects on the ovary and rest of the body. Girls experience breast budding (*thelarche*) as the first outward sign of puberty, which occurs under estrogen stimulation. Average age of initiation of thelarche has decreased over time. As discussed earlier, there is variability between studies as to the mean age of thelarche. Thelarche does occur nearly one year earlier in Blacks compared to Whites. The mean age of thelarche in Blacks ranges from 8.87 to 9.5 years, for Whites between 9.96 years and 10.38 years,[1,3] and for Mexican Americans 9.8 years. Practically for the clinician, one can use about $9\frac{1}{4}$ for Blacks and about 10 for Whites as the mean age of initiation of thelarche. Around 96% of Whites and 99% Blacks have breast development by age 12. Delayed puberty should be evaluated if there are no signs of breast development by age 13. SMR or Tanner staging is a way to assess normal and abnormal breast development (Figs. 1-1 to 1-3).

Additional changes of puberty include estrogenization of the vaginal mucosa, leading to cellular changes from a predominant columnar epithelium to a squamous epithelium. The vaginal mucosa changes from reddish in color to paler pink. Girls eventually begin to develop physiologic leukorrhea, a thin white discharge resulting from the rapid turnover of the vaginal mucosa. Vaginal fluid becomes acidic with the progression of puberty compared to an alkaline or neutral pH, prepubertally.

The vagina elongates and the uterus begins to develop and enlarge as well, under the influence of estrogen stimulation. Prepubertally, the size of the uterus and cervix exist in a 1:1 ratio. As the uterus grows, it doubles in size from 3.3 cm (SD 1.3 cm) to a final adult size of 6.98 cm (SD 1 cm), representing a 3:1 size ratio compared to the cervix.

Adrenarche

On an average, adrenal activity begins between ages 6 and 8. The mean age of pubic hair development is 8.8 years for Black girls and 10.5 years for White girls. Axillary hair appears later—the mean age of onset being 10.1 years for Black girls and 11.8 years for White girls. Some have proposed classifying axillary hair by stage as well. Stage 1 would be no axillary hair, stage 2 sparse hair, and stage 3 full adult hair (Fig. 1-2). Hormones contributing to

adrenarche are DHEA, DHEAS, androstenedione, and testosterone.

Menarche

As puberty progresses, FSH and LH continue to increase, resulting in subsequent increases in estrogen that is present not only at night but throughout the day. Cycling estrogen promotes the growth of the endometrium, leading to initial uterine bleeding, which is menarche. The average age for menarche has decreased over time. Studies show that the average age of menarche determined by data collected in the 60s was 12.76 years,[12] compared to NHANES data collected during 1988–94 that showed the average age of menarche to be 12.54 years.[13] Black girls begin menses earlier than White girls; 12.1 years compared with 12.6 years. Using NHANES data, the time from onset of thelarche to menarche is 2.6 years for Blacks and 2.2 years for Whites. Commonly, anovulatory cycles exist for the first one or two years post menarche. During this time, the uterus, vagina, ovaries, and fallopian tubes continue to grow. Eventually, the negative feedback loop of estrogen on the hypothalamus changes to being positive. Rising estrogen levels trigger the surge of both FSH and LH, leading to follicular growth and eventual ovulation. Females are born with approximately 2–4 million primordial follicles, though only 400,000 remain at menarche.

The menstrual cycle consists of three stages— the follicular phase, the ovulatory phase, and the luteal phase[14] (Chap. 28). During the follicular phase, estradiol levels begin to increase, causing proliferation of the endometrium. Coinciding with the estradiol increase, FSH rises, stimulating follicular development. Often four follicles begin to grow, but one becomes the dominant follicle and the others become atretic. During the ovulatory phase the surge of LH causes the follicle to release the ovum. Estrogen levels start to diminish and the remaining corpus luteum produces progesterone that prepares the uterine lining for implantation. If fertilization does not happen, then progesterone levels decrease, signaling the uterus to shed, leading to menstruation. The cycle begins again with rising estrogen that leads to the follicular phase.

Male Physiology

Initiation of Puberty

The same hormonal process occurs initially for males as well as females—GnRH appears signaling the activation of the hypothalamic-pituitary-testicular axis. The first outward sign of puberty that the adolescent appreciates will be pubic hair growth. The first detectable pubertal change assessed by clinicians is change in testicular volume. Both FSH and LH induce testicular changes.[15] LH induces Leydig cells to develop and produce testosterone, while FSH stimulates Sertoli cells to produce sperm. FSH binds to the outer membrane of Sertoli cells, activating the seminiferous tubules within the Sertoli cells to grow and begin spermatogenesis. Cellular growth leads to the increase in testicular volume. Pubertal initiation is evident when the testes are 4 cc in volume, measured by an orchiometer, or have a longitudinal axis of 2.5 cm, representing SMR 2 (Fig. 1-3). On an average, this occurs around age 11. Biro[5] and others have proposed an additional genital stage, stage 2A, indicating a volume of 3 cc testicles without pubic hair, which represents a clinically significant change from prepubertal size and the initiation of puberty. This may be clinically useful in evaluating boys for delayed puberty. Black boys enter SMR 2 at an average age of 10.78, slightly earlier than White and Mexican-Americans, who enter SMR 2 at the age of 11.08 years.[2] As puberty progresses, LH causes the evolution of adult-type Leydig cells. The seminal vesicle enlarges and eventually holds 3.4–4.5 cc of seminal fluid. Spermatogenesis can be detected between 11 and 15 years, with sperm being detected in first morning urine specimen at a mean age of 13.3 years.[16] This occurs at an average of SMR 2.5, though sperm concentration, motility, and morphology do not reach adult levels until 17 years of age. On an average, 3 million sperm are produced daily. First conscious ejaculation occurs at a mean age of 13.5, roughly SMR 3.

Testicular volume continues to increase throughout puberty. Shortly after testicular changes begin, phallus growth occurs under the influence of dihydrotestosterone. Genital growth can be categorized by using SMR staging (Fig. 1-3). SMR 1—prepubertal appearance; SMR 2—slight growth of the penis; SMR 3—lengthening of the penis, with slight broadening; SMR 4—further overall growth, broadening of the shaft, and development of the glans penis; SMR 5—adult appearance. The penis usually doubles in size during puberty. Penis size is a common concern among adolescent boys. There is minimal correlation between flaccid penis size and erect size. The average adult erect size is 6 in, with 75% of men in the range of 5–7 in.[17] Most erections are straight and can exist in between the horizontal or vertical axis to the body. Occasional variations in penis shape include curvatures to erections in any direction. This typically does not represent a medical concern unless intercourse is difficult or painful due to anatomy. Teenagers should be reassured about normal variations in genital size.

Pubic hair growth is under the influence of androgens, both adrenal and gonadal. Pubic hair appears within 6 months of the change in testicular volume in 90% of boys. Pubic hair is evaluated by SMR rating as well (Fig. 1-2). Black boys enter pubic hair SMR 2 at an average age of 11.5, slightly earlier than White and Mexican-American boys, who enter SMR 2 at the age of 11.8 years and 12.2 years, respectively.[2] Pubic hair maturation usually takes approximately 3.5–4 years.

Additional physical changes that occur include nocturnal emissions, which begin around age 14 (SMR 4), voice change due to lengthening of the vocal cords (SMR 3), axillary hair growth, increase in muscle mass, and beard development.

Gynecomastia is a common finding in boys, specifically in the earlier stages of puberty (Chap. 27). Estradiol stimulates breast gland growth. Breast enlargement may be minimally visible, similar to SMR 2, but can grow significantly, causing the teen much embarrassment and concern. The teen usually experiences discomfort along with breast growth, which may last for 6 months. Approximately 50% of adolescent boys develop gynecomastia—50%

unilateral and 50% bilateral. Regression usually happens over a 2-year period. If the gynecomastia does not regress or is causing significant psychologic sequelae, then referral to a surgeon may be appropriate.

Skeletal Growth

A hallmark of the physical part of adolescence in addition to the development of secondary sex characteristics is the growth spurt and attainment of final adult height.

Growth hormone (GH), insulin-like growth factor (IGF-1), and estradiol appear to be the main contributors to the adolescent growth spurt as well as achieving peak bone mass.

GH increases during puberty, which in turn stimulates IGF-1 production. GH alone, as well as IGF-1, potentiates bone growth. In addition, increasing sex steroids influence growing cartilage as well as indirectly stimulating GH production. Estrogen mediates increased GH response in males and females.[18] Estrogen in lower concentrations contributes to growth, but in higher doses is the major contributor to the final stages of epiphyseal fusion.

Increased height velocity compared to latency begins on an average at age 9 in girls and 11 in boys, coinciding with the initiation of puberty. Nearly 25% of adult height is achieved during puberty. Linear growth first occurs in the limbs, before truncal growth. This explains the "all hands and feet" appearance of many teenagers. Peak height velocity, at a rate of 8 cm per year, is achieved at age 11.5 in girls, corresponding to SMR stage 2 to 3 breast development. Height growth decelerates once menarche begins, but girls may have 5–7 cm growth remaining after menarche. Peak height velocity in boys occurs at 13.5 years at a rate of 9 cm per year, corresponding to SMR stage 3 to 4 (Figure 1-2). Growth will be completed in 95% of boys when in SMR stage 5. Average adult female height is 163 cm and average adult male height is 177 cm. Final height differences between males and females can be attributed to longer time of prepubertal growth, greater rate of growth, and longer duration of puberty. Teenagers who have early onset puberty have a more pronounced growth spurt compared to those who undergo late onset puberty.[19] There is data to suggest that greater growth occurs during the springtime.[20] Racially, Whites and Blacks are significantly taller than Mexican-Americans.[2]

A recent study from Sweden,[21] tracking peak height velocity and its relationship to BMI and height from birth through infancy, childhood, and adolescence, revealed interesting associations. The growth pattern in early life is strongly associated with subsequent growth. Longer length as well as higher BMI at birth are associated with later onset of puberty. However, a significant increase in BMI during childhood is associated with earlier onset of puberty. Higher BMI during childhood is also associated with less height gain during puberty.

Clinically, it is important to use growth curves to follow adolescent growth. Crossing major percentile lines can indicate a disease process or may represent either early or delayed puberty. Often teenagers, or their parents, are concerned about their stature. Combined with knowing their SMR staging (Figs. 1-1 to 1-3),[22] pubertal development, and parental height, the clinician can assess whether they are on a healthy trajectory, and hence, guesstimate a final height (Chap. 15).

Bone accretion during adolescence is critical. Teenagers accrue 40% of their bone mass during puberty. Bone deposition is greatest during puberty than any other time in life aside from infancy. Peak bone mineral density (BMD) deposition occurs after peak height velocity is achieved—15.8 years for girls and 17.5 years for boys. Increase in BMD is associated with increasing BMI, height, weight, age, and pubertal development.[23] Calcium intake is essential for achieving healthy BMD. Adolescents often lack sufficient calcium (Chap. 29). Girls need 1500 mg (5 dairy servings) and boys need 1200 mg of calcium per day to achieve peak bone mineralization. Blacks retain more calcium than Whites and bone density is higher in Blacks.[24] Another factor that increases BMD includes impact loading sports such as running/jumping that cause strain on the skeleton and stimulates bone deposition. The presence of estradiol[25] in both boys and girls contributes positively to bone accretion.

Delayed puberty, interruption of puberty with a subsequent decrease in estradiol (anorexia nervosa), Klinefelter syndrome with lack of gonadal hormones, and growth hormone deficient individuals are all at risk for decreased BMD and subsequent osteopenia.

Body Composition

Body composition changes significantly during growth and puberty. Prepubertally, girls and boys are similar in their body composition makeup. Lean body mass starts to increase at age 6 in girls and age 9.5 in boys. For girls, lean body mass decreases from 80% to 75% during puberty and body fat increases from 16% to 27%. Hips enlarge for girls, decreasing the waist/hip ratio, contributing to increased fat deposition and the typical "pear-shaped" appearance of girls. Muscle mass accounts for 42% of body weight for girls and 54% in boys. Overall, boys have 1.5 times the lean body mass and half the body fat of girls.

Obesity has become epidemic in children and adolescents, especially in the United States (Chap. 31). It is paramount that clinicians use BMI growth curves to assess obesity. The best current definition of overweight and obesity are based on the BMI growth curves. As body composition changes, BMI—weight in (kg) and height (m^2)—increases during puberty. A BMI between 85th and 94th percentile is considered overweight and 95% or greater is considered obese. Feedback and counseling about the risks of being overweight to both patients and their family is essential.

Additional Physical Changes

Mean blood pressure naturally increases slowly during adolescence. Mean blood pressure is influenced by age, sex, and height. It is important for health care providers to reference blood pressure tables when assessing vital signs, paying particular attention to the 95th percentile for diastolic and systolic pressures, which will determine when an assessment for high blood pressure is necessary. Red blood cell volumes as well as hematocrits tend to increase during adolescence. Teenagers, particularly

females, are at risk of developing anemia, and should be screened once during puberty after their menarche has started.

ADOLESCENT DEVELOPMENT

Paralleling physical growth and puberty is cognitive and psychosocial development. There is an equally intense process occurring in the brains of teenagers that rival the physical change that occurs. During the span of about a decade, individuals evolve from being concrete thinking generally dependent on adults, 10-year-old preadolescents, to self-sufficient, aware of their identity, abstract-thinking individuals, who can survive in the world independently. Recognizing the ebbs and flows of this developmental process allows the practitioner to truly understand the teenager, assess individual behavior, and place into context the risk-taking that occurs along the way.

Cognitive Development

Understanding cognitive development will help the practitioner evaluate some of the capabilities and limitations of their patients. Cognitive development involves the interplay of neuropsychologic maturation, environmental stimulation, environmental responsiveness, and constant internal cognitive reorganization.[26] Piaget defined the process of cognitive development. The important issue for adolescence is the transition from concrete thinking to formal operational thinking or abstract reasoning. Piaget describes this transition as beginning to occur around age 11, though the transition can happen at any point in early to middle adolescence, or not at all. Concrete thinkers view the world as black and white, right and wrong. They can understand logical math and science problems but cannot yet think abstractly. The concrete thinker lacks the ability to extract general principles from one experience and to apply them to a whole new experience. The future cannot be appreciated except as a direct projection of clearly visible current situations and known options. Moral concepts are limited to co-opting existing societal rules.[27] With the transition to abstract thinking, teenagers begin to think about things in a hypothetical sense and can reason about the "what-ifs" and the contrary-to-fact concepts in life. Formal operations allow adolescents to think about their own and other people's thinking. It allows them to enter a realm of moral and ethical reasoning—an essential ability needed to live in society. They begin to grasp long range consequences of their actions and consider delaying immediate gratification for longer term goals. Concrete thinkers may choose to not smoke marijuana because they will get in trouble with the law—a black and white choice, while abstract thinkers may not smoke because they realize that if they get high, they may drive under the influence and harm themselves.

Identity Formation

Erik Erickson[28] developed a theory of eight psychosocial stages that occur during one's lifespan. The key stage that describes adolescence is Erickson's fifth stage of development, identity versus identity confusion. Teenagers face the task of finding out who they are and what they are all about. They ask "Who am I? How am I different from my peer group? Where am I going with my life?" They are confronted by a wide variety of roles, culturally, vocationally, and sexually for example, and need to ascertain for themselves what fits for them in relation to defining their identity. They try out different personalities and roles—being neat one day, sloppy the next; argumentative one day, cooperative the next, mimicking their peer group one day, being different the next. During this experimentation, they define for themselves what feels comfortable and what does not. Adolescents who successfully cope with these conflicting identities emerge with a new, healthy sense of self. Those who do not resolve this identity crisis may end up in a state of identity confusion, either withdrawing from peers and family, or immersing themselves in the world of peers, losing much of their individual identity. Identity formation is complex, with multiple societal, cultural, and family

influences, that span the course of adolescent development.

A key component to self-identity is developing a sexual identity. As pubertal changes occur, teenagers develop sexual feelings. They begin to integrate feelings of sexual arousal with how they perceive societal and gender stereotypes. Teens need to determine both, sexual roles—perceiving themselves in the role of either male or female sexual beings (most often similar to gender identity which is usually determined at a young age) and sexual orientation—their physical and erotic attraction to males, females, or both. This process is often complex and confusing. Initial awareness of sexual urges often results in masturbation, which allows the teenager a healthy outlet to explore feelings of arousal as well as attraction. Frequently same sex experimentation in the form of mutual masturbation takes play in early adolescence, most often with boys. Romantic games such as "spin the bottle" allow teenagers the opportunity to begin to model sexual roles of their older peers and adults. As teens continue to define their sexual identity, they experiment with more serious sexual interaction, which obviously puts them at a risk of sexually transmitted infections (STIs) and pregnancy. As teens emerge into adulthood, hopefully they have determined their sexual identity and integrated that self-concept into the greater construct of self-identity.

Stages of Adolescence

It is important to understand that stages of adolescence are based on many theories as well as scientific psychologic observations that generally concur with evolving development. It is difficult to put an exact age on any of the stages. Few, if any, of the psychosocial theories incorporate true pubertal development in regard to SMR ratings. As the initiation of puberty is occurring earlier, one could hypothesize that adolescent development will then start earlier. It is recognized that the earlier puberty starts, the more risk-taking an adolescent may engage in.[29] For example, early developers initiate sexual intercourse at a younger age compared to late developers. The clinician should take this into account when providing anticipatory guidance, adjusting pubertal development to psychologic theories of development. Early as well as late initiators of puberty may be out of sync with the average stage of development.

Early Adolescence

Early adolescence is generally defined as occurring between ages 10 and 13. Dominant during this time period are the physical changes that teens need to incorporate into their view of themselves and the world. They are acutely aware and often self-conscious about their physical appearance and how others view them. They may begin testing their parents, experimenting with more independence. Though parents remain the most important influence in an adolescent's life, peer interaction becomes important. Frequently they imitate their peer group in interests, dress, and style, conforming to the norm. They are most comfortable with same sex friendships, though they may begin to have opposite sex friendships as well. They start to become at risk for experimentation with drugs and alcohol. They often are still concrete thinkers but begin to move towards formal operational thinking.

Middle Adolescence

Middle adolescence is generally defined as happening between ages 14 and 17. Teens have become more comfortable with their bodies and on an average, are no longer undergoing rapid physical change. They have started to think abstractly and have tested many different roles in helping determine their identity. Working towards independence has becomes a major task. Society permits middle adolescence to begin working and driving, which create more responsibility. Teens continue to explore their identity. In the sexual realm, more one-on-one dating occurs as teens begin to experience intimacy. Same sex and opposite sex experimentation may occur as adolescents work at determining their sexual orientation.

Roughly 50% of teens will have had sexual intercourse by their senior year in high school (Chap. 22). This is the period of highest risk-taking for adolescents. Teens have a sense of omnipotence and invincibility during this period. Teens may recognize risk for others but do not always apply it to themselves because the bad outcomes "won't happen to me." Peer pressure continues throughout this time with a high proportion of adolescents trying alcohol (80%) or marijuana (50%) by their senior year (Chap. 34). Adolescents' need for emancipation from parents becomes a struggle as teens attempt to relinquish parents as their primary love object in preparing for future intimacy. Most adolescents transition through this phase smoothly, though 20% experience a tempestuous and stormy transition.[30]

Late Adolescence

Late adolescence is typically defined by ages between 18 and 21. If development has taken a typical course, then teens in this stage are entering young adulthood. They have largely formed their identity and are becoming independent individuals who should be able to sustain themselves in the world without parental support, though the average young adult still relies on parents for financial support. Erickson's sixth stage of development, intimacy versus isolation, occurs during this time. The older adolescents want to fuse their new identity with another and develop a sense of intimacy. They have the need to commit to multiple types of relationships—intellectual, social, or sexual. Empathy as well as burgeoning idealism develops during this time.

Society holds those who are 18 fully responsible for their actions and decisions. They are treated as adults in the judicial system, have the right to vote, and can serve our country in a variety of ways. The only remaining adult privilege yet to be given is the right to drink alcohol. Older adolescents have fully developed the ability to think abstractly and can think more realistically about both their present and future. Risk-taking tends to decrease throughout this period.

References

1   Herman-Giddens ME, Slora EJ, Wasserman RC, et al. Secondary sexual characteristics and menses in young girls seen in office practice: a study from the Pediatric Research in Office Settings network. *Pediatrics* 99(4): 505–512, 1997.

2   Sun SS, Schubert CM, Chumlea WC, et al. National estimates of the timing of sexual maturation and racial differences among US children. *Pediatrics* 110(5): 911–919, 2002.

3   Wu T, Mendola P, Buck GM. Ethnic differences in the presence of secondary sex characteristics and menarche among US girls: the Third National Health and Nutrition Examination Survey, 1988–1994. *Pediatrics* 110(4):752–757, 2002.

4   Herman-Giddens ME, Kaplowitz PB, et al. Navigating the recent articles on girls' puberty in Pediatrics: what do we know and where do we go from here? *Pediatrics* 113(4):911–917, 2004.

5   Biro FM, Lucky AW, Huster GA, et al. Pubertal staging in boys. *J Pediatr* 127(1):100–102, 1995.

6   Garcia-Mayor RV, Andrade MA, et al. Serum leptin levels in normal children: relationship to age, gender, body mass index, pituitary-gonadal hormones, and pubertal stage. *J Clin Endocrinol Metab* 82(9): 2849–2855, 1997.

7   Ahmed ML, Ong KK, Morrell DJ, et al. Longitudinal study of leptin concentrations during puberty: sex differences and relationship to changes in body composition. *J Clin Endocrinol Metab* 84(3):899–905, 1999.

8   Kaplowitz PB, Slora EJ, Wasserman RC, et al. Earlier onset of puberty in girls: relation to increased body mass index and race. *Pediatrics* 108(2):347–353, 2001.

9   Halvorson LM, DeCherney AH. Inhibin, activin, and follistatin in reproductive medicine. *Fertil Steril* 65(3):459–469, 1996.

10 Burger HG, McLachlan RI, Bangah M, et al. Serum inhibin concentrations rise throughout normal male and female puberty. *J Clin Endocrinol Metab* 67(4): 689–694, 1988.

11 Palmert MR, Hayden DL, Mansfield MJ, et al. The longitudinal study of adrenal maturation during gonadal suppression: evidence that adrenarche is a gradual process. *J Clin Endocrinol Metab* 86(9): 4536–4542, 2001.

12 MacMahon B. Age at Manarche, United States. Series 11. Report No. 133NCHS. DHEW Pub. No. (HRA) 74-1615. Washington DC: National Center for Health Statistics, Vital and Health Statistics, 1973.

13 Anderson SE, Dallal GE, Must A. Relative weight and race influence average age at menarche: results from two nationally representative surveys of US girls studied 25 years apart. *Pediatrics* 111(4 Pt 1): 844–850, 2003.

14 Laufer MR. The physiology of puberty. In: Emans SJ, Laufer MR, Goldstein DP (eds.), *Pediatric and Adolescent Gynecology,* 4th ed., Philadelphia, PA: Lippencott-Raven, 1998, pp.109–140.

15 Griffin JE, Wilson JD. Disorders of the testes and the male reproductive tract. In: Wilson JD, Foster DW, Kronenber HM, et al. (eds.), *Williams Textbook of Endocrinology,* 9th ed., Philadelphia, PA: WB Saunders, 1998, pp. 819–837.

16 Grumbach MM, STyne DM. Pubert: Ontogeny, neuroendocrinology, physiology and disorders. In: Wilson JD, Foster DW, Kronenber HM, et al. (eds.), *Williams Textbook of Endocrinology,* 9th ed., Philadelphia, PA: WB Saunders, 1998, pp. 1509–1549.

17 Lee PA, Reiter EO. Genital size: a common adolescent male concern. *Adolescent Medicine State of the Art Reviews* 13(1):171–180, viii, 2002.

18 Veldhuis JD, Metzger DL, Martha PM, et al. Estrogen and testosterone, but not a nonaromatizable androgen, direct network integration of the hypothalamo-somatotrope (growth hormone)-insulin-like growth factor I axis in the human: evidence from pubertal pathophysiology and sex-steroid hormone replacement. *J Clin Endocrinol Metab* 82(10):3414–3420, 1997.

19 Juul A, Bang P, Hertel NT, et al. Serum insulin-like growth factor-I in 1030 healthy children, adolescents, and adults: relation to age, sex, stage of puberty, testicular size, and body mass index. *J Clin Endocrinol Metab* 78(3):744–52, 1994.

20 Tanner JM, Davies PS. Clinical longitudinal standards for height and height velocity for North American children. *J Pediatr* 107(3):317–29, 1985.

21 Luo ZC, Cheung YB, He Q, et al. Growth in early life and its relation to pubertal growth. *Epidemiology* 14(1):65–73, 2003.

22 Hofmann AD, Greydanus DE. *Adolescent Medicine.* 3d ed., Stamford, CT: Appleton & Lange, 1997, pp. 14–16.

23 Bonjour JP, Theintz G, Law F, et al. Peak bone mass. *Osteoporos Int.* 4 (Suppl 1):7–13, 1994.

24 Anderson JJ, Pollitzer WS. Ethnic and genetic differences in susceptibility to osteoporotic fractures. *Adv Nutr Res* 9:129–149, 1994.

25 Wickman S, Kajantie E, Dunkel L. Effects of suppression of estrogen action by the p450 aromatase

inhibitor letrozole on bone mineral density and bone turnover in pubertal boys. *J Clin Endocrinol Metab* 88(8):3785–3793, 2003.

26 Ford CA, Coleman WL. Adolescent development and behavior: implications for the primary care physician. In: Levine MD, Carey WB, Crocker AC (eds.), *Developmental-Behavioral Pediatrics,* 3d ed., Philadelphia, PA: WB Saunders, 1999, pp. 69–75.

27 Hoffman A. Adolescent growth and development. In: Hofmann AD, Greydanus D (eds.), *Principles of Adolescent Health Care*, 3d ed., Stamford, CT: Appleton & Lange, 1997, pp. 17–18.

28 Erickson EH. *Identity, Youth, and Crisis.* New York, NY: Norton, 1968.

29 Martin CA, Kelly TH, Rayens MK, et al. Sensation seeking, puberty, and nicotine, alcohol, and marijuana use in adolescence. *J Am Acad Child Adolesc Psychiatry* 41(12):1495–1502, 2002.

30 Ford CA, Coleman WL. Adolescent development and behavior: implications for the primary care physician. in Levine MD, Carey WB, Crocker AC(eds.), *Developmental-Behavioral Pediatrics,* 3d ed., Philadelphia, PA: WB Saunders, 1999, pp. 69–75.

CHAPTER

2

CARING FOR ADOLESCENTS IN THE OFFICE

Paritosh Kaul and David W. Kaplan

INTRODUCTION

Adolescence is a period of transition from childhood to adult life and is a dynamic stage of development. Taking care of adolescents can be a rewarding experience since the clinician has the opportunity to change the course of the adolescent's life in potentially significant ways. This chapter discusses concepts of caring for adolescents in the office setting. The "office" is defined broadly to include a wide range of health care settings, from primary community health center clinics to tertiary adolescent health clinics. Clinical settings also include school based health clinics, juvenile detention facilities, mobile vans, and private practice offices. The office décor and personnel differ greatly from one setting to another but they all exist to deliver health care to the adolescent.

DEMOGRAPHY

In 2002, there were 18.8 million adolescents between the ages 15 and 19 years and 18.6 million between the ages 20 and 24 years in the United States; together, adolescents' ages 15–24 years constituted a little over 13% of the United States'

population. Hispanics are the second most populous racial/ethnic group. It is projected that by 2040, the proportion of adolescents from racial and ethnically minority groups will increase and the percentage of non-Hispanic Whites will drop below 50%.

MORTALITY AND MORBIDITY

The three leading causes of death in adolescents aged 15–24 in 2002 were accidents (unintentional injuries) (45.5%), homicide (15.3%), and suicide (11.3%). Among accidents, motor vehicle accidents accounted for 75% of the unintentional injuries (34%) (Kochanek, 2004). These three violent and preventable causes of death among youth account for 72.8% of all deaths among this age group. Other causes of death in 2002 among this age group in decreasing order were malignancies, heart disease, congenital diseases, human immunodeficiency virus (HIV), respiratory disease, cerebrovascular disease, and diabetes mellitus.

Health behaviors established in adolescence can have a significant effect on adult morbidity and mortality. For example, cigarette smoking increases the risk of lung cancer, heart disease, asthma, and other respiratory diseases (Chap. 34). Obesity increases the risk of diabetes and heart disease and lack of regular physical activity increases the risk of heart disease and obesity (Chap. 31). Use of alcohol and other illicit drugs increase the risk of unintended and intended injuries. Unsafe sexual behaviors may result in acquiring sexually transmitted diseases (STDs) and HIV, as well as unintended pregnancies (Chaps. 24 and 26).

The major causes of morbidity among teens are psychosocial and behavioral in origin. There are over 870,000 pregnancies among 15–19 year-old females and an estimated 4 million cases of STDs that occur each year among teenagers. Substance abuse, smoking, dropping out of school, depression, running away from home, physical violence, and juvenile delinquency are all frequent issues in this age group that need to be addressed.

Violence among adolescents leads to one-fourth of all deaths in this age group. In 2003 (Youth Risk Behavior Survey—YRBS), about one in six high school students carried a weapon or a gun (17.1%) and one in three were involved in a physical fight (33%). The rates are higher among males than females and among Black youth as compared to White or Hispanic youth. Overall, the prevalence of weapon carrying decreased significantly from 26.1% to 18.3% during 1991–1997 and leveled off in 2003 at 17.1%. Physical fighting decreased significantly from 42.3% to 33% and physical fighting on school property declined significantly from 16.2% to 12.8% during 1991–2003.

GENERAL GUIDELINES FOR THE OFFICE VISIT

The Office Setting

The ambiance of the office sets the tone for the visit. Adolescent are extremely sensitive to nonverbal cues and they do not like to be treated like young children. The offices where teens are seen with pediatric patients should be designed so that a separate area or corner is reserved for teens. Another alternative is to have a separate session in the evening or afternoon dedicated only to adolescents. In the clinics where separate space is not an option, posters or magazines should be present that acknowledge and welcome the adolescent to the clinic. The front-office personnel that check-in the patient should be teen-friendly and accepting of adolescent demeanor. Posters and educational material around the office should reflect to the teen that the office is a safe, supportive, and accepting place to discuss sensitive issues.

Scheduling Patients

Taking care of adolescents is a time-intensive process. In some offices, a 40%–50% no-show rate is not unusual and this financial concern can result in pressure to schedule less time for the adolescent, which may be insufficient to deal with complex psychosocial issues. Forty-five minutes to 1 hour is usually necessary for the initial appointment. Follow-up visits can be scheduled for shorter duration of 30 minutes or less, depending on the nature of the problem. Depending on the adolescent's age, the parents should gradually transition the adolescent to take responsibility for their own health care needs like making appointments, calling for refills of asthma medications or contraceptive needs. This does not imply that parents are not important. They should be involved as partners in the health care of their teenager (Chap. 3).

Health care providers should always be alert to a hidden agenda. It is not unusual for a young adolescent girl to present with a sore throat, but actually be worried that she is pregnant. Adolescents may present with vague symptoms, symptoms without any positive findings on clinical examination, or symptoms with findings not consistent with the extent of their complaints. Such concerns should alert the clinician to look for other issues. When multiple problems exist, the clinician should prioritize the issue depending on the seriousness and urgency of the situation. In an adolescent girl, who is smoking cigarettes, doing poorly in school, smoking marijuana, and having frequent unprotected sexual intercourse, the health care provider needs to prioritize the issues and at that visit address the lack of contraception and the risk of unintended pregnancy or STDs. Future appointments can deal with other issues.

Confidentiality

The initial visit should address issues of confidentiality (Chap. 3). The parent and the adolescent should be aware of what they can expect from the visit. Clinicians should be familiar with their state laws for consent for care of minors regarding issues of STDs, pregnancy, mental health, and substance abuse. The Center for Adolescent Health & the Law has produced a monograph (English, 2003) that summarizes the state laws that allow minors to give their own consent for health care.

Screening Questionnaires

The American Medical Association (AMA) guidelines for adolescent preventive services (GAPS) have screening questionnaires for adolescents and their parents/guardians. There are two forms for the patients; a younger adolescent questionnaire and an older questionnaire both of which are available in English and Spanish from the AMA website *http://www.ama-assn.org*. A screening questionnaire that is used at The Children's Hospital in Denver, Colorado, is provided by Kaplan and Love-Osborne (2005).

Billing

Reimbursement for adolescents' health care continues to be a challenge (Bradley and Blythe, 2003). Reimbursement rates for the amount of time spent are usually not adequate because of the time required to care for adolescents with complicated psychosocial issues. The other significant contributing issue is the high no-show rates among the teens, which leads to loss of valuable clinical time. In some situations it is necessary to double-book the clinician when they are seeing adolescents. The issue of confidentiality is another factor resulting in complex billing issues in adolescents (Chap. 3). For teens with health insurance who are seen for confidential problems, such as suspected pregnancy or contraception, the visit might not be billable if the adolescent's parents get a copy of the insurance payment listing tests, procedures, and medications. The health care provider might keep

a list of resources of school-based health centers, community-based organizations, and subsidized hospital-based clinics that provide confidential and free services to adolescents. A more detailed discussion on billing and billing codes are provided by the American Academy of Pediatrics (AAP, 2003).

THE ADOLESCENT INTERVIEW

The initial introduction and interaction with the adolescent is extremely important, as it may set the success of establishing trust with this patient. When the teen patient is accompanied by an adult, the clinician should introduce himself/herself to the adolescent first and then to the accompanying adult. This sets the tone and sends a message both to the teen and the adult that the primary person in the room is the adolescent. Clinicians should avoid making assumptions that the accompanying adult is the parent, since various adults may accompany adolescents on their visit.

Once introductions are made, the clinician should describe the manner in which the encounter will take place. The provider should state that both the parent/guardian and the adolescent would be interviewed together. Then, as part of the visit, the adolescent would be interviewed alone. Parents should be informed that interviewing the adolescent alone is a routine, and not a reflection of them as parents, or something unusual the clinician has noticed in the teen and/or parent. In some cases, the parents could be concerned that the interview solely with the adolescent would reveal "family secrets" like alcoholism or psychiatric illness in the family. The parent should feel included and not isolated, and an easy technique to foster positive parental rapport is to solicit information from them on topics like the family history, past medical and surgical history, and others. There might be occasions where the parent would like to talk to the clinician alone and that request should be respected. In situations where the adolescent is angry and upset, the clinician should ask the parent to leave the room sooner, which would give time to the provider and the teen to establish a positive therapeutic relationship and address the issues with the adolescent.

As mentioned above, the provider should initiate the conversation with non-threatening questions regarding past medical and surgical history, allergies, and medications; then, progress to more intimate issues. As an aid for eliciting an adolescent psychosocial history, the acronym HEADSS was developed by Henry Berman, MD in 1972 and later refined by Eric Cohen, MD in 1985. Since then it has been used and recently has been expanded from HEADSS to become HEEADSSS or HE²ADS³ with an additional E for eating and S for safety (Goldenring and Rosen, 2004) (see Table 2-1).

Not all questions or areas need to be explored in the first interview. These screening questions should serve to gain an insight into the adolescent's life. In cases of crises, safety issues should be the immediate concern. Complex patients, such as those with an eating disorder or a high-risk juvenile delinquent, may require more than one visit to elicit a complete history. Three visits of shorter duration of 30 minutes are better than one interview of 90 minutes (Coupey, 1997). The multiple visits give both the patient and the provider time to reassess the situation and reflect on what was expressed during the interview. These multiple visits also serve to strengthen the relationship between the primary care provider and the patient.

TABLE 2-1

HE²ADS³: AN ACRONYM FOR ADOLESCENT PSYCHOSOCIAL HISTORY

H	Home
E	Education
E	Eating
A	Activities
D	Drugs
S	Sexuality
S	Suicide and depression
S	Safety

Source: Adapted from Goldenring JM, Rosen DS. Getting into adolescent heads: An essential update. Contemp Pediatr 21:64, 2004.

Home

The home environment is vital in the teen's life and a not-so-controversial place to start. It is essential not to make any assumptions regarding the patient's living conditions or members of the family. It is safe to start with the question, "Whom do you all live with at home?" Inquire from the teen regarding missing family members, especially parents, along with questions regarding how the teen is coping with the fact and situation.

Patient A: I live with my mother, two sisters and one younger brother.
Clinician: You live with your mother, brother, and two sisters? Right?
Patient A: Yes.
Clinician: And where is your father?
Patient A: I don't know.
Clinician: When was the last time you had contact with him?
Patient A: I don't know. He left when I was little.
Clinician: Some people might feel angry about not having a father around. How do you feel about it?
Patient A: I guess it's OK. I never knew him, so I really don't care.

This is in contrast to another patient who could respond very differently:

Clinician: Some people might feel angry about not having a father around. How do you feel about it?
Patient B: I feel very bad and wish he were around.
Clinician: I can understand that. It's not easy to grow up without a father. How have you dealt with this since your childhood?

Apart from immediate family members, inquiries should be made regarding extended family members (such as grandparents, uncles, aunts, and cousins) to gauge the support system that exists around the adolescent. Connection with supportive adults has been shown to be a protective factor against high-risk behavior (Resnick et al, 1997). The health care provider should confirm if there has been a recent change in the living situation and also, if the patient has ever thought of running away from home.

Education and Employment

The adolescent spends a great amount of time at school among his peers and the school environment has a strong influence on the teen. Instead of asking "How is school?" it is preferable to ask more specific questions like, "How are your grades in school this year as compared to last year?" Some other questions to ask the teen regarding school are, "What is your favorite subject?" or "In which subjects do you have the most difficulty?" A decline in school performance could correlate with other high-risk behaviors, especially substance abuse and truancy.

The clinician should not presume that the student attends regular class and is not special in education. Asking the patient if he/she has ever been sent to the principal's office or the dean's office will give an idea regarding discipline issues at school. Older adolescents should have a plan regarding their future career goals and employment. If they do not, this issue needs to be explored. An open-ended, yet insightful question to ask the teen is, "Where do you see yourself 5 years from now?"

Eating

This *E* is a new addition to the HEADSS acronym. The primary care provider should screen the patient regarding unhealthy dietary behaviors. The pattern of disordered eating which occurs in both ends of the spectrum with obesity, anorexia nervosa, and bulimia nervosa and their variations, should be explored during the interview with the adolescent (Chaps. 29–31). A simple question, "What do you think about your weight?" opens the door to a more extensive evaluation.

Activity

An excellent approach to eliciting additional information and obtaining a clearer picture of teen behavior is inquiring about activities that the teen enjoys. Asking the teen about his friends and what they do for fun, can lead to further questions regarding high-risk behaviors when the patient is not at school or at home. The adolescent should also be questioned regarding involvement in sports and other physical activities (Chaps. 32 and 33). This is an opportunity to talk about using protective gear, seat belts, and helmets. Developmentally, many adolescents are concrete thinkers and are sometimes unable to understand the consequences of their actions. The goal during the interview process is to provide anticipatory guidance so that adolescents come to the same conclusion as the clinician regarding safety issues and consequences of their actions.

In the example below, the teen has admitted to drinking and driving.

> *Clinician*:   What do you think happens when someone drinks?
> *Patient*:   You feel happy, high, and dizzy.
> *Clinician*:   Exactly, the alcohol affects the brain. You do feel happy but unfortunately you are unable to make correct decisions. The dizziness means you can't coordinate or move correctly. So what do you think could happen to someone who drives when intoxicated?
> *Patient*:   He could get into an accident since he can't control the car well.
> *Clinician*:   That's right and teen accidents are the number one reason for deaths among teenagers.

When asked what they do for fun, the teen often responds, "I hang out with my buddies." The adolescent should be further questioned as to what do they do when they "hang out." Do they play some games or go to the mall or watch movies? The clinician should also inquire about the duration of TV the teen watches, including the programs she/he watches. Apart from TV, adolescents also spend a great deal of time playing video games, and primary care providers should elicit a history regarding duration and content of the video games. Adolescents who spend a considerable amount of their time with the TV and video games are exposed to inappropriate messages regarding drugs and sexuality. (Strasburger, 2004).

Drugs

Substance abuse is a problem that affects many individuals with over 50% of teens consuming alcohol before they complete high school (Johnston, O'Malley, and Bachman, 2003). In an atmosphere of trust and confidentiality, health care providers must ask routine questions to all patients. The CRAFFT questionnaire is an office-based brief tool for initial assessment of the substance abusing teen (Knight, 2002). More information about drug use is provided in Chap. 34.

Suicide and Depression

Inquiring from the adolescent about his/her mood as well as signs and symptoms of depression is important (Chap. 36). Adolescents will often not present with the classic adult signs of depression, but may present with symptoms of irritability and sleep disturbances (i.e., too little or excessive amounts—Chaps. 14 and 36). When making inquiries about suicide, the question should be asked in an accepting manner with no blame on the patient who might have thought about it.

> *Clinician*:   Sometimes things get very rough for teens and the pain is so unbearable that they wish they could end it all. Have you ever had such thoughts?

If the patient acknowledges significant suicidal ideation, the provider needs to contact the mental health provider and refer the patient. Adolescent depression and suicide is discussed in Chap. 36.

Sexuality

The sexual history is one of the most intimate parts of the interview. Questions should be asked in gender-neutral terms with no presumptions regarding the sexual orientation of the adolescent. Sexuality and sexual abuse are both sensitive topics and need to be approached in a careful but supportive fashion (Chaps. 22 and 23).

Safety

This *S* for safety is an addition to the original acronym HEADSS. Since violence is prevalent in our twenty-first century society, it is imperative that the clinician inquires about safety issues both at home and school; this includes asking about being victims of bullies. Some adolescent girls may

be victims of dating violence and the health care provider should be sensitive to their needs (Chaps. 22 and 23). This type of violence is prevalent in all sections of society irrespective of race, economic, and social boundaries (Rickert, Wiemann, 1998).

PRINCIPLES OF INTERVIEWING ADOLESCENTS

Communicating with adolescents and eliciting information from them is an art. The following are suggestions that may be helpful to clinicians taking care of adolescents.

Patient Issues

Primary care providers should keep in mind that many adolescents are brought to the clinic against their will and are angry to be there, while others are shy and feel awkward about being present in a medical setting. These patients need to be reassured and starting the interview with general comments may help to break the ice.

Provider Issues

Adolescents are usually honest with their health care provider once trust is established. It is critical that health care providers who take care of teens are also honest with them, since the adolescents know if a provider is insincere, almost as if they had an internal radar to sense it. For most adolescents, an authoritative style of interaction does not work well. They respond poorly to a provider who they see as dishonest, overpowering, or authoritative.

While each provider has her/his own style and approach to the patient, the provider should avoid playing the role of a parent. At the same time, the health care provider should correct the misperceptions that the teen may have regarding issues, both medical and behavioral. Clinicians need to be supportive toward the adolescent, but this does not imply that the provider should support inappropriate behavior or downplay high-risk behavior.

Health care providers need to be themselves and not try to talk or behave like teens. This includes the avoidance of inappropriate dressing or using street or explicit language on the part of the clinician. The teenager has come to the office and is looking for a professional who will provide medical care. They are not seeking a person who behaves like their peers. There is a difference in being friendly or being a friend to the patient and in behaving like a teen.

Open-Ended Questions

These types of questions initiate conversation and allow the teen to express themselves and paint the complete picture regarding current issues or symptom complexes. Open-ended questions such as, "Tell me more about your headache," will elicit a response about the headache. However, to get more information the health care provider will need to ask specific and concrete questions such as, "When you have the headache, do you feel any nausea?" This type of questioning is inappropriate when trying to elicit specific information, specifically when dealing with adolescents. As mentioned previously, if the provider is concerned about the grades at school, instead of asking, "How is school?" or "How are you doing in school" (which are open-ended questions and their response will be "good"), the more appropriate line of questioning would be, "What are your grades in school as compared to last year?"

Time Frame

When inquiring about the timing of the present symptom, it is helpful to relate the symptom as a complex or issue around an event, rather than dates. "Did your chest pains start after your first quarter grades?" Health care providers can also use holidays to remind their patients about contraception refills, "You need to come in for your next shot before Halloween."

Scales

Adolescents may have difficulty in describing the severity of a symptom and a scale may help them to quantify it. An adolescent who is depressed can be asked, "On a scale from 1 to 10, with 10 being the worst you feel, feeling down, sad, and hoping things would end, and 1 being feeling great, happy, and positive, what would you rate your mood as?" Sometimes the teen may respond better to a grading system resembling that in school with which they are more familiar.

> *Clinician*: What kind of grade do you think your mood has been these days on an A to F scale?
> *Patient*: I feel like a B these days.
> *Clinician*: And would that be a B plus or a B minus?
> *Patient*: I feel like a B plus.
> *Clinician*: And when you started your medications, what would you say, your mood was?
> *Patient*: That time was real bad; I was like a C minus.
> *Clinician*: I am glad you are feeling so much better after you started taking the medications.

Insight Questions

In situations where the primary care provider would like information which ask the adolescent to look within and translate abstract feelings/concepts into concrete issues, clinicians should use this type of questioning. The translation of these issues should be easy for the teen to follow. They should be approached in a nonthreatening style and the questions should not intimidate them.

When the clinician would like information regarding the patient's self-worth or how he thinks his peers or the world perceives him, a simple question suggested is, "If I were to come to your class and ask your friends, what kind of a person Joe (patient's name) is, what do you think they would tell me?"

In some situations, the clinician may need to gather more information about the exact situation at home or at school. For example, in an adolescent who is constantly having arguments with his mother at home and the clinician is unable to elicit the basis for these arguments, the primary care provider could ask the patient, "If I were invisible and in the room when you and your mother are having an argument, what would I hear?"

Another question which opens the door to the hopes and aspirations or the pain that exists in the life of the adolescent is, "If you had three wishes, what would they be?" or, "If there was one thing you would like to change in your life, what would it be?"

Restatement and Summation

The health care provider can restate what the patient has just mentioned and summarize the adolescent's feelings. This results in the clinician confirming what the teen has expressed and also encouraging him/her to make additional remarks and opening the door to other issues that affect his/her life. The scenario below is of a 16-year boy who presents to the office for lack of sleep.

> *Clinician*:   So, let me see if I understand your sleep pattern. You work the night shift and get home at 11 pm, watch TV till 3 am and then go to sleep?
>
> *Patient*:   No. I don't watch TV. I play in my room with my Playstation because I feel so agitated.
>
> *Clinician*:   What gets you agitated? Something at work, at home, or when you ride the bus while coming home?
>
> *Patient*:   No, it's at home. My dad comes home at that time from the bar and he is drunk and starts fighting with my mom and yelling at all of us.
>
> *Clinician*:   That would be a difficult situation for anyone to handle. I understand it must be for everyone at home and especially you. Are you sure you feel safe at home?

Clarification

When a youth uses words or concepts that are unfamiliar to the provider, the clinician should ask for clarification. Apart from clarification, the teen realizes that the provider is actively listening to him or her. The adolescent is also pleased about the fact that the provider does not know everything, and now she/he is in a position to educate the provider.

Nonverbal Cues

Observation of nonverbal cues will help a clinician understand the emotions that the adolescent is experiencing. The health care provider should look for cues such as body language, eye movement, poor eye contact, signs of nervousness or fear, and hand movements. Often during sensitive topics the patient may have his/her eyes brimming with tears. The clinician should acknowledge those emotions and reassure the patient that the office is a safe place for the adolescent to express these emotions.

THE PHYSICAL EXAMINATION

The age of the patient and the situation should determine if the clinician should perform the physical examination with or without the parent. Many adolescents are extremely modest and this discomfort may be increased when the provider is of the opposite sex. The patient should be given privacy to undress and change into a gown and also a choice regarding the presence of parents and/or a chaperone. The younger the adolescent, the more likely she/he will be to prefer a parent or a chaperone to be present during the physical examination. The best approach to address this discomfort is to verbalize the patient's concern and reassure him or her by explaining the process and purpose of the examination. In most cases the teens do respond to this reassurance.

The adolescent is reassured if the provider continues to talk to him or her during the clinical examination. Remarks regarding normalcy of the adolescent reassure the teen who is concerned about the changes that are occurring in his or her body. Normal physical growth and development is addressed in Chap. 1 and details about disorders of various systems are provided in the appropriate chapters in this book.

Adolescents should be offered to have a chaperone. The examination of the genitourinary system in boys and the gynecologic examination in girls need to be carried out with sensitivity. During the examination of the breast and a gynecologic examination, a male provider should always have a female chaperone present with him. It is essential that the male clinician be respectful, sensitive, empathetic, and non-threatening to ensure that the adolescent girl is as comfortable as possible. (Brown, 2000) (Chap. 27).

PREVENTIVE SERVICES FOR ADOLESCENTS

The goal of the primary care provider taking care of adolescents is to promote optimal physical and mental health and support healthy behaviors among adolescents as they transition into adulthood. In the 1990s, five national organizations developed clinical practice guidelines and recommendations for preventive services to adolescents. These guidelines include GAPS published by the AMA and are a set of comprehensive recommendations (Elster and Kuznets, 1992; Elster, 1998). These recommendations were developed to provide a framework for the organization and content of clinical preventive health services for adolescents. Bright Futures (BF) is a national health promotion initiative sponsored by the National Center for Education in Maternal and Child Health that has a unique set of guidelines for health professionals to promote the developmental health and well-being of their patients in partnership with the parents. These guidelines are available as a book or are available from their website *http://www.brightfutures.org.*

The U.S. Preventive Services Task Force (USPSTF) was convened by the Office of Disease Prevention and Health Promotion, U.S. Department of Health and Human Services and published recommendations for periodic health examinations from infancy to old age, which addressed the health problems of each population group. The second edition of these recommendations was published in 1996. These guidelines are available at the USPSTF website *http://www.ahrq.gov/clinic/uspstfix.htm.*

In 1995, the AAP revised its recommendations and published its set of guidelines for different stages during the pediatric age group including those for adolescents. They also adapted Guidelines for Health Supervision III, which described in detail the components of routine health examinations. The American Academy of Family Physicians (AAFP) recommended contents for periodic health examinations in 1994. Comparisons among the five sets of recommendations are found in the reference by Elster, 1998. Research has noted that many of the recommended services to adolescents are provided by pediatricians in their practice at a rate less than those recommended (Halpern-Felsher, 2000). Female physicians and fresh medical school graduates provide more preventive services than their colleagues.

GAPS consists of 24 recommendations that address those issues that are of the greatest medical or psychologic burden of suffering to the adolescent population (Elster and Kuznets, 1992; Elster, 1998). These recommendations address issues for the delivery of health care, health guidance to teens and their parents, screening, and immunizations. The AMA has also developed materials to assist clinicians in implementing these recommendations. Annual adolescent visits are recommended for routine screening and counseling for future cardiovascular disease and universal screening for health risk behaviors like sexual behavior and contraception, alcohol, and substance use.

Screening guidelines, specifically for laboratory tests, are revised regularly. GAPS recommends that adolescents should be screened annually for STDs. Guidelines for treatment of STDs have been published by the Centers for Disease Control and Prevention (CDC), which are addressed in Chap. 24. Adolescents with a previous history of STDs should be screened for STDs every 6 months. Studies have documented relatively short periods of time until STD reinfection occurs (Orr, 2001). Annual Pap smears are also recommended. The American College of Obstetricians and Gynecologists has recommended that screening for cervical cancer should start 3 years after initiation of sexual intercourse.

IMMUNIZATIONS

It is vital that all adolescents who come in contact with the health care system be immunized against vaccine preventable diseases. Although most states require a second dose of measles-mumps-rubella

(MMR) and hepatitis B vaccines, not all adolescents are up-to-date with their immunizations. The rates for immunizations increased after the legislation required seventh grade students for their MMR and hepatitis B vaccine (Averhoff et al, 2004). However, the rates for immunization of adolescents are at 64% for MMR and 38% for Hepatitis B, well below the Healthy People 2010 goal of 90%. (Rickert et al, 2004). The AAP recommends a routine preadolescent appointment at 11–12 years (AAP Red Book 2003). The purpose of these visits is, if needed, (a) to immunize all adolescents with two doses of MMR; (b) varicella and/or hepatitis B as indicated; (c) booster dose of Td; (d) other immunizations as needed.

The American College Health Association (ACHA) has also published their recommendations for institutional prematriculation immunizations (ACHA, 2003). They have mandated immunizations against measles, mumps, rubella, tetanus, hepatitis B, polio, and varicella. Students at risk should be immunized against hepatitis A, pneumococcal disease, and influenza. Immunization of college students with meningococcal vaccine is recommended by ACHA and required by the state law for college students in many states. It is also recommended for high-risk groups, such as those with complement deficiency or asplenia.

CONCLUSION

Adolescents are unique as is their relationship with their health care providers; both undergo transformation. Parents are no longer the only historians. The patients now have their own stories along with a different perspective as well. Clinically caring for adolescents is exhilarating but demanding and seeing their transformation into mature adults can be a source of considerable delight to all clinicians who take care of these unique individuals.

Bibliography

Akinbami LJ, Gandhi H, Cheng TL. Availability of adolescent health services and confidentiality in primary care practices. *Pediatrics* 111:394–401, 2004.

American Academy of Family Practice. Age charts for periodic health examinations. Kansas, MO: American Academy of Family Physicians, 1994.

American Academy of Pediatrics, Committee on Practice and Ambulatory Medicine. Recommendations for pediatric preventive health care. *Pediatrics* 96:373, 1995.

American Academy of Pediatrics. *Coding for Pediatrics 2004*, 26th ed., Elk Grove Village, IL: American Academy of Pediatrics, 2003.

American Academy of Pediatrics. Immunizations in special clinical circumstances. In: Pickering LK (ed.), *Red Book: 2003 Report of the Committee on Infectious Diseases*, 26th ed., Elk Grove Village, IL: American Academy of Pediatrics 2003, p 88.

American College Health Association. *Recommendations for Institutional Prematriculation Immunizations*, March 2003, *www.acha.org*.

American College of Obstetricians and Gynecologists. *Cervical Cytology Screening*, Washington DC: American College of Obstetricians and Gynecologists, 2003; *Practice Bulletin* 45: p 1, 2003.

Averhoff F, Linton L, Peddecord M, et al. A middle school immunization law rapidly and substantially increases immunization coverage among adolescents. *Am J Public Health* 94(6):978, 2004.

Bradley J, Blythe M, (eds.). *Quick Reference Guide to Pediatric Coding and Documentation for Adolescent Medicine: A Companion to Coding for Pediatrics*, Elk Grove Village, IL: American Academy of Pediatrics, 2003.

Brener N, Lowry R, Barrios L, et al. Violence related behaviors among high school students—United States, 1991–2003. *MMWR Morb Mortal Wkly Rep* 53(29): 651, 2004.

Brown RT. Issues for the male clinician. In: Coupey SM (ed.), *Primary Care of Adolescent Girls*, Philadelphia, PA: Hanley & Belfus, 2000, p 81.

Callahan ST, Cooper WO. Gender and uninsured among young adults in the United States. *Pediatrics* 113: 291–297, 2004.

Centers for Disease Control and Prevention. Improving the health of adolescents and young adults: A guide for states and communities. *Healthy People 2010*, Division of Adolescent and School Health, Health Resources and Services Administration, Maternal and Child Health Bureau, Office of Adolescent Health, Rockville, MD, 2004.

Cohall AT, Cohall R, Ellis JA, et al. More than heights and weights: What parents of urban adolescents want from health care providers. *J Adolesc Health* 34:258–261, 2004.

Committee on Infectious Diseases. Recommended childhood and adolescent immunization schedule—United States, 2004. *Pediatrics* 113:1448, 2004.

Coupey SM. Interviewing adolescents. *Pediatr Clin North Am* 44:1349, 1997.

Elster AB. Comparison of recommendations for adolescent clinical preventive services developed by national organizations. *Arch Pediatr Adolesc Med* 152:193, 1998.

Elster AB, Kuznets NJ. *AMA Guidelines for Adolescent Preventive Services (GAPS):Recommendations and rationale.*, Baltimore, MD: Williams & Wilkins, 1992.

English A, Kenney KE. *State Minor Consent Laws: A Summary*, 2d ed., Chapel Hill, NC: Center for Adolescent Health & the Law, 2003.

Goldenring JM, Rosen DS. Getting into adolescent heads: An essential update. *Contemp Pediatr* 21:64, 2004.

Green M, ed. Guidelines for health supervision of infants, children, and adolescents. *Bright Futures*, Arlington, VA: National Center for Education in Maternal and Child Health, 1994.

Grunbaum JA, Kann L, Kinchen S, et al. Youth risk surveillance—United States, 2003. *MMWR Morb Mortal Wkly Rep* 53: SS-2, 2004.

Guttmacher AE, Collins FS, Carmona RH. The family history-more important than ever. *N Engl J Med* 2333–2336, 2004.

Halpern BL, Ozer EM, Millstein SG, et al. Preventive service in a health maintenance organization. How well do pediatricians screen and educate adolescent patients? *Arch Pediatr Adolesc Med* 154:173, 2000.

Handal GA. Adolescent immunization. *Adolesc Med* 11:439–452, 2000.

Hoffman AD. Communicating with adolescents and their parents. In: Hoffman AD, Greydanus DE (eds.), *Adolescent Medicine*, 3d ed., Stamford, CT: Appleton & Lange, 1997, p 40.

Johnston LD, O'Malley PM, Bachman JG. *Monitoring the Future National Survey results on Adolescent Drug Use: Overview of Key Findings.* (NIH Publication No. 04-5506), Bethesda, MD: National Institute on Drug Abuse, 2003.

Kaplan DW, Love-Osborne K. Adolescence. In: Hay WH, Hayward AR, Levin MJ, et al. (eds.), *Current Pediatric Diagnosis and Treatment*, 17th ed., New York: McGraw Hill, 2005, p 102.

Kaul P, Alderman EA. Teen sexuality: Patient Care. *Adolesc Med* 41, 2003.

Kaul P, Coupey SM. Clinical evaluation of substance abuse. *Pediatr Rev* 23(3):85, 2002.

Kaul P, Stevens SC. Substance abuse. In: Hay WH, Hayward AR, Levin MJ, et al. (eds.), *Current Pediatric Diagnosis and Treatment*, 17th ed., New York: McGraw Hill, 2005, p 147.

Knight J, Sherritt L, Shrier L, et al. Validity of the CRAFFT substance abuse screening test among adolescent clinic patients. *Arch Pediatr Adol Med* 156:607, 2002.

Kochanek KD, Smith BL. Deaths: Preliminary data for 2002. *Natl Vital Stat Rep* 52(13), 2004.

Orr DP, Johnston K, Brizendine E, et al. Subsequent sexually transmitted infection in urban adolescents and young adults. *Arch Pediatr Adol Med* 155:947, 2001.

Resnick MD, Bearman PS, Blum RW, et al. Protecting adolescent from harm: Findings from the national longitudinal study on adolescent health. *JAMA* 278: 823, 1997.

Rickert D, Deladisma A, Yusuf H, et al. Adolescent immunizations. Are we ready for a new wave? *Am J Prev Med* 26(1):22, 2004.

Rickert VI, Wiemann CM. Date rape among adolescents and young adults. *J Pediatr Adolesc Gynecol* 11:167, 1998.

Steele RW. Prevention and management of sexually transmitted diseases. *Adolesc Med* 11:315–326, 2000.

Strasburger VC. Children, adolescents, and the media. *Curr Probl Pediatr Adolesc Health Care* 34(2):54, 2004.

US Preventative Services Task Force. *Guide to Clinical Preventive Services:An Assessment of the Effectiveness of 169 Preventive Interventions*, 2d ed., Baltimore, MD: Williams & Wilkins, 1996.

3

CONSENT, CONFIDENTIALITY, AND OTHER RELATED ISSUES IN THE CARE OF ADOLESCENTS:

Medical, Legal, Ethical, and Practical Considerations

Anne Lyren and Tomas Jose Silber

INTRODUCTION

As adolescents navigate the passage from childhood to adulthood, they face many complex challenges. Clinicians eager to optimize adolescent health may play a pivotal role in this process.[1–3] Whether struggling with issues of body image, sexuality, substance abuse, school performance, relationships, or acute or chronic health issues, teens often need professional guidance. Many times, unfortunately, adolescents either forgo needed healthcare or do not share important information out of fear that their parents "might be told."[3–8]

Interactions with adolescent patients can sometimes be difficult, particularly when the conversation is in regard to sensitive topics that may resonate with the professional's own life experience.[9] To be most effective, the physician must approach these exchanges with skill, care, self-awareness, and appropriate knowledge of important ethical and legal considerations.[10–13] The predominant and the most controversial theme, not surprisingly, becomes the balancing of the medical rights of minors with parental rights. The goal becomes the art of delivering family-centered care while respecting the developing adolescent autonomy.[14,15]

The purpose of this chapter is to provide a practical, yet well-researched approach to the dilemmas, "gray areas," and difficulties involved in caring for teenagers, without losing sight of the profound satisfaction that such work can provide. It highlights

TABLE 3-1

DEFINITIONS

- *Confidentiality* in a health care setting is defined as an agreement between patient and provider that information discussed during or after the encounter will not be shared with other parties without the explicit permission of the patient. It is best classified as a rule of biomedical ethics that derives from the moral principle of autonomy and accompanies other rules like promise-keeping, truthfulness, and privacy.
- *Privacy* means freedom from unsanctioned intrusion. In a health care setting, it involves psychologic, social, and physical components in addition to confidentiality.
- *Informed consent* describes the process during which the patient learns the risks and benefits of alternative approaches to management and freely authorizes a course of action proposed by the clinician.
- *Assent* describes the process during which a minor who is not entitled to give informed consent, receives the same information as above and freely agrees to the action proposed. (This is an ethical, not a legal obligation).

medical, legal, and ethical considerations as well as their application. Table 3-1 contains the necessary definitions.

MEDICAL CONSIDERATIONS

In taking care of teenagers, clinicians come across situations every day that may involve confidentiality and/or the request to be seen without parental consent. Moreover, professionals are constantly faced by dilemmas, ranging from uncertainty about the adolescent's role in decision making, to dealing with an adolescent's refusal of a recommended treatment. Less frequently, but more poignantly, physicians have to give advice under more extreme circumstances, such as counseling the dying adolescent and his/her family, assessing a newly diagnosed HIV positive youth, or, increasingly, being asked about an adolescent's participation in research. What follows is a conceptual summary of current knowledge on all these issues.

Confidentiality for Adolescents

As part of the process of individuation, most adolescents desire more privacy in their personal lives. At the same time that they begin to exercise their autonomy, they also encounter increasingly complex and dangerous health threats. To be effective, the physician must respect the adolescent's participation and encourage a mature approach to his or her health care.[1–8,10–15] To go one step further, any health care system that intends to serve adolescents must be especially careful not to establish unnecessary barriers for a population that historically has not appropriately accessed health care.[6–8,16] Several studies have demonstrated that many adolescents clearly have concerns they do not want to discuss with their parents and suggest they will not seek health care if confidential services are not available.[4–8] Social forces that advocate for parental notification for all forms of adolescent health care suggest that involving parents may help deter high-risk activities. Research, however, has demonstrated that the main effect of mandatory parental notification would be to induce hesitance in adolescents to seek health care without any change in their participation in high-risk behaviors.[3,7,8] Confidentiality matters to adolescents and is a critical part of establishing a safe and trusting relationship—an essential ingredient for the adolescent to receive optimal care.[11–13]

Decision Making for Adolescents

The question of who makes decisions for adolescents is not as simple as it may appear at first glance. Decisions are routinely made by parents, who make appointments, accompany their adolescent children to the medical office, and pay the bills. Through infancy and childhood, parents have always come with their children to doctor's visits and have taken a primary role in all health related issues. Indeed, parents have the right and responsibility to act as surrogate decision makers for their children, as long as they do not have adequate decision-making capacity. The assumption is that, unless proven otherwise, parents are the most appropriate surrogate decision makers because they know their children well and are in the ideal position to decide what is in the child's best interest. Only once children reach the age of majority do they legally assume this responsibility. In the United States, an informed adult patient, acting without undue influence, who is able to understand risks, benefits, and alternatives of testing and treatment options, is considered the ultimate decision maker and may consent in matters of health care. All this seems clear-cut and yet the transfer of decision-making authority from parents to their adolescent children can be quite complex. Teenagers do not necessarily need to wait to reach adult status in order to be able to consent to treatment. In most jurisdictions, if deemed "mature minors," adolescents are entitled to give consent for the assessment and treatment of a variety of conditions, such as substance abuse and mental health care, as well as wide areas of care, such as reproductive health (visits for presumed pregnancy, concerns regarding sexually transmitted disease, contraception, and so forth) (Table 3-2). Moreover, a special category of adolescents fit the category of "emancipated minors" and therefore, can give consent for all care, as they are legally recognized as adults (Table 3-3).

A growing body of interdisciplinary literature has examined the concept of decision making in adolescence.[12,13] While there is agreement that this capacity develops variably, thus requiring individual evaluation for each adolescent patient, there is also a consensus that most children by the age of 14 have reached a developmental level that allows for medical decision making with a level of sophistication similar to that of an adult.[17,18]

Frustration over the elusiveness of exact or even unified standards of competence necessary for adolescent decision making, and the lack of a precise instrument to measure when adolescents are capable to provide informed consent, should not cause physicians to lose sight of the primary goal of getting every adolescent involved in his or her own health care. The reality is that in most instances, instead of decisions resting exclusively in the hands of a parent, decision-making responsibilities are shared among the triad of clinician, parents, and adolescent patient. In this model, the three parties communicate openly to determine the adolescent's best interest. The physician provides necessary medical data, the parents provide cultural context and family perspective, and the patient is empowered to share relevant questions, facts, and opinions. Ideally, the triad then comes to a consensus on a decision that is in the patient's best interest. Following this, the parent, who is legally empowered, gives informed permission for the intervention. Equally important is that the adolescent patient provides assent to the intervention.[19]

The standards for assent are identical to those of informed consent, an indicated willingness, after careful evaluation of relevant facts, to participate in the offered treatment. As is the case for those circumstances in which adolescents can give informed consent, the physician must always assess the patient's developmental ability to understand and agree (or disagree). In any case, the spirit of the informed consent doctrine, wherein patients are given the greatest opportunity to make their own well-informed decisions, should remain the ideal in discussions of decision making and/or assent for adolescent patients at every age and level of development.[12,13]

Treatment Refusal

Occasionally, the triad of physician, parent, and patient will not agree on the decision that is in the best interest of the adolescent. A parent who refuses to allow permission for treatment, e.g., antidepressant medication, may be making a reasonable choice. If however, the physician believes that the parental

MINORS' RIGHT TO CONSENT TO HEALTH CARE AND TO MAKE OTHER IMPORTANT DECISIONS

State	Contraceptive Services	Prenatal Care	STD/HIV Services	Treatment for Alcohol and/or Drug Abuse	Outpatient Mental Health Services	General Medical Health Services	Abortion Services	Drop Out of School	Marriage	Medical Care for Child	Medical Placing child for Adoption
Alabama	NL	MC	MC	MC	MC	MC	PC	MD	PC	MC	MC
Alaska	MC	MC	MC	NL	NL	MC	NL	MD	PC	MC	NL
Arizona	MC	NL	MC	MC	NL	NL	NL	MD	PC	NL	MC
Arkansas	MC	MC	MC	NL	NL	MC	PN	NA	PC	MC	MC
California	MC	MC	MC	MC	MC	NL	NL	NA	PC	NL	MC
Colorado	MC	NL	MC	MC	MC	NL	NL	MD	MD	MC	MC
Connecticut	NL	NL	MC	MC	MC	NL	MC	PC	PC	MC	MC
Delaware	MC	MC	MC	MC	NL	MC	PN	MD	MD	MC	MC
Dist Columbia	MC	MC	MC	MC	MC	NL	MC	NA	PC	MC	MC
Florida	MC	MC	MC	MC	MC	NL	NL	PC	MD	MC	NL
Georgia	MC	MC	MC	MC	NL	NL	PN	MD	MD	MC	MC
Hawaii	MC	MC	MC	MC	NL	NL	NL	MD	MD	NL	MC
Idaho	MC	NL	MC	MC	NL	MC	PN	MD	PC	MC	MC
Illinois	MC	MC	MC	MC	MC	MC	NL	MD	PC	MC	MC
Indiana	NL	NL	MC	MC	NL	NL	PC	PC	MD	NL	NL
Iowa	NL	NL	MC	MC	NL	NL	PN	MD	PC	NL	MC
Kansas	NL	MC	MC	MC	NL	MC	PN	MD	PC	MC	MC
Kentucky	MC	MC	MC	MC	MC	MC	PC	PN	MD	MC	MC
Louisiana	NL	NL	MC	MC	NL	MC	PC	MD	PC	MC	PC
Maine	MC	NL	MC	MC	NL	NL	MC	MD	PC	NL	NL
Maryland	MC	MC	MC	MC	MC	MC	PN	MD	MD	MC	MC
Massachusetts	NL	MC	MC	MC	MC	MC	PC	MD	PC	MC	NL
Michigan	NL	MC	MC	MC	MC	NL	PC	MD	PC	MC	PC
Minnesota	MC	MC	MC	MC	NL	MC	PN	PC	PC	MC	PC
Mississippi	MC	MC	MC	MC	NL	PC	PC	MD	PN	MC	MC

State											
Missouri	NL	MC	MC	MC	NL	MC	PC	PN	PC	MC	MC
Montana	MC	MC	MC	MC	MC	MC	NL	MD	PC	MC	MC
Nebraska	NL	NL	MC	MC	NL	NL	PN	MD	MD	NL	NL
Nevada	NL	NL	MC	MC	NL	MC	NL	MD	PC	MC	MC
New Hampshire	NL	NL	MC	MC	NL	MC	NL	PC	PC	NL	MC
New Jersey	NL	MC	MC	MC	NL	MC	NL	MD	PC	MC	MC
New Mexico	MC	NL	MC	NL	NL	NL	NL	PC	PC	NL	MC
New York	NL	MC	MC	MC	MC	MC	NL	MD	PC	MC	MC
North Carolina	MC	MC	MC	MC	MC	NL	PC	MD	PC	NL	NL
North Dakota	NL	NL	MC	MC	NL	NL	PC	MD	PC	NL	MC
Ohio	NL	NL	MC	MC	MC	NL	PN	NA	PC	NL	MC
Oklahoma	MC	MC	MC	MC	NL	MC	NL	PC	MD	MC	MC
Oregon	MC	NL	MC	MC	MC	MC	NL	MD	PC	NL	NL
Pennsylvania	NL	MC	MC	MC	NL	MC	PC	MD	PC	MC	PN
Rhode Island	NL	NL	MC	MC	NL	NL	PC	MD	PC	MC	MC
South Carolina	MC	MC	MC	NL	NL	MC	PC	MD	PC	MC	PC
South Dakota	NL	NL	MC	MC	NL	NL	PN	MD	PC	NL	MC
Tennessee	MC	MC	MC	MC	MC	NL	PC	MD	PC	NL	NL
Texas	NL	MC	MC	MC	MC	NL	PN	NA	MD	NL	MC
Utah	MC	MC	MC	NL	NL	PC	PN	NA	PC	MC	NL
Vermont	NL	NL	MC	MC	NL	NL	PN	NA	PC	NL	MC
Virginia	MC	MC	MC	MC	MC	NL	NL	MD	PC	MC	MC
Washington	NL	NL	MC	MC	MC	MC	NL	MD	PC	NL	MC
West Virginia	NL	NL	MC	MC	MC	NL	PN	MD	PC	NL	MC
Wisconsin	NL	NL	MC	MC	MC	NL	PC	NA	PC	NL	NL
Wyoming	MC	NL	MC	NL	NL	NL	PC	MD	PC	NL	MC
Total MC/MD	26	28	51	45	21	22	3	34	11	30	35
Total PC/PN	0	0	0	0	0	2	31	9	40	0	5
Total NL/NA	25	23	0	6	30	27	17	8	0	21	11

MC = minor explicitly authorized to consent; MD = minor allowed to decide; PC = parental consent explicitly required; PN = parental notice explicitly required; NL = no law or policy found.

Note In all but four states, the age of majority is 18. In AL and NE, it is 19, and in PA and MS it is 21; however, in MS 18 is the age of consent for health care.

TABLE 3 - 3

MINORS AUTHORIZED TO GIVE CONSENT

Emancipated Minors[*] (equivalent to reaching the age of majority)

- Married
- Incarcerated
- Enlisted in armed forces
- Proof of financial self-sufficiency

Mature Minors[†] (applicable only to limited circumstances, e.g. reproductive health)

- Can understand the condition for which care will be provided
- Capable of comprehending alternatives to the treatment offered
- Considered to be able to make decisions free of coercion

Emergency Situation, Medical Urgency

- *Always*

[*]Varies by jurisdiction.
[†]It is the treating clinician who makes the determination.

dissent puts the adolescent at significant risk of imminent harm, such as in the case of abuse, neglect, and idiosyncratic beliefs, e.g., refusal of life-saving antibiotics in a patient with meningitis, the physician is obligated to request help from the judicial system. The courts are the place of last recourse to a case and determine what is in the best interest of the child.

Adolescent dissent or treatment refusal is to be given the same importance as parental refusal.[19] Despite what may appear to be an inappropriate disagreement with the doctor and/or parent, e.g., refusing initiation of contraception even though sexually active, dissent should be taken seriously, especially if there is evidence that the patient has adequate knowledge and understanding and thus satisfies the criteria for medical decision making. If the physician only honors assent when the adolescent patient agrees with the intervention or physician's recommendation, and would not have accepted dissent if voiced, the process intended to empower the adolescent would be nothing more than a sham offer,

sometimes refusal only indicates that further discussion and reflection may be needed. Motivational interviews can help in this conundrum.[20] In all cases where the intervention is optional or can be deferred until the situation is clearer for all parties, an adolescent patient's dissent should be respected. In cases where the situation is too urgent and dangerous to accept a refusal, e.g., hospitalization of an adolescent with sepsis, it is still possible to inform the adolescent what will be done and openly explain that he/she has no choice in the matter.

Issues of dissent often arise in cases of anorexia, substance abuse, and mental health conditions. In these situations, the delicate balance between respecting adolescents' burgeoning autonomy and protecting them from their own poor choices must be inclined toward an intervention of "justified paternalism."[21] Since treatment refusal is a well-described symptom in patients with anorexia nervosa and substance abusing adolescents, physicians and parents may justify mandatory treatment intervention by arguing that the decision-making capacity of the adolescent is impaired by the very nature of the disease process or condition.

Nonetheless, clinicians should impose treatment against a patient's wishes only with tremendous caution, because paternalistic actions, such as the privation of freedom, are suspect and morally wrong unless they can be carefully justified. This justification involves not only that a potentially dreadful outcome could be prevented, but also that the danger was greater than the wrong caused by the violation of the patient's autonomy, and that from a wider perspective, such intervention can be generalized to others in similar circumstances.[21]

End-of-Life Decisions

Life-threatening or terminal illness decisions in adolescence can be especially challenging because of the finality of death. Parents and physicians feel more comfortable permitting an adolescent patient to participate in relatively mundane or low-risk medical decisions, such as whether to undergo nevus removal or treatment for primary nocturnal enuresis. Decisions involving withholding or withdrawal of life-sustaining treatments are exponentially more critical. When considering an adolescent's ability to make these particular decisions, physicians must consider the idea that decision-making capacity may vary depending on the specifics of the particular decision in question. While it is true that the standards for evaluating decision-making capacity are no different for life-threatening situations than for the usual illness situations, the care and stringency with which they are to be scrutinized need to be rigorous, transparent, and well documented. Again, the most important elements include whether the adolescent understands the nature of the decision, the risks, benefits, alternative, and likely or potential consequences of his decisions.[22]

When end-of-life issues can be contemplated in advance, advanced directives may be useful to empower adolescents before the incredible stress of acute health decompensation (Chap. 6).[23] In addition, hospice services can provide experienced individuals from multiple disciplines trained to assist with decision making and care coordination for adolescents and their families.[24]

Emerging Issues: HIV/AIDS

The rates of HIV and AIDS are rapidly increasing in the adolescent age group (Chap. 24). Because an asymptomatic period exists between infection and diagnosis, the incidence of HIV infection in the adolescent population is likely underestimated. Prompt diagnosis is critical for HIV as well as other sexually transmitted infections (STIs), particularly in a population that is sexually active with many partners. Little direct empiric evidence is available regarding confidentiality policies for adolescents seeking HIV testing specifically, and legal protections vary widely and wildly among the states. Nonetheless, analogous evidence from the areas of contraceptive health and other STI testing and treatment suggests that adolescents who are not assured confidential testing and counseling for HIV may eschew seeking care for this concern.[6–8,25,26]

Research on Adolescents

Research involving adolescents is seminal to the advancement of adolescent health. A regulatory framework exists which stratifies risk incurred by child research subjects.[27] The categories include (1) no more than minimal risk, which is considered to be that experienced in everyday life; (2) more than minimal risk but with potential for direct benefit to the research subject; (3) minor increase over minimal risk with no direct benefit, but where the research results are likely to result in generalizable knowledge about the research subject's disorder or condition; and (4) not otherwise approvable but presenting an opportunity to understand, prevent, or alleviate a serious problem affecting the welfare of children. Research in this category is reviewed by a special committee, under the discretion and responsibility of the secretary of the Department of Health, Education, and Welfare. All categories require both the assent of the adolescent participant, thereby acknowledging the emerging capacity for informed consent, and the permission of at least one parent, thereby offering another layer of protection for a potentially vulnerable population of research subjects. Dissent on the part of the adolescent is considered binding.

Parental permission may be waived under certain limited circumstances, such as when the involvement of the parents would explicitly affect the results of the research.[27] Part of the regulatory framework for research subject protection is a system of local Institutional Review Boards that play a pivotal role in applying these general principles to individual research protocols. In this way, specific issues such as compensation for participation, wording of consent and assent forms, and assignment of risk can be reviewed and appropriately applied.

As the body of adolescent research grows, adolescent research subjects must be carefully protected from both overcautious limitations and from entrepreneurial exploitation of their developing decision-making abilities. The physician needs to guide the adolescent and his/her parents in the understanding and questioning of research projects to ensure that indeed they aim to strike a balance between facilitating much needed research in adolescent health and protecting this potentially vulnerable group of research subjects.

LEGAL CONSIDERATIONS

A lot has been written about the medical rights of minors.[10–13, 28–34] Nevertheless, since there are variations in legal requirements from one jurisdiction to another (Table 3-2), and since the law evolves through time, we urge our readers to become familiar with what is legally permissible in their area of practice. In practices that cover more than one jurisdiction, the law that applies is not that of the area from which the patient comes, but rather where the services are being delivered. The following section concentrates on the key legal concepts relating to confidentiality, informed consent, the mature minor doctrine, the Health Insurance Portability and Accountability Act (HIPAA) privacy rules, and the medical record.

Confidentiality

Confidentiality is a legal construct that may be broadly defined by the concept that information about health care treatment and services cannot be disclosed without the permission of the person who agreed to such care.[29–31] The law's mandates, complemented by the application of ethical principles, and the information available from research may all offer perspectives on the appropriate handling of medical information regarding adolescent patients.[35]

The sources of the confidentiality obligation in the law are embedded in federal and state statutes, regulations, policies, and protocols of federal and state agencies. Many, though not all of these provisions, have been interpreted in court decisions.[30,31] However, the effectiveness of laws depends on how they might be interpreted in the future and of their understanding by patients, parents, and providers.[12,13] For instance, research in this area has shown that adolescents have a better understanding of the limits of confidentiality and substantially poorer understanding of the protections offered, which

may limit discussions of sensitive topics.[36] When confidentiality is extended to adolescents, it often cannot be complete and it certainly needs to be conditional.[12,13] The former is usually the case whenever consent for care is required from a parent or other third party, such as a court or child welfare agency. The latter is determined by state law (such as sexual abuse) and clinician's judgment (e.g., suicidal depression). In circumstances when adolescents can give informed consent for their treatment, confidentiality is implied.[12,13,28–34]

Consent

The doctrine of informed consent represents the ideal in medical decision making and corresponds to legal decision-making entitlements. In order for a person to give informed consent, he or she must be both competent and have sufficient information to have a solid understanding of the proposed intervention, including the risks, benefits, and available alternatives. The person must also be free of manipulative or coercive forces that may unduly or inappropriately influence the decision. The role of the physician is to provide the necessary information, assess the patient's understanding, and answer questions. For adolescent patients, application of the adult model of the informed consent doctrine can be confusing because no simple empiric standards exist on how to appropriately assess the equivalent of legal competence or decision-making capacity of adolescents.

Many states have provisions that take into account the medical rights of minors[37] (Table 3-2). These range from establishing the characteristics required to qualify as an "emancipated minor," to describing circumstances in which mature minors are allowed to give consent (Table 3-3). Emancipated minors may include minors who are married, incarcerated, enlisted in the armed services, or having shown proof of self-sufficiency. These individuals can legally consent to all medical care and treatment. Most states acknowledge as mature minors those adolescents who are felt by their doctor to have decision-making capacity and they can give consent if they are seeking care for particular medical conditions.[38] Usually these include drug and alcohol abuse, sexually transmitted diseases, prevention of pregnancy, and mental health care. An adolescent can also give consent for the treatment of a medical emergency. This concept can also be extended to include medical urgencies, such as severe pain.

Consent and confidentiality are quite intertwined. Adolescents, who by virtue of being an emancipated minor or mature minor status have the legal authority to consent to their own care, have the most complete protection of confidentiality. However, many ambiguities exist. Confidentiality for pregnant teens, teen parents, and abortion options remains an evolving area, and in many states, still little or no statutory law exists for guidance. Hence, the importance of the mature minor doctrine.

The Mature Minor Doctrine

In the latter half of the twentieth century, following in the steps of the civil rights movement, thoughts began to be given to the civil rights of adolescents. This interest led to legislation on freedom of speech in schools, the transformation of the juvenile justice system, and the acknowledgment of the minor's rights to obtain contraceptives.[10] In this climate, it did not take long to realize that many adolescents were deprived of services because they would rather forgo the care than tell their parents. The next step was the enactment in many jurisdictions of the medical rights of minors.[30] They were built on the concept that the determining rule for an adolescent's consent to treatment was the level of the developmental capacity of the adolescent rather than any arbitrary legal disposition. That was when the concept of the mature minor was born. Today we can be grateful for the most important feature of the mature minor doctrine; it is clinical. It is the treating physician who determines who is a "mature minor," not a legislator, judge, committee, or psychiatrist.[38] The only test needed to pass the mature minor threshold is—does the patient understand the doctor's explanations, does the patient have the capability to consider the consequences of all the alternatives proposed, and is the

patient making the decision free of coercion?[29,30] It is now several decades since the "mature minor" doctrine has become firmly established and has clearly withstood challenge in court.[39]

Health Insurance Portability and Accountability Act and Adolescents

The HIPAA privacy rule creates new regulations guaranteeing patient access to protected medical information and to exercise control on the disclosure of such information.[40] The provisions of the HIPAA privacy rules for the care of competent adults preempt state law unless state law is stronger. HIPAA did not develop strong and uniform confidentiality protections for adolescents at the federal level; however, it does leave all the current state protections in place. Thus, HIPAA privacy rules defer to the states on the issue of confidentiality for minors. Therefore, if a state law permits an adolescent to consent to confidential care, under HIPAA this information cannot be released to anybody, including a parent, without the adolescent's consent. In those cases, the confidentiality protections apply to the written information contained in medical records as well as to information communicated verbally.[13,40]

Medical Records

A wide range of civil liability and criminal penalties may apply to the unauthorized disclosure of medical records. While basic rules of confidentiality apply to medical records, there are many exceptions requiring disclosure to a variety of funding entities such as Medicare and Medicaid, to other governmental agencies such as law enforcement, or to peer review organizations. Only parents, not adolescents, can authorize release of their child's medical records. However, some states have enacted specific provisions that give minor patients the right to decide whether or not to release medical records that pertain to care for which they can give their own consent.[37]

ETHICAL CONSIDERATIONS

The principle of respect for persons as well as the principle of autonomy, recognize the developmental advances that occur during adolescence. Other ethical constructs, such as the principles of justice, beneficence, and nonmaleficence address and argue for increasing extension of the rights to give consent and maintain confidentiality to this age group.[41]

An ethically guided approach to consent and confidentiality in adolescent health care clearly involves concern for allowing an appropriate exercise of autonomy and a fair evaluation of the adolescent's decision-making capacity. Indeed, the capacity to act as one's own decision maker, especially as it relates to one's body, is usually attained earlier than is legally recognized, and once this occurs the patient has increasing claims to private communication and care. In this model, the parents play a progressively diminishing role in information processing and decision making as their adolescents assume this responsibility. Such a model does not preclude efforts to strengthen the relationship between parent and teenager.[41] Efforts to strengthen communication between the parent and adolescent can and should take place even when confidential services are available to adolescents who need or want it. Unfortunately, not all teens and parents can communicate effectively and the fact that adolescents may not seek some important services without the assurance of confidentiality is an important ethical justification for the explicit provision of confidential care.[2,5–8]

Confidentiality, put simply, is the physician's assurance that whatever a patient will share in his office visit will not be disclosed without the patient's permission. Following the Hippocratic tradition, the conversations between a physician and an adult patient are kept confidential. The transition from childhood to adolescence, is sometimes abrupt, often not anticipated, and occasionally not welcomed. The question arises as to when and under what circumstances can confidentiality be extended to teenagers. This not only may be a source of confusion and conflict, but more worrisome, it may jeopardize the quantity or quality of physician visits and the health care the physician can provide to adolescent patients.[2,5–8]

A crucial concept that can come to the rescue of clinicians is the distinction between conditional and unconditional confidentiality, as the latter cannot be extended to minors. For the protection of adolescents from imminent and serious harm, circumstances exist when disclosure must occur. This exception applies to cases of physical or sexual abuse, acute suicidal, or homicidal ideation, and similar dangerous situations.[12,13,21] Such disclosures should be preceded when possible by a discussion between the adolescent and physician that the parents or other authority will be notified, and the justification for this action.

It is obvious that the debate on the adolescent's right to consent and confidentiality is only one component in a larger struggle now going on in our culture, involving the social sciences, political theory, moral philosophy, and the like. Our society stands at the crossroads at which a number of different ethical systems are converging. Each is the carrier of a highly particular kind of moral tradition, as evidenced by the appearance of "parental sovereignty," "child welfare," and "adolescent rights." Of course, when such moral traditions encounter each other, they are, to some large degree, hurt and fragmented in the process. Thus, it is no surprise that the confusions of pluralism are often expressed in issues that are related to the status of adolescents. Though guidelines and statutory regulations are clarifying some of the confusions, the issues require, above all else, the conscientious reflection by all clinicians regarding themselves and the nature of their commitments to adolescent patients and their parents.[41]

For all of the reasons discussed, it behooves every clinician to establish policies in their practice that are based on ethical principles and incorporate accurate information about the legal requisites in their jurisdiction, and then educate their practice and their community about these issues.

PRACTICAL CONSIDERATIONS

While it has been necessary in this chapter to delve into the medical, legal, and ethical considerations relating to the medical care of adolescents, there is a need to move beyond theory, as messy reality has a habit of intruding into the most lofty plans. Therefore, this chapter ends by addressing ways in which all of the above considerations may be incorporated into a practice. This last section will address issues ranging from how to introduce the idea of adolescent consent and confidentiality to the difficult topics of payment and handling of medical records.

The first step is to recognize that the appropriate care of adolescents requires a strong commitment.[12,13] One way of establishing that a practice is intent on serving teens is to set forward a contract, either verbal or written, so that the adolescent patient and parent understand and interact around the concept of confidentiality. This conversation should clarify the basic meaning of confidentiality. It has been proposed to state this in clear or simple language: "What we talk about will be private; I will not discuss it with anyone else."[12] Some adolescents may wrongly assume that a discussion of confidentiality implies misconduct or that they have secrets. Therefore, it is useful to clarify, "Our discussion will be private, even if you don't mind your parents knowing about anything that we talk about."[12]

Patients and parents need to be educated to the conditional nature of confidentiality. They have to understand that the risk of imminent physical harm or suspected abuse is a necessary exception to the assurance of confidentiality. It is helpful to use examples that make this understandable. For example, "Everything will be confidential unless something serious happens, such as if you become suicidal."[12] When confidentiality needs to be waived, the clinician needs to let the patient know that this will happen and plan together the best way to do so.[12,13,35] Confidentiality, of course, needs to be extended to parents as they might wish to give information to the clinician without the teenager in the room.[12] Doctors often learn important information from an adult about a behavior that the teen is minimizing, hiding, or denying.[42]

Cultural competencies are a fundamental ingredient for respectful and successful policy implementation. While autonomy, independence, and self-reliance are classical Anglo-American values, other communities value more obedience, interdependence, and collaboration. The current movement toward family-centered care may be a fortunate development allowing for improved communication. Thus, there does not need to be a contradiction between the health professional's attempts to communicate with the parents and setting up a separate relationship with the adolescent. The aim that always remains is to establish a process that helps adolescent patients recognize that the care is centered on their needs and that they will never be excluded.[41] A practice can always request assent to medical treatment, a clear indication that the adolescent's views and opinions are to be respected. Seeking the assent of a minor who is not legally authorized to consent is also educational and can stimulate decision-making skills. Assent should only be obtained when there is a genuine choice and refusal would be accepted.[21]

Some of the difficulties in providing confidential care and implementing adolescent consent regulations are often institutional and systemic. Institutions frequently adopt their own policies based largely on protecting the legal and financial interests of the institution. These often tend toward an interpretation that ignores the medical rights of minors. Physicians who practice in such institutions are troubled by the fallibility in the system that deems promises of adolescent confidentiality, either ineffective or outright false. Parents and others may then easily access the medical record and insurance or billing statements, which can undermine efforts of confidentiality and jeopardize the confidential adolescent patient/doctor relationship. Nowhere is this more clearly noticeable than in issues related to appointment making, payment for services, and the handling of medical records.[43,44]

Laws which authorize minors to consent to their own care generally do not address payment for services, and in some cases actually relieve parents of financial liability. It may be difficult, even impossible, to assure full confidentiality unless an adolescent has a way to pay for services, or unless the services are provided without charge. Payment for services, often through parental health insurance, is a significant obstacle to confidential care, as billing may indicate the reason for consultation (e.g. pregnancy test). It is, therefore, crucial to alert adolescents that one can help with referrals to a variety of settings, such as health departments and family planning clinics. Thus, eligible adolescents, who otherwise would be lost, could learn about programs that can offer confidential treatment at very low or no cost, such as the Title X class and the State Children's Health Insurance Program (SCHIP).[45]

In the same vein, how one handles medical records needs to be acknowledged as an important component in the medical care of adolescents.[12] Clinicians need to be aware that protecting the confidentiality of medical records for their young patients is far more difficult than protecting verbal communications. In some cases, such as legally-mandated reporting of child abuse, the physician may not have discretion to refuse disclosure. However, in such cases of mandatory release of information, this needs to be explained to the patient. All requests for disclosure of records related to their adolescent patients need to be reviewed, taking into account sensitive or damaging information that might be revealed if records are transferred. If that is the case, permission from the adolescent should also be obtained and legal counsel should be sought.[12]

CONCLUSION

Adolescence is a remarkable period of growth and transition, as it encompasses the acquisition of the biologic capacity to reproduce, the psychological capacity to develop abstract thought, the spiritual capacity to form value systems, and the legal capacity recognized in the "mature minor" doctrine.[7,13] Nevertheless, parents, the primary providers in infancy and childhood, still have a significant role to play in the lives of their adolescent children. During this transitional time, the caring physician must be able to acknowledge and address issues of decision-making capacity and confidentiality, in order to empower and prepare the adolescent for the next transition, to young adulthood, when the productive exercise of full autonomy will take place. To do this effectively, clinicians also need to convey to parents that the judgments they

make, the policies they follow, and the regulations they abide by are intended to promote the well-being of all adolescents.

The approach outlined in this chapter is intended to facilitate dealing with adolescent consent, confidentiality, and other ethical issues relating to the care of teenagers. Based on sound ethical-legal principles and current bio-psycho-social considerations, it allows for flexible adaptation to different socio-cultural environments and to different styles of practice. The treatment of teenagers can then proceed unencumbered and provide great professional satisfaction.

References

1   Silber TJ. The physician-adolescent patient relationship: the ethical dimension. *Clin Pediatr* 1980;19: 50–55.

2   Schuster M, Bell R. Communication between adolescents and physicians about sexual behavior and risk prevention. *Arch Pediatr Adolesc Med* 1996; 150:906–913.

3   Ford CA, Millstein SG, Halpern-Felsher BL, Irwin CE. Influence of physician confidentiality assurances on adolescents' willingness to disclose information and seek future health care. *JAMA* 1997;278: 1029–1034.

4   Cheng TL, Savageau JA, Sattler AL, DeWitt TG. Confidentiality in health care: A survey of knowledge, perceptions, and attitudes among high school students. *JAMA* 1993;269:1404–1407.

5   Ginsburg KR. Factors affecting decision to seek health care: The voice of adolescents. *Pediatrics* 1997;100:922–930.

6   Klein J, Wilson K, McNulty M, et al. Access to medical care for adolescents: Results from the 1997 Commonwealth Fund Survey of the health of adolescent girls. *J Adolesc Health* 1999;25:120–130.

7   Ford CA, Bearman PS, Moody J. Foregone health care among adolescents. *JAMA* 1999;282:2227–2234.

8   Reddy DM, Fleming R, Swain C. Effect of mandatory parental notification on adolescent girls' use of sexual health care services. *JAMA* 2002;288: 710–714.

9   Silber TJ. Approaching the adolescent patient: Pitfalls and solutions. *J Adol Health Care* 1986; 7:315–405.

10 Hofmann AD. Toward a rational policy for consent and confidentiality. *J Adolesc Health Care* 1980; 1:9–17.

11 Society for Adolescent Medicine. Reproductive health and adolescents: Position paper. *J Adolesc Health* 1991;12:649–661.

12 Society for Adolescent Medicine. Confidential health care for adolescents: Position paper. *J Adolesc Health* 1997;21:408–415.

13 Ford C, English A, Sigman G. Confidential health care for adolescents: Position Paper of the Society for Adolescent Medicine. *J Adolesc Health* 2004;35: 160–167.

14 American Medical Association, Elster A (ed.). *AMA Guidelines for Adolescent Preventive Services (GAPS). Recommendations and Rationale.* Baltimore, MD: Williams and Wilkins, 1984.

15 Levenberg P, Elster A. *Guidelines for Adolescent Preventive Services (GAPS): Implementation and Resource Manual.* Chicago, IL: American Medical Association, 1995.

16 Society for Adolescent Medicine. Access to health care for adolescents: Position paper. *J Adolesc Health* 1992;13:162–170.

17 Weithorn LA, Campbell SB. The competency of children and adolescents to make informed treatment decisions. *Child Dev* 1982;52:1589–1598.

18 McCabe MA. Involving children and adolescents in medical decision making: Developmental and clinical considerations. *J Pediatr Psychol* 1996;4: 505–516.

19 Leikin SL. Minors' assent or dissent to medical treatment. *J Pediatr* 1983;102:169–176.

20 Baer JS, Peterson PL. Motivational interviewing with adolescents and young adults. In: Miller WR, Rollnick S (eds.), *Motivational Interviewing. Preparing People for Change,* New York: The Guilford Press, 2001; pp. 320–332.

21 Silber TJ. Justified paternalism in adolescent health care. *J Adolesc Health Care* 1989;10:449–453.

22 Lantos JD, Miles SH. Autonomy in adolescent medicine: A framework for decisions about life-sustaining treatment. *J of Adolesc Health Care* 1989; 10: 460–466.

23 Weir RF, Peter C. Affirming the decisions adolescents make about life and death. *Hastings Cent Rep* 1997;27:29–40.

24 Freyer DR. Care of the dying adolescent: Special considerations. *Pediatrics* 2004;113:381–388.

25 Society for Adolescent Medicine. HIV infection and AIDS in adolescents: Position paper. *J Adolesc Health* 1994;15:427–434.

26 Jackson S, Hafemeister TL. Impact of parental consent and notification policies on the decisions of adolescents to be tested for HIV. *J of Adolesc Health* 2001;29:81–93.

27 Department of Health and Human Services, National Institutes of Health, Office for Protection from Research Risks. Code of Federal Regulations: Title 45—Public Welfare. Part 46: Protection of Human Subjects. 11/13/01.

28 Melton GB, Koocher GP, Saks MJ. *Children's Competence to Consent,* New York: Plenum Press, 1983.

29 Morrisey JM, Hofmann AD, Thrope JC. *Consent and Confidentiality in the Health Care of Adolescents. A Legal Guide,* New York: The Free Press, 1986.

30 Holder A. *Legal Issues in Pediatrics and Adolescent Medicine,* 2d ed., New Haven, CT: Yale University Press, 1985.

31 English A. Treating adolescents: Legal and ethical considerations. *Med Clin North Am* 1990;74: 1097–1112.

32 AMA Council on Scientific Affairs. Confidential health care for adolescents. *JAMA* 1993;269: 1420–1424.

33 AAP Committee on Bioethics. Informed consent, parental permission and assent in pediatric practice. *Pediatrics* 1995;95:314–317.

34 English A, Morreale M. A legal and policy framework for adolescent health care: Past, present, and future. *Houst J Health Law Policy* 2001;1: 63–108.

35 Silber TJ. *Ethical Issues in the Treatment of Children and Adolescents,* Thorofare, NJ: Slack, 1983.

36 Ford CA, Thomsen SL, Compton B. Adolescents' interpretations of conditional confidentiality assurances. *J Adolesc Health* 2001;29:156–159.

37 English A, Kenney KE. *State Minor Consent Laws: A Summary,* 2d ed., Chapel Hill, NC: Center for Adolescent Health & the Law, 2003.

38 Sigman AS, O'Connor C. Exploration for physicians of the mature minor doctrine. *J Pediatr* 1991;119: 520–525.

39 Carter v. Cangello 164 Cal. Rptr. 363. Cal. Ap. May 1, 1980.

40 English A, Ford CA. The HIPAA privacy rule and adolescents: Legal conundrums and clinical challenges. *Perspect Sex Reprod Health* 2004;36: 80–86.

41 Silber TJ. Ethical considerations in the medical care of adolescents and their parents. *Pediatr Ann* 1981; 10:408–410.

42 Ross LF. *Children, Families, and Health Care Decision Making*, Oxford: Clarendon Press, 1998.

43 Klein J, McNulty M, Flatau C. Teenagers' self-reported use of services and perceived access to confidential care. *Arch Pediatr Adolesc Med* 1998;152: 676–682.

44 Akinbami LJ, Gandhi H, Cheng TL. Availability of adolescent health services and confidentiality in primary care practices. *Pediatrics* 2003;111: 394–401.

45 Brindis C, Morreale MC, English A. The unique health care needs of adolescents. *Future Child* 2003; 13:117–135.

46 Society for Adolescent Medicine. Confidential health care for adolescents: Position paper. *J Adolesc Health* 2004;35:160–167.

4

CULTURAL DIVERSITY IN ADOLESCENT HEALTH CARE

David L. Bennett, Melissa Kang, and Peter Chown

INTRODUCTION

Adolescent health care is a multicultural challenge. All clinical encounters have a cultural dimension and we are all cultural beings whose own understanding of adolescence is influenced by our cultural background. An awareness of the interplay of cultures involved in primary health care for adolescents not only helps avert problems and misunderstandings, but also improves satisfaction for all concerned and leads to better outcomes. This chapter explores the knowledge, skills, and behaviors that practitioners need to provide a culturally sensitive and effective service. In this discussion, the terms "adolescents" and "young people" are used interchangeably to refer to the age group 12–24 years.

CONCEPTS OF CULTURE AND ETHNICITY

Culture may be defined as "shared learned meanings and behaviors that are transmitted from within a social activity context for purposes of promoting individual/societal adjustment, growth, and devel-opment. Culture has both external (i.e., artifacts, role activity contexts, institutions) and internal (i.e., values, beliefs, attitudes, activity contexts, patterns of consciousness, personality styles, epistemology) representations. The shared meanings and behaviors are subject to continuous change and modification in response to changing and external circumstances."[1] Ethnicity, on the other hand, is a sense of shared "peoplehood" and while ethnicity can be based on a shared culture, it can also be based on other factors such as language, country of origin, or physical features.[2]

Health professionals, like all other people, view the world through the parameters of their own cultural framework. However, because this is largely unconscious, we may not see ourselves as cultural beings, rather culture is seen as something that only "ethnic" people have. Because of its all-pervasiveness, we are for the most part, unaware of the extent to which our own culture influences our own way of thinking, seeing things, and judging others. It is essential to recognize, therefore, that culture is always an issue in health, illness, and health care, and that the medical systems in which we work are a product of the cultures in which they occur.[2]

For primary health care professionals working with adolescents, the challenge is to go beyond just awareness of these factors and to achieve "cultural competency" in their practice. This concept embodies the ability to identify and challenge one's own cultural assumptions, values, and beliefs, and to be able to develop empathy for those viewing the world through a different cultural lens.[3] Cultural competence also involves the application of communication and interaction skills that can be learned and integrated into clinical encounters.

ADOLESCENCE—DEVELOPMENT AND DIVERSITY

Pubescence is a biologically universal phenomenon (Chap. 1). However, broader concepts of adolescence, the accompanying psychosocial phenomena, differ between cultures and the expectations, roles, and duration of adolescence can vary greatly. Cultural norms and life experiences (such as being a refugee or migrant, having a chronic illness or disability) can affect the timing of developmental milestones (including the physical changes of puberty), and shape expectations of what is considered "normal."

Development has been defined as the "unfolding of an individual's full potential within a given cultural context."[4] In some traditional societies, adulthood is reached abruptly with a rite of passage at or around puberty. In most societies, however, concepts of adolescence are evolving and not all societies view young people in the same way. In particular, the age range covering adolescence has changed over time, as have the traits attributed to young people and the nature of their position and function within society.

Culture and Adolescent Development

Adolescence is a developmental period in which the young person must negotiate fundamental psychosocial tasks in their progression toward maturity (Chap. 1). The nature of these tasks and the importance placed on their achievement, can vary

greatly between Western and non-Western cultures. For example, in Western culture, the individual is paramount and young people are encouraged to develop independence from an early age. In non-Western collective cultures, however, ethnic identity and allegiance to the family and community are more greatly valued and play a central role in shaping the development of the adolescent's identity.[5] The term "adolescence," as a psychosocial concept, may not be understood or even be familiar among some societies where a young person may continue to be seen as a dependent child until they marry.

Cross-Cultural Issues in Identity Formation

Many Australian adolescents from non-English speaking backgrounds face the challenge of dealing with the tasks of adolescence while growing up between two cultures. This involves not only two languages, but also different behavioral and social expectations.[6] Subtle stressors (personal, peer, family, and social) influence decisions about ethnic identity and working out how they can remain affiliated to their culture of origin and also determine their place within the new culture.[7]

This identity struggle (for example, "Am I Australian?", "Am I Chinese?" or "Can I be both?") can also give rise to potential conflict with their family who may fear losing control of the adolescent through their own confusion about the social norms of the adopted culture. The adolescent may be torn between the family's expectations about maintaining the values and customs of their old culture and experience extreme parental restrictions and close monitoring, while striving to adopt the norms of the new culture in order to fit in with their peers. Girls in particular may be subject to stricter controls, especially if parents feel threatened by their exposure to the values of the new culture.

Those young people who manage to retain the most important elements of their ethnic culture, while developing the skills to adapt to the new culture, appear to cope best in their psychosocial adjustment.[6] Often these young people may be seen as having a dual identity—the one they present to their family and community and the other to their peers and others to whom they relate in the new society.

Traditional family roles may change due to the influence of the new culture. Young people may have to adopt an adult role in the family because of their greater competence with the English language and familiarity with the social norms of their new country than have their parents. They may affiliate more with the families of friends who are native to their new culture. These developments may also create conflict within the family where the parents fear the erosion of their control.

Health practitioners also need to be aware of the health issues and needs of indigenous young people and the impact of culture on the presentation, diagnosis, and treatment of their health problems.[8] These critically important issues are beyond the scope of this chapter.

Cultural Assumptions and Stereotypes

While culture plays a central role in shaping people's identity, values, beliefs, social roles, and behaviors:

- Within any given culture, there can be enormous diversity and range of variables relating to ethnicity, language and religion, socio-cultural and educational backgrounds, rural or urban background, and so forth.
- It is misleading to assume that a definitive set of cultural attributes, attitudes, values, and practices apply to all people from a particular cultural background.

For migrants and refugees a range of issues need to be taken into consideration, including circumstances related to migration or refugee experience, time spent in a refugee camp, resettlement experience in the new country, reception of the host society, racism, length of time in the new country, and level of acculturation. It is important for health practitioners to avoid making cultural assumptions based on stereotypes. The focus must always be on young persons as individuals and their own perception, their cultural identity and its relevance to their life.

CULTURAL FACTORS AFFECTING YOUNG PEOPLE'S HEALTH

In Australia, young people aged 15–24 years born overseas have lower mortality and morbidity rates than Australian-born youth.[9] These findings may be partly due to the protective influence of family and cultural factors. A young person's experience of belonging to or identifying with a particular culture can enhance their resilience and promote overall well-being.[7] That is, the sense of belonging, identity, and support involved in cultural affiliation can enable young people and their families not only to survive the hardships, traumas, and losses associated with migration and resettlement, but in fact to be strengthened by these experiences.

On the other hand, young people from non-English speaking backgrounds may be at risk of poor mental health as a result of the stresses associated with the experience of migration, resettlement, and acculturation, as well as exposure to traumatic experiences.[6] Stressors include adaptation difficulties, English language difficulties, intergenerational conflict related to differences between traditional cultural values and those of the new society, and exposure to racism or discrimination and isolation. Even second- or third-generation children of migrants may still have an affiliation with their parents' culture of origin and may therefore face issues related to ethnicity, language, parents' cultural mores, and other factors.

The Refugee Experience

Some young people from refugee backgrounds may have experienced torture or trauma themselves or witnessed violence perpetrated against members of their family. Being forced to flee from one's country, when conditions become intolerable, is a process fraught with danger, taking place in the contexts of war, violence, invasions, and political repression.[10] Many family members may become separated from each other before and during the period of flight, a time that can be highly traumatic and perilous, with ongoing health consequences. Prolonged periods may be spent in refugee camps where the effect of poor nutrition and living in unsanitary conditions may also have a long lasting impact on health. Loss of extended family, friends, and home, combined with long periods of insecurity and anxiety about the future, also impact on mental health. Even when resettled safely in a new country, the effects of the refugee experience are long-term. Young people from refugee backgrounds often find themselves without the support of an emotionally available adult, as their parents struggle to cope with their own trauma and loss.

Research suggests that there are higher rates of mental health problems among migrant and refugee teenagers, compared with the general population.[6] For example, post-traumatic stress disorders are common, ranging from vague symptoms of depression, school failure, and eating and sleeping problems to high-risk behaviors such as drug abuse and sexual promiscuity. Psychotic breaks also occur in young people exposed to uncontrollable violence in terrifying ethnic wars. Failure to seek treatment early and lack of access to culturally appropriate early intervention services may severely reduce the quality of life for these young people. However, it is also important for the health professional not to make generalized assumptions and to bear in mind that many young people from non-English speaking backgrounds may have coped well with the experience of migration and resettlement.

CULTURAL SENSITIVITY IN PRIMARY HEALTH CARE

Young people are generally reluctant to seek professional help for their concerns[11] and there are additional barriers to care related to a lack of confidence and skills by service providers.[12] Ethnic minorities may have particular problems accessing treatment; for example, Asian and Black patients are less likely to have their psychological problems identified in primary care settings.[13] In this context, primary health care providers (including their ancillary staff) need to have an appreciation of the range of cultural, ethnic, and social diversity among adolescents and create a welcoming environment for young people from different cultural backgrounds. Specific measures can include providing multilingual pamphlets on different health topics, and displaying posters, artifacts, or photographs that reflect specific cultural groups. Effective health care involves:

- Understanding that one's own assumptions, attitudes, and beliefs about culture and different cultural groups are shaped by one's own cultural background and values
- Learning about the cultural background of their patients and considering how this may impact on their developing adolescent identity (as discussed earlier)
- Ensuring that the young person is perceived first and foremost as an individual and being careful not to make assumptions based on cultural stereotypes, for example, categorizing a young person as having particular cultural characteristics based solely on their parents' country of birth. (In the first place, it is misleading to assume that people from a particular cultural or language background share the same set of cultural attributes, beliefs, and practices, and in the second, it cannot be assumed that the young person necessarily relates to the cultural identity of the parents)
- Consulting with specialist services or workers if unsure about cultural issues in people from another culture
- Using a professional health care interpreter when there are language difficulties (see "Effective Communication"). This also has legal implications, as consent can only be given by patients if they are properly informed, which includes understanding the language used

Effective Communication

The single most crucial role of a primary health care provider caring for adolescents, regardless of their presenting complaint or cultural background, is to foster and develop a relationship of trust.

The skills required to communicate in a culturally appropriate manner are the same generic skills that apply to consultation with any young person, namely, an open, sensitive, empathic, and non-judgmental approach; a positive regard and respect for differing values and practices; reassurance about confidentiality; an open-ended questioning style and avoidance of medical jargon; reassurance of normality and the allaying of fears and anxieties.[14] However, it is important to bear in mind that engaging with a young person from a non-English speaking background may take considerably longer than for a young person from the mainstream. Providers need to consider the cultural context of the young persons in order to understand their presenting problems and behavior and communicate effectively with them. The style of communication and reticence to express feelings openly or discuss private family matters are often culturally determined. Some practical approaches to consultation include:

- Ask the young persons how they would like to be addressed and do your best to pronounce their names correctly; do not give them nicknames because their names are difficult to pronounce (as this is disrespectful to them and their heritage).
- Treat each patient as an individual and engage them in a dialogue about their cultural beliefs, health practices, and family history but be prepared that in some cases it may take considerable time and sensitivity to overcome a culturally bound reticence.
- Adopt a respectful, open, and nonjudgmental approach in dealing with differing cultural norms and practices. For example, assumptions about the role of verbal and nonverbal behavior (such as eye contact) may not be transferable from one culture to another (in Australian Aboriginal culture, it can be considered disrespectful to maintain eye contact).
- Ask sensitively about experiences that may have adversely affected their development, health, and attitudes to illness, for example, migration, refugee experience, exposure to war and trauma, language difficulties, discrimination, and racism. Again, be aware that the young person may be especially reticent about discussing these experiences.

- Be aware that it may not always be appropriate to see an adolescent unaccompanied by a parent and an attempt to have a private consultation with the young patient alone may be met with suspicion (although the provider can explain that seeing adolescent patients alone is considered "routine, good health practice" and suggest this as a possibility). Attempting to force this issue may risk alienating the parents and consequently losing the young person as a patient.
- Enquire about acculturation and identity issues when taking a history or conducting a psychosocial assessment: How do they view themselves within the context of their culture? "Thuy, you said that your parents were born in Vietnam and that you grew up here in Australia. What is it like to be you, a Vietnamese in Australia?" In which ways do they follow/not follow the norms of their culture?
- How do they feel about their own/parents' culture/host culture? What has changed, if anything, since they became adolescents? Are they treated differently by parents, siblings, and relatives?

Cultural Issues around Diagnosis and Treatment

- Ask about the meaning of the young person's symptoms, where relevant, within their culture (for example, mental health symptoms related to depression, anxiety, or eating disorder).
- Check their understanding of the diagnosis and treatment instructions.
- Learn which cultural differences might affect treatment (for example, attitudes to sexuality).
- Show the patient that you respect the differences between the two of you; find out if there are similarities in ideas and expectations and build on them.
- Explain that you will give the best medical care possible, but that you are not an expert on their culture so encourage them to explain this to you if they would like to.
- Be sensitive to gender issues, particularly the needs of young women when conducting physical examinations or investigating sexual

health problems; where possible provide a female practitioner or offer to conduct the examination in the presence of a female nurse or family member (if acceptable to the young person).

- Develop a management plan that addresses the impact of cultural issues and is culturally acceptable, without compromising the quality of care provided to the patient.

Understanding the Role of Family in Different Cultures

In families of non-English speaking background, parents are usually the first point of contact for reaching adolescents, so their support and participation are essential. They may have very different expectations and attitudes about health, help-seeking behavior, and the role of the doctor. For example, there may be a cultural perception that a family physician's role is to deal only with physical complaints and provide medical treatment, rather than spend time engaging the young person in conversation and exploring psychosocial issues. Approaches that would normally be adopted with adolescent patients such as ensuring confidentiality, seeing the young person alone, and encouraging independent decision making by the young person may contradict family and cultural values and risk alienating the parents. The young person also may not be comfortable about talking to a health care provider alone. This needs to be handled carefully and not rushed.

It is important to engage the parents when consulting with a young person of non-English speaking background in the following ways:

- Providing information to both the parents and young persons to help them understand issues of adolescence and adolescent development in the context of their new culture
- Explaining the doctor's role in treating the young person and respecting the parents' need to remain actively involved, should they wish to do so

Addressing Language Difficulties

Where there are language difficulties, it is important to use a professional health care interpreter. Friends and relatives should not be used as interpreters for parents. Even when a child or teenager is the most language competent person, ethical, cultural, informational, and/or familial problems can occur if they are used in this way because:

- Young people are emotionally involved and can filter information in both directions.
- There may be uncertainty about their community language, even if their apparent fluency impresses the health professional.
- They are not bound by a Professional Code of Ethics, as interpreters are, and confidentiality may become a big issue (where communities are small, the word can spread quickly).

Be aware that informed consent can only be obtained if the individual understands what is being presented in a language with which they are fluent. While there are laws in relation to the ages at which adolescents can give their own consent (for example, for prescription of birth control pills or a surgical procedure), for underage teens, parental consent may also be required. Whatever the young person's English language abilities in such a situation, a health care interpreter will be needed to ensure that the parent has a full understanding of what is being proposed.

In framing questions for people who are functionally competent in English, but not sophisticated speakers, consider the importance of the following: volume, clarity, pace of speech (speaking slowly), use of simple, nontechnical language, avoiding idioms or slang, attending behavior (i.e., importance of nonverbal indicators of respect), questioning and clarifying, and the use of open-ended questions.[15]

CONCLUSION

Young people are not a homogeneous group—there is enormous diversity, regardless of their country of birth, language, or ethnicity.[10] Diversity among adolescent patients represents a significant challenge for primary health care providers. It has been the goal in this chapter to highlight the integral relationships between culture, development and health, key knowledge, skills, and behaviors needed by practitioners to deliver culturally sensitive care to young people and their families. An approach which

TABLE 4-1

CULTURALLY SENSITIVE CONSULTATION—PRACTICE POINTS

- Be prepared to spend a longer time than usual in engaging and developing a relationship of trust with the young person from non-English speaking background.
- Treat each young person as an individual, in the first instance within the context of their cultural background; ask about their cultural beliefs, health practices, and family history.
- Be mindful that it may be culturally unacceptable for young persons to discuss family matters or to talk openly about their feelings. This reticence needs to be understood and addressed in a sensitive and respectful manner.
- Assess the degree to which cultural factors may play a role in diagnosis and treatment. Do not assume that culture is always an issue.
- Where language is an issue, check out whether the young person/parents have clearly understood the questions/information given to them; check their understanding of the diagnosis and treatment instructions, for example, by asking them to repeat the instructions back to you in their own words (do not assume that they have understood just because they say they have—in some cultures it may be considered impolite to disagree with or question an older person or someone in authority).
- Where there are language difficulties, use a professional interpreter. Do not rely on members of the family who may also have limited English or have an interest in presenting their own point of view; be aware of medico-legal issues.
- Be sensitive to gender issues, particularly the needs of young women when conducting physical examinations or investigating sexual health problems.
- Develop a management plan that addresses the influence of cultural issues and is culturally acceptable.
- Where the young person is accompanied by a parent, try to spend some time alone with the adolescent. Explain to the parents your reasons for doing this; however, respect parents' wishes to be involved and actively encourage their participation.

incorporates respect for young persons as individuals within their cultural framework and sensitivity to the issues they and their families may face as migrants or refugees settling in a new country will go a long way toward ensuring that they receive appropriate and effective health care. For a list of important points to keep in mind during a culturally sensitive consultation, see Table 4-1.

ACKNOWLEDGMENTS

The authors wish to thank Ms. Jan Kang, Coordinator of Planning and Operations, Diversity Health Institute, Sydney, Australia; Richard G. MacKenzie, MD, Director, Division of Adolescent Medicine, Children's Hospital of Los Angeles; and Donald E. Greydanus, MD, Program Director, Pediatrics and Adolescent Medicine, Kalamazoo, Michigan, for their helpful comments in the preparation of this chapter.

Note: This chapter on cultural diversity in adolescent health is written from a non-U.S. perspective; thus, the terminology that refers to people of color in this chapter differs from the rest of the book. For example, the term "black" in England and Australia can include Asian Indians, Aborigines, and African Americans. The term "black" from the U.S. perspective is used primarily to refer to African Americans. The most important aspect of the chapter's contributions is to illustrate the concept of cultural diversity from a multidimensional perspective. Regardless of terminology, the concepts are basically universal.

References

1   Marsella AJ, Yamada AM. An introduction and overview of foundations, concepts, and issues. In: Cuellar I, Paniagua F (eds.), *Handbook of Multicultural Mental Health Assessment and Treatment of Diverse Populations*. New York: Academic Press, 1999; pp. 3–24.

2 Fitzgerald MH. Gaining knowledge of culture during professional education. In: Higgs J, Tichen A (eds.), *Practice Knowledge and Expertise in the Health Professions*, Oxford: Butterworth Heinemann, 2001; pp. 149–156.

3 Fitzgerald MH. Establishing cultural competency for health professionals. In: Skultans V, Cox J (eds.), *Anthropological Approaches to Psychological Medicine*, London: Jessica Kingsley, 2000; pp. 184–200.

4 Friedman HL. Culture and adolescent development. *J Adolesc Health* 1999;25:1–61.

5 Lau A. Psychological problems in adolescents from ethnic minorities. *Br J Hosp Med* 1990;44: 201–205.

6 Bashir M. Immigrant and refugee young people: Challenges in mental health. In: Bashir M, Bennett DL (eds.), *Deeper Dimensions—Culture, Youth, and Mental Health*, Sydney, Australia: Transcultural Mental Health Centre, 2000; pp. 64–74.

7 Bevan K. Young people, culture, migration, and mental health: A review of the literature. In: Bashir M, Bennett DL (eds.), *Deeper Dimensions—Culture, Youth, and Mental Health*. Sydney, Australia: Transcultural Mental Health Centre, 2000; pp. 1–63.

8 Cox L. Young Indigenous people in Australia: issues for the GP. In: *The Missing Link—Adolescent mental health in general practice*, Darlinghurst, NSW: Alpha Biomedical Communications, 2001; pp. 21–33.

9 Al-Yaman, F., Canberra, Australia: Australian Institute of Health and Welfare, 2004 (personal communication).

10 Bennett DL, Eisenstein E. Adolescent health in a globalized world: A picture of health inequalities. In: Alderman EM, Brown RT (eds.), *Adolescents, Families and Societies in the New Millennium, Adolescent Medicine: State of the Art Reviews*, Philadelphia, PA: Hanley and Belfus, 2001;12(3): 411–426.

11 Booth ML, Bernard D, Quine S, et al. Access to health care among Australian Adolescents: Young people's perspectives and their socio-demographic distribution. *J Adolesc Health* 2004;34:97–103.

12 Kang M, Bernard D, Booth M, et al. Access to primary health care for Australian young people: service provider perspectives. *Br J Gen Pract* 2003;53: 947–952.

13 Odell SM, Surtees PG, Wainwright NW, et al. Determinants of general practitioner recognition of psychological problems in a multi-ethnic inner-city health district. *Br J Psychiatry* 1997;171:537–541.

14 Bennett DL, Kang M. Adolescence. In: Oates K, Currow K, and Hu W (eds.), *Child Health: a Practical Manual for General Practice*, Australia: McLennan and Petty, 2001; pp. 104–120.

15 Lloyd M, Bor R. Managing the cross-cultural interview "Advice on cross-cultural communication with patients." In: Lloyd M, Bor R (eds.), *Communication Skills for Medicine*, 2d ed., London: Churchill Livingstone, 2004.

5

TRANSITION TO ADULTHOOD:

Adolescents with Disabilities

Patience Haydock White

INTRODUCTION

Transitions are a part of everyone's experience as they move through life. Dreaming about the future and planning that future along with persistent hard work are essential to be successful at the next step in one's life as an adult. Children and adolescents with special health care needs and disabilities (SHCN/D), along with their peers without special health care needs, must move through a transition from childhood to adulthood. Continuity of services becomes essential if regular services are needed to support a young person's life. Many young adults with SHCN/D, such as asthma or spina bifida, move into adulthood without assistance; however, many need careful guidance to become independent adults fully participating in adult systems and adult society and not dependent on welfare and living in poverty. Youth with SHCN/D are more likely to require the use of services (such as medical, educational, and vocational) and are also more likely to be less successful in adulthood than their peers without disabilities. Today people with SHCN/D are more likely to be unemployed, have poorer health status, live in households with an income less than $15,000 per year, and be more isolated without a network of friends and available transportation.[1] In addition, caretakers of youth with SHCN/D have become more interested in the issue of transition services because in the United States over 90% of children with disabilities now survive into adulthood.[2]

Youth with SHCN/D have all the challenges in transitioning to adult-oriented systems of postsecondary school, work, and independence; however, due to their chronic illness/disability, they more frequently require constant involvement with the health care system. This chapter will discuss the definition and general principles of transition, transition needs expressed by youth with SHCN/D, the barriers and hurdles that youth with SHCN/D face as they move into adulthood, and conclude with what a health care professional can do to facilitate the transition process along with an up-to-date list of resources. In this chapter, Perrin's definition for disability and chronic illness will be used: *disability* is the inability to carry out age appropriate daily activities as a result of a health condition or impairment and *chronic condition* is a health problem, such as asthma or diabetes, that at the time of diagnosis, is predicted to be present for more than 3 months.[3]

TRANSITION DEFINITION AND GENERAL PRINCIPLES

Transition has been defined as "a multifaceted, active process that attends to the medical, psychosocial, and educational/vocational needs of adolescents as they move from Child to Adult centered care."[4] The goal of transition is to maximize the young person's potential in adulthood. This transition process includes four major components: (1) early preparation and letting go; (2) movement from pediatric to adult healthcare systems, including skill building in communication, decision making, assertiveness, self-care and funding issues; (3) graduation from school to work, including education, jobs/careers, finances, and community supports; and (4) self-determination/ interdependence. The optimal goal of transition planning is to provide services that are patient centered, flexible, responsive, uninterrupted, coordinated, developmentally and age appropriate, psychologically sound, and comprehensive. No matter how the model of transition care is organized, there are certain general principles that apply.[5] They are listed as follows:

1. Transition is often confused with transfer. Transition for youth with disabilities should be a process, not an event, and should involve the entire family. This process must be planned and take into account not only chronological age, but also the developmental stage, level of maturity, type, activity, and severity of the medical illness.
2. The transition process should begin at diagnosis. The plan should include goals for independence and self-management that are centered on a flexible time schedule to recognize the young person's increasing capacity for making choices and growing independence.
3. Different possibilities for moving into adult-oriented systems should be discussed with the

adolescent, who should be an integral part of the decision-making process. Self-advocacy skills are a key component to growing up and must be fostered throughout this process. Families need to understand their changing role as the focus shifts toward a confidential relationship between the adolescent and his or her teachers, physicians, and other care providers. The young person with SHCN/D must develop skills to negotiate the gap between the pediatric and adult health care systems.

The young person will have to adjust to the different approaches of pediatric and adult health care providers. Pediatric health providers are oriented to team approaches to care, child development, communicating with the family members more than the child, and are less focused on independence and adult issues such as employment and adult relationships. Around transition, pediatric providers can feel that they are deserting patients and that their adult counterparts lack the knowledge and skills to care for the young adult. The adult provider is oriented to aging and slow decline, patient autonomy resulting in communication with the young adult that often leaves the family out of the loop. Around transition issues, the busy adult provider may find it difficult to work with an emotionally demanding adolescent, find there are fewer support systems such as social services, and there is less financial reimbursement in the United States compared to older patients on Medicare. In addition, the adult provider may feel poorly trained in adolescent developmental issues or in diseases that, until recently, did not present to adult physicians. Thus, the adolescent who sometimes wants to be treated as an adult and at other times like a child, is faced with systems that have two different approaches, leaving the adolescent with SHCN/D needing assistance to navigate these two systems.[6,7]

4. Pediatricians, other health care providers, and the family must also prepare for this transition and understand that "letting go" is in the best interests of their patient/child. Some of the major barriers to this process result from fears about the unknown and the level of environmental and family stress. Many times, the philosophy of "why change if there is not a problem?" becomes

the operating mode. As a result, the process of transition occurs in a crisis, when the young adult is forced by age, insurance, or life plans to move to another facility and/or provider. Choosing a new provider when the youth is well and involved in the choice, usually has better psychologic and medical outcomes than being forced to move during a time of illness or crisis.

As many youth with SHCN/D interface with the medical system, health professionals can play a significant role in the development of youth with disabilities. Studies have demonstrated that health professionals tend to focus on finding a way to "fix" the disability in the individual and the youth with a disability often does not share this approach. A study showed that the longer the youth had had their orthopedic disability, the less likely they were to opt for a surgical "cure." Recently, the community of people with disabilities has articulated several observations about the medical model, in which most health professionals are trained and work. They feel it should be changed to a more interactive model, as outlined in Table 5-1.[8] The following quote from a psychiatrist with a disability, who is chair of a large rehabilitation department, demonstrates the need to change from a medical model to an interactive model for health professionals and society: "Most of the negative consequences of having a disability are not the result of the disabling condition, but rather by

the way those without disabilities related to their disabled peers."[9] Throughout the process of transition, young persons with SHCN/D must feel that they have some control of their future (self-determination) and can feel comfortable asking for or rejecting help when needed (interdependence).

5. Coordination between health care, educational, vocational, and social service systems is essential. This concept of care coordination is so essential to quality outcomes that it has been identified as one of the 20 most important areas for quality improvement by the Institute of Medicine.[10] An example of coordination between education and health is the attention that may need to be paid to the medical needs of the youth with SHCN/D as they move to postsecondary schooling. Many youth with SHCN/D drop out of postsecondary education due to health reasons. As obtaining as much education is necessary to obtain the best job, keeping these youth in school is key.

6. Adolescents in all countries reach an age of majority when society expects them to make decisions concerning their lives, work, and medical care. At this point, the adolescent should have been prepared by the planned process of transition to assume this responsibility. The maturational process during adolescence focuses on basic tasks that are not only sequential, but also overlapping. Addressing a later task before mastering an earlier one can increase the risk of

TABLE 5-1

TWO MODELS OF DISABILITY

Medical Model	Interactional Model
Disability is a deficiency or abnormality	Disability is a difference
Being disabled is a negative	Being disabled is, in itself, neutral
Disability resides in the individual	Disability derives from the interaction between the individual and society
The remedy for disability-related problems is cure or normalization of the individual	The remedy for disability-related problems is a change in the interaction between the individual and society
The agent of remedy is the professional	The agent of remedy could be the individual, an advocate, or anyone who effects the arrangements between the individual and society

Source: Gill C Vocational Development Institute of Disability Research, Rehabilitation and Training Research Center, 1996, Chicago, Ill.

failure. An example is that it is difficult to find and keep a satisfying job without prior work experience and career exploration.

What Young People with SHCN/D Want from Transition Services/Providers

Youth with SHCN/D have ideas as to what they are looking for when they think of their future. In 2002, the Bureau of Maternal and Child Health asked youth with SHCN/D what they wanted for their future. Being valued as a human being and treated with dignity, having opportunities for social experiences, dating, community involvement, recreation and worship, obtaining education and/or job training, becoming independent, and finding meaningful work for reasonable pay were stated as the most important aspects of their future.[11]

In a recent exploratory study, adolescents with nonprogressive physical disabilities were also asked how they defined success in life and what they identify as precursors for present and future success. For them success meant "being happy" or getting and doing what one wants in life. They said that being successful meant having a job, getting an education, and living on one's own. The adolescents also indicated that being believed in was a key factor in being successful. They felt that others' expectations of them were too low and limited their opportunities.[12] The literature points to the important role of significant others whose guidance, support, and encouragement are critical to success in life.[13] Adolescents with SHCN/D state that being accepted by others is important. They are similar to all adolescents who want to be accepted as part of the group. Because youth with SHCN/D often face pervasive negative attitudes,[14,15] being accepted by others give them the strength needed to cope with the adversities in life.[16] With regards to transition services, an American survey of 1300 teenagers aged 14–18 years (range 14–25 years) with a variety of disabilities (i.e., learning disabilities, chronic illness, mental health problems, physical disabilities, arthritis, and sensory impairments), was conducted in 1995 by the Parent Advocacy Coalition for Educational Research (PACER) Center in Minneapolis, Minnesota.

It pointed out that only 45% had had someone discuss with them how to make medical decisions, less than half had been asked about their work plans, and 50% had heard of transition planning.[17]

In another study, the main concern of young people with SHCN/D was that they wanted their adult health care provider to feel comfortable with people with disabilities. Other barriers/perceptions of transition outlined by adolescents and young adults were:

1. Not beginning transition planning soon enough
2. Lack of availability of a medical summary
3. Difficulty finding an adult provider
4. Excessive use of medical jargon
5. Determining how to pay for medical care
6. Concerns as to whether adult providers would understand how their illness/condition affects them as individuals

In another study, young people commented that pediatric caregivers are more caring than adult medical providers and parents do not want to "let go." In particular, young adults commented that they were burned out on health care in pediatric settings, wanted to be more involved in decisions related to their own health care, and felt no one seemed to be planning for transition.[18]

Youth with SHCN/D suggested the following ideas as helpful approaches for a successful transition: have an attentive health care provider who listens; be allowed to make decisions related to health care; have providers communicate about the transition process; have the health care provider's gender match the young person's; introduce the young person to an adult provider at age 14 or 15; and be given options of care with rationale for each option.

Transition Needs of and Barriers for Youth with SHCN/D

Youth with SHCN/D are a diverse group and have a changing epidemiology; however, there are several generalizations that can be made about their health care transition needs.[19] Youth with SHCN/D require primary and subspecialty care to maintain and improve their functioning. Because youth with SHCN/D may already have a chronic illness, secondary health conditions and other health conditions that would have minor effect on a youth without SHCN/D, can result in major functional impairments. Youth with SHCN/D often do not have the same opportunities for health maintenance or prevention. For example, someone with limitations in mobility or congenital heart disease may not be able to exercise. Youth with SHCN/D may develop secondary chronic illnesses sooner due to their illness or its treatment and experience secondary functional losses. For example, asthmatics that are treated with steroids may develop severe osteoporosis with fractures. Youth with SHCN/D may require prolonged and more complicated treatment for a particular health problem than youth without SHCN/D. Many youth with SHCN/D, such as youth with HIV/AIDS, require prolonged drug treatment and these drugs may be the reason they can survive into adulthood. Youth with SHCN/D may need durable medical equipment, assistive technologies, and long-term services, such as personal assistance and continuous medical supervision.

The hurdles to a smooth transition are multiple, as outlined in Table 5-2. In particular, barriers to

TABLE 5-2
HURDLES TO SUCCESSFUL TRANSITION

Hurdles to Successful Medical Transition	
The young person	Lack of familiarity with adult clinic and team
	Reluctance to leave pediatric team especially if long disease duration
	Immaturity–lack of social skills
	Dependence on parents
	Nonadherence
	Not yet independent in managing their own health-care
	Prevention and management of comorbidities
The parents	Lack of familiarity with adult clinic and/or team
	Dislike of individual approach of adult care
	Over-protectiveness
	Negative preconceptions of adult care
	Awareness of lack of confidence of pediatric team in adult service
The pediatric health professional	Reluctance to let go long-term patients
	Lack of confidence in adult system
	No pediatric-adult interface
	Lack of knowledge of transition issues/resources
The adult health professional	Lack of confidence in pediatric illnesses
	Lack of training in adolescent healthcare
	Individual rather than family-centered approach
	Negative attitudes of paternalistic style of pediatric care
	Lack of knowledge of transition issues/resources
The delivery system	Lack of planning
	Lack of preparation of young person, their family, and the adult team
	Suitable clinic space
	Difficulties in administrative transfer of patient notes and x-rays
	Consensus regarding management guidelines between pediatric and adult specialty services
	Lack of health care insurance availability
Time and money	Lack of available time for the full spectrum of transitional care
	Lack of funding

Source: With permission, from Janet L. Donayh, MD, 2005.

health care access can be physical (i.e., facilities inaccessible, lack of transportation), social (communication challenges), system (lack of coordinated care, lack of subspecialists within a reasonable distance), and financial (lack of medical insurance or lack of coverage for special services such as specialized therapies, primary or subspecialty care). A major concern in the United States is how young people with SHCN/D can pay for their medical care. Thirty percent of all young adults between 18 and 24 years of age are uninsured, making them the largest group of uninsured Americans. The health care financing for young adults with SHCN/D is a maze of systems that have different qualifying criteria. The majority is covered by employer-sponsored health insurance through their parents, and those who are poor or on social security income receive Medicaid health insurance coverage. Yet, when the young people with SHCN/D between the ages 18 and 23 age out of Medicaid coverage and their parents' health care policies, many find themselves with no available coverage and can not get a job that will offer them or allow them to afford health care coverage. Similarly, those who have qualified for social security income and Medicaid as a child will have to go through a redetermination for social security income as an adult at age 18. Because the qualifying criteria are different for adults on supplemental security income (SSI), many young adults with SHCN/D lose their SSI and Medicaid. Thus, young people with SHCN/D who become young adults with SHCN/D, find little availability of health insurance and health providers that were an essential part of why they survived and now are looking to participate in adult society.[20,21]

School to Work

The majority of people in the United States obtain their health insurance from the employer. Youth with SHCN also want a satisfying job, but their problem of not obtaining a job as adults with SHCN/D begins in adolescence. American data on participation in the workforce of adolescents with disabilities shows that they are twice as likely as their peers without disabilities to be unemployed. In addition, research shows that youth with disabilities are more likely to

drop out of school, live with parents, and be socially isolated compared to their peers without disabilities. Based on data from the National Health Interview Survey on Disabilities (NHIS, 1884–95), Scal et al found that graduation rates declined based on severity of condition. Those without disabilities between ages 18 and 30, 82.6% graduated; in contrast, graduation rates for those with disabilities were: 79.5% for mild, 76.1% for moderate, and 61.4% for severe. When Scal et al looked at employment, they reported that 78.8% of those 18–30 years of age were in the labor force, but only 72.4% with mild and 38.7% with severe disabilities were employed.[22] This lack of education and work experience delays one of the most important developmental tasks of adolescence, finding a vocation.

A key part of the equation to becoming employed is that all who interact and guide the youth with disabilities and the youth themselves, need to understand the future workplace. What does a future employee need to know to survive in the workplace of the future? The world of work today is undergoing a monumental change that, social scientists say, is equivalent to the disrupting changes that came with the industrial revolution.

The Bureau of Labor Statistics in the United States forecasts that by the year 2006 nearly one in every two jobs added to the economy will be in the service industry (health, business, and social). Most jobs requiring high skill levels will increase, whereas the low-skill jobs will decline. There will be labor efficiency, with better technology, better processes, and fewer better-educated workers. The employee of the future with continual retraining can expect lifelong employability, not employment. The employee, like business, must be reinvented to keep up with new technology. The technology explosion makes the workplace friendlier for people with disabilities, allowing flexible hours and locations for work. In this fast-changing global economy, the United States Department of Labor suggests that workers will need to:

- Get as much education as possible—be skilled not stuck
- Keep upgrading their skills (retrain)—be prepared not *jobsolete*

- Sharpen career exploration/development skills to remain employed in this changing global economy
- Change careers—not just jobs—three to four times during their working years[23,24]

Education is essential in today's knowledge-based economy. Current studies still show that the level of education attained is directly related to lifetime earnings and who becomes employed.[24] The relationship holds up for those with disabilities as well. This means that in the United States, in order for individuals with disabilities to not live in poverty and have access to health insurance, they must be employed in a high-skilled job that requires education beyond high school. Thus, counseling to make postsecondary education a reality for young people with disabilities is central to their success.

While in high school, youth with SHCN/D may have an Individual Education Plan (IEP) or if they are not eligible for an IEP, they may have services under Section 504 of the Rehabilitation Act. Transition provisions were outlined in the 1990 reauthorization of Individuals with Disabilities Education Act (IDEA) that required schools to develop individualized transition plans for students with SHCN/D. Students with 504 plans do not have legal mandates for transition plans as do students with IEPs. Primary care providers may need to advocate for appropriate school-based services for transition. Plans for a transition from high school to postsecondary education (either college or vocational school) should be reflected in the IEP or 504 plan. Almost all colleges and universities have an office of disabled student services. The student should contact this office even before applying to determine available services and after they are accepted. A major source of information for postsecondary education is the HEATH Resource Center,[35] which is a national clearinghouse on postsecondary education for people with disabilities.

The medical provider can assist the youth by encouraging that the youth with SHCN/D: (1) obtain postsecondary education, (2) learn any accommodations they might need, and (3) have an early consultation with Division of Rehabilitation Services to determine if a student is eligible for any educational or support services. Table 5-3 offers a set of questions to consider as the youth with SHCN/D prepares to go on to further schooling without the protection of an IEP that they had in high school.[34]

Early work experience is equally important. A 1996 survey from *The New York Times* of 300 employers revealed the top three qualities that counted with employers were—attitude, communication skills, and previous work experience. In the United States, a study was conducted that showed over 53% of 13-year olds without disabilities were involved in a work experience outside their homes once a week. The average age at which parents felt children without disabilities should start work was 13 years (SD 1.9 years).[25] The recent US Department of Labor publication, *Futurework*, states that today young people hold an average of nine jobs between the ages of 18 and 32 with more than half of the job changes occurring before the age of 23. Youth with SHCN/D need to start work experiences at similar ages as their peers without disabilities so they can be competitive in the fast changing job market. Research shows part-time work experience is important, but it needs to be done in association with careful counseling that asks what the adolescent is learning, about his or her likes and dislikes, and abilities as they think of their future work choices.

Dreaming about future roles is essential in shaping the directions that one takes in adulthood. Expanding the horizons of a child with a disability can be limited by physical and social isolation. This isolation and lack of a peer group can hinder the person with SHCN/D in finding a job because the majority of jobs today are still obtained via the family/friend network. This has been found to be equally true for people with disabilities. Few found lasting jobs through a rehabilitation agency.[26,27] The health care provider can assist this process by asking if the youth is completing chores at home and finding out if the family is treating the youth as they do other members of the family. This expectation to be part of the family is an excellent way to start the process for the youth with SHCN/D to take on responsibility like others in their family and is good training for expectations in the workplace.[28]

TABLE 5-3

ELEMENTS OF EFFECTIVE TRANSITION PLANNING TO POSTSECONDARY EDUCATION ASSESS THE IMPACT OF ILLNESS ON THE STUDENT

Educationally

Has the illness necessitated any special accommodations at school?

Was class missed at certain times of day to perform a health care routine?

Did the illness affect attendance?

Did medication affect ability to concentrate or participate in school? (i.e., was the student more alert at certain times of the day? Were frequent breaks from class required to take medications or rest?)

Was extra time necessary to complete class work, tests, or homework?

Was technology, such as computers, used in the classroom or at home to fulfill academic requirements?

Was in-class assistance required, such as a person to take notes?

Medically

Are any activities restricted?

Does the student require specialized medical care (for example, dialysis)?

Does the student require the coordinated care of many health care providers?

Does the student have a care routine which must be performed at a specific time of day?

Does the student have a care routine which can only be done by a specially trained individual, such as a physical therapist, respiratory therapist, or nurse?

Is there a medication schedule which must be strictly adhered to?

Are required drugs difficult to find?

Is the care of a medical specialist required? How frequently?

Environmentally

Do certain environmental factors such as heat, cold, molds, dust, odors, and humidity affect the student's health and well-being?

Does the student need to limit exposure to noise and distractions?

Does the student require a special living environment?

Are certain activities such as walking long distances or climbing stairs difficult?

Activities of Daily Living

Is assistance getting out of bed required?

Is assistance with food preparation/eating needed?

Does the student require a special diet?

Does the student need assistance bathing or using the bathroom?

Is assistance with dressing necessary?

Is assistance with mobility required?

Excerpt from a forthcoming resource paper written by the Adolescent Employment Readiness staff for the HEATH Resource Center, 1997. Source: A consensus statement on health care transitions for young adults with special health care needs. *Pediatrics* 2002, 110:1304–1306.

Transition to Independent Living

Moving to living on one's own can be difficult for many youth with SHCN/D, especially those with cognitive, physical, and emotional disabilities. This is due to the fact that many of the necessary support systems are not readily available. Youth with chronic health conditions that are unstable can find this task very difficult if they have not developed the necessary skills to manage their condition and solve problems related to their condition. Two amendments to the Medicaid program provide funding mechanisms to support community living for young adults with SHCN/D. One is the Home and Community Based Services (HCBS) waiver that supports case management, homemakers, home health aides, personal care residential habilitation, transportation, supported employment, adaptive equipment, and home modification. The other is the Community Supported Living Arrangements (CSLA) that supports state wide systems of individualized supported living. Learning to be as independent as possible really means that young adults with SHCN/D have learned to be interdependent. They have learned when and how to ask for assistance which demonstrates mature decision-making skills. These skills along with the appropriate social skills are essential for youth to transition to independent living and self-care.[29]

Medical Care and the Role of the Health Care Provider in Transition

Guiding young people with SHCN/D who need assistance toward a productive adulthood can be accomplished by many different people who are involved with the adolescent with SHCN/D; these include their family, community, educators, and health care providers. The health care provider is in an excellent position to support and potentially lead the transition process for the family and young person with SHCN/D. Over the past several years, the American Academy of Pediatrics (AAP),[30,31] the Society of Adolescent Medicine,[32] and the American Medical Association (AMA)[33] have developed statements confirming the important role of the physician and other health care professionals in this process. Though these statements focus on the health transition, the health care professionals should not work in isolation from other professionals and networks that affect these young people.

Recently, a consensus document has been approved by the AAP, the American Academy of Family Physicians (AAFP), and the American College of Physicians-American Society of Internal Medicine (ACP-ASIM).[34] This consensus statement is a call to action of the critical first steps needed to ensure the successful transition of young people with SHCN/D to the adult health care system. The statement is outlined in Table 5-4 and includes policy

TABLE 5-4

A CONSENSUS STATEMENT ON HEALTH CARE TRANSITIONS FOR YOUNG ADULTS WITH SHCN/D FROM THE AAP, AAFP, AND THE ACP-ASIM

1. Ensure that all young people with SHCN/D have an identified health care professional who attends to the unique challenges of transition and assumes the responsibility for current health care, care coordination, and future health care planning
2. Identify the core knowledge and skills required to provide developmentally appropriate health care transition services to youth with SHCN/D and make them part of training and certification requirements for primary care residents and physicians in practice.
3. Prepare and maintain an up-to-date medical summary that is portable and accessible.
4. Create a written health care transition plan by age 14 together with the young person and family. At a minimum, this plan should include what services need to be provided, who will provide them, and how they will be financed. This plan should be reviewed, updated, and available when transfer of care occurs.
5. Apply the same guidelines for primary and preventive care for all adolescents and young adults with and without SHCN/D recognizing that youth with SHCN/D may require more resources and services than those without SHCN/D to optimize their health. See references 35, 36, and 37 for examples of guidelines.
6. Ensure affordable, continuous health insurance coverage for all youth with SHCN/D throughout adolescence and adulthood. This insurance should cover appropriate compensation for healthcare transition planning and care coordination for those who have complex medical conditions.

Source: Council on Adolescent Development: Facilitating the transition of adolescence. *JAMA* 1987, 24:2405–3406.

suggestions to ensure better transition outcomes for youth with SHCN/D.[33]

Table 5-5 lists a series of suggested tasks for health care providers to assist the youth with SHCN/D with their transition toward adulthood.

Care coordination across all the systems, including the family and youth in the decision-making process, and encouraging the youth to move from assent to consent in the medical and other spheres of their life, can be challenging and complex. The

TABLE 5-5

TEN EASY STEPS TO WHAT HEALTH CARE PROVIDERS CAN DO TO FOSTER A SUCCESSFUL TRANSITION TO ADULTHOOD FOR A YOUNG PERSON WITH SPECIAL HEALTH CARE NEEDS

1. Communicate at the age appropriate level and early that you want their involvement in their medical care and that they will be transferring to an adult provider in the future. Speak directly with the children and when they become adolescents, spend part of the visit without the adolescents' parents when developmentally appropriate. Respect their desire for privacy. Reinforce their competence and competent behaviors.

2. At the appropriate level for youths' age, teach and reteach about their illness/condition. Ask if they understand their condition and listen closely to their response.

3. Discuss choices. Let adolescents be active participants in planning and solving problems in their medical and transitional care. (How would you like to take your medication–by pill or liquid?) Guide them on how to find all those needed for their adult health care team and assist them in understanding their health care insurance.

4. Be a catalytic consultant by guiding adolescents to their next developmental milestone toward more independent behavior, and their family to a new, less controlling role. Communicate that transition planning is a process not just the day they go to an adult provider. Start the transition process at an early age reminding them each year of the milestones to be attained.

5. Take responsibility yourself or identify someone to lead the transition process. In consultation with adolescents/families prepare a written transition plan by the age of 14 and compile summaries of their medical records that can be continuously updated. (AAP/ACFP/ACP transition Policy 2002). Review the possible health insurance options with families and youth.

6. Coordinate their care and assure that someone is providing basic preventive care (send a letter to the primary care physician, if appropriate, asking if they are using GAPS or other adolescent health guidelines) Ask about healthy behaviors such as exercise, eating calcium, and a good diet. Strategize with them ways to keep their weight appropriate for their height. Assist them to develop healthy habits so they can be part of the action.

7. Encourage resilient behavior and assist adolescents to dream about their future (What do they want to be when they grow up? What does it take to obtain that favorite job? What job or volunteer experience will they do this summer? What did they think of their last volunteer or paid work experience? Do they need a referral to a college/vocational counselor? Do they understand their legal rights as a person with a disability?)

8. Have high expectations for them in the future and treat them as you would others without special health care needs (Do they do chores around the home like others in their household? Do they have friends? What social and recreational activities do they participate in? If none, brainstorm with them how it could happen).

9. Assist them to attain the highest level of education possible for their capacity (How are they doing in school? Are they missing a lot of school? Would they benefit from a 504 or an IEP (Individual Education Plan)? What subjects do they like and are good at? Do they plan to go on to postsecondary school? Do they need accommodations for postsecondary school educational experiences? Develop a transition plan for college or postsecondary school.

10. Try to shift from a medical model (see Table 5-1) where health care professionals mainly talk of curing the illness or making youth more "normal" with treatments (problem is in the youth) to a more interactive model where young persons accept who they are and at the appropriate levels work to interact in an interdependent manner with their environment/society (problem is in the interaction with society and being amenable to change with the assistance of others).

TABLE 5-6

KEY ELEMENTS TO AN EFFECTIVE TRANSITION PROGRAM

1. A policy on timing of transfer
2. A period of preparation and deliberate education program that focuses on skills so that the young person is able to function in the adult clinic (understanding of the disease, treatment rationale, source of symptoms, recognizing deterioration and taking appropriate action, how to seek help from health professionals and how to operate with the medical system)
3. Creation of a coordinated transfer process (including detailed written plan, pretransfer visit to adult clinic with introduction to adult provider, and designated coordinator, such as a clinic nurse)
4. An engaged and capable adult provider/service
5. Administrative support
6. Primary care involvement

Source: US Preventive Services Task Force, Public Health Service, *Guidelines to Clinical Preventive Services,* 2d ed., Washington DC: US Public Health service, 1996.

leadership of the provider for the transition process will vary according to the capacity of the family to handle the process. As "letting go" by the family can be full of anxiety, the provider may need to lead the process by showing the next step and carefully planning this process. Similarly, health care providers can create a transition policy in their practice/service and/or hospital to facilitate the process. The key elements to an effective transition program are outlined in Table 5-6. A list of resources is attached in Table 5-7 to assist all involved. There are many tools and guides available as well as a wealth of information to help everyone through this transition planning process.[35–39]

TABLE 5-7

SELECTED NATIONAL WEB RESOURCES ON TRANSITION

Transition issues

*AAP Medical Home *www.aap.org.advocacy/medhome/aap.htm*

ABLEDATA A database of technology products *http://www.abledata.com*

Adolescent Employment Readiness Center *www.dcchildrens.com/about/abt2b.htm*

HEATH Provides specialized educational information *www.heath.gwu.edu*

*Illinois Chapter of the AAP ICAAP @ MSN.com

Institute for Community Inclusion at Children's Hospital in Boston, Mass *www.communityinclusion.org/transition*

*Institute for Child Health Policy www.hctransition.ichip.edu

Join, leave, search & post to the Health Care Transition, available at:
 http://mchenet.ichp.edu/scripts/lyris.pl?enter=transition

*MCHB Healthy and Ready to Work National Center-web site with tools, guides,
and check lists *www.hrtw.org*

National Information Center for Children and Youth with Disabilities *www.nichcy.org*

National Organization on Disability *www.nod.org*

National Transition Network *www.ici2.umn.edu/ntn*

Transition Research Institute *www.edu.uici.edu/sped/tri/internet*

University centers on disability *www.aucd.org*

*Transition check lists

(Continued)

SELECTED NATIONAL WEB RESOURCES ON TRANSITION (*CONTINUED*)

Vocational web sites

www.teenleader.org/teenleader/alumni/cyber_jobs.shtml

www.hhs.gov/kids

http://cando.lancs.ac.uk

Web sites for Kids

Family Voices KASA (kids as self advocates) *www.kasa.org*

National Youth Leadership Network *www.nyln.org*

www.disabilitycentral.com/activteen

Starbright Foundation *http://starbright.org/*

Girl Power *http://www.health.org/gpower*

Australian Youth Site *www.rch.unimelb.edu.au/ChIPS/*

Family Related

Exceptional Parent Magazine *www.eparent.com*

Family Village *http://www.familyvillage.wisc.edu/*

Family Voices *http://www.familyvoices.org/*

Parents Helping Parents *http://www.php.com/*

The Consortium for Appropriate Dispute Resolution in Special Education (CADRE) *www.directionservice.org/cadre*
  or call 541-686-5060

Family Education Network *http://www.familyeducation.com/*

Institute for Child Health Policy *www.ichp.edu*

Institute for Family-Centered Care *http://www.familycenteredcare.org*

America's Promise *www.americaspromise.org/*

Fathers Network *www.fathersnetwork.org/*

National Parent Network on Disabilities *www.npnd.org/*

National Information Center for Children and Youth with Disabilities (NICHCY)

http://www.nichcy.org

Federal Government Related

Social Security Online *http://www.ssa.gov/*

President's Committee on Employment of People with Disabilities *http://www.pcepd.gov/*

Children's Defense Fund *www.childrensdefense.org*

IDEA Practices *www.ideapractices.org*

National Dissemination Center for Children with Disabilities *www.nichcy.org*

Other Transition Centers (generic):

ONTRAC transition programme

British Columbia Children's Hospital

Room 2 D20 4480 Oak St

Vancouver BC

Canada 3V4

Tel: (604) 875-3472

(Continued)

TABLE 5-7

SELECTED NATIONAL WEB RESOURCES ON TRANSITION (*CONTINUED*)

Parent Training and Information Centre

PACER Centre Inc.

4826 Chicago Avenue South

Minneapolis MN 55412

USA

Tel: (612) 827-2966

National Centre for Youth with Disabilities

University of Minnesota

PO Box 721

420 Delaware St SE

Minneapolis MN 55455

USA

Tel: (612) 626 2931

Adolescent Employment Readiness Centre

Children's National Medical Centre

111 Michigan Ave NW

Washington DC 20010-2970

Tel: (202) 884 3203

Fax: (202) 884 3385

CONCLUSION

Youth with SHCN/D desire to become independent members of society and attain the same education, jobs, careers, health, and well being that all youth seek. Yet, youth with SHCN/D have needs for greater medical supports throughout this transition process and their needs are delineated. Transition as it is defined by the medical community and its general principles are outlined. Also covered are the issues and hurdles for youth with SHCN/D for their movement from school to work and home to independence, as well as suggestions to health care professionals as to what they can do individually and in their workplaces to assist in this important process of transition.

References

1 NOD/Harris Survey of People Disabilities Study, No. 942003, Louis Harris Association: Washington, DC, 1998.

2 Blum RW. Transition to adult health care: Setting the stage. *J Adol Health* 1995;17:3–5.

3 Perrin JM. Health services research for children with disabilities. *Milbank Q* 2002; 80:303–324.

4 Blum RW (ed.). Improving transition for adolescents with special health care needs from pediatric to adult-centered health care. *Pediatrics* 2002;110:1301–1335.

5 Conference Proceedings. Moving on—transition from pediatric to adult health care. *J Adol Health* 1995; 17:3–36.

6 Viner RM. Transition from pediatric to adult care. Bridging the gaps or passing the buck? *Arch Dis Child* 1999;81:271–275.

7 Rosen D. Between two worlds: Bridging the cultures of child health and adult medicine. *J Adoles Health* 1995;17:10–16.

8 Gill C. Vocational Development. Institute of Disability Research, Rehabilitation and Training Research Center, Chicago, IL, 1996.

9 Strax TE. Psychological issues faced by adolescents and young adults with disabilities. *Pediatr Ann* 1991;20:501–506.

10 Adams K, Corrigen J (eds). Committee on Identifying Priority Access for Quality Improvement. Washington,

DC: National Academy Press, p. 5, 2003. Priority Areas for National Action: Transforming Health Care Quality. Available at: *www.nap.edu.*

11 Blum RW, Garell D, Hodgma CH, et al. Transition from child centered to adult health care-systems for adolescents with chronic conditions. *J Adol Health* 1993;14:570–576.

12 King G, Cathers T. What adolescents with disabilities want in life: implications for service delivery Keeping Current 96-2, 1996. Available at: *www.fhs.mcmaster. ca/canchild/publications/keepingcurrent/KC96-2.*

13 Spekman J, Goldberg RJ, Herman KL. An exploration of risk and resilience in the lives of individuals with learning disabilities. *Research and Practice* 2000;8:11–18.

14 Doyle Y, Moffat P, Corlett S. Coping with disabilities: the perspective of young adults from different ethnic backgrounds in inner London. *Soc Sci Med* 1994;38:1491–1498.

15 Law M. Changing disabling environments for children with physical disabilities: A research study completed with participating families—Cambridge. Working Paper Series No. 31, University of Waterloo: Waterloo, IA, 1993.

16 Brooks RB. Children at risk: Fostering resilience and hope. *Am J Orthopsychiatry* 1994, 64:545–553.

17 Wright B. Teens say jobs training their top need. In: *Point of Departure.* Minneapolis, MN: Act Project, PACER Center, 1996;2:8.

18 Patterson D, Lanier C. Adolescent health transitions: Focus group study of teens and young adults with special health care needs. *Fam Community Health* 1999;22(2):42–58.

19 Dejong G, Palsbo SE, Beatty PW. The organization and financing of health services for persons with disabilities. *The Milbank Q* 2002;80:261–301.

20 White PH. Access to health care: Health insurance considerations for young adults with special health care needs/disabilities. *Pediatrics* 2002;110 (suppl. 6):1328–1335.

21 Vladeck BC. Where the action really is: Medicaid and the disabled. *Health Aff* 2003;22:90–100.

22 Scal P, Larson S, Ireland M, Blum R. Young adults with childhood onset disability making their way into adulthood. *Pediatr Res* 2003;53 (abstract).

23 Hammonds KH, Kell K, Thurston K. Rethinking work. *Bus Week* 1994;76–87.

24 Futurework—Trends and Challenges for work in the 21st century. A report of the United States Department of Labor, Labor Day, 1999.

25 Philips S, Sandston KL. Parental attitudes towards work. *Youth Soc* 1990;22:160.

26 Benz MR, Doren B, Yovanoff P. Crossing the great divide: Predicting productive engagement for young women with disabilities. *Career Development for Exceptional Individuals*, 1998;21(1):3–16.

27 Crudden A, McBroom LW, Skinner AL, Moore JE, *Comprehensive examination of barriers to employment among persons who are blind or visually impaired*, Mississippi, MS: Rehabilitation Research & Training Center on Blindness & Low Vision, Mississippi State University, 1998.

28 White PH. Transition: A future promise for children and adolescents with special health care needs and disabilities. *Rheum Dis Clin North Am* 2002;28: 687–703.

29 Hallum A. Disability and the transition to adulthood: issues for the disabled child, the family and the pediatrician. *Curr Probl Pediatr* 1995;25:12–50.

30 American Academy of Pediatrics, Council on children with disabilities and committee on adolescents. Transition care provided for adolescents with special health care needs. *Pediatrics* 1996;98: 1203–1206.

31 American Academy of Pediatrics Committee on children with disabilities. The role of the pediatrician in transitioning children and adolescents with developmental disabilities and chronic illnesses from school to work or college. *Pediatrics* 2002;106: 854–856.

32 Blum RW, Garell D, Hodgma CH, et al. Transition from child centered to adult health care-systems for adolescents with chronic conditions. *J Adol Health* 1993;14:570–576.

33 Council on Adolescent Development: Facilitating the transition of adolescence. *JAMA* 1987;24: 2405–3406.

34 A consensus statement on health care transitions for young adults with special health care needs. *Pediatrics* 2002;110:1304–1306.

35 Edelman A, Schuyler VE, White PH. Maximizing Success for Young Adults with Chronic Health-related Illnesses: Transition Planning for Education After High School White Paper in conjunction with HEATH Resource Center of the American Council on Education, 1998.

36 American Medical Association, Dept. of Adolescent Health Guidelines for Adolescent Health services (GAPS), *Clinical Evaluation and Management Handbook*, Chicago, IL: American Medical Association, 2000.

37 Green M, Palfrey JS (eds.), *Bright Futures: Guidelines for Health Supervision of Infants, Children, and Adolescents*, 2d ed., Arlington, VA: National Center for Education in Maternal and Child Health, 2000.

38 US Preventive Services Task Force, Public Health Service, *Guidelines to Clinical Preventive Services*, 2d ed., Washington DC: US Public Health service, 1996.

39 Britto MT, DeVellis RF, Hornung RW, et al. Health care preferences and priorities of adolescents with chronic illnesses. *Pediatrics* 2004;114: 1272–1280.

6

END-OF-LIFE ISSUES IN ADOLESCENT HEALTH CARE

David R. Freyer and David S. Dickens

INTRODUCTION

Thou hast nor youth nor age, but, as it were,
an after-dinner's sleep, dreaming on both.

William Shakespeare, *Measure for Measure*

Poised between the dependency of childhood and the self-reliance of adulthood, adolescents with life-threatening illness face extraordinary challenges in laying full claim to neither but, in turns, longing for both. As noted recently by Himelstein and colleagues, "A unique aspect of pediatric palliative care is that the complex experience of life-threatening illness occurs, by the very nature of the child as patient, within the context of growth and development—physical, emotional, social, psychologic, and spiritual."[1] Nowhere do the truth and force of this statement become more apparent than during the care of adolescents at the end of life.

In the United States alone, approximately 3000 adolescents succumb annually to chronic illnesses such as malignant neoplasms, congenital malformations and syndromes, cardiac disease, chronic pulmonary disorders, renal failure, acquired immunodeficiency syndrome, and cerebrovascular conditions.[2] The management of these individuals

is not only medically and emotionally challenging, but is further complicated by a unique combination of ethical, legal, and psychosocial issues associated with their emerging maturity. This chapter will review these issues as they apply to medical decision making and clinical management of adolescents at the end of life.

DECISION MAKING BY ADOLESCENTS

The fundamental decision facing adolescents with a chronic, life-threatening illness is whether to continue treatments intended to cure or alter the course of the underlying condition. Depending on the diagnosis, such treatments may include renal dialysis, antiretroviral medications, chronic ventilator support, cancer chemotherapy, irradiation, or major surgery. In some circumstances, they may include life-prolonging measures such as antibiotic treatment for pneumonia, transfusions of blood products, correction of metabolic disturbances, or resuscitation efforts. In addition to that most basic decision, choices must be made concerning the use of various palliative care interventions intended to alleviate symptoms, such as analgesics, sedatives, stool softeners, supplemental oxygen, or oral suction. Palliative care has been defined as the active, total care of patients with life-threatening illness, focused on controlling pain and other symptoms and addressing psychologic, social, and spiritual concerns.[3] It should be noted that for most patients, the transition to palliative care is gradual; the need for effective symptom control increases as the patient's condition deteriorates despite continued disease-directed treatment. Rather than forcing patients and families to choose in all-or-none fashion between either continued treatment or palliative care, a more clinically useful approach is one that melds elements of both beginning early in the patient's course.[3,4]

Decision-Making Competence: Ethical, Legal, and Developmental Aspects

A critical notion in adolescent decision making is that of *competence* or *capacity*. In this respect alone, medical decision making is more complex in adolescents than it is in adults or young children. In the United States, persons who are 18 years of age or older and possess appropriate mental capacity are empowered to make medical decisions for themselves, including those pertaining to discontinuation or forgoing of life-sustaining treatment. This right is based on respect for personal autonomy or self-determination. Prerequisites for exercising autonomy include being able to receive and understand all relevant information, to foresee the implications of a decision, and to be free from controlling influences.[5]

Adolescents less than 18 years old in the United States ordinarily are not considered legally competent to make their own medical decisions (Chap. 3). At the same time, it is not uncommon for some adolescents, especially those who are older and medically experienced, to demonstrate autonomy and desire to make their own decisions. This has led to efforts to define the essential elements of *functional competence* in minors (Table 6-1).

With these conditions in mind, there is now a broad agreement that adolescents aged approximately 14 years and older should be presumed, unless there is contravening evidence, to have the functional competence or capacity for making binding medical decisions for themselves, including those related to end-of-life issues.[6–8] Yet, experienced clinicians have observed that children substantially younger than 14 years also may meet criteria for functional competency, especially those who are medically experienced and knowledgeable as the result of chronic illness.[9] Furthermore, research indicates that a mature conception of death can be developed by children 10 years of age or younger.[1,10,11] Therefore, it has been proposed that, barring evidence to the contrary, decision-making capacity should be presumed for terminally ill, cognitively normal adolescents aged approximately 10 years and older.[12] If there is uncertainty

TABLE 6-1

CRITERIA FOR FUNCTIONAL COMPETENCE IN ADOLESCENTS

Criterion	Functional Correlate
To reason	To consider multiple factors in predicting future consequences
To understand	To comprehend essential medical information
To choose voluntarily	To be free from coercive influence of authority figures, such as parents and physicians
To appreciate the nature of the decision	To grasp the gravity, immediacy and permanence of the choice
To conceptualize death appropriately	To conceive of death as universal, unalterable, and permanent

Source: Foley GV, Whittam EH. Care of the child dying of cancer: Part I. *CA Cancer J Clin* 40:327–354, 1990.
Leiken S. A proposal concerning decisions to forgo life-sustaining treatment for young people. *J Pediatr* 115:17–22, 1989.
King NMP, Cross AW. Children as decision-makers: guidelines for pediatricians. *J Pediatr* 115:10–16, 1989.

about the patient's capacity, a formal assessment of developmental level and cognitive function needs to be obtained by an experienced child psychologist or psychiatrist.[7] Younger adolescents without sufficient capacity for full decisional authority should be given choices over other important aspects of their care. Their values and preferences should be taken into account by responsible adults even as the adults make the final decision according to a "best interest" standard (what they judge to be in the best interest of their child).[7] Additional considerations that may be useful in decision making by dying adolescents have been published recently.[12,13]

The competence-based decisional standard described above is generally accepted as appropriate for minors in the context of chronic and life-threatening or terminal illness. The situation is more controversial for functionally competent adolescents with acute life-threatening illnesses who refuse treatment despite the high probability of a favorable outcome (e.g., a teenager diagnosed with low-stage Hodgkin's disease). These situations—which fortunately seem to be rare—are beyond the scope of this discussion. They require a sensitive, highly individualized approach and sometimes legal intervention.[7,8,14]

In the United States, the legal status of end-of-life decision making by adolescents is inconsistent.[6,14] Some states have "emancipated minor statutes" that allow binding medical decisions if the minor is married, a parent, or financially independent. Some states have allowed application of the "mature minor doctrine" through the courts to endow competent adolescents with medical decision-making authority on a case-by-case basis.[15] (A much different legal framework is used in the Canadian province of Ontario, where, according to the Health Care Consent Act of 1996, patients are deemed to have capacity according to their ability to understand relevant information and to appreciate reasonably foreseeable consequences of the decision, rather than their age).[16] In the United States, legal intervention should be necessary only when there is serious disagreement between the functionally competent minor and responsible adults about a major treatment decision. In most cases, the responsible

adult will be willing to enact the wishes of the minor by making the legally valid treatment decision according to a modification of the "substituted judgment" standard (the application of a patient's previously expressed values and preferences in a medical decision made on his or her behalf).[7,17] For fully competent adolescents, advance treatment directives may be useful for clearly delineating their decisional preferences, but currently these instruments are not legally binding as they are for adults.[1,6,7]

Decision Making: Role of the Care Provider

In caring for adolescents and their families faced with end-of-life issues, a critical role for the care provider is to assist them in the difficult task of making medical care decisions. Hinds and colleagues have published their research findings concerning the factors rated as important by adolescents, parents, and physicians in making end-of-life decisions.[18] For the adolescents participating in those studies, important factors were being well-informed and the opinions and recommendations of their treatment team and parents. For the parents, key factors were information from the health care team regarding their child's health and disease status, trust in the health care team, and feelings of support they received from that team. For physicians, major factors taken into account were the preferences of the adolescents and parents, a desire to limit suffering, and other input from medical professionals.[18] Religion was frequently cited by both adolescents and parents as being important in making decisions. In the international component of their prospective studies, an awareness of their child's preference was rated as important more often by American parents than by those from the other cultures.[18]

These findings, combined with broad clinical experience, help point the way to providing optimal care to adolescents and their families faced with life-threatening illness. Clearly, excellent communication is essential, arguably the most important aspect of good decision making. At a minimum, this needs to involve the patient, parents, and physician. Three-way dialogue is extremely important, but time spent alone with the patient or parents can provide valuable insights. Optimal communication at end-of-life represents an extension of good practices that are established much earlier, ideally at the time of initial diagnosis. Care providers should attempt to create a communication milieu that favors candor and willingness to listen. Throughout the course, the adolescent should be encouraged to express opinions and feelings, and should participate in ordinary medical choices in order to cultivate the insight and skills needed later for major end-of-life decisions. Over time, this process will assist physicians and parents in assigning a decisional role that is commensurate with a given adolescent's capacity. Momentous clinical developments and the decisions associated with them are sometimes best discussed in the context of a formal care conference involving the adolescent, parents and other key support figures, and the health care team.[9,19] This provides a forum for communicating essential information, including disease status, prognosis, expected clinical course, treatment options, and role for palliative care.

SYMPTOM MANAGEMENT

Consistent with the definition of palliative care given earlier, the primary clinical goal for dying adolescents is to relieve suffering and maximize quality of life. In general, the appropriateness of any intervention, whether disease- or symptom-directed, is judged according to that goal. Thus, any intervention that enhances comfort, satisfaction, dignity, and personal fulfillment should be considered, whereas treatments that are ineffective or overly burdensome (from the patient's perspective) should be discontinued.[20] In general, when disease-directed treatment is discontinued and care becomes exclusively palliative, invasive monitoring (e.g., arterial blood gases) and "routine" monitoring (e.g., daily serum chemistry profiles) are discontinued. Rather, simple clinical parameters (e.g., respiratory character and skin turgor) are used to determine whether to employ interventions that will

contribute meaningfully to quality of life (e.g., nasal oxygen or intravenous fluids).

Evaluating Symptoms in Adolescents

Suffering has been defined as the enduring of pain or distress.[21] The ability to recognize suffering is dependent on the highly individualized and subjective manner in which it is experienced and then communicated to the clinician. To decipher symptoms, especially in their early stages, a comprehensive awareness is needed for the adolescent's medical status, developmental level, cognitive function, and psychologic history. Also critical are familial, cultural, and spiritual influences. In adolescents, symptoms may be under-reported to reduce feelings of dependency, or they may be magnified as a manifestation of anxiety. Care is needed to interpret symptoms and understand their meaning, in order to address the contributing causes, which may be physical or otherwise.[13] Scales for symptom assessment have been validated in children and adolescents with life-limiting illness and are helpful for identifying and tracking control of symptoms and for palliative care research.[22,23]

Once a particular symptom is identified as a source of suffering, the adolescent should be reassured it will be addressed. Management options should be discussed. Most medical interventions, including those of a palliative nature, are accompanied by benefits and burdens, which may be weighted differently by individual teenagers. For example, some adolescents choose high doses of opiate analgesics for optimal pain relief, while others forgo them in order to avoid sedation that interferes with their participation in desired activities. It is important for adolescents and their families to have realistic expectations for the terminal course, including the relative difficulty certain symptoms pose for control. Educational materials can be offered to help prepare them, such as those obtained through Children's Hospice International.[24] Unfortunately, some symptoms at the end of life may be incompletely controlled despite maximal intervention. Honest sharing of these possibilities may assist adolescents and their families during decision making and also bereavement, when comfort may be found in knowing that everything appropriate was done to relieve their child's suffering.

Pain

Pain is the principal cause of suffering at the end of life.[25,26] In some ways, pain is paradigmatic of suffering and its relief embodies the fundamental commitment of palliative care. The World Health Organization (WHO) has established guidelines for the management of cancer pain in children.[27] These guidelines have been validated in prospective analyses and translated to the general palliative care setting.[28,29] The WHO guidelines emphasize the concepts of treating pain "by the ladder" (sequential use of analgesic drugs of increasing potency to match the patient's level of pain); "by the clock" (use of analgesics on a scheduled rather than as-needed basis to minimize breakthrough pain); "by the appropriate route" (use of the least invasive and most appropriate route of administration); and "by the patient" (recognition that there can be variability in response among different patients). Nonnarcotic pain medications are generally to be considered prior to narcotic use. If narcotics become necessary, the WHO recommends escalating from least to most potent as deemed indicated (Table 6-2). Adjuvant therapy may be necessary to augment the analgesic effect of narcotics. The identification of contributing factors, such as anxiety or neuropathic components to the pain, may assist in selecting appropriate adjuvant therapies (Table 6-3).

As with any symptom at the end of life, the adequacy of pain control interventions needs to be regularly reassessed and the measures modified as required. Side effects from the analgesics themselves, such as opiate-induced constipation, need to be addressed, if not prevented. Pain that is refractory to the WHO approach may benefit from opiate rotation or may require sustained escalation of the opiate dose until pain relief is achieved, sometimes to doses much higher than those used in acute care settings.[30] In those situations, reluctance is sometimes encountered in increasing the opiate dose to the necessary level, due to physician and family concerns about addiction or hastening death through respiratory depression. These can usually be surmounted through education and reassurance. Families may be reminded that addiction is irrelevant to a dying patient. Also, there is an established consensus that it is ethically permissible for opiates to be used in whatever doses are necessary to control pain as their intended effect, even if doing so results in an unintended effect of hastening death through respiratory depression.[20] In actual practice, this rarely seems to be operative, as the dose escalation curve is so incremental that patients become tolerant of large doses that would not be possible in opiate-naïve patients. This consensus is consistent with palliative care recommendations from the American Academy of Pediatrics (AAP), which does not support physician-assisted suicide or euthanasia for adolescents or younger children.[4]

Finally, while it is true that pain management is a high priority in palliative care, it is important to recognize that not every patient experiencing pain suffers and not all who suffer do so because of pain. Adolescents should be allowed to use pain control interventions to a degree that is compatible with other life priorities. Suffering caused by non-pain symptoms needs remedies other than or in addition to analgesics.

Other Symptoms

Additional symptoms that can cause substantial distress at the end of life include fatigue, dyspnea, nausea and vomiting, and depression or anxiety.[22,25] Each of these may result from one or more underlying conditions, requiring a thorough, up-to-date clinical assessment in order to determine appropriate management. As with pain control, potential interventions should be discussed with the adolescent to respect personal autonomy. In general, the palliative care philosophy favors approaches that maximize efficacy but minimize invasiveness and diminution of quality of life. A partial list of common symptoms other than pain is shown with etiologies and interventions to be considered (Table 6-4). For a more complete discussion of symptom management, the reader is referred to recent sources.[31–33]

TABLE 6-2

NARCOTICS COMMONLY USED IN PALLIATIVE CARE

	Usual Starting Dose			
Medication	Parenteral (Dose for >50 kg)	Oral (Dose for >50 kg)	Oral: Parenteral Conversion Ratio	Half-life (H)
Codeine[a,b]	NA	0.5–1 mg/kg q 3–4 h (30 mg q 3–4 h)	1.5:1	2–4
Oxycodone[a]	NA	0.1–0.2 mg/kg q 3–4 h (5–10 mg q 3–4 h)		2–3
Oxycodone-SR	NA	0.1–0.2 mg/kg q 12 h (10 mg q 12 h)		4–6
Morphine[c]	0.05–0.1 mg/kg iv/sc q 2–4 h bolus (5–10 mg iv/sc q 2–4 h) 0.03 mg/kg/h ci (1 mg/h)	0.15–0.3 mg/kg q 4 h (5–10 mg q 4 h)	3:1	2–4
Morphine-SR	NA	0.3–0.6 mg/kg 8–12 h (15–30 mg q 12 h)		
Hydromorphone	0.015 mg/kg 2–4 h (1–1.5 mg q 2–4 h)	0.06 mg/kg q 3–4 h (2 mg q 3–4 h)	5:1	2–3
Fentanyl[d]	1–2 mcg/kg iv/sc/im q 1–4 h bolus (50–100 mcg iv/sc/im q 1–4 h) 0.5–2 mcg/kg/h ci (25–75 mcg/h) 25 mcg/h patch td; change q 3 days	NA (poorly tolerated)		3
Methadone	0.1 mg/kg iv/sc q 4–8 h (5–10 mg iv/sc q 4–8 h)	0.1–0.2 mg/kg q 4–8 h (5–10 mg q 4–8 h)	2:1	12–50

Note: Nonstandard abbreviations used: ci =continuous infusion; NA =not applicable; sc =subcutaneous; SR =sustained release; td =transdermal.

[a]Prodrug that is inactive in 1%–7% of patients; inhibited by certain medications

[b]Ceiling effect at 30 mg

[c]Delayed clearance with severe renal insufficiency: consider hydromorphone, fentanyl, or methadone

[d]Approximate transdermal dose (mcg/h): 24-h morphine dose (mg per day) divided by 3.5

Source: World Health Organization. *Cancer Pain Relief and Palliative Care in Children*, Geneva, IL: World Health Organization, 1998. Initiative for Pediatric Palliative Care. Available at: *http://www.ippcweb.org* (accessed May 12, 2004).

TABLE 6-3
MEDICATIONS COMMONLY USED AS ADJUVANTS TO NARCOTICS FOR PAIN CONTROL

Class	Medication	Typical Starting Dose (Dose for >50 kg)	Advantages	Disadvantages
Antidepressants	Amitriptyline[a]	0.2–0.5 mg/kg per dose po qhs (10–25 mg po qhs; 300 mg per day max)	Helpful for insomnia, depression	Anticholinergic
Anticonvulsants[b]	Gabapentin	5–10 mg/kg per dose po tid; titrate up to effect (100 mg po tid; 3600 mg per day max)	Helpful for neuropathic pain	Sedation, ataxia, nystagmus, dizziness
	Carbamazepine	2–5 mg/kg per dose po bid; titrate up to effect (100–200 mg po bid; 1.6 g per day max)	Helpful for neuropathic pain	Cytopenias, ataxia
Anxiolytics[c]	Lorazepam	0.02–0.1 mg/kg per dose po/iv q 4–6 h (0.5–2 mg po/iv q 4–6 h)	Helpful for anxiety, muscle spasm	Monitor levels (target 4–12 mcg/mL) Sedation
Antihistamines	Diphenhydramine	0.5–1 mg/kg per dose q 4–6 h (25–50 mg po/iv; 400 mg per day max)	Antipruritic; helpful for anxiety, muscle spasm	Sedation, anticholinergic
	Hydroxyzine	0.5–1 mg/kg per dose q 6–8 h (12.5–25 mg po; 600 mg per day max)	Antipruritic, helpful for anxiety, muscle spasm	Sedation, anticholinergic
Psychostimulants[d]	Methylphenidate	0.1–0.5 mg/kg per dose po bid (5 mg po q 2 h prn; 20 mg per day max)	Improves fatigue	Sleep disturbances, anorexia
Corticosteroids[e]	Dexamethasone	0.25–0.5 mg/kg per dose po/iv q 6–24 h (4–16 mg po qd; 16 mg per day max)	Helpful for pain due to nerve compression, increased intracranial pressure, bone metastases. Also nausea and vomiting, fatigue, anorexia	With chronic use gastritis, sleep disturbance, hyperglycemia, osteopenia

[a]Bryson HM, Wilde MI. Amitriptyline. A review of its pharmacological properties and therapeutic use in chronic pain states. *Drugs Aging* 8:459–476, 1996.

[b]Ingelmo PM, Locatelli BG, Carrara B. Neuropathic pain in children. *The Suffering Child* 2:1–11, 2003.

[c]Reddy S, Patt RB. The benzodiazepines as adjuvant analgesics. *J Pain Symptom Manage*, 9:510–514, 1994.

[d]Bruera E, Driver L, Barnes EA, et al. Patient-controlled methylphenidate for the management of fatigue in patients with advanced cancer: a preliminary report. *J Clin Oncol* 21:4439–4443, 2003.

[e]Hardy JR, Rees E, Ling J, et al. A prospective survey of the use of dexamethasone on a palliative care unit. *Palliat Med* 15:3–8, 2001;: Mercadante S, Fulfaro F, Casuccio A. The use of corticosteroids in home palliative care. *Support Care Cancer* 9:386–9, 2001.

TABLE 6-4

SELECTED NONPAIN SYMPTOMS: COMMON CAUSES AND TREATMENT OPTIONS

Symptom	Common Causes	Treatment Options
Fatigue	Muscular weakness	For general improvement: dexamethasone, methylphenidate[a]
	Sleep disturbances	Benzodiazepine, tricyclic antidepressant
	Dyspnea	See below
	Depression	See below
	Chronic pain	See text
	Anemia	Erythropoietin, red blood cell transfusion[b]
	Malnutrition	Supplemental nutrition, megestrol, cyproheptadine[c]
	Dehydration	Supplemental hydration[d]
Nausea/vomiting	Medication side effect	General measures: 5-hydroxytryptamine antagonist, phenothiazine, diphenhydramine, anxiolytic[e]
	Gastritis	Histamine (H2) blocker, proton pump inhibitor
	Intestinal obstruction	Surgical intervention often not indicated
	Constipation	Fiber, stimulant, osmotic, cathartic
	Ileus	Review of medications; stimulant or prokinetic agent
	Increased intracranial pressure	Dexamethasone
Dyspnea	Anatomical obstruction	General measures: attention to environmental conditions, supplemental oxygen (may help even in absence of hypoxemia), opioid and anxiolytic (may help even in absence of pain or anxiety)[f]
	Neuromuscular weakness	
	Pulmonary metastases	
	Infection	Appropriate antibiotics
	Hypersecretion	Anticholinergic: atropine, glycopyrrolate [g]
	Fluid overload	Diuretic
	Anemia	See above
Depression/Anxiety	Situational	Counseling; selective serotonin reuptake inhibitor, tricyclic antidepressant, psychostimulant, benzodiazepine[h]

[a]Bruera E, Driver L, Barnes EA, et al. Patient-controlled methylphenidate for the management of fatigue in patients with advanced cancer: a preliminary report. *J Clin Oncol* 21:4439–4443, 2003; Hardy JR, Rees E, Ling J, et al. A prospective survey of the use of dexamethasone on a palliative care unit. *Palliat Med* 15:3–8, 2001; Mercadante S, Fulfaro F, Casuccio A. The use of corticosteroids in home palliative care. *Support Care Cancer* 9:386–389, 2001; Rozans M, Dreisbach A, Lertora JJ, et al. Palliative uses of methylphenidate in patients with cancer: a review of depression with psychomotor retardation: diagnostic challenges and the use of psychostimulants. *J Clin Oncol* 20:335–339, 2002.

[b]Crawford J, Cella D, Cleeland CS, et al. Relationship between changes in hemoglobin level and quality of life during chemotherapy in anemic cancer patients receiving epoetin alfa therapy. *Cancer* 95:888–895, 2002; Monti M, Castellani L, Berlusconi A, et al. Use of red blood cell transfusions in terminally ill cancer patients admitted to a palliative care unit. *J Pain Symptom Manage* 12:18–22, 1996.

[c]Jatoi A, Kumar S, Sloan JA, et al. On appetite and its loss. *J Clin Oncol* 21:S79–S81, 2003.

[d]Bruera E, MacDonald N. To hydrate or not to hydrate: How should it be? *J Clin Oncol* 21:S84–S86, 2003.

[e]Ferris FD, VonGunten CF, Emanuel LL. Ensuring competency in end-of-life care: controlling symptoms. *BMC Palliat Care* 1:1–14, 2002.

[f]Booth S, Kelly MJ, Cox NP, et al. Does oxygen help dyspnea in patients with cancer? *Am J Respir Crit Care Med* 153:1515–1518, 1996; Allard P, Lamontagne C, Bernard P, et al. How effective are supplementary doses of opioids for dyspnea in terminally ill cancer patients? A randomized continuous sequential clinical trial. *J Pain Symptom Manage* 17:256–265, 1999.

[g]Ripamonti C, Fulfaro F, Bruera E. Dyspnoea in patients with advanced cancer: incidence, causes, and treatments. *Cancer Treat Rev* 24:69–80, 1998.

[h]Ly KL, Chidgey J, Addington-Hall J, et al. Depression in palliative care: a systematic review. Part 2. Treatment. *Palliat Med* 16:279–284, 2002.

PSYCHOSOCIAL SUPPORT FOR THE DYING ADOLESCENT AND FAMILY

Active psychosocial support is indicated for both adolescents and their families, taking into account the underlying diagnosis, current physical condition, trajectory of the illness, developmental maturity, established behavioral patterns, and background of cultural and religious life.[12,34–36] Like any patient, teenagers need to be reassured early that pain and other symptoms will be approached aggressively. Emotional reactions such as sadness and anxiety are expected and may vary during the course of illness, sometimes in response to changes in physical condition or external events. Although these can usually be addressed through supportive interactions with the health care team, formal behavioral or pharmacologic intervention may be considered if the problems are severe, persistent, or seriously interfere with the patient's preparatory work before dying. Many adolescents set proximate survival goals (even if not acknowledged as such) around prominent events, such as graduation, social functions, and family celebrations. Likewise, it is not uncommon for them to discuss future plans far beyond their expected survival time. Such apparent denial is common even in patients who demonstrate a good intellectual understanding of their illness. A period of preparation for dying is common among adolescents, though the practices vary individually. These may include visits to reach closure with certain family or friends, writing poetry or music, planning their funerals, and distributing cherished possessions. Depending on their personalities and preexisting communication patterns, some teenagers may share their feelings with family members, while others prefer to confide in another special person. In those cases, families should be encouraged to be patient and quietly convey their continued willingness to talk.

Psychosocial support is also important for parents and siblings during this time.[35,37] Formal referrals for counseling or similar services from hospice professionals can supplement the support many families find through their networks of family, friends, and religious communities. The findings of Hinds and colleagues indicate the importance of spiritual issues and religious support for many adolescents and families.[18] Grief experienced by parents and siblings following death of the adolescent is profound, complex, and long-lasting.[38,39] Active bereavement care for the family is strongly recommended,[1,38] even though limited controlled studies have not yet documented overall benefit from the interventions.[40] A role for the pediatrician in bereavement care has been described.[41]

THE DELIVERY OF PALLIATIVE CARE SERVICES

While relief of a symptom is always appropriate beginning immediately with the diagnosis of a chronic disease, palliative care as the dominant, unifying mode of management for a given patient becomes indicated when the goal of comfort supercedes other treatment end points. The ideal scenario for palliative care delivery would be the provision of all needed interventions in a timely, developmentally appropriate way in the setting of a patient's choice. This could be achieved by the optimal home care service defined by Goldman.[37] Unfortunately, seldom are all these criteria actually met for adolescents and younger children due to the presence of multiple barriers, including the relative scarcity of pediatric palliative care or hospice services; deficits in relevant training, experience, and competency for health care professionals; and serious reimbursement challenges in the United States.[42] The AAP has described a model for comprehensive palliative care that is appropriate for adolescents and children.[4] Although some studies indicate that for children, home is their preferred location to receive care, patients and families should be offered the option of either home or the inpatient setting.[43] Occasionally, hospitalization late in the course becomes indicated to manage severe, accelerating symptoms or family anxiety, and families may be comforted knowing in advance that inpatient care remains available. Depending on the acuity and needs of the adolescent, care at home can be provided with or without the help of a home care team from a local hospice organization or visiting nurse agency. A hospice team offers the advantage of comprehensive services that include in-home nursing assessments with round-the-clock physician access, social work, assistance with arranging respite care, spiritual care if desired, and bereavement care for parents and siblings.[44]

CONCLUSIONS

Adolescents at the end of life pose medical, ethical, legal, and psychosocial challenges to their physicians and other health care professionals.[1,12,63] Even though most are minors, adolescents should make medical decisions to the full extent their functional competence allows, including discontinuation of disease-directed therapy where applicable. When palliative care begins, suffering should be minimized and quality of life maximized, as perceived by the adolescent. Psychosocial, spiritual, and bereavement concerns of the patient and family need to be addressed. If available, pediatric hospice care may be beneficial. The adolescent care team must play an active role throughout the patient's course, as studies indicate that their continued involvement is meaningful to families and improves coordination of palliative care services.[43]

References

1 Himelstein BP, Hilden JM, Boldt AM, et al. Pediatric palliative care. *N Engl J Med* 350:1752–1762, 2004.

2 Anderson RN, Smith BL. Deaths: leading causes for 2001. Natl Vital Stat Rep 52:1–88, 2003. Available at: *http://www.cdc.gov/nchs/data/nvsr/nvsr52/nvsr52_09 .pdf.* (accessed May 8, 2004)

3 Frager G. Pediatric palliative care: building the model, bridging the gaps. *J Palliat Care* 12:9–12, 1996.

4 American Academy of Pediatrics—Committee on Bioethics and Committee on Hospital Care. Palliative care for children. *Pediatrics* 106:351–357, 2000.

5 Beauchamp TL, Childress JF. *Principles of Biomedical Ethics,* 5th ed. New York: Oxford University Press, 2001.

6 Weir RF, Peters C. Affirming the decisions adolescents make about life and death. *Hastings Cent Rep* 27: 29–40, 1997.

7 American Academy of Pediatrics—Committee on Bioethics. Guidelines on forgoing life-sustaining medical treatment. *Pediatrics* 93:532–536, 1994.

8 American Academy of Pediatrics—Committee on Bioethics. Informed consent, parental permission, and assent in pediatric practice. *Pediatrics* 95:314–317, 1995.

9 Nitschke R, Meyer WH, Sexauer CL, et al. Care of terminally ill children with cancer. *Med Pediatr Oncol* 34:268–270, 2000.

10 Bluebond-Langner M. *The Private World of Dying Children.* Princeton, NJ: Princeton University Press, 1980.

11 Foley GV, Whittam EH. Care of the child dying of cancer: Part I. *CA Cancer J Clin* 40:327–354, 1990.

12 Freyer DR. Care of the dying adolescent: special considerations. *Pediatrics* 113:381–388, 2004.

13 George R, Hutton S. Palliative care in adolescents. *Eur J Cancer* 39:2662–2668, 2003.

14 Traugott I, Alpers A. In their own hands: adolescents' refusal of medical treatment. *Arch Pediatr Adolesc Med* 151:922–927, 1997.

15 Sigman GS, O'Connor C. Exploration for physicians of the mature minor doctrine. *J Pediatr* 119:520–525, 1991.

16 Ontario Health Care Consent Act of 1996. Available at: *http://192.75.156.68/DBLaws/Statutes/English/96h02_ e.htm* (accessed May 8, 2004).

17 Freyer DR. Children with cancer: special considerations in the discontinuation of life-sustaining treatment. *Med Pediatr Oncol* 20:136–142, 1992.

18 Hinds PS, Oakes L, Furman W, et al. End-of-life decision making by adolescents, parents, and healthcare providers in pediatric oncology. *Cancer Nurs* 24: 122–136, 2001.

19 Nitschke R, Humphrey GB, Sexauer CL, et al. Therapeutic choices made by patients with end-stage cancer. *J Pediatr* 101:471–476, 1982.

20 The Hastings Center Guidelines on the Termination of Life-Sustaining Treatment and Care of the Dying. Briarcliff Manor, NY: The Hastings Center, 1987.

21 *American Heritage Dictionary*, 4th ed. Boston, MA: Houghton Mifflin, 2000.

22 Collins JJ, Byrnes ME, Dunkel IJ, et al. The measurement of symptoms in children with cancer. *J Pain Symptom Manage* 19:363–377, 2000.

23 Collins JJ, Devine TD, Dick GS, et al. The measurement of symptoms in young children with cancer: the validation of the memorial symptom assessment scale in children aged 7–12. *J Pain Symptom Manage* 23:10–16, 2002.

24 Children's Hospice International. Available at: *http://www.chionline.org* (accessed May 12, 2004).

25 Wolfe J, Grier HE, Klar N, et al. Symptoms and suffering at the end of life in children with cancer. *N Engl J Med* 342:326–333, 2000.

26 Drake R, Frost J, Collins JJ. The symptoms of dying children. *J Pain Symptom Manage* 26:594–603, 2003.

27 World Health Organization. *Cancer Pain Relief and Palliative Care in Children*, Geneva, IL: World Health Organization, 1998.

28 Grond S, Radbruch L, Meuser T, et al. Assessment and treatment of neuropathic cancer pain following WHO guidelines. *Pain* 79:15–20, 1999.

29 Meuser T, Pietruck C, Radbruch L, et al. Symptoms during cancer pain treatment following WHO guidelines: a longitudinal follow-up study of symptom prevalence, severity and etiology. *Pain* 93:247–257, 2001.

30 Mercadante S. Recent progress in the pharmacotherapy of cancer pain. *Expert Rev Anticancer Ther* 1:487–494, 2001.

31 Hanks G, Doyle D. *Oxford Textbook of Palliative Medicine.* 3d ed. Oxford: Oxford University Press, 2003.

32 Initiative for Pediatric Palliative Care. Available at:*http://www.ippcweb.org* (accessed May 12, 2004).

33 Wolfe J, Friebert S, Hilden J. Caring for children with advanced cancer: integrating palliative care. *Pediatr Clin N Am* 49:1043–1062, 2002.

34 Easson WM. The seriously ill or dying adolescent: special needs and challenges. *Postgrad Med* 78:183–189, 1995.

35 Carr-Gregg MRC, Sawyer SM, Clarke CF, et al. Caring for the terminally ill adolescent. *Med J Aust* 166:255–258, 1997.

36 Klopfenstein KJ. Adolescents, cancer, and hospice. *Adolesc Med* 10:437–443, 1999.

37 Goldman A. Home care of the dying child. *J Palliat Care* 12:16–19, 1996.

38 Whittam EH. Terminal care of the dying child: psychosocial implications of care. *Cancer* 71:3450–3462, 1993.

39 Davies AM. Death of adolescents: parental grief and coping strategies. *Br J Nurs* 10:1332–1342, 2001.

40 Rowa-Dewar N. Do interventions make a difference to bereaved parents? A systematic review of controlled studies. *Int J Palliat Nurs* 8:452–457, 2002.

41 Wessel MA. The role of the primary pediatrician when a child dies. *Arch Pediatr Adolesc* 152:837–838, 1998.

42 Hilden JM, Himelstein BP, Freyer DR, et al. End-of-life care: special issues in pediatric oncology. In: Foley K, Gelband H (eds.), *Improving Palliative Care for Cancer*. Washington, DC: National Academy Press, 2001, pp. 161–198.

43 Collins JJ, Stevens MM, Cousens P. Home care for the dying child: a parent's perception. *Austr Fam Phys* 27:610–614, 1998.

44 Boling A, Lynn J. Hospice: current practice, future possibilities. *Hosp J* 13:29–32, 1998.

45 Leiken S. A proposal concerning decisions to forgo life-sustaining treatment for young people. *J Pediatr* 115:17–22, 1989.

46 King NMP, Cross AW. Children as decision-makers: guidelines for pediatricians. *J Pediatr* 115:10–16, 1989.

47 Bryson HM, Wilde MI. Amitriptyline. A review of its pharmacological properties and therapeutic use in chronic pain states. *Drugs Aging* 8:459–476, 1996.

48 Ingelmo PM, Locatelli BG, Carrara B. Neuropathic pain in children. *The Suffering Child* 2:1–11, 2003.

49 Reddy S, Patt RB. The benzodiazepines as adjuvant analgesics. *J Pain Symptom Manage*, 9:510–514, 1994.

50 Bruera E, Driver L, Barnes EA, et al. Patient-controlled methylphenidate for the management of fatigue in patients with advanced cancer: a preliminary report. *J Clin Oncol* 21:4439–4443, 2003.

51 Hardy JR, Rees E, Ling J, et al. A prospective survey of the use of dexamethasone on a palliative care unit. *Palliat Med* 15:3–8, 2001.

52 Mercadante S, Fulfaro F, Casuccio A. The use of corticosteroids in home palliative care. *Support Care Cancer* 9:386–9, 2001.

53 Rozans M, Dreisbach A, Lertora JJ, et al. Palliative uses of methylphenidate in patients with cancer: a review of depression with psychomotor retardation: diagnostic challenges and the use of psychostimulants. *J Clin Oncol* 20:335–339, 2002.

54 Crawford J, Cella D, Cleeland CS, et al. Relationship between changes in hemoglobin level and quality of life during chemotherapy in anemic cancer patients receiving epoetin alfa therapy. *Cancer* 95:888–895, 2002.

55 Monti M, Castellani L, Berlusconi A, et al. Use of red blood cell transfusions in terminally ill cancer patients admitted to a palliative care unit. *J Pain Symptom Manage* 12:18–22, 1996.

56 Jatoi A, Kumar S, Sloan JA, et al. On appetite and its loss. *J Clin Oncol* 21:S79–S81, 2003.

57 Bruera E, MacDonald N. To hydrate or not to hydrate: How should it be? *J Clin Oncol* 21:S84–S86, 2003.

58 Ferris FD, VonGunten CF, Emanuel LL. Ensuring competency in end-of-life care: controlling symptoms. *BMC Palliat Care* 1:1–14, 2002.

59 Booth S, Kelly MJ, Cox NP, et al. Does oxygen help dyspnea in patients with cancer? *Am J Respir Crit Care Med* 153:1515–1518, 1996.

60 Allard P, Lamontagne C, Bernard P, et al. How effective are supplementary doses of opioids for dyspnea in

terminally ill cancer patients? A randomized continuous sequential clinical trial. *J Pain Symptom Manage* 17:256–265, 1999.

61 Ripamonti C, Fulfaro F, Bruera E. Dyspnoea in patients with advanced cancer: incidence, causes and treatments. *Cancer Treat Rev* 24:69–80, 1998.

62 Ly KL, Chidgey J, Addington-Hall J, et al. Depression in palliative care: a systematic review. Part 2. Treatment. *Palliat Med* 16:279–284, 2002.

63 Hurwitz CA, Duncan J, Wolfe J. Caring for the child with cancer at the close of life. *JAMA* 292:2141–2149, 2004.

MEDICAL HEALTH

7

DISORDERS OF THE EYES, EARS, NOSE, THROAT, AND NECK

Carter D. Brooks, Charles F. Koopmann, Jr., and Donald E. Greydanus

THE EYE[1]

The Red Eye

A primary care practice will frequently see adolescents with red eyes. The majority of these will have a nonthreatening, self-limited process—most often conjunctivitis—readily handled by the non-eye specialist. For a few, the problem will be more serious, and identifying these constitutes the major challenge in the differential diagnosis of the red eye. Symptoms and signs beyond local inflammation, irritation, and discharge are the best indicators of more serious underlying causes. Table 7-1 lists possible additional features of a red eye-generating condition and the underlying causes that one should consider when presented with a red eye plus something else. The majority of the entities listed in Table 7-1 should be managed by an eye specialist, and in many cases, the referral is urgent. Acute narrow-angle glaucoma

represents a special emergency as irreversible loss of vision can occur within hours of onset of this condition.

Discrete Lesions Associated with Red Eyes

A number of localized processes can produce generalized redness. In most cases, recognition of the condition is straightforward and in some, management is not complex. For example, red eyes in an adolescent may reflect ocular intolerance to contact lenses, lens solutions, or other ocular medicaments, cosmetics, or other materials applied near, though not in the eye.

Blepharitis: This may result from chronic infection at the lid margins or may be associated with a generalized skin problem, such as seborrhea. This can cause secondary inflammation of the conjunctiva and cornea requiring ophthalmologic consultation.

---

[1]The authors appreciate the critical review of the EYE Section by Kurt Haller, MD (Ophthalmologist, Kalamazoo, Michigan).

TABLE 7-1

ENTITIES SUGGESTED BY A RED EYE PLUS
ADJUNCTIVE SIGNS/SYMPTOMS IN MORE
SERIOUS CAUSES OF ACUTE RED EYE

Pain (quality)	Cloudy cornea
Episcleritis (dull ache)	Keratitis
Scleritis (moderate to	Uveitis
severe, deep)	Acute Glaucoma
Keratitis (sharp)	Contact lens overwear
Iritis (sharp)	**Pupils unequal,**
Acute, narrow-angle	**immobile, irregular**
glaucoma (sharp,	Iritis
stabbing, headache,	Trauma
vomiting)	Acute glaucoma
Foreign body	**Cornea stains with**
Photophobia	**fluorescein**
Epidemic keratoconjunc-	Corneal abrasion
tivitis (adenovirus)	Keratitis
Keratitis	Corneal ulcer
Uveitis	(viral—including
Acute Glaucoma	herpes, fungal)
Contact lens overwear	**Redness greatest**
Visual loss	**near limbus**
Keratitis	Keratitis
Scleritis	Uveitis
Uveitis	Acute glaucoma
Acute glaucoma	

Hordeolum (stye): The equivalent of a small furuncle on the lid margin, this may cause considerable local swelling and redness. Manage the primary lesion by local moist heat application; topical antibacterials dosed into the conjunctiva may help localize the infection. If incision and drainage become necessary, refer the adolescent.

Chalazion: This is a granuloma of the eyelid, which can present acutely with swelling, redness, and pain or chronically as an indolent lump. Surgical removal may become necessary if the chalazion persists or is large enough to compromise vision.

Subconjunctival Hemorrhage: Bleeding under the conjunctiva presents a dramatic picture, usually with innocent implications. In some cases the cause of the problem is obscure; sometimes it can be tied to Valsalva-like pressure elevation associated with vomiting, coughing, or sneezing. In the absence of other eye complaints the problem should clear spontaneously.

Pterygium: A fleshy nodule with satellite vessels, this lesion typically takes many years to develop and is unlikely to present a problem in adolescents. It is most often located in the nasal portion of the bulbar conjunctiva and is mostly a cosmetic blemish unless it overgrows the cornea.

Orbital Cellulitis

In its more superficial form, preseptal or periorbital cellulitis requires cultures, close surveillance, topical decongestant, and systemic antibiotics. A deeper, retrobulbar cellulitis may produce proptosis, marked swelling, pain, and damping of extraocular movements. This condition requires urgent consultation, inpatient care, adequate antibiotic coverage, and sometimes surgical drainage. The infection often begins in the adjacent paranasal sinuses; *Haemophilus influenzae, Streptococcus pneumoniae,* and *Staphylococcus aureus* are common causes. Among possible sequelae are cavernous sinus thrombosis, meningitis, and blindness.

Systemic Illnesses which Include Red Eyes as Part of the Presentation

Many conditions, especially those involving infectious and autoimmune mechanisms, will show reddened eyes as part of the clinical picture. In many of these conditions, the nonocular features of the condition will predominate and provide most of the diagnostic evidence. Those related to infection could include pharyngoconjunctival fever (adenovirus), leptospirosis (perhaps acquired from exposure to contaminated water), and (mostly in another age) measles. Among sexually active patients, consider

Reiter syndrome (*Chlamydia*-induced urethritis, arthritis, conjunctivitis) and *gonococcal ophthalmia.*

Autoimmune diseases inducing eye inflammation include rheumatoid arthritis with or without Sjögren's keratoconjunctivitis sicca. Pauciarticular juvenile arthritis has a high risk of uveitis, often without red eyes. Sarcoidosis and inflammatory bowel disease may also cause uveal tract inflammation. Primary skin diseases which may produce red eyes include acne rosacea, psoriasis, and seborrhea. Again, nonocular features should establish the diagnosis.

Conjunctivitis

If no danger signals indicate more threatening eye disease, no systemic clues suggest a generalized process, and there is no recent history of trauma, the diagnosis of exclusion will be conjunctivitis. In adolescents, various forms of conjunctivitis will cause the majority of red eye complaints. Given a patient in whom this diagnosis seems likely, separating the probable causes of conjunctivitis is the next step. Features of the history that may help include:

- Any known or suspected precipitating factor?
- Contact with people with a similar syndrome?
- Bilateral onset, persistently unilateral, or unilateral becoming bilateral?
- Respiratory symptoms? Suggesting allergy or infection?

Table 7-2 contrasts major forms of conjunctivitis. Establishing a firm etiologic diagnosis based on these findings may be uncertain as a good deal of overlap exists among the several categories. Treatment principles presented in Table 7-2 and the text below represent examples and not a definitive list of management possibilities.

Overall, most conjunctivitis will have a viral cause. Two agents, *herpes simplex virus* and adenovirus, deserve special attention. Herpes simplex can cause corneal, conjunctival, and periocular disease. Usually the adolescent will show unilateral involvement, and vesicles adjacent to the eye,

TABLE 7-2

COMMON CAUSES OF CONJUNCTIVITIS: DIFFERENTIAL DIAGNOSIS AND TREATMENT

Agent	Appearance	Circumstances
Bacterial (N. gonorrhoeae)	Very inflamed, copious purulent discharge, swelling, tenderness	Possible genital gonorrhea or exposure to infected sex partner
Bacterial (S. pneumoniae, H. influenzae, S. aureus, and others)	Red with sticky, purulent discharge, lid matting especially in the morning	
Viral (ECHO, coxsackievirus, adenovirus)	Red, edematous, sometimes hemorrhagic, watery discharge. Occasionally preauricular node, feels scratchy, itchy	Very contagious, especially epidemic keratoconjunctivitis (adenovirus type 8, 18, 37)
Chlamydia	Mild irritation, mucopurulent discharge, follicular response (seen magnified) lower lid	Usually hand to eye inoculation from genital source
Allergic (Aeroallergen—pollen, mold, mite, dander)	Conjunctival edema, redness, itching, discharge sticky. Vernal conjunctivitis has cobblestone appearance	Occurrence in season or circumstance of exposure, often other allergic respiratory symptoms
Chemical/Irritation	Red, variable	Known or suspected irritant exposure

if present, suggest the diagnosis. A special hazard here is a dendritic corneal ulcer, demonstrable with fluorescein staining. Patients with this problem require topical antiviral treatment (i.e., trifluridine ophthalmic) and possibly, systemic treatment (i.e., acyclovir) as well, depending on the extent of the problem. This management is best left to an ophthalmologist.

Epidemic keratoconjunctivitis, caused by certain adenovirus strains, presents special problems because of its extreme infectivity. Patients with this problem shed virus for two weeks during which they must avoid hand to eye contact, wash hands frequently, avoid using towels or other possible virus transmitters in common with others, and stay out of swimming pools which might transmit the virus passively. Virus transmission can occur readily in a clinic if hands and instruments are inadequately sterilized between patients. No effective chemotherapy exists for non-herpes viral conjunctival infection. Physical measures, such as cool compresses, may make the patient more comfortable while cleansing the lid margins. If the process does not show definite improvement in 7–10 days, the adolescent should be reevaluated by an eye specialist.

Bacterial conjunctivitis, if diagnosed accurately, should respond to topical antibiotics, though without antibacterial treatment, the process is self-limited and clears completely. Numerous effective antibacterial eye preparations, old and new, are available. Older preparations (aminoglycosides, polymyxin/trimethoprim) can adequately treat uncomplicated superficial bacterial infection. Fluoroquinolones should be reserved for those whose infections have developed under contact lenses. A red eye may also signal a sexually transmitted infection. Where circumstances warrant, inquire about sexual contacts and genitourinary symptoms.

Bibliography

Greenberg MF, Pollard ZF. The red eye in childhood. *Pediatr Clin N Am* 50:105, 2003.

Greydanus DE. Disorders of the ears, eyes, nose, and throat. In: Hofmann AD, Greydanus DE, *Adolescent Medicine*, 3d ed., Stamford, CT: Appleton & Lange, 1997, Chap. 8, pp. 93–118.

Leibowitz HM. The red eye. *New Engl J Med* 343: 345–351, 2000.

New drugs for allergic conjunctivitis. *Med Lett* 42:39–40, 2000.

Patel SJ, Lundy DC. Ocular manifestations of autoimmune diseases. *American Fam Physician* 66:991, 2002.

Ophthalmic Moxifloxacin and Gatifloxacin. *Med Lett* 46:25–27, 2004.

Sheikh A, Hurwitz B, Cave J. Antibiotics for acute bacterial conjunctivitis. *Cochrane Database Syst Rev* (2): CD001211, 2000.

Shingleton BJ, O'Donoghue MW. Blurred vision. *N Engl J Med* 343:556–562, 2000.

EYE INJURIES

Males aged 11–15 years experience the highest relative incidence of eye injuries, about half of which occur during sports involvement. Thus, a physician caring for adolescents should be prepared to care for eye injuries at several levels:

- Recognize serious injuries; determine urgency of referral
- Render immediate care before and during referral, assuring that time-sensitive matters (e.g., chemical burns) are addressed immediately, and no further damage occurs during the initial examination and transfer of the patient.
- Recognize and care for less serious problems.
- Promote eye safety in sports and avoidance of activities (i.e., BB pellet, airgun, and unprotected paint ball use) which pose a particular threat to the eye.

Bibliography

Catalano RA. Eye injuries and prevention. *Pediatr Clin N Am* 40:827, 1993.

Duma SM. The effect of frontal air bags on eye injury patterns in automobile crashes. *Arch Ophthalmol* 120:1517, 2002.

Harlan JB Jr, Pieramici DJ. Evaluation of patients with ocular trauma. *Ophthalmol Clin N Am*. 15:153, 2002.

Levine LM. Pediatric ocular trauma and shaken infant syndrome. *Pediatr Clin N Am* 50:137, 2003.

Mester V, Kuhn F. Intraocular foreign bodies. *Ophthalmol Clin N Am* 15:235, 2002.

Refractive Errors and Use of Contact Lenses

The role of the primary care physician in the management of refractive error lies largely in recognizing possible problems and initiating appropriate referrals. In adolescents, the commonest diagnosis will be myopia. The incidence of this problem varies in different populations ranging from about 20% in the United States adolescents to 80% among Chinese in Singapore. Aside from ethnic influences, development of myopia occurs more commonly with a positive family history and among better students, those who spend more time studying, reading, or doing close work, and less time engaging in sports. Myopia can be present from an early age, but will be less apparent in small children whose world lies close at hand. The process typically progresses through adolescence, stabilizing as the patient reaches maturity.

Management options include eyeglasses, hard or soft contact lenses, or surgical reshaping of the cornea such as laser-assisted in-situ keratomileusis (LASIK). Though often useful when applied appropriately, LASIK surgery should not be attempted until the patient has demonstrated at least a year of no change in lens prescription requirement. This essentially precludes its use in adolescents. Many myopes find eyeglasses a perfectly satisfactory solution to their vision problem. Among reasons for choosing contact lenses instead of spectacles, cosmetic considerations and convenience for sports participants rank high. Patients typically find that contact lenses provide better peripheral vision; no evidence supports the proposition that contact lens use improves central vision or arrests myopic progression. Since many adolescents will base their eye care choices on cosmetic considerations, the question around a move to contact lenses will be when rather than if. Use of any contact lens requires continuing maintenance and attention to detail, so the adolescent must have sufficient maturity to care for the selected lens system. The eye care professional and the patient will choose the lens type. Because of greater expected comfort, most will opt for some form of soft lens.

Several preexisting eye problems can predispose to poor tolerance of contact lenses and could affect the decision to use this form of correction. Allergic conjunctivitis occurring as part of a wider seasonal upper respiratory process may preclude comfortable use of contact lenses. If the allergy season is limited, lenses may be used safely and comfortably "out of season." Vernal keratoconjunctivitis can run a longer and more severe course, interfering with contact lens use much of the time. Atopic conjunctivitis (allergic eye inflammation occurring with atopic dermatitis) is a chronic and often severe form of ocular allergy requiring active treatment—sometimes corticoids—and precluding comfortable use of contact lenses. In addition, patients afflicted with blepharitis or chronic dry eye may not be able to use contact lenses successfully so long as the process remains active.

Chronic use of contact lenses can result in a variety of presentations of intolerance. Ability to recognize and advise concerning these problems will be a major contribution to eye care in the clinician's office. Table 7-3 lists and contrasts major contact lens-induced problems as a diagnostic aid to the clinician looking at an inflamed eye in a lens wearer. These lens-induced problems fall into three major categories—infections, allergic/immune inflammation, and irritation (mechanical and chemical). Most lens intolerance results from a combination of factors, and distribution of syndromes among the categories in Table 7-3 has been based on a judgment of the most important of the several factors.

Corneal hypoxia contributes as a major or minor cause to many of the lens-induced problems, but is identified as a primary problem only in corneal edema and the tight lens syndrome. Factors common to many of the problems include poor lens hygiene with accumulation of bacteria or other biologic debris, poor lens fit leading to distortion and mechanical problems, and less-than-optimal lens change schedules resulting in hypoxia and accumulation of biologic waste on or under the lens. For the non-eye care specialist, encountering an inflammatory eye problem in a lens wearer, the conservative approach would attribute the problem to the lens. Recommend

TABLE 7-3

PATTERNS OF CONTACT LENS INTOLERANCE

	Presentation	Mechanisms	Management
Infection			
Contact lens-induced acute red eye (CLARE)	Red eye, foreign body sensation, corneal infiltrate, typically present on awakening	Bacterial toxins accumulate under extended wear lens while the eye is closed	Discontinue lens use until problem has remitted. May recur
Peripheral corneal infiltrates	Single or multiple, small grey ulcers at corneal periphery, mild discomfort	Multiple staphylococcal toxin, hypoxia	Discontinue lens use, treat with topical antibiotic, critique lens management
Microbial keratitis	Pain, tearing, photophobia, single large infiltrate	Bacterial infection enabled by extended lens coverage, hypoxia, contaminated lens, or lens care materials	Serious problem, culture lesion, and eye care materials, treat with topical and systemic antibiotic. Refer
Allergic/immune			
Giant papillary conjunctivitis	Conjunctival injection, increased mucus production, itching, 0.3 mm or larger papillae especially on superior tarsal conjunctiva	Immune-mediated inflammation facilitated by lens-induced irritation. More common with extended wear lens	Discontinue use of lens until acute problem subsides Avoid longer-term extended wear lenses
Allergic conjunctivitis	Irritation, conjunctival injection, punctate keratopathy, infiltrates	Allergy to lens care solutions, especially thimerosal	Improve lens care technique, more thorough rinse or use another lens care system
Irritation—chemical			
Toxic conjunctivitis	Conjunctival redness, follicles, corneal erosions, infiltrates	Irritation from residual antiseptic (chlorhexidine, benzalkonium), enzymes or incidentals (e.g., hair spray) on lens	Improve lens care technique, watch outside contaminants on lens, try alternative lens care system
Corneal edema	If acute, pain, tearing, reduced vision, photophobia, redness Chronic similar but more subtle	Lens system and mode of use allow insufficient oxygen to the cornea	Discontinue contact use until resolved, replace with lens and usage pattern which allow better oxygen diffusion
Irritation—mechanical			
Superficial punctate keratitis	Burning, irritation, punctate lesions on the cornea	Multiple mechanisms, hypoxia, mechanical injury, chemical toxicity, dry eye	Improved cleaning of lens, replacement with better fitting lens
Tight lens syndrome	Irritation, pain, blurred vision, light sensitivity	High water content lenses dry and distort, tightness can induce hypoxia	Discontinue lens use, treat inflammation or infection, use more appropriate lens

lens removal until the eye improves, a specific diagnosis can be confirmed, and a strategy for avoiding recurrence developed.

Bibliography

Corneal surgery for correction of refractive errors. *Med Lett* 41:122–123, 1999.

Donshik PC. Extended wear contact lenses. *Ophthalmol Clin N Am* 16:79, 2003.

Greydanus DE. Papilledema. In: AD Hofmann, DE Greydanus, *Adolescent Medicine*, 3d ed., Stamford, CT: Appleton & Lange, 14:261–262, 1997.

Greenwald MJ. Refractive abnormalities in childhood. *Pediatr Clin N Am* 50:197, 2003.

Mutti DO. Parental myopia, near work, school achievement, and children's refractive error. *Invest Ophthalmol Vis Sci* 43:3633, 2002.

Shingleton BJ, O'Donoghue MW. Blurred vision. *N Engl J Med* 343:556–562, 2000.

Suchecki JK, Donshik P, Ehlers WH. Contact lens complications. *Ophthalmol Clin N Am* 16:471, 2003.

THE EAR

Approach to Ear Disorders

The first aspect of evaluating ear problems is a good history, including such important concerns as: date of onset of symptoms, precipitating factors (upper respiratory infections [URIs], allergic symptoms, recent swimming activity), redness and/or tenderness of the auricle, presence and nature of ear drainage, and changes in auditory acuity. Ear piercing may induce auricular chondritis due to *Pseudomonas aeruginosa* requiring removal of the foreign body, antibiotic therapy (as ciprofloxacin) and surgery (debridement and drainage). The most important aspect of diagnosing external and middle ear problems is adequate visualization. Thus, the clinician should have adequate means for removing obstructing wax or exudates—a soft cotton fluff (not cotton swab) for mopping liquid exudates, loop, curette, or spoon (soft plastic may be safest but not always the most effective), a suction source and tip, and a means of irrigation where it seems certain that the tympanic membrane (TM) is intact. Adequate otoscopes,

including a pneumatic model for assessing TM mobility and a simple means of measuring hearing are necessary as well.

The External Ear

Ceruminosis

Ceruminosis (excessive cerumen formation) is usually idiopathic and familial. It is often an insignificant physiologic variant, unless it impacts and occludes the ear canal. Foreign body, dermatosis, infection, or canal stenosis are potential causes which should either be ruled out or, if present, considered in the management plan. Signs and symptoms of ceruminosis vary from none-at-all to fluctuating hearing levels or consistent hearing loss and popping sounds when swimming or washing the ear.

Management consists of softening and lysing the impaction by one of several methods. The least expensive is the twice-daily instillation of acetic acid (white household vinegar to water at 1:1) or mineral oil, using a wick of cotton or gauze to keep the impaction moist. It will gradually soften after 5–7 days and can be flushed out with gentle tepid water irrigation using a bulb syringe. More rapid results can be obtained by gently flooding the ear with 10–15 drops of a lytic agent (Cerumenex or Debrox drops), allowing them to stand for 15–30 minutes and then irrigating as above. This procedure can be repeated once or twice a day for 3–4 days if needed. A few individuals may develop contact dermatitis with the use of these agents (Cerumenex in particular), and proper caution should be given. Some clinicians prefer to use 3% hydrogen peroxide because it is inexpensive, readily available, and also provides an effervescence which helps to debride the ear canal. Resistant cases may need to be treated by direct removal with a curette under magnification.

Otitis Externa

Otitis externa most commonly presents as local pain with increased discomfort on manipulation of the pinna; pain on chewing may also occur. Examination may disclose redness, swelling, and exudate in the ear canal. In severe cases, inflammation may spread beyond the canal itself to include the postauricular crease and in the most severe cases, the skin overlying the mastoid tip and/or the auricular skin. "Swimmer's ear," which develops in chronically wet ears, is a common mechanism but one should consider other possibilities as well. Table 7-4 below lists alternative causes of external otitis.

Management consists of cleaning the external auditory canal of debris, drainage, and cerumen plus the application of ototopical antibiotic drops; this usually suffices unless the cellulitis has spread beyond the canal itself. In this circumstance, an antibiotic appropriate to treat *S. aureus* or *Pseudomonas sp.* (causing necrotizing otitis externa) is used. Local management begins with thorough, gentle cleansing of the canal with suction or mopping with a cotton wisp to remove all accessible exudate. When there is appreciable edema of the external auditory canal, a wick (cotton or Merocel compressed cellulose) should be inserted and left in place for 2 or 3 days. Ototopical antibiotic (e.g., Floxin Otic or Ciprofloxin) or a combination of antibiotic-steroid (Cipro-Dex) should be used. Alcohol/acetic acid may also be efficacious but can cause pain in a sensitive external auditory canal. Burow's solution may be better tolerated. The older triple antibiotic preparations (e.g., Neosporin) may work well but can

TABLE 7-4

SOURCES OF EXTERNAL EAR INFECTION

Lesion	Causative Agents
Otitis externa (bacterial)	*Staphylococcus* sp., *Pseudomonas* sp.
Otitis externa (fungal)	*Aspergillus* sp., *Candida* sp.
Otitis externa (viral)	Zoster, Ramsay Hunt syndrome
Ear canal furuncle	Various
Otitis media with perforation and drainage	Various, often *Pseudomonas* sp.
Necrotizing otitis externa	*Pseudomonas* sp. (diabetes or other immune suppression)

TABLE 7-5

CONDITIONS WHICH PREDISPOSE TO OTITIS EXTERNA

Opportunities for Prevention
External
Water exposure—Swimming, diving, showering
High humidity
Heat
Foreign bodies—ear plugs, hearing aids, Q-tips
Drainage from the middle ear space
Allergic reactions (hair spray, other chemicals)
Cerumen impactions
Endogenous
Dermatologic—Seborrhea, contact dermatitis, atopic dermatitis, psoriasis
Immune deficiency—hematologic, chemotherapy, diabetes

lead to neomycin sensitization. Avoid topical aminoglycosides if there exists a possibility of TM perforation.

Patients can prevent many cases of external otitis if they recognize predisposing factors and apply simple hygienic measures. Table 7-5 lists circumstances which favor development of infection in the ear canal. A simple preventative program aims toward maintenance of a dry, acidic, cerumen-covered canal. After swimming, diving, or showering, the patient should dry the canal noninvasively and treat with Burow's solution or acid alcohol to reduce the risk of developing otitis externa. Instrumentation by the adolescent (i.e., use of Q-tips, hair pins, and the like) should be totally avoided.

Bibliography

Dohar JE. Evolution of management approaches for otitis externa. *Pediatr Infect Dis J*22:299–308, 2003.

Jones RN, Milazzo J, Seidlin M. Ofloxacin otic solution for treatment of otitis externa in children and adults. *Arch Otolaryngol Head Neck Surg* 123:1193–2000, 1997.

Sander R. Otitis externa: a practical guide to treatment and prevention. *Am Fam Physician* 63:927–936, 2001.

THE MIDDLE EAR

Otitis Media

Acute suppurative otitis media (AOM) is among the most frequent diagnoses made by primary care physicians in children aged 3 or less. However, this diagnosis should be reserved for those patients with purulent middle ear effusion, and not for those with red tympanic membranes with no effusion or in patients with serous middle ear effusion. With growth, upper airway anatomy becomes less conducive to infection ascending from the nasopharynx; by adolescence middle ear infections occur much less often. AOM in this age group should lead one to consider predisposing factors such as residua from infection at an earlier age, eustachian tube dysfunction, upper airway allergy, frequent URIs, and possibly immunodeficiency. Otitis media with effusion (OME), also primarily a disease of the very young, often reflects the sterile remains of a treated AOM, or can develop when eustachian tube blockage prevents aeration of the middle ear cavity. In this circumstance, a serous transudate replaces absorbed air producing the effusion. Table 7-6 contrasts features of these two forms of middle ear disease.

Studies comparing primary care practitioners with otolaryngology specialists have found that, in a common test population, primary care deliverers diagnose AOM more often than specialists. This results in more prescription of antibiotics and ultimately more bacterial resistance. Factors contributing to this include failure to obtain a good view of the tympanic membrane due to cerumen in the external auditory canal and patient motion. Evaluation of the TM position and movement with the pneumatic otoscope will aid in diagnosing otitis media and differentiating its forms.

AOM is an infectious process with up to 40% due to virus infection. Bacterial pathogens include *S. pneumoniae* and *H. influenzae* in roughly equal numbers with fewer infections due to *Moraxella catarrhalis*. Several studies have examined the impact of antibiotic treatment on the natural course and cure rate of otitis media and agree that the antibiotics confer only marginal benefit. Not all medical groups employ antibiotics freely in AOM. Physicians in northern Europe use antibiotics very sparingly in this disease, apparently with satisfactory results. Guidelines from the American Academy of Pediatrics and the American Academy of Family Practice also suggest withholding antibiotics in those with less severe disease and assurance of good follow-up. Many of these patients show improvement by 48–72 hours and ultimately cure the process without the need for antibacterial treatment.

It is not surprising, given the free use of antibiotics in AOM in many places, that the causative organisms have become more resistant to drug treatment. This has led to the modified antibiotic dosage recommendations noted below.

TABLE 7-6

CONTRAST BETWEEN ACUTE OTITIS MEDIA (AOM) AND OTITIS MEDIA WITH EFFUSION (OME)

	Acute Otitis Media	*Otitis Media with Effusion*
Presentation	Ear pain, full feeling	Ear full feeling, little pain
Appearance	TM bulging, decreased mobility, possibly red	TM retracted or flat, decreased mobility, abnormal color (not red), opaque (not scarred)
Cause	Infection—bacterial, viral	Residual from infection, eustachian tube blockage, allergy
Treatment	Antibiotics in selected cases	Patience, tube placement with persistent effusion

Most research directed at causes, treatment, and sequelae of both AOM and OME has considered only small children, forcing clinicians to extrapolate findings and recommendations to adolescents who are largely unstudied in this regard.

Given a diagnosis of AOM, clinicians should remember that a substantial fraction have a viral process (as evidenced by serous middle ear effusion) and thus, should not be placed on antibiotic therapy. A significant number of patients with bacterial disease will also clear the infection by themselves and not require antibiotics. Delaying antibiotic treatment in a patient who has modest local disease and little systemic toxicity, while treating with local and systemic analgesics leads to a satisfactory outcome most of the time. If the problem seems to demand antibiotics, remember that the causative bacteria will very likely be *S. pneumoniae* (with intermediate antibiotic resistance) or *H. influenzae* (with a high likelihood of beta lactamase production). Current dosing recommendations would begin with high dose amoxicillin (80–90 mg/kg per day orally in small children up to a maximum of 2 gm twice daily in mature adolescents) with a 5 day treatment course except in compromised patients. If no improvement occurs after three days, switch to a beta-lactamase resistant drug—amoxicillin-clavulanate (orally, with the same amoxicillin dose); cefuroxime axetil (250–500 mg orally, twice daily) or ceftriaxone (1 g intramuscularly, single dose) are also effective. Fluoroquinolones will manage AOM satisfactorily but should not be used as first-line treatment at this time.

Otitis media with effusion typically runs a self-limited course over weeks to two or three months. Systemic or upper airway topical corticoids will hasten disappearance of fluid from the middle ear but do not improve the long-term outcome. Antihistamines and/or decongestants provide no benefit and some evidence suggests that they inhibit clearing of middle ear fluid. Surgical placement of pressure-equalizing tubes is used to clear fluid from the middle ear; it is rarely needed in adolescents unless they have severe eustachian tube dysfunction with atelectasis, adhesive changes in the tympanic membrane, or there is a conductive hearing loss attributed to the presence of middle ear effusion.

Bullous myringitis may complicate or confuse the diagnosis of otitis media. Bullae form on the TM and can cause severe pain. Formerly attributed to *Mycoplasma pneumoniae*, this appears rather to be a non-specific reaction of the drumhead. The spectrum of causative organisms is about the same as is seen with AOM. Auralgan drops may be useful in managing pain in this condition. In cooperative patients, rupturing the bullae yields rapid pain relief and is an accepted mode of therapy to obtain patient comfort. Sensorineural hearing loss may occur as a sequela of bullous myringitis and thus, a formal audiogram is warranted. A temporary conductive hearing loss may also occur due to serous middle ear effusion, which usually resolves with time.

Otorrhea

Otorrhea may occur in acute suppurative otitis media (when the TM ruptures), in patients with a chronic TM perforation, or in patients with tympanostomy tubes in place. The treatment in each case is usually the same: use oto-topical ear drops for 5–10 days (Floxin, Ciprofloxacin, or Cipro-Dex). Systemic antibiotics are rarely necessary for acute otorrhea. Adolescents with suppurative otorrhea (often with suppurative rhinorrhea) due to viral URIs usually do not require systemic antibiotic therapy for the otorrhea. Subsets of patients that need special consideration are those who have tympanostomy tubes and who have otorrhea along with granulation tissue (a foreign body reaction) around the tube. These patients benefit from the use of topical drops containing steroids. One can use ciprofloxacin/dexamethasone (Cipro-Dex) or two sets of drops (Floxin for antibiotic coverage and Inflamase Forte for steroids).

Bibliography

Glasziou PP, Del Mar CB, Hayem M, Sanders SL. Antibiotics for acute otitis media in children. *Cochrane Database Syst Rev* 2:CD000219, 2000.

Keene WE, Markum AC, Samadpour M. Outbreak of *Pseudomonas aeruginosa* infections caused by commercial piercing of upper ear cartilage. *JAMA* 291: 981–985, 2004.

McCormick DP, Saeed KA, Pittman C, et al. Bullous myringitis: a case controlled study. *Pediatrics* 112: 982–986, 2003.

McCracken GH Jr. Diagnosis and management of acute otitis media in the urgent care setting. *Ann Emerg Med* 39:413–421, 2002.

Roland PS, Dohar JE, Lanier BJ, Hekkenburg R, Lane EM, Conroy PJ, Wall GM, Dupre SJ, Potts SL, and the Ciprodex AOMT Study Group. *Arch Otolaryngolo-Head Neck Surg* 130:736–741, 2004.

Rosenfeld RM, Bluestone DC (eds.). *Evidence-based Otitis Media,* 2d ed., Hamilton, Ontario: B.C. Decker, 2003.

Rovers MM, Schilder AGM, Rosenfeld RM. Otitis media, *Lancet* 363:465–473, 2004.

White CB, Foshee WS. Upper respiratory tract infections in adolescents. *Adolesc Med* 11:225–249, 2000.

THE MIDDLE EAR—TRAUMA

Pressure injuries to the TM including rupture can result from claps on the ear, high-speed falls on water (as in water skiing), or uncompensated changes in pressure (due to diving, sudden ascent or descent in altitude). Penetration injuries may occur with small foreign bodies in the canal. Head injuries can cause petrous bone fracture or affect middle ear contents including the oval or round windows producing a perilymphatic fistula resulting in sensorineural hearing loss. Any trauma to the head or tympanic membrane may result in a discontinuity of the middle ear ossicles resulting in a conductive hearing loss (up to 50–60 dB) when the perforation of the TM heals. Most TM ruptures will heal without help but need surveillance during the repair phase. For those that do not improve after several weeks, or any suspected of having middle or inner ear damage, referral to an otolaryngologist is advisable.

THE INNER EAR

Hearing Loss and Acoustic Injury

General Approach

Given an adolescent with hearing loss, important points in the history include time of onset of the hearing loss (recent or remote), rapidity of onset (acute or gradual), circumstances surrounding acute onset (injury, infection, other neurologic problems), and any family history of deafness. Evaluate for features of conductive hearing loss (impacted cerumen, middle ear fluid) and stigmata of syndromes, which include deafness (e.g., Waardenburg syndrome, neurofibromatosis). Examination should include pure tone audiometry done in quiet surroundings. The Rinne's test done with a 512-Hz tuning fork compares bone conduction (fork stem on the mastoid process) with air conduction. A normal examination will show air conduction lasting about twice as long as bone. A deficit in air conduction suggests conductive hearing loss, which is usually correctable with the appropriate surgical correction.

Differential Diagnosis

Conductive hearing loss will account for most of the correctable processes seen in adolescents. In addition to middle ear fluid and wax, other conditions that may interfere with sound wave conduction include TM damage, otosclerosis, cholesteatoma, ear canal swelling from otitis externa, and canal exostoses. The differential diagnosis of sensory neural hearing loss (SNHL) is extensive and will usually require consultation (Table 7-7). Most cases of SNHL in children will not have a specific, discernible cause. Among inducers of SNHL are drugs (aminoglycosides, anticancer agents—especially cisplatin, quinine, salicylates, loop diuretics, and deferoxamine). Much of SNHL is inherited making the family history critical to obtain. Identifiable syndromes include Alport's (nephritis and hearing loss), Waardenburg's (iris heterochromia and white forelock), Friedreich's ataxia, and neurofibromatosis. Infectious causes of SNHL include meningitis, numerous viral diseases, and possibly Lyme and Kawasaki diseases, while several tumors, most notably acoustic neuroma, may cause nerve deafness as well. A definitive listing of all categories and sources of SNHL is beyond the scope of this discussion.

Noise-induced hearing loss has long threatened those with loud occupations, avocations, or experiences. These include loud industrial and military

TABLE 7-7

CAUSES OF SENSORINEURAL HEARING LOSS

Congenital	Isolated idiopathic defect
	Rubella syndrome
	Syphilis
Postnatal nongenetic	*Infectious:* Chronic or recurrent otitis media including a variable complication of viral infections such as measles, mumps, influenza. Complication of meningitis
	Metabolic: As a variable manifestation of hypothyroidism, hyperparathyroidism, hyperlipoproteinemia, chronic renal disease
	Trauma: Acoustic nerve injury from continuous loud noise, fractures
	Neoplasm: Acoustic neuroma, other ear tumors, leukemia, lymphoma
	Ototoxic drugs: Aminoglycosides, furosemide, aspirin, lead, mercury, others
	Neurologic disorders: Multiple sclerosis, Friedreich's ataxia
	Ménièare's disease
	Anatomic: Perilymphatic fistula (rupture can lead to sudden loss on that side)
Postnatal genetic	Familial progressive sensorineural deafness
	Otosclerosis (usually not manifested until third decade or later)
	As a variable component of many syndromes: Waardenburg, Pendred, progressive retinitis pigmentosa (Usher), glomerulonephritis with nerve deafness (Alport), albinism, Alström, Hurler, Refsum, von Recklinghausen, trisomy 13–15, and trisomy 18

Source: Used with permission from: Greydanus DE. Disorders of the ears, eyes, nose, and throat. *Adolescent Medicine*, 3d ed., Stamford, CT: Appleton & Lange, 1997, Chap. 8, p. 97.

settings, recreational shooting, auto air bag deployment, and nearby lightning strikes. Where the insult is acute, recovery in several hours to days may be expected. Chronic exposure leads to irreversible loss. Of considerable interest to those caring for adolescents is the impact of loud music on hearing. This has been extensively studied with variable findings. Most research concludes that personal tape or disc devices do not cause much problem. Studies of rock musicians have demonstrated temporary threshold changes, which though significant, are usually temporary unless exposure to the loud noise is chronic and repetitive. The follow-up on these series is relatively short leaving one to wonder what impact, if any, this may have on hearing when the ex-rockers move on to presbycusis.

Meniere's disease typically presents with severe vertigo but causes aural fullness, tinnitus, and hearing loss as well. These may be accompanied by nausea, vomiting, and sweating. A hallmark of the process is its episodic course. The underlying cause seems to be hydrops of inner ear structures; this has led to recommendations that it be treated with salt restrictions and diuretics.

Bibliography

American College of Occupational and Environmental Medicine. ACOEM Evidence-based statement: Noise-induced hearing loss. *J Occup Environ Med* 45:579–581, 2003.

Greydanus DE. Disorders of the Ears, Eyes, Nose, and Throat. In: Hofmann AD, Greydanus DE, *Adolescent Medicine*, 3d ed., Stamford, CT: Appleton & Lange, 1997, Chap. 8, pp. 93–118.

Isaacson JE, Vora NM. Differential diagnosis and treatment of hearing loss. *Am Fam Physician* 68:1125–1132, 2003.

Lockwood AH, Salvi RJ, Burkard RF. Tinnitus. *N Engl J Med* 347:904–910, 2002.

Mostafapour SP, Lahargoue K, Gates GA. Noise-induced hearing loss in young adults: the role of personal listening devices and other sources of leisure noise. Laryngoscope 108:1832–1839, 1998.

NOSE/SINUSES/THROAT DISORDERS

General Approach

History and physical examination of the patient with upper respiratory complaints should focus on acuteness (or chronicity) of the process, and whether the source of the problem seems to be a virus (for which little specific treatment is available), a bacterial infection (which may benefit from an antibiotic), or an allergic process which might respond to environmental controls or antiallergic drugs. Viral respiratory diseases will occur more commonly in colder months, may include fever and systemic indisposition after a relatively acute onset and may result from exposure to others with similar problems, or in a setting of a community epidemic. Purulent infections will often develop as sequelae to viral disease, will have a more gradual onset, more fever, and localization. Viral infections may have an associated purulent rhinorrhea, which should resolve within 7–10 days. Allergic processes will show chronicity, a seasonal or situational pattern of recurrence, and a family history of atopy.

The history should include questions appropriate to establish a most-likely category for the cause of the presenting complaint. Physical examination includes examination of the interior of the nose, looking especially for frankly purulent nasal discharge where bacterial sinusitis is suspect. A classic allergic nose shows substantial pale, boggy mucosal swelling with clear watery or mucous discharge. The examiner should assess the pharynx, fauces, and oral mucosa for redness, swelling, exudate, enanthem, or ulceration. Evaluation of lymph nodes above the shoulders for swelling and tenderness will also help direct the diagnostic search, as might examination of ears, eyes (conjunctiva especially), and chest.

Epistaxis

The most common cause of nosebleeds is local trauma or irritation of the Kiesselbach's plexus in the anterior nasal septum. Epistaxis is more common in the male teenager. Nose picking, excessive drying due to low humidity, and rhinitis from any cause are the usual precipitants. Rhinitis may be due to upper respiratory tract infections, allergies, excessive use of vasoconstrictive nose drops with rebound hyperemia, or sniffing cocaine or glue. Trauma is another frequent but usually obvious cause. Rarely, staphylococcal infections of the nasal vestibule, deformed septum, juvenile polyps (often associated with allergic disorders), adolescent nasopharyngeal angiofibromas, hereditary hemorrhagic telangiectasia, malignant melanoma, lymphoma, rhabdomyosarcoma, hypertension, or bleeding disorders (usually in the male) may be implicated.

Diagnosis usually can be established by the history and physical examination alone. Local causes commonly produce hyperemia of the septal mucosa, with or without a demonstrable bleeding point or scab. If suggested by severe, protracted, or recurrent nose bleeds, evaluation for nasal tumors may require special techniques to visualize the posterior nasal cavity. Angiofibromas develop from vascular structures supplied by branches of the external or, less commonly, internal carotid artery in the nasopharynx and pterygomaxillary areas; they produce nasal obstruction, sinusitis with purulent rhinitis, and severe recurrent epistaxis. Bleeding disorders and hypertension should be suggested by additional relevant findings.

Acute epistaxis usually can be arrested simply by applying pressure through pinching the nares together for several minutes. Resistant cases may be treated by packing with petroleum jelly gauze or cotton soaked in a solution of 1%–2% cocaine plus 1:1000 epinephrine. Other methods include using a cotton ball soaked with 0.25% phenylephrine or 1% lidocaine, following by chemocautery with silver nitrate (Argyrol), as well as packing with Gelfoam or topical thrombin. Posterior nasal packing (gauze pad or balloon tampon) may be required for more proximal bleeding. Preventive measures for local causes include cutting finger nails, discouraging nose picking, application of petroleum jelly to the anterior nares at night, and increased humidification. Attention also should be given to any coexistent rhinitis.

Acute Viral Rhinosinusitis

The "common cold" produces more illness in more individuals more often than any other disease process. Because it is common, uncomfortable but not life-threatening, and not so far amenable to specific curative therapy, it has not attracted research interest to commensurate with its overall personal and societal impact. A 2001 survey assessed productivity loss attributable to the common cold and estimated that the total United States economic loss associated with colds at $26 billion a year. In the study sample, mean duration of the cold was 6.4 days with one cold in five lasting more than 8 days. About 15% of the cold sufferers visited a physician seeking help in caring for the infection.

Numerous viruses can cause a common cold syndrome. Overall, picornaviruses (notably the human rhinovirus [HRV]) cause the greatest number of colds—around half in most large series and up to 80% in some seasonal outbreaks. Other viruses which

may produce a URI include respiratory syncytial virus, influenza, parainfluenza, coronavirus, adenovirus, and probably others. Many of these viruses induce a poor immune response allowing reinfection. HRV in contrast produces good immunity but possesses 100+ serotypes, overwhelming much immune protection through diversity. All of the cold-causing viruses, including HRV, infect new subjects through large and small droplet spread. HRV, unlike many other respiratory viruses, is fairly hardy outside the body and spreads efficiently through a finger to eye or finger to nose route. This provides an opportunity to interdict virus spread through improved personal hygiene. In a study carried out in university residence buildings, dispensers containing an alcohol-gel hand cleaner were placed in dormitory rooms, bathrooms, and dining halls, presumably with a directive for use. Compared with dormitories not so equipped, users of this simple treatment had 20% fewer illnesses and 40% less missed school or work days. Frequent hand washing and care not to allow contact between fingers and eyes or nose should reduce transmission of HRV-caused colds.

Frequency of infection varies depending on age and social circumstances. Young children, especially those in larger daycare settings may have up to a cold a month in fall, winter, and spring. With acquisition of immunity and perhaps better hygiene habits, frequency falls to 2–4 per year by young adulthood. Though colds may occur throughout the year, they are most frequent in fall and spring. The fall increase in URI incidence may relate to return to school and increased social mixing as well as more time spent in indoor environments. Whether colder air *per se* favors infection through host or viral factors is unknown; total body chilling does not facilitate respiratory infection.

Virus inoculation studies using HRV have shown that volunteers can be infected via the mucosa of the eye or nose but not mouth. The incubation period is 10–16 hours and viral shedding peaks at about 3 days. Duration of infectivity can last more than two weeks. Initial symptoms in the induced infections consisted of sore or scratchy throat. CT imaging studies during naturally-acquired colds have demonstrated maxillary and/or ethmoid sinus abnormalities in 60%–90% of those scanned.

Most physicians and patients ultimately accumulate a war chest of favorite remedies for the common cold. These may include chicken soup, herbal remedies, ethanol in various forms, inhalation of steam with or without eucalyptus and menthol, plus rest and fluids. Some of these probably work. Faced with infectious rhinitis, it is very important that our management at least does not make things worse. Thus, we coordinate folk remedies and emphasize hygiene (containing coughs and sneezes, hand washing, and keeping fingers away from eyes and nose). Patients with rhinitis will feel a need to blow their noses occasionally and they should do this gently. A study, which looked at the dynamics of nose blowing, found that good blows generated intranasal pressures averaging 66 mmHg (versus 4.6 mmHg for sneezing) and propelled up to 1 mL of nasal contents into the sinuses.

Among herbal treatments, Echinacea has received the most attention for common cold management. The Cochrane database concluded that Echinacea could probably benefit those with viral URI and the risk of adverse effect was small. A recent American university-based trial, designed to circumvent shortcomings in earlier work, concluded that Echinacea provided no detectable harm or benefit. Apparently the case for Echinacea has yet to be made. Steam inhalation usually feels comforting during a cold and some have claimed it might provide an antiviral benefit. Studies looking at this have failed to confirm this attractive possibility. Zinc-containing lozenges and nasal sprays have elicited some interest but yielded inconsistent results in clinical trials.

Numerous antivirals have been considered for URI prevention or treatment. Intranasal interferon exerted a useful effect but produced a side effect profile including common-cold-like symptoms. Pleconaril showed modest but significant protective effect. It reached a late stage of FDA review but was rejected because of an unfavorable risk/benefit ratio. After numerous disappointments this field seems relatively inactive. Consumer cold remedies typically contain a systemic decongestant and a first generation antihistamine. The latter probably provide symptom relief through their anticholinergic side action. Though vasoconstrictor nose sprays (oxymetazoline and others) have a deservedly bad reputation because of rebound congestion, they can provide substantial relief safely if used for a period not exceeding 3–5 days.

Bibliography

Barrett BP, Brown RL, Locken K, et al. Treatment of the common cold with unrefined Echinacea. A randomized, double-blind, placebo-controlled trial. *Ann Intern Med* 137:939–946, 2002.

Belongia EA, Berg R, Liu K. A randomized trial of zinc nasal spray for the treatment of upper respiratory illness in adults. *Am J Med* 111:103–108, 2001.

Bramley TJ, Lerner D, Sarnes M. Productivity losses related to the common cold. *J Occup Environ Med* 44:822–829, 2002.

Echinacea for prevention and treatment of upper respiratory infections. *Med Lett* 44:2930, 2002.

Hayden FG, Herrington DT, Coats TL, et al. Efficacy and safety of oral pleconaril for treatment of colds due to picornaviruses in adults: results of 2 double-blind, randomized, placebo-controlled trials. *Clin Infect Dis* 37:1722, 2003.

Jefferson TO. Antivirals for the common cold. *Cochrane Database Syst Rev* 3:CD002743, 2001.

Melchart D, Linde K, Fischer P, Kaesmayr J. Echinacea for preventing and treating the common cold. *Cochrane Database Syst Rev* 1:CD000530, 2004.

Monto AS. Epidemiology of viral respiratory infections. *Am J Med* 112(Suppl 6A): 4S–12S, 2002.

Singh M. Heated, humidified air for the common cold. *Cochrane Database Syst Rev* 1 CD001728, 2004.

White CB, Foshee WS. Upper respiratory tract infections in adolescents. *Adolesc Med* 11:225–249, 2000.

White C. The effect of hand hygiene on illness rate among students in university residence halls. *Am J Infect Control* 31:364–370, 2003.

CHRONIC RHINOSINUSITIS

Rhinosinusitis symptoms that last beyond two to three weeks probably do not represent a single viral URI. Some surveys suggest that nearly 40% of patients have chronic rhinitis, not clearly attributable to infection. Though data vary, most series suggest that about half of these individuals have allergic upper airway disease. Considering and trying to establish this diagnosis is worthwhile as it can lead to an effective, organized treatment approach. Given a patient with chronic rhinitis, the following features should be considered.

- Seasonal or situational (e.g., animal exposure) occurrence
- Family history suggesting atopy
- Personal history suggesting atopy (infantile eczema, asthma)
- Characteristic physical findings (chronic mouth breathing, allergic shiners, swollen, pale, boggy nasal mucosa). Itching of nose, throat, and eyes
- Immunodeficiency or gastroesophageal reflux—especially if associated with recurrent ear infections

These findings may occur in conjunction with asthma; well over half of asthmatics also have chronic rhinitis (Chap. 8). Allergic asthma and allergic rhinitis are increasingly viewed as different manifestations of a unitary airway disease sharing common pathophysiologic mechanisms and, to some extent, common treatments. Some evidence suggests that effective rhinitis management favorably affects the course of asthma, reducing the need for emergency room care and hospital admission.

Substantial numbers of allergic rhinitis patients diagnose their own condition and treat themselves using nonprescription remedies. The primary care physician can contribute to treatment by identifying patterns associated with seasonal allergens in their part of the country (e.g., trees in early spring, grass in early summer and ragweed in late summer in the Northeast and upper Midwest). Winter or perennial allergens could include dust mites, animal dander, or perhaps indoor molds. With a suspect allergen in mind, one can suggest tactics for minimizing allergen exposure, though the clinician may choose to delegate extensive counseling of this type to specialists in allergy/immunology. Most adolescents with allergic rhinitis will respond satisfactorily to treatment with topical nasal corticoids (Table 7-8) and nonsedating antihistamines.

TABLE 7-8

TOPICAL NASAL CORTICOIDS

Beclomethasone (Vancenase, others)—1 spray per nostril 2–4 times per day
Budesonide (Rhinocort)—2 sprays per nostril 2 times a day or 4 sprays per nostril once per day
Flunisolide (Nasalide, others)—2 sprays per nostril 2 times a day; maximum 8 sprays per nostril per day
Fluticasone (Flonase)—2 sprays per nostril once per day
Mometasone (Nasonex)—2 sprays per nostril once per day
Triamcinolone (Nasacort, others)—2 sprays per nostril once a day or 2 times a day

They should use pharmacologic suppression continuously in season; intermittent dosing in response to symptom flares produces inferior results.

Allergen immunotherapy, a form of treatment whose origin antedates the era of modern antiallergic pharmacology, occasionally adds a useful dimension. Though time-consuming and expensive, some patients seem to prefer this approach. For those not responding satisfactorily to environmental or pharmacologic control, it provides an additional treatment option.

Some patients present with a clinical picture that suggests upper airway allergy, but show no skin test positivity. Though some of these results may reflect failure to administer the inciting antigen tests, many have a nonallergic process. This pattern is more common in people at middle age and beyond, but will occasionally appear at any age. In such a patient, it is useful to look for nasal eosinophilia. Its presence suggests the NARES syndrome (nonallergic rhinitis with eosinophilia), while failure to find eosinophils would be more consistent with vasomotor rhinitis. This endpoint can be capricious and diagnosis and treatment should not be based on a single finding. Generally NARES patients respond well to antihistamine/nasal steroid management, while those without eosinophilia are resistant to treatment. Very rarely chronic rhinitis can result from drug or hormonal influences, including nasal use of street drugs.

Bibliography

Ayars G. Nonallergic rhinitis. *J Allergy Clin Immunol* 20:283–302, 2000.

Bachert KC, Vignola AM, Gevaert P, et al. Allergic rhinitis, rhinosinusitis, and asthma: one airway disease. *J Allergy Clin Immunol* 24:19–43, 2004.

Colton R, Zeharia A, Karmazyn B, et al. *Exserohilum* sinusitis presenting as proptosis in a healthy adolescent male. *J Adolesc Health* 30:73–75, 2002.

Corren J, Manning BE, Thompson SF, et al. Rhinitis therapy and the prevention of hospital care for asthma: A case-control study. *J Allergy Clin Immunol* 113:415–419, 2004.

Dolor RJ, Witsell DI, Hellkamp AS et al. Comparison of cefuroxime with or without intranasal fluticasone for the treatment of rhinosinusitis. *JAMA* 286:3097–3105, 2001.

Newer antihistamines. *Med Lett* 43:35, 2001.

Plaut M. Immune-based, targeted therapy for allergic diseases. *JAMA* 286:3005–3006, 2001.

Simons FER. Advances in H₁-antihistamines. *N Engl J Med* 351:2203–2217, 2004.

Virant FS. Allergic rhinitis. *J Allergy Clin Immunol* 20:265–282, 2000.

PURULENT SINUSITIS

While a mild degree of sinusitis will accompany many uncomplicated viral URIs, this should clear as the primary infection recedes. Persistent, recurrent, or unusually severe sinus symptoms or signs suggest that the process has proceeded into another phase. A chronic cough, especially nocturnal, suggests chronic sinusitis or gastroesophageal reflux. Sinus disease does not typically occur in isolation. It may be a sequel of a viral URI, or of a previous sinus infection, may reflect sinus drainage problems resulting from allergy, anatomic abnormality or functional problems such as cystic fibrosis or ciliary dyskinesia, or could result from gastrointestinal reflux or an immune deficiency state. Most series divide their cases according to duration into acute, sometimes subacute, chronic, and recurrent cases. Suggested time frames vary but acute usually implies continuation or worsening of symptoms at the end of atypical URI course while chronic implies persistence of the problem beyond 90 days.

A defining standard for diagnosing sinusitis would be culture-positive returns from a sinus puncture and aspiration, a procedure that does not lend itself well to routine use. Sinus x-rays can demonstrate fluid or mucosal thickening but lack sensitivity. Most guidelines do not recommend basing the diagnosis on findings from plain sinus films. CT scan images are much more sensitive and can demonstrate abnormal anatomy about the sinus ostia. Screening sinus CT scans (limited coronal views) are useful for diagnostic purposes. Three millimeter cut axial and coronal sinus CTs should be reserved to demonstrate fine anatomy where surgery is contemplated. Screening sinus CTs should not be obtained during the acute episode (unless one is concerned about a complication of sinusitis such as orbital cellulitis or meningitis) since over 90% of sinus CTs taken during a viral URI will be interpreted as sinusitis. Sinus transillumination, performed by placing a bright point source of light against the cheek over the antra and examining the degree of transmission through the hard palate (after adequate dark adaptation), suggests opaque fluid in the maxillary sinuses, if no light transmits or there is notable asymmetry. More subtle changes are not helpful and overall the technique is relatively insensitive.

The clinical diagnosis of purulent sinusitis depends on assembling a convincing array of signs and symptoms, none of which are invariably present. Suggestive signs and symptoms include:

- Purulent nasal discharge
- Facial pain or tenderness on pressure or percussion over sinuses
- Maxillary toothache
- Fever
- Cough, especially at night
- Suggestive symptom sequence with URI to possible sinusitis
- Prior history

One should consider sinus disease when evaluating a patient with chronic cough, and remember that incompletely treated sinusitis may trigger worsening of asthma. Sinus disease occurs in a sensitive area and can proceed to eye or intracranial complications if severe and unchecked.

Infectious agents with potential to invade the sinuses can include viruses, bacteria, and fungi. Virus-induced processes should be self-limited and fungi will mostly infect patients with underlying immune deficiencies. In considering the bacteriology of sinus infections, recall that both the sinuses through their ostia and the middle ear through the eustachian tube are in effect adjunctive nasal cavities. Thus, bacterial causes of sinusitis mirror those which cause otitis media, most commonly nontypable *H. influenzae, S. pneumoniae,* and *M. catarrhalis.* The issues with antibiotic treatment of sinusitis parallel those with otitis media—penicillin resistance among *S. pneumoniae* and beta-lactamase production by *H. influenzae* and *M. catarrhalis.* Antibiotic strategy should be similar, with high dose amoxicillin first up followed by a beta lactamase protected product (amoxicillin/clavulanate) or a second generation cephalosporin for poor responders. Antibiotics penetrate inefficiently into sinus cavities so patients should receive a treatment course of adequate duration. There are many recommendations—at least 10 days seems wise, or treat until symptoms have resolved plus an additional 7 days.

Adjunctive treatments of sinusitis offer marginal benefit. Wet or dry heat over painful sinuses often seems to relieve symptoms as may inhalation of steam. No evidence exists to confirm benefit. Combination antihistamine/ decongestant/ analgesic products can provide pain relief but have no demonstrated efficacy beyond that.

Bibliography

American Academy of Pediatrics. Subcommittee on management of sinusitis and subcommittee on quality improvement. Clinical practice guideline: Management of sinusitis. *Pediatrics* 108:798–808, 2001.

Goldsmith AJ, Rosenfeld RM. Treatment of pediatric sinusitis. *Pediatr Clin N Am* 50:413–426, 2003.

Hickner JM, Bartlett JG, Besser RE, et al. Principles of appropriate antibiotic use for acute rhinosinusitis in adults: Background. *Ann Intern Med* 134:498–505, 2001.

Leggett JE. Acute sinutitis. *Postgrad Med* 115:13–17, 2004.

Piccirillo JF. Acute bacterial sinusitis. *N Engl J Med* 351:902–910, 2004.

White CB, Foshee WS. Upper respiratory tract infections in adolescents. *Adolesc Med* 11:225–249, 2000.

Pharyngitis and Tonsillitis

Sore throat has multiple causes, a broad spectrum of clinical presentations, and a wide range of severities from trivial to threatening. For most adolescents with a significant degree of pharyngeal pain, the diagnosis is "strep throat" until proven otherwise. In adults, *Streptococcus pyogenes* causes 5%–15% of troublesome sore throats; in children it causes 15%–25%. Thus the majority of even moderate or severe sore throats will derive from causes other than streptococci and it is incumbent on the thoughtful practitioner to keep in mind the extensive list of possible alternative agents and mechanisms. Table 7-9 lists numerous infectious causes of pharyngitis/tonsillitis organized by adjunctive features (exudates or membrane, conjunctivitis, rash, adenopathy, and vesicles or ulcers) seen with throat infection caused by that agent. In Table 7-10 appear a number of noninfectious mechanisms and infectious agents associated with pharyngitis, which is usually nonspecific and mild or moderate in severity.

Special attention to Group A *S. pyogenes* is legitimate as it is the commonest readily treatable cause of pharyngitis/tonsillitis. Timely treatment will slightly shorten the adolescent's discomfort and prevent the (very rare) nonsuppurative complications, rheumatic fever, and glomerulonephritis. Every clinician has a good idea of what strep tonsillitis looks like—beefy red, swollen tonsils and fauces, petechiae on the soft palate, white or yellowish exudates, cervical adenopathy, fever, systemic toxicity, and possibly a scarlatiniform rash. Unfortunately in practice things are rarely so clear and diagnosis of streptococcal throat infection on clinical grounds fails frequently. Culture from a carefully and aggressively obtained throat swab constitutes the standard for diagnosis. However, this approach does not provide an answer for 18 to 24 hours and does not discriminate between infected patients and those with a carrier state. Rapid tests, based on detection of

TABLE 7-9

CAUSES OF PHARYNGITIS (CLINICAL SYNDROME) WITH SPECIAL FEATURES

Exudate

Streptococcus pyogenes, groups A, C, G

Corynebacterium diphtheriae

Arcanobacterium haemolyticum

Yersinia enterocolitica

Herpes simplex

Fusobacterium sp. (Vincent's angina)

Adenovirus

Epstein-Barr (EB) virus (infectious mononucleosis)

Skin Rash

S. pyogenes

A. haemolyticum

EB virus

Human immunodeficiency virus

Conjunctivitis

Adenovirus (pharyngoconjunctival fever)

Enterovirus

Vesicles/Ulcers

Herpes simplex

Candida sp.

Coxsackievirus (herpangina)

Aphthous stomatitis

Adenopathy

S. pyogenes

Y. enterocolitica

Cytomegalovirus

EB virus

TABLE 7-10

INCIDENTAL OCCURRENCES OF SORT THROAT: INFECTIOUS OR NONSPECIFIC CAUSES

Neisseria gonorrhoeae	Dry air
Mycoplasma sp.	Systemic lupus erythematosus
Chlamydia sp.	Behçet syndrome
Influenza	Rhinovirus (common cold)
Sinusitis with drainage	Neutropenia
Upper airway allergy	

immunologic markers of the Group A streptococci (GAS), provide answers in minutes with a high degree of specificity. However, sensitivity seems to run from 80% to 90%, leaving a substantial fraction of those tested in diagnostic limbo.

Attempts to standardize clinical criteria for diagnosis have led to standardized diagnostic criteria such as the Centor score. This scoring scheme assigns one point for each of the following criteria:

- History of fever
- Absence of cough
- Presence of exudates on pharynx or tonsil
- Presence of enlarged, tender anterior cervical lymph nodes

One series looked at the diagnostic sensitivity of this scoring system correlating serologic or culture evidence of GAS infection with Centor score levels:

Score 0, 1	14% streptococci positive
Score 2	20% positive
Score 3	43% positive
Score 4 (maximum)	52% positive

A logical approach might exclude those with Centor scores of 0 or 1 from further diagnosis or specific treatment. Patients with scores of 3 or 4 and probably 2 should have rapid screening. Negative outcomes on the rapid screen should have culture confirmation. Those testing positive on the rapid screen or follow-up culture would receive treatment consisting of penicillin V, 500 mg twice or three times a day for 10 days. Alternatives include benzathine penicillin, one dose of 1.2 million units intramuscularly or, for those with penicillin sensitivity, erythromycin 40 mg/kg per day in 2–4 divided doses for a 10 day course (Table 7-11). Cephalosporins may be more effective then penicillin for GAS tonsillopharyngitis (Casey, 2004).

Most sore throat sufferers who test negative for strep will have a viral process, some of which will present a characteristic picture (Table 7-9). However, *Arcanobacterium haemolyticum* is a gram-positive to gram-variable rod that can cause pharyngitis similar to GAS; approximately two-thirds have a nonproductive cough and a scarlatiniform-like rash (see Chap. 19). *A. haemolyticum* is often missed on a sheep blood agar for GAS that is read at 24 hours.

TABLE 7-11

EFFECTIVE ANTIBIOTICS FOR STREPTOCOCCAL PHARYNGITIS*

Antibiotic*	Dose
Bicillin L-A	1.2 m units IM
Bicillin C-R 900/300	900,000 units benzathine penicillin G with 300,000 units procaine penicillin G IM
Penicillin V potassium	250 mg q.i.d. × 10 days. (Variations of b.i.d. or t.i.d. have been reported to be effective)
Erythromycin	250 mg q.i.d. × 10 days
Clindamycin	75 mg q.i.d. × 10 days
Cefaclor	250 mg t.i.d. × 10 days
Cefadroxil	500 mg b.i.d. × 10 days
Cephalexin	250 mg q.i.d. or 500 mg b.i.d. × 10 days
Cefprozil	250 mg b.i.d. or 500 mg once a day × 10 days

*This is not an exhaustive list

Source: Used with permission from: Greydanus DE. Disorders of the ears, eyes, nose, and throat. In: Hofmann AD, Greydanus DE (eds.), *Adolescent Medicine*, 3d ed., Stamford, CT: Appleton & Lange, 1997, Chap. 8, p. 106.

Erythromycin is the antibiotic of choice, since penicillin often does not work. Azithromycin and clarithromycin are also effective. In addition, it is important not to forget potentially serious causes of sore throat such as peritonsillar abscess (apparent mass adjacent to the tonsil, trismus) or diphtheria (adherent grey membrane). Among socially and sexually active adolescents some infectious causes of pharyngotonsillitis will occur more frequently. Potential sources include infectious mononucleosis (EB virus, cytomegalovirus), *Chlamydia, Neisseria gonorrhea*, and human immunodeficiency virus.

Bibliography

American Academy of Pediatrics. Group A streptococcal infections. In: Pickering LK, (ed.), *Red Book Report of the Committee on Infectious Diseases*, 26th ed., Elk Grove Village, IL: American Academy of Pediatrics, 2003, p. 573.

Bisno AL, Gerber MA, Gwaltney JM, Jr, et al. Practice guidelines for the diagnosis and management of Group A streptococcal pharyngitis. *Clin Infect Dis* 35:113–125, 2002.

Casey JR, Pichichero ME. Cephalosporins better than penicillin for childhood streptococcal tonsillopharyngitis. *Pediatrics* 113:866–882, 2004.

McIsaac WH, Kellner JD, Aufricht P, et al. Empirical validation of guidelines for the management of pharyngitis in children and adults. *JAMA* 291:1587–1595, 2004.

Pichichero ME. Group A streptococcal vaccines. *JAMA* 292:738–739, 2004.

Swedo SE, Leonard HL, Rapoport JL. The pediatric uutoimmune neuropsychiatric disorders associated with streptococcal infection (PANDAS) subgroup. *Pediatrics* 113:907, 2004.

White CB, Foshee WS. Upper respiratory tract infections in adolescents. *Adolesc Med* 11:225–249, 2000.

DENTAL CONDITIONS

Gingivitis and *periodontitis* are common dental disorders in youth. Pubertal gingivitis can present in young female teenagers as a generalized gingival inflammation persisting through adolescence. Juvenile periodontitis can be noted in a localized form in young teenagers, possibly due to immunologic reaction to Actinobacillus actinomycetemcomitans. Generalized juvenile periodontitis can occur in older teenagers and resemble periodontitis seen in adults. Juvenile periodontitis can be seen in a variety of disorders, including diabetes mellitus, acute lymphoblastic leukemia, sickle cell anemia, histiocytosis, pregnancy, hypophosphatasia, trisomy 21, and others.

The highest rate of cavity formation occurs in adolescence. The normal oral flora, especially *Streptococcus mutans*, produce sticky compounds that lead to plaque formation and if unchecked, eventual tooth damage. The use of fluoridation and dental sealants have led to some decrease in the rate of dental caries. However, inadequate childhood care and poor oral hygiene leave many teenagers with major dental and periodontal problems, including severely carious, broken, and missing teeth as well as chronic gingivitis. Malocclusion requiring orthodontic treatment also becomes more prominent at this time due to maturation of facial features. Impacted wisdom teeth (third molars) with eruption gingivitis or pericoronitis are another frequent dental condition in adolescents.

Oral manifestations of sexually transmitted diseases include those seen in HIV infection (Candida infections, periodontitis, gonorrhea, tonsillitis, and pharyngitis), syphilis (pharyngitis, chancre mucous patch), herpes labialis (recurrent ulcers) and oral condylomata acuminate (human papillomavirus). Leukoplakia from the use of tobacco, other tissue damage from smokeless tobacco, effects of oral contraceptives on periodontal structures, athletic-induced injuries to dental structures, and the perimolysis noted in bulimia are also noted in adolescents. Recent studies note a beneficial effect of 13-cis-retinoic acid on leukoplakia, a potentially premalignant condition. Cigarette smoking can lead to mucosal irritation and stained teeth. Smokeless tobacco can induce gingivitis, loss of gum tissue, mucosal hyperkeratosis, and increased risk for oral carcinoma. Perimolysis refers to the hydrochloric acid effects on enamel and dentin which leads to loss of enamel and increased susceptibility to caries. Attention to these issues, institution of good oral hygienic practices, and regular evaluation by a dentist are important elements of health maintenance to be reinforced by the primary care clinician.

Bibliography

Greydanus DE. Disorders of the ears, eyes, nose, and throat. In: Hofmann AD, Greydanus DE (eds.), *Adolescent Medicine*, 3d ed., Stamford, CT: Appleton & Lange, 1997, Chap. 8, pp. 93–118.

Mouradian WE, Wehr E, Crall JJ. Disparities in children's oral health and access to dental care. *JAMA* 284: 2625–2631, 2000.

Sonis A, Zaragoza S. Dental health for the pediatrician. *Curr Opin Pediatr* 13:289, 2001.

Stookey GK. Caries prevention. *J Dent Educ* 62:803–811, 1998.

NECK DISORDERS

Temporomandibular Joint Syndrome

Temporomandibular joint (TMJ) syndrome is characterized by pain on motion of the jaw and frequently, a "locking" of the temporomandibular joint on opening. Various organic factors may be involved including arthritis, malocclusion, subluxation of the TMJ meniscus (this is the only joint other than the knee to have a meniscus), inflammation, and others. Adolescents, however, infrequently evidence underlying pathology other than malocclusion or subluxation. Rather, most cases seem to be due to spasm and fatigue of the muscles of mastication. Emotional tension reflected in unconscious clenching of the jaw or bruxism is thought to be a significant contributing factor. Adolescents who undergo orthodontia or extraction for orthognathic treatment may be at increased risk of the TMJ syndrome later in life.

Symptoms are usually unilateral and include pain and tenderness in and around the joint on the affected side along with difficulty in chewing. Limited jaw motion, clicking sounds, crepitation, otalgia, and headaches may also occur. Physical examination corroborates these complaints. A click alone, however, is not diagnostic, as it may be a normal physiologic finding. X-ray films including tomography are usually either normal or demonstrate restriction of forward condylar motion; rarely, actual bone disease may be detected. The TMJ syndrome often is misdiagnosed as migraine or tension headache, otitis media, sinusitis, impacted wisdom tooth, or dental abscess.

Management consists of putting the jaw at rest. Soft foods, local heat, ibuprofen (analgesic and anti-inflammatory agent), muscle relaxants, gentle massage, biofeedback relaxation techniques (to minimize jaw clenching and bruxism), and avoiding opening the jaw widely can be helpful. Other therapeutic modalities include orthotics, restorative dental procedures, correction of occlusion, orthodontics, and surgical orthognathics. Treatment may be required for a number of weeks and the condition may recur. In resistant cases more vigorous investigation for meniscus dislocation, malocclusion, or emotional tension is indicated; if present, these conditions must be dealt with appropriately. Unless specific pathology is identified requiring operative intervention, surgery should be avoided because it is rarely helpful and bears a significant risk of inadvertent facial nerve injury.

Bibliography

Greydanus DE. Disorders of the ears, eyes, nose, and throat. In: Hofmann AD, Greydanus DE (eds.), *Adolescent Medicine*, 3d ed., Stamford, CT: Appleton & Lange, 1997, Chap.8, pp. 93–118.

Guidelines for temporomandibular disorders in children and adolescents. *J Pediatr Dent (Special Issue: Reference Manual)* 21(5):66–67, 1999–2000.

NECK MASSES

Many diseases are manifested by enlarged cervical lymph nodes, either localized or part of a generalized lymphadenopathy. Other extralymphatic conditions also may present as a cervical mass. Table 7-12 cites the differential diagnosis relevant to the adolescent. Refer to the index for discussions of specific issues.

Bibliography

Greydanus DE. Disorders of the ears, eyes, nose, and throat. In: Hofmann AD, Greydanus DE (eds.), *Adolescent Medicine*, 3d ed., Stamford, CT: Appleton & Lange, 1997, Chap. 8, pp. 93–118.

Haberman TM, Steensma DP, Lymphadenopathy. *Mayo Clin Proc* 75:723–732, 2000.

Kelly CS, Kelly RE, Jr. Lymphadenopathy in children. *Pediatr Clin N Am* 45:875–888, 1998.

TABLE 7-12

DIFFERENTIAL DIAGNOSIS OF CERVICAL MASSES*

Lymphatic, Infectious Masses

Viral upper respiratory tract infections (adenovirus, *herpes simplex virus*, enterovirus)

Infectious mononucleosis (also consider toxoplasmosis and cytomegalovirus infection)

Reactive to infections of ears, pharynx, teeth, scalp

Suppurative adenitis (usually secondary to conditions cited above); *streptococcus* and *staphylococcus* most common (also consider anaerobic bacteria and *H. influenzae*)

Tuberculosis; atypical mycobacteria

Fungi (histoplasmosis, coccidioidomycosis)

Cat scratch fever

Lymphatic, Noninfectious Masses

Hodgkin's disease

Lymphoma

Leukemia

Sarcoidosis

Extralymphatic Masses

Bronchial cleft cyst

Hygroma

Enlarged thyroid gland; thyroiditis, colloid goiter, hyperthyroidism, tumor

Ectopic parotid gland; parotitis (mumps, bacterial), parotid duct stone, tumor

Lipoma, fibroma, dermoid cyst; lymphoma; carcinoma

*Used with permission from: Greydanus DE. Disorders of the ears, eyes, nose, and throat. In: Hofmann AD, Greydanus DE (eds.), *Adolescent Medicine*, 3d ed., Stamford, CT: Appleton & Lange, 1997, Chap. 8, p. 107.

8

DISORDERS OF THE THORAX AND LUNGS

Douglas N. Homnick

Although physiology and diseases of the thorax and lung are ultimately tied, it is convenient to think of syndromes that affect each as somewhat distinct. For example, the thorax consisting of bone, cartilage, striated muscle, and supporting parenchymal structures is more easily traumatized but less prone to infection than the lung. The lung maintains an intimate connection between the external physical and internal physiologic environments and is therefore affected by conditions stemming from contact with biologic or organic foreign material. The following chapter discusses more common conditions that affect both lung and thorax with consideration of physical signs that may indicate disease in either. Consistent with the theme of the text, the emphasis will be on the adolescent and illustrative cases are occasionally provided.

Reference

Homnick DN, Greydanus DE. Pulmonary disorders in the adolescent. *Adolesc Med* 11:483–704, 2000.

CASE STUDY 8-1

Chest Pain (Chronic)

R.J. is a 15-year old presenting to the clinic with a 3-month history of sharp, intermittent chest pain occurring primarily at rest and lasting for about 1 minute. The patient localizes the pain to the left lower sternal border and your subsequent examination is normal. There is no associated syncope, light headedness, or palpitations. The pain may be relieved somewhat by change of position.

There are many causes of chest pain in adolescents (see Table 8-1) but among the most common is that with no apparent etiology (idiopathic 12%–85%) and pain with a musculoskeletal origination (15%– 31%) (see Chap. 9). Case 1 represents a case of precordial catch syndrome (Texidor's twinge), a not infrequent cause of idiopathic benign chest pain in teens. Typically teens with precordial catch syndrome present with sharp stabbing, localized precordial pain, occurring most frequently at

TABLE 8-1

CAUSES OF CHEST PAIN

Pulmonary	Mitral valve prolapse
Asthma	Coronary artery disease
Infection	**Gastrointestinal**
Bronchitis	Gastroesophageal reflux
Pneumonia	Esophageal foreign body
Pleural disease	Achalasia
Pleurisy	**Musculoskeletal**
Pleural effusion	Muscular injury
Pneumothorax	Rib fracture
Cystic fibrosis	Spinal deformities
Diaphragm irritation	Vertebral injury
Gallbladder disease	Scoliosis
Subphrenic abscess	Costochondritis
Psychogenic	Tietze syndrome
Hyperventilation	Slipped rib syndrome
Anxiety	Herpes zoster
Unresolved mourning	Exercise-induced stitch
Association with ill	or cramp
family member	**Systemic diseases**
Cardiac	Leukemia
Arrhythmia	Sickle cell anemia
Myocarditis	Connective tissue
Cardiac tumor	disorders
Structural lesions	**Miscellaneous**
(acquired or	Breast development
congenital)	Mastitis
Idiopathic hyper-	Cocaine abuse
trophic subaortic	
stenosis	

Source: Adapted from Howenstine MS, Eigen H. Medical Care of the Adolescent with Asthma. *Adolesc Med* (3):505, 2000. With permission

rest, often exacerbated by deep breathing and lasting no more than a minute or two. It is self-limited over months and is often relieved by change in position. There are no associated findings on physical examination.

Proper diagnosis of chest pain should include historical information on the duration of pain (chronic if greater than 3 months), location, nature (e.g., sharp stabbing, dull aching, burning, intermittent, persistent), and associated systemic symptoms (cough, fever, night sweats, weight loss, and so forth). Pain causing primary sleep disturbance is almost always of organic origin. Pain of cardiac origin is rare (4%–6%) but may accompany congenital anatomic or acquired lesions and arrhythmias. Mitral valve prolapse produces pain in about 30% of those affected (Chap. 9). Cardiac pain may be accompanied by fatigue, exertional dyspnea, syncope, and a heart murmur may be noted on physical examination. Suspected pain of cardiac origin should be evaluated by a pediatric cardiologist.

Inspection of the chest wall and thorough palpation, including the breasts, is essential to identify the origin of thoracic pain. Benign gynecomastia with small, moveable, tender nodules may occur in either sex in early adolescence. Concern, particularly among males as to abnormal breast development can easily be laid to rest by a careful examiner. Pain of pulmonary origin (see discussion of lung conditions) is most often accompanied by shortness of breath (e.g. spontaneous pneumothorax), wheeze, or cough. Pleurodynia accompanying Coxsackie B infection is sharp persistent pain. Sharp, stabbing pain associated with pleuritis occurs during deep inspiration. Chronic pulmonary, cardiac, and rarely, hepatic disease is accompanied by digital clubbing and this plus growth failure or malnutrition, suggests a serious underlying disease.

Gastrointestinal pain, particularly that associated with gastroesophageal reflux disease (GERD), occurs relatively uncommonly in adolescents (<5%). However, if present, may be described as burning, often localized to the epigastrium or lower substernal chest wall. Chronic cough may be associated with severe GERD. Chest pain of psychologic origin is often described as chest discomfort; it commonly accompanies the hyperventilation associated with panic disorder. Evaluation by a clinical psychologist with appropriate intervention will often relieve the pain.

Chest pain of musculoskeletal origin may emanate from muscle (trauma), nerve (e.g. herpes zoster), or cartilage/bone (infection, inflammation, or trauma). Chest wall pain may be due to several conditions encountered in the adolescent. More common conditions include costochondritis, rib stress fracture, and slipping rib syndrome.

References

Disla E, Rhim HR, Reddy A, et al. Costochondritis: a prospective analysis in an emergency department setting. *Arch Int Med* 154(21):2466, 1994.

Gregory PL, Biswas AC, Batt ME. Musculoskeletal problems of the chest wall in athletes. *Sports Med* 32(4): 235, 2002.

Homnick DN, Pratt HD. Respiratory diseases with a psychosomatic component. *Adolesc Med* 11(3):547–566, 2000.

Kocis KC. Chest pain in pediatrics. *Ped Clin N Amer* 46(2):189, 1999.

DISORDERS OF THE CHEST WALL

Costochondritis

Up to 30% of patients presenting to the emergency department with chest wall pain have this condition. It occurs commonly in youth of either gender, often in those undertaking stressful activity of the upper body such as weight lifting and gymnastics. The etiology is unknown although there is soft evidence of localized inflammation of the costochondral junction. Localized, palpable pain over the costochondral junction without systemic symptoms is typical. If there is a localized, nonsuppurative nodule, usually located at the second or third costochondral junction, the condition is termed Tietze syndrome. The etiology of this condition is likewise unknown although inflammation is also implicated. Diagnosis of either condition is dependent on history and clinical examination as radiographs are usually normal. Soft tissue swelling and occasionally partial calcification of the costal cartilage may be evident. Treatment of these self-limited conditions consists of reassurance, mild analgesics, such as oral nonsteroidal anti-inflammatory agents, and discontinuation of any aggravating activity. Severe pain may respond to local injection of corticosteroid, especially with Tietze syndrome.

Stress Fractures of the Ribs

Stress related rib fracture, especially that of the first rib, occurs in athletes engaged in strenuous activity, particularly those involving overhead activity such as baseball, basketball, tennis, or weight lifting. With first rib fracture, pain occurs in the shoulder, cervical triangle or clavicular region. Fracture may occur in other ribs including the so called floating ribs (eleventh and twelfth ribs) in cases of extreme chest wall and abdominal muscle contraction. Baseball pitching, golf, and surfing have all been associated with traumatic rib fracture. Collegiate rowers appear to be at particular risk with 12% of a national rowing team diagnosed with rib fracture over about a 1-year period (Christiansen, 1997). Pain is insidious in onset progressing from ill defined to sharp pain over days to weeks. Pain may be felt in the back as the fracture site is often at the posterolateral rib angle. Examination often reveals local rib tenderness and plain chest x-ray most often is diagnostic. Treatment for first rib fracture includes sling immobilization of the shoulder and use of a soft cervical collar. Prognosis is good with return to normal activity within 3 months.

Slipping Rib Syndrome (Painful Rib, Clicking Rib Syndrome)

This occurs in up to 3% of patients presenting with rib pain. Sharp pain is often described in the lower chest or upper abdomen along with a tender spot on palpation of the lower costal margin. The etiology is thought to be due to hyper mobility of the anterior ends of ribs 11 and 12 with a tendency of one rib to slip under the other. The development of this condition may follow chest trauma. Pain is likely due to impingement on the intercostal nerve or strain of the lower costal cartilage. The excess rib movement may be accompanied by a snap, click, or pop associated with sharp intermittent pain. The hooking maneuver (the examiner hooks his/her fingers under the lower costal margin and pulls anteriorly) will reproduce the pain accompanied by a typical click. There is no specific radiologic diagnostic test. Conservative management consists of rib strapping, avoidance of precipitating activities, and use of mild analgesics. Occasionally local nerve block and injection of corticosteroid may be necessary to relieve severe pain. Excision of the anterior end of the rib and costal cartilages may provide definitive relief in extreme cases.

CHEST DEFORMITY

Pectus Excavatum

Pectus deformities (pectus excavatum and carinatum, Fig. 8-1) occur in about 1% of the population with boys affected in a 4:1 ratio to girls. Pectus excavatum (funnel chest) is most common with inward indentation of the sternum readily apparent on chest inspection. With adolescent growth acceleration, the defect becomes more severe but stops progressing once adult growth is attained. Dystrophic growth of the costal cartilages appears to be the cause of the sternal depression. There is often a familial tendency toward this defect. Although specific symptoms are not routinely associated with pectus excavatum, adolescents may complain of fatigue, decreased exercise tolerance, and chest and back discomfort. Mitral valve prolapse may occur in up to 20% of children with pectus excavatum and resolves about half the time with repair. Pectus deformities are also seen in connective tissue disorders including Marfan and Ehlers-Danlos syndromes. Embarrassment as a result of the cosmetic nature of the deformity most often leads to the patient seeking medical or surgical evaluation of the deformity. Surgery is indicated primarily for cosmetic purposes. Although mild restrictive defects in pulmonary function may accompany severe pectus excavatum deformities, functional improvement in lung function and exercise tolerance is quite variable after surgery. Subjective improvement may be noted by patient and family.

Pectus Carinatum (Pigeon Chest)

This defect characterized by anterior protrusion of the sternum, with or without torsion, is less common than pectus excavatum. It also occurs more commonly in males than in females and progresses during adolescent growth. It has not been associated with consistent cardiorespiratory symptoms and, like pectus excavatum, surgery is primarily

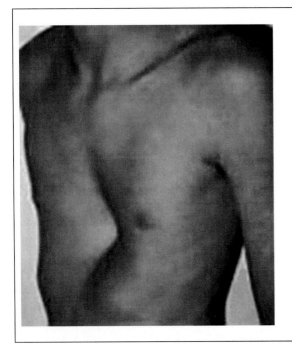 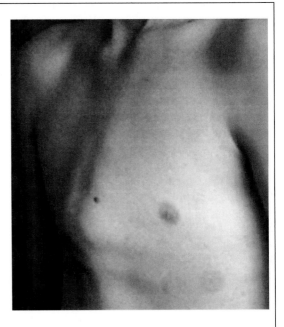

FIGURE 8-1

PECTUS EXCAVATUM (LEFT) AND PECTUS CARINATUM (RIGHT).

for cosmetic reasons. Several different surgical techniques have been developed for the pectus deformities (Goretsky, 2004).

CASE STUDY 8-2

Chest Pain (Acute)

T.S. is an 18-year-old male with known diagnosis of cystic fibrosis (CF). He has moderate pulmonary disease with exacerbations of chronic *P. aeruginosa* bronchitis/pneumonia requiring antibiotic therapy 3–4 times per year. He presents to the emergency department complaining of acute, sharp, left-sided chest pain associated with shortness of breath of about 4 hours duration. On examination there are decreased breath sounds on the left and a slight shift of cardiac point of maximum intensity to the right. Cardiac sounds are more distant than his last exam.

Causes of acute chest pain in CF patients include pleurisy associated with infectious exacerbation (see section on CF) and acute, secondary pneumothorax. Five to eight percent of all CF patients and 16%–20% of CF adults over 18 years will experience at least one episode of pneumothorax. Up to 50% will experience a recurrence and local thoracoscopic apical resection and pleurodesis is the definitive treatment. The cause is often the rupture of emphysematous portions of the lung apex during severe cough or Valsalva. Primary spontaneous pneumothorax is, however, not uncommon in normal adolescents, the cause of which is often unknown.

References

Arroyo JF, Vine R, Reynaud C, et al. Slipping rib syndrome: don't be fooled. *Geriatrics* 50(3):46, 1995.

Christiansen E, Kanstrup IL. Increased risk of stress fractures of the ribs in elite rowers. *Scand J Med Sci Sports* 7(1):49, 1997.

Goretsky MJ, Kelly RE, Croitoru D, Nuss D, Chest wall anomalies: pectus excavatum and pectus carinatum. *Adolsc Med* 15:455–472, 2004.

Gumbiner CH. Precordial catch syndrome. *S Med J* 96(1):38, 2003.

Honda N, Machida K, et al. Scintigraphic and CT findings of Tietze syndrome: report of a case and review of the literature. *Clin Nucl Med* 14(8):606, 1989.

Scott EM, Scott BB. Painful rib syndrome-a review of 76 cases. *Gut* 34(7):1006, 1993.

Williams AM, Crabbe DCG. Pectus deformities of the anterior chest wall. *Ped Resp Rev* 4:237, 2003.

PRIMARY SPONTANEOUS PNEUMOTHORAX

The incidence of primary spontaneous pneumothorax is estimated at about 18/100,000 population in men and 6/100,000 in women (Sahn, 2000). The typical patient is an otherwise normal, tall, thin male between 10 and 30 years. Smoking increases the risk of spontaneous pneumothorax by up to a factor of twenty. Subpleural emphysematous bullae or blebs are commonly found when patients proceed to thoracoscopic surgery. This contrasts with the infected, fibrotic, and cystic lung apex found in patients with CF.

Most episodes of spontaneous pneumothorax occur at rest with the sudden onset of pleuritic (sharp) chest pain and dyspnea. The exam may be normal with small pneumothoraces. Those with air occupying more than 15% of the pleural cavity are accompanied by decreased movement of the chest wall, decreased breath sounds, distant cardiac tones, and hyper resonance on percussion. Tachycardia is common and if accompanied by cyanosis and hypotension indicates tension pneumothorax.

Diagnosis is made with a combination of physical examination and upright chest x-ray (Fig. 8-2). Treatment depends on the size of the pneumothorax, the clinical presentation, and whether it is recurrent. With a pneumothorax that is less than 15% of the hemithorax volume and minimal symptoms, simple observation may be sufficient. The addition of supplemental oxygen hastens the reabsorption of the pleural gas by a factor of 4 by replacing less well absorbed nitrogen with more diffusible oxygen. A larger primary pneumothorax,

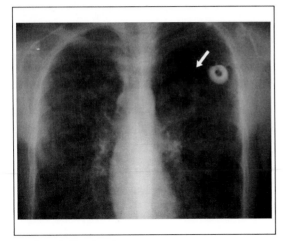

FIGURE   8 - 2

LEFT PNEUMOTHORAX (UNDER PORT-A-CATH) IN A PATIENT WITH CYSTIC FIBROSIS.

especially when accompanied by symptoms, requires evacuation of the intrapleural air. Simple aspiration of air with a small-bore catheter, with or without water seal, may be sufficient with a one-time leak. With reaccumulation of intrapleural air or with development of a tension pneumothorax, placement of a thoracostomy tube will be necessary either under radiographic guidance by an interventional radiologist or at the bedside by skilled pulmonary or critical care staff. The tube is then attached to a water seal device or Heimlich valve for a day or two until the persistent leak is resolved. Persistent leaks of greater than about 4–5 days require surgical intervention.

Recurrence of pneumothorax is quite common occurring in 30%–50% of patients (Sahn, 2000). Thoracoscopy with resection of bullae and local pleurodesis by pleural abrasion or instillation of a sclerosing agent, such as talc, has generally replaced the administration of sclerosing agents through a chest tube. The recurrence rate for primary pneumothorax with this method is 5%–9%. In secondary pneumothorax such as in CF, the recurrence rate appears to be somewhat higher probably due to forceful cough and extreme lung and airway inflammation. A consensus document on the management of spontaneous pneumothorax was published by the American College of Chest Physicians in 2001 (Bauman, 2001).

References

Bauman MH, Strange C, Heffner JF, et al. Management of spontaneous pneumothorax-consensus conference. Chest 119:590, 2001.

Oxcan C, McGahren ED, Rodgers BM, Thoracoscopic treatment of spontaneous pneumothorax in children. *J Pediatr Surg* 38(10):1459, 2003.

Sahn SA, Heffner JE. Spontaneous pneumothorax: *N Engl J Med* 342(12):868, 2000.

Yim AP, Ng CS. Thoracoscopy in the management of pneumothorax. *Curr Opin Pulm Med* 7(4):210, 2001.

CASE STUDY 8-3

Chronic Cough

L.L. is a 13-year-old female who presents to your clinic with a 3-month history of dry, hacking cough. This occurs at night and exacerbates with physical activity. There has been no history of congestion, headache, or wheeze and no constitutional symptoms. Spirometry done in the clinic reveals a forced expiratory volume over 1 second (FEV_1) of 72% predicted. You give her 2 puffs of an albuterol inhaler in the clinic and 20 minutes later repeat the spirometry. There is an 18% improvement in forced FEV_1 to 85% predicted accompanied by subjective improvement in cough.

There are many causes of chronic cough in children and adolescents (Table 8-2). Cough as the primary presenting symptom of asthma is not uncommon and is sometimes referred to as cough equivalent or cough variant asthma. Cough associated with asthma often occurs upon retiring and also exacerbates with physical activity and during upper respiratory tract infections. As physical findings of wheeze are usually absent, spirometry can be diagnostic with greater than a 12% increase in the FEV_1 indicating reversible airway obstruction. Alternatively, an asthma diagnosis may be accomplished by bronchial challenge (bronchoprovocation) with cold air, exercise, methacholine or histamine, often performed in a hospital pulmonary

TABLE 8-2
CAUSES OF CHRONIC COUGH IN ADOLESCENTS

Upper airway	Postnasal drip/nasal allergy
	Sinusitis
	Foreign body in external
	auditory canal
Lower airway	Asthma
	Infection (tuberculosis,
	mycoplasma, chlamydia)
	Cystic fibrosis
	Primary ciliary dyskinesia
	Irritation (primary smoking,
	environmental tobacco smoke,
	indoor air pollution)
Other	Psychogenic
	Gastroesophageal reflux disease

Source: Adapted from Homnick D, Pratt H. Respiratory diseases with a psychosomatic component. *Adolesc Med* 11(3):547, 2000. With permission

function laboratory. A drop in FEV_1 of 10%–20% during bronchoprovocation also indicates reversible airway obstruction and most often indicates a suspected diagnosis of asthma. The treatment of cough variant asthma is the same as for chronic asthma, i.e., anti-inflammatory medications, long-acting bronchodilators, and short-acting broncho-dilators for acute care (see discussion of asthma management).

Other causes of chronic cough include postnasal drip from chronic sinusitis or allergic rhinitis, airway irritation from smoke or other particulates and toxic chemicals, chronic infection (e.g., tuberculosis [TB]), chronic bronchitis from primary ciliary dyskinesia or cystic fibrosis, GERD, and foreign body aspiration, among others. Psychogenic cough is not uncommon among adolescents and presents with a dry, loud, repetitive, honking cough. The cough is disruptive to social interaction but is absent during sleep. Treatment for psychogenic cough centers mainly on behavioral therapy. Treatment for other causes of chronic cough depends on defining the underlying etiology. For a discussion of upper airway etiologies, see Chap. 7.

DISORDERS OF THE LUNG

Bronchitis

Acute bronchitis (tracheobronchitis), caused by bacteria, or more commonly viruses, is a common condition in adolescence. As this inflammatory condition usually affects both the trachea and bronchi, tracheobronchitis is a more accurate description. It can usually be subdivided into acute and chronic or recurrent forms by duration and frequency of symptoms. Acute tracheobronchitis is usually a consequence of viral infection and resolves in less than 3 weeks. Common viral etiologies include respiratory syncytial virus, adenovirus, rhinovirus, influenza, and enteroviruses. Bronchitis associated with bacterial infection often follows an initial viral infection. Causes of bacterial bronchitis in adolescence include *Mycoplasma pneumoniae*, *Chlamydia pneumoniae (TWAR)*, *Moraxella catarrhalis* and *Bordetella pertussis*.

Chronic tracheobronchitis, defined as symptoms lasting more than 3 weeks, is rare and usually associated with a known chronic disease or toxic exposure leading to defective mucus clearance. Etiologies include conditions such as CF and primary ciliary dyskinesia, ongoing irritant exposure (e.g., cigarette smoke), or undiagnosed chronic airway inflammation (e.g., asthma). True chronic bronchitis, defined by the American Thoracic Society (ATS, 1962) as a productive cough occurring for 3 months per year for two consecutive years without evidence of other respiratory disease, probably does not apply to children and adolescents. Recurrent bronchitis is defined as four or more episodes during a year. Common causes of acute and chronic/recurrent tracheobronchitis are outlined in Table 8-3.

Tracheobronchitis occurs most often during the winter months. It begins initially as a dry, hacking, nonproductive cough that progresses gradually to a cough productive of variable types and quantities of mucus. In the case of bacterial infection this tends to be purulent and occasionally blood tinged and with viruses, thin, and clear or white. Coarse rhonchi are heard on auscultation of the chest, particularly in the midline, and wheezing is not uncommon. Sternal chest pain or discomfort may be present and exacerbated by cough.

TABLE 8-3

CAUSES OF ACUTE AND CHRONIC/RECURRENT
BRONCHITIS

Acute Infection

Viral—Respiratory syncytial virus, parainfluenza,
  1, 2, influenza

A and B, adenovirus, rhinovirus

Bacterial—*S. pneumoniae, S. aureus, H. influenza,*
  M. catarrhalis, M. pneumoniae, C. pneumoniae
  (TWAR), B. pertussis, C. diphtheria, M. tuberculosis

Chemical exposures—Aspiration of gastric contents,
  smoke inhalation

Chronic/Recurrent

Cystic fibrosis

Asthma

Primary ciliary dyskinesia

Tuberculosis

Retained foreign body

Aspiration-anatomic abnormalities
  (tracheoesophageal fistula, laryngeal cleft);
  dysfunctional swallowing with and without
  gastroesophageal reflux

Immunodeficiency—IgG, IgA, IgG subclasses,
  common variable, immune deficiency, inability
  to respond to polysaccharide antigen

Inhalation injury
  Smoking—active
  Indoor air pollution—environmental tobacco
    smoke, wood stoves, chemicals
  Outdoor air pollution—soot, SO_2, ozone, NO_2

Chronic airway damage—following infection
  or traumatic airway injury with delayed
  or incomplete healing

Airway compression—dynamic (tracheobroncho-
  malacia) or extrinsic
  (vascular or nodal compression)

Source: Adapted from Loughlin GM. Bronchitis. In: Chernick
and Boat (eds), *Disorders of the Respiratory Tract in Children.*
Philadelphia, PA: W.B. Saunders, 1997. With permission

Chest radiography is usually unremarkable or
may occasionally show perihilar bronchial thickening or cuffing. Typical viral infection produces
minimal nonpurulent sputum, low grade or absent
fever, normal or low white blood cell counts, and
normal erythrocyte sedimentation rate. Bacterial etiologies produce more fever and elevated white blood
cell counts.

Diagnostic studies may be helpful in determining
etiology of tracheobronchitis. Cold hemagglutinins
are usually positive with *M. pneumoniae* infection
and along with specific IgM, leads to appropriate
therapy. *C. pneumoniae* is an under appreciated frequent cause of lower respiratory symptoms in children, teens, and adults and is found in up to 18% of
cases of respiratory infection in large studies. It is difficult to isolate on culture but acute and convalescent
sera may be revealing.

Treatment of acute tracheobronchitis is symptomatic with liberal intake of fluids, mild analgesics,
humidification, and mild cough suppressants if
sleep is disturbed. Antibiotics are reserved for
proven bacterial infection or chronic symptoms
associated with mucopurulent sputum, fever, and
elevated white blood cell count. Macrolides such as
erythromycin, clarithromycin, and azithromycin are
often prescribed. Fluoroquinolones can be used for
patients over 18 years and tetracyclines as an alternate to macrolides for children over 9 years.

Pneumonia

Community acquired pneumonia (CAP) is defined
as pneumonia which is acquired outside of the hospital setting. The annual incidence of CAP is
unknown but estimated to be about 6–12 cases per
1000 older children and adolescents. It is not
uncommon to see increases in bacterial pneumonia
in young individuals following significant viral
epidemics with influenza A or B.

Viral pneumonia is most common and usually
associated with milder symptoms than those of
bacterial origin (Table 8-4). Causes of viral and
bacterial pneumonias include those agents found in
tracheobronchitis and frequently originate from the
upper airway. Bacterial pneumonia following a
significant viral infection such as influenza is
likely due to aspiration of upper airway bacteria,
which establishes infection in inflammation damaged
lower airways. Less common bacterial organisms

TABLE 8-4

CLINICAL FEATURES OF VIRAL VS. BACTERIAL PNEUMONIA

	Viral Pneumonia	*Bacterial Pneumonia*
Incidence	Frequent	Comparatively infrequent: mycoplasma and pneumococcal pneumonias predominate
Symptoms and signs	Often begins with an upper respiratory tract infection that gradually worsens. Cough may be protracted, but symptoms are relatively mild; pneumonia due to measles or varicella, however, can be severe, as can any of the viral infections in immunologically deficient individuals	Abrupt onset with more severe symptoms. Cough may produce blood-streaked, purulent sputum. Mycoplasma pneumonia tends to be milder than other bacterial forms and more like viral disease
Chest x-ray	May be negative or demonstrate patchy, diffuse, or interstitial infiltrates	Often more signs of consolidation. Lobar involvement common in pneumococcal pneumonia
Treatment	Symptomatic	Antibiotics. Drainage of pleural effusion if present
Complications	Rarely myocarditis, pericarditis, encephalitis	Empyema, lung abscess relatively common; less commonly, septicemia, endocarditis, or meningitis

Source: Adapted from Greydanus DG, Homnick DN (eds). Disorders of the lung-pneumonia. In: *Adolescent Medicine*. Stamford, CT: Appleton & Lange, 1997. With permission

such as *Pseudomonas aeruginosa* are found in individuals with long standing defects in mucociliary clearance such as cystic fibrosis, primary ciliary dyskinesia, individuals with tracheostomies and bronchiectasis (see discussion of cystic fibrosis).

In CAP, atypical pneumonia is probably an inaccurate term as it is recognized that infection with atypical organisms (mycoplasma, chlamydia, legionella, and pertussis) may have presentations and radiographic findings indistinguishable from the common bacterial etiologies. Bacterial pathogens, most commonly *Streptococcus pneumoniae, Haemophilus influenza* (including nontypable varieties), *Staphylococcus aureus, Streptococcus pyogenes, and Neisseria meningitidis*, usually present with high fever, malaise and myalgias, chest pain, and sputum production that is purulent and sometimes blood tinged. Diagnostic studies

primarily include culture of expectorated sputum and blood counts commonly show polymorphonuclear leukocytosis.

Lobar consolidation with or without pleural effusion is the usual chest radiographic finding with these organisms (Fig. 8-3). If pleural fluid is present, ultrasound is of benefit in determining the quantity and quality of the effusion—i.e., is the fluid free flowing or has it begun to organize with fibrin loculations? In the case of effusion, obtaining fluid through needle thoracentesis can be helpful in determining the need for, and the timing of, thoracostomy tube placement.

Pleural effusions are generally divided into two types, transudative and exudative. Transudative fluid is generally of noninfectious origin, e.g., the ultrafiltrate of congestive heart failure, nephrotic syndrome, or hypoproteinemia. Exudative fluid is most often of infectious, neoplastic, or collagen-vascular disease

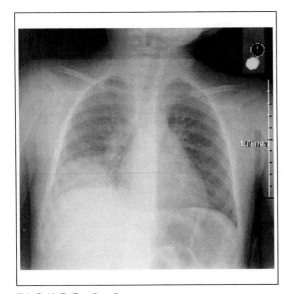

FIGURE 8-3

RIGHT LOWER LOBE CONSOLIDATION IN *S. PNEUMONIAE* PNEUMONIA.

origin and has different cellular and biologic properties from transudates. Exudates associated with pneumonia are termed parapneumonic and with ongoing inflammation, increase in inflammatory cell content and decrease in pH and organization may become empyema that is difficult to evacuate. Generally pH < 7.2, low glucose concentration (<80 mg/dL), and high lactate dehydrogenase

(LDH > 2000 IU/L) indicates the need for a chest tube. With extensive organization of the effusion, thoracoscopy, to break up loculations or for pleural decortication, can aid in recovery and a shorter hospital stay. Criteria for diagnosis of pleural effusion are outlined in Table 8-5.

Atypical bacterial and viral pathogens generally present with more insidious onset, lower fever and more variable radiographic findings including patchy bronchopneumonic infiltrates (Fig. 8-4). Both *C. pneumoniae* and *M. pneumoniae* are frequent causes of wintertime pneumonia in older children, adolescents, and adults, occurring in mini epidemics. Up to 20% of patients may be coinfected with both organisms. Infection with *M. pneumoniae* often presents with headache, paroxysmal cough productive of thin white mucus, and low grade fever. Rashes including simple maculopapular, erythema multiforme and Stevens-Johnson syndrome may accompany infection. Lobar consolidation and effusion (up to 25%) can occur with *M. pneumoniae* but patchy pneumonia is more usual. *C. pneumoniae* presents in a similar manner to *M. pneumoniae* infection with cough and sore throat with or without low grade fever.

Bedside cold agglutinins can be done to rapidly detect disease caused by mycoplasma when IgM titers are over about 1:64. One takes $^{1}/_{4}$–$^{1}/_{2}$ mL of whole blood and puts it in an anticoagulant tube. By tilting the tube, a uniform layer of blood spreads across the side and at room temperature

TABLE 8-5

PLEURAL FLUID CHARACTERISTICS

Fluid Characteristics	Transudate	Exudate
Predominant cell type	Mononuclear	Polymorphonuclear
WBC	<10,000/µL	>10,000/µL
pH	≥serum (7.40)	<7.30*
Pleural/serum protein	<0.5	≥0.5
Pleural/serum LDH	<0.6	≥0.6
LDH > upper serum normal level	–	+

*pH < 7.20 = high risk of location, pH < 7.10 high risk of surgical intervention

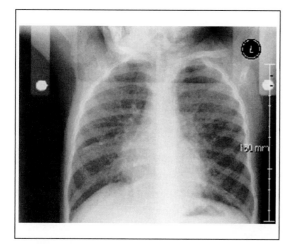

FIGURE 8-4

PERIHILAR, DIFFUSE INFILTRATES TYPICAL FOR VIRAL OR "ATYPICAL" BACTERIAL PNEUMONIA.

should show no granulations. The tube is then placed in ice water for several minutes and the same maneuver undertaken. If cold hemagglutinins are present one will see dark granulations resembling minute coffee grounds in the blood layer. Warming to body temperature will cause disappearance of the granules and recooling, their reappearance. Useful diagnostic tests and recommended antimicrobial therapy for these and common bacterial agents are found in Table 8-6.

References

American Thoracic Society, Committee on Diagnostic Standards for Nontuberculous Respiratory Diseases: Definitions and classification of chronic bronchitis, asthma, and pulmonary emphysema. *Am Rev Respir Dis* 85:762, 1962.

Gordon RC. Community-acquired pneumonia in adolescents. *Adolesc Med* 11(3):681–695, 2000.

Hammerschlag MR. Chlamydia trachomatis and Chlamydia pneumoniae infection in children and adolescents. *Ped Rev* 25:43, 2004.

Thomas CF Jr., Limper AH. Pneumocystis pneumonia. *N Engl J Med* 350:2487–2498, 2004.

Ward MA. Lower respiratory tract infections in adolescents. *Adolesc. Med* 11(2):251–262, 2000.

CASE STUDY 8-4

Abnormal Chest X-Ray and Positive Tuberculin Skin Test

R.C. is a 17-year old with cough, fever, and congestion for about 1 week. Because of some question of decreased breath sounds in the bases of both lungs, a chest x-ray is obtained. A 1.5–2.0 cm round lesion with some calcification is noted in the right lower lung along with some right hilar adenopathy in an otherwise normal study. You obtain an HIV titer that is negative and query other family members for TB and HIV disease. At a follow up visit 72 hours later, the cough, congestion, and fever are improved but a tuberculin skin test (TST) applied to R.C.'s right forearm reveals induration of 8 mm at 72 hours. You make a diagnosis of latent tuberculosis infection (LTBI) and recommend therapy.

PULMONARY TUBERCULOSIS

Since the mid 1980s the incidence of pulmonary TB has been rising and is the most common presentation of this disease. This has closely paralleled the HIV epidemic and it is no wonder that regions with a high TB prevalence are also those with high HIV rates. All patients presenting with active TB infection should be screened for HIV infection no matter what age or perceived risk factors.

Pulmonary TB can be divided into primary and postprimary (secondary or reactivation disease). In the primary form, airborne organisms enter the lung in an aerosol form in association with close contact to a patient with active TB. This is most often a primary relative in the case of pediatric and adolescent infection. The TB bacillus is contained in a primary granuloma in the lung parenchyma and enlargement of a regional (usually hilar) lymph node accompanies the asymptomatic infection (Fig. 8-5). The chest x-ray demonstrates this primary lesion (Ghon complex) several weeks after initial infection. Calcification of the lesion indicates infection has occurred some time in the past.

TABLE 8-6

COMMUNITY ACQUIRED PNEUMONIA—TESTING AND TREATMENT

Pathogen	Test	Comments	Treatment
Pyogenic bacteria	Sputum Gram stain	Done on sputum in acute illness and is highly specific for *S. pneumoniae, S. aureus, H. influenzae, N. meningitidis,* and *M. catarrhalis*, but patients may produce no sputum	According to specific culture and sensitivity IV cefuroxime, cefotaxime. Resistant *S. pneumoniae* IV high dose penicillin, IV vancomycin
	White blood count and differential	Count increased with concomitant increase in polymorphonuclear leukocytes	Resistant *S. aureus* IV vancomycin, PO or IV linezolid
	Blood culture	Sensitivity low but highly specific	
Mycoplasma pneumoniae	Cold agglutinin titer	Elevated at 1:32 after several days of illness. False-positive lower titers may be seen in pneumonias due to viruses and some bacteria	PO or IV erythromycin, azithromycin, clarithromycin Alternate if >18 years, PO fluoroquinolones
	Mycoplasma-specific IgM titer	May be positive after 1 week but persists for several weeks	
	IgG titer	May remain positive for months	
	Mycoplasma complement fixation titers	Definite diagnosis can only be made with a 4-fold rise in titers	
	Mycoplasma culture	Not widely available	
	Polymerase chain reaction	Not widely available	
Chlamydia pneumoniae	Microimmunofluorescence IgM and IgG titers	Sensitivity and specificity vary with the laboratory. Time of rise in titers also may be variable	Same as mycoplasma
	Chlamydia complement Fixation titers	Because of recurrent nature of illness useful only in children	
	Polymerase chain reaction	Not widely available	
Influenza A and B	Three rapid tests available on respiratory secretions	Sensitivity varies with test but all are highly specific	Consider amantidine, rimantadine if during first 48 hours and influenza A
Respiratory syncytial virus	Antigen testing on respiratory specimens	Rapid and highly specific	
Legionella pneumoniae	Urine specimen	Rapid and highly specific for *L. pneumophila*, the most common pulmonary infection isolate	Same as mycoplasma

Source: Adapted from Gordon RC. Community—acquired pneumonia in adolescents. *Adolesc Med* 11(3):685, 2000. With permission

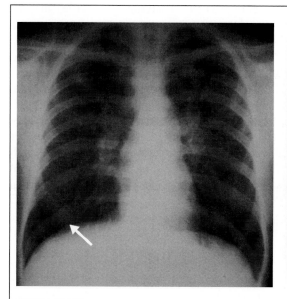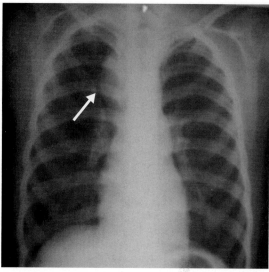

FIGURE 8-5

A PRIMARY TB LESION (LEFT) AND RIGHT HILAR ADENOPATHY (RIGHT).

The tuberculin skin test (TST) becomes positive 2–12 weeks after initial infection with a median interval of about 3–4 weeks. The interpretation of the TST in patients with a normal chest x-ray depends on the individual's risk factors and exposure history and is independent of BCG vaccine history (Table 8-7). However, any degree of TST reaction in a patient with x-ray findings consistent with tuberculosis disease should be interpreted as positive and treated. LTBI is defined as infection in a person with positive TST and normal x-ray findings or those of a healed primary complex (calcification) and will require treatment different than active disease. The case presented of LTBI requires treatment with 9 months of isoniazid (INH) therapy as outlined in Table 8-7.

Postprimary or secondary disease occurs when a primary complex is reactivated resulting in active lobar TB pneumonia, cavitary disease, or endobronchial disease. Because hematogenous spread may occur, any organ system may be affected including cervical lymph nodes, kidney, meninges, and joints. Miliary disease rarely occurs in immunocompetent adolescents. Hemoptysis and secondary

pneumothorax are both risks of cavitary and endobronchial disease.

An attempt to obtain a sputum specimen for *Mycobacterium tuberculosis* culture and antibiotic susceptibility testing should be made on all patients with suspected active pulmonary or endobronchial disease. The exception may be made when culture and sensitivities of the organism obtained from the index case is known. The best specimen, especially on the nonexpectorating child or adolescent with nonproductive cough, is obtained from gastric washings done on three successive mornings. Bronchoscopy may be used to assess the degree of bronchial obstruction and obtain specimens in the case of endobronchial disease.

AFB (acid-fast bacillus) smears on gastric aspirates are often negative but cultures positive. Ziehl-Neelsen or auramine-rhodium staining with fluorescent microscopy should be performed on all specimens obtained. Polymerase chain reaction (PCR) with the use of DNA probes can be done on sputum and other fluids obtained and has comparable sensitivity and specificity to culture of AM gastric washings; however, a diagnosis may be

T A B L E   8 - 7

INTERPRETATION OF TUBERCULOSIS SKIN TESTS

Induration ≥5 mm

Children in close contact with known or suspected
  contagious cases of tuberculosis disease

Children suspected to have tuberculosis disease:

- Findings on chest radiograph consistent with
  active or previously active tuberculosis
- Clinical evidence of tuberculosis disease

Children receiving immunosuppressive therapy or
with immunosuppressive conditions, including HIV
infection

Induration ≥10 mm

Children at increased risk of disseminated disease:

- Those younger than 4 years of age
- Those with other medical conditions, including
  Hodgkin disease, lymphoma, diabetes mellitus,
  chronic renal failure, or malnutrition

Children with increased exposure to tuberculosis
disease:

- Those born, or whose parents were born, in high-
  prevalence regions of the world
- Those frequently exposed to adults who are HIV
  infected, homeless, users of illicit drugs, residents
  of nursing homes, incarcerated or institutionalized,
  or migrant farm workers
- Those who travel to high-prevalence regions of
  the world

Induration ≥15 mm

Children 4 years of age or older without any risk
factors

Source: Adapted from the American Academy of Pediatrics.
Tuberculosis. In: Pickering IK (ed), Red Book: 2003 Report of the
Committee on Infectious Diseases, 26th ed. ELK Grove Village, IL:
American Academy of Pedaitrics, 2003, p. 643. With permission

provided in a few days versus the up- to- 8 weeks
that TB cultures typically take.

Standard culture using media such as
Lowenstein-Jensen and Middlebrook are positive
within several weeks up to 10 weeks. The advantage

to culture is that bacterial sensitivities may be
obtained, which is particularly important in areas
where a high degree of antibiotic resistance has
been determined and the use of four drug regimens
is contemplated.

Treatment should be guided by culture and sensitivities of the index case, often a primary relative,
or specimens directly obtained from the adolescent
as outlined above. HIV infected individuals are
treated with the same regimen as HIV negative individuals, however, HIV patients should not be treated
with thioacetazone due to a small incidence of fatal
skin reactions.

Treatment of LTBI includes INH given as a single
daily dose for 9 months. Efficacy in preventing activation of latent infection approaches 100% in children
and substantial percentages in adults (54%–88%).
Rifampin may be given for at least 6 months where
the index case is known to have bacteria with INH
resistance. Treatment of postprimary disease includes
three drugs (usually INH, rifampin, and pyrazinamide
for the first 2 months, INH and rifampin for an additional 4 months) for antibiotic susceptible bacterial
isolates. Where drug resistance is known or suspected, a fourth drug is added such as ethambutol or
an aminoglycoside. Endobronchial disease is treated
with oral corticosteroids to reduce airway obstruction.
Drug regimens and dosing schedules are summarized
in Table 8-8.

Clinical monitoring of response to therapy
should be undertaken in all patients with follow up
x-rays done periodically. Directly observed therapy
(DOT) regimens are used where adherence to medical therapy cannot be guaranteed.

References

De la Rosa JM, Escobedo M. Tuberculosis and other
    infectious diseases in the adolescent immigrant.
    Adolesc Med 11:453–466, 2000.

Frieden TR, Sterling TR, Munsiff SS, et al. Tuberculosis.
    Lancet 362:887, 2003.

Treatment Regimens for Primary and Postprimary
    Tuberculosis. American Academy of Pediatrics.
    Summaries of infectious diseases. Pickering LL,
    (ed.), *Red Book: 2003 Report of the Committee on
    Infectious Diseases,* 26th ed., Elk Grove Village, IL:
    American Academy of Pediatrics, 2003, p. 643.

TABLE 8-8

TREATMENT REGIMENS FOR PRIMARY AND POST PRIMARY TUBERCULOSIS

Infection or Disease Category	Regimen	Remarks
Latent tuberculosis (positive TST result, no disease)		
• Isoniazid-susceptible	9 months of isoniazid, once a day	If daily therapy is not possible, DOT twice a week can be used for 9 months
• Isoniazid-resistant	6 months of rifampin, once a day	
• Isoniazid-rifampin-resistant	Consult a tuberculosis specialist	
Pulmonary and extrapulmonary (except meningitis)	2 months of isoniazid, rifampin, and pyrazinamide daily, followed by 4 months of isoniazid and rifampin	If possible drug resistance is a concern, another drug (ethambutol or an aminoglycoside) is added to the initial 3-drug therapy until drug susceptibilities are determined. DOT is highly desirable If hilar adenopathy only, a 6-months course of isoniazid and rifampin is sufficient Drugs can be given 2 or 3 times per week under DOT in the initial phase if nonadherence is likely
Meningitis	2 months of isoniazid, rifampin, pyrazinamide, and an aminoglycoside or ethionamide, once a day, followed by 7–10 months of isoniazid and rifampin, once a day or twice a week (9–12 months total)	A fourth drug usually an aminoglycoside, is given with initial therapy until drug susceptibility is known For patients who may have acquired tuberculosis in geographic areas where resistance to streptomycin is common, capreomycin, kanamycin, or amikacin may be used instead of streptomycin

tst = tuberculin skin test, dot = direct observed therapy.

Source: Adapted from the American Academy of Pediatrics. Summaries of infectious diseases. In: Pickering LL (ed), *Red Book:2003 Report of the Committee on Infectious Diseases*, 26th ed., ELK Grove Village, IL: American Academy of Pediatrics, 2003, p. 649. With permission

CYSTIC FIBROSIS

Although, about three-fourths of CF children and adults with CF receive their specialty care in Cystic Fibrosis Foundation (CFF) accredited pediatric and adult care centers; primary care practitioners continue to play an important role in their care. CF patients, particularly in rural areas, often have their first contact with primary care providers during pulmonary exacerbations. Also CF patients require all the routine maintenance care, participate in sports, and experience common ailments, just as their normal peers.

CF, however, continues to be the most common lethal genetic disease in the United States with a median age of death at 25.1 years in 2002. About 90% of patients succumb to respiratory failure due to progressive lung damage from inflammation associated with retained, thick airway secretions and chronic infection, most often with *P. aeruginosa*. The primary defect in CF involves an abnormal copy of a gene in a homozygous or compound heterozygous state coding for a defective membrane transport protein, CF transmembrane regulator (CFTR) protein. This leads to abnormal water, sodium, and chloride transport across epithelial membranes leading to thick, tenacious secretions. In the gut, blockage of pancreatic exocrine glands leads to malabsorption of nutrients, including fat and fat soluble vitamins. This leads to malnutrition, and may lead to inspissation of stool leading to intestinal obstruction termed distal intestinal obstruction syndrome (DIOS).

The gold standard for diagnosis of CF continues to be the sweat test. When done in duplicate in a CF center monitored laboratory by pilocarpine iontophoresis per CFF and National Committee for Clinical Standards guidelines, the sweat test will detect about 99% of patients with CF. Genetic testing is available through several laboratories and tests for the most common mutations of CF with an accuracy approaching 98%. The advantage of genetic testing includes the ability to detect some rare mutations that may have associated borderline or normal sweat tests, for prenatal testing in high-risk patients, and to detect the carrier state, important for siblings as they approach reproductive years. CF is an autosomal recessive disorder and carriers do not show evidence of the disease. The most common mutation is ΔF508/ΔF508 representing 50%–67% of US mutations. It should be noted that sweat tests done in non CF approved laboratories and by unapproved methods may give high numbers of false negative and false positive results leading to psychologically traumatic misdiagnosis and missed medical diagnoses with excess morbidity. A nomogram for interpretation of sweat testing results and genetic analysis is found in Fig. 8-6.

As CF is a multiorgan disease, therapy is directed both at the overall patient and at specific organ systems as summarized below:

Nutrition

CF patients require up to 150% of the RDA of calories and additional fat-soluble vitamins including A, D, E, and K. Methods to supplement calories include high calorie, high protein food bars or milkshakes.

Enteral tube feedings including nasogastric, gastric, and jejunal tube feedings are accomplished overnight in many patients particularly those with moderate to severe disease. Appetite stimulants such a megestrol acetate and cyproheptadine hydrochloride have been used with some success. The goal, as defined by the CFF, is to have all patients at least 90% of ideal body weight for height. Distal intestinal obstruction syndrome occurs with greater frequency in teens, most often due to refusal to take pancreatic enzymes. Treatment protocols including oral or NG administration of balanced electrolyte solutions (e.g., Golytely) are available.

Infection

Sinopulmonary infection is the single most frequent problem in CF often beginning in early childhood. By teen years, infections with multidrug resistant *P. aeruginosa*, methicillin resistant *S. aureus*, and *Burkholderia cepacia* are often well established and are a challenge to control, requiring multiple IV and PO (oral) antibiotics. Those with specific activity against *P. aeruginosa* include ceftazidime, aminoglycosides such as tobramycin, semisynthetic penicillins such as ticarcillin and piperacillin, carbapenems, and the fluoroquinolones (ciprofloxacin and levofloxacin).

Airway clearance with manual chest percussion and specific devices such as the flutter device (Fig. 8-7), the percussion vest, and high-frequency oscillatory nebulizer devices (Intrapulmonary Percussive Ventilator, Percussive Neb) are essential adjuncts to care and are done on a daily basis.

Problems occurring with increasing frequency in adolescence include CF related diabetes (CFRD) and osteopenia and osteoporosis. CFRD has features of both type I and type II diabetes and is likely due to gradual fibrosis of the endocrine portion of the pancreas. Screening for CFRD, which can contribute to poor nutrition and frequent infections leading to more rapid lung function decline, should begin in late childhood and continue through adolescence and adulthood.

Malnutrition, malabsorption of vitamins and calcium, and reduced physical activity contribute to the development of osteopenia and osteoporosis. Screening with dual energy x-ray absorptiometry

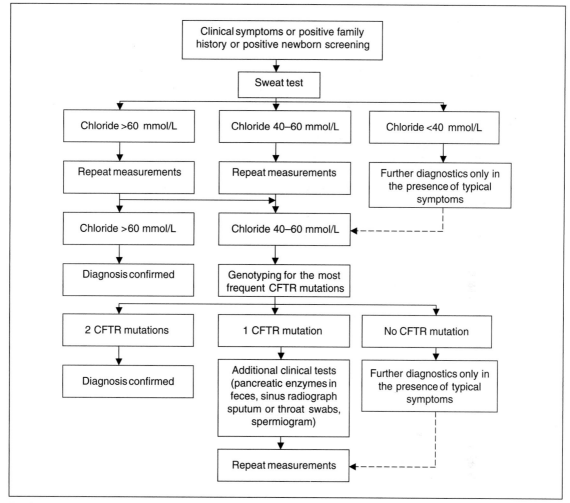

FIGURE 8-6

FLOW DIAGRAM FOR DIAGNOSIS OF CYSTIC FIBROSIS.
(Source: Adapted from Ratjen F, Doring G. Cystic Fibrosis: *Lancet* 361:681, 2003. With permission)

(DEXA) scans begins in late childhood. Encouraging weight bearing, exposure to sunlight, and adequate supplementation with calcium and vitamin is essential to bone health in CF. With osteopenia, bisphosphonates have been used with success in CF teens and adults.

New Therapies

Newer therapies intended to slow decline in lung function by reducing inflammation, controlling chronic infection, and thinning mucus have been introduced over the last few years. All reduce lung decline or improve lung function by a modest amount but collectively are in part responsible for the increase in longevity that CF adults have today (median age at death 25.1 years in 2002 and 18.7 in 1985). These therapies include inhaled antibiotics such as colistin (Coly-Mycin) and tobramycin (Tobi), dornase alpha (human recombinant, DNase, Pulmozyme) which thins mucus, and high dose ibuprofen and azithromycin (Zithromax) which have anti-inflammatory effects, among others. Some of these commonly used in current practice are listed in Table 8-9.

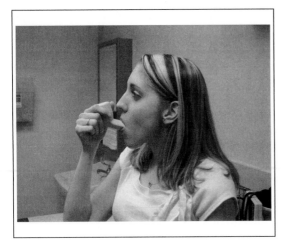

F I G U R E   8 - 7

THE FLUTTER VALVE IS A CONVENIENT AND
EFFECTIVE MEANS OF INDEPENDENT AIRWAY
CLEARANCE FOR CF ADOLESCENTS AND ADULTS.

T A B L E   8 - 9

NEW THERAPIES FOR TREATMENT
OF CYSTIC FIBROSIS

Therapy	Indication
Inhaled tobramycin (TOBI) 300 mg bid 28 days on, 28 days off	Chronic treatment of established *P. aeruginosa* colonization/infection
Inhaled colistin (Coly-Mycin) 150 mg bid aerosol daily	Acute treatment: may be used as part of *P. aeruginosa* eradication program
Dornase alpha (human recombinant DNase, Pulmozyme) 2.5 mg qd or bid aerosol daily	Mucolytic for enhancement of airway clearance in CF pulmonary disease
Azithromycin 250, 500 mg PO 3x/week	Used as chronic anti-inflammatory agent in CF
Ibuprofen 20–30 mg/kg/day (serum levels necessary)	Used as chronic anti-inflammatory agent in CF

Lung transplantation is a salvage procedure and not a cure for CF. Only 133 transplants were done in the United States in 2002 representing about 0.4% of CF patients. Survival is approximately 80% in the first year and drops to about 60% by year 5. Complications post transplant include breakdown of anastomoses, infection, obliterative bronchiolitis, and tissue rejection and patients must stay on lifelong immunosuppressive therapy.

Transition to Adult Care

With about 40% of CF patients currently over the age of 18 years, transition to adult care becomes an important issue (Chap. 5). The CFF has recognized this with the development of a CF adult care center program mirroring pediatric centers in terms of team care but with adult care practitioners. The CFF has recommended transitioning patients between 16 and 18 years through gradual joint contact with adult care providers, adult and pediatric care team meetings, and so forth. The American Academy of Pediatrics (AAP), in its 1996 statement on transition of care for adolescents with special health care needs recommends that transitioning:

1. Begin early, with special attention to maximizing opportunities for independence and for the necessary health, educational, and social services.
2. Include active participation of the family and patient in the process.
3. Consider the patient individually, realistically, and positively, as well as encourage functional independence and appropriate attitudes toward self-worth and interpersonal relationships (including issues of sexuality).
4. Encourage the patient's willingness to accept the plan.
5. Consider having the pediatrician and the adult care practitioner as comanagers for a period of time (e.g., 1 or 2 years) and include recommendations by the pediatrician for referral to adult health care providers (especially subspecialists) who are sensitive to and have an interest in families that include adults with special health care needs.

Innovations in care allowing for independent functioning of adults, such as mechanical airway clearance devices and the use of home IV and inhaled antibiotics, have facilitated transitioning to independent adult living from a medical care delivery perspective.

References

American Academy of Pediatrics Committee on Children with Disabilities and Committee on Adolescence. Transition of care provided adolescents with special health care needs. *Pediatrics* 98:1203, 1996.

Cystic Fibrosis Foundation. *Consensus Conferences—Gastrointestinal Problems in CF*. Vol. II, Sec. II. Bethesda, MD, June 3–4, 1991.

Cystic Fibrosis Foundation. *Consensus Conferences—Guide to Bone Health and Disease in Cystic Fibrosis*. Vol. X, Sec. 4. Bethesda, MD, June 2002.

Hand WL. Current challenges in antibiotic resistance. *Adolesc Med* 11:427–438, 2000.

Nasr SZ. Cystic fibrosis in adolescents and young adults. *Adolesc Med* 11:589–603, 2000.

CASE STUDY 8-5

Chronic Wheezing and Cough

A.J. is a 14-year-old male with wheezing and cough. This occurs on most days, particularly in the morning. He awakes with cough and wheezes at least two nights per week and has difficulty participating in sports activities because of chest tightness, cough, and wheeze. When seen in the office he was noted to be afebrile with a respiratory rate of 24. Saturation was 96% on room air and he had bilateral wheezing with fair air exchange but a prolonged expiratory phase. FEV_1 was 67% of predicted in the office with normal forced vital capacity. Twenty minutes after giving two puffs of albuterol his FEV_1 had risen to 75% of predicted. His therapy at home consists of an albuterol MDI (metered dose inhaler) given up to four times per day and he has required five "bursts" of oral corticosteroids during the last year. You grade his asthma and start additional therapy.

Asthma is a chronic, inflammatory disease that includes bronchospasm (increased airway hyper reactivity), increased mucus production, cellular infiltration into airway and airway submucosa, airway edema and narrowing, and in some cases, deposition of submucosal collagen. It involves increased airway responsiveness to a variety of both immunologic (e.g., animal dander, pollen, and dust mite) and nonimmunologic stimuli (e.g., viruses, cold air, and exercise).

Asthma is the most common chronic disease of children and adolescents numbering about 5 million under the age of 18 years in the United States. Children and adolescents miss about 10 million school days per year and parents often miss work caring for these youngsters. This has significant social and economic loss (about 6 billion dollars per year in direct and indirect costs).

Asthma management protocols and guidelines have been available in the United States since the 1991 publication of the Expert Panel Report 1, Guidelines for the Diagnosis and Management of Asthma, National Institutes of Health, National Heart, Lung, and Blood Institute. Additional evidence based guidelines including updates were published in 1997 as the Expert Panel Report 2 (with a further update in 2002) (Guidelines, 1997; 2002), and the joint AAP and American Academy of Allergy, Asthma, and Immunology, Pediatric Asthma, Guide for Managing Asthma in Children in 1999. Basic asthma management consists of classifying asthma according to severity, a stepwise approach to therapy, instituting environmental controls, and arranging for follow-up care.

ASTHMA CLASSIFICATION

Asthma in adolescents can be classified as severe, moderate, or mild persistent asthma, and mild intermittent asthma according to symptom frequency and pulmonary function (Table 8-10). Severity is usually assigned at first contact before optimal asthma control is achieved and patients are assigned to the most severe classification that either symptoms or pulmonary function (peak expiratory flow rate [PEFR] or FEV_1) indicates.

STEPWISE THERAPY FOR ASTHMA MANAGEMENT (≥5 YEARS)

Classify severity: Clinical features before treatment or adequate control			Medications required to maintain long-term control
	Symptoms/day Symptoms/night	PEF or FEV$_1$ PEF variability	Daily medications

Step 4
Severe persistent
	Continual
	Frequent
		≤60%
		>30%
			• **Preferred treatment:**
			  • **High-dose inhaled corticosteroids**
			    AND
			  • **Long-acting inhaled beta$_2$-agonists**
			  • Corticosteroid tablets or syrup long term (2 mg/kg/day, generally not to exceed 60 mg/day). (Make repeat attempts to reduce systemic corticosteroids and maintain control with high-dose inhaled corticosteroids.)

Step 3
Moderate persistent
	Daily
	>1 night/week
		>60%–<80%
		>30%
			• Preferred treatment:
			  • Low-to-medium dose inhaled corticosteroids and long-acting inhaled beta$_2$-agonists
			• Alternative treatment (listed alphabetically):
			  • Increase inhaled corticosteroids within medium-dose range
			  OR
			  • Low-to-medium dose inhaled corticosteroids and either leukotriene modifier or theophylline

Step 2 Mild persistent	>2/week but < 1x/day >2 nights/months	≥80% 20–30%	• Preferred treatment: • Low-dose inhaled corticosteroids • Alternative treatment (listed alphabetically): cromolyn, leukotriene modifier, nedocromil, OR sustained-release theophylline to serum concentration of 5–15 mcg/mL
Step 1 Mild intermittent	≤2 days/week ≤2 nights/month	≥80% <20%	• No daily medication needed • Exacerbations may occur, separated by long periods of normal lung function and no symptoms. A course of systemic corticosteroids is recommended
Quick relief All patients			• Short-acting bronchodilator: 2–4 puffs short-acting inhaled beta$_2$-agonists as needed for symptoms • Intensity of treatment will depend on severity of exacerbation; up to three treatments at 20 minute intervals or a single nebulizer treatment as needed. Course of systemic corticosteroids may be needed • Use of short-acting beta$_2$-agonists >2 times a week in intermittent asthma (daily, or increasing use in persistent asthma) may indicate the need to initiate (increase) long-term-control therapy

Source: Adapted from the Guidelines for the Diagnosis and Management of Asthma. Update on Selected Topics 2002. NIH/NHLBI. NIH Publication No. 02-5075, June 2002.

According to this, the adolescent presented in case 5 is classified as having moderate persistent asthma.

Environmental Controls

Controlling aggravating factors both immunologic and nonimmunologic is an essential part of asthma control. Environmental tobacco smoke (ETS) exposure, also known as side stream or second hand smoke exposure, and primary smoking are both clearly detrimental to an adolescent's health. In young children, ETS is associated with at least twice the risk of lower respiratory tract infection as well as upper airway problems such as otitis media. In the adolescent, besides the emerging risks of lung cancer, cardiac disease and the development of chronic obstructive pulmonary disease with emphysema, immediate problems include chronic hoarseness, nasal congestion, halitosis, chronic cough, deconditioning, and asthma instability. Lung function does improve upon smoking cessation and appears to be dose dependent. Reduced dust mite and animal exposure can lead to reduced atopic symptoms including allergic rhinitis and asthma. Patient friendly brochures are useful to provide information on this important aspect of asthma and allergy prophylaxis and are available through organizations such as the American Lung Association or in the guidelines mentioned earlier.

Stepwise Approach to Managing Asthma

Matching therapy to severity not only provides for asthma control but prevents overtreatment with potentially toxic drugs. It has been our practice to provide a short course or "burst" (e.g., 1–2 mg/kg divided bid for 5–7 days) of a corticosteroid such as prednisone or prednisolone on first contact with an asthmatic with decreased lung function and unstable asthma symptoms. Distribution of aerosol medications is dependent on many factors including particle size and flow rate but also airway caliber. Even a delivery system that provides optimal particle size used with optimal technique may not provide sufficient drug to inflamed, narrowed lower airways. Reducing some of that inflammation with associated improvement in airway caliber will optimize drug delivery and hasten attainment of asthma control. This is done while starting a comprehensive program of anti-inflammatory maintenance or controller medications and short acting beta-adrenergic or rescue medications. Common asthma medications and doses are found in Tables 8-11a and 8-11b.

A stepwise approach using a step down scheme of reducing medication as asthma control is achieved seems a wise management approach (Table 8-10). An additional strategy that is without evidence based support but is found by many to be clinically useful is to double the dose of inhaled corticosteroid with exposures known to cause asthma flare ups such as upper respiratory infections or animal exposures. This appears to obviate the need for short courses of oral corticosteroids in some patients.

The medication basis for asthma control at all persistent asthma severity levels includes inhaled corticosteroids (ICS). Additional control includes the addition of a long acting bronchodilator such as formoterol, or salmeterol, or a leukotriene modifier (zafirlukast, montelukast). We have routinely used leukotriene modifiers as "add-on" agents in asthma patients to help keep down doses of inhaled corticosteroids and maintain asthma control.

In the case presented, a reasonable approach to initial management would be as follows:

1. A short burst of oral prednisone or prednisolone at 1–2 mg/kg/day divided every 12 hours for 5–7 days to a maximum of 40 mg bid
2. Addition of an ICS in standard doses
3. Addition of a leukotriene modifier to provide complimentary effects to the ICS and to keep ICS dose down
4. Close follow-up and monitoring

TABLE 8-11
ASTHMA CONTROL MEDICATIONS

(a) Inhaled Corticosteroids

Medication	Dosage Form	Adult Dose	Child Dose
Systemic corticosteroids			
Methylprednisolone	2, 4, 8, 16, 32 mg tablets	7.5–60 mg daily in a	0.25–2 mg/kg daily in a
Prednisolone	5 mg tablets,	single dose in a.m. or	single dose in a.m. or
	5 mg/5 cc,	every other day as	every other day as
	15 mg/ 5 cc	needed for control	needed for control
Prednisone	1, 2.5, 5, 10, 20,	Short-course "burst" to	Short-course "burst" 1–2
	50 mg tablets;	achieve control; 40–60 mg	mg/kg/day, maximum
	5 mg/cc, 5 mg/5 cc	per day as single or 2	60 mg/kg/day, doses
		divided doses for 3–10 days	for 3–10 days
Long-acting inhaled beta$_2$-agonists *(Should not be used for symptom relief or for exacerbations. Use with inhaled corticosteroids.)*			
Salmeterol	MDI 21 mcg/puff	2 puffs q 12 h	1–2 puffs q 12 h
	DPI 50 mcg/blister	1 blister q 12 h	1 blister q 12 h
Formoterol	DPI 12 mcg/single-use capsule	1 capsule q 12 h	1 capsule q 12 h
Combined medication			
Fluticasone/Salmeterol	DPI 100, 250, or	1 inhalation bid; dose	1 inhalation bid; dose
	500 mcg/50 mcg	depends on severity	depends on severity
		of asthma	of asthma
Cromolyn	MDI 1 mg/puff	2-4 puffs tid-qid	1–2 puffs tid-qid
	Nebulizer 20 mg/ampule	1 ampule tid-qid	1 ample tid-gid
Nedocromil	MDI 1.75 mg/puff	2-4 puffs bid-qid	1–2 puffs bid-qid
Leukotriene modifiers			
Montelukast	4 or 5 mg chewable tablet	10 mg qhs	4 mg qhs (12 months–
	10 mg tablet		2 years)
			4 mg qhs (2–5 years)
			5 mg qhs (6014 years)
			10 mg qhs (>14 years)
Zafirlukast	10 or 20 mg tablet	40 mg daily (20 mg	20 mg daily (7–11 years)
		tablet bid)	(10 mg tablets bid)
Zileuton	300 or 600 mg tablet	2,400 mg daily	
		(give tablets qid)	
Methylxanthines *(Serum monitoring is important [serum concentration of 5–15 mcg/mL at steady state])*			
Theophylline	Liquids, sustained-release	Starting dose 10 mg/kg/day	Starting dose 10 mg/
	tablets, and capsules	up to 300 mg max; usual	kg/day; usual max: <1
		max 800 mg/day	year of age: 0.2 (age in
			weeks) +5 = mg/kg/day
			≥1 year of age: 16 mg/
			kg/day

TABLE 8-11

ASTHMA CONTROL MEDICATIONS (*CONTINUED*)

(b) Estimated Comparative Daily Dosages for Inhaled Corticosteroid (Applies to all three Corticosteroids)						
	Low daily dose		Medium daily dose		High daily dose	
	Adult	Child	Adult	Child	Adult	Child
Medication	(mcg)	(mcg)	(mcg)	(mcg)	(mcg)	(mcg)
Beclomethasone CFC 42 or 84 mcg/puff	168–504	84–336	504–840	336–672	>840	>672
Beclomethasone HFA 40 or 80 mcg/puff	80–240	80–160	240–480	160–320	>480	>320
Budesonide DPI 200 mcg/inhalation	200–600	200–400	600–1200	400–800	>1200	>8000
Budesonide inhalation suspension for nebulization (child dose)	0.5		1.0		2.0	
Flunisolide 250 mcg/puff	500–1000	500–750	1000–2000	100–1250	>2000	>1250
Fluticasone MDI: 44,110, or 220 DPI: 50,100, or 250 mcg/inhalation	88–264 100–300	88–176 100–200	264–660 300–600	176–440 200–400	>660 >600	>440 >400
Triamcinolone acetonide 100 mcg/puff	400–1000	400–800	1000–2000	800–1200	>2000	>1200

Source: Adapted from the Guidelines for the Diagnosis and Management of Asthma. Update on Selected Topics 2002. NIH/NHLBI. NIH Publication No. 02-5075, June 2002.

Long-acting bronchodilators have trivial anti-inflammatory activity but help maintain asthma control through long acting bronchodilation (8–12 hours). They may be particularly useful as add-on therapy where patients show a great deal of bronchodilator responsiveness during bronchodilator challenges. It should be emphasized, however, that salmeterol *not* be used for acute relief of bronchoconstriction because of its slow (up to 1 hour) onset of activity. Formoterol may be useful for acute as well as chronic use because of its much more rapid onset of activity, 5–15 minutes, similar to albuterol sulfate. There has also been some concern with salmeterol of sudden death with its use in some patients and an FDA "black box" warning has been placed on this drug in the medication brochure. This occurred as a result of

a long-term placebo control trial of salmeterol compared to placebo as add-on therapy to usual asthma therapy in which a small, but greater number of deaths occurred in the treatment group (SMART, Perera, 2003). The risk may be greater for Black patients. Severe asthmatics usually require all three controller drug classes (ICS, leukotriene modifiers, and long-acting bronchodilators) for optimal control.

Side effects associated with chronic use of inhaled corticosteroids, especially effects on growth, are of considerable concern to parents, particularly those of children and early or prepubertal adolescents. Although mild growth delay may occur in the first one to two years of using ICS, especially in steroid naïve patients, there is sufficient data to show that with standard doses long-term growth delay does not occur and that patients normally reach predicted adult height.

Exercise Induced Asthma

Up to a third of athletes may be at risk or developing exercise asthma (EIA). Typical symptoms include chest tightness, wheeze, or cough during sustained aerobic exercise, or often at the end of a vigorous exercise period. Triggers that enhance the risk of developing EIA include cold and dry air. A refractory state may be induced by slow and thorough warming up prior to onset of vigorous activity and failure to do this may lead to increased EIA symptoms. Conditioning is also important as increased aerobic fitness with optimal exercise efficiency decreases EIA risk.

Management consists of a careful warm up prior to exercise and medical prophylaxis as outlined in Fig. 8-8. It is important to control underlying asthma with anti-inflammatory medications to raise an individual's threshold to induction of EIA. A short-acting bronchodilator such as albuterol or a rapid onset long-acting bronchodilator such as formoterol should be given 20–30 minutes prior to beginning the activity. If this does not completely control symptoms then additional benefit may be obtained through daily administration of a leukotriene modifier or addition of inhaled nedocromil sodium to the bronchodilator prior to the exercise period.

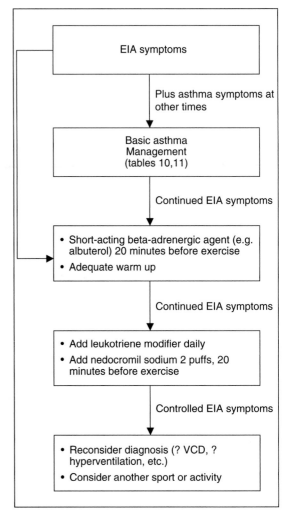

F I G U R E   8 - 8

FLOW DIAGRAM FOR THE TREATMENT OF EXERCISE INDUCED ASTHMA.

Special Circumstances in Adolescent Asthma

Those who care for adolescents should be aware of special circumstances that aggravate asthma and are not uncommon in adolescence. Females may experience exacerbations of asthma with menstrual periods. This may be due to lowered resistance to stress with resultant increased airway hyperreactivity. The use of oral contraceptive pills (OCPs) may exacerbate menstruation-associated asthma in some teens but improve it in others (Chap. 25). It is important to note that OCPs are not contraindicated in teens with asthma but monitoring of symptoms and peak expiratory flow after starting these medications and around the time of menstruation is indicated.

Particulates and chemicals in the form of perfumes, hair sprays, and cigarette smoke are all significant asthma triggers often encountered in adolescence. Smoking and exposure to environmental tobacco smoke are clearly related to unstable asthma (Chap. 34). Direct questioning of even young adolescents about primary smoking or second hand exposures should be part of any teen evaluation.

Obesity, besides its negative effects on body image and self-esteem can lead to unstable asthma. In part, this is due to poor conditioning and increased ventilatory load for a given level of activity but also for yet undefined reasons (Chap. 31). Obesity is an independent predictor for the persistence of asthma symptoms from childhood into adolescence.

References

Agertoft L, Pedersen S. Effect of long-term treatment with inhaled budesonide on adult height in children with asthma. *N Engl J Med* 343(15):1064, 2000.

Guerra S, Wright AL, Morgan WJ, et al. Persistence of asthma symptoms during adolescence: role of obesity and age at onset of puberty. *Am J Respir Crit Care Med* (Epub ahead of print), 2004.

Guidelines for the Diagnosis and Management of Asthma. Expert Panel Report 2. NIH/NHLBI. NIH publication 97–4051, April 1997.

Guidelines for the Diagnosis and Management of Asthma. Update on Selected Topics 2002. NIH/NHLBI #5074, 2002.

Howenstine MS, Eigen H. Medical care of the adolescent with asthma. *Adolesc Med* (3):501–519, 2000.

Kelly HW, Strunk RC, Donithan M, et al. Growth and bone density in children with mild-moderate asthma: A cross-sectional study in children entering the Childhood Asthma Management Program (CAMP). *J Pediatr* 142(3):286, 2003.

Patel DR, Homnick DN. Pulmonary effects of smoking. *Adolesc Med* 11:567, 2000.

Pediatric Asthma-Promoting Best Practice. *Guide for Managing Asthma in Children.* AAAAI/AAP. Milwaukee, WI. 1999.

Perera BJ. Salmeterol multicenter asthma research trial (SMART): interim analysis shows increased risk of asthma related deaths. *Ceylon Med J* 48(3):86, 2003.

CASE STUDY 8-6

Throat Tightness in an Athlete

L.M. is a 16-year-old female with known history of moderate persistent asthma. She has been treated successfully with inhaled corticosteroids and has little difficulty with her asthma in general. She uses an inhaled albuterol 20 minutes before exercise and is careful to warm up before full participation in competitive tennis. Despite this she often has to stop in the middle of games because of feelings of throat and upper chest tightness. A couple of times during competitions she could no longer participate. Stopping exercise causes quick (within minutes) resolution of her symptoms. A few times her coach has noted coarse inspiratory breath sounds during these episodes.

Although an upper airway problem in adolescence, vocal cord dysfunction (VCD) may be confused with EIA and patients may receive unnecessary treatment for lower airway disease. A typical episode of VCD consists of sudden onset of inspiratory stridor with accompanying throat tightness, hoarse voice, cough, and occasional wheeze. Exercise, particularly during the stress of high performance often precipitates the attacks. About half the patients may also have co-existent asthma leading to confusion in the diagnosis. Spirometric evaluation may show a typical flat inspiratory curve and symptoms may be elicited during vigorous exercise testing in an exercise laboratory, confirming the diagnosis. Direct laryngoscopy may show paradoxical but not complete closure of the vocal cords particularly during the stressful event, such as exercise. Successful treatment of VCD includes evaluation by a speech pathologist skilled in diagnosis and treatment of hyper functional voice disorders. Other methods that have been successful include relaxation therapy and hypnosis. Prognosis is good unless there is significant underlying psychopathology. A comparison of the features of EIA and VCD is found in Table 8-12.

TABLE 8-12

VOCAL CORD DYSFUNCTION (VCD) VERSUS EXERCISE-INDUCED BRONCHOSPASM (EIB)

	VCD	EIB
Women > men	+	−
Associated psychiatric diagnosis	+	±
Exercise-induced	+	+
Very short duration of symptoms	+	−
Improves with bronchodilator	−	+
Eosinophilia	−	±
Hypoxia	−	+
Syncope	−	+
Dyspnea	+	+
Stridor	+	−
Wheeze	Inspiration	Expiration > inspiration
Spirometry	Blunted inspiration portion of flow-volume loop	Normal inspiration portion of flow-volume loop
Laryngoscopy	Tonic adduction of vocal cords during inspiration or inspiration/expiration	
Chest x-ray	Normal	Hyperinflation

Source: Adapted from Homnick DN, Pratt HD. Respiratory diseases with a psychosomatic component. *Adoles Med* 11(3):547, 2000. With permission.

Reference

Homnick DN, Pratt HD. Respiratory diseases with a psychosomatic component. *Adolesc Med* 11(3): 547, 2000.

ACKNOWLEDGMENTS

The author thanks Ms. Cori Edgecomb for her expert administrative assistance in the preparation of this manuscript and Dr. John H. Marks for his careful and thoughtful review of its content.

9

CARDIOVASCULAR DISORDERS IN THE ADOLESCENT

Eugene F. Luckstead, Sr., and H. Noubani

INTRODUCTION

This chapter focuses on some of the common cardiovascular problems seen in the adolescent age group. Congenital and acquired heart disease concerns are addressed from the adolescent perspective. This practical approach should help physicians medically manage adolescents with problems of chest pain, syncope, dysrhythmia, shock, hypertension, hyperlipidemia, mitral valve prolapse and congenital or acquired heart anomalies. Surgically and/or interventionally treated adolescents with congenital and acquired cardiac-related management issues and their follow-up needs are discussed. Physician guidance for short term, obstetrical and lifetime cardiac concerns may be needed for adolescents with surgically corrected or palliated congenital and/or acquired heart lesions. The use of new and evolving interventional techniques such as angioplasty, advancing trends in pacemaker technology, electrophysiologic dysrhythmia detection, and improved ablation techniques are some of the exciting recent developments for treatment of the adolescent cardiac patient.

The Patient Population

It is estimated that ~90% of adults with a history of congenital heart problems are functioning at a normal or near normal cardiac level. Since adolescence does bridge the gap between childhood and adulthood, one must be cognizant of the fact that today's youth with congenital heart disease often have a near normal or normal long-term life outlook. Actually most former congenital cardiac patients as adolescents are entirely asymptomatic with less than 4% on any cardiac medications. However, one should be aware of those patient exceptions that do have significant residual congenital and acquired heart issues! How should physicians anticipate, manage, or follow this group of adolescent cardiac patients?

The patient's physician should be keenly aware of the overall impact any cardiac problem has on other aspects of patient care; this includes social and psychologic issues. Typically, these patients will need follow-up periodically by their cardiologist at least on a yearly basis or as needed in some cases. There have been documented significant noncompliance issues occurring in this population with large time gaps noted in follow-up care. Patients often need reminders regarding endocarditis precautions, school activity-level guidance, and other restrictions when indicated; this is especially true for those youth that are in denial. Gersony documented a 30%–40% noncompliance factor in his large long-term follow-up series where he monitored over 2000 patients with known aortic stenosis (AS), pulmonic stenosis (PS), and/or ventricular septal defects (VSD). Some patients in the series had gone ten years without a cardiologist repeat follow-up or any evaluation! (Gersony, 1993).

There is a need for cardiologists who can bridge the gap for the over one million cardiac patients during the transition from the pediatric to the adult age group (Chap. 5). Additional training and a higher priority must be placed on both pediatric and adult fellowship training programs for such patients. Another solution could be a team approach between selected pediatric and adult cardiology colleagues. Also, good communication between the cardiologist and the patient's physician is critical for accurate information and guidance. Unfortunately, managed care has added another obstacle between such ideal physician-specialist communications; changing network demands affects their primary care physicians aggravating further noncompliant issues. Because poor memory or lack of knowledge concerning the degree and type of congenital heart problem has been frequently noted in these patients, accurate past information must be available from both prior specialists and hospital sources when indicated.

Most patients in the adolescent congenital heart population will fall into one of two groups. Doroshow (2001) described three types of such groups for follow-up purposes. Her Group 3 adolescent cardiac patients needed closer monitoring and more attention than the patients with short- and long-term cardiac management issues did in her Group 1 or 2. Group 1 had mild congenital heart anomalies or well tolerated defects such as small VSD, small patent ductus arteriosus (PDAs), mild AS or PS, and mitral valve prolapse (MVP). Group 2 was comprised of surgically or interventionally corrected VSD, atrial septal defect (ASD), PDA, PS, or aortic coarctation patients. Those patients with prior surgical or interventional management for tetralogy of Fallot, transposition of

great vessels (TGV), AS or A/V (Atrioventricular) canal defects were placed in the Group 3 category. Additional information on recommended follow-up can be provided from resources such as the 22nd Bethesda Conference and other publications relevant to the adolescent with known cardiac disease (Perloff, 1991).

ASD do have the potential for paradoxical emboli in adolescents and adult age patients, resulting in a stroke or brain abscess. However, such embolic complications are rare in children and much less likely to occur with smaller defects or in patients without the adult age atrial arrhythmias of atrial fibrillation or atrial flutter. An increased incidence of atrial dysrhythmias and "sick sinus syndrome" postsurgical is known and possibly may occur with interventional ASD closure. Aortic valve stenosis is not typically a completely correctable congenital heart lesion. These aortic valve stenosis patients may require further intervention later in life; many will need an eventual surgical artificial valve replacement or a Ross procedure. Similarly, A/V canal defects (*endocardial cushion defects*) will require short and long term monitoring of their A/V mitral or tricuspid valve insufficiency residual defects. Chronic afterload reduction with drugs like captopril or enalapril is helpful; however, many will remain asymptomatic.

Excellent surgical results are now the expected norm from most timely cardiac surgery for congenital heart anomalies. Current surgical techniques are successful in over 90% of cases, but continued periodic monitoring of the cardiac pathophysiology, such as residual abnormally elevated right ventricular pressure, residual VSD, and significant degrees of pulmonary insufficiency is necessary. Ventricular arrhythmias, pacemaker implantation when surgical complete heart block occurs, and the possible greater risk for sudden death, warrant a guarded long-term prognosis for this postsurgical patient care group. Patients with prior surgical treatment for TGV need close scrutiny and monitoring particularly those patients who have had atrial switch (Senning) or Mustard procedures. Over the past decade, the arterial switch (Jatene) corrective surgery for TGV continues to provide excellent outcomes in both early and long-term natural history studies, once patients are past the earlier high-risk perioperative period.

Other forms of cyanotic and single ventricle necessitated palliative operative procedures with most patients having a Fontan or veno-caval operation; these will need individual or specific physician monitoring and long-term guidance.

Although growth failure is a definite problem for younger children and infants with cardiac anomalies, this is not typical for adolescents since most adapt or attain normal growth when puberty occurs. Obesity now seems to be a greater problem for both these cardiac adolescents and their noncardiac adolescent peer group (Chap. 31). Other complaints such as chest pain and dyspnea are more commonly seen in the adolescent cardiac patients when compared with their noncardiac peer group but are usually just as benign.

Endocarditis and realistic exercise limitations must be specific and patient care individualized depending on their type of congenital heart problem especially for those in the higher risk groups. Over 75% of the endocarditis cases do occur in patients with cardiac abnormalities. There was a reported 35-fold increase in endocarditis in children with VSD, AS, or PS documented by a large natural history study (Gersony, 1993). Endocarditis does *not* occur in secundum ASD, or six months after complete repair without residual defects for VSD or PDA and is uncommon after PS repair. However, be suspicious with a known cardiac patient when assessing for fever without a source, unexplained weight loss, malaise, chronic myalgia, and joint pain; obtain 2–3 blood cultures prior to any antibiotic use. An echocardiogram can be helpful in subtle cases particularly for right sided heart lesions, VSD, and aortic valve lesions.

Bibliography

Allen HD, Gersony WM, Tauert KA. Insurability of the adolescent and young adult with heart disease: Fact or artifact? *Circulation* 86:703–710, 1992.

Doroshow RW. The Adolescent with simple or corrected congenital heart disease. *Adol Med* 12(1):1, 2001.

Gersony WM, Hayes CJ, Driscoll DJ, et al. Second natural history study of congenital heart defects. *Circulation* 87:152–165, 1993.

Greydanus DE, Patel D, Pratt H, Bhave S, (eds.). Cardiovascular disorders. *India Manual of Adolescent Medicine, Review of Adolescent Medicine*, New Delhi, India: Cambridge Press, 2002, 6:34–57.

Luckstead EF. Cardiovascular evaluation of the young athlete. *Adol Med* 9:441–455, 1998.

Luckstead EF. Cardiovascular disorders in the college student. *Pediatr Clin N Am* 52: 243–278, 2005.

McInerny T. The role of the general pediatrician in coordinating the care of children with chronic illness. *Pediatr Clin N Am* 31:199–209, 1984.

Perloff JK. 2nd Bethesda Conference: Congenital heart disease after childhood: An expanding patient population. *Circulation* 84:1881–1890, 1991.

Rowlett JD, Greydanus DE. *The Cardiovascular System in Adolescent Medicine*, 3d ed., Hoffmann AD, Greydanus DE (eds.) Stamford, CT: Appleton & Lange, 1997, Chap. 12, pp. 147–173.

Walsh CA, Doroshow RW. Adolescent cardiology. *Adolesc Med* 12:1–180, 2001.

PSYCHOLOGIC OVERLAY

Psychosocial dysfunction involves emotional adjustment similar to adolescents with other chronic diseases. Anxiety, isolation, poor self-esteem, and depression can be noted similar to other adolescents with chronic diseases. Sport participation must be individualized; most can safely participate in some form of sport or exercise-related activity including elite-level athletics (Luckstead, 1998). Intellectual function and levels of educational school attainment are similar to their noncardiac adolescent peers. Their school attendance and involvement is the same as adolescents without cardiac issues if they had only mild or corrected heart disease. However, other studies have noted minimal differences or similar school attendance patterns for patients with more severe forms of heart disease (Manning, 1983).

References

Luckstead EF. Cardiovascular evaluation of the young athlete. *AdolMed* 9:441–455, 1998.

Manning JA. Congenital heart disease and the quality of life. In: ME Engle and JK Perloff (eds.), *Congenital Heart Disease After Surgery: Benefits, Residua, Sequelae*. New York:York Medical Books, 1983, pp. 347–361, 1983.

CHEST PAIN IN THE ADOLESCENT

The primary care physician often refers adolescents with chest pain to the pediatric cardiologist for fear that there is a life threatening underlying cardiac etiology for the chest pain. Generally, there are two types of such chest pain. The first type of chest pain is cutaneous in origin and the other type is visceral. The typical features of the cutaneous type is that pain is initiated by stimulating the richly innervated skin, localized, of brief duration, and is described as sharp or stabbing in nature. This type can also be provoked by touching the area, changing position, or after eating. However, the second type of pain is often vague, poorly innervated cutaneously, diffuse, and described as oppressive or dull. The causes of chest pain can be divided into the following major categories: noncardiac types that account for the majority (~95%) and those that are cardiac in origin. Among the major noncardiac causes are chest wall syndrome (Chap. 8), pulmonary (Chap. 8), gastrointestinal, psychogenic, and cardiac.

Gastrointestinal Pain Sources

Patients with upper gastrointestinal problems like esophagitis, gastritis, or duodenal ulcers may present with chest pain (Sabri, 2003). Typically these patients will have their pain at night, often exacerbated by eating and on physical exam have demonstrated epigastric tenderness. In these cases, the patient needs further evaluation by a gastroenterologist. Most of these patients will have a family history of peptic ulcers.

Psychogenic Chest Pain

Psychogenic chest pain accounts for one-fourth of adolescent patients referred because of chest pain complaints. Two-thirds of these cases are associated with deaths in the family, separation anxiety, aggression, or physical disability. About 47% of these patients have a family history of a similar condition. Some of these patients have chest pain associated with hyperventilation syndrome or adolescent depression.

Chest Pain of Cardiac Etiology

There are several cardiac disease entities where one of the clinical symptoms is chest pain. For example, syncope, presyncope, palpitations, and a family history of sudden death in middle aged relatives should alert the clinician to the possible seriousness of the chest pain complaint. Moreover, there are certain syndromes (i.e., Marfan syndrome, Friedreich's ataxia syndrome, Turner syndrome, Noonan syndrome) that may present with a chief complaint of chest pain. These cases should be further investigated and managed properly.

The pericardium itself can be another source of chest pain and secondary to either an infection (i.e., viral, bacterial, or fungal) or inflammatory reaction. Typically these patients present with chest pain that is exacerbated when lying down and decreases after sitting. They may have a friction rub on physical cardiac exam; however, the absence of a friction rub does not rule out pericardial disease. The pericardium can also have air displacing pericardial fluid. This is called pneumopericardium and may be secondary air from the contiguous organs.

Patients following open-heart surgery must be considered for postpericardiotomy syndrome in their differential of chest pain; this manifests a few weeks after surgery. It is characterized by fever, leukocytosis, possible friction rub, and a high sedimentation rate. Postpericardiotomy effusion is usually diagnosed by echocardiogram. Most cases are managed with aspirin or nonsteroidal anti-inflammatory drugs; occasionally, indomethacin or steroids are needed. Although uncommon, if a patient becomes hemodynamically unstable and pericardial tamponade occurs, then pericardiocentesis is indicated.

Some teenagers are born with subtle congenital abnormalities of their coronary arteries. They are asymptomatic until presenting as chest pain or worse; sudden death occurs during exercise or while active in sports. Such anomalies include anomalous left coronary artery with the left coronary artery originating from the pulmonary artery. Single coronary arteries and other anomalies can also exist; some are recognized only after exercise and sudden death. Other less common abnormalities include coronary artery fistula.

Abnormal coronary arteries can also be acquired. The most commonly acquired heart disease in America is Kawasaki disease. This involves the coronary arteries in 20%–25% of untreated cases. It occurs typically after the first or second week of the illness or possibly later. Patients who are diagnosed with homozygous type II hypercholesterolemia are at high risk for developing coronary artery disease; they also may present with chest pain.

The myocardium can be the target of many diseases. This can be from infectious agents, (diphtheria, *Coxsackie B virus*, or rickettsia as well as fungal or parasitic infections), drugs (cocaine), autoimmune disorders or malignancies. Such patients usually will present with congestive heart failure; chest pain can be the presenting symptom.

Some patients may have a family history of hypertrophic cardiomyopathy. When these adolescents present with significant exercise-related chest pain or severe chest pain, cardiac possibilities should be further investigated. Arrhythmias occasionally present as a manifestation of chest pain; this is seen mostly in patients with supraventricular or ventricular tachycardia episodes. Patients with cardiac valve anomalies can present clinically with chest pain, as for example adolescents with severe AS or mitral valve prolapse. About 10%–15% of patients with MVP will complain of recurrent episodes of chest pain but the etiology appears to be idiopathic.

Bibliography

Lam JC, Tobias JD. Follow-up survey of children and adolescents with chest pain. *South Med J* 94:921, 2001.

Luckstead EF, Greydanus DE. In: *Cardiac Evaluation: Medical Care of the Adolescent Athlete,* Los Angeles: Practice Management Information Corporation, 1993.

Luckstead EF. Cardiovascular disorders in the college student. *Pediatr Clin N Am* 52:243–278, 2005.

Owens TR. Chest pain in the adolescent. *Adolesc Med* 12: 95–104, 2001.

Sabri MR, Ghavanini AA, Haghighat M, et al. Chest pain in children and adolescents: Epigastric tenderness as a guide to reduce unnecessary workup. *Pediatr Cardiol* 24:3, 2003.

Selbst SM, Ruddy RM, Clark BJ, et al. Pediatric chest pain: A prospective study. *Pediatrics* 82:319, 1988.

ATHEROSCLEROSIS, HYPERLIPIDEMIA, AND HYPERTENSION IN YOUTH

Adolescent Cardiac Risk Factors

Many of the risk factors for cardiovascular death in adults begin and can be modified during the adolescent years. These risk factors include obesity, smoking, sedentary lifestyle, and dietary fat intake. Essential hypertension may also begin in adolescence or young adulthood and increase the risk of cardiovascular death later in adulthood. Thus, clinicians caring for such youth can detect factors that may lead to considerable morbidity and even mortality later in life. Therefore, careful evaluation and effective education that promotes healthy adult life styles could pay tremendous dividends to the adolescent patient for many decades to come.

One challenge concerns the important medical question: "At what age does atherosclerosis actually have its origins?" Does this cardiac process begin at birth, infancy, childhood, adolescence, or only when we become older adults? Not only is this important but it is a medical concern to discern the actual medical facts and particularly note that children and adolescents do not follow known adult profiles. We do know that the actual clinical expression of atherosclerosis in children is rare. Exceptions are those rare homozygote genetic lipoprotein diseases like familial hypercholesterolemia (FH). Children and youth do not develop actual "fixed" signs of clinically significant atherosclerosis until reaching their third decade of life; however, diabetes mellitus may play a catalytic intermediary earlier role in these areas.

FH has high levels of low-density lipoprotein-cholesterol (LDL-C), which causes premature development of atherosclerosis. Studies on FH families can provide important information on how other children and youth may develop atherosclerosis. Such affected children (FH) are typically initially asymptomatic despite their high levels of LDL-C from this inherited autosomal dominant lipoprotein disorder resulting from defective LDL receptor gene mutations. Endothelial dysfunction has been shown in children to be an early predictor and a reversible stage of atherosclerosis that can be measured by flow-mediated techniques using the brachial artery (de Jongh, Atherosclerosis, 2002).

An accurate understanding of the natural history of the process of atherosclerosis itself is important, from tracking the first stage of highly reversible "fatty streak" in children to the later second stage of irreversible harmful "atheromatous plaques" seen in young and older adults. Older clinicians caring for children and adolescents often ask if one can actually medically prevent or alter the course and progression of pediatric age patient atherosclerosis? Will diet changes, life-style changes, or selected drugs be effective? At what age and stage of the atherosclerosis process intervention can clinicians intervene and document a positive effect? A review of the known important risk factors for developing pediatric age atherosclerosis includes the following:

1. Plasma lipids changes in children and youth
2. Hypertension
3. Smoking
4. Abdominal girth obesity
5. Physical inactivity
6. High dietary fat intake

Recent prospective studies of children with known FH were treated with statin medications to investigate their effect on endothelial dysfunction; this study provides the first well-documented evidence of improved endothelial dysfunction in pediatric age FH patients by administering statins (de Jongh, J Am Coll Cardiology, 2002). If shown to be safe, use of statin medications could possibly allow earlier intervention for atherosclerosis abnormalities in non-FH children and other youth. A few cases of lupus-like syndromes have been noted and this needs further evaluation.

Regular exercise reduces high blood pressure and improves overall glucose metabolism, while also apparently decreasing LDL-C and increasing high-density lipoprotein-cholesterol (HDL-C). Regular, sustained exercise may actually cause a mild regression of atherosclerosis progression or even possibly a mild reversal. However, direct or confirmatory experimental evidence demonstrating the beneficial effect of such exercise training slowing the process of atherosclerosis remains lacking. Physical activity or exercise definitely has been documented to have a known positive effect on obesity factors and decreasing systemic hypertension levels (Morrison, 1999). Since obesity is at least partially responsible for the clustering of many of these cardiovascular risk factors, one must have increased physical activity as a central part of any obesity management program for youth. Otherwise, significant diet-induced weight loss alone without exercise and/or weight-training typically results in both fat and actual undesired fat-free muscle loss.

Lipoprotein values are known to change markedly from birth to early infancy. Further, lipoprotein changes continue into childhood and early adolescence until young adults reach 35 years of age (Table 9-1). The apparent effects of diet, exercise, drugs, and genetics on these parameters provide interesting results, which are viewed differently by physicians, cardiovascular experts, nutritionists, and other international groups (Writing Group, 1995;

TABLE 9-1

NORMAL LIPOPROTEIN VALUES: PEDIATRIC AGE (1–17 YEARS)

Birth

Total cholesterol: 70 mg/dL (average)

Low density lipoprotein-cholesterol (LDL-C): 30 mg/dL (average)

High density lipoprotein-cholesterol (HDL-C): 35 mg/dL (average)

Age: 1–12 years

Total cholesterol: 150 mg/dL (average)

Low density lipoprotein (LDL-C): 100 mg/dL (average)

High density lipoprotein (HDL-C): 55 mg/dL (average)

After 17 years

Adult values typical for both boys and girls

Age 15 years (with +/− one year) is transition to adult values

    Separates adult from childhood values

    Tanner stage 4 in both girls and boys

Source: Olson RE. Atherosclerosis in children: Implications for the prevention of atherosclerosis. *Adv Pediatr* 47:55–78, 2000.

Kwiterovich, 1997; Newman, 1995; Olsen, 1995). Most children actually are at low risk for modifiable atherosclerosis risk factors such as hypercholesterolemia, hypertension, hyperhomocysteinemia, smoking, and obesity. However, the actual earlier existence of such risk factors has been reported in a recent Greek adolescent study (Bouziota, 2003).

Atherosclerosis begins as a disease in childhood in the large and middle-sized arterial blood vessels. (e.g., aorta, iliac, femoral, carotid, cerebral, and coronary arteries) The two basic lesions are the reversible fatty streak or spot present in all infants and children and the nonreversible atheromatous plaque that is noted after puberty. The lipid deposit of the actual fatty streak itself is largely intracellular and composed of cholesterol ester, free cholesterol, and triglycerides in the arterial intima. Most fatty streaks will remain unchanged or can disappear during adolescence but some may instead progress to become precursors of the atheromatous plaques. By contrast, most atheromatous plaques are extracellular and are derived from plasma lipoproteins and not reversible (Olson, 2000).

A recent multicenter cooperative study of pathological determinants of atherosclerosis in youth (PDAY) (McGill, 1997) performed autopsies on 2876 accident victims from 15 to 34 years of age; one-half were Black and one-fourth were women. The findings were as follows: adolescent boys aged 15–19 had about 20% fatty streaks in the aorta; plaques were only 0.35% in the aorta. The right coronary artery had fatty streaks in 1.8% in boys; plaques were noted in 0.2% of girls and 0.5% of boys. There was no difference in atheromatous plaque development between boys or girls until they reached 15 years of age. There was no correlation between their serum cholesterol levels and their aortic or right coronary atheromatous plaque presence between the ages of 15 and 24. It appears that between birth and 15 years of age atherosclerosis development does not occur except possibly in the form of fatty streaks, most of which apparently are reversible (Strong, 1999).

The actual modifiable risk factors for atherosclerosis (i.e., high cholesterol levels, hypertension,

hyperhomocysteinemia, smoking, and being overweight) have been typically low-risk factors for most children. There is now concern that this is changing worldwide with obesity, smoking, less physical activity, and type II diabetes mellitus becoming more prevalent in the preadolescent and adolescent age groups (Luckstead, 2002). The average cholesterol level between ages 1 and 15 in both girls and boys is 150 mg/dL; LDL-C levels average 100 mg/dL; the HDL-C average is ~50 mg/dL. Blood pressure is typically lower in children than the youth and young adult ages (Olson, 2000). Children have lower homocysteine levels; however, pediatric age obesity has increased ~30% over the last decade and smoking is increasing in the preadolescent and adolescent. Efforts to reduce these trends for youth-age obesity and smoking need urgent attention and aggressive health education measures and programs that are effective. Additionally, what role does inflammation have as an important factor in coronary artery atherosclerosis development needs critical study (Ross, 1998).

One must challenge and educate the medical community, schools, parents, media, and others to promote reputable and accurate information. Of particular concern are the actual risks and benefits of significantly limiting fat intake in growing children and the "fast-food mentality" of today's culture. Well-documented evidence is lacking that feeding low-fat diets to growing children will either prevent or alter their atherosclerosis development from adolescence to young adulthood. The prevalence of fatty streaks in childhood does not correlate with atheromatous plaque development in later adulthood. Girls actually have a greater number of aortic fatty streaks and higher serum cholesterol than boys during childhood, but less atheromatous plaques than boys. It has been shown that a significant number of atheromatous plaques do not occur in the coronary arteries of boys until after 19 years of age. Although high blood cholesterol levels do enhance fatty streak formation, they do not enhance atheromatous plaque formation. Actual progression from arterial large vessel fatty streaks to nonreversible atheromatous plaques does not occur until after puberty in males and until after menopause in most females. Therefore, stating that atherosclerosis actually begins in childhood may be semantically correct but is otherwise at the least definitely misleading (Olson, 2000).

Well-meaning parents and some physicians believing that dietary fat intake will cause atherosclerosis problems with their children's hearts may impose strict dietary restrictions on them with adverse consequences. This has resulted in a higher incidence of infants and children showing nonorganic failure to thrive or growth and nutritional abnormalities (McCann, 1994); some children develop over-eating issues when they later reach adulthood. There remains concern about whether long-term low-fat diets are safe for children. Most dietary studies were in medical centers and were not performed in the actual long-term home care environments of ordinary families. Children can consume about 30% of their daily energy from fat and apparently will do quite well. Controversy persists over the American Heart Association, National Cholesterol Education Program, and American Academy of Pediatrics (AAP) recommendations for a lower dietary fat percentage during the first 2–3 years of life (Olson, 1995; Third Report, 2001). Pediatricians in Canada continue to recommend decreasing the dietary fat percentage intake from 40% at the age 2 to 30% by the middle of adolescence (such as Tanner stage 4) when significant growth decreases (Park, 2001). European pediatricians have made similar recommendations by proposing parents feed a 30%–35% total fat dietary intake until after 2–3 years of age (Berenson, 1998). Both groups state that any type of diets with less than 30% total fat content simply are *not* desirable for children.

Another Viewpoint

Controversy continues regarding the best way to screen for hyperlipidemia in adolescence. Levels of total cholesterol and triglycerides are of interest, especially LDL and HDL cholesterol. In the United States, a multistep process has been recommended by the Expert Panel on Blood Cholesterol Levels in Children and Adolescents (Third Report, 2001). Health assessment involves obtaining a family history for hyperlipidemia (as one or both parents

with a cholesterol level at or over 240 mg/dL) and premature cardiovascular events; if there is a positive family history, the youth is screened with total cholesterol or a fasting lipoprotein profile. The results of two fasting profiles can be averaged. A positive family history refers to a parent or grandparent with documented coronary artery disease before age 55; this includes a documented history of myocardial infarction, sudden death, cardiac catheterization documenting coronary artery disease, angina pectoris, peripheral vascular disease, or cerebrovascular disease. Some clinicians screen those with an unknown family history, those with risk factors for secondary hyperlipidemia (Table 9-2) and those with other cardiovascular risk factors (i.e., hypertension or obesity). Many clinicians also screen a young adult over age 19 who has never been screened before.

All adolescents should be advised to eat a healthy diet, whether they have hyperlipidemia or

TABLE 9 - 2

CAUSES/ASSOCIATIONS OF SECONDARY HYPERLIPIDEMIA

Alcohol
Anabolic steroids
Anorexia nervosa
Antihypertensive medications
Chronic renal disease (including hemolytic uremic
   syndrome and renal failure)
Diabetes Mellitus
Gaucher's disease
Glucocorticoids (hypercortisolism)
Glycogen storage disease
Hypothyroidism
Hypopituitarism
Isotretinoin
Klinefelter syndrome
Nephrotic syndrome
Obesity (Major factor)
Oral contraceptives
Obstructive liver disease
Pregnancy
Progeria syndrome
Systemic Lupus Erythematosus

Source: Stone NJ. Secondary causes of hyperlipidemia.
Med Clin No Amer 78:117–142, 1994.

not (Krauss, 2000). For example, youth should seek to keep their total cholesterol intake at or below 300 mg a day and their total dietary fats should constitute no more than 30% of their caloric intake while saturated fats (as well as trans-unsaturated fats) are no more than 10%. This is the American Heart Association Step I diet. All youth should also be counseled about proper exercise as well as avoidance of smoking and obesity. If he or she has a total cholesterol of 170–199 mg/dL or a LDL of 110–129 mg/dL, then further dietary counseling is recommended. Youth are advised and to stay on the Step I diet. The lipid pattern is followed on an annual basis. If the total cholesterol is 200 mg/dL or higher and/or the LDL is over 129 mg/dL, stricter dietary guidelines are indicated. The total daily cholesterol can be restricted below 200 mg and saturated fats no higher than 7%. This is the American Heart Association Step II diet.

Management of elevated lipids in adolescence usually involves dietary education alone. Mild elevations of LDL cholesterol and triglycerides are usually due to secondary hyperlipidemia and attention should be given to the underlying disorder along with dietary counseling. Primary hyperlipidemia is essentially a genetic disorder leading to alterations in the patient's lipoprotein metabolism. An example is common FH, an autosomal dominant condition with very high LDL levels, decreased HDL levels, and typically normal triglyceride levels. Other such lipoprotein variations are described in more detail in the literature (Carter, 1997; Domanski, 2004).

Pharmacotherapy is often suggested if these measures are not working, especially if the LDL stays over 190 mg/dL; use 160 mg/dL when other cardiovascular risk factors exist. These medications are usually started in adulthood, but severe disease may warrant their initial use during the adolescent years. HMG-CoA reductase inhibitors (Lovastatin, Simvastatin, Fluvastatin, Pravastatin, Atorvastatin, and Cerivastatin) affect hepatic LDL receptors while inhibiting the production of cholesterol; cholesterol (total and LDL) is lowered while HDL cholesterol is raised and triglycerides lowered. Side effects may include myalgia, rash, and headache. These statin-type medications are often the primary medications now used for adults with abnormal lipid profiles.

Other medications that have been used in adults and not recommended for adolescents include bile acid sequestrants, nicotinic acid, and fibric acid. Bile acid sequestrants (Cholestyramine or Colestipol) bind bile acids in the intestine and induce hepatic LDL receptors; they reduce total cholesterol and LDL cholesterol. Common side effects include constipation and abdominal discomfort. Nicotinic acid (Niacin and the extended-release niacin, Niaspan) reduces VLDL synthesis in the liver; it also reduces total cholesterol, LDL cholesterol, and triglycerides while increasing HDL cholesterol. Side effects commonly include abdominal discomfort and flushing; the flushing may be lessened with aspirin. Fibric acid (Gemfibrozil) increases lipoprotein lipase activity while decreasing hepatic triglyceride production; cholesterol (total and LDL) is reduced and HDL cholesterol increased and triglycerides lowered. Frequent side effects include increased appetite, loose stools, abdominal discomfort, and myalgias.

Bibliography

Berenson GS. For the Bogalusa heart study: Association between multiple cardiovascular risk factors and atherosclerosis in children and young adults. *N Engl J Med* 338:1650–1666, 1998.

Carter GA. Hypercholesterolemia in children. *Pediatric Ann* 26:122, 1997.

Bouziota C, Koutedakis V. A three year study of coronary heart disease risk factors in Greek adolescents. *Ped Exerc Sci* 15:9–18, 2003.

Domanski M, Proschan M. The metabolic syndrome (*editorial comment*). *J Am Coll Cardiol* 43(8): 1396–1398, 2004.

de Jongh S, Lilien MR, Roodt J, et al. Early statin therapy restores endothelial function in children with familial hypercholesterolemia. *J Am Coll Cardiol* 40:2117–2121, 2002.

de Jongh S, Lilien MR, Bakker HD, et al. Family history of cardiovascular events and endothelial dysfunction in children with familial hypercholesterolemia. *Atherosclerosis* 163:193–197, 2002.

Gotto AM Targeting high-risk young patients for statin therapy. *JAMA* 292:377–378, 2004.

Hognestad A, Aukrust P, Wergeland R, et al. Effects of conventional and aggressive statin treatment on markers of endothelial function and inflammation. *Clin Cardiol* 27:199–203, 2004.

Luckstead EF. Cardiac risk factors and participation guidelines for youth sports. *Pediatr Clin N Am* 49: 681–707, 2002.

Luckstead EF. Cardiovascular disorders in the college student. *Pediatr Clin N Am* 52:243–278, 2005.

Knopp RH. Drug treatment of lipid disorders. *N Engl J Med* 12: 498–511, 1999.

Krauss RM, Eckel RH, Howard B, et al. AHA dietary guidelines. Revision 2000: A statement for healthcare professionals from the Nutrition Committee of the American Heart Association. *Circulation* 102: 2284–2299, 2000.

Kwiterovich PO, Barton BA, McMahon RP, et al. Effects of diet and sexual maturation on low-density lipoprotein cholesterol during puberty: The dietary intervention study in children (DISC). *Circulation* 96:2526–2533, 1997.

McCrindle BW. Cardiovascular risk factors in adolescents: Relevance, detection, and intervention. *Adolesc Med* 12:147–162, 2001.

McGill HC for the PDAY Research Group. Effect of serum lipoproteins and smoking on atherosclerosis in young men and women. *Arterioscler Thromb Vasc Biol* 17:95–106, 1997.

Morrison JA, Barton BA, Biro FM, et al. Overweight, fat patterning, and cardiovascular disease risk factors in Black and White boys and girls. *J Pediatr* 135: 451–464, 1999.

Newman TB, Garber AM, Holtzman NA, et al. Problems with the report of the expert panel on blood cholesterol levels in children and adolescents. *Arch Pediatr Adolesc Med* 49:241–247, 1995.

Olson RE. The dietary recommendations of the American Academy of Pediatrics. *Am J Clin Nutr* 101:141–147, 1995.

Olson RE. Atherosclerosis in children: Implications for the prevention of atherosclerosis. *Adv Pediatr* 47: 55–78, 2000.

Park MK, Menard SW, Yuan C. Comparison of auscultatory and oscillometric blood pressures. *Arch Pediatr Adol Med* 155:50–53, 2001.

Ross R. Atherosclerosis: An inflammatory disease. *N Engl J Med* 340:115–126, 1998.

Safety of aggressive statin therapy. *Med Lett* 46:93–95, 2004.

Stone NJ. Secondary causes of hyperlipidemia. *Med Clin No Amer* 78:117–142, 1994.

Strong JP. The PDAY Research Group: Prevalence and extent of atherosclerosis in adolescents and young adults: Implications for prevention from the pathobiological determinants of atherosclerosis in youth studies. *JAMA* 281:727–735, 1999.

The Writing Group for the DISC Collaborative Research Group. Efficacy and safety of lowering dietary intake of fat and cholesterol in children with elevated low-density lipoprotein cholesterol; The dietary intervention study in children (DISC). *JAMA* 273:1429–1435, 1995.

Third Report of the National Cholesterol Education Program (NCEP) on Detection, Evaluation, and Treatment of High Blood Cholesterol in Adults (Adult Treatment Panel III). NIH Publication No. 01–3770, 2001. Available at *http://www.nhlbi.nih.gov/guidelines/cholesterol/profmats.htm.*

HYPERTENSION

Accurate diagnosis and using appropriate treatment methods is very important in adolescents with systemic hypertension. One should use the national standardized blood pressure reference values and guidelines (Luckstead, 2002; Wells, 2001). These diagnostic blood pressure guidelines are standardized from ages 1 to 17 for female and male patients. The blood pressure systolic, diastolic >90% and >95% blood pressure percentile are plotted against their 5%–10%–25%–50%–75%–90%–95% referenced age height standard percentiles during the pediatric and adolescent growth years. Blood pressure measurements above 130 systolic and above 90 diastolic are suspect for hypertension in the older age groups and above 120 systolic and 80 diastolic are suspect at younger ages assuming proper blood pressure measurement techniques are used. Management factors will depend on the adolescent patient's diagnosis of mild, moderate, or severe hypertension.

Whether it is acute, subacute, or chronic systolic and/or diastolic systemic hypertension will further influence treatment measures. Anxiety, illness, drug side effects and/or abuse, obesity factors renal, cardiac, and endocrine related hypertension etiologies will need study. Essential hypertension that occurs in families comprises a high percentage of those not caused by the listed known target-organ etiologies. Ambulatory blood monitoring may unmask some of the labile or anxiety related sources of hypertension. Severe levels of hypertension will require close observation and treatment in a hospitalized setting; potent beta-blockers, vasodilators, and other intravenous medications and close monitoring can be used in such instances. An individualized antihypertensive approach to each case is now preferred by most physicians instead of the previous use of a step-type medication sequence with diuretics, beta-blockers, ace inhibitors, calcium channel blockers, and others.

Exercise, Diet, and/or Drugs

Since diet alone is not the answer for hypertension treatment, what directions should physicians be actively pursuing for such children and youth? One obvious answer is to highlight the importance for increased and sustained physical activity options particularly for the preadolescent and adolescent age patients. Youth should strive for at least 60 minutes of moderate to vigorous physical activity per day; this need not be sport-related. Such heightened physical activity levels when coupled with prudent dietary habits will also enhance weight control issues, help reduce marginal or higher blood pressure problems, and promote long-term healthy lifestyle behaviors. Concepts of dealing with atherosclerosis have been previously covered. Chapter 31 reviews concepts of obesity in the adolescent.

Bibliogrpahy

Conti CR. Obesity is not only an adult problem (editorial). *Clin Cardiol* 27:183–184, 2004.

Domanski M, Proschan M. The metabolic syndrome (editorial comment). *J Am Coll Cardiol* 43(8): 1396–1398, 2004.

Inge TH, Zeller M, Garcia VF, et al. Surgical approach to adolescent obesity. *Adolesc Med* 15:429–454, 2002.

Luckstead EF. Cardiac risk factors and participation guidelines for youth sports. *Pediatr Clin N Am* 49:681–707, 2002.

Luckstead EF. Cardiovascular disorders in the college student. *Pediatr Clin N Am* 52:243–278, 2005.

McCrindle BW. Cardiovascular risk factors in adolescents: Relevance, detection, and intervention. *Adolesc Med* 12:147–162, 2001.

National High Blood Pressure Education Program Working Group on Hypertension Control in Children and Adolescents. Update on the 1987 Task Force report on high blood pressure in children and adolescents: A working group report from the National High Blood Pressure Education Program. *Pediatrics* 98:649–658, 1996.

Wells T, Stowe C. Approach to use of antihypertensive drugs in children and adolescents. *Curr Ther Res Clin Exp* 62:329–350, 2001.

MURMURS ASSOCIATED WITH ADOLESCENT HEART ANOMALIES

One can detect a heart murmur in about 50% of adolescents; however, significant congenital or acquired heart disease is present in only 1% of those with murmurs. A large number of benign or "innocent" murmurs may be detected (Table 9-3). The two most commonly noted are the pulmonary or early systolic medium to high pitched right ventricular outflow murmur and the vibratory or musical sounding early and midsystolic left ventricular outflow murmur (Still's murmur). Usually, both murmur types are grade 2 or 3 based on the 1–6 Levine murmur scale; thrills are not usually associated with these murmurs.

Additional conditions causing murmurs include aortic stenosis, atrial septal defects, coarctation of the aorta, mitral valve prolapse, PDA, pulmonic stenosis, and tetralogy of Fallot (the prototype lesion for the cyanotic congenital cardiac disorders and VSD). Advances in cardiac surgery over the past 30 years have significantly altered the natural history of many infants and children with congenital cardiac disorders; most children are now healthy and surviving into the adolescent and adult years. In addition, some congenital cardiac disorders will

TABLE 9-3

INNOCENT MURMURS OF ADOLESCENCE

Still's murmur (vibratory systolic ejection or early systolic murmur)
Jugular venous hum
Pulmonary ejection systolic murmur
Carotid bruit
Coronary artery *diastolic* murmur

TABLE 9-4

CONGENITAL HEART DISEASE: ADOLESCENT AGE

Anomalous coronary arteries
Atrial septal defect
Aortic stenosis (most are bicuspid aortic valves)
Coarctation of the aorta
Ebstein's anomaly
Mitral valve prolapse
Pulmonary valve stenosis
VSD (ventricular septal defects)
PDA (patent ductus arteriosus)
Endocardial cushion defects (A/V canal types)

continue to escape childhood detection and not be diagnosed until adolescence or later. (Table 9-4).

Aortic Stenosis

AS is noted in 3%–6% of all congenital heart disease series. Youth with AS present with grade 2 or 3/6 systolic ejection murmurs noted over the aortic area at the second right and third left intercostal space. The murmur usually is referred over the precordium, cardiac apex and to the neck vessel areas. If AS occurs at the valve level, usually an early systolic ejection click is noted at the valve site, cardiac apex, and/or suprasternal notch areas. A thrill is noted in the valve areas and the neck with grade 4 or greater murmurs; this is most likely with subaortic stenosis. Isolated AS is noted in ~3–5% of congenital heart anomalies and AS occurs in ~20% associated with other heart defects. The adolescent may present with symptoms of chest pain, syncope, dyspnea, and fatigue if moderate or severe AS is present; left ventricular hypertrophy as noted on an electrocardiogram (ECG) is uncommon and most have normal chest x-rays and ECGs. Progressive valve stenosis is typical and moderate or severe disease may lead to exercise-related sudden death in ~1%. Most youth with AS may participate in some sports when provided with guidance from cardiologists and clearance by experts in cardiology and sports medicine using national guidelines (The 26th Bethesda Conference, 1994; Basilico, 1999). Surgical and medical issues include early accurate

diagnosis, subacute bacterial endocarditis (SBE) prophylaxis, interventional palliative measures, and/or surgery (e.g., surgical valvotomy, balloon angioplasty, and valve replacement), or the eventual use of the Ross surgical procedure.

Atrial Septal Defect

ASDs do not have their own murmur but instead will amplify the physiologic pulmonary flow murmur at the left second intercostal space resulting from right ventricular volume overload. When the pulmonary blood flow is greater than 2:1, a late diastolic tricuspid (scratchy) murmur or diastolic flow rumble from a functional tricuspid stenosis is heard by experienced physicians. The heralding clinical sign is a widely split and fixed second heart sound. Secundum ASDs are seen in the majority of adolescents with incomplete endocardial cushion (ostium primum); ASD defects following at a distant second. A superior ECG QRS-axis (LAD) and mild RVH (right ventricular hypertrophy) are more often seen with ostium primum defects than secundum atrial defects; echocardiograms will usually delineate the ASD type. Occasionally sinus venosus type ASDs are encountered. Mild right ventricular enlargement on chest x-ray with increased venous vascularity (Kerley B lines) and a prominent pulmonary artery segment are typically seen in moderate to large size defects; many of these secundum types are now closed interventionally. There have been reports of occasional dysrhythmias with interventional and surgical atrial defect closures. Except for bicuspid aortic valves, secundum atrial defects remain the most common unrecognized defect in adolescent, young, and older adult.

Coarctation of the Aorta (C/A)

This congenital cardiac anomaly has a slight male predominance when mild or moderate in degree; it may go undetected until adolescence. It is frequently associated with other heart defects such as a bicuspid aortic valve and VSD. There may be complaints of pain, weakness, or cramps in the legs during or after exercise. On cardiac examination one can detect a systolic ejection murmur over the back interscapular area and left chest supraclavicular regions. One detects hypertension in the arms, hypotension in the legs, and delayed or absent femoral pulses. Increased upper extremity musculature is noted along with "stork-like" or thin legs; this phenotype has been described more often on clinical physical examination in older patients. Patients with C/A may have systolic bruits over the chest from the presence of collateral vessel circulation; the chest x-ray depicts a dilated aorta and posterior rib notching. When not recognized, premature death in adulthood results from C/A complications such as dissecting aortic aneurysm rupture or cerebrovascular complications like a Circle of Willis aneurysm rupture.

Management involves surgical and/or interventional palliation or correction at both the aortic coarctation site itself and for associated defects like bicuspid aortic valve stenosis when possible. Extreme precaution to avoid massive collateral vessels bleeding at surgery is warranted and spinal cord selective perfusion techniques are needed in the older adolescent and adult coarctation patient. C/A is not an experienced surgeon's favorite operation because of these extensive collateral bleeding challenges.

Mitral Valve Prolapse

MVP is diagnosed by echocardiographic studies in 5%–10% of the general population and about 20% of female adolescents and young women. However, when recently revised MVP criteria are used, the MVP incidence was decreased to ~2% in the population. This abnormality is usually identified after 10 years of age either as an isolated finding or associated with other cardiac anomalies or conditions (Table 9-5). MVP is noted in infancy when patients have Marfan or Ehlers-Danlos syndrome. A midsystolic click is associated with prolapse of the posterior mitral valve leaflet into the left atrium. The associated late systolic murmur of mitral regurgitation follows the mid-systolic click in most patients. Examining the adolescent in an upright or standing position or by performing the Valsalva maneuver decreases the left ventricular volume and enhances the MVP. Some cardiologists, although a

TABLE 9-5

CONDITIONS AND CARDIAC ANOMALIES SEEN WITH MVP

Anorexia nervosa (from decreased left ventricular volume)
Anxiety and anxiety disorders
Atrial septal defects (primum defects)
Ehlers-Danlos syndrome
Hurler syndrome
Marfan syndrome
Osteogenesis imperfecta
Pectus carinatum or excavatum
Pseudoxanthoma elasticum
Rheumatic fever
Rheumatoid/collagen vascular diseases
Scoliosis
Skeletal joint hyperextensibility
Straight Back syndrome

Source: Rowlett JD, Greydanus DE. *The Cardiovascular System in Adolescent Medicine*, 3d ed., Hoffmann AD, Greydanus DE (eds.), Stamford, CT: Appleton & Lange, 1997, Chap. 12, pp. 147–173 Greydanus DE, Patel D, Pratt H, Bhave S, (eds.). Cardiovascular disorders. *India Manual of Adolescent Medicine, Review of Adolescent Medicine*, New Delhi, India: Cambridge Press, 2002, Vol. 6, pp. 34–57.

minority, insist that the MVP diagnosis should not be made unless there is actual evidence of myxomatous degeneration of the mitral valve. A loud holosystolic murmur suggests the presence of moderate to severe degeneration with mitral regurgitation; this is similar to the acute rheumatic fever (ARF) Carey-Coombs murmur. A careful evaluation including ECG, two- and three-dimensional echocardiography, and three-dimensional MRI are the current diagnostic methods used to identify mitral valve dysfunction and clinically significant mitral valve regurgitation (MR).

MVP may present without symptoms and be noted only on cardiac examination. At least one-third has a history of chest pain, tachycardia, palpitations, or fainting spells. Theories for the origin of the chest pain include chordate tendineae stretching, myocardial ischemia, or arrhythmias; the chest pain is often a stabbing, precordial pain lasting hours to days. Severe pain and even cardiac arrhythmias may develop.

Less than 1% present with central nervous system symptoms (i.e., cerebrovascular accident or transient vision loss) or endocarditis.

Management is dependent on the severity and extent of the disorder. Youth without clinical mitral insufficiency and symptoms have a benign course and simply need periodic evaluation for the development of mitral insufficiency. If chest pain develops, evaluate for other causes (see the discussion on chest pain in this chapter). Beta-blockers may control chest pain in MVP when it is associated with arrhythmias. Patients with mitral valve insufficiency do need SBE prophylaxis while the presence of significant arrhythmias (dysrhythmias) warrants careful cardiologic evaluation and anticipatory management. Long-term studies have shown MVP to be a mild or benign condition unless serious arrhythmias occur or significant myxomatous valve degeneration is noted (Nisimura, 1985). Sudden death may develop in those with severe ventricular arrhythmias. Most athletes with MVP can participate safely in sports with minimal restrictions. Females with MVP should not be on estrogen-containing contraceptives, because of increased risk of embolism.

Patent Ductus Arteriosus

PDA, if small or moderate in size, may go undiagnosed until later childhood, adolescence, or the adult years. Clinically, patients have a continuous murmur that peaks or "spills over" the second heart sound in the second left intercostal space or left upper chest region; occasionally it is heard over the back. It may be associated with C/A or aortic valve stenosis or both. If an isolated lesion, pulses are usually in both the arms and legs. If the pulmonary blood flow is over twice the systemic blood flow, one can hear a diastolic flow rumble or murmur; this indicates the presence of a resultant functional mitral stenosis from left ventricular volume overload from the PDA. The ECG may be normal or show left ventricular hypertrophy and echocardiograms are usually diagnostic. Treatment can be interventional or surgical, but risk of SBE or shortened life span results without treatment.

Pulmonic Valve Stenosis

Pulmonic stenosis at the valve, infundibulum and supravalvar levels may go undetected until later childhood, adolescence, or adulthood. Pulmonic valve stenosis is most common and often has a systolic ejection click preceding the systolic ejection murmur of pulmonic stenosis; no click is heard with the nonvalve types of pulmonic stenosis. The murmur will refer to the upper chest and both axilla if it is at the valve level. It is usually loudest at the pulmonic valve site (second left intercostal space) and louder on referral to the left axilla. Good correlation exists between increasing right ventricular hypertrophy on ECG and increased pulmonic stenosis gradients when contrasted with aortic valve stenosis where such ECG correlation is poor. Echocardiography offers excellent correlation for pulmonic stenosis severity at subpulmonic, valve, and supravalvar levels. Clinical murmur intensity also correlated well with the degree of stenosis. Balloon angioplasty is very effective in children and adolescents at the valve stenosis level. Some may require surgical relief but the more severe are usually recognized in early childhood. PS often occurs with other heart lesions and related to specific syndromes when the stenosis occurs at the pulmonary artery and subpulmonic (infundibular) levels.

Tetralogy of Fallot

Adolescents with previously treated complex cyanotic congenital heart disorders now survive well into their adolescent and young adulthood years. Some have had Blalock-Taussig (subclavian artery to pulmonary artery) or other arterial shunts; however, most had repair of the ventricular septal defect and relief of the right ventricular outflow infundibular pulmonic stenosis. One of the best predictive factors for long-term survival in such patients is the residual degree of right ventricular hypertension and/or dysfunction and the amount of pulmonary insufficiency present. As adolescents, such patients have a systolic ejection murmur at the left upper sternal border radiating to the axilla and sometimes the back. These findings are consistent with infundibular PS from mild to moderate residual outflow dynamics after repair. They often also will have pulmonary valve regurgitation, resulting in an early or proto-diastolic murmur at the left upper sternal border. Both murmurs occur often in youth after tetralogy of Fallot repair.

Major late postoperative problems for these patients include ventricular arrhythmias, sudden death, endocarditis, and myocardial failure. There is a greater risk of ventricular arrhythmias when there is trifascicular block (LAD and CRBBB). These youth should be encouraged to have an active lifestyle and follow SBE prophylaxis according to published standards (Dajani, 1997; Prevention, 2001). Adolescents with cyanotic congenital heart disease have an increased risk for thromboembolism. Low dose estrogen oral contraception is a safe option for such sexually active youth who wish effective contraception. The female adolescent with a good hemodynamic repair has a risk of pregnancy complications similar to the general population. However, she has a higher risk of having a child with congenital heart disease than the general population and genetic counseling is recommended. She could have fluorescent in-situ hybridization (FISH) for microdeletion on chromosome 22 (22 q11-). Fetal echocardiography is highly recommended during the second trimester and newborn pediatric cardiology consultation at birth.

Ventricular Septal Defects

Most VSDs are holosystolic or pansystolic in timing. The smaller defects are actually louder than the bigger defects because of their restrictive nature or VSD pressure differences between their left ventricle and right ventricle. When VSDs become smaller they will have late attenuation of the murmur and a higher pitch just before spontaneous closure. Most are heard best at the left lower sternal border, some are heard best at the base of the heart. Larger defects will have a diastolic flow rumble at the apex when the pulmonary blood flow is over twice the systemic blood flow; this represents functional mitral stenosis from left atrial volume overload. Apical ventricular muscular defects are reportedly least likely to close spontaneously. About 70% of small and medium sized VSDs will

close by 5–6 years of age and another 10%–20% by adolescence.

Other Cyanotic Cardiac Anomalies

Adolescents with surgically treated cyanotic lesions such as TGV, total anomalous pulmonary venous return (TAPVR), tricuspid atresia, truncus arteriosus, and single ventricle variants are now seen regularly in adolescents. Those with the arterial switch corrective procedure for TGV are doing very well; similarly, patients with TAPVR are also typically doing well. Other patients will be at various stages of palliation and will need individual management guidelines and modification as they proceed through adolescence into their adult years.

Bibliography

Basilico FC. Cardiovascular disease in athletes. *Am J Sports Med* 27(1):108–120, 1999.

Brickner ME, Hillis LD, Lange RA. Congenital heart disease in adults. *N Engl J Med* 342:256–263, 2000.

Dajani AS, Taubert KA, Wilson, et al. Prevention of bacterial endocarditis: Recommendations by the American Heart Association. *JAMA* 277:1794–1801, 1997.

Doroshow RW. The adolescent with simple or corrected congenital heart disease. *Adolesc Med* 12:1–22, 2001.

Etchells E, Bell C, Robb K. Does this patient have an abnormal systolic murmur? *JAMA* 277:564, 1997.

Greydanus DE, Patel D, Pratt H, Bhave S (eds.). Cardiovascular disorders. In: *India Manual of Adolescent Medicine, Review of Adolescent Medicine*, Cambridge Press, Delhi, India, 2002, Chap. 6, pp. 34–57.

Hagler DJ. Palliated congenital heart disease. *Adolesc Med* 12:23–34, 2001.

Hannoush H, Younes H, Arnaout S, et al. Patterns of congenital heart disease in unoperated adults: A 20-year experience in a developing country. *Clin Cardiol* 27:236–240, 2004.

Luckstead EF, Greydanus DE. The sport-specific physical examination and cardiovascular examination. In: *Medical Care of the Adolescent Athlete*. Los Angeles, CA: Practice Management Information Corporation, 1993.

Luckstead EF. Cardiovascular evaluation of the young athlete. *Adolesc Med* 9:441–455, 1998.

Luckstead EF. Cardiovascular disorders in the college student. *Pediatr Clin N Am* 52:243-278, 2005.

Nisimura RA, McGoon MD, Shub C, et al. Echocardiographic documented MVP: Long term follow-up of 237 patients. *N Engl J Med* 313:305–309, 1985.

Prevention of bacterial endocarditis. *Med Lett* 43:98, 2001.

Rowlett JD, Greydanus DE. *The Cardiovascular System in Adolescent Medicine*, 3d ed., Hoffmann AD, Greydanus DE (eds.), Stamford, CT: Appleton & Lange, 1997, Chap. 12, pp. 147–173.

The 26th Bethesda Conference. Recommendations for determining eligibility for competition in athletes with cardiovascular abnormalities. *J Am Coll Cardiol* 24:845–899, 1994.

Walsh CA, Doroshow RW (eds.). Adolescent cardiology. *Adolesc Med* 12:1–180, 2001.

SYNCOPE, DIZZINESS, AND SUDDEN DEATH

The evaluation of the adolescent with syncope must be thorough (Chap. 13). An accurate description of the syncope event is very helpful; prior cardiac problems, family history of syncope, associated illnesses, medication, or drug use/abuse must be accurately obtained from the history. There is a definite association of syncope with exercise and sudden death in both adolescent athletes and nonathletes. Syncope has been associated with sudden death in nearly 25% of such cases. Although most instances of syncope are neurocardiac or vasovagal in etiology, one must search diligently for those potentially lethal cases that are more likely from a cardiac origin.

ECG, Holter, and event monitors may be helpful with dysrhythmia-related syncope; echocardiographic studies, MRI or angiographic examinations will help diagnose muscle function, valve and abnormal coronary, systemic and pulmonary vessel abnormalities. Exercise stress testing, electrophysiologic conduction mapping and cardiac catheterization as well as angiography are useful in the higher risk syncope diagnostic dilemmas. Adolescents with exercise-related severe dizziness or syncope warrant further cardiovascular evaluation. This is especially true if planning to participate actively in sport or exercise-related activities.

Suggested Readings

Kosinski DJ. Syncope in the athlete. *Syncope: Mechanisms, and Management.* Armonk, NY: Futura Publishers, 2001, pp. 317–336.

Luckstead EF. Cardiovascular disorders in the college student. *Pediatr Clin N Am* 52:243–278, 2005.

Moak JP, Bailey JJ, Makhlouf FT. Simultaneous heart rate and blood pressure variability analysis: Insight into mechanisms underlying neurally mediated cardiac syncope in children. *J Am Coll Cardiol* 40:1466–1472, 2002.

Narchi H. The child who passes out. *Pediatr Rev* 21: 384–389, 2000.

Ross R, Grubb BP. Syncope in the child and adolescent. *Syncope: Mechanisms and Management.* Armonk, NY: Futura Publishers, 2001, pp. 305–316.

Walsh CA. Syncope and sudden death in the adolescent. *Adolesc Med* 12:105–132, 2001.

HYPOTENSION

Hypotension associated with dizziness episodes are relatively common in the adolescent but most are orthostatic in nature. Table 9-5 lists some of the underlying factors that may lead such phenomena in youth; the most common factor is syncope or near-syncope episodes. Neurocardiogenic syncope often is diagnosed by history; some may need confirmation by a positive Tilt-Table test. The evaluation includes a thorough history, including specifics such as amount of sleep, type of fluid intake, medication taken, and eating patterns. A careful physical examination and a urine specific gravity test help to assess fluid volume status; other tests are indicated by the findings. Management is directed by the underlying etiology.

Syncope during exercise is very different from syncope that occurs after extreme exercise or aerobic activities. One must diligently search for underlying cardiac, central nervous system, or metabolic causes when syncope occurs during exercise, since there is a higher risk of life-threatening events (see Tables 9-6 and 9-7). Exercise induced syncope without structural heart disease has been shown by Tilt-Table testing to

TABLE 9-6

PRECIPITANTS/CAUSES OF HYPOTENSION AND DIZZINESS IN YOUTH

Anorexia nervosa

Arrhythmias

Diabetes mellitus

Dysautonomias

Glucocorticoid deficiency (intrinsic or after removal of exogenous glucocorticoids)

Hypothyroidism

Hypovolemia

Medication induced:

    Beta-adrenergic blockers

    Calcium channel blockers

    Diuretics

    Tricyclic antidepressants

Normal variant

Orthostatic hypotension (as medication-induced)

Post-micturition syncope

Seizure disorders

Shock/congestive heart failure

Subclavian steal syndrome

Syncope (Neurocardiogenic syncope)

Vasovagal stimuli

Others

Source: Rowlett JD, Greydanus DE. *The Cardiovascular System in Adolescent Medicine*, 3d ed., Hoffmann AD, Greydanus DE (eds.), Stamford, CT: Appleton & Lange, 1997, Chap. 12, pp. 147–173.

Greydanus DE, Patel D, Pratt H, Bhave S, (eds.). Cardiovascular disorders. *India Manual of Adolescent Medicine, Review of Adolescent Medicine*, New Delhi, India: Cambridge Press, 2002, Vol. 6, pp. 34–57.

be hypotension-related and correctable by medical measures alone. The recently described Brugada syndrome has a high risk of sudden death with exercise and has been preceded by a syncope event in ~80% of cases; pediatric and young adult cases have been reported (Priori, 2001).

Reference

Priori SG, Aliot E, Blomstrom-Lundquist C, et al. Task force on sudden death of the European society of cardiology. *Eur Heart J* 22:1418, 2001.

DYSRHYTHMIAS, PALPITATION, AND ANXIETY-PANIC ATTACKS

Cardiac rhythm disorders can range from anxiety with cardiac palpitations to paroxysmal supraventricular tachycardia or atrial flutter or fibrillation in the adolescent patient. Ventricular dysrhythmias, such as ventricular tachycardia and ventricular fibrillation, are the most feared but fortunately are uncommon, unless associated with long and/or short QT syndromes or cardiomyopathy-related to exercise precipitation of sudden death events. (Table 9-7). Preexcitation syndromes and other types of aberrant conduction abnormalities and second or third degree heart block can also present with cardiac syncope or cardiac symptoms. Documentation in such patients is by ECG, Holter monitor, event monitor studies or electrophysiologic mapping. When studies are not abnormal, this helps manage the adolescent's cardiac concerns.

Hypertrophic cardiomyopathy, coronary artery anomalies, long QT syndromes, and Marfan syndrome remain the top four causes of sudden cardiac death for adolescents and young adults. Syncope and chest pain may be the only presenting symptoms or they may be entirely asymptomatic until their sudden cardiac demise. Sport participation, training, and other exercise-related activities often can precipitate the symptoms of severe dizziness or syncope; unfortunately some will have only their sudden unexpected death.

Exercise-related tachyarrhythmias occur with preexcitation syndromes, long and short QT syndromes, Brugada syndrome, coronary artery anomalies, and other cardiac entities. Only about 20% of the coronary artery anomalies are diagnosed prior to sudden death. Exertional chest pain or syncope with exercise-related ECG changes was the only early warning sign in these patients. Basilico's review of multiple sudden cardiac death studies in athletes demonstrated that between 42% and 57% of the sudden deaths were cardiomyopathy related (Basilico, 1999). Patients with long QT syndrome have a QTc of over 460 milliseconds, preferably over 500 milliseconds for the diagnosis. Once diagnosed, it can have significant reduction in the

TABLE 9-7

PATHOPHYSIOLOGY OF ADOLESCENT SYNCOPE

Vasomotor CV	Cardiac Structural	Noncardiac Causes
Neurocardiac	**Obstructive Anomalies**	**Central Nervous System**
vaso-vagal	Aortic stenosis	Seizures
(*most common*)	HCM (Cardiomyopathy)	Migraine
Increased Vagal Tone	Coarctation of Aorta	**Metabolic-Endocrine**
Fear, anxiety	**Dysrhythmias**	Hypoglycemia
Adolescents	Long or short QTc interval	Hyperglycemia
Athletes	SVT; VT; AF	Toxins-Poisoning
Reflex	W-P-W; Heart block	**Psychiatric/Psychological**
Cough, hair grooming	Pacemaker dysfunction	Hyperventilation/ Hysterical
Positional, micturition	**Cardiac LV Dysfunction**	Drug abuse
Orthostatic	CHF	
Dehydration	Coronary artery anomalies	
Blood loss		

(Abbreviations: HCM = Hypertrophic cardiomyopathy; SVT = Supraventricular tachycardia; VT = Ventricular tachycardia; AF = Atrial fibrillation; WPW = Preexcitation syndrome or Wolff-Parkinson-White syndrome; CHF = Congestive heart failure)

sudden death risk with the use of beta-blocker medications. Several series have reported reductions from a 60% to 70% sudden death to ~6% in long QT syndrome patients (Luckstead, 2002). Unfortunately, some undiagnosed youth with long QT syndrome will have sudden death as their first and last symptom. Routine ECG's will only diagnose about 10% of long QT individuals; long QT syndrome patients most often present with syncope (30%), palpitations (15%), seizures (10%), and cardiac arrest (9%). There is a 30% positive family history for long QT syndrome. Intense aerobic activity and competitive sports can be lethal but if on medication recreational activities are selectively usually permissible.

Bibliography

Basilico FC. Cardiovascular disease in athletes. *Am J Sports Med* 27(1):108–120, 1999.

Luckstead EF. Cardiac risk factors and participation guidelines for youth sports. *Pediatr Clin N Am* 49: 681–707, 2002.

Luckstead EF. Cardiovascular disorders in the college student. *Pediatr Clin N Am* 52:243–278, 2005.

Priori SG, Aliot E, Blomstrom-Lundquist C, et al. Task force on sudden death of the European Society of Cardiology. *Eur Heart J* 22:1418, 2001.

Wever EFD, Robles de Medina EO. Sudden death in patients without structural heart disease. *J Am Coll Cardiol* 43:1137–1144, 2004.

ACQUIRED HEART PROBLEMS IN THE ADOLESCENT

Rheumatic Fever and Rheumatic Heart Disease

Rheumatic fever is the leading cause of acquired heart disease in the world for children, adolescents, and young adults; however, it is now second to Kawasaki disease in the United States. The peak incidence of rheumatic fever occurs in late childhood (ages of 7–10) and late adolescence, between ages of 18 and 21. ARF is a collagen vascular disease involving multiple body systems in the body, but the highest risk is the degree of cardiac involvement. An antigen-antibody immunologic hypersensitivity reaction occurs within 2 to 3 weeks after an untreated or partially treated pharyngitis due to Group A, beta-hemolytic streptococcus; this causes the clinical presentation of acute rheumatic fever. Those with an acute rheumatic fever episode are at a greater risk for recurrent disease, especially in the first year and for the following five years. Rheumatic fever does not occur following streptococcal skin diseases such as impetigo. Approximately 2%–3% of untreated pharyngitis caused by Group A, beta-hemolytic streptococcus will result in the sequelae of ARF; it has been reported to be higher during certain high "streptococcal exposure" periods. A suggested list for the differential diagnosis for ARF is shown in Table 9-8.

According to the revised Jones criteria, major clinical manifestations for rheumatic fever are

TABLE 9-8

DIFFERENTIAL DIAGNOSIS OF RHEUMATIC FEVER

Infective endocarditis

Infectious mononucleosis

Chorea (see Table 9-7)

Kawasaki syndrome (uncommon in patients over age 5 years)

Henoch Schönlein purpura

Lyme disease

Myocarditis

Mixed collagen—vascular disease

Pericarditis

Rheumatoid arthritis

Rubella arthritis

Septic arthritis

Serum sickness

SLE (systemic lupus erythematosus)

Uremia

Others

Source: Rowlett JD, Greydanus DE. *The Cardiovascular System in Adolescent Medicine*, 3d ed., Hoffmann AD, Greydanus DE (eds.) Stamford, CT: Appleton & Lange, 1997, Chap. 12, pp. 147–173.
Greydanus DE, Patel D, Pratt H, Bhave S, (eds.). Cardiovascular disorders. *India Manual of Adolescent Medicine, Review of Adolescent Medicine*, New Delhi, India: Cambridge Press, 2002, Vol. 6, pp. 34–57.

carditis, polyarthritis, chorea, erythema marginatum, and subcutaneous nodules. Minor manifestations include the presence of arthralgia, fever (over 39°C), and positive laboratory tests (i.e., increased erythrocyte sedimentation rate, increased C-reactive protein, or prolonged PR interval on an ECG). The presence of two major manifestations or one major (with the exception of subcutaneous nodules or erythema marginatum alone) with two minor manifestations strongly suggests ARF as the diagnosis. Additional clinical features may include epistaxis, precordial pain, pneumonia, pulmonary edema, atelectasis, abdominal pain, and/or anemia. Supportive evidence of a preceding Group A beta-hemolytic streptococcal infection includes a positive throat culture for this organism (or a positive rapid streptococcal antigen test) with increased or rising streptococcal antibody titers of antistreptolysin O (ASO: above 250–300 Todd units), anti-streptokinase, anti-hyaluronidase, anti-Dnase B (antideoxyribonuclease B) or anti-DPNase (antidiphosphopyridine nucleotidase).

Carditis

Approximately 50% of rheumatic fever patients develop carditis; younger children and adolescents develop this complication more often than older patients do. The endocardium is most commonly involved, followed in order of frequency by the myocardium and pericardium. Carditis develops within 3 weeks of the infection and may follow the presentation of arthritis. If both major manifestations occur, one is typically more severe than the other. When chorea occurs, carditis (sometimes mild) is present ~30% of the time. Rheumatic fever patients with severe carditis may have tachycardia and moderate to severe valvulitis, usually with the murmur suggestive of moderate to severe mitral regurgitation (Carey-Coombs murmur) or mild to moderate aortic valve regurgitation. Both aortic valve and mitral valve insufficiency, when seen together clinically or by echocardiographic studies, strongly suggest the diagnosis of ARF. ARF is easily diagnosed when it is moderate to severe in degree, particularly in the 7–10-year old or adolescent–young adult age ranges. When ARF occurs between ages 3 and 5, it is typically severe and has a carditis presentation.

Congestive heart failure occurs when the myocardium is primarily involved; however, pericardial friction rubs and rapidly developing pericardial effusion with possible tamponade present the highest ARF lethal risk factor. Myocarditis can present with a broad range of clinical features, ranging from minimal findings (such as prolonged PR interval) to severe clinical myocarditis with congestive heart failure. Pericarditis also varies in symptoms, with decreased heart sounds, friction rub, chest pain and significant ECG ST-T wave changes. Pericardial effusion can lead to cardiac tamponade and should be aggressively treated. Youth with findings of pericardial effusion and no valvulitis may not have rheumatic fever, but other disorders instead such as systemic lupus erythematosus (SLE), mixed collagen vascular disease, infectious pericarditis, or juvenile rheumatoid arthritis. Usually such non-rheumatic fever disorders with pericardial effusions are less severe and less likely to have tamponade. Subcutaneous nodule and erythema marginatum (or annulare) can accompany severe carditis in ARF patients.

Arthritis

The most common major manifestation of ARF is arthritis, developing in at least 80% of adolescents and 95% of adults. Typically, one or more joints become swollen, tender, and warm; large joints are involved (i.e., knees, ankles, elbows, wrists) in a classical migratory fashion. Back pain and a preference not to be moved around in bed are common clinical ARF presentations. Abdominal pain may accompany the clinical symptoms with arthritis or other complaints. Any major joint can be involved, but less than six are typically involved at any one time. Joint symptoms may evolve over several days to weeks if not treated; however, salicylates or non-steroidal medication can dramatically improve the clinical symptoms and signs within 1–2 days. The arthritis of rheumatic fever is essentially a benign condition and permanent joint damage is not seen. When salicylates or nonsteroidal medications do not cause major and rapid joint symptom improvement

consider other diagnoses, such as *Neisseria gonorrhea* arthritis, septic arthritis, and reactive arthritis. If a septic joint is suspected, arthrocentesis is needed to obtain a joint cell count, Gram's stain, and bacterial cultures.

Chorea (Sydenham's Chorea; St. Vitus Dance)

Chorea may develop several months after the throat infection and is characterized by choreiform movements of the extremities and trunk. There are involuntary, sudden, and purposeless motions that stop during sleep and can be unilateral. Muscle weakness and emotional liability are common. Snapping or hyper-reactive deep tendon knee reflexes are noted. Chorea may be an isolated manifestation but does occur in 25%–30% with mild carditis; the cardiac involvement is usually characterized by mild mitral regurgitation appearing with the chorea or up to 2 or 3 months after the chorea develops. An echocardiogram may reveal evidence of the associated chronic mild rheumatic heart disease. Those with isolated chorea will not have serologic evidence of a recent streptococcal infection. A cross reaction of antibodies directed at both brain tissue and streptococci is identified as causing the CNS changes; an MRI may reveal changes in the patient's basal ganglia. Table 9-9 lists the differential diagnosis of chorea. Chorea can be a serious manifestation of rheumatic fever and last many weeks to months, ultimately resolving without complications. Chronic psychologic behavior changes and minor relapses are not uncommon.

Physicians should have orders simplifying the sleeping and hospital environment by minimizing external stimuli, limiting visitors, and limiting activities, such as TV watching. Severe cases may need medications such as haloperidol to treat, modify, and shorten the chorea signs. Sedation and joint padding to prevent injury are other helpful management principles. The family and particularly the school and teachers, need guidance as these patients go through their recovery period. Handwriting deterioration is often an early school sign of Sydenham's chorea along with their changing emotional lability; teachers often recognize symptoms before the parents and

TABLE 9-9

DIFFERENTIAL DIAGNOSIS OF CHOREA

Ataxia/athetosis
Benign familial chorea
Chorea
Conversion Reactions
Drug Reactions
Gilles de la Tourette syndrome
Habit tics
Huntington's chorea
Hyperthyroid chorea
Simple restlessness
SLE (systemic lupus erythematosus)
Wilson's disease

Source: Rowlett JD, Greydanus DE. *The Cardiovascular System in Adolescent Medicine*, 3d ed., Hoffmann AD, Greydanus DE (eds.) Stamford, CT: Appleton & Lange, 1997, Chap. 12, pp. 147–173.
Greydanus DE, Patel D, Pratt H, Bhave S, (eds.). Cardiovascular disorders. *India Manual of Adolescent Medicine, Review of Adolescent Medicine*, New Delhi, India: Cambridge Press, 2002, Vol. 6, pp. 34–57.

friends. Recovery may be monitored to some degree by the handwriting and emotional lability improvement, since erythrocyte sedimentation rate and other tests are not helpful.

Erythema Marginatum

Less than 10% of those with rheumatic fever develop this dermal manifestation characterized as a fleeting, pink, macular rash involving the trunk and proximal extremities; the face is not involved. It may disappear even as one looks at it. Erythema marginatum is a nonpruritic rash that is nonindurated, blanches with pressure, and may be noted with heat. It is probably a vasomotor phenomenon and may appear in a migratory fashion for several weeks or months. When circular, it is called *erythema annulare*. It should never be used as the sole major criteria for the diagnosis of ARF.

Subcutaneous Nodules

These nodules are firm, usually nontender (can be tender) and are freely mobile in the subcutaneous tissue; the skin is not involved. They range in size from 0.1 to 2.0 cm and may be single or multiple; they usually disappear in 1–2 weeks. The subcutaneous nodules of rheumatic fever are typically located over the extensor regions of the wrists, elbows, and knees; other locations include the back vertebral spinous processes (thoracic or lumbar), the occiput, buttocks, and Achilles tendons. Subcutaneous nodules are an uncommon feature of rheumatic fever, but when present, are typically found only with acute carditis or subacute carditis; they may not be seen until several weeks after the carditis appears. If these nodules are isolated without carditis and do not disappear in a few weeks, other disorders should be suspected, such as rheumatoid arthritis, sarcoidosis, collagen-vascular disorders, and neoplastic disease.

Summary: Rheumatic Fever

The major long-term complication of rheumatic fever is the development of chronic rheumatic heart disease, especially from those patients with acute carditis or chorea. Prevention of rheumatic heart disease is most successful by the appropriate treatment of Group A beta-hemolytic streptococcal pharyngitis in all patients (Chap. 7). Recurrence rates of rheumatic heart disease are the greatest during the first year and the succeeding five years after the first episode. Highest risk periods are from 5 to 15 years with peaks at 7–10 years and 18–21 years. Children between the ages 3 and 5 will typically have severe carditis as their acute disease. ARF has not been seen below 3 years of age. There is a known familial predisposition for ARF. Those with rheumatic valvular heart disease will need SBE prophylaxis for life.

Suggested Readings

Berrios X, del Camp E, Guzman B, et al. Discontinuing rheumatic fever prophylaxis in selected adolescents and young adults. *Ann Intern Med* 118:401, 1993.

Danjani A, Taubert K, Ferrieri P, et al. Treatment of acute streptococcal pharyngitis and prevention of rheumatic fever: A statement for health professionals. *Pediatrics* 96:758, 1995.

Luckstead EF. Cardiovascular disorders in the college student. *Pediatr Clin N Am* 52:243–278, 2005.

Jones TD. Diagnosis of rheumatic fever. *JAMA* 126:481, 1944.

Newburger JW, Takahashi, M, Gerber MA, et al. Diagnosis, treatment, and long-term management of Kawasaki disease. *Pediatrics* 114:1708–1733, 2004.

Sondheimer HM, Lorts A. Cardiac involvement in inflammatory disease: Systemic Lupus Erythematosus, Rheumatic fever and Kawasaki disease. *Adolesc Med* 12:69–78, 2001.

Special Writing Group of the Committee on Rheumatic Fever, Endocarditis, and Kawasaki Disease of the Council on Cardiovascular Disease in the Young of the American Heart Association. *JAMA* 268:2069, 1992.

Vincent MV, Demers DM, Bass JW. Infectious exanthems and unusual infections. (Kawasaki syndrome). *Adolesc Med* 11:327–358, 2000.

OTHER INFECTIOUS CARDIAC DISEASES

Infective Endocarditis

Infective endocarditis occurs after bacterial vegetations infect heart tissue, typically endothelial valves (damaged or prosthetic) or a site opposite a ventricular septal defect. Underlying factors do include congenital heart disease, intravenous drug use, central venous catheters, mitral valve prolapse with mitral insufficiency, and others. Acute endocarditis may develop rapidly in heart tissue and present as a toxic-appearing patient with fever and evidence of embolic phenomena. Subacute endocarditis may occur in a youth with preexisting heart disease and the subtle presentation may take weeks or months; minimal fever and occasional embolic events may be seen. However, the line between clinical presentations of acute versus subacute disease may be mixed. Infective endocarditis in youth is most often due to *Streptococcus viridans, Staphylococcus epidermidis* or *Staphylococcus aureus. Candida albicans* is most often the offender at the tricuspid valve from those using drugs intravenously. Many other organisms may be implicated in specific cases, including pneumococci, enterococci, Gram-negative bacilli, anaerobes, fungi, and others. Infective endocarditis symptoms are listed in Table 9-10. The differential diagnosis includes rheumatic heart disease and SLE. Blood cultures taken during periods of elevated temperature increase the chances of identifying the causative organism; multiple (at least three)

TABLE 9-10

SIGNS AND SYMPTOMS: INFECTIVE ENDOCARDITIS

Fever
Fatigue and malaise
Nail bed splinter hemorrhages
Osler's nodes (tender subcutaneous embolic lesions in distal extremities)
Janeway and Roth nodes
Changing heart murmurs (mitral, aortic and tricuspid valve sites)
Retinal hemorrhages
Splenomegaly
Clubbing
Abscesses or infarctions due to septic embolic to the brain, lungs or kidneys
Congestive heart failure
Cerebrovascular accident

Source: Rowlett JD, Greydanus DE. *The Cardiovascular System in Adolescent Medicine*, 3d ed., Hoffmann AD, Greydanus DE (eds.) Stamford, CT: Appleton & Lange, 1997, Chap. 12, pp. 147–173.

Greydanus DE, Patel D, Pratt H, Bhave S, (eds.). Cardiovascular disorders. *India Manual of Adolescent Medicine, Review of Adolescent Medicine*, New Delhi, India: Cambridge Press, 2002, Vol. 6, pp. 34–57.

cultures are recommended. Echocardiography usually diagnoses the valve or septal defect lesions of infective endocarditis. There can also be anemia, leukocytosis, elevated erythrocyte sedimentation rate, and microscopic hematuria. Aggressive bacterial-sensitive antibiotic treatment is important to sterilize the blood and reduce the vegetative lesion; occasionally surgical removal of the vegetations may be necessary. Complications such as embolization are frequent and the mortality rate can approach 20%.

Clinicians need to follow published SBE standards for endocarditis prophylaxis when patients at risk have various invasive-type procedures (Dajani, 1997; Prevention, 2001). High risk populations for endocarditis include those with previous endocarditis, prosthetic valves, complex forms of cyanotic congenital heart disease, high pressure left to right shunts (i.e., ventricular septal defects and A/V canal), aortic or pulmonic valve stenosis, and surgical aortic-pulmonary shunts (such as Blalock-Taussig shunts). Those at moderate risk include patients with acquired valvular dysfunction (i.e., chronic rheumatic heart disease), hypertrophic cardiomyopathy, mitral valve prolapse, and other congenital heart disease.

Those with similar risks as the general population and not requiring SBE precautions include youth with repaired atrial septal defects, patent ductus arteriosus or ventricular septal defects without residual after 6 months endothelization of the cardiac operative site. Others anomalies include nonoperative isolated secundum atrial septal defects, mitral valve prolapse without mitral insufficiency, pacemakers, and those with Kawasaki disease or rheumatic fever without valvular heart disease. Not all procedures require SBE prophylaxis; filling cavities, local dental anesthesia, incision, or biopsy of surgically scrubbed skin does not need SBE precautions. However, other procedures need SBE precautions, including teeth cleaning and/or extraction, and any type of body piercing.

Bibliography

Bayer AS, Bolger AF, Taubert KA, et al. Diagnosis and management of infective endocarditis and its complications. *Circulation* 98:2936–2948, 1998.

Ceatta F, Podlecki CD, Bell TJ. Adolescent knowledge of bacterial endocarditis prophylaxis. *J Adolesc Health* 14:540, 1994.

Danjani A, Taubert K, Ferrieri P, et al. Treatment of acute streptococcal pharyngitis and prevention of rheumatic fever: A statement for health professionals. *Pediatrics* 96:758, 1995.

Luckstead EF. Cardiovascular disorders in the college student. *Pediatr Clin N Am* 52:243–278, 2005;

Prevention of bacterial endocarditis. *Med Lett* 43:98, 2001.

Wilson WR, Karchmer AW, Dajani AS, et al. Antibiotic treatment of adults with infective endocarditis due to streptococci, enterococci, staphylococci, and HACEK microorganisms. *JAMA* 274:1706–1713, 1995.

MYOCARDITIS

Myocarditis in the adolescent patient is often caused by a viral infection. Most are enteroviruses but one also now finds adenovirus, cytomegalovirus, and other viruses. Other etiologies may be toxins, bacteria

(*Corynebacterium diphtheria* in nonimmunized youth), syphilis (*Treponema pallidum*), Rickettsial (Q fever; Rocky Mountain spotted fever), protozoal (Chagas'; malaria), collagen vascular disorders (SLE, JRA), sarcoidosis, rheumatic fever, dilated cardiomyopathy, mitochondrial disorders, storage disorders, and others. Myocarditis has a wide spectrum from the asymptomatic patient to severe manifestations such as congestive heart failure, arrhythmias, and sudden death. One should suspect myocarditis in any adolescent presenting with congestive heart failure or ventricular tachycardia of an unknown etiology. The erythrocyte sedimentation rate, C-reactive protein (CRP) and cardiac isoenzymes are usually increased; viral cultures, IgM and IgG studies may later occasionally isolate the specific virus. The chest x-ray and EKG are often abnormal in myocarditis; echocardiograms help document the myocardial dysfunction. An endomyocardial biopsy increases the likelihood for a specific myocardial causative agent. Management includes anti-arrhythmic drugs, pericardiocentesis, analgesics, and high-dose intravenous gamma globulin. The long-term prognosis varies, ranging from full recovery in most; eventual heart transplantation may be needed in severe cases.

PERICARDITIS

Infectious causes of pericarditis include viral (as with myocarditis), tuberculosis, other bacteria from a focus (*S. aureus, Hemophilus influenza, Neisseria meningitidis, Neisseria gonorrhoeae*, Salmonella), and fungal (Histoplasmosis and others with immune compromised hosts). Noninfectious causes of pericarditis include rheumatic fever, (during an acute attack), post-pericardiotomy syndrome (postoperative in cardiac patients 5–14 days after surgery), collagen vascular disorders (SLE, JRA), uremia, and malignant lymphoma as well as metastatic diseases. Pericarditis may also occur from medications used to manage collagen vascular disorders; another form of this disorder is idiopathic autoimmune pericarditis.

Symptoms include fever, chest pain (worse when supine), respiratory distress, abdominal pain, and if tamponade is present, shock. On physical examination one can detect a friction rub (may be absent in larger effusions), pulsus paradoxus (over 13 mmHg), jugular venous distension, and distant heart sounds. The chest x-ray shows a globular or dilated left ventricle while the EKG reveals ST segment elevation and/or T wave changes and decreased voltages. The echocardiogram shows pericardial effusion when it is present.

Treatment depends on the etiology and severity of the pericarditis. Pericardiocentesis is used for cardiac tamponade, diagnosis, and treatment for bacterial or mycobacterial disease. Nonsteroidal anti-inflammatory drugs (NSAIDs) or steroids are given after pericardiotomy; aspirin, or steroids are indicated for rheumatic fever. Intravenous immune globulin is given for Kawasaki myocarditis while NSAIDs are given for idiopathic autoimmune pericarditis. Dialysis is used for pericarditis resulting in uremia. Any underlying malignancy must be treated when this is the cause of the pericarditis.

Suggested Readings

Luckstead EF. Cardiovascular disorders in the college student. *Pediatr Clin N Am* 52:243–278, 2005.
Towbin JA. Myocarditis and pericarditis in adolescents. *Adolesc Med* 12:47–68, 2001.

SUDDEN DEATH

Causes of sudden death in adolescents are listed in Table 9-11; an incidence of 1:100,000 to 1:300,000 is described. Family and personal history for cardiac disease helps identify youth with cardiac-induced sudden death potential. A careful medical examination is also important, especially with a history of dyspnea, syncope, angina, or a family history of sudden death. The most common cause of sudden death in the adolescent or young adult athletes in the United States is hypertrophic cardiomyopathy (HCM) (36%); an echocardiogram will help make the diagnosis. Coronary artery anomalies include coronary artery aneurysms and abnormal left coronary artery (absence or anomalous origin); they represent 24% of sudden death

TABLE 9-11

CARDIAC CAUSES OF SUDDEN DEATH IN YOUTH

Aortic valve stenosis (~1%)
Arrhythmias
Atrial septal defect (post-surgical or post-interventional closure)
Blunt trauma (Commotio Cordis)
Brugada syndrome
Coarctation of aorta
Congenital heart block (third degree, Mobitz type II)
Drug-induced arrhythmias (cocaine with or without heroin)
Ehlers-Danlos Syndrome
Hypertrophic cardiomyopathy (CHM) (36%)
Increased cardiac mass (not CHM) (10%)
Kawasaki disease (prior history of disease as infant or child; later youth manifestation)
Long QT syndrome (congenital; acquired)
Marfan syndrome with ruptured aorta (4%)
Mitral value prolapse
Myocarditis
RV arrhythmogenic cardiomyopathy
Short QT syndrome
Tetralogy of Fallot (postoperative arrhythmias)
Transposition of Great Vessels (postoperative arrhythmias)
Wolff-Parkinson-White syndrome

Luckstead EF. Cardiac risk factors and participation guidelines for youth sports. *Pediatr Clin N Am* 49:681–707, 2002.

cases. Increased cardiac mass (not HCM) causes 10% of cases while a ruptured aorta in Marfan syndrome (see next topic) represents about 5% of sudden death cases. Those with AS (4%) usually have a classic loud systolic murmur at the right sternal border with radiation to the neck. Various lethal arrhythmias may occur, as noted with the long QT syndrome, short QT syndrome and the Wolff-Parkinson-White syndrome. Cocaine is a classic illicit drug that can invoke lethal cardiac arrhythmias especially when combined with alcohol or heroin to enhance the euphoria (Chap. 34).

Suggested Readings

Liberthson RR. Sudden death from cardiac causes in children and young adults. *N Engl J Med* 334:1039, 1996.

Luckstead EF. Cardiovascular disorders in the college student. *Pediatr Clin N Am* 52:243-278, 2005.

Maron BJ, Shirani J, Poliac LC, et al. Sudden death in young competitive athletes. *JAMA* 1276:199, 1996.

Maron BJ, Thompson PD, Puffer JC, et al. Cardiovascular preparticipation screening of competitive athletes. A statement for health professionals from the Sudden Death Committee (Clinical Cardiology) and Congenital Cardiac Defects Committee (Cardiovascular Disease in the Young), American Heart Association. *Circulation* 94:850–856, 1996.

Shaddy RE. Cardiomyopathies in adolescents: dilated, hypertrophic, and restrictive. *Adolesc Med* 12:35–45, 2001.

Walsh CA. Syncope and sudden death in the adolescent. *Adolesc Med* 12:105–132, 2001.

SYNDROMES WITH CARDIAC FEATURES

Marfan Syndrome

This autosomal dominant connective tissue disorder has a wide phenotypic expression and a prevalence of 4–10 per 100,000. A mutation in the glycoprotein fibrillin gene on chromosome 15 has been identified; spontaneous mutation is the cause in 25% (Chap. 21). These are tall (compared to first-degree relatives) and slender youth with very long extremities in which the arm span is longer than the height. A classic feature is arachnodactyly or spider fingers along with dolichostenomelia (long, narrow head) and a high arched palate with dental crowding. The joints are hyperextensible and joint dislocations are common, especially in the hip joint. As many as 75% have scoliosis with or without kyhphosis. In addition to the classic cardiac defects (see Table 9-12), a wide variety of features may be found: eye defects (ectopia lentis, myopia with retinal detachment, strabismus, nystagmus, megalocornea, cataracts, coloboma, iris tremor), chest wall defects (pectus excavatum or carinatum), pulmonary defects (spontaneous pneumothorax,

TABLE 9-12

CARDIAC DEFECTS OF MARFAN SYNDROME

Abdominal aortic aneurysm (can be dissecting)
Aortic dissection
Aortic insufficiency
Aortic root dilatation (due to medial cystic necrosis)
Arrhythmias (such as ventricular types, Long Q-T syndrome, others)
Calcification of mitral annulus (under 40 years of age)
Endocarditis
Mitral regurgitation
Mitral valve prolapse (often first sign in pediatric age or infants)
Pulmonary artery dilation
Thoracic aortic aneurysm (can be dissecting)

Source: Rowlett JD, Greydanus DE. *The Cardiovascular System in Adolescent Medicine*, 3d ed., Hoffmann AD, Greydanus DE (eds.) Stamford, CT: Appleton & Lange, 1997, Chap. 12, pp. 147–173.

Greydanus DE, Patel D, Pratt H, Bhave S, (eds.). Cardiovascular disorders. *India Manual of Adolescent Medicine, Review of Adolescent Medicine*, New Delhi, India: Cambridge Press, 2002, Vol. 6, pp. 34–57.

apical blebs), hernias (inguinal, diaphragmatic, umbilical, incision), striae cutis distensae, pes planus, renal ectopy, and others.

Marfan syndrome is diagnosed by physical examination of the youth and the family history. Diagnosis requires one major criterion in one organ system and one minor criterion in another organ system if there is a positive family history. Without a positive family history, one major criteria is required in two different organ systems and another minor criteria in a third organ system; major organ systems include the cardiovascular, ophthalmologic, central nervous, and musculoskeletal systems. The differential diagnosis includes homocystinuria, Ehlers-Danlos syndrome, Marfanoid hypermobility syndrome, and familial mitral valve prolapse syndrome. An echocardiogram, chest x-ray, and slit lamp examination are important parts of this diagnostic assessment; these procedures are repeated periodically in patients with Marfan syndrome. The most recent mean survival age for males with Marfan syndrome in the United States is 43 and 46 years for females. However, age ranges may be increased significantly from earlier and increased use of beta blockers in children and adolescents along with earlier aggressive aortic arch surgery, thus decreasing vascular complications.

Comprehensive management for these youth is required for such maximal longevity. For example, surgical correction of aortic root dilation when it reaches 6 cm measured by echocardiography has been shown to prevent premature death. Beta-blocker medications are recommended early before significant aortic dilation occurs and after prophylactic graft replacement for aortic dilation; many use these medications when the aortic root is questionably enlarged. Aortic rupture during sports-related exertion can occur, especially in sports with high static demand (isometric) activities and those with possible acceleration-deceleration impact injury. Marfan syndrome remains the fourth leading cause of sudden death in athletes. Pregnant adolescents with Marfan syndrome who have aortic dilatation and chest pain need careful evaluation to rule out dissecting aortic aneurysms. Yearly ophthalmologic evaluation is mandatory to detect minor lens dislocation and other eye abnormalities. SBE prophylaxis is important if structural aortic, mitral, and tricuspid valve defects are present. Genetic counseling is important for all families since this is an autosomal dominant disorder.

Suggested Readings

De Paepe A, Devereux RB, Dietz HC, et al. Revised diagnostic criteria for the Marfan syndrome. *Am J Med Genet* 62:417, 1996.

Luckstead EF. Cardiovascular disorders in the college student. *Pediatr Clin N Am* 52:243–278, 2005.

Kainulainen K, Pulkkinen L, Savolainen A, et al. Location on chromosome 15 of the gene defect causing Marfan syndrome. *N Engl J Med* 323:935, 1990.

Pyeritz RE. Disorders of vascular fragility: Implications for active patients. PSM 29(6):53–60, 2001

Shores J, Berger KR, Murphy EA, et al. Progression of aortic dilatation and the benefit of long-term beta-adrenergic blockage in Marfan syndrome. *N Engl J Med* 330:1335, 1994.

NOONAN SYNDROME

Noonan syndrome was initially described by Noonan and Emke in 1963 (Chap. 21). Many were included in Turner's original series as "male Turner syndrome" and have similar phenotypic physical appearances with short stature, webbed neck, and broad shield-shaped chests. The most common cardiac anomaly is pulmonic valve stenosis or pulmonic valve dysplasia. Additional anomalies include ASDs and new reports over the past several years that 34% of Noonan cases have HCM.

Suggested Readings

Feit LR. Genetics of congenital heart disease. *Adv Pediatr* 45:267–292, 1998.

Luckstead EF. Cardiovascular disorders in the college student. *Pediatr Clin N Am* 52:243–278, 2005.

TURNER SYNDROME

Turner syndrome also known as ovarian dysgenesis occurs in one in 2000 female births and presents most commonly in 30% with C/A (Chap. 21). Other commonly associated cardiac anomalies are bicuspid aortic valve and AS. This syndrome may present with systemic hypertension and recently reports have shown an increased risk for aortic dissection and rupture. All patients with documented Turner syndrome should have a baseline echocardiogram even if they do not have heart disease.

Suggested Readings

Cunniff C. Turner syndrome. *Adolesc Med* 13:359–366, 2002.

Luckstead EF. Cardiovascular disorders in the college student. *Pediatr Clin N Am* 52:243-278, 2005.

WILLIAMS SYNDROME

One in 20,000 live births has Williams syndrome; they have a deletion of 7q11.23 (Chap. 21). It is characterized by mental retardation (I.Q. between

40 and 80), cocktail or highly social personality, elfin facies, and patients with Williams syndrome look more like each other than actual family members in many cases. Other problems include dental problems (malocclusion, microdontia), early puberty, obesity, central hypotonia, orthopedic defects (with joint limitations), osteoporosis, ocular, and auditory problems (hyperacusis), structural genitourinary anomalies, enuresis, soft lax skin, anxiety, attention-deficit/hyperactivity disorder, and other medical and/or behavioral problems.

This is also a disorder of hypercalcemia with calcium deposition for unexplained reasons. Approximately 80% have cardiovascular defects and typical heart lesions seen in Williams syndrome are supravalvar AS and peripheral pulmonary artery stenosis. Other cardiovascular lesions include renal artery stenosis and systemic hypertension. Any artery can become narrowed due to the structural protein elastin abnormalities. Guidelines for growth-weight curves as well as guidelines for health supervision have been developed by the AAP.

Suggested Reading

Committee on Genetics. American Academy of Pediatrics. Health care supervision for children with Williams syndrome. *Pediatrics* 107:1192–1204, 2001.

THE DISABLED OR MENTALLY CHALLENGED ADOLESCENT WITH HEART DISEASE

Down Syndrome

This is due to trisomy of chromosome 21 and occurs in approximately 1 in 750 births; 3% have congenital cardiac disorders, including A/V canal, VSD, and tetralogy of Fallot. Early development of pulmonary hypertension occurs with high-pressure shunts. Table 9-13 lists classic features of Down syndrome (Chap. 21). As with other youth who have mental retardation and physical defects, comprehensive medical care is important along with special education, psychosocial interventions as needed, and a supportive family milieu.

TABLE 9-13

FEATURES OF DOWN SYNDROME

Atlanto-axial dysplasia
Alzheimer's disease in adults (premature onset)
Cardiac anomalies (50%; different profile of cardiac lesion frequency than non-Down children)
Cataracts and other vision difficulties
Typical facies
  Mild microcephaly
  Box-like shaped head; mandibular hypoplasia
  Upward slanting palpebral fissures and epicanthal folds
  Depressed nasal bridge
  Protruding tongue
Clinodactyly
Dental disorders
Duodenal atresia (and other gastrointestinal disorders) (15%)
Hearing difficulties
Hypogonadism (in males; normal onset of puberty)
Infertility (males)
Leukemoid reaction and leukemia (higher risk)
Mental retardation (varying levels)
Respiratory tract infections (upper and lower)
Seizure disorders
Simian crease (single transverse palmar crease)
Skin infections
Spondylolisthesis
Thyroid dysfunction (Hypothyroid > Hyperthyroid)

Source: Roizen NJ. Medical care and monitoring for the adolescent with Down syndrome. *Adolesc Med* 13:345–358 2002.

Adults with Down syndrome have a decreased life expectancy when compared with the general population.

Down syndrome adolescent age patients have various congenital cardiac anomalies. Their spectrum includes atrial septal and ventricular septal defects, patent ductus arteriosus, endocardial cushion defects, tetralogy of Fallot and Eisenmenger syndrome. For some reason, aortic valve stenosis, pulmonic valve stenosis, coarctation of aorta, TGV and total anomalous pulmonary venous return are rarely seen in Down syndrome patients. There is definitely an earlier and higher risk of secondary pulmonary hypertension in un-operated high pressure left to right shunts. Surgical correction before 6 months of age usually prevents secondary pulmonary hypertension (Eisenmenger syndrome) from developing later in the adolescent and young adult Down syndrome patient.

Suggested Readings

Curry C. Rational evaluation of the adolescent with mental retardation. *Adolesc Med* 13:331–343, 2002.
Down syndrome. Patient page. *JAMA* 285:1112, 2001.
Roizen NJ. Medical care and monitoring for the adolescent with Down syndrome. *Adolesc Med* 13:345–358 2002.

FRAGILE X SYNDROME

This is an X-linked dominant disorder of reduced penetrance with a marker on the distal long arm of the X chromosome (Xq27.3). Approximately one in 1400 males and one in 2500 females are affected and the Fragile X syndrome represents the most common cause of mental retardation (Chap. 21). Other conditions associated with mental retardation include Down syndrome, Williams syndrome, Prader-Willi syndrome, neurofibromatosis, meningomyelocele, cerebral palsy, and autism (Chap. 21). Features of the Fragile X syndrome are listed in Table 9-14. Cardiac

TABLE 9-14

FEATURES OF FRAGILE X SYNDROME

Antisocial features with gaze aversion, turning the body away to avoid social interaction)
Attention-deficit/hyperactivity disorder
Autistic-like features
Cardiac defects (see text)
Craniofacial dysmorphism (relative macrocephaly, large ears, prominent chin)
Finger-joint hypermobility and other connective tissue defects
Hyperactivity
Language deficit
Macro-orchidism (can be prepubertal)
Noise sensitivity
Speech features (high-pitched, jocular, retarded)
Tantrums

Source: Rowlett JD, Greydanus DE. *The Cardiovascular System in Adolescent Medicine*, 3d ed., Hoffmann AD, Greydanus DE (eds.) Stamford, CT: Appleton & Lange, 1997, Chap.12, pp. 147–173.
    Greydanus DE, Patel D, Pratt H, Bhave S, (eds.). Cardiovascular disorders. *India Manual of Adolescent Medicine, Review of Adolescent Medicine*, New Delhi, India: Cambridge Press, 2002, 6:34–57.

defects include mitral valve prolapse and dilatation of the ascending aorta. Table 9-14 also lists behavioral aspects of Fragile X syndrome in males; behavioral aspects in girls include being shy and having social anxiety as well as depression.

10

THE GASTROINTESTINAL TRACT, PANCREAS, AND LIVER

Michael Stephens, Lisa A. Feinberg, Arthur N. Feinberg, and Steven Werlin

GASTROESOPHAGEAL REFLUX

Gastroesophageal reflux (GER), the passage of gastric contents into the esophagus, is a common physiologic event occurring multiple times each day in all individuals. *Gastroesophageal reflux disease* (GERD) occurs when there are symptoms or complications of GER. The most common symptoms in adolescents are heartburn, chest pain, regurgitation, dysphagia, vomiting, and odynophagia. Recently extra-esophageal symptoms, such as asthma and cough, have received increasing attention (Chap. 8). Complications of GERD include bleeding, stricture formation, Barrett's esophagus, and esophageal carcinoma. The usual mechanism of GER is transient lower esophageal sphincter relaxations and, not as is commonly thought, weak lower esophageal sphincter pressure.

The diagnosis of GERD is usually based on the clinical picture. The upper gastrointestinal (GI) series will detect anatomic lesions but is rarely helpful in the patient with suspected GERD. An abnormal esophageal pH probe test predicts the likelihood that a patient has esophagitis, not whether the patient has reflux. Endoscopic gastro-duodenoscopy can be useful to determine whether or not there is esophagitis and to rule out other conditions such as eosinophilic esophagitis, peptic ulcer disease, and strictures, in patients unresponsive to therapy. Clinicians may use the "treat and test" strategy, that is, test only following failure of acid suppression.

Treatment consists of acid suppression and avoidance of acidy and spicy foods, caffeinated as well as alcoholic beverages, and smoking. Nothing should be eaten for 2 hours prior to bedtime. The patient with occasional heartburn can be treated with antacids or over the counter H_2 receptor antagonists (H_2RA). Most adolescents with frequent or chronic heartburn respond to H_2RAs. Those that do not can be treated with proton pump inhibitors (PPIs); PPIs are safe and effective for long term use. For maximum effectiveness PPIs should be taken 15–30 minutes before the morning meal. Adolescents can be given full adult doses of acid suppressants. A typical course of acid suppression is 4–8 weeks. If a patient fails acid suppression or needs repetitive courses of therapy, then a gastroenterology consultation is indicated. Surgical therapy is rarely indicated.

Suggested Readings

Hassal E, Israel D, Shepherd R, et al. Omeprazole for treatment of chronic erosive esophagitis in children: A multicenter study of efficacy, safety tolerability and dose requirements. *J Pediatr* 137:800, 2000.

Hillemeier C. Gastroesophageal reflux in the adolescent. *Adolesc Med* 11:647–662, 2000.

Rudolph CD, Mazur LJ, Liptak GS, et al. Guidelines for the evaluation and treatment of gastroesophageal reflux in infants and children: Recommendations of the North American Society for Pediatric Gastroenterology and Nutrition. *J Pediatr Gastro Nutr* 32(Sup 2):S1, 2001.

Sood MR, Rudolph CD. Gastroesophageal reflux in adolescents. *Adolesc Med* 15:17–36, 2004.

ACHALASIA

Achalasia is a rare motility disorder of the esophagus, occurring in about 0.1/100,000 children per year; only 5% of achalasia patients present during childhood. The underlying mechanism of achalasia is damage to both the intrinsic and extrinsic esophageal innervation (particularly loss of the myenteric plexus), causing lack of esophageal peristalsis and lack of relaxation of the lower esophageal sphincter (LES). The resultant obstruction at the LES leads to dysphagia, odynophagia, and chest pain. At first the dysphagia is mild and intermittent. Eventually polydipsia may develop as the patient increases fluid intake in an attempt to empty the obstructed esophagus. Regurgitation of undigested food, particularly at night, is common. The differential diagnosis of dysphagia is found in Table 10-1.

The diagnosis of achalasia is often suspected on chest x-ray; a megaesophagus and fluid column is frequently visible. The diagnosis can only be made by esophageal manometry. The typical findings include aperistalsis of the esophagus, lack of or incomplete relaxation of the LES, and elevated

TABLE 10-1

DYSPHAGIA IN ADOLESCENTS

Gastroesophageal reflux
Anatomic
Epidermolysis bullosa
Foreign body
Paraesophageal hernia
Stricture
Vascular ring

Collagen vascular disorders
Dermatomyositis/polymyositis
Mixed connective tissue disease
Rheumatoid arthritis
Scleroderma

Disorders of neuromuscular coordination
Cerebral palsy
CNS injury such as anoxic encephalopathy
  and head trauma
Muscular dystrophy
Myasthenia gravis

Esophageal motor disorders
Achalasia
Chagas disease
Diffuse esophageal spasm
Intestinal pseudo-obstruction

Infections
Candida
Cytomegalovirus esophagitis
Herpes simplex esophagitis
Human immunodeficiency virus

Inflammatory
Behçet's disease
Crohn's disease
Eosinophilic esophagitis
Graft vs. host disease
Pill esophagitis

basal LES pressure. Endoscopy should be done to evaluate for other types of obstructing lesions. The treatment of choice is now laparoscopic myotomy to relieve the obstruction. Other treatments include open myotomy and pneumatic dilatation. Injections of botulinum toxin may give relief and are useful as a temporizing treatment in the severely malnourished patient prior to definitive treatment.

Suggested Readings

Hirano I. Achalasia. *Clin Perspect Gastro* 165, 2002.

Vaezi MF, Richter JE. Practice guidelines: Diagnosis and management of achalasia. *Am J Gastroenterol* 94: 3406, 1999.

PEPTIC ULCER DISEASE AND *HELICOBACTER PYLORI*

Primary *peptic ulcer disease* (PUD) occurs in the absence of systemic conditions including inflammatory bowel disease, eosinophilic gastroenteritis, autoimmune gastritis, trauma, sepsis, burns, ingestion of aspirin and NSAIDs (nonsteroidal anti-inflammatory drugs), corticosteroids, antibiotics, and others. It occurs when there is a disturbance in the equilibrium between cytotoxic (i.e., acid, pepsin, bile acids, *Helicobacter pylori* infection) and cytoprotective factors (i.e., mucous layer, bicarbonate secretion, prostaglandins, and mucosal blood flow). Both pepsinogen secretion and the proton pump of the parietal cell, the final common pathway for acid secretion, are influenced by histamine, acetylcholine, and gastrin production. Pepsinogen is converted to pepsin in an acidic medium. The association of *H. pylori* (then known as *Campylobacter pylori*) and PUD was first described in 1983. *H. pylori* produces urease, which breaks urea down into bicarbonate and ammonia, which may be cytotoxic. *H. pylori* produces inherent virulence factors (i.e., vacA, cagA, and cagE), which act to destroy the gastric mucosa. NSAIDs and acetazolamide inhibit bicarbonate secretion, thus predisposing toward ulcer formation. There is an association between *H. pylori* infection and subsequent malignancy (carcinoma, MALT lymphoma).

H. pylori is transmitted person to person (humans are the only known reservoir) by oral-oral or fecal-oral contact; poverty and overcrowding predispose to transmission. It is estimated that 50% of the world population has been infected with *H. pylori* and asymptomatic colonizing is common. The host immune response plays a role in the development of symptomatic disease versus colonization.

Clinical manifestations of PUD include recurrent or chronic epigastric abdominal pain, which may be nocturnal or preprandial. There may be vomiting, with or without blood, and frank or occult blood in the stool. The differential diagnosis of these symptoms includes gastritis, GERD, functional dyspepsia, hepatobiliary disease, and lactose intolerance.

Definitive diagnosis is by endoscopy and biopsy. Imaging studies such as barium contrast radiography are neither sensitive nor specific. Other tests to infer the presence of *H. pylori* such as breath hydrogen tests and serologic studies lack sensitivity and specificity in children. A breath urea test using labeled isotopic urea with recovery of labeled CO_2, indicating the presence of urease-producing *H. pylori*, is helpful for diagnosis. Stool antigen enzyme immunoassay is another noninvasive test with high sensitivity and specificity.

In patients with the above symptoms, laboratory studies are done to rule out pancreatitis, inflammatory bowel disease, hepatobiliary disease, and parasites. A 4–8-week course of acid suppression therapy with either an H_2RA or a proton pump inhibitor is given. Endoscopy and biopsy are performed if there is no symptomatic improvement. Previous acid suppressive therapy decreases the sensitivity of subsequent *H. pylori* tests.

Acid suppression will typically heal an *H. pylori* induced ulcer, but the ulcer will always recur unless the *H. pylori* is eradicated, which requires triple therapy for 7–14 days. Most regimens include a proton pump inhibitor or an H_2RA and two antibiotics. Three commonly used triple therapies employing twice-daily dosages, which contain a proton pump inhibitor and two antibiotics are listed in Table 10-2. Antibiotic resistance and treatment failure may occur in up to 20% of patients.

Suggested Readings

Chelmisky G, Czinn S. Peptic ulcer disease in children. *Pediatr Rev* 20:349, 2001.

Chelmisky G, Blanchard SS, Czinn SJ. Helicobacter pylori in children and adolescents. *Adol Med Clin* 15: 53–66, 2004.

TABLE 10-2
FIRST LINE TRIPLE THERAPY FOR *H. PYLORI*

1. Amoxicillin 50 mg/kg bid for 14 days + clarithromycin 15 mg/kg bid for 14 days + proton pump inhibitor bid for 10–14 days
2. Amoxicillin 50 mg/kg bid for 14 days + metronidazole 20 mg/kg bid for 14 days + proton pump inhibitor bid for 10–14 days
3. Clarithromycin 15 mg/kg bid for 14 days + metronidazole 20 mg/kg bid for 14 days + proton pump inhibitor bid for 10–14 days

Drumm B, Koletzko S, Oderda G. Helicobacter pylori infection in children: A consensus statement. *J Pediatr Gastroenterol Nutr* 30:207, 2000.

Marsh WM. Infectious diseases of the gastrointestinal tract in adolescents *Adolesc Med* 11:263–278, 2000.

INFLAMMATORY BOWEL DISEASES—CROHN'S DISEASE, ULCERATIVE COLITIS

Etiology/Epidemiology

Ulcerative colitis (UC) and *Crohn's disease* (CD) are chronic inflammatory disorders that are classified as inflammatory bowel diseases. Current thinking suggests that patients with a genetically determined predisposition develop an immune mediated response to an environmental trigger, which leads to chronic dysregulated inflammation. The recent discovery of several genes, including *CARD15*, *DLG5*, and the OCTN cation transporter, associated with CD, lends support to this hypothesis. Inflammatory bowel diseases (IBD) are divided into CD and UC based on clinical characteristics (Table 10-3), though at diagnosis 5%–10% of patients do not clearly fit into either category and are termed indeterminate colitis. In the future, genetic factors may help categorize IBD patients more accurately, predicting the likely clinical course and appropriate therapies for individual patients. The incidence of IBD in industrialized countries is increasing more so for CD than UC. Reports range from 5 to 7 cases per 100,000 per year for IBD, 0.2 to 5.3 per 100,000 for CD, and 0.5 to 2.1 per 100,000 for UC.

Signs/Symptoms

Patients with IBD can present with a diverse constellation of signs and symptoms depending on the area of involvement, including abdominal pain, hematochezia, diarrhea, anorexia, nausea, weight loss, fatigue, and oral ulcerations. Signs can include abdominal tenderness, perianal skin tags or fistulae, other fistulae, delayed puberty, iron deficiency anemia, hypoalbuminemia, and signs of extra-intestinal complications. Laboratory tests frequently include an elevated erythrocyte sedimentation rate (ESR) and C reactive protein. IBD is a systemic disease with many extra-intestinal manifestations (Table 10-4).

Evaluation

The diagnosis of IBD is usually confirmed by a combination of clinical observations, and laboratory, radiographic, endoscopic, and histologic findings. The most appropriate diagnostic approach often includes: complete blood count, ESR, CRP,

TABLE 10-3
CHARACTERISTICS OF CROHN'S DISEASE AND ULCERATIVE COLITIS

Crohn's Disease	Ulcerative Colitis
Parenteric	Colon only
Skip lesions	Pancolitis, beginning
Transmural (fistulizing,	at rectum and moving
perforating, structuring)	more proximally
Noncaseating granulomas	Superficial (mucosal)

TABLE 10-4

EXTRA INTESTINAL MANIFESTATIONS OF IBD

Skin	Anemia of chronic
Erythema nodosum	disease
Pyoderma gangrenosum	Thrombocytosis
Perianal disease	Autoimmune
Joints	hemolytic anemia
Arthralgia	**Vascular**
Arthritis	Vasculitis
Ankylosing spondylitis	Thrombosis
Eye	**Kidney**
Uveitis	Nephrolithiasis
Episcleritis	Obstructive
Conjunctivitis	hydronephrosis
Liver	Enterovesical fistula
Primary sclerosing	Urinary tract
cholangitis	infection
Hepatitis	Amyloidosis
Cholelithiasis	**Pancreas**
Bone	Pancreatitis
Osteoporosis	**Lung**
Mouth	Pulmonary vasculitis
Cheilitis	Fibrosing alveolitis
Stomatitis	**Growth**
Aphthous ulcerations	Delayed growth
Blood	Delayed puberty
Iron deficiency anemia	

albumin, and stool specimens to rule out bacterial and protozoal pathogens. Upper endoscopy and colonoscopy with biopsies are key components to confirm the diagnosis. An upper GI series with small bowel follow-through is the primary tool for evaluation of the jejunum and proximal ileum; however, enteroclysis, CT scan, MRI, and WBC scanning show usefulness in selected patients. Capsule endoscopy, a new technique, may prove to be the most sensitive way to assess the small bowel.

Management

Recent advances in immunomodulatory therapy have made the management of IBD mainly the purview of the sub-specialist. As with any chronic disease, a cooperative approach between the sub-specialist and primary care physician is critical. Since there is no cure, the goal of therapy is to achieve sustained remission from disease activity. This is uniquely important in the adolescent as the patient's self-esteem and social functioning can be significantly damaged by uncontrolled disease and complications; these complications include chronic pain, frequent school absences, urgency, short stature, delayed development of secondary sexual characteristics, osteoporosis, need for surgery, and possibly ostomy. Careful monitoring of growth and sexual development is an important component of long-term IBD management.

Medical management includes the use of 5-aminosalicylate (5-ASA) agents such as mesalamine, corticosteroids, antibiotics such as metronidazole, immunomodulating agents including thiopurines (azathioprine or 6-mercaptopurine), methotrexate, infliximab (a monoclonal antibody that binds free and receptor bound TNF-α), cyclosporine, tacrolimus, and mycophenolate. Ensuring adequate nutrition is critical to promote healing and growth. Nutritional therapy, using elemental or polymeric formula as the primary source of nutrition, has been shown to reduce inflammation and is the "frontline" therapy in many Canadian and European IBD centers. Corticosteroids are typically reserved only for brief, acute therapy to control symptoms and are avoided for maintenance therapy because of their long-term side effects. Budesonide, a newer generation corticosteroid, that may have fewer adverse effects, is effective in ileocolonic CD. Since 5-ASA agents provide sustained remission in only a minority of patients, the thiopurines are now the drugs of choice for maintenance of remission.

Surgical management remains an important component of IBD therapy. UC can be cured with colectomy and must be considered in the patient with colitis unresponsive to medical management, steroid dependant, or long-standing disease given the risk of malignancy. Emergent colectomy can be necessary in patients who develop toxic megacolon. Surgery may be required in patients with CD who develop strictures, fistulae, abscesses, and intestinal perforation. There is a high risk of recurrence following surgery for CD and medical therapy should not be discontinued following a surgically created state of remission.

Suggested Readings

Fish D, Kugathasan S. Inflammatory bowel disease. *Adolesc Med* 15:67–90, 2004.

Hanauer SB, Dassopoulos T. Evolving treatment strategies for inflammatory bowel disease. *Annu Rev Med* 52:299, 2001.

Kim SC, Ferry GD. Inflammatory bowel diseases in pediatric and adolescent patients: Clinical, therapeutic, and psychosocial considerations. *Gastroenterology* 126:1550, 2004.

Mamula P, Markowitz JE, Baldassano RN. Inflammatory bowel disease in early childhood and adolescence: Special considerations. *Gastroenterol Clin North Am* 32:967, 2003.

Stephens M, Batres LA, Ng D, et al. Growth failure in the child with inflammatory bowel disease. *Semin Gastrointest Dis* 12:253, 2001.

DIARRHEA

Diarrhea is defined as excess loss of fluid via the intestine, due to increased frequency of stooling, increased volume of stool, or both. Stool output is >10 g/kg per 24 hours in children and >200 g per 24 hours in adults. Mechanisms are secretory, osmotic, inflammatory, or increased/decreased motility. Secretory diarrhea is manifested by increased electrolyte transport stimulated by external secretagogues such as cholera toxin, toxigenic *Escherichia coli*, carcinoid syndrome, vasoactive intestinal polypeptide (VIP), *Clostridium difficile, Cryptosporidium*, and bile salt malabsorption. The diarrhea is watery and the osmolarity is similar to that of serum. Osmotic diarrhea is caused by transport defects, malabsorption or ingestion of solutes, and may be caused by lactase deficiency, complex sugar malabsorption, or excessive ingestion of hyperosmolar laxatives. The diarrhea is watery, acidic, and has an osmolarity greater than that of serum. Diarrhea due to increased intestinal motility is caused most commonly by irritable bowel syndrome (IBS), hyperthyroidism, and infection. Diarrhea

associated with decreased motility is commonly associated with bacterial overgrowth. Inflammatory diarrhea is associated with stool leukocytosis and is seen most commonly in IBD, celiac disease, and bacterial or viral infections.

Differential Diagnosis

The differential diagnosis is broad and may be subdivided into anatomic, infectious, inflammatory/immune/allergic, toxic/metabolic, neoplastic, and functional etiologies. A clinical approach is also outlined (Tables 10-4 to 10-6). Although "short-gut" syndrome typically follows neonatal surgery, an occasional adolescent will develop the short gut syndrome following extensive bowel resection as treatment for a volvulus or Crohn's disease. The lack of surface area leads to malabsorption of fat, including fat soluble vitamins, carbohydrates, protein, and electrolytes. Vitamin B_{12} malabsorption and deficiency may occur if there is loss of the terminal ileum.

Many older children and adolescents are able to compensate for loss of mucosal surface with an increase in the height of the intestinal villi, thus increasing the surface area available for absorption. The mainstay of treatment is total parenteral nutrition (TPN), which accounts for the 90% survival rate from childhood. TPN should be used when necessary, but elemental enteral feedings, should be encouraged with advancement to more complex feedings as tolerated. Complications of TPN include catheter infection, gallstones, cirrhosis and liver failure, and thromboembolism. Abnormal intestinal lymphatic drainage may contribute to long chain fatty acid malabsorption, protein-losing enteropathy, and edema. It may be congenital but in adolescents is often acquired as a consequence of IBD, lymphatic and other neoplasms, radiation enteritis, and mycobacterial infections. Treatment consists of a diet high in medium chain triglycerides, which are absorbed directly and dietary sodium restriction to treat edema.

Bacterial Overgrowth

Bacterial overgrowth syndrome may be due to disorders of peristalsis (scleroderma, intestinal pseudo-obstruction), mechanical stasis due to prior surgery, and short bowel syndrome. Steatorrhea may occur

TABLE 10-5

DIFFERENTIAL DIAGNOSIS OF DIARRHEA IN THE ADOLESCENT

Anatomic

Short bowel syndrome

Fecal impaction with overflow diarrhea

Meckel's diverticulum

Protein losing enteropathy due to intestinal angiectasia

Chronic cholestasis

Infectious agents

Bacterial: *Salmonella, Shigella, E. coli, Campylobacter, Yersinia,* cholera, *Staphylococcus* food poisoning, *Clostridium perfringens, C. difficile* (antibiotic-associated colitis), and so forth

Viral: rotavirus, Norwalk agent, adenovirus, cytomegalovirus, astrovirus, calicivirus, others

Parasitic: *Giardia, Entamoeba, Isospora, Cryptosporidium, Trichuris,* and so forth

Post-gastroenteritis malabsorption syndrome

Bacterial overgrowth secondary to stasis, functional or mechanical

Inflammatory/immune/allergic

IBD: ulcerative colitis, Crohn's disease

Pancreatitis

Celiac disease

Collagen vascular disease: lupus, scleroderma

Henoch-Schönlein purpura (HSP) and hemolytic uremic syndrome (HUS)

Immunodeficiency (HIV, congenital, DiGeorge syndrome)

Allergy (cow milk and soy protein intolerance)

Eosinophilic gastroenteritis

Endocrinopathy (thyrotoxicosis, Addison's disease)

Toxic/metabolic

Pancreatic insufficiency: cystic fibrosis, chronic pancreatitis, Schwachman-Diamond,

Johannson Blizzard, Pearson, pancreatic enzyme deficiencies

Bile acid disorders: primary malabsorption, overuse of bile acid sequestrants, chronic liver disease

Enzyme deficiency: lactase, sucrase, monosaccharide malabsorption, enterokinase deficiency

Drug effects: many drugs, especially antibiotics, laxative abuse

Poisoning: heavy metals

Neoplastic

Secretory tumors: carcinoid, vasoactive intestinal peptide (VIP)

Functional

Recurrent abdominal pain, irritable bowel syndrome, functional dyspepsia

Abbrev: HIV = human immunodeficiency virus

due to bacterial de-conjugation of bile salts. These bacteria also bind and prevent the absorption of vitamin B_{12} causing a megaloblastic anemia. The bacteria may cause damage to the intestinal mucosa with sub-sequent carbohydrate malabsorption. Treatment consists of antibiotic decontamination, with 2–4 weeks of metronidazole or Augmentin with an 8-week course if symptoms recur. In adolescents, tetracycline or

TABLE 10-6

APPROACH TO THE PATIENT WITH ACUTE DIARRHEA (SYMPTOMS <2 WEEKS)

Historical points

Mostly infectious. Also may be ingestion, abscess, intussusception, Meckel's diverticulum

Vomiting + diarrhea. Most likely viral—may be *Staphylococcus, Giardia* or *Cryptosporidium*

Fever—not parasitic, but amebae can -> fever

Voluminous watery stools—vibrio or rotavirus

Bloody stools—*Salmonella, Shigella, Campylobacter, Yersinia*

Tenesmus—*Shigella colitis*

Farm animal exposure—*Campylobacter* or *Yersinia*

Reptiles and poultry—*Salmonella sp.*

Physical exam

Evaluate hydration status

Abdominal and rectal examinations—look for peritoneal and obstructive findings + blood or mucus in stool

Extraintestinal manifestations:

    Neurological—paresthesias (toxins from fish or mushrooms), muscle weakness (*C. botulinum*), meningismus
    (*Salmonella* or *Shigella*)

    Immune—reactive arthritis (*Salmonella, Shigella, Campylobacter, Yersinia, C. difficile*); Guillain-Barré syndrome—
    Campylobacter; nephritis or IgA nephropathy—*Campylobacter, Yersinia* or *Shigella*; erythema nodosum—
    Campylobacter, Yersinia or *Salmonella*; Dermatologic—pallor and petechiae for *E. coli* 0157:H7, *Shigella* (HUS),
    lower extremity purpura and arthritis for HSP

Laboratory

Fecal leukocytes >5/hpf, occult blood, bacterial cultures, ova and parasites, viral antigens (mainly to establish an
    outbreak—not routinely necessary).

Toxicology studies if suspicious of ingestion

Imaging studies and surgical consult if suspicion merits

Treatment

E. coli: trimethoprim-sulfamethoxazole (TMP-SMX). Do not treat for 0157:H7 (ineffective, may increase risk of HUS)

Shigella: amoxicillin, third-generation cephalosporin or quinolone

Vibrio: tetracycline

C. difficile: metronidazole or vancomycin

Yersinia (immunodeficient patients): TMP-SMX, third-generation cephalosporin, aminoglycoside

Campylobacter (immunodeficient patients): erythromycin

Salmonella (immunodeficiency, typhoid fever or metastatic infection) TMP-SMX, third-generation cephalosporin
    or chloramphenicol. Antibiotic treatment may prolong carrier state.

Abbrev: HUS =hemolytic uremic syndrome, HSP =Henoch-Schönlein purpura

ciprofloxacin may be used. Surgical resection of stenotic areas may be helpful.

Celiac Disease

Celiac disease (gluten-sensitive enteropathy, non-tropical sprue) occurs due to sensitivity to the gliadin fraction of gluten found in wheat, rye, and barley. It is common worldwide, with a high incidence in people of northern European ancestry. Hereditary factors are evidenced by concordance in twins as well as the presence of HLA DQ2 or DQ8 in almost all patients. Association with disorders such as insulin-dependent diabetes mellitus, arthritis, and vasculitis suggests an autoimmune component. Malabsorption of all nutrients is present. Stools are typically fatty or greasy. Megaloblastic anemia due to folate or vitamin B_{12} deficiency may be found. Anti-endomysial and anti-tissue transglutaminase antibodies are excellent screening tests with high sensitivities and specificities. Because of the high association in the range of 5%–10% all adolescents with type 1 diabetes, hypothyroidism, and Down syndrome should be screened for celiac disease. Definitive diagnosis is by intestinal biopsy, which reveals villous atrophy of the intestinal mucosa with lymphocytic infiltration and hyperplasia of the crypts. Treatment is a lifetime gluten-free diet.

Except for cystic fibrosis and as a sequela of chronic pancreatitis, malabsorption due to pancreatic insufficiency is rare in the adolescent. Treatment with pancreatic enzymes is based the lipase content of the supplement. The requirement is about 1000 U/kg per meal. It is important to note that the FDA is only now requiring standardization of pancreatic enzyme products. New drug applications (NDA) for all pancreatic enzyme preparations must be submitted within four years. Because of poor reliability and consistency of the products generic pancreatic enzyme preparations are frequently ineffective.

Suggested Readings

Marsh WM. Infectious diseases of the gastrointestinal tract in adolescents. *Adolesc Med* 11:263–278, 2000.

Musher DM, Musher BL. Contagious acute gastrointestinal infections. *N Engl J Med* 351:2417–2427, 2004.

Pietzak MM, Thomas DW. Childhood malabsorption. *Pediatr Rev* 24:195, 2003.

Rossi T. Celiac disease. *Adolesc Med* 15:91–104, 2004.

Vanderhoof JA, Lagnas AN. Short bowel syndrome in children and adults. *Gastroenterol* 113:1767, 1997.

POLYPS AND POLYPOSIS SYNDROMES

A gastrointestinal polyp is a tumor that visibly protrudes into the bowel. Appearance, location, and histologic features can characterize polyps. Polyps are generally asymptomatic, but when symptomatic may be the source of significant bleeding, abdominal pain, or obstruction. There is increased risk of malignancy associated with some hereditary forms of polyposis. A polyp may serve as the lead point for an intussusception.

Solitary juvenile polyps, the most common type of polyp found in adolescents, typically present with painless rectal bleeding between the ages 2 and 10. Polyps that are located in the more proximal colon can present with melena. Approximately 75% of juvenile polyps are located in the distal 25 cm of the colon. When seen endoscopically, juvenile polyps are usually large (1–3 cm), erythematous with a friable surface, and pedunculated. Histologically they consist of mucus filled cystic glands and inflammatory cells in a prominent lamina propria. The risk of malignant transformation of isolated juvenile polyps is low. Endoscopic polypectomy is curative.

More than three juvenile polyps in the gastrointestinal tract characterize the juvenile polyposis syndrome (JPS). The incidence is <1/100,000. Symptoms at presentation can include abdominal pain, gastrointestinal bleeding, diarrhea, or in severe cases, protein losing enteropathy. A family history of multiple juvenile polyps is suggestive of JPS. As the condition progresses there can be hundreds of polyps throughout the gastrointestinal tract. Mutations of the *SMAD4* and *BMPR1A* genes are found in 20%–50% of patients and when present, can be used to screen other family members. Dysplasia may be seen in JPS polyps. The risk of colorectal carcinoma in patients with JPS is up to 15% in patients less than 35 years old. Malignancies of the stomach, duodenum, and pancreas have also been reported. There is currently no consensus on screening of asymptomatic patients, but annual fecal occult blood testing is recommended in patients with a family history of JPS. Other syndromes associated with juvenile polyps include Cowden syndrome (multiple hamartomas, macrocephaly, and breast cancer) and Bannayan-Riley-Ruvalcaba syndrome (macrocephaly, pigmentation of the genitalia, and developmental delays).

Familial adenomatous polyposis (FAP), an autosomal dominant disorder, due to mutation in the *APC* (adenomatous polyposis coli) gene, located on chromosome 5q21–22 is the most common of the adenomatous polyposis syndromes; penetrance is 80%. Patients typically present during late childhood or early adolescence with greater than 100 colonic polyps, which may be tubular or villous. Histologically dysplasia is always present, and the risk of cancer is nearly 100% by the fifth decade. Extracolonic malignancies, associated with FAP include duodenal ampullary carcinoma, thyroid cancer, hepatoblastoma, gastric carcinoma, and central nervous system tumors. The diagnostic criterion for FAP is the presence of greater than 100 adenomatous colorectal polyps. Genetic testing, which may reveal a mutation in the *APC* gene, is not necessary for diagnosis as all the mutations have not yet been discovered.

Gardner syndrome is distinguished from FAP by the presence of extra intestinal manifestations including dental anomalies, osteomas, lymphomas, fibromas, and a tendency to form desmoid tumors. Gardner syndrome is caused by the same mutations in the *APC* gene as FAP. Turcot syndrome refers to the association between brain tumors and FAP. If a mutation in the *APC* gene is detected then genetic screening of first degree relatives is indicated.

Family members who are positive for the gene mutation should undergo surveillance colonoscopy at intervals of every 1–2 years. If the probands mutation is not identified then screening colonoscopy is recommended for first degree relatives and should be repeated at 1–2 year intervals. Family members should receive genetic counseling before any gene testing is undertaken. Total colectomy with ileoanal pouch formation is the recommended treatment for such patients. Esophagogastroduodenoscopy should be performed at 1–3 year intervals with multiple biopsies of the papilla even if it is visually normal.

Multiple, sessile or pedunculated, hamartomatous polyps throughout the gastrointestinal tract characterize Peutz-Jeghers syndrome (PJS), an autosomal dominant disorder, due to a mutation in the *STK11* gene on chromosome 6. Histologically there are elongated branching glands lined by epithelium and arborizing smooth muscle. The most common presenting complaint in patients is recurrent, intermittent, colicky abdominal pain. Patients can also present with microcytic anemia due to chronic blood loss. Patients often have melanocytic macules of the lips, buccal mucosa, and digits, which may fade as the patient approaches adulthood. Gastrointestinal complications of PJS include bleeding, intussusception, and obstruction. The risk of malignant transformation of the polyps is thought to be low, but these patients are at risk for extra-intestinal malignancies including ovarian granulosa cell tumors, Sertoli cell tumors, cervical cancer, and breast cancer. The overall risk of cancers in patients with PJS is 18 times greater than that of the general population.

Suggested Readings

Barnard JA. Gastrointestinal polyps and polyp syndromes in adolescents. *Adolesc Med* 15:119–130, 2004.

Desai DC, Murday V, Phillips R, et al. A survey of phenotypic features in juvenile polyposis. *J Med Genet* 25: 476, 1998.

Hyer W, Beveridge I, Domizio Peet al. Clinical management and genetics of gastrointestinal polyps in children. *J Pediatr Gastroenterol Nutr* 31:469, 2000.

ANORECTAL DISEASE

An *anal fissure* is a tear in the epithelium and superficial tissue of the anal canal. Adolescents will present with pain upon defecation and bright red blood is often seen when wiping. Most fissures are due to trauma; caused by over-stretching of the anal canal due to constipation. Trauma, including possible sexual abuse must be considered when constipation is not present. Predisposing factors include hypertonicity of the internal anal sphincter and decreased blood flow to the mucosa. Secondary fissures may be caused by Crohn's disease or other underlying pathology. Acute fissures will heal with minimal intervention consisting of stool softeners and warm Sitz baths. Chronic fissures are defined by the persistence of symptoms beyond 6 weeks and the presence of fibrotic tissue at the base of the fissure. Nonsurgical approaches to treatment of chronic fissures are aimed at reducing resting anal sphincter pressure. Treatments include nitric oxide donors (glyceryl trinitrate applied topically), topical calcium channel blockers, or botulinum toxin injection. However, cure rates are only marginally better than placebo. Surgical treatment options include manual dilation of the anus or internal sphincterotomy, which may be effective in treatment of fissures associated with increased sphincter tone. The major complication of surgical intervention is incontinence.

Solitary rectal ulcer syndrome presents as rectal bleeding, mucous discharge, straining, tenesmus, and pain localized to the rectal area. On colonoscopy discrete rectal lesion(s) are seen surrounded by normal mucosa. The appearance of the lesion can vary from hyperemic mucosa to ulcerations. Polypoid lesions may be seen as well. Histologically there is fibromuscular obliteration of the lamina propria, which differentiates it from inflammatory bowel disease. Solitary rectal ulcer syndrome is caused by rectal prolapse, in most cases secondary to excessive straining. The anterior rectal mucosa may be forced into the anal canal, causing congestion, edema, and ulceration. Treatment includes avoidance of straining, softening of stools, and topical treatment with sulfasalazine or steroid enemas. Patient's refractory to medical management may require rectopexy to prevent further prolapse.

Proctitis in the adolescent is often infectious in etiology. Common pathogens include sexually transmitted diseases such as *Neisseria gonorrhoeae, Chlamydia trachomatis*, herpes simplex, or *Treponema pallidum*. Other pathogens may include (but are not limited to) *Campylobacter, Shigella*, and *Entamoeba histolytica*. A thorough history, including sexual history, is necessary in determining the appropriate cultures to send. Other possible causes of proctitis include radiation exposure in oncology patients and inflammatory bowel disease.

Hemorrhoids are uncommon in adolescents. Hemorrhoids are distended veins arising from either the internal or external rectal plexus and thus are classified into two subgroups, internal and external. Internal hemorrhoids arise from above the dentate line and are covered by mucosa. External hemorrhoids arise from below the dentate line and have a cutaneous covering. Hemorrhoids are graded on a scale of one to four. First degree hemorrhoids do not prolapse below the dentate line. Second degree hemorrhoids reduce spontaneously. Third degree hemorrhoids may be manually reduced. Fourth degree hemorrhoids are not reducible. Visual exam and digital rectal exam are an appropriate first step in diagnosing hemorrhoids. Flexible sigmoidoscopy may also be helpful in ruling out other sources of bleeding. Hemorrhoids arise when the connective tissue supporting the anal cushions is compromised. This may occur with chronic constipation and repetitive straining. Straining also produces an increase in venous pressure and leads to engorgement. Internal hemorrhoids can also be associated with portal hypertension and underlying liver disease should be considered and ruled out in patients presenting with hemorrhoids. Treatment of isolated hemorrhoids may vary from dietary modification with increased fiber to surgical intervention. Generally stool softeners and bulking agents are sufficient treatment for grades one through three. Topical analgesics may provide short-term relief from discomfort. Grade four hemorrhoids generally require banding or hemorrhoidectomy.

Suggested Readings

Ertem D, Acar Y, Karaa EK, et al. A rare and often unrecognized cause of hematochezia and tenesmus in childhood: Solitary rectal ulcer syndrome. *Pediatrics* 110:e79, 2002.

Lindsey I, Jones OM, Cunningham C, et al. Chronic anal fissure. *Brit J Surg* 91:270, 2004.

Nisar PJ, Scholefield JH. Managing haemorrhoids. *BMJ* 32:847, 2003.

CONSTIPATION

Constipation can be best defined as a decrease in the frequency, an increase in the hardness of stools, or difficulty in passing hard stools, typically at infrequent intervals. Most episodes of constipation in adolescents are acute self-limited events easily treated with laxatives for 1 or 2 days. These episodes often follow a viral illness. In contrast chronic constipation, often associated with encopresis, typically follows untreated or unsuccessfully treated constipation in younger children. This cycle is frequently initiated by stool withholding in toddlers. Stools then become hard and painful to pass, thus triggering a cycle of pain and withholding. Encopresis may develop from chronic rectal distension and overflow incontinence. The fecal mass may partially obstruct the bladder leading to recurrent urinary tract infections, especially in girls.

Typically the adolescent eats a low fiber diet, high in dairy products, both of which promote hard stools. Other conditions which may lead to chronic constipation are found in Table 10-7. While chronic constipation is uncommon in adolescents its recognition and treatment can be at times challenging as many patients present with the complaint of abdominal pain and deny constipation. On physical examination a large abdominal mass is commonly palpated. On rectal examination a hard fecal mass is present unless a large stool has been recently passed; there may be perianal soiling. An empty rectal vault suggests the possibility of Hirschsprung's disease. The diagnosis is based on a history and physical examination, while laboratory tests are needed infrequently. In the appropriate clinical setting, thyroid function should be measured; a plain abdominal film will demonstrate the fecal mass.

Treatment of chronic constipation is based on several principles. The fecal impaction must be eliminated, using a regimen of phosphate enema followed by a high dose of a potent laxative, such as magnesium sulfate, phosphosoda, or polyethylene glycol. An appropriate high fiber, high fluid, and low dairy product diet is recommended. Maintenance laxative therapy is prescribed for a minimum of several months and then slowly tapered. Effective maintenance preparations include milk of magnesia, senna, lactulose, and polyethylene glycol. Biofeedback is not usually beneficial and relapses are frequent.

Suggested Readings

Baker SS, Liptak GS, Colletti RB, et al. Medical position statement: The North American Society for pediatric gastroenterology and nutrition: Constipation in infants and children: Evaluation and treatment. *J Pediatr Gastroenterol Nutr* 29:612, 1999.

TABLE 10-7

CONSTIPATION IN ADOLESCENTS

Anatomic
Imperforate anus
Pelvic tumor
Spina bifida
Drugs
Antacids
Anticholinergics
Antidepressants
Antihypertensives
Opiates
Phenobarbital
Sucralfate
Sympathomimetics
Metabolic/endocrine
Celiac disease
Cystic fibrosis
Diabetes mellitus
Hypercalcemia
Hypokalemia
Hypothyroidism
MEN type 2B
Motor disorders
Hirschsprung's disease
Pseudo-obstruction
Miscellaneous
Constitutional
Colonic inertia
Depression
Down syndrome
Genetic predisposition
Lead ingestion
Low fiber diet
Neurological injury
Sexual abuse

Higgins PDR, Johanson JF. Epidemiology of constipation in North America: A systematic review. *Am J Gastroenterol* 99:750, 2004.

Van Ginkel R, Reitsma JB, Buller HA, et al. Childhood constipation: Longitudinal follow-up beyond puberty. *Gastroenterology* 125:357, 2003.

Youssef NN, Sanders L, Di Lorenzo C. Adolescent constipation and management. *Adolesc Med* 15:37–52, 2004.

ACUTE ABDOMINAL PAIN

Acute abdominal pain originating from the gastrointestinal tract usually has an infectious/inflammatory or an obstructive etiology; however, other systemic origins are not rare. (Tables 10-8 and 10.9).

Diagnostic Approach

A thorough history including family, occupational, traveling, dietary, social, and sexual history is of paramount importance. Is the onset of pain acute or gradual? Where is the pain localized? Does it radiate, or is it referred? What is the quality of the pain? Most pain is of acute onset, though pain due to intestinal obstruction may be more gradual. Are there other symptoms such as anorexia, nausea, vomiting, or diarrhea? Pain in the left upper quadrant may indicate constipation or pancreatitis. Unremitting right lower quadrant (RLQ) pain and anorexia suggests appendicitis. Severe lower quadrant pain on either side may be diagnostic of ovarian pathology, pelvic inflammatory disease, intussusception, or volvulus. Back pain may be indicative of pancreatitis, nephrolithiasis, intestinal obstruction, diskitis, or appendicitis (retrocecal). Pain radiating to the groin and leg is seen in urolithiasis and in ovarian torsion. Sharp shooting pain may be pleuritic or peritoneal in nature, while severe

TABLE 10-8

GI TRACT ETIOLOGIES OF ACUTE ABDOMINAL PAIN

Infections/inflammatory

Gastroenteritis (viral, bacterial, parasitic, food poisoning)

Pancreatitis

Hepatitis

Diverticulitis

Peritonitis

Gastritis/peptic (post-viral, *H. pylori*, peptic ulcer, GERD)

Vasculitis (HSP, HUS, Kawasaki, sickle-cell disease)

Inflammatory bowel disease

Appendicitis

Mesenteric adenitis

Obstructive

Constipation

Traumatic (hematoma, foreign body)

Intussusception

Volvulus

Incarcerated hernia

Post-surgical adhesions

Biliary causes (stone, cyst, hydrops)

Abbrev: GERD = gastroesophageal reflux disease, HSP = Henoch-Schönlein purpura, HUS = hemolytic uremic syndrome

TABLE 10-9

NON-GI ETIOLOGIES OF ACUTE ABDOMINAL PAIN

Female reproductive tract: imperforate hymen, pelvic inflammatory disease (PID), tubo-ovarian abscess, Fitz-Hugh-Curtis perihepatitis, endometriosis, ectopic pregnancy, mittelschmerz, ovarian cyst, ovarian torsion.

Male reproductive tract: testicular torsion, orchitis, prostatitis

Renal: nephro/urolithiasis, UTI, hydronephrosis, abscess, uremia

Cardiopulmonary: pulmonary infarction/embolism, pericarditis, pleuritis, mediastinitis, pneumothorax, acute rheumatic fever

Toxic-metabolic: diabetic ketoacidosis, hypercalcemia, multiple endocrine adenomatosis, acute intermittent porphyria, familial Mediterranean fever, hyperlipidemia, hereditary angioneurotic edema, heavy metal poisoning, narcotic withdrawal

Vasculitis: collagen vascular diseases, HUS, HSP

Musculoskeletal: abdominal wall abscess, hematoma, strain.

Other: intraabdominal mass (abscess, tumor), vertebral disk infection, abdominal epilepsy, abdominal migraine, streptococcal infections, EBV, psychologic disorders

Abbrev: UTI = urinary tract infection, EBV = Epstein-Barr virus

colicky pain suggests cholelithiasis, nephrolithiasis, or intussusception. The pain of pancreatitis is described as "dull" and "boring." Vomiting is frequent in appendicitis, obstruction, pancreatitis, gall bladder disease, and urolithiasis. Dysuria and frequency suggest a urinary tract infection.

A thorough physical examination, including rectal and pelvic evaluation, is obligatory. Ear-nose-throat examination may reveal tonsillitis due to *Streptococcus* or Epstein-Barr virus causing abdominal pain from mesenteric adenitis (Chap. 7). The chest exam may reveal rales, rubs, egophony, or splinting (pneumonia, pleuritis, or pericarditis) (Chaps. 8 and 9). Abnormal findings on abdominal exam include distension, (obstruction), increased (obstruction, gastroenteritis) or decreased (appendicitis) bowel sounds, tenderness, masses, organomegaly, and costovertebral angle tenderness. Findings on rectal exam are most helpful to diagnose appendicitis (RLQ pain), functional constipation (hard stool mass), ulcerative colitis, or intussusception (blood). Findings on pelvic exam include cervical motion tenderness (pelvic inflammatory disease.) and adnexal tenderness (tubo-ovarian abscess, ectopic pregnancy, ovarian cyst, tumor).

Suggested Readings

Hirsh MP, McKenna CJ. Abdominal pain in children: Surgical considerations. *Topics Emer Med* 18:49, 1999.

Lavalle JM. A practical approach to non-traumatic, non-gynecologic abdominal pain in the adolescent patient. *Adoles Med* 4:35, 1993.

Leung AK, Sigalet DL. Acute abdominal pain in children. *Am Fam Physician* 67:2321, 2003.

Plescow RG, Berhane R, Grand RJ. Gastrointestinal disorders in adolescents. *Adoles Med* 2:485, 1991.

Functional Gastrointestinal Disorders
Nonorganic Recurrent Abdominal Pain

The term recurrent abdominal pain (RAP) should be viewed as a symptom, not a diagnosis; thus, it is incumbent upon the clinician to determine which patients fall into that 10%–15% with a definable organic cause. Years of accumulated knowledge and experience enable the clinician to utilize a careful history with special attention to pain radiating away from the umbilicus, nocturnal pain, persistent vomiting

with presence of blood or bile, bloody diarrhea, fever, weight loss, or family history of inflammatory bowel disease (IBD) or peptic ulcer disease. Significant physical findings may include poor growth, delayed puberty, organomegaly, abdominal tenderness away from the umbilicus, perianal disease, recurrent aphthous stomatitis, and joint swelling.

The mechanism of organic abdominal pain is based on either inflammation (e.g., IBD) or distension due to obstruction of a hollow viscus. Sensory receptors (e.g., heat, stretch, or chemoreceptors connect to the enteric nervous system) often referred to as the "gut brain"; this is a complex system including the myenteric (or Auerbach's plexus) involving motility and the submucosal (or Meissner's plexus) involving secretory function. The interstitial cells of Cajal are intermediaries between the nerve terminals and the smooth muscle, involving peristalsis. The gut brain then communicates with the autonomic nervous system, which relays information to the central nervous system.

Nonorganic RAP in childhood and adolescence is poorly understood, but is thought to be due to visceral hyperalgesia or hypersensitivity. Certainly emotions and conditioned responses are present in recurrent nonorganic abdominal pain; however, research has not substantiated a psychogenic origin in all cases. Thus, RAP is best divided into three categories: (1) organic etiology, (2) psychogenic (e.g., depression, school avoidance), and (3) functional gastrointestinal disorders (FGIDs). FGIDs consist of IBS, nonulcer dyspepsia (NUD), and nonorganic abdominal pain. The Rome II criteria, the most current diagnostic tool in use, are found in Table 10-10.

Irritable Bowel Syndrome

Etiology and Pathogenesis

Patients with IBS have lower visceral perception thresholds to thermal and pressure stimuli delivered to the colon, without demonstrable anatomic or inflammatory changes. IBS may follow an event involving infection, inflammation, trauma or allergy, with subsequent increase in proinflammatory cytokines (interleukins and prostaglandins), increased numbers of colonic mast cells, and degenerative changes in the myenteric plexus. As the gut brain carries stimuli to the CNS (central nervous system),

TABLE 10-10

ROME II CRITERIA FOR DIAGNOSIS OF FUNCTIONAL GASTROINTESTINAL DISORDERS

	Abdominal Pain <12 weeks out of the Year	*Bowel Pattern*	*Organic Pathology*	*Miscellaneous*
Irritable bowel syndrome (IBS)	Upper or lower abdominal pain	<3 stools/week, or >3 stools/day, Relief with defecation Change in stool consistency	no	Straining Urgency Feeling of incomplete evacuation Mucus in stool Bloating
Functional dyspepsia (FD)	Upper abdominal pain	No association with change in patterns	no	
Functional abdominal pain	Upper or lower abdominal pain	Occasional relation to defecation	no	No evidence of feigning No evidence of IBS or FD

positron emission tomography studies in adults have shown increased activation in the prefrontal cortex region.

Diagnosis

Diagnosis is made by the Rome criteria (Table 10-10). Supportive findings may include straining, urgency or feeling of incomplete evacuation, passage of mucus, and bloating. IBS has frequently been subdivided into a constipation-predominant (IBS-C, 25%) or a diarrhea-predominant (IBS-D, 25%), and a pain-gas-bloat-predominant (IBS-PBG, 50%), with some overlap. A complete history and physical examination usually readily distinguishes those with organic pain from those with functional pain. Useful laboratory studies include a complete blood count (CBC), ESR, and a stool test for occult blood. In the appropriate setting, further workup includes serology for celiac disease, urinalysis and urine culture, stool for ova and parasites, and abdominal ultrasound.

Treatment

The hallmark of treatment for IBS is education; unfortunately, many parents harbor misperceptions such as patient malingering or physician misjudgment. The family must be reassured that the pain is real. It is incumbent upon the clinician to spend time with families exploring conditions with which they may have had some peripheral experience, and also to allay their anxiety with evidence that the history and physical findings do not support these diagnoses.

Nutritional counseling is important, as adolescents tend to consume low fiber diets, caffeine, and poorly absorbed carbohydrates. Any medication use is symptomatic and should be tailored to the individual patient's needs. Anticholinergics, such as dicyclomine or hyoscyamine, are frequently used, but their effectiveness has not been demonstrated in controlled studies. Symptomatic treatment with laxatives, loperamide, and fiber is helpful in some adolescents. Tricyclic antidepressants in low doses are very beneficial in many patients. Tricyclics may be given only to those with a normal QTc, so an ECG must be obtained prior therapy. Selective serotonin reuptake inhibitors (SSRIs) have also been used, and psychologic counseling may be beneficial as adjunctive therapy. It is critical to impress upon these adolescent patients that even if they have symptoms, they must minimize school and work absenteeism. A newer medication is tegaserod, a serotonin receptor agonist, that may be used in females with IBS-C, rare cases of severe diarrhea and death have been reported as adverse reactions. Alosetron, a serotonin receptor antagonist, may be used for IBS-D in females over age 19. Alosetron was withdrawn from the market briefly because of deaths due to ischemic colitis. This agent may only be prescribed by physicians approved by the manufacturer.

Suggested Readings

Hyams JS. Irritable bowel syndrome, functional dyspepsia, and functional abdominal pain syndrome. *Adolesc Med* 15:1–16, 2004.

Li Y, Zuo X, Guo Y, et al. Visceral perception thresholds after rectal thermal and pressure stimuli in irritable bowel syndrome patients. *J Gastroenterol Hepatol* 19:187, 2004.

Mertz HR. Irritable bowel syndrome. *N Engl J Med* 349:2136–2146, 2003.

Talley NJ, Dennis EH, Schletter-Duncan VA, et al. Overlapping upper and lower gastrointestinal symptoms in irritable bowel syndrome patients with constipation or diarrhea. *Amer J Gastroenterol* 98:2454, 2003.

Thiessen PN. Recurrent abdominal pain. *Pediatr Rev* 23:39, 2002; Disorders. *J Pediatr Gastroenterol Nutr* 28:187, 2002.

Nonulcer Dyspepsia

Diagnosis

The Rome II criteria for functional dyspepsia are found in Table 10-10. Because clinical presentation is less reliable than in RAP or IBS, endoscopy is often performed to rule out organic etiologies.

Treatment

The treatment for functional dyspepsia is symptomatic educational and supportive measures. NSAIDs, caffeine, and spicy foods are discontinued. A trial of acid suppression with an H_2 receptor antagonist or a proton pump inhibitor should be considered. Prokinetic agents are not generally effective except in the rare patient with gastroparesis; amitriptyline may be helpful.

Nonorganic Abdominal Pain Syndrome

The Rome II criteria for this diagnosis are in listed Table 10-10. Basic laboratory and imaging studies are often helpful. The CBC and ESR are elevated in infectious/inflammatory conditions. A chemistry profile is frequently helpful; this includes calcium and amylase (for pancreatitis), liver function studies (for hepatobiliary disease), and stool for occult blood (for colitis, bacterial enteritis, intussusception, volvulus). Pregnancy test, urinalysis, and culture should be obtained when indicated. If diarrhea is present, stool culture as well ova and parasites should be obtained. Gram stains and cultures from a pelvic examination should be done in female adolescents. Chest x-ray, abdominal flat plate, and ultrasound are valuable adjuncts for diagnosis. When indicated the gastroenterologist or gynecologist may perform further studies, such as endoscopy and laparoscopy. Management is similar in adolescents to that described in IBS above.

PANCREAS

Acute pancreatitis is the most common pancreatic disorder in adolescents. Blunt abdominal injuries, mumps, and other viral illnesses, multisystem disease, congenital anomalies, biliary stones microlithiasis (sludging), and drug toxicity account for most known etiologies; other causes are uncommon. Many cases are of unknown etiology. Most pediatric series report fewer than 10 cases per year at large children's hospitals. Recently we and others have reported more than 30 cases per year; the median age in our series was 12.5 years at the Medical College of Wisconsin, Milwaukee.

The patient with acute pancreatitis has steady epigastric pain, persistent vomiting, fever, and appears acutely ill. The differential diagnoses of acute and chronic abdominal pain are found elsewhere in this chapter. The abdomen may be distended and tender with a palpable mass. The pain increases in intensity for 24–48 hours, during which time vomiting may increase; this adolescent patient may require hospitalization for dehydration and may need intravenous hydration as well as narcotic analgesics. The prognosis for the acute uncomplicated case is excellent.

Severe acute pancreatitis, the most severe form of acute pancreatitis, is rare in adolescents. In this life-threatening condition, the patient is acutely ill with severe nausea, vomiting, and abdominal pain. Shock, high fever, jaundice, ascites, hypocalcemia, and pleural effusions may occur. The pancreas becomes necrotic and may be transformed into an infected inflammatory hemorrhagic mass. The mortality rate is 25% and is due to the *systemic inflammatory response syndrome* with multiple organ dysfunctions.

The pathophysiology of pancreatitis is due to the colocalization of digestive enzymes in organelles with lysosomal enzymes causing activation of trypsinogen into trypsin, which then activates other proenzymes. The diagnosis of pancreatitis is usually made by the elevation of the serum amylase or lipase in the appropriate clinical setting. However, elevated enzymes are neither sensitive nor specific for the diagnosis of pancreatitis. The serum amylase is elevated for up to 4 days. Initially, levels are normal in 10%–15% of patients. The serum lipase typically remains elevated 8–14 days longer than serum amylase. While ultrasound and CT scanning have major roles in the diagnosis and follow-up of adolescents with pancreatitis, at least 20% initially have normal imaging studies. ERCP or magnetic resonance cholangiopancreatography (MRCP) are essential in the investigation of recurrent pancreatitis, pancreas divisum, sphincter of Oddi dysfunction, and disease associated with gallbladder pathology. Endoscopic ultrasonography is a new technique for the visualization of the pancreatobiliary system.

The aims of medical management are to relieve pain and restore metabolic homeostasis. Analgesia should be given in adequate doses, while fluid, electrolyte, and mineral balance should be restored and maintained. Nasogastric suction is useful in patients who are vomiting. Prophylactic antibiotics are useful in severe cases to prevent infected pancreatic necrosis. The response to treatment is usually complete over 2–5 days. Refeeding may commence when vomiting has resolved, the serum amylase is falling, and clinical symptoms are resolving. Endoscopic therapy may be of benefit when pancreatitis is caused by anatomic abnormalities, such as strictures or stones. When pancreatitis is associated with trauma or systemic disease, the prognosis is related to the associated medical conditions. Prognostic systems widely used in adults such as *Ranson's criteria* and the *APACHE score* are inappropriate for use in adolescents.

The treatment of severe acute pancreatitis may involve enteral or total parenteral nutrition, antibiotics, gastric acid suppression, and peritoneal lavage to reduce the risk of secondary infection. Surgical therapy of acute pancreatitis is rarely required in adolescents, but may include drainage of necrotic material or abscesses. Chronic, relapsing pancreatitis

in children is frequently hereditary or due to congenital anomalies of the pancreatic or biliary ductal system. Hereditary pancreatitis (HP) is transmitted as an autosomal dominant trait with incomplete penetrance but variable expressivity. Symptoms frequently begin in the first decade but are usually mild at the onset. The gene for HP has been identified as the cationic trypsinogen gene and is found on the long arm of chromosome 7. Mutations of other genes including *cystic fibrosis* gene *(CFTR)* in the 5T promoter region and the *SPINK 1* gene *(pancreatic trypsin inhibitor)* have also been associated with recurrent of chronic pancreatitis

A thorough diagnostic evaluation of every patient with more than one episode of pancreatitis is indicated. Serum lipid, calcium, and phosphorus levels are determined. Stools are evaluated for *Ascaris*, and a sweat test is performed. Evaluation of the *HP*, *SPINK 1*, and the *CFTR* genes is performed. Plain abdominal films are evaluated for the presence of pancreatic calcifications, and abdominal ultrasound or CT scanning is performed to detect the presence of a pseudocyst. The biliary tract is evaluated for the presence of stones. ERCP is performed and bile is analyzed for the presence of cholesterol crystals.

Suggested Readings

Lopez MJ. The changing incidence of acute pancreatitis in children: A single institution perspective. *J Pediatr* 140:622, 2002.

Werlin SL, Kugathasan S, Frautchy BC. Pancreatitis in children. *J Pediatr Gastroenterol Nutr* 37:591, 2003.

Witt H. Chronic pancreatitis and cystic fibrosis. *Gut* 52(Supp 2):31, 2003.

GALLBLADDER DISEASE

As many as 25 million adults in North America have cholelithiasis. Sparse epidemiologic evidence is available in adolescent patients, but an ultrasound screening study found that 0.13% of Italians age 6–19 had gallstones. Much higher prevalences are seen in specific ethnic groups (Native Americans, Swedish, and Czechs) and females out number males. Stones are categorized by content; cholesterol stones contain greater than 50% cholesterol, while pigmented stones contain mixtures of various calcium salts in addition to smaller amounts of cholesterol. Many conditions can predispose to cholelithiasis including pregnancy, obesity, hemolytic disease, abdominal surgery, malabsorption, ileal resection, rapid weight loss, medications including oral contraceptives, trauma, burns, sepsis, and underlying hepatobiliary disease. Complications include choledocholithiasis, pancreatitis, and cholecystitis. Treatment is primarily surgical and is almost always performed laparoscopically. ERCP can be useful in acute settings such as choledocholithiasis. Nonsurgical treatments, such as lithotripsy or ursodeoxycholic acid, are effective in only limited situations and there is a very high rate of recurrence following therapy. These agents are typically used only in high-risk patients.

Acalculous cholecystitis is rare in adults but more common in younger patients. It is characterized by distension of the gallbladder without stones and with evidence of inflammation (usually sonographic evidence of wall thickening). Hydrops of the gallbladder is characterized by distension but no inflammation. Both have been associated with trauma, burns, sepsis (infectious hepatitis, gastroenteritis, *Leptospira*, group B streptococci, *Shigella, Salmonella, E. coli*), periarteritis nodosa, Kawasaki syndrome, and familial Mediterranean fever. Treatment is controversial, and in many situations, expectant management is all that is necessary. Surgery may be needed; gangrene of the gallbladder is a significant risk in adult patients but is rare in younger patients.

Suggested Reading

Trowbridge RL, Rutkowski NK, Shojania KG. Does this patient have acute cholecystitis? *JAMA* 289:80–86, 2003.

VIRAL HEPATITIS, A–G

Hepatitis is a clinical syndrome, including malaise, fever, myalgia, right upper quadrant abdominal pain, hepatomegaly, anorexia, nausea and vomiting, jaundice and dark urine, due to hepatic inflammation. Acholic stools are a presentation of biliary obstruction. There may be extrahepatic manifestations including pruritus, urticaria, serum sickness, arthritis, acrodermatitis (Gianotti-Crosti syndrome), and erythema nodosum. Hepatocellular damage is confirmed in the laboratory by elevated hepatic enzymes such as aspartate transaminase (AST) and alanine aminotransferase (ALT). Biliary obstruction may be demonstrated by elevated alkaline phosphatase or γ-glutamyltransferase (GGT) levels and absence of urine urobilinogen. Multiple etiologies include hepatotropic viruses A-G, Epstein-Barr virus, cytomegalovirus, HIV, varicella-zoster virus, rubella, enterovirus, adenovirus, and others. Viral hepatitis must also be distinguished from other causes of similar symptoms such as bacterial illness (i.e., sepsis, syphilis, tuberculosis, leptospirosis, brucellosis, Fitz-Hugh-Curtis syndrome), parasitic infestations (i.e., schistosomiasis, malaria, ascariasis, liver flukes), Gilbert syndrome, gall bladder disease, Wilson's disease (WD), cystic fibrosis, α_1 antitrypsin deficiency, chronic hemolytic disease, autoimmune hepatitis, collagen vascular disease and hepatitis induced by drugs, toxins, or hypoxia. The clinical course of hepatitis may be asymptomatic, acute, chronic, or fulminant (see Table 10-11).

Suggested Readings

Hochman JA, Balistreri WF. Chronic viral hepatitis: Always be current! *Pediatr Rev* 24:399, 2003.
O'Connor JA. Acute and chronic viral hepatitis. *Adolesc Med* 11:279–292, 2000.
Suskind DL, Rosenthal P. Chronic viral hepatitis. *Adolesc Med* 15:145–158, 2004.

CHRONIC HEPATITIS

Patients with elevated liver enzymes lasting more than 6 months have chronic hepatitis. Chronic liver disease can present insidiously. Symptoms include fatigue, anorexia, weight loss, jaundice, pruritus, easy bruising, and persistent bleeding. The liver may be enlarged, normal, or small. Splenomegaly may be present if significant cirrhosis has developed. Other findings include pallor or flushing, muscle wasting,

SPECIFIC ASPECTS OF HEPATOTROPIC VIRUSES A-G

	General Comments	Clinical Diagnosis	Laboratory	Treatment	Prevention
Hepatitis A	Picornavirus 48% of hepatitis A-G Incubation 4 weeks	No prodrome Self-limiting (1 month) Rarely fulminant unless associated with hepatitis C	Elevated AST, ALT +HAV IgM at 4-20 weeks +HAV IgG at 8 weeks that lasts indefinitely	Supportive	χglobulin 0.2 mL/kg HAV vaccine 2 doses 6-12 months apart Give both for exposures <2 weeks ago
Hepatitis B	DNA virus 34% of hepatitis A-G Incubation 6-25 weeks Transmission vertical, blood-borne or sexual	Prodrome: acrodermattitis, hives Fulminant course with 30% mortality rate Chronic in 6%-10% susceptibility to hepatocellular ca	+HBs antigen +HBe antigen-active viral replication Lose +Ag in recovery Chronic—persistent +HBs Ag and +HBe Ag is ominous	Supportive Acute liver failure-lactulose, fresh frozen plasma Chronic: lamivudine and interferon (IFN) α2b, transplantation	HB vaccine at exposure, then doses 1 and 6 months post-exposure HB vaccine + HBIg in newborn exposures by age 12 hours
Hepatitis C	RNA Flavivirus Prevalence: 0.4% of adolescents age 12-19 Transmission vertical, blood-borne, rarely sexual	Insidious presentation 20%-40% self-limited 60%-80% chronic 80% of chronic with hepatic dysfunction Chronic pts develop cirrhosis—20% liver ca	HCV RNA anti-HCV, IgM, IgG Antibodies not protective Hepatic dysfunction	Avoid hepatotoxins Pegylated IFN Chronic: ribavirin	Screen blood products No vaccine—mutagenicity of virus
Hepatitis D	RNA virus Accompanies hepatitis B, asymptomatic alone Transmission similar to hepatitis B	Similar to hepatitis B	IgG anti hepatitis D	Supportive or treatment for accompanying hepatitis B	See hepatitis B No vaccine for hepatitis D
Hepatitis E	RNA calicivirus transmission similar to hepatitis A	Similar to hepatitis A, but more severe High fatality rate in pregnancy	HEV RNA IgM anti hepatitis E	Supportive+	Precautions similar to hepatitis A
Hepatitis G	RNA Flavivirus Co-infects hepatitis B and C	Does not worsen hepatitis B or C	None available commercially	See hepatitis B and C	See hepatitis B and C

Abbrev: IFN = interferon HAV-HEV = hepatitis A virus – hepatitis E virus

palmar erythema, spider angiomata, digital club-bing, caput medusa, ascites, gynecomastia, mental status changes, asterixis, prolonged relaxation phase of deep tendon reflexes, and Babinski's sign. Laboratory findings can include elevated amino-transferases, bilirubin, alkaline phosphatase, ammo-nia, and γ-glutamyltransferase. Serum proteins normally synthesized by the liver can be low includ-ing albumin and coagulation factors, resulting in prolongation of the PT and PTT tests; thrombocy-topenia, anemia, and leukopenia may be present.

Unrecognized chronic liver disease can present with fulminant hepatic failure. Complications of ful-minant liver failure include encephalopathy, cerebral edema, coagulopathy and hemorrhage, aplastic anemia, hypoglycemia, electrolyte and acid-base disturbances, renal insufficiency (hepato-renal syn-drome), ascites, hemodynamic instability, hepato-pulmonary syndrome, and infection (including sepsis, spontaneous bacterial peritonitis, pneumo-nia). Fulminant hepatic failure can also represent an acute process especially when caused by infections, toxins, or drugs. The causes of chronic liver disease are listed in Table 10-12.

Therapy of liver failure is primarily supportive until the inciting agent is removed or resolves. Although specifics are beyond the scope of this text, treatment of liver failure includes correction of metabolic derangements, cardiorespiratory support, replacement of fat soluble vitamins and coagulation factors as needed, management of ascites, and clearance of toxins with binding agents or dialysis where appropriate (e.g., acetaminophen, ammonia, ethanol) and treatment of infection when present. If improvement is not seen or expected with support-ive care, liver transplantation becomes necessary.

Drugs/toxins/illicit drugs must always be consid-ered in the adolescent presenting with liver disease. Early identification of the offending agent and inter-action with the local or regional poison control center is key to assure optimal care. Acetaminophen over-dose represents the rare situation where effective treatment is available (using N-acetylcysteine). The indication to treat is determined by plotting the blood level on a widely available nomogram. "Huffing" halogenated hydrocarbons or toluene can cause severe liver damage; cocaine, Ecstasy (a synthetic amphetamine) and mushrooms can also cause

TABLE 10-12

ETIOLOGY OF CHRONIC LIVER DISEASE IN ADOLESCENTS

Nonalcoholic steatohepatitis
Infection
Viral hepatitides: hepatitis B, C, CMV, EBV, HSV, echovirus
Parasitic infection
Cystic fibrosis
Autoimmune liver disease
Primary sclerosing cholangitis
Autoimmune hepatitis
Primary biliary cirrhosis
Drugs/toxins
Wilson's disease
Hemochromatosis
α_1-antitrypsin deficiency
Total parenteral nutrition
Budd-Chiari syndrome
Neoplasm
Primary: hepatocarcinoma, hemangioendothelioma
Infiltrative: leukemia, lymphoma
Fatty liver of pregnancy
Veno-occlusive disease

hepatic injury (Chap. 34). Many other drugs are also associated with hepatotoxicity.

In an era of epidemic obesity (Chap. 31), non-alcoholic steatohepatitis (NASH) is becoming a much more common problem seen in adolescent patients. NASH is a significant cause of liver dis-ease and can lead to fibrosis and cirrhosis. Hyperinsulinism and insulin resistance are risk fac-tors. The primary intervention is to address under-lying obesity; a transient worsening of the hepatitis can occur early in weight loss but improvement is usually seen with long-term success.

WD is an important cause of chronic liver dis-ease and liver failure in childhood and adolescence. The classic triad of WD is liver disease, neuropsy-chiatric manifestations, and Kayser-Fleischer rings. WD is a defect in copper metabolism involving autosomal recessive mutations of ATP7B. The result is copper overload and toxicity. Other mani-festations may include renal insufficiency, hemoly-sis, diabetes mellitus, pancreatic insufficiency, hypoparathyroidism, dysrhythmia, increased skin pigmentation (especially on the anterior lower legs), and acanthosis nigricans. The prevalence of WD is approximately 1 in 30,000 and 1 in 90 are carriers. WD must be considered in all children and adolescents with chronic liver disease even in the absence of obvious neuropsychiatric manifestations. The serum ceruloplasmin is often, but not always low. An elevated 24-hour urinary copper is more specific but may also be present in other chronic liver diseases. The diagnosis is usually confirmed by measuring the copper concentration in a liver biopsy. The presence of Kayser-Fleischer rings is pathognomic for WD in the absence of other cholestatic disorders. Typically Kayser-Fleischer rings can only be seen on slit lamp examination. Treatment is chelation of copper using D-penicillamine. Recently zinc acetate has been used to prevent intestinal absorption and it may also increase metallothionein binding of Cu in the liver. Zinc is unlikely to be useful without chelation in patients who present with Cu overload, but may be helpful for maintenance and in asymptomatic family members diagnosed prior to the onset of Cu overload. When WD presents with fulminant hepatic failure liver transplantation is usually necessary.

Autoimmune liver diseases are probably the most common cause of chronic liver disease in North American adolescents. These include autoimmune hepatitis (AIH), and primary sclerosing cholangitis (PSC). These diseases are differentiated based on the pattern of autoantibodies and histologic appearance. Significant overlap can occur. The diagnosis of AIH is based on elevated liver function tests and the pattern of piecemeal necrosis on liver biopsy; cirrhosis is often present at the time of diagnosis. Two types of AIH are currently recognized based on autoantibody profiles. Type 1 patients have anti-smooth muscle antibody (SMA) or anti nuclear antibody (ANA). Type 2 patients have anti-liver kidney microsomal antibodies. Type 2 AIH is seen mainly in Europe and Canada but less commonly in other parts of North America, South America, or Japan. Type 2 AIH, typically a more severe condition, is rarely seen in adults. AIH may be associated with many other autoimmune or immune mediated diseases including ulcerative colitis and diabetes mellitus. It is also associated with HLA DR3, DR4

and DR6. Immunosuppressive therapy employing corticosteroids and azathioprine is very effective.

Primary sclerosing cholangitis (PSC) results in chronic inflammation of the intra- and extra-hepatic biliary tree, leading to focal narrowing and dilatation and ultimately biliary cirrhosis. Most adolescents with PSC also have other immune mediated diseases, particularly IBD or celiac disease. The diagnosis requires cholangiography to demonstrate typical irregular narrowing of the biliary tree often with dilatation of other areas. Liver biopsy findings are often nonspecific. Patients often have an elevated antinuclear cytoplasmic antibody level with a perinuclear pattern (pANCA). An increased risk of cholangiocarcinoma has been seen in adult patients. No medical therapy has proven effective, and management is supportive; many patients ultimately require transplantation.

α_1-*antitrypsin* (α_1-AT) deficiency is the most common genetic cause of liver disease in children, affecting 1 in 1600 to 1 in 2000 live births. The disease is autosomal dominant and involves mutations of the gene for α_1-AT, a protein that inhibits neutrophil proteases. The disease can present with liver disease in infancy or may present later in childhood or adolescence. Lung disease (emphysema) affects up to 65% of patients but does not present until later in life. α_1-AT deficiency can be screened for with protein inhibitor ZZ typing (usually referred to as the Pi type).

Suggested Readings

D'Agata ID, Balistreri WF. Evaluation of liver disease in the pediatric patient. *Pediatr Rev* 20:376, 1999.

Ferenci P, Caca K, Loudianos G, et al. Diagnosis and phenotypic classification of Wilson disease. *Liver Int* 23:139, 2003.

Hyams JS, ed. Gastrointestinal Disorders in Adolescents. *Adolesc Med* 15: 1–199, 2004.

Jonas MM. Nonalcoholic fatty liver disease. *Adolesc Med* 15:159–174, 2004.

Li DY, Schwarz KB. Autoimmune hepatitis. *Adolesc Med* 15:131–144, 2004.

Neimark E, Schilsky ML, Shneider BL. Wilson's disease and hemochromatosis. *Adolesc Med* 15:175–194, 2004.

O'Connor JA. Acute and chronic viral hepatitis. *Adolesc Med* 11:279–292, 2000.

Pineiro-Carrero VM, Pineiro EO. Liver Disorders. *Pediatrics* 113:1097, 2004.

Poupon R. Autoimmune overlapping syndromes. *Clin Liver Dis* 7:865, 2003.

Sathya P, Martin S, Alvarez F. Nonalcoholic fatty liver disease (NAFLD) in children. *Curr Opin Pediatr* 14:593, 2002.

Suchy, FJ, Sokol, RJ & Balistreri, WF, *Liver Disease in Children*. Philadelphia, PA: Lippincott Williams & Wilkins, 2001

Suskind DL, Rosenthal P. Chronic viral hepatitis. *Adolesc Med* 15:145–158, 2004.

Wyllie R, Hyams JS. *Pediatric Gastrointestinal Disease*. Philadelphia, PA: W.B. Saunders, 1998.

11

MUSCULOSKELETAL DISORDERS

Dilip R. Patel and Donald E. Greydanus

TORTICOLLIS

Torticollis, or wry neck, refers to restricted neck motion with abnormal head posturing, usually involving the sternocleidomastoid, trapezius, or scalenus muscles. It is often bilateral and lasts for varying lengths of time. A slow, twisting, tilting head motion occurring intermittently is called *spasmodic torticollis*. *Retrocollis* refers to forceful neck extension, and *antecollis* implies forward flexion. Chronic torticollis can result in muscular hypertrophy or atrophy and usually affects the sternocleidomastoideus, although facial muscles can be involved as well.

The most common cause of torticollis is congenital muscle anomaly, trauma, or rotary (atlantoaxial) subluxation, though a variety of other factors may be involved (Table 11-1). Often, the patient awakens with a tilted head and painful unilateral spasm of the neck muscles. There may be a history of recent neck strain, sleeping near a draft, or edema caused by acute pharyngitis, tonsillitis, or regional adenitis. Cervical spine imaging studies are indicated to rule out osseous structural anomalies. Atlantoaxial instability is common in individuals with Down syndrome and they should be screened by appropriate imaging studies and neurologic assessment.

Treatment depends on the etiology of torticollis. Nonsteroidal anti-inflammatory analgesics, moist heat, cervical traction, and/or a cervical collar may be helpful for symptomatic relief. Resolution of acute torticollis usually occurs in 7–10 days. Spasmodic torticollis may be benefited by various medications including trihexyphenidyl (Artane), benztropine (Cogentin), amantadine, and haloperidol. The torticollis sometimes seen with phenothiazine toxicity may be reversed by diphenhydramine hydrochloride (Benadryl), 2 mg/kg intravenously (IV). Treatment with local Botox injection is also used effectively in cervical dystonia.

SCOLIOSIS

Scoliosis is defined by the Scoliosis Research Society as a lateral curvature of the spine greater than 10 degrees as measured by the Cobb method on a standing posteroanterior radiograph of the spine, associated with vertebral rotation.

Epidemiology

Idiopathic scoliosis is divided into three age-related groups. Infantile idiopathic scoliosis is present at birth or develops during the first three years of life. Although common in Europe, it is infrequent in the

TABLE 11-1

CAUSES OF TORTICOLLIS

Osseous or ligamentous

Odontoid process defects

Congenital vertebral anomalies (Klippel-Feil syndrome
  [fusion of cervical vertebra with short neck, low posterior hair line and limited neck motion]; scoliosis,
  renal anomalies or Sprengle's scapulae elevation
  may also be noted)

Juvenile rheumatoid arthritis

Osteoid osteoma

Eosinophilic granuloma

Rotary subluxation (may follow upper respiratory tract
  infections, wrestling, tumor, or edema secondary to
  pharyngitis, tonsillitis, syphilis, tuberculosis)

Muscular

Congenital sternocleidomastoid or other muscular
  anomaly

Dystonia musculorum deformans

Neurologic

Posterior fossa tumor

Phenothiazine toxicity (with extrapyramidal signs due
  to haloperidol, chlorpromazine, and others)

Myasthenia gravis

Syringomyelia

Postencephalitic extrapyramidal involvement

Ocular

Fourth cranial nerve palsy

Congenital nystagmus

Traumatic

Functional (psychogenic disorders)

United States. Juvenile idiopathic scoliosis develops after age three but before puberty, and also is
relatively uncommon. In contrast, idiopathic scoliosis is a frequent condition in adolescents, accounting for 80%–85% of all cases of scoliosis in the
teenage years. It is particularly prevalent in adolescent girls with a female to male ratio of 8:1 (7:1 in
curves greater than 20 degrees). Estimates of the
incidence in this age group vary, but most studies
find that 3%–5% of all adolescent girls are affected
to some degree, although only 15% of these develop
curvatures serious enough to require treatment.

Etiology

The cause of idiopathic scoliosis is unknown.
Hormonal factors have been implicated because of
the increased incidence of severe curves in girls,
but no definite relationship has been established.
Some studies have demonstrated abnormalities of
proprioception and vibratory sense in patients with
even small degrees of idiopathic scoliosis, possibly
implicating abnormalities of posterior column
function. Genetic influences are thought to be an
important determinant of idiopathic scoliosis,
transmitted as an autosomal dominant trait in some
families and often appearing in more than one sibling. Further, up to 80% of newly diagnosed cases
have parents with at least mild degrees of curvature, as determined by the forward bending test of
Adams.

Structural scoliosis (as contrasted to compensatory scoliosis secondary to paravertebral muscle
spasm or leg length inequality) is grouped into three
etiologic categories: congenital, neuromuscular or
paralytic, and idiopathic, with the latter being the
most common in the adolescent age group.
Congenital malformations of the spine, such as
hemivertebrae and unsegmented vertebral bars,
often produce structural curves which are present
at birth. Paralytic and spastic disorders (either as
the result of primary muscle or primary nerve
pathology), also may manifest in scoliosis. This
usually begins as a flexible deformity, but progresses rapidly with growth when permanent structural changes develop. Severe cardiopulmonary
compromise consequent to progressive compression of the thoracic cavity as the scoliosis advances,
is a common outcome in untreated cases. Scoliosis
in myelomeningocele may result from either vertebral abnormalities, associated paralysis, or both,
posing particularly difficult management problems.
Causes of scoliosis are listed in Table 11-2.

Clinical Features

The most dominant characteristic of idiopathic
scoliosis is a painless thoracic curve with a right
convexity. About 30% of adolescents present with

TABLE 11-2

TYPES OF SCOLIOSIS

Infantile idiopathic scoliosis (ages 0–3; left thoracic curve; mostly males; 20% are progressive)

Juvenile idiopathic scoliosis (ages 3–10; equal male-female ratio)

Adolescent idiopathic scoliosis

Functional scoliosis (compensatory spinal curve due to structural defect other than in the spine, e.g., a shortened leg)

Congenital scoliosis (congenital vertebral anomalies- hemivertebrae, failure of segmentation; 25–50% also have renal anomalies; cardiac anomalies also noted)

Neuromuscular scoliosis (cerebral palsy, poliomyelitis, spinal muscle atrophy, muscular dystrophy, child- hood paraplegia, arthrogryposis, amyotonia con- genita, diastematomyelia, myelomeningocele, others)

Neurofibromatosis (short, anular thoracic scoliosis that may produce paraplegia)

Miscellaneous

   Spinal cord tumor (osteoid osteoma, lipoma, others)

   Marfan syndrome

   Morquio's disease

   Ehlers-Danlos syndrome

   Juvenile rheumatoid arthritis

   Fractured vertebra

   Post-irradiation

   Postburn

insidious onset back pain. It is usually first noted at the onset of puberty and progresses to variable degrees during the period of maximum spinal growth (sexual maturity rating [SMR] stages 2–3 in females and stages 3–4 in males). The risk of significant progression is greatest in those who present with a high degree of curvature at a low SMR stage.

The outcome of untreated scoliosis is dependent on the ultimate degree of curvature. There is no spe- cific way to predict which adolescents will progress to a significant degree and which ones will not; how- ever, those who present with scoliosis early in the growth spurt and have rapid progression, are at

greatest risk of significant change. Long term seque- lae of significant curves include chronic back pain, degenerative arthritis, hunch back deformity, poor adolescent body-image, and, in advanced cases, seri- ous cardiorespiratory compromise. Decreased forced vital capacity and decreased total lung capacity are commonly found in adolescents with curves of 50–60 degrees, even if asymptomatic; also, some individuals with even relatively mild curves (i.e., under 35 degrees) may show abnormal ventilatory patterns in response to exercise. Untreated severe scoliosis (40–50 degrees) and some lesser cases (even under 30 degrees) will con- tinue to progress in adulthood, leading to com- paction of the thoracic cavity, further impairment of respiration, alveolar hypoventilation, polycythemia, and increased pulmonary vascular resistance. Death from advanced severe scoliosis (curves over 90 degrees) can occur in adults in their 30s and 40s secondary to deteriorating pulmonary function, pul- monary hypertension, and cor pulmonale.

Diagnosis

Careful screening of all teenagers for idiopathic scoliosis is an essential aspect of any complete health evaluation and is particularly important during early adolescence and the period of rapid growth. Scoliotic curves less then 25 degrees are particularly difficult to detect without careful inspection. The patient should first be examined from both the back and side (to rule out kyphosis) while standing upright with feet together, and then by the forward bending test of Adams. The latter is conducted by having the standing patient bend over 90 degrees or more with arms hanging downward in a relaxed position, elbows extended and palms together. Measurement of the angle of trunk rota- tion via an inclinometer also may be employed.

Significant findings in the standing position include a thoracic spinal curve in combination with a compensatory lumbar curve, pelvic tilt, and asym- metry of the flanks, scapulae, shoulders, and rib cage. One hemithorax may appear larger than the other, breasts may appear asymmetric, and rib flar- ing may be seen. A positive forward bending test will reveal one paravertebral area to be more elevated than the other (usually the right side is higher than the left) and a winging upward of the right scapula. Compensatory and postural curves will disappear during this maneuver. True structural scoliosis may be further differentiated from compensatory curves due to leg length inequality by comparing the heights of the right and left iliac crests or by measuring leg lengths from the anterior superior iliac spine to the ipsilateral medial malleoli. Findings of café au lait spots, nerve root irritation, paravertebral muscle spasm, a dermal sinus over the spine, hemangiomas, nevi, painful curvatures, and/or unequal leg length all suggest some other cause. Other signs indicating an alternative diagnosis include thoracic curves with a left instead of a right convexity; short, sharp, angular deformities in the mid thoracic region; long, sweeping, poorly compensated curves; and rapidly progressive deformities in spite of treatment. Even when examination suggests that the curvature is of the idiopathic form, the adolescent also should be carefully evaluated for other associated conditions. For example, the combination of scoliosis, hypoestrogenism, amenorrhea, hypomastia and mitral valve prolapse has been reported in adolescent ballet dancers.

Diagnosis is confirmed by x-ray evaluation of the entire spine. This can be limited to a single standing anteroposterior film of the spine. In idiopathic scoliosis, the x-ray usually demonstrates a right thoracic curvature from approximately T5-T6 to T11-L1 and a left lumbar curve from approximately T11-T12 to L-4. Curves are measured by the method of Cobb in which straight lines are first drawn across the top of the uppermost vertebrae of both the thoracic and lumbar curves. Perpendiculars are then drawn downward from the thoracic line and upward from the lumbar line. The number of degrees of the more acute angle of intersect between these perpendiculars is taken as the degree of scoliosis.

Management

Treatment of idiopathic scoliosis depends upon the degree of curvature, rate of the patient's growth, rate of curvature change, associated symptomatology, and the ability of the adolescent to comply with treatment regimens. Curve progression occurs in about 10% of adolescents with idiopathic scoliosis, with females 10 times at greater risk. Curves less then 30 degrees at skeletal maturity generally do not show progression. The greatest risk of curve progression is at SMR stages 2–3. One method of assessing skeletal maturity is Risser grading, which is based on the degree of ossification of iliac crest apophysis: grade 1 = up to 25% ossification; grade 2 = 26%–50%; grade 3 = 51%–75%; grade 4 = 76%–100%; and grade 5 = complete bony fusion of the apophysis. The higher the magnitude of the curve and the lesser the Risser grade, the greater the potential for curve progression.

No treatment is indicated for physically mature adolescents who have all but completed their growth (SMR stages IV–V) with minimal, asymptomatic and cosmetically acceptable curves less than 20 degrees, and no indication of underlying neurologic or musculoskeletal disease. Immature adolescents (SMR stages II-IV) with curves of 25 degrees or less may not need treatment, but should be followed with periodic clinical and radiographic assessment according to the following schedule:

- Curves less than 15 degrees; follow at 6–12-month intervals
- Curves between 15 and 20 degrees; follow at 5–6-month intervals
- Curves of 25 degrees or more; follow at 4-month intervals

Curves of 30 degrees or more and progressive curves of lesser magnitude in rapidly growing younger adolescents, require referral to an orthopedic surgeon experienced in the management of scoliosis. Bracing (either Milwaukee or Boston brace) is generally indicated for 25–40 degree curves in skeletally immature individuals; such braces are usually worn for 22–23 hours a day until the spine matures. Part-time bracing for 12–16 hours a day is less effective in preventing curve progression than full-time bracing. Weaning from the brace is initiated when the curve has been stable for at least a year and skeletal maturation has occurred. This usually takes 2–3 years to complete, with many patients wearing their braces at night until aged 17 or 18. Closure of the vertebral end-plate epiphyseal centers is the most reliable indicator of spinal maturation. This begins in the lumbar spines, progresses cranially and is complete by age 17–18 in girls and 18–19 in boys. If the curve progresses during the weaning process, a return to full-time use may be indicated. Patients undergoing bracing should be encouraged to be as active as possible. Almost all routine school and athletic activities can be continued with some restriction on contact/collision sports and no trampoline exercises. Swimming is permitted if the adolescent wears the brace to the locker room and promptly reapplies it when finished with the swim.

Surgery is indicated in advanced cases (curves over 45–50 degrees) or in cases refractory to conservative measures. These patients should be referred to an orthopedic surgeon with expertise in management of scoliosis. Electrical stimulation of back muscles and exercise therapy program are ineffective in correction of the spinal curve. Spinal manipulation, diet manipulation, or megavitamins have no proven role in the treatment of scoliosis.

Suggested Readings

Committee on Sports Medicine and Fitness. Atlantoaxial instability in Down syndrome: Subject review. *Pediatrics* 1995;96(1):151–154.

Betz RR. Kyphosis of the thoracic and thoracolumbar spine in the pediatric patient: normal sagittal parameters and scope of the problem. *Instruc Course Lect.* 2004;53:479–484.

Greydanus DE. The musculoskeletal system. In: Hofmann AD, Greydanus DE, eds. *Adolescent Medicine.* 3d ed.Stamford, CT: Appleton & Lange, 1997; Chap. 15, pp. 289–313.

Herring JA, ed. *Tachdjian's Pediatric Orthopaedics*, 3d ed. Philadelphia, PA: W. B. Saunders, 2002.

Lonstein JE. Adolescent idiopathic scoliosis. *Lancet* 1994;344:1407–1412.

Reamy BV, Slakey JB. Adolescent idiopathic scoliosis: review and current concepts. *Am Family Phys* 2001; 64(1):111–116.

Sponseller PD. Sizing up scoliosis. *JAMA* 2003;289: 608–609.

Weinstein ST, Dolan LA, Spratt KF, et al. Health and function of patients with untreated idiopathic scoliosis: a 50-year natural history study. *JAMA* 2003;289: 559–567.

KYPHOSIS

Kyphosis, identified in 4% of the general population, refers to an abnormally increased curve of the spine in the saggital plane; it commonly affects the thoracic spine. The normal thoracic curve in the saggital plane is 20–45 degrees. Two main types of kyphosis are seen in adolescents, namely, postural kyphosis and Scheuermann's disease.

Postural kyphosis accounts for 95% or more of all cases, and primarily occurs in youth who chronically slouch to a marked degree. Slouching may be simply habitual, in response to particularly rapid statural growth, to achieve an affected pose, to hide developing breasts, or for some other reason. Postural lordosis, with an increased anterior lumbar convexity and exaggerated protrusion of the sacrum and buttocks, is a frequent concomitant finding in patients with kyphosis. Postural kyphosis is flexible, and is corrected or disappears when the patient hyperextends the back while in the prone position. If uncorrected, postural curves may become chronic, resulting in a protuberant abdomen, low back pain, and, possibly, degenerative changes in the spine. Underlying vertebral structural abnormalities should be ruled out by plain films. Management involves an exercise program (e.g, weight lifting, track, ballet, modern dance) to strengthen back and abdominal muscles as well as promote good posture, along with attention to proper positioning while sitting and standing. Counseling also is indicated for any associated psychological factors.

Scheuermann's disease (dorsum rotundum), seen in 0.4%–10% of adolescents between ages 10 and 14, is characterized clinically by a fixed kyphotic deformity, most commonly affecting the thoracic spine; it is radiographically characterized by anterior wedging of 5 degrees or more in three adjacent vertebrae. It usually first appears in young adolescents during their period of accelerated growth and is believed to be due to rapid skeletal maturation with vertebral body compression. The ultimate consequences of this disease include considerable cosmetic deformity and a painful round back. Chronic low back pain can develop in adulthood if the curvature extends to the lumbar spine. Lateral x-rays of the spine show intravertebral disk space narrowing, anterior vertebral wedging, Schmorl's nodes, and abnormal vertebral body end plates in the mid-thoracic and thoracolumbar regions; such radiographic findings differentiate Scheuerman's disease from postural kyphosis or other structural abnormalities. Management of mild disease is limited to thoracic hyperextension exercises, while bracing or surgery may be necessary for a progressive deformity of more than 45 degrees. Surgery may be needed for curves of over 70 degrees or for sharply angulated kyphosis of any extent which is painful and progressive.

Suggested Readings

Pizzutillo PD. Nonsurgical treatment of kyphosis. *Instruc Course Lect* 2004;53:485–491.

Wenger DR, Frick SL. Scheuermann's kyphosis. *Spine* 1999;15(24):2630–2639.

SPONDYLOLYSIS

Anatomic lesion or defect of the pars interarticularis of the vertebra is referred to as *spondylolysis*. The lesions are classified in Table 11-3. Type 2(A) is the most common type seen in adolescents and most common lesion seen in athletes and will be

T A B L E   1 1 - 3

CLASSIFICATION OF SPONDYLOLYSIS

Type 1: Dysplastic: Dysplasia of L5 pars interarticularis with subluxation of L5 over S1; pars may be elongated.

Type 2: A. Fatigue or stress fracture of the pars
      B. Elongated pars
      C. Acute fracture of the pars

Type 3: Degenerative secondary to intersegmental instability

Type 4: Traumatic: Acute fracture other than pars

Type 5: Pathologic associated with bone disease.

discussed here. The lesion most commonly affects L5 with an overall prevalence of 4%–6%, and 8%–15% in athletes, with significantly higher prevalence in certain high risk sports in which repetitive hyperextension of the spine occurs such as gymnastics, dancing, rowing, football, wrestling, and soccer. In addition to the high risk sports, other risk factors include a positive family history, male gender, and underlying spina bifida occulta.

Most athletes with spondylolysis are asymptomatic. Gradual onset of lower back pain, especially associated with hyperextension of the spine, is the common initial symptom. There may be paraspinal muscle tightness and localized tenderness in acute lesions. Athletes typically have exaggerated lumbar lordosis and tight hamstrings. Neurological examination of lower extremities is normal. Plain films of the lumbosacral spine in AP, lateral, and oblique views, may show the pars defect as radiolucency, giving the characteristic Scotty dog with collar sign on the oblique views. SPECT is more sensitive in localizing the lesion of spondylolysis. Normal plain films, and negative SPECT rule out spondylolysis. CT scan of the spine is more definitive in localizing the lesion as well as in assessing the potential for healing; the characteristic sign on CT scan is the incomplete ring. Recent, though limited, studies suggest the utility of MRI in this condition.

Symptom-free patients do not need treatment. Bracing initiated within 1 month of pain onset, and lasting from 6 to 8 months, has been shown to promote osseous or fibrous union of the pars interarticularis in some cases. Rehabilitation exercises that specifically focus on hamstrings, quadriceps, abdominals, and back extensors, are the mainstay of conservative management. When the adolescent has a full range of pain-free lumbosacral spine movements with good core strength and stability, returning to sports activities can be allowed.

Spondylolisthesis refers to slippage of one vertebra over the one below, with bilateral spondylolysis at the same level; typically, there is slippage of L5 over S1. The lesions are graded based on the degree of slippage: grade 1 = slippage of less then 25%; grade 2 = 25%–50%; grade 3 = 50%–75%; grade 4 = 75%–100%; grade 5 = complete or 100% plus (spondyloptosis). The adolescent with spondylolisthesis presents with clinical finding similar to that of spondylolysis. Additionally, depending on the level and degree of slippage, patients may have lower extremity neurologic findings with high degree of slippage. Management of grades 1 and 2 is similar to that of spondylolysis. Patients with grade 3 and above should be referred to an orthopedic surgeon for further evaluation and treatment.

Suggested Readings

Lim MR, Yoon SC, Green DW. Symptomatic spondylolysis: diagnosis and treatment. *Curr Opin Pediatr* 2004;16(1):37–46.

Mc Timoney CA, Micheli LJ. Current evaluation and management of spondylolysis and spondylolisthesis. *Curr Sports Med Rep* 2003;2(1):41–46.

LOW BACK PAIN

Most cases of low back pain in adolescents have no discernible basis other than paravertebral muscle spasm, and are due to traumatic or postural strain. Various exogenous factors should be investigated; such as a recent change from high-heeled to low-heeled shoes or vice versa, the wearing of poorly fitting shoes, cramped study or working conditions, a poorly supportive bed, or simply being overweight. Participation in sports or other activities involving stress to the back without proper prior conditioning, lifting or pushing heavy objects, and the like, also are possible contributors. Spondylolysis or spondylolisthesis is the most frequent structural abnormality causing low back pain in adolescents. A psychogenic cause should be considered, particularly if the adolescent also complains of various ill-defined aches and pains in other parts of the body or the symptoms appear to provide significant secondary gain, as noted in school avoidance. The differential diagnosis of back pain in adolescents includes many conditions as listed in Table 11-4. A thorough history and physical examination will help narrow down the diagnostic considerations in most cases. A complete blood count, erythrocyte sedimentation rate, and plain films of the spine are most useful investigations that will help delineate the cause of back pain in most cases. Only a few patients will need further imaging studies, such as CT or MRI scans.

TABLE 11-4

CAUSES OF LOW BACK PAIN

Mechanical disorders
Muscle strain
Disk herniation
Apophyseal ring fracture
Slipped vertebral apophysis
Spinal facture
Hypermobility syndrome
Postural kyphosis
Developmental disorders
Spondylolysis and spondylolisthesis
Scheuermann's kyphosis
Idiopathic scoliosis
Syringomyelia
Tethered spinal cord
Idiopathic juvenile osteoporosis
Lumbarization
Sacralization
Spina bifida occulta
Infections
Diskitis
Vertebral osteomyelitis
Inflammatory conditions
Spondyloarthropathy
Ankylosing spondylitis
Juvenile rheumatoid arthritis
Benign neoplasms
Osteoid osteoma
Osteoblastoma
Eosinophilic granuloma
Aneurysmal bone cyst
Malignant neoplasms
Spinal cord astrocytoma
Spinal cord ependymoma
Malignant Neoplasms
Acute lymphocytic leukemia
Ewing's tumor
Osteogenic sarcoma
Metastasis
Intra-abdominal conditions
Inflammatory bowel disease
Hydronephrosis
Urinary tract infection
Ovarian cyst
Intra-abdominal neoplams
Psychosomatic

Slipped Disk

A slipped or herniated disk in adolescents is most likely a result of cumulative trauma rather than acute injury to the spine. There is a history of trauma in about half the patients; the most affected levels being L4-5 and L5-S1. Unlike adult patients, adolescents do not present with neurologic signs. Typically there is intermittent or chronic low back pain, especially associated with activities. In fact, the most common symptoms are back pain, stiffness, and leg pain. Associated conditions found in some cases of disk herniation in adolescents include transitional vertebra, spina bifida occulta, and congenital spinal stenosis. In these cases, MRI is the diagnostic study of choice. Initial treatment in the absence of neurologic signs is conservative, with back rehabilitation exercises in consultation with a physical therapist and modification of activities. The prognosis with conservative therapy is very good in most adolescents. Patients who do not respond to physical therapy or have neurologic signs should be referred to an orthopedic surgeon for further evaluation. A lesion unique to adolescents is a slipped vertebral apophysis, which can present with signs and symptoms similar to a slipped disk. It most commonly involves displacement of the inferior rim of the fourth lumbar vertebra (L4) and may cause nerve root pressure or stenosis of the canal. MRI is the study of choice and the patient should be referred to an orthopedic surgeon; excision of this lesion produces excellent results.

Diskitis

Diskitis, caused by a bacterial infection of the intervertebral disk space, usually is consequent to bacteremia (particularly with *Staphylococcus aureus*) complicating a respiratory or urinary tract infection. Vertebral osteomyelitis may present with similar symptomatology. Both conditions have a similar pathogenesis with specific manifestations dependent on other contributory factors; for example, vertebral osteomyelitis is more likely in those with sickle cell disease and in those who are intravenous drug abusers. The spectrum of disk space infection and osteomyelitis is often referred to as infectious spondylitis.

Presenting symptoms of diskitis and vertebral osteomyelitis are similar and include back pain (often with radiation to the hip or leg), local tenderness, abdominal pain, involuntary muscle spasm, and limping due to back pain and spasm. Fever, elevated white blood cell count, and elevated ESR, may be present. Standard spine x-rays usually do not reveal any abnormalities for the first 10–14 days; however, x-rays will demonstrate disk space narrowing followed by end plate erosions or irregularity with or without soft tissue changes. Late radiographic findings include vertebral body fraying and eventual collapse. A much earlier diagnosis can be established through radionuclear bone scans and/or MRI, as either of these procedures will detect pathology well before ordinary films. A needle or open biopsy of infected tissue for culture and antibiotic sensitivities is also important, since blood cultures tend to be positive in only about half of all cases.

Rarely, patients with severe diskitis and vertebral osteomyelitis may need bed rest and cast immobilization of the spine. Antibiotics are indicated, based on the organisms identified and sensitivity reported. Some clinicians recommend starting out with oral antibiotics in diskitis, only switching to an intravenous agent (along with disk space aspiration) if the infection does not respond. Antibiotic therapy may be needed for several weeks depending on the clinical response. Surgical consultation is indicated in patients who do not respond to conservative treatment.

Suggested Readings

Bono CM. Low-back pain in athletes. *JBJS* 2004;86A(2): 382–396.

Greydanus DE. The musculoskeletal system. In: Hoffman AD, Greydanus DE, eds. *Adolescent Medicine*. 3d ed. Stamford, CT: Appleton & Lange, 1997; Chap. 15, pp. 289–313.

Lim MR, Yoon SC, Green DW. Symptomatic spondylolysis: diagnosis and treatment. *Curr Opin Pediatr* 2004;16(1):37–46.

Mc Timoney CA, Micheli LJ. Current evaluation and management of spondylolysis and spondylolisthesis. *Curr Sports Med Rep* 2003;2(1):41–46.

Richards BS, McCarthy RE, Akbarnia BA. Back pain in childhood and adolescence. *Instruc Course Lect* 1999;48:525–542.

SLIPPED CAPITAL FEMORAL EPIPHYSIS

Epidemiology

Slipped capital femoral epiphysis (also called *adolescent coxa vera*) is characterized by an anterolateral displacement of the femoral neck in relation to the femoral head, with the latter retaining a normal position relative to the acetabulum. This condition has a prevalence of 1 in 100000 adolescents, with 75% of all cases occurring in tall, obese, early pubertal adolescents (SMR II-III) or obese preadolescents. It also can be seen in somewhat older, thin teenagers at the peak of their growth spurt. Males are affected more often than females, with a male to female ratio of between 2:1 and 3:1; also, it is more common in African Americans than Caucasians. The peak incidence is in spring or during summer months. The condition tends to be unilateral more often than bilateral (unilateral to bilateral ratio of 3:1), though a third of all patients with unilateral disease will have involvement of the opposite side at a later date. It also tends to be chronic (80%) rather than acute (20%), though an acute slip may develop over a chronic slip. Chronic disease is characterized by the development of severe pain and difficulty in weight bearing in a patient known to have mild disease. A severe acute slip in the absence of weight bearing and without previous symptoms is relatively uncommon. As slippage is through the hypertrophic zone of the growth plate with vascular disruption, significant complications include vascular necrosis of the femoral head, degenerative osteoarthritis of the hip and chondrolysis.

Etiology

The precise cause of slipped capital femoral epiphysis is unknown, but increased stress on a wide and rapidly growing epiphyseal plate has been postulated. Obesity, in combination with physiologic maturational events, appears to be a significant factor. In early puberty, the epiphyseal angle relative to the femoral shaft shifts from the horizontal to the oblique, and it is conjectured that an overweight condition increases the stress on this now disadvantageously positioned growth plate. Trauma can be contributory and plays a definite role in 10% of all cases. Genetics and autoimmune factors also may be involved. On rare occasion, an association has been noted between slipped femoral epiphysis and a number of other conditions including hypothyroidism, hypopituitarism, rickets, renal osteodystrophy, and radiotherapy in combination with chemotherapy using actinomycin D. Those with renal osteodystrophy and secondary hyperparathyroidism, however, are more likely to develop pathologic fractures than slipped epiphysis.

Clinical Features

Symptoms of a slipped epiphysis often first begin with an aching sensation in the groin, buttocks, lateral hip, or knee; the discomfort may or may not increase in severity over time. Referred knee pain can be the only sign and a slipped epiphysis must always be considered in the absence of obvious knee pathology. In some cases, several weeks or months of mild discomfort is followed by the acute onset of marked pain when a slight degree of slippage suddenly gives way and becomes severe. Findings on physical examination vary from being relatively unrevealing to demonstrating pain on hip motion, a limp with an externally rotated foot, limited internal rotation, abduction, and flexion of the hip. Occasionally, the patient's only complaint is of a painless limitation of hip rotation or an externally rotated leg and foot.

Diagnosis

Early diagnosis is essential because treatment at this stage offers an excellent prognosis in most cases, while delay can result in permanent hip deformity and traumatic arthritis. Hip x-rays (frog-leg or lateral as well as anteroposterior views) will distinguish a slipped capital epiphysis from other diagnostic considerations for hip pain (Table 11-5). Early in the course, lateral films show apparent displacement of the femoral head posteriorly and inferiorly, together

TABLE 11-5

DIFFERENTIAL DIAGNOSIS OF HIP PAIN IN TEENAGERS

Trauma/strain
Slipped capital femoral epiphysis
Transient synovitis
Monoarticular arthritis
Septic hip arthritis
Osteochondritis dissecans
Idiopathic chondrolysis
Late-onset Legg-Calve-Perthes disease
Osteoid osteoma
Sickle cell anemia
Collagen vascular disorders
Iliopsoas abscess
Stress fracture of the femoral neck
Meraligia paresthetica
Snapping hip syndrome
Trochanteric bursitis
Neoplasm

with an increased width of the epiphyseal plate with irregular margins. In more advanced cases, the femoral head becomes further displaced in relation to the femoral neck; in chronic slips, remodeling of the femoral neck can be seen.

Management

Patients with SCFE should be referred to an orthopedic surgeon. All weight bearing should be avoided from the moment this condition is suspected. Initially, traction is applied to prevent further slippage and relieve associated muscle spasm as well as synovial inflammation. However, surgery either by surgical pinning or epiphysiodesis, is the definitive treatment. Delayed treatment with significant slippage may require a corrective osteotomy to return the femoral head to a more normal weight-bearing position. Occasionally, an adolescent or parent will refuse surgical correction; in these instances a bilateral leg cast with cross bars or spica cast is an alternative.

In severe cases, the outcome of surgery unfortunately is often unsatisfactory. If adequate surgical correction is not possible, the patient faces the probability of either partial or total vascular necrosis of the femoral head, chondrolysis (particularly in females and African Americans), and/or traumatic arthritis with persistent hip pain, stiffness and limp. Total hip replacement may be required. It also needs to be kept in mind that slippage of the opposite femoral head occurs in about one-third of all youths with unilateral disease. Each patient should have periodic x-rays of the noninvolved side until growth is complete and epiphyses closed to detect possible delayed involvement of the opposite joint.

Suggested Readings

Greydanus DE. The musculoskeletal system In: Hoffman AD, Greydanus DE, eds. *Adolescent Medicine,* 3d ed. Stamford, CT: Appleton & Lange, 1997; Chap. 15, pp. 289–313.

Hamer AJ. Pain in the hip and knee. *BMJ* 2004;328(7447): 1067–1069.

Hollingworth P. Differential diagnosis and management of hip pain in childhood. *Br J Rheumatol* 1995;34(1): 78–82.

Hurley JM, Betz RR, Loder RT, et al. Slipped capital femoral epiphysis. *JBJS* 1996;78A(2):226–230.

Loder RT, Aronsson DD, Dobbs MB, et al. Slipped capital femoral epiphysis. *Instruc Course Lect* 2001;50: 555–570.

ACUTE TRANSIENT SYNOVITIS OF HIP

Acute transient synovitis of the hip is characterized by the sudden onset of limp or refusal to bear weight. It typically occurs in children, especially males, aged between 3 and 12 years. Proposing factors include viral infections, allergic reactions, and trauma, with half of all patients having a history of an antecedent upper respiratory tract infection. Laboratory data reveals a normal white blood cell count and, sometimes, a slight increase in the erythrocyte sedimentation rate. X-rays of the hip are normal and ultrasound may show fluid in the joint space. If a joint aspirate is done, it is sterile. The differential diagnoses include septic arthritis, Legg-Calve-Perthes disease, slipped femoral capital epiphysis, and juvenile rheumatoid arthritis, among others. Treatment is symptomatic. The condition usually resolves spontaneously within 1–2 weeks and recurrences are rare.

Avascular Necrosis of Femoral Head

Avascular necrosis of the femoral head (Legg-Calve-Perthes disease) is most common in children aged 2–12, but can be seen in early adolescence. Proposed etiologic factors include genetic predisposition, trauma, recurrent hip synovitis, immature bone, and abnormal venous constriction in the hip. Symptoms include hip pain which may radiate to the anterior thigh, decreased range of motion of the affected hip (particularly on abduction with the hip flexed and on internal rotation in the prone position), limp, muscle atrophy in the buttocks and thighs, and hip synovitis with tenderness to palpation. As in all hip disorders, pain may be referred and exclusively felt in the knee and distal medial thigh. X-rays are diagnostic with the earliest sign being a decrease in epiphyseal height. As the condition advances, a subchondral fracture and avascular necrosis may be seen. A technetium bone scan will be positive. Treatment aims to minimize distortion of the femoral head during the active stage of disease and includes bed rest, limb traction, and analgesics. An orthopedic consultation is indicated in all cases of avascular necrosis of the femoral head. Bracing to reduce weight bearing may be tried as well. Eventually, surgery may be necessary to improve the abnormal position of the femoral head or to remove necrotic bone. In general, the younger the age of onset, the better the prognosis, regardless of the treatment.

Suggested Reading

Thompson GH, Price CT, Roy D, et al. Legg-Calve-Perthes disease. *Instruc Course Lect* 2002;51:367–384.

OSTEOCHONDRITIS DISSECANS OF KNEE

Osteochondritis dissecans most commonly occurs in the knee, but also may be seen in the hip, elbow, and ankle. The presumptive etiology is trauma to a partially flexed joint, leading to a fracture of the involved metaphysis. In the knee, the condition is

TABLE 11-6

PAPPAS CLASSIFICATION OF OSTEOCHONDRITIS DISSECANS

Category I
Seen in early puberty
Often bilateral
Good prognosis
Category II
Seen in teenagers with Tanner Stages 3–5
Often seen with specific sports (at knees in soccer or elbows in pitching a baseball)
Need orthopedic consultation
Category III
Seen in skeletally mature individuals (Tanner Stage 5), usually over age 20
Symptoms often develop suddenly, secondary to the bony fragment detachment
May be a consequence of Category I or II
Requires orthopedic evaluation

characterized by the gradual separation of a fragment of subchondral metaphysis and associated cartilage from the medial femoral condyle. On occasion, the lateral femoral condyle, the femoral head, and the patella can be involved.

Osteochondritis dissecans is classified into three categories according to age of onset, manifestations, management and prognosis (Table 11-6). Most commonly, the disease appears in athletic males during late childhood or adolescence and is unilateral in 90% of all cases. The patient usually reports an aching sensation over the affected knee after exercising as well as a giving-way or locking sensation; however, there may be no symptomatology at all in some cases. Physical examination often reveals a mild knee effusion and local condylar tenderness, particularly when the knee is flexed. Knee x-rays show a characteristic radiolucent lesion of subchondral bone. If the fragment is not loose (*in situ* lesion), management simply consists of rest and nonsteroidal anti-inflammatory agents with healing expected in approximately 8–12 weeks.

If the diagnosis is delayed, the lesion may progress to full separation of the fragment of subchondral bone and articular cartilage, with dislodgement into the joint space. A limp, swelling, limited knee motion and locking episodes suggest this possibility. In some cases, flexion of the knee to 30 degrees from an extended position with the tibia fully internally rotated elicits pain, with relief on external tibial rotation (the Wilson sign). X-rays of the knee demonstrate the displaced fragment in the joint space. MRI is the imaging study of choice and helps delineate the exact nature of the lesion. Orthopedic consultation is indicated in all cases with advanced lesions of osteochondritis dissecans of the knee as these lesions need surgical intervention.

Suggested Readings

Greydanus DE. The musculoskeletal system In: AD Hofmann, DE Greydanus, eds. *Adolescent Medicine*, 3d ed. Stamford, CT: Appleton & Lange, 1997; Chap. 15, pp. 289–313.

Robertson W, Kelley BT, Green DW. Osteochondritis dissecans of the knee in children. *Curr Opin Pediatr* 2003;15:38–44.

BLOUNT DISEASE

Growth disturbance of the posterior and medial portions of the proximal tibia may result in a severe bow leg deformity in childhood known as Blount disease, or *tibia vara*. Occasionally a mild unilateral form occurs in early adolescence during growth. Consequent shortening of leg length on the involved side may necessitate surgical correction and these patients should be referred to an orthopedic surgeon.

Popliteal Cyst

Popliteal cyst (Baker's cyst) is a benign lesion consisting of a painless cystic mass of variable size (1–4 cm or more) most commonly arising from the gastrocnemius or semimembranosus bursa; it communicates with the knee joint. It is a smooth, firm, nonpulsatile, slow-growing lesion in the back of the knee, rarely causing symptoms unless it becomes very large. Rupture of the cyst into the calf may produce symptoms mimicking thrombophlebitis. Pain or motion restriction as well as pressure on nerve branches, also may be seen. Aspiration reveals gelatinous fluid similar to a wrist ganglion cyst. The differential diagnosis includes muscle tears, vascular aneurysms, and benign tumors. Baker's cyst resolves over a few months to sometimes years and treatment usually is not necessary. Rarely surgical excision may be performed if it is symptomatic. Postoperative recurrences or occurrence on the opposite side is not unusual.

Leg Aches

Leg aches, or intermittent aches or pains in the lower leg or thigh muscles, are usually easily distinguished from specific knee or hip disorders. Occasionally, pain in other areas, including the groin and in or behind the knees, is noted as well. There is no known etiology, and this condition has been linked to such diverse etiologies as puberty, rapid growth, overexertion with lactic acid buildup, excessive caffeine intake, and even acne! Typically the pain is bilateral; occurs in the late afternoon or early evening, or awakens the patient from sleep. Older children and young teenagers seem particularly prone to this complaint, which also has been called idiopathic myalgia or growing pains. No specific disorder has been found. X-rays and laboratory tests, including erythrocyte sedimentation rate and creatine phosphokinase, are normal. Resolution occurs over several months or years and there are no sequelae. When pain exists on dorsiflexion or plantar flexion of the foot and ankle, a diagnosis of anterior or posterior compartment syndrome should be considered.

Hallux Valgus

Hallux valgus or bunion is common in adolescents; the female to male ratio is 3:1. Most cases are idiopathic, while some are associated with other anomalies, such as metatarsus primum varus, pes planus, and short first metatarsal; it may also be seen in patients with neuromuscular disorders and cerebral palsy. Bunion is more commonly seen in girls who wear shoes with narrow toe box and high heels. On examination, a localized prominence over the medial aspect of great toe with erythema and callus from friction is noted. X-rays of the foot confirm the diagnosis of hallux valgus. Conservative treatment consists of wearing wide shoes with a decreased heel height; corrective surgery is needed in many cases.

Pes Planus

Pes planus or flat feet are common, usually asymptomatic, and considered to be a normal anatomic variation that requires no treatment. Flexible flatfeet maintain the medial longitudinal arch in a nonweight bearing position. On weight bearing, the medial arch is flattened and the heel goes into a valgus position with forefoot pronation. This results in a shift of weight bearing from the lateral column of the foot to the medial column. Very rarely patients with flexible flatfeet present with activity related foot pain; this includes running or jumping activities. Management is conservative with pain control, medial arch support, and leg and ankle strengthening.

Sever's Disease

Sever's disease is characterized by traction apophysitis at the insertion of the Achilles tendon with bilateral (sometimes unilateral) chronic heel pain exacerbated by running or walking, particularly on hard surfaces; this may be observed in athletes wearing cleated shoes or working out on paved surfaces. It is particularly liable to occur in 10–14-year olds and its etiology is unknown. Examination reveals medial-lateral heel tenderness, tenderness at the insertion of the Achilles tendon, decreased ankle dorsiflexion, and an absence of swelling. X-rays usually are normal, but there may be increased radiodensity or even fragmentation of the calcaneal epiphysis. Differential diagnosis includes other causes of foot pain listed in Table 11-7. Treatment involves activity modification, 1/2 inch heel lifts, ice, physical therapy to stretch the Achilles tendon, and nonsteroidal anti-inflammatory medications. The adolescent may return to sports activities when pain free. This is a benign, self-limiting condition with no long-term sequelae, and overzealous treatment or restriction of activities should be avoided.

TABLE 11-7

CAUSES OF FOOT AND ANKLE PAIN IN ADOLESCENTS

Poorly fitting shoes
Ankle sprain
Occult fracture (ankle or foot) due to specific trauma
 or chronic stress
Achilles tendonitis (with or without hypermobile
 flat feet)
Pes cavus (high arched feet)
Ingrown toe nails
Ganglion cyst
Osteomyelitis (including Brodie's abscess)
Infection from puncture wound of the plantar surface
 with or without retained foreign body
Accessory navicular bone
Tarsal coalition
Osteochondroses
  Sever's disease
  Freiberg's disease
  Kohler's disease
Tumors
  Synovial sarcoma
  Ewing's sarcoma
Metatarsalgia
Hallux valgus
Plantar faciitis
Peroneal tendon tendonitis/subluxation
Retrocalcaneal bursitis
Reflex sympathetic dystrophy
Tarsal tunnel syndrome

Tarsal Coalition

A tarsal coalition may present with a rigid, painful spastic foot and peroneal muscle spasm. In this often autosomal dominant condition, there is a calcified or fibrocartilaginous connection between two or more tarsal bones (usually at the calcaneonavicular joint or the talocalcaneal joint) resulting in rigid flat feet. The estimated prevalence is 1% in the general population and in almost half of the individuals, this is a bilateral condition. Symptoms typically develop during adolescence with sport activity, such as prolonged walking especially on uneven ground. AP and lateral weight bearing as well as oblique X-rays are diagnostic. Most symptomatic patients will need corrective surgery and should be referred to an orthopedic or foot surgeon.

Suggested Readings

Bohne WH. Tarsal coalition. *Curr Opin Pediatr* 2001;13(1):29–35.

Greydanus DE. The musculoskeletal system In: AD Hofmann, DE Greydanus, eds. *Adolescent Medicine.* 3d ed. Stamford, CT: Appleton & Lange, 1997; Chap. 15, pp. 289–313.

Mann RA, Mann JA. The bunionette deformity. *Instruc Course Lec* 2004;53:303–309.

Mizel MS, Hecht PJ, Marymont JV, Temple HT. Evaluation and treatment of chronic ankle pain. *Instruc Course Lec* 2004;53:311–321.

Scherl SA. Lower extremity problems in children. *Pediatrics In Review* 2004;25(2):52–62.

Thometz J. Tarsal coalition. *Foot and Ankle Clinics* 2000;5(1):103–118.

HYPERMOBILITY SYNDROME

Individuals with this condition have marked hyperextensibility and hypermobility of their joints and are sometimes referred to as being "double-jointed." It occurs in 4%–8% of the population as an isolated finding, often with a positive family history. Hyperextensibility also may be a component of various congenital connective tissue disorders, such as Marfan syndrome (Chaps. 9 and 21), osteogenesis imperfecta (Chap.21), and Ehlers-Danlos syndrome (Chap. 21).

Hypermobility of the upper extremities usually is asymptomatic and may even be advantageous in sports (as basketball, ballet and gymnastics) or playing musical instruments (as the flute, piano, and violin). On the other hand, hyperextensibility of weight bearing joints, such as the knees and spine, may be a contributory factor for overuse injuries. The diagnosis is established by finding hyperextensibility in at least three of the following joints: spine, knees, elbows, metacarpophalanges, wrists and thumbs. The Beighton scoring system is often used for objective assessment. Two points are given for each of the following findings: (1) hyperextension of both fifth metacarpophalangeal joints to 90 degrees; (2) apposition of both thumbs to the volar aspect of the forearm; (3) hyperextension of both elbows to 10 degrees or more; and (4) hyperextension of both knees to 10 degrees or more. An additional point is given if the patient can place his or her hands flat on the floor with the knees extended. At least 6 points are required for the diagnosis. Asymptomatic patients with idiopathic hypermobility need no treatment, while in some patients, appropriate exercises and pain control is needed.

Suggested Readings

Baum J, Mudholkar GS, et al. Benefits and disadvantages of joint hypermobility among musicians. *N Engl J Med* 1993;329(15):1079–1082.

Hakim A, Grahame R. Joint hypermobility. *Best Practice and Research Clinical Rheumatol* 2003;17(6): 989–1004.

OSTEOID OSTEOMA

Osteoid osteoma is a relatively common benign bone tumor usually seen in those aged 10–30 years; there is a 2:1 male to female ratio. It should be suspected when pain localizes to a bone or joint, increases during rest and at night (often awakening the individual from sleep), and diminishes with exercise. Seventy five percent of all cases also will obtain relief with aspirin administration. The pain varies in intensity, but often is exceptionally severe. Usually there is no history of trauma and no pain on weight bearing. Most tumors are solitary and located in the femur or tibia; however, multiple tumors have been reported on rare occasions and almost any bone may be a site. Physical findings may be absent or variably include (depending on the tumor's location) localized swelling, muscle atrophy, favoring of the affected extremity, and degenerative joint changes. If close to a joint, a reactive synovitis may develop. Osteoid osteoma of the spine may cause a painful scoliosis due to paravertebral muscle spasm.

X-rays classically show a small radiolucent, rounded nidus, usually less than 1 cm in diameter and sometimes only 2–3 mm, surrounded by reactive sclerotic bone. Calcium deposits may or may not be noted within the central area. Sometimes, however, the tumor is not readily visible on standard films, as the lesion can be easily obscured by normal, overlying, dense bone; in these instances, a CT scan is indicated. This is particularly likely to occur in the spine.

An osteoid osteoma over 2 cm is termed an *osteoblastoma*. Pain may be less acute and is more likely to recur after surgical removal. X-rays also may not be classic as with osteoid osteoma. The differential diagnosis (Table 11-8) also includes fibrous dysplasia which is an intramedullary bone disease involving one or several bones. The McCune-Albright syndrome is a form of polyostotic fibrous dysplasia and may be accompanied by characteristic café au lait spots with irregular borders ("Coast of Maine") as compared to the typically smooth borders of those seen in neurofibromatosis ("Coast of California"). Polyostotic fibrous dysplasia may present with skeletal deformities in growing adolescents. Aneurysmal bone cysts may also occur in this age

TABLE 11-8

DIFFERENTIAL DIAGNOSIS OF OSTEOID OSTEOMA

Osteoid osteoma
Fibrous dysplasia
Aneurysmal bone cyst
Giant cell tumor
Osteochondroma, osteoblastoma (benign exostosis)
Malignant tumors
Osteogenic sarcoma
Ewing's tumor
Soft-tissue sarcoma
Leukemia
Stress fracture with callus formation
Osteomyelitis
Non-ossifying fibroma
Enchondroma
Chondroblastoma
Chondromyxoid fibroma
Eosinophilic granuloma

group. Usually located in long bones, they may present simply with pain and swelling or with a pathologic fracture. X-rays are diagnostic. Simple surgical excision is curative for an osteoid osteoma, although recurrences are possible if removal is not complete. Surgical curettage is also used to cure aneurysmal bone cysts.

Suggested Readings

Baum J, Mudholkar GS, et al. Benefits and disadvantages of joint hypermobility among musicians. *N Engl JMed* 1993;329(15):1079–1082.

Greydanus DE. The musculoskeletal system In: Hofmann AD, Greydanus DE, eds. *Adolescent Medicine*, 3d ed. Stamford, CT: Appleton & Lange, 1997; Chap. 15, pp. 289–313.

Hakim A, Grahame R. Joint hypermobility. *Best Practice and Research Clinical Rheumatol* 2003;17(6): 989–1004.

PILONIDAL CYST AND SINUS

Pilonidal cyst and sinus is a common embryonic defect due to failure of the distal end of the neurenteric canal to close completely and has a greater prevalence in males than females. Although present at birth as an asymptomatic sinus tract, it often becomes infected in adolescence or adulthood. Factors which may precipitate an infectious episode include recurrent trauma from such activities as horseback riding, trail riding on a motorcycle or jeep, and foreign body irritation from hair tufts. *S. aureus* and coliform organisms are most commonly involved. In the noninfected state, the only evidence of the sinus is a small dimple located at the upper end of the gluteal crease over or just below the coccygeal region. Some cases may be further marked by a small tuft of hair, in which case the coexistence of spina bifida occulta should be ruled out. Infectious complications initially include local pain, erythema, and swelling with progression to a variably sized chronic or recurring cyst or abscess. There also may be one or more draining, often foul smelling, sinus tracts. Rupture of a cyst or abscess into the cerebrospinal fluid with resultant meningitis is a rare complication.

Management of an infected pilonidal sinus consists of oral or intravenous antibiotics, local warm-hot soaks several times a day, attention to hygiene, and surgical consultation for definitive treatment—incision and drainage or surgical excision of the sinus tract.

Suggested Readings

Greydanus DE. The musculoskeletal system In: Hofmann AD, Greydanus DE, eds. *Adolescent Medicine*, 3d ed. Stamford, CT: Appleton & Lange, 1997; Chap. 15, pp. 289–313.

Hull TL, Wu J. Pilonidal disease. *Surg Clin North Am* 2002;82(6):1169–1185.

SEPTIC ARTHRITIS

Eighty percent of all cases of *septic arthritis* occurs in the lower extremities with the knee most frequently involved, followed by the hip, and then ankle in that order. Predisposing factors include bacteremia, septicemia, penetrating wounds, and, sometimes, local cellulitis. Bacterial infection of the synovial space should be suspected when there is rapid onset of joint pain, together with swelling, erythema, increase warmth, tenderness, and limited motion; also, there may be a limp or an inability to bear weight in the absence of trauma. Fever, malaise and other systemic signs also may be present. Septic arthritis should be considered in the differential diagnosis in any instance of acute joint disease. Irreversible damage to the joint can result if the treatment is delayed. It also is important to note that partial treatment can obscure symptoms.

Etiology

Gonococcal Arthritis

Neisseria gonorrhoeae is the predominant causal agent of septic arthritis in adolescence. Its spread is presumed to be hematogenous after genital involvement occurs. Affected males frequently have a history of urethral gonorrhea marked by a purulent, painful, penile discharge. Females, however, tend to be asymptomatic carriers with arthritis occurring in the absence of antecedent genital signs and often during menstruation.

In any sexually active youth (known or suspected) who exhibits several hot, painful joints with or without fever and chills, a gonococcal origin always should be considered. It is particularly likely to be the cause when septic arthritis closely follows genital gonorrhea in males or occurs in females with positive endocervical cultures, particularly if menstruating. Migratory polyarthritis and tenosynovitis, particularly of wrist and Achilles tendon sheaths, are other classic findings. A gonococcal dermatitis also may be seen and is characterized by scattered vesiculopustules on a markedly erythematous base, sometimes resembling true purpura. Gonorrheal arthritis should not be confused with *N. meningococcus* infection. This is a significant differential consideration in that meningococcemia also may present with migratory arthritis and, while the associated skin lesions are typically petechial, they can be maculopapular or manifest as subcutaneous nodules in subacute and chronic forms.

Approximately 90% of all cases of bacterial arthritis due to organisms other than *N. gonorrhoeae*, are monoarticular. If the patient presents with polyarticular disease which is thought to be nongonococcal in origin, some other underlying cause should be entertained (Table 11-9). Reiter syndrome and Behçet syndrome also should be considered because these diseases also are associated with arthritis and genital infection (Table 11-10).

TABLE 11-9

DIFFERENTIAL DIAGNOSIS OF SEPTIC ARTHRITIS

Bacterial septic arthritis

Nonbacterial infectious arthritis (viral, mycoplasma, Lyme disease, mycobacterial, and fungal).

Cellulitis

Traumatic injury

Acute rheumatic fever

Juvenile rheumatoid arthritis and other collagen vascular disease

Toxic synovitis

Serum sickness

Acute lymphocytic leukemia

Henoch-Schönlein purpura

Psoriatic arthritis

Arthritis associated with inflammatory bowel disease

TABLE 11-10

ARTHRITIS ASSOCIATED WITH GENITAL INFECTIONS

Disease	Description	Type of Arthritis
Gonoccal arthritis	Arthritis is a complication of gonococcal urethritis in males or cervicitis in females and one of the many complications seen in the 1%–3% of patients Local disease progress to septicemia. Coexistent dermatitis (erythematous pustule with a necrotic, umbilicated center) assists in diagnosis.	Two types: 1) Polyarthritis (and tenosynovitis) with fever, chills, and dermatitis. Joints are swollen, painful and warm. Blood cultures are positive. Joint cultures may be negative. Develops about 2 weeks after sexual exposure. 2) Monoarthritis (often knee or wrist) with minimal effusion, no dermatitis, negative blood culture, and (often) positive joint culture.
Reiter syndrome	Triad of urethritis, conjunctivitis (iritis), and arthritis predominating in males. Minority have complete type. Can follow bacterial dysentery (shigella salmonella, yersinia campylobacter) or be sexually acquired (chlamydia and mycoplasma have both been implicated). Bacterial antigens (including Chlamydia) may be demonstrable in involved joints. Buccal ulceration, balanitis circinata, keratoderma blennorrhagicum, Achilles tendonitis, increased ESR and HLA-B27 also may be noted. Arthritic symptoms usually self-limited.	Variable arthritis picture. Often, acute, self-limiting involvement of the lower extremity joint developing 10–14 days after urethritis. Inflammation of ligament-tendon insertions, dactylitis and even severe joint destruction can occur. Sacroiliitis is a less common complication resembling ankylosing spondylitis. Early treatment with tetracycline or other anti-chlamydial agents may reduce arthritic symptoms and pain relieved by NSAIDs.
Behçet syndrome	Triad of recurrent aphthous stomatitis, genital ulcerations and iritis in association with other features including polyarthritis. Also thrombophlebitis, meningoencephalitis, erythema multiforme, vasculitis, pyodermas, epididymitis, and others. Seen especially in Japan and Mediterranean countries. Increased HLA-B5 reported. Placed in a group of spondyloarthroses; seronegative for rheumatoid factor with peripheral arthritis and sacroiliitis.	Variable pattern. Transient arthritis of various joints that resolves without sequelae. Aspirin used as treatment.

Other Causes

S. aureus is the next most common infecting agent and the most frequent cause of septic arthritis in older children and nonsexually active adolescents (60% of all cases). Heroin addicts are particularly likely to develop staphylococcal arthritis of the sternoclavicular or sacroiliac joint. Gram-negative organisms (other than *N. gonorrhoeae*) and anaerobes also may be seen, particularly in cases of illicit parenteral drug use and penetrating trauma. In the latter instance, the infection also is likely to be polymicrobial. Other organisms are reviewed in Chap. 20.

Diagnostic Studies

In addition to positive clinical findings, laboratory tests in acute septic arthritis commonly reveal a peripheral leukocytosis (over 15000 WBC per mm^3) with a shift to the left, elevated C-reactive protein, and an elevated erythrocyte sedimentation rate. The synovial fluid (obtained by arthrocentesis) is whitish, opaque and thick with a friable mucin clot, low glucose content (as compared to blood glucose), absence of crystals, and a white blood cell count ranging from 20000 to 200000 per microliter (usually >50000 per microliter) of which 75% are polymorphonuclear cells. Synovial leukocytosis in and of itself, however, is not diagnostic of septic arthritis; rheumatoid, crystal-induced, and reactive arthritis also may have a synovial fluid leukocytosis of over 50000 per microliter.

The diagnosis of septic (bacterial) arthritis is established by the presence of intracellular bacteria on synovial fluid, Gram's stain, and positive synovial fluid and/or blood cultures. Such studies, however, are not always positive. The Gram stain will demonstrate characteristic intracellular organisms in only 50%–75% of cases due to *S. aureus* and in 40% of cases due to *N. gonorrhoeae*. Single synovial fluid and blood cultures also are often negative. Multiple blood cultures, however, may increase the likelihood of recovering an organism when associated bacteremia is present. In cases of suspected gonococcal arthritis, appropriate endocervical or penile cultures also should be taken and cultures of saline aspirates from the margins of vesicular skin lesions may be positive as well. Immunoelectron microscopy and polymerase chain reaction studies of synovial biopsies can identify such organisms as *N. gonorrhoeae*, *Ureaplasma urealyticum*, and *Borrelia burgdorferi*. Other laboratory tests are less helpful. The rheumatoid factor is positive in many disorders, including subacute bacterial endocarditis and rheumatoid arthritis. Tests for HIV antibodies and Lyme antibodies are not conclusive as single tests.

Joint x-rays early in the course of septic arthritis also are not diagnostic; often, only nonspecific changes and widening of the synovial space are seen. In arthritis of the hip, a bilateral film in the frog-leg position may show joint capsule swelling and displacement of the femoral head upward and laterally. After 2–4 weeks, however, X-rays become classic with rarefaction and erosion of subchondral bone. Hopefully, the diagnosis already will have been considered and treatment started well before this time. However, early X-rays are important in excluding other causes of joint pain and in providing a baseline for future comparisons. Other useful diagnostic procedures include computerized tomography, technetium-99m-methylene diphosphonate or gallium bone scanning, and MRI.

Management

General principles of treatment for septic arthritis include appropriate antibiotics, symptomatic management and, in some cases, periodic joint aspiration or open drainage in consultation with an orthopedic surgeon (Chap. 20). While the latter is variably required in other joints, drainage is always indicated in septic arthritis of the hip as long as fluid is present. This may be by daily closed aspiration or by open drainage, if the fluid cannot be aspirated, or if there is a slow response to antibiotics. Arthroscopic drainage is another alternative used by some clinicians.

Gonococcal arthritis usually responds promptly to ceftriaxone (1 g IM or IV, once per day for 7 days). Alternatives include cefotaxime (1 g IV, three times a day for 7 days), ciprofloxacin (400 mg IV twice daily), others; if allergic to beta-lactam drugs, spectinomycin (2 g IM, twice a day for 7 days) can be used. Parenteral therapy can be discontinued in 1-2 days when improvement begins and the 7-day course completed with an oral antibiotic, such as ciprofloxacin

(500 mg twice daily), cefixime (400 mg twice daily) or ofloxacin (400 mg twice daily). Quinolone antibiotics should not be used in individuals under age 18, in those of any age who are nursing or pregnant, and in areas where quinolone-resistant *N. gonorrhoeae (QRNG)* is prominent. Specific antibiotic treatment of septic joint due to nongonococcal agents should be planned based on specific organisms identified and antibiotic sensitivity, preferably in consultation with infectious disease specialist. Generally a third generation cephalosporin can be started initially in most cases (Chap. 20).

Suggested Readings

Braverman PK, Rosenfeld WD, eds. Sexually transmitted diseases. *Adolesc Med Clin* 2004;15:201–428.

Bardin T. Gonococcal arthritis. *Best Pract Res Rheumatol* 2003;17(2):201–208.

Garcia-De La Torre I. Advances in the management of septic arthritis. *Reuma Dis Clin North Am* 2003; 29(1):61–75.

Greydanus DE. The musculoskeletal system In: Hofmann AD, Greydanus DE, eds. *Adolescent Medicine*, 3d ed. Stamford, CT: Appleton & Lange, 1997; 15, pp. 289–313.

Miller JC. Infectious causes of arthritis in adolescents. *Adolescent Medicine* 1998;9(1):115–126.

Nade S. Septic arthritis. *Best Pract Res Rheumatol* 2003;17(2):183–200.

Parker CT, Thomas D. Reiter syndrome and reactive arthritis. *J Am Osteopathic Assoc* 2000;100(2): 101–104.

Shirtliff ME, Madler JT. Acute septic arthritis. *Clinical Microbiology Reviews* 2002;15(4):527–544.

Szer IS. Arthritis in adolescence. *Adoles Med* 1991;2(3):547–548.

Waagner DC. Musculoskeletal infections in adolescents. *Adolesc Med* 2000;11:375–400.

Workowski KA, Levine WC. Sexually transmitted diseases treatment guidelines, 2002. *MMWR* 2002;51/RR-6:38039.

Yurdakul S, Hamuryudan V, Yazici H. Behçet syndrome. *Curr Opin Rheumatol* 2004;16(1):38–42.

LYME DISEASE ARTHRITIS

Lyme disease is caused by the spirochete, *Borrelia burgdorferi*, and transmitted by the bite of an *Ixodes* carrier tick. This condition should be considered in the differential diagnosis of any chronic arthritis which occurs in areas where infected ticks are endemic. This includes New England, the mid-Atlantic states, Wisconsin, upper Michigan, Minnesota, New Jersey, and the northwestern United States.

Joint manifestations vary over the course of the disease (Table 11-11). Early in the disease (Stage 1),

TABLE 11-11

LYME DISEASE: CLINICAL COURSE

Stage	Time after Bite	Predominant System Involved & Manifestations
1	1 day to 4 weeks	Constitutional: flu-like/fatigue
		Dermatological: erythema chronicum migrans
2	3 weeks to 5 months	Cardiac: AV block (syncope)
		Congestive heart failure
		Neurological: meningoencephalitis, cranial neuritis (Bell's palsy), polyradiculitis
		Ophthalmological: uveitis/blindness
		Musculoskeletal: migratory joint and muscle pain
3	5 months to years	Musculoskeletal: monoarthritis/oligoarthritis
		Neurological: demyelination, psychiatric
		Dermatological: acrodermatitis chronica atrophicans

there may be only migratory arthralgias with little or no joint swelling. About 60%–80% of all patients also will demonstrate erythema chronicum migrans; this begins as a red macule or papule at the site of the bite, expands to form a large erythematous ring with central clearing, and then gradually fades over a period of three to four weeks. Other symptoms which may be seen include fever, fatigue, myalgias, and regional adenopathy. Stage 2 of the disease occurs weeks to months later (with an average of 6 months), when overt arthritis of both large and small joints (including the temporomandibular joint) may appear. Even later (Stage 3), there may be intermittent episodes of monoarthritis of the lower extremities with large, mildly painful knee effusions, but without fever, and lasting from several weeks to several months. Other variable symptoms which may be seen in Stages 2 and 3 include neurological symptoms, such as peripheral neuritis, headache, meningitis, and/or facial palsy (15%–20%); there can also be subtle memory impairment, behavioral changes and/or somnolence (4%), atrioventricular block (4%–8%), and keratitis (4%). Boys with HLA-DR4 or DR2 phenotypes tend to be more seriously affected than others and may develop severe, refractory arthritis.

Laboratory Studies

Significant laboratory data include elevated IgM and IgG titres to *B. burgdorferi*, although these generally do not rise until Stage 2 disease. The finding of elevated antibodies, however, is not absolutely diagnostic because serologic testing methods are not yet completely reliable, particularly in the face of such problems as attenuation by antibiotic treatment or infection with *Treponema pallidum*.

Management

Treatment in early Stage 1 disease consists of oral penicillin V, amoxicillin or tetracycline for 10–30 days. Treatment in late disease or in early disease which fails to respond to oral antibiotics, is by intravenous therapy with ceftriaxone or penicillin G for 2–3 weeks. Symptomatic management of arthritic symptoms is with nonsteroidal anti-inflammatory agents. Particularly severe and prolonged arthritis may require intra-articular steroid injections.

Suggested Readings

Greydanus DE. The musculoskeletal system In: Hofmann AD, Greydanus DE, eds. *Adolescent Medicine*, 3d ed. Stamford, CT: Appleton & Lange, 1997; Chap. 15, pp. 289–313.

Massarotti EM. Lyme arthritis. *Med Clin North Am* 2002;86(2):297–309.

VIRAL ARTHRITIS

Etiology

Some generalized viral illnesses may manifest synovial inflammation in addition to their other clinical signs. Deposition of immune complexes within the synovial space is thought to be responsible. In adolescents, rubella (either with wild virus or with the attenuated virus used in rubella vaccine) and hepatitis B are most frequently involved. Epstein-Barr virus (mononucleosis), mumps, chicken pox, adenovirus, and coxsackievirus also have been implicated on occasion, as have the herpetoviridae (e.g., herpes simplex, varicella-zoster, cytomegalovirus) and parvovirus B19 (erythema infectiosum).

Clinical Features

Regardless of etiology, most cases evidence either a pauciarticular arthritis involving 1 or 2 large joints or a migratory polyarthritis involving multiple small joints with morning stiffness. Symptoms may or may not be preceded by fever which also can occur with Lyme disease, reactive arthritis, subacute bacterial endocarditis, and Still's disease.

In the usual course of arthritis in hepatitis B infection, migratory joint symptoms occur during the prodromal period before symptoms of liver involvement appear and resolve when jaundice develops. An urticarial or maculopapular rash and/or fever can develop at the same time. Arthritis associated with rubella (wild or attenuated virus) and parvovirus B19 infections occur almost exclusively in young women and most often presents as a symmetric, polyarticular disease of the fingers and hand.

Laboratory Studies

Synovial fluid cultures are negative for viral arthritis and the erythrocyte sedimentation rate often is normal. Peripheral white blood cell counts reflect the underlying disease, often showing a lymphocytosis or leukopenia. A positive rheumatoid factor also may be found, confusing the diagnosis. Laboratory tests will reveal the presence of hepatitis B surface antigen along with increasing levels of aminotransferase in hepatitis B infection.

Management

Treatment is symptomatic. With few exceptions, all cases of viral arthritis are self-limited and spontaneously resolve in 2–5 days without sequelae. Exceptions to this usually benign course may be seen in hepatitis B and rubella. Hepatitis B arthritis can present with more severe polyarticular involvement resembling rheumatoid arthritis. Wild rubella virus has been implicated in some cases of chronic disease.

Suggested Readings

Greydanus DE. The musculoskeletal system In: Hofmann AD, Greydanus DE, eds. *Adolescent Medicine*, 3d ed. Stamford, CT: Appleton & Lange, 1997; Chap. 15, pp. 289–313.

Masuko-Hongo K, Kato T, Nishiok K. Virus-associated arthritis. *Best Pract Res Rheumatol* 2003;17(2): 309–318.

ACKNOWLEDGMENTS

The authors thank Ms. Cori Edgecomb for assistance in preparation of this manuscript.

12

RHEUMATIC DISORDERS

Mary D. Moore

OVERVIEW

Rheumatic disorders (Table 12-1) are a diverse group of complex, chronic inflammatory conditions of unknown causes, with peak onset in early adult life. The hallmark is arthritis of the peripheral joints and axial skeleton; however, the inflammatory process can affect other organ systems such as skin, eye, kidneys, lungs, heart, and central nervous system. There is considerable overlap in the clinical features of the rheumatic disorders and it can be quite difficult to establish an accurate diagnosis early, as specific clinical features may not be evident at the onset. The causes of most rheumatic diseases remain unknown, but there has been an explosion in information on the role of the immune response in chronic inflammation, as well as the development of new immunotherapies that target specific immunologic sites and inflammatory mediators. The morbidity and mortality of these disorders have improved significantly in the past decade, and future advances are anticipated.

Adolescents with these conditions represent many challenges for clinicians, not only in diagnosis and treatment, but also in the prevention of severe secondary complications, such as opportunistic infections and glucocorticoid-induced osteopenia. The development of a severe, potentially fatal disorder causes tremendous stress to the adolescent and the family, as they adjust to the limitations and uncertainties imposed by these complicated and unpredictable conditions. It is imperative that clinicians treating adolescents have a general awareness of these disorders and recognize features that can suggest the presence of a rheumatic disorder.

EPIDEMIOLOGY AND ETIOLOGY

In children and adolescents, the most common rheumatic disorders are juvenile idiopathic arthritis (JIA) and the spondyloarthropathies, both occurring at frequencies of 0.5–2 per 1000 individuals. At any time, half of the children with JIA will have an inactive disease. Epidemiologic studies of JIA have been mainly descriptive and are further complicated by the differences in diagnostic criteria, the marked heterogeneity in disease expression, as well as the inability to identify specific etiologic agents. Despite major advances in understanding of the inflammatory response, the etiology of most rheumatic diseases remains unknown. Stress, infection, and trauma can all play a role in triggering the onset of arthritis, as well as causing exacerbations of existing disease. However, the actual contribution of each factor is not known. Genetic factors also contribute to the development of JIA, but the association is much less consistent than the strong

TABLE 12-1
RHEUMATIC DISORDERS

Juvenile idiopathic arthritis (JIA)
Spondyloarthropathies
  Ankylosing spondylitis
  Reactive arthritis (also called Reiter syndrome)
  Psoriatic arthropathy
  Enteropathic arthropathy (arthritis associated with
    inflammatory bowel disease).
Systemic lupus erythematosus (SLE)
Dermatomyositis
Systemic vasculitides
  Kawasaki disease
  Henoch-Schönlein purpura (HSP),
  Serum sickness
  Polyarteritis nodosa (PAN)
Others

association of HLA B27 in the spondyloarthropathies. JIA probably encompasses several diseases of differing etiologies.

Systemic lupus erythematosus (SLE) and dermatomyositis are much less common, with an approximate incidence of 4–6 per 100,000 children and adolescents. Scleroderma has an incidence of 4 per million overall and is extremely rare in childhood and adolescence. The systemic vasculitides are distinctly uncommon in childhood and adolescence, with the exception of Kawasaki disease (Chap. 9) and Henoch-Schönlein purpura (HSP) (Chap. 16), conditions which have a much more favorable outcome than the other vasculitides. However, systemic vasculitis can occur in adolescence, but is extremely rare and most large pediatric rheumatology centers have a handful of cases at most. Like most rheumatic disorders, the etiology of systemic vasculitis is still unknown. The one exception is polyarteritis nodosa where 50% of cases are associated with hepatitis B infection. Similar to adults, there is a female predominance in most rheumatic disorders, except for some of the vasculitides and the spondyloarthropathies.

EVALUATION OF THE ADOLESCENT WITH A SUSPECTED RHEUMATIC DISORDER

The importance of a detailed history and physical examination, including a comprehensive family history, cannot be overemphasized. The working impression from the history and examination will guide in the development of a thoughtful, logical, and appropriate diagnostic and treatment plan. The family and adolescent need education on the disease process, its treatment, and a realistic assessment of disease outcome. Nonorganic musculoskeletal pain is a therapeutic challenge. It is important to identify these individuals early to avoid putting the patient through an extensive and unnecessary evaluation; more importantly, one can then focus on symptom control and facilitate a prompt return to school and normal function. Table 12-2 provides a differential diagnosis of arthritis.

Musculoskeletal complaints are extremely common and are the third most common reason for patients to see a physician; only infections and routine physical exams are more common. Between 10% and 20% of healthy adolescents have chronic or recurrent limb pain, and most of these patients will not have a rheumatic disorder. Most youths presenting with a musculoskeletal complaint will have a transient cause of their symptoms, such as trauma, overuse syndromes, joint hypermobility, or a reactive process from an intercurrent infection. Evaluation begins with careful history-taking, a thorough physical examination, and a few simple laboratory investigations. A more comprehensive investigation should be reserved for those patients with more serious or persistent symptoms, or in whom the screening studies suggest an underlying inflammatory or systemic condition.

History and Physical Examination

Details should be obtained on the timing and progression of symptoms, pain characteristics, and conditions that relieve symptoms. Relief of symptoms with one of the ubiquitous nonsteroidal anti-inflammatory drugs (NSAIDs) does not confirm

TABLE 12-2

DIFFERENTIAL DIAGNOSIS OF ARTHRITIS IN ADOLESCENCE

1. Rheumatoid arthritis: juvenile (JIA) or adult form (RA)
2. Rheumatic fever
3. Spondyloarthropathies
   a. Ankylosing spondylitis
   b. Psoriatic arthropathy
   c. Reactive arthritis (Reiter syndrome)
   d. Enteropathic arthropathy (arthritis associated with inflammatory bowel disease)
   e. Unclassified (undifferentiated) spondyloarthropathy
4. Infectious joint disease
   a. Septic arthritis
   b. Viral arthropathy
   c. Complication of osteomyelitis
   d. Sexually transmitted disease arthritis
   e. Lyme arthritis
5. Other rheumatoid disorder
   a. Systemic lupus erythematosus (SLE)
   b. Dermatomyositis
   c. Scleroderma
   d. Mixed connective tissue disease (MCTD)
6. Vasculitis
   a. Henoch-Schönlein purpura (HSP)
   b. Polyarteritis nodosa (PAN)
   c. Kawasaki disease
   d. Serum sickness
   e. Sjögren syndrome
   f. Wegener's granulomatosis
   g. Churg-Strauss disease
7. Generalized disorders often complicated by arthritis
   a. Hemophilia
   b. Sickle cell disease
   c. Serum sickness
   d. Secondary gout and pseudogout
   e. Neoplastic disease
      • Leukemia
      • Lymphoma

   • Primary bone and synovial tumors as villonodular synovitis
   • Neuroblastoma (in children)
   f. Polychondritis
   g. Hypertrophic osteoarthropathy
8. Diseases sometimes complicated by arthritis
   a. Psoriasis
   b. Inflammatory bowel disease
   c. Acne fulminans
   d. Hyperlipidemia
   e. Acromegaly
   f. Hyperparathyroidism
   g. Hemochromatosis
   h. Sarcoidosis
   i. Alkaptonuria
   j. Whipple's disease
   k. Familial Mediterranean fever
   l. Hypogammaglobulinemia
   m. Behçet syndrome
   n. Bacterial endocarditis
9. Chronic pain syndromes
   a. Joint hypermobility syndrome
   b. Reflex sympathetic dystrophy (RSD) (complex regional pain syndrome I)
   c. Fibromyalgia
10. Traumatic arthritis
    a. Slipped femoral epiphysis
    b. Legg-Calvé-Perthes disease
    c. Congenital dislocation of the hip
    d. Any poorly healing fracture or inadequately treated infection
11. Nonrheumatologic disorder of bone/joints
    a. Osteochondritis
    b. Chondromalacia patellae
    c. Idiopathic tenosynovitis and tendonitis

Source: From Greydanus DE. Rheumatoid disorders and other miscellaneous disorders. In: Hofmann AD, Greydanus DE, eds. *Adolescent Medicine*. 3d ed. Stamford, CT: Appleton & Lange, 1997; Chap. 20, p. 433. (with permission)

the presence of a rheumatic disease, as the NSAIDs are also analgesic. Arthralgia refers to pain in a joint and is often from a less serious process, while arthritis refers to clinical signs of inflammation, such as palpable joint swelling. Inflammatory joint pain tends to be chronic and relatively indolent with a vague progressive onset and course. Migratory arthritis resolves in one joint as it appears in the next joint; this is classically seen in acute rheumatic fever (Chap. 9) and gonococcal arthritis (Chaps. 11 and 20), but can occur in a number of other conditions. The arthritis of JIA tends not to migrate but to take on an additive pattern; the adolescent may present with joint pain and morning stiffness first, and note obvious joint swelling weeks later. Inflammatory pain is typically worse in the morning and improves with exercise. In contrast, mechanical pain is usually relieved by rest and tends to be worse at the end of the day and after strenuous activity. The patient should be asked about prior episodes of musculoskeletal disease and the presence of precipitating factors, such as trauma, sports activities, recent immunizations, travel, exposures, or intercurrent illnesses.

The presence or absence of systemic symptoms should be determined. Symptoms of possibly serious or chronic underlying inflammatory conditions would include weight loss, progressive weakness or immobility, growth failure, fever, chills, bruising, pallor, and chest pain. Signs and symptoms suggestive of a rheumatic disorder include mouth ulcers, Raynaud's phenomenon, morning stiffness, and photosensitivity. Nighttime pain, in particular pain that awakens the patient from sleep, is unusual and suggests a more serious condition such as musculoskeletal infection, malignancies, or fractures. A tactful inquiry into social factors and school absences is vital, as this can provide clues to establishing nonorganic causes of symptoms. It can be difficult in the initial visit to establish sufficient rapport to elicit sensitive information. The youth might not feel comfortable enough with the practitioner or might not consider a problem (such as bullying or family discord) to be related to the musculoskeletal symptoms. Information should be obtained about sleep quality, depressive symptoms, and social functioning.

The family history is often overlooked and this omission can delay the establishment of the correct diagnosis. For example, an older boy with intermittent episodes of inflammatory arthritis and a positive family history of back arthritis in males will often have a spondyloarthropathy.

The physical examination begins with obtaining growth parameters, body temperature, and blood pressure. It is useful to watch the patient and family before they are aware of being observed, as this can provide clues about family functioning or symptom exaggeration. The entire musculoskeletal system should be examined, as occult sites of involvement can be uncovered, which can redirect the clinical evaluations. For example, a stiff, tender back in an adolescent with a swollen knee or the individual with monoarticular complaints may have further sites of inflammation. Similarly, referred pain must be considered. The joints should be examined for swelling, warmth, tenderness, restriction of motion, and pain on motion, as these signs usually indicate inflammatory arthritis. The degree of discomfort should be determined. In inflammatory arthritis, the joints are not usually red; pain and tenderness will be mild to moderate and joint contracture as well as muscle atrophy may be prominent. It would be uncommon for a child or adolescent with a rheumatic disease to have extreme pain or be unable to bear weight. In these cases, consider other conditions, such as malingering, infection, fracture, neurologic disorders, or malignancy. The articular examination is usually normal in children with overuse syndromes, nonorganic diseases, and simple arthralgia.

Laboratory Investigation

The choice of diagnostic testing is guided by the information provided in the history and physical examination. A complete blood count (CBC) and an erythrocyte sedimentation rate (ESR) or C-reactive protein (CRP) should be obtained. Normal physical examinations and laboratory studies rule out a serious underlying inflammatory condition in the vast majority of patients. Other initial studies to consider would include urinalysis, appropriate cultures (blood, synovial, urogenital, and stool), serologic tests for infectious agents (such as Lyme or parvo virus), and studies of renal and hepatic function. The CRP and ESR are nonspecific indicators of inflammation and can be completely normal in children or adolescents with inflammatory arthritis, particularly in those with involvement of only a few joints. Many JIA patients, especially those with pauciarticular JIA, will have a low titer of antinuclear antibody (ANA). Similarly, low titer ANA are seen in most rheumatic diseases and the titer does not correlate with disease severity. A positive ANA occurs in over 95% of patients with autoimmune thyroid disease (Chap. 15).

In contrast to adult rheumatoid arthritis,RF is present in only 10% of JIA cases. ANA and RF can occasionally be present in healthy individuals or in other systemic conditions, and are only helpful in distinguishing the type of JIA after the diagnosis is already established. More specific serologic tests (ie, complement levels, anti-double-stranded DNA, antinuclear cytoplasmic antibodies) should be obtained in those suspected of having SLE or a systemic vasculitis. Histocompatibility locus antigen (HLA) testing is not a useful screening tool, except for testing for HLA B27 in a youngster with inflammatory symptoms suspected of having a spondyloarthropathy. However, approximately 10%–30% of patients with a spondyloarthropathy are negative for B27. Also, 8%–10% of the general population are positive for this antigen; and most of these individuals will not develop a spondyloarthropathy.

Arthrocentesis is mandatory in any patient with a swollen joint who is suspected of having an infectious arthritis (Chaps. 11 and 20). Results of a synovial fluid test can also be helpful in establishing noninflammatory arthritis such as trauma. Synovial fluid should be examined for cell count, differential, gram stain, glucose, and culture. Serologic studies and determination of total protein concentration of the synovial fluid are not helpful. The presence of ANA or RF in the joint fluid is merely a reflection of the serum level and measurement of synovial ANA or RF are not necessary or useful. In most types of inflammatory arthritis, the synovial fluid will have cell counts ranging from 1000 to 50,000 cells/mm^3 and a predominance of polymorphonuclear leukocytes. In infectious arthritis, the synovial glucose is usually lower and the cell count is often more than 50,000 cells/mm^3. However, there is considerable overlap, and the diagnosis of infectious arthritis will usually be confirmed by a positive blood or synovial fluid culture. Synovial fluid examination is not helpful in distinguishing the type of inflammatory arthritis in a patient with a suspected rheumatic disorder. Rather, the main utility of a joint tap is to rule out infection or trauma. Gout and pseudogout are extremely rare in childhood or adolescence, but where appropriate, synovial fluid should be examined for crystals.

Radiographs of the involved area will be normal in patients with new onset of inflammatory arthritis and are used to exclude other conditions, such as infections, tumors, and orthopedic conditions. Referred pain (e.g., hip disease presenting with knee complaints) should be considered when ordering radiographs. It can be helpful to also obtain radiographs of the uninvolved side for comparison. Radionuclide scans, CT scans, and MRI studies can be considered in children with severe or more chronic symptoms where further investigation is necessary.

JUVENILE IDIOPATHIC ARTHRITIS

The term JIA refers to a heterogeneous group of diseases of unknown cause characterized by chronic inflammatory arthritis in those younger than age 16. For decades, juvenile rheumatoid arthritis (JRA) was the standard designation in the U.S. and Canadian centers. European centers commonly referred to this condition as juvenile chronic arthritis (JCA) and the clinical classification was different from JRA. The term JIA has recently replaced JRA and JCA at the recommendation of the International League of Associations for Rheumatology (ILAR), which released the JIA classification criteria in 1997. The intent of the new ILAR classification is to provide internationally standardized terminology in order to facilitate basic and clinical research. These classification categories will no doubt be revised, as further insights into the etiology and pathogenesis of chronic arthritis become available.

TABLE 12-3

ILAR CLASSIFICATION OF JIA

Systemic arthritis
Oligoarthritis
Polyarthritis (RF negative)
Polyarthritis (RF positive)
Psoriatic arthritis
Enthesitis related arthritis
"Other" arthritis category

The ILAR classification of JIA includes seven groups: systemic arthritis, oligoarthritis, polyarthritis (RF negative), polyarthritis (RF positive), psoriatic arthritis, enthesitis related arthritis, and an *other* arthritis category (Table 12-3). Psoriatic arthritis, enthesitis, and other arthritis are discussed in further detail in the section on Spondyloarthropathy. Group type is determined by the type of joint involvement in the first 6 months of disease. It is important to correctly classify the subgroup of arthritis as the differential diagnoses, prognoses, and the complications vary with the types of JIA (Table 12-4). Common to all forms of JIA are the challenges involved in therapy of a chronic inflammatory condition occurring in growing, developing individuals. A multidisciplinary approach, including a physical therapist, occupational therapist, medical social worker, orthopedist, ophthalmologist, and rheumatologist, is necessary to ensure the best possible outcome.

The etiology and pathogenesis of JIA remains unknown and evidence suggests that both genetic and environmental factors likely play a role. The strongest evidence is for linkage with certain HLA alleles (such as HLA-B27 in spondylitis and HLA-DR4 in classic RA), but there is increasing evidence that non-HLA genes are important as well. Any chronic arthritis beginning in adolescence

TABLE 12-4

COMPARISION OF JIA SUBTYPES AND SPONDYLOARTHROPATHY

	Systemic	Pauciarticular	Polyarticular	Spondyloarthropathy
Gender	M = F	F ≫ M	F > M	M ≫ F
Age of onset (year)	1–6	1–4	1–8	8–18
Laboratory studies				
Rheumatoid factor	−	−	+	−
Antinuclear antibody	−	+++	++	−
HLA B27	−	−	−	+++
Sites of joint disease				
Peripheral arthritis	+++	++	+++	+
Cervical spine	+	−	+	−
LS spine/sacroiliac disease	−	−	−	++
Extra-articular manifestations				
Chronic iritis	−	+++	+	−
Acute iritis	−	−	−	+
Fever, weight loss, leukocytosis	++	−	+	−
Rashes	+++	−	−	++

−, not found; +, occasional; ++, frequent; +++, often.

Source: Petty RE: Classification of child arthritis: A work in progress. *Baillieres Clin Rheumatol* 1998;12:181–190.

Gare RA: Epidemiology. *Baillieres Clin Rheumatol* 1998;12:191–208.

will most likely be one of the polyarticular JIA subtypes or a spondyloarthropathy. Systemic and oligoarticular JIA generally begins in the preschool ages.

Differential Diagnosis

JIA probably encompasses several diseases of differing etiologies. In addition, other types of inflammatory arthritis, such as reactive arthritis and Lyme arthritis can be difficult to distinguish from oligoarticular JIA. Another difficulty is that inflammatory conditions evolve over time and it might be decades later that another rheumatic disease becomes evident. The typical example of this process would be a boy diagnosed with oligoarticular JIA who develops typical spinal involvement, intestinal disease, or psoriasis in adult life, and is then correctly diagnosed as having a spondyloarthropathy.

The diagnosis of JIA is made on the presence of chronic arthritis (longer than 6 weeks duration), onset before the 16th birthday, and the exclusion of other conditions that can mimic JIA. The possibility of malignancy must always be considered in the evaluation of a patient with joint pain prior to instituting therapy for the arthritis. Neuroblastoma and lymphoid malignancies are the most common childhood neoplasms that can present with arthritis. Up to 10% of children with acute leukemia will have frank arthritis, and many more will have bone and/or joint pain at onset. Clues that malignancy may be the cause of the joint symptoms include pain out of proportion to physical findings, bone pain, cytopenias, elevated acute phase reactants with a normal or low platelet count, elevations in uric acid and/or LDH, and radiographic abnormalities. Use of corticosteroids in unsuspected malignancy can dramatically worsen outcome and should absolutely be avoided. Consultation with an oncologist and an examination of the bone marrow may be indicated prior to starting treatment, especially if corticosteroids or a cytotoxic medication are to be used.

Infection must also be considered in a patient with arthralgia or arthritis. Analysis of synovial fluid is mandatory in cases in which septic arthritis is suspected. Pyogenic causes of arthritis include bacteria (usually *S. aureus or N. gonorrhoeae*), Lyme arthritis, and rarely, fungal infections, tuberculosis, and other pathogens. Unusual and/or opportunistic pathogens should be considered in patients with suspected infectious arthritis who are immune suppressed. In addition to infection and malignancy, the differential diagnosis of arthralgia and arthritis in childhood is extensive and includes trauma, reactive arthritis, acute rheumatic fever, hemophilia, inflammatory bowel disease, bacterial endocarditis, viral infections, serum sickness, lupus, dermatomyositis, hereditary connective tissue and metabolic disorders (Table 12-1). Because of the disruption in the normal immune system regulation, those with primary or acquired immune deficiencies can present with inflammatory arthritis or arthralgia. A careful, detailed history and physical examination is crucial to planning an appropriate evaluation for the patient.

Clinical Characteristics of JIA Subgroups

Several features distinguish JIA from adult RA. Children, especially younger children, are much less likely to present with complaints of pain, even when there is easily demonstrable inflammatory arthritis on examination. The typical complaints are morning stiffness and/or limp. Systemic signs and symptoms such as fever, weight loss, lymphadenopathy, and anemia, are seen only in patients with systemic JIA or RF positive polyarticular JIA. Although less striking than in adult RA, where the male:female ratio is 1:10, JIA is also more common in females, with an overall ratio of about 5:1.

Oligoarthritis

Also known as pauciarticular JIA, this is the most common subgroup (30%–40% of cases of JIA) and is utilized for children and adolescents with up to four affected joints. Typically, the large joints are affected. In about half of the patients, disease is limited to a single joint, most often the knee. Elbows and ankles are also commonly involved.

This subtype is most common in young girls, with a peak age of onset at about 2 years. There is a high incidence of concomitant inflammatory eye disease (uveitis, also called iridocyclitis or iritis) as well as the presence of ANA in sera. The uveitis of JIA is typically asymptomatic at first and usually requires a slit lamp examination for diagnosis. The uveitis can lead to vision loss and ocular damage if not recognized and promptly treated.

Joint symptoms in oligoarticular disease are often mild and of insidious onset. The patient may present to the clinician for evaluation of abnormal gait or a reluctance to walk or play. The patient may experience a minor trauma and then the warm stiff joint is noted; they do not appear systemically ill. Undiagnosed or untreated disease may result in muscular atrophy and joint contractures, particularly of the knee. It is not unusual for the patient to already have atrophy and a contracture at the time the diagnosis of JIA is even considered. Most patients in this subgroup experience a full remission of their arthritis. However, approximately 10% may go onto to develop additional joint involvement over time and have joint involvement similar to the polyarticular JIA types. This subset is referred to as extended oligoarthritis.

Polyarthritis (RF Negative)

This category refers to children and adolescents with five or more joints involved during the first 6 months of their illness and a negative serum rheumatoid factor. Patients will present with a gradual onset of symptoms: decreased activity, morning stiffness, joint swelling, and occasionally joint pain. Girls are more commonly affected, and both large and small joint involvement may be seen. Systemic symptoms occur, but are generally milder than those seen in the systemic or RF positive subtypes. Chronic uveitis occurs less frequently than in the oligoarthritis category. The prognosis for this subtype is better than the prognosis for RF positive individuals; however, the two subtypes share many clinical features and both can be associated with significant morbidity.

Polyarthritis (RF Positive)

These patients also present with a gradual onset of symptoms, but occasionally the onset may be one of a dramatic acute polyarthritis. Again, girls are most commonly affected and the arthritis is widespread and symmetric. Low-grade fever, fatigue, and poor appetite are often present. Examination reveals proliferative synovitis, joint effusions, often with decreased range of motion. Mild adenopathy or hepatosplenomegaly may be present; chronic uveitis is rare. These patients often have a persistent destructive arthropathy and may have associated subcutaneous rheumatoid nodules. This small group of patients represents the onset in childhood of classic adult RA and the course and prognosis is similar to RA.

Systemic Arthritis

Systemic onset JIA (Still's disease) occurs in approximately 10% of cases. This diagnosis can be quite difficult to make as the inflammatory arthritis is not usually present on initial evaluation, and may not be evident for weeks, months, and rarely, years. These patients present with high fever, malaise, and rash. The fever pattern typically occurs with one or more fever spikes in 102°F to 105°F range, followed by a return to normal or occasionally subnormal temperatures. The rash is often present only during fever spikes or after a hot bath, when it transiently appears as a fine, salmon-colored, macular eruption of the trunk, proximal extremities, and skin overlying affected joints. Most patients have adenopathy and hepatosplenomegaly and are found to have moderate to severe anemia as well as a striking neutrophilic leukocytosis. Other manifestations of systemic onset disease may include pericarditis, myocarditis, pleural effusion, and interstitial lung disease. Renal disease is rare. Other important considerations in the differential diagnosis include infections, inflammatory bowel disease, and malignancy. RF and ANA are usually absent, and diagnosis is made on clinical findings. With the lack of specific laboratory studies, establishing the diagnosis of systemic JIA can be quite difficult, especially when the chronic arthritis is not yet evident. In contrast to oligoarticular and polyarticular subtypes, systemic JIA occurs equally in boys and girls, and usually has onset in the pre-school ages.

Psoriatic Arthritis

For the purpose of arthritis classification, children and adolescents with psoriatic arthritis either have psoriasis (Chap. 19) and arthritis or arthritis plus two of three other features (i.e., dactylitis, nail involvement, or psoriasis in a first-degree relative that has been confirmed by a dermatologist). Generally, there are no associated systemic symptoms, and both the prognosis and number of involved joints are quite variable. RF is absent by definition. Psoriatic arthritis has a variable course, but can be quite destructive, and is discussed further in the section on spondyloarthropathy.

Enthesitis-Related Arthritis

Enthesitis refers to inflammation in an enthesis—the site of attachment of connective tissue (i.e., tendons, fascia, and ligaments) to bone. Enthesitis is the hallmark of the spondyloarthropathies. These patients are generally older boys and often have a family history of a spondyloarthropathy in a first or second degree relative. For JIA classification purposes, the patient must have both enthesitis and arthritis, or arthritis or enthesitis alone plus two of five additional features (i.e., sacroiliac joint tenderness, positive HLA-B27, a relative with spondyloarthropathy, symptomatic anterior uveitis or be a male with initial onset of arthritis after age 8). However, these distinctions are somewhat arbitrary, and it is expected that the majority of youngsters with enthesitis-related arthritis will, over time, have a diagnosable spondyloarthropathy. The clinical manifestations and management of the spondyloarthropathies are discussed later in this chapter.

Other Arthritis

This subgroup encompasses patients who do not fit into any of the other six categories or who have features from more than one category in whom precise classification is not possible. Further revisions of the ILAR criteria will be likely as specific etiologic agents are identified and as the results of ongoing epidemiologic studies become available. It is important to remember that these conditions evolve over time and the precise diagnosis may not be evident for decades.

Laboratory and Radiographic Findings

In general, routine laboratory studies will be normal in individuals with inactive disease or oligoarthritis. The degree of lab abnormality will correlate with disease activity and severity. Abnormalities include elevations in serum proteins involved in the acute phase reaction, such as CRP, fibrinogen (the main cause of an elevated ESR), immunoglobulins (Ig), complement, and transferrin. In inflammatory states, the platelet count can also be elevated (affectionately called "the poor man's sed rate" by rheumatologists). CBC usually shows a mild normocytic anemia and the white blood count (WBC) is mildly elevated. Patients with systemic JIA can have profound anemia, thrombocytosis, leukocytosis, and elevation in hepatic enzymes. Neuromuscular, renal, pancreatic, and pulmonary involvement is distinctly rare in JIA and corresponding laboratory studies should be normal. If there are such abnormalities, another rheumatic disorder or a drug-induced reaction should be considered. Because of nonspecific elevations in serum immunoglobulins, caution must be used in trying to interpret increases in specific types of immunoglobulin G (IgG) (such as elevated streptococcal antibodies). Similarly, the presence of high titer RF can give falsely positive results on immunoglobulin M (IgM) based tests.

As discussed earlier, specific serologic abnormalities in JIA include positive ANA. The titers are usually low (under 1:640) and in speckled or diffuse patterns–the least specific ANA patterns. JIA patients will not have the more specific autoantibodies of other rheumatic disorders, such as anti-DNA or antineutrophil cytoplasmic antibodies (ANCA). Ten percent of the general population has positive HLA B27, hence the results of such a test in a JIA patient needs to be considered on an individual basis. Synovial fluid is usually examined in JIA to establish the diagnosis or to rule out a secondary infection in a patient with established JIA. Fluid results will be typical for inflammatory arthritis and there are no pathognomonic features in JIA.

Standard radiographs are usually normal at onset of JIA joint disease. Typical destructive changes may take years to develop, if ever. Radiographs are obtained at onset for baseline studies for comparison and more importantly, to rule out other causes of the articular symptoms. The first radiographic changes are soft tissue swelling and juxta-articular osteoporosis, followed by bone erosion and later, loss of articular cartilage, decreased joint space, and bone destruction. A distinct feature in the developing child or adolescent is regional overgrowth or undergrowth in joints with persistent disease. The most common example of this feature is a leg length discrepancy in a child or adolescent with oligoarthritis involving only one knee, while radiographs show advanced epiphyseal development in the involved joint. Wrist films in patients with polyarthritis can show advanced bone age and later more specific and destructive changes. Over time, severe arthritis will lead to a dramatic bone overgrowth and impressive bony fusion at involved sites; generalized osteoporosis is evident on radiographs in severe JIA patients with longstanding disease.

The most common radiographic findings of cervical spine disease in JRA are calcification of the anterior aspect of the first cervical vertebra, anterior erosion of the odontoid, and ankylosis of the apophyseal joint. Other radiographic features include growth disturbances of the vertebral bodies, spondylitis of the cervical spine, and micrognathia. To evaluate for suspected neurologic impingement or cervical spine fractures, radionuclide scanning or MRI can be particularly useful. Radionuclide scanning is not a useful tool to diagnosis peripheral inflammatory arthritis or to screen for occult sites of inflammation, as the specificity and sensitivity are too low. The major use of scanning is to evaluate for nonrheumatic conditions.

Clinical Course and Prognosis

The hallmark of the rheumatic diseases is inflammation of synovial tissue. There is a marked increase in macrophages and T lymphocytes, local production of inflammatory mediators, recruitment of neutrophils into the joint space leading to synovial hypertrophy, increased vascularity, and joint fluid secretion. Over time, the inflammatory process extends from the synovium with local invasion of cartilage, then erosion of bone. If inflammation does not remit or cannot be controlled by treatment, the final result will be end-stage joint destruction and ankylosis.

The natural course of JIA is extremely variable. However, most children do quite well with early recognition and management. Remission rates vary from 26% to 65% and severe disability occurs in 20%–45%. This marked variation in outcome is due to differences in clinical criteria, length of follow-up, and types of treatment. There is considerable variability in the severity and clinical course in JIA. Patients with oligoarticular disease generally have milder synovitis and a better prognosis. However, 10%–15% of patients with oligoarthritis later progress to polyarticular disease (the group called *extended oligoarthritis*). Children and adolescents with oligoarthritis may develop significant disability due to joint contractures and muscular atrophy, which often persist even when the inflammation has subsided. One cannot over emphasize the importance of physical therapy in managing these complications. Although oligoarticular JIA is associated with milder arthritis, this subtype is at high risk of inflammatory eye disease and the possibility of severe vision loss or even blindness, if eye disease is not treated. Patients with systemic onset generally recover from the acute systemic illness without major sequelae, but these patients often develop severe polyarthritis that can be quite challenging to control.

Children and adolescents with more severe outcomes are systemic JIA patients with persistent polyarthritis and those who have positive rheumatoid factor. Persistent inflammatory arthritis for greater than 5 years is also predictive of more severe disability. Better understanding of drug combinations and the new anticytokine therapies have brightened the long term outcome for patients with polyarticular disease (both RF positive and RF negative). Another important consideration is that children initially diagnosed with JIA may, years later, be rediagnosed with a different rheumatic disease. This was seen in one series of JIA patients followed for decades where 22% were rediagnosed with another condition, and most of those children were ultimately diagnosed with a spondyloarthropathy.

Musculoskeletal Complications

Growth Abnormalities

Children with chronic inflammatory disease of any type may have generalized inhibition of growth and subsequent short stature, either from the disease itself or from chronic administration of corticosteroids; the resultant psychological distress can be severe (Chap. 15). Many JIA patients will have localized sites of altered growth or deformity. Muscle spasm and disuse results in flexion contracture. Leg length discrepancies are the most common orthopedic sequelae of JIA and can be severe. Usually this problem occurs in the knee and is due to peri-articular hyperemia leading to accelerated growth in the affected leg. Occasionally, the end result can be premature epiphyseal fusion with resultant shortening as the uninvolved limb achieves normal growth. Associated leg length discrepancy and hip disease can lead to development of contracture as well as genu valgus. Secondary scoliosis may occur.

Hip disease is unusual at onset of JIA, but is common in polyarticular disease, and correlates with a worse prognosis and high risk of long-term disability. Hip involvement in early childhood may contribute to valgus deformity of the femoral neck, persistent femoral anteversion, and dysplasia of both femoral head and acetabulum. Joint replacement can be successful in patients with disabling, end-stage disease who have failed medical and conservative management. In the hand and wrist,

deformities similar to adult rheumatoid disease are seen. Additionally, some patients develop extensive fusion of carpal bones. Ankles and feet are similarly prone to fusion, particularly at the subtalar joint. Complex foot deformities may be seen as a result of soft tissue damage and growth disturbances and lead to chronic foot pain. Coordination of care with the orthopedic surgeon is important in any JIA patient with significant chronic arthritis. Chronic arthritis in the temporomandibular joint (TMJ) can result in a shortened mandible and micrognathia. Also, TMJ disease can lead to chronic pain, disturbances of speech and chewing in addition to the cosmetic alteration.

Cervical Spine Disease

The inflammatory process in the cervical spine is similar to that in the peripheral joints. The normal cervical spine has 32 synovial articulations. There is a synovial lined bursa between the odontoid process and transverse ligament. The three most common lesions that result in cervical instability are atlantoaxial subluxation, basilar invagination, and subaxial subluxation, or a combination. Expansion from synovitis may lead to distention and finally, to rupture of the transverse ligament or to odontoid fracture resulting in cervical instability; the atlas then slides anteriorly and atlanto-axial subluxation is considered when the distance between the odontoid process and the anterior arch of the atlas exceeds 4 mm in adults.

Although cervical spine involvement is more common in JIA than in adult RA, children and adolescents have less pain and a much lower incidence of neurologic involvement and complications. Historically, in adult RA, subaxial subluxation occurs in 20%–25%, with neurologic progression in up to a third of untreated cases. The incidence of cervical spine complications in JIA is less than that of adult RA. As therapeutic management of inflammatory arthritis has improved significantly over the past decade, the incidence of C-spine complications, as well as other musculoskeletal complications of JIA, should decrease.

Mortality in JIA and the Macrophage Activation Syndrome

Mortality from JIA is quite rare but does occur. The vast majority of the deaths occur in children and adolescents with systemic onset disease, either from infections, complications of pharmacologic therapy, traumatic C-spine injuries, or a rare syndrome called macrophage activation syndrome (MAS). MAS is a form of the hemophagocytic lymphohistiocytosis syndrome and is a potentially fatal complication. Viral infections and drugs have been implicated in the onset of MAS. These patients become rapidly ill with fever, worsening adenopathy, organomegaly, petechiae and bleeding. The sedimentation rate rapidly falls and pancytopenia is present. The ferritin level is often markedly elevated. This complication needs prompt recognition and treatment. Supportive care, management of any concurrent infection, and treatment with high dose corticosteroids can control MAS. There are reports of clinical response to agents such as cyclosporine A and tumor necrosis factor inhibitors when given with large doses of corticosteroids. MAS patients presenting with renal or pulmonary failure have a particularly poor prognosis.

Ocular Complications

Eye involvement occurs in nearly a quarter of children and adolescents with JIA and is typically asymptomatic at onset. Eye disease is present in 40%–50% of oligoarticular JIA, 10% of polyarticular patients, and rare in systemic-onset JIA. Early detection and treatment are essential to improving the outcome of JIA-associated uveitis. Uveitis (also called iridocyclitis or iritis) is the most common ocular process and typically occurs in girls with oligoarthritis and a positive ANA. However, uveitis has been reported in all subtypes of JIA. Usually eye involvement develops within a few years of the chronic arthritis, but eye disease can occasionally predate the onset of arthritis. Similarly, there are case reports of JIA patients showing their first bout of eye disease decades into their JIA.

The uveitis is typically a painless and insidiously progressive disease. Complications include posterior synechiae with resultant pupillary abnormalities, secondary glaucoma, cataracts, band keratopathy, and vision loss (even blindness). There is no correlation between the severity of arthritis and risk for development of uveitis. In addition, children with a spondyloarthropathy may develop chronic anterior uveitis; however, in these cases, they more typically present with an acute uveitis with a red, painful eye with photophobia. All patients with JIA need regular evaluations for eye disease, at least yearly. Oligoarticular patients, because of their higher risk of eye disease, need screening visits 2–3 times yearly for the first several years of their disease. All patients with a rheumatic disease (including JIA) with ocular symptoms should be promptly referred for evaluation of an inflammatory cause of their symptoms. The under-recognition and under treatment of inflammatory eye disease can result in permanent eye damage.

MANAGEMENT OF INFLAMMATORY ARTHRITIS

The past decade has seen major advances in the understanding and treatment of chronic inflammatory arthritis. There is increasing emphasis on early identification of patients at risk of severe disease and aggressive control of inflammation, often using several pharmacologic agents simultaneously. Medications include methotrexate, leflunomide, hydroxychloroquine, sulfasalazine, and novel biologic agents that specifically inhibit inflammatory mediators, specifically interleukin-1 and tumor necrosis factor. Essential to optimal outcome is the early diagnosis and prompt institution of treatment. As our arsenal of therapeutic agents grow and are utilized appropriately, we are likely to continue to see long-term outcomes improve. Treatment of JIA and the spondyloarthropathies are similar and management has been combined into this section.

General Guidelines

All children and adolescents with chronic arthritis need an individualized treatment plan and should be managed by a practitioner skilled in the treatment of these disorders. Pain should be controlled, using appropriate nonnarcotic analgesics and narcotics are reserved for severe pain. Conservative therapies should not be overlooked and include moist heat, splinting or casting for comfort, crutches or canes, sufficient rest, and an appropriate exercise program. Younger children generally do not like topical medications and find the burning sensation or texture of many of these agents unacceptable. However, these agents can be useful in adolescents. Referral to the occupational and physical therapists is important and should be considered in all patients with extensive disease of significant local conditions, such as atrophy or contractures. Sleep disturbances are quite common in arthritis patients. It can be difficult to fall asleep or stay asleep due to joint pain and stiffness. Also, many patients have mood disorders and anxiety from the stress of having an unpredictable and chronic condition.

Medications

NSAIDs

Nonsteroidal anti-inflammatory drugs (NSAIDs) are the most commonly used drugs in the treatment of inflammatory arthritis, and virtually all patients will be tried on NSAIDs first (Table 12-5). NSAIDs are also used extensively in many other disorders, including noninflammatory musculoskeletal conditions (Chap. 11). They control pain, fever, swelling, and stiffness, but have no effect on long-term outcome. Traditional NSAIDs include aspirin, indomethacin, ibuprofen, naproxen, sulindac, and tolmetin sodium and many are available over the counter (Table 12-5). The traditional NSAIDs nonselectively inhibit cyclooxygenase 1 and 2 (COX-1 and COX-2), which contributes to the risk of NSAID side effects and toxicity. The COX-1 enzyme is expressed constitutively in most organ systems, including the kidney, the gastrointestinal tract and in platelets. Newer, selective COX-2 inhibitors (celecoxib, rofecoxib, and valdecoxib) are associated with less renal and gastrointestinal side effects.

Aspirin has a long historical record of use in JIA, but its use has decreased markedly due to the risk (though very slight) of Reye syndrome, the

TABLE 12-5

NONSTEROIDAL ANTI-INFLAMMATORY DRUGS (ADULT DOSES)

Tolmetin sodium (Tolectin): 15–30 mg/kg/day; 400 mg t.i.d. or q.i.d. (max: 1800 mg/day)

Naproxen (NaProsyn): (250–500 mg b.i.d)

Ibuprofen (Motrin): 600 mg q.i.d. or 800 mg t.i.d.

Fenoprofen calcium (Nalfon): 300–600 mg t.i.d. or q.i.d. (max: 3200 mg/day)

Diflunisal (Dolobid): 250–500 mg b.i.d. (max: 1500 mg/day)

Ketoprofen (Orudis): 75 mg t.i.d. or 50 mg q.i.d. (max: 300 mg/day)

Sulindac (Clinoril): 150–200 mg b.i.d. (max: 400 mg/day)

Piroxicam (Feldene): 10 mg b.i.d. or 20 mg once per day

Oxaprozin (DayPro): 1200 mg once per day; max: 1800 mg/day

Others

potential for drug toxicity and the availability of other NSAIDs. Salicylates should be promptly discontinued in patients with concomitant influenza or varicella infections. Salicylates, aspirin in particular, are the only NSAIDs that have clinically relevant effects on platelet function. In addition to the effect on prostaglandin synthesis, aspirin acetylizes platelet COX-1, irreversibly leading to diminished platelet aggregation; this is an effect that clinically lasts 4–6 days after a dose as small as 80 mg.

All NSAIDs can cause side effects in the gastrointestinal tract, central nervous system, and other systems (i.e., renal, hepatic, and hematopoietic); there are also cutaneous reactions. NSAID side effects are related to duration of use, dose, chemical structure, degree of COX-1 inhibition, concurrent use of other pharmacologic agents, as well as the presence of any preexisting comorbid disease. There is considerable variability in frequency and severity of side effects among the NSAIDs. Aspirin and the other salicylates are associated with more frequent side effects and with a much higher risk of toxicity in overdoses. Many patients will have vague dyspepsia on virtually all

NSAIDs. Significant gastrointestinal complications include gastric or duodenal ulceration, occult blood loss, esophagitis, perforation and rarely, massive bleeding. These complications are more prevalent in older patients and the overall risk is 2%–5% of patients on these agents for more than a year. The selective COX-2 inhibitors have a significantly lower risk of gastrointestinal side effects when compared to the other NSAIDs. Concomitant use of misoprostol or a proton pump inhibitor (Chap. 10) can mitigate the gastrointestinal toxicity of NSAIDs and the use of these agents should be considered in patients at higher risk, such as patients also on corticosteroids, and those with a prior history of gastrointestinal disease or on more than one NSAID.

NSAIDs can be associated with a variety of rashes, from urticaria to severe Stevens-Johnson syndrome. NSAIDs should be avoided in asthmatics who are aspirin sensitive. Chronic naproxen can cause a photosensitive rash, called pseudoporphyria, particularly in fair complexion individuals. This rash can lead to chronic scarring. Persistent elevations in hepatic transaminases occur in 3% of patients on chronic NSAIDs; the frequency is about 5% with aspirin. Rarely, hepatic toxicity can be severe and even fatal. Renal effects are less common in younger patients, but can occur. Patients most at risk include those with lupus, kidney disease, and other health problems. Renal toxicity includes decreased renal function, interstitial disease, hyperkalemia, and proteinuria (Chap. 16). Hematologic effects are rare and include cytopenias, which usually are mild and resolve with stopping the NSAID. However, permanent and severe cytopenia can occur. The nonselective NSAIDs, but not the COX-2 agents, reversibly inhibit platelet aggregation. All NSAIDs can cause headache, mental confusion, drowsiness, and dizziness; these symptoms resolve promptly with stopping the drug. Rarely, some NSAIDs (i.e., ibuprofen, sulindac, tolmetin, naproxen) can cause an aseptic meningitis, especially in lupus patients.

Choice of NSAID is based on many factors–cost, ease of administration, projected length of therapy, half-life, tolerability, and risk factors for toxicity. For adolescents, a NSAID that can be given once or twice daily is preferable, as it eliminates disruption to the school day and is easier to remember. Ibuprofen, naproxen, rofecoxib and several salicylate preparations are available in liquid form. Ketorolac and indomethacin are the only NSAIDs that can be given parenterally. Concomitant administration of one of the antiulcer medications should be considered for high risk patients. All patients on chronic NSAID therapy should be monitored every few months for hematopoietic, renal, and hepatic toxicity, as well as screened for any suspicious gastrointestinal symptoms, such as melena and persistent abdominal pain. Except for determining salicylate levels in patients on chronic salicylate therapy, serum levels of the other NSAIDs are not useful clinically.

Corticosteroids

Corticosteroids are a group of powerful anti-inflammatory medications that are invaluable agents in the control of inflammation. However, the side effects can be significant and specific to youth, such as the risk of severe growth failure. The decision to use corticosteroids is made on a case by case basis. Oral or parenteral corticosteroids are reserved for refractory cases of inflammatory diseases and are indicated in the treatment of severe systemic JIA (i.e., profound anemia, pericarditis, MAS). The lowest possible dose needed for disease control should be utilized and for the shortest amount of time. For patients with significant corticosteroid toxicity and/or those on long-term and high doses, alternate inflammatory agents (steroid sparing drugs) should be started in order to allow reduction or elimination of the corticosteroid dose.

There are significant side effects with systemic corticosteroids. The severity and frequency of side effects are directly related to the duration of therapy and the dose of corticosteroid. Corticosteroids increase the risk of infection, from typical bacterial pathogens, to an increased risk of tuberculosis and increased frequency of infection with opportunistic organisms, especially with long-term administration. Acute effects of corticosteroids include fluid retention, weight gain, changes in mood, aggravation of acne, sleep disturbance, and rarely, psychosis or severe muscle weakness. The physical effects can be quite distressing to adolescents and can lead to non-compliance. Chronic corticosteroids lead to osteoporosis, dyslipidemias, altered glucose regulation, and accelerated atherogenesis. Overall the risk of osteonecrosis of the hips is 2% in any patient on chronic corticosteroids. In lupus patients, this risk can be as high as 25%. All patients on corticosteroids need to be counseled about adequate calcium and vitamin D intake, as well as appropriate weight bearing exercise. In patients anticipated to need long term corticosteroids, bone density determinations should be done yearly and consideration given to starting a bisphosphonate to prevent osteoporosis.

Intra-articular corticosteroids are particularly useful in a patient with only a few symptomatic joints, and can obviate the need for systemic corticosteroids or regular NSAID use. An injection can effectively control synovitis for several months. Virtually any synovial joint can be injected and the amount to inject depends on the joint size. Most joints can be injected in the outpatient setting using appropriate sterile technique and local anesthetic. However, for joints such as the hip and sacroiliac joints, injection is done under fluoroscopy or via needle guided ultrasound. In adolescents with significant anxiety, a short acting sedative can be given. Occasionally, general anesthesia may be necessary, particularly if more than six joints will be injected. In longstanding and severe arthritis, joint injection can be difficult due to fibrosis, bony changes, and contracture. With significant synovial hypertrophy, it might be difficult to get adequate dispersal of the corticosteroid through the joint; in these cases, ultrasound guided injection can be helpful. The risk of joint infection or structural injury is extremely rare with intra-articular injections. Occasionally, minor atrophy along the needle tract can occur due to the corticosteroid leaking into adjacent tissue.

Disease Modifying AntiRheumatic Agents (DMARDs)

For most children with JIA, methotrexate is the most commonly used first line DMARD. Historically, other agents considered as first line DMARDs include D-penicillamine, intramuscular gold salts, hydroxychloroquine, and sulfasalazine. Leflunomide has similar efficacy and toxicity to methotrexate, but has a very long half-life and significant risk of teratogenicity. Because of the teratogenicity and the higher chance of unplanned pregnancy in teens, leflunomide is not used as often as methotrexate. Methotrexate is commonly started in children and adolescents with polyarthritis, in the oligoarticular patients with significant refractory arthritis, and in chronic uveitis that is severe and refractory to corticosteroids. Combination therapies using moderate doses of DMARDs are more effective in controlling inflammatory arthritis than use of single agents alone. Often, methotrexate is combined with hydroxychloroquine or sulfasalazine. There is also increased use of methotrexate with one of the biologic agents designed to block specific cytokines (discussed below). The choices and doses to be used must be determined on a case by case basis, and by a physician with experience in the management of complex inflammatory disorders.

Cytotoxic and Immune Modulating Agents

Cytotoxic medications include cyclophosphamide, chlorambucil, and azathioprine. These agents are used infrequently and reserved for patients with life-threatening disease who have failed management with other agents. There are ongoing registries of JIA patients in the United States and Europe, who have received autologous bone marrow transplantation with good control of their disease. Most patients referred for transplantation are severe systemic JIA patients in whom the disease cannot be adequately controlled with the usual DMARDs. Cytotoxic medications and bone marrow transplantation have significant risk and should only be recommended after other agents have failed to control disease. Immune modulating agents include cyclosporine and mycophenolate; these agents are reserved for severe inflammatory disorders unresponsive to the usual DMARDs.

There are now several biologic agents available that specifically target individual cytokines or certain inflammatory cells. In addition, further agents are being investigated in clinical trials. Because of their unique specificity for inflammatory mediators, these agents have relatively few adverse effects. They are quite expensive, must be given parenterally, and the long-term safety is not known. However, they show tremendous potential for the control of severe inflammatory disorders. In addition to controlling inflammatory arthritis, they have efficacy in the control of inflammatory eye disease and other conditions. Etanercept (Enbrel), infliximab (Remicade), and adalimumab (Humira) inhibit tumor necrosis factor (TNF) and all three have been shown to be effective in JIA patients. Infliximab is also approved for the treatment of inflammatory bowel disease. Anakinra (Kineret) is a biologic agent with specific effects against the Interleukin-1 receptor.

Surgical Management

Up to 10% of children with JIA seen in a pediatric rheumatology centers require surgical intervention. Children with severe JIA have significant osteoporosis and can experience spontaneous fractures. JIA patients require surgical intervention when medical and physical therapy (e.g., splinting and casting) are not sufficient to control pain, improve contracture, or correct deformity. The most common procedure in JIA patients is soft tissue release, particularly of the knee or hip. Occasionally, synovial biopsy may be necessary for diagnostic reasons. Therapeutic synovectomy can be helpful for the patient with severe pain or loss of function, and is most commonly performed on the knee. When feasible, synovectomy is best performed via arthroscopy, because recovery time and complications are less. Arthroscopy may be impossible in the presence of severe pericapsular contracture which will decrease distensibility and visibility of the joint. Severe bone ankylosis may require a corrective osteotomy to improve joint position and relieve pain. In rare cases, leg length discrepancy is so severe that surgical correction is needed. Joint replacement is a well established treatment of end-stage JIA. Children and adolescents with severe JIA are often smaller and lighter than other children and adolescents of the same age, and the joint prosthesis may need to be custom made.

SPONDYLOARTHROPATHIES

The spondyloarthropathies are a group of overlapping disorders, characterized by male predominance, absence of RF and ANA (seronegative), involvement of the axial skeleton and enthesitis. The majority of these conditions have in common the presence of HLA-B27 (overall about 75%–90%). An earlier term for the spondyloarthropathies was seronegative arthritis. However, RA and JIA patients can also be seronegative and this designation is now used infrequently. The typical patient is a young male presenting with inflammatory arthritis in a large peripheral joint or in the lower back and sacroiliac joint. The disorder is often not accurately diagnosed for decades.

The current American College of Rheumatology classification includes the following subcategories: ankylosing spondylitis, reactive arthritis (also called Reiter syndrome), psoriatic arthropathy, and enteropathic arthropathy (arthritis associated with inflammatory bowel disease). There is also a subset called *unclassified* or *undifferentiated* spondyloarthropathy, for patients who do not yet meet diagnostic criteria for definite diagnosis. Classic ankylosing spondylitis does not occur in adolescents. The patient may present with an asymmetric pauciarthritis and only later in adult life be correctly diagnosed; children presenting with isolated hip arthritis are particularly likely to evolve into a spondyloarthropathy. Some investigators define juvenile spondyloarthropathy as disease occurring in youngsters less than 16 years old.

Epidemiology and Etiology

The spondyloarthropathies are ancient disorders– ankylosing spondylitis has been described in skeletal remains dating to the thirtieth century B.C. In contrast, adult RA and SLE appeared in the Renaissance period. The incidence of ankylosing spondylitis is 2.1/1000, with a male:female ratio ranging from 3:1 to 9:1. Ankylosing spondylitis represents about half of all cases of spondyloarthropathy. In children and adolescents, the spondyloarthropathies account for one-third of the cases of chronic arthritis and most of these children will also fulfill JIA criteria as well.

The etiology of the spondyloarthropathies is still unknown. There have been tremendous advances in the last two decades in the understanding of the immune response, in identification of microbial triggers of inflammation, and delineation of the contributions of HLA antigens and enteric infections in these diseases. The actual role of HLA B27 is still not entirely clear. Patients can have a spondyloarthropathy without the presence of this antigen. Theories of the role of HLA B27 include molecular mimicry (where a bacterial antigen is similar in structure to B27), posttranslational modification of the B27 molecule (resulting in an altered structure and subsequent autoimmune response); or the B27 molecule might be associated with a deficient or altered host response to various infectious agents; this results in the triggering of a chronic immune response. A transgenic HLA B27 rat model has also contributed to our understanding of these disorders.

Clinical Features

The hallmark of the spondyloarthropathies is enthesitis–inflammation at the sites of connective tissue attachment to bone. Typical sites of involvement include the lower extremities (e.g., heel and plantar fascia) and the sacroiliac joints. Pathologically, sites of enthesitis show nonspecific inflammatory changes with lymphocyte inflammation and destructive changes in adjacent bone. In addition to enthesitis, the spondyloarthropathies are also associated with synovitis, tendonitis, axial disease (sacroiliac joint in particular), as well as mucocutaneous features. Enthesitis, especially of the lower extremities, is often misdiagnosed as an overuse syndrome and it may be decades before the youngster is identified as having a spondyloarthropathy. In one large series, the diagnosis of a spondyloarthropathy was made at a mean of 7.3 years from first onset of symptoms.

For many young children, the initial presentation may be hip involvement. Indeed, isolated hip involvement is distinctly uncommon in JIA. In general, youngsters with a spondyloarthropathy will usually be older males. Other clinical features useful to distinguish spondyloarthropathy from JIA

are the presence of enthesitis, tarsal disease, and back pain. In children and adolescents later diagnosed with a spondyloarthropathy, the discriminative value of either enthesitis or tarsal disease approached that of the gold standard of diagnosis. Back involvement in children and adolescents with a spondyloarthropathy usually originates from inflammation of the sacroiliac joints. Symptoms may be bilateral or unilateral. Pain is inflammatory in nature; worse in the morning, associated with morning stiffness, and often relieved by exercise and improved by the end of the day. Pain is usually mild to moderate and persists for months. A careful and thorough physical examination should be done. The mouth should be inspected for lesions and the skin examined for psoriasis (especially the nape of the neck, elbows, knees, and umbilicus). Shoes should be removed and the feet examined carefully for nail pits, sausage toes (dactylitis) and signs of enthesitis. In addition to the standard examination of the back, a useful procedure is the Schober's test, which can indicate spinal limitation and suggest a spondyloarthropathy. In this procedure, marks are placed 10 cm apart over the patient's lower spine and the distance is remeasured with the patient flexing forward. Normally, there should be an increase of 5 cm in the measured distance.

The differential diagnosis is similar to conditions mimicking JIA, such as trauma, overuse syndromes, septic arthritis, and hemoglobinopathies. In evaluating patients with a suspected spondyloarthropathy, the importance of a careful history and physical examination cannot be over stated. The patient should be asked about symptoms of inflammatory pain, such as morning stiffness, night time and early morning pain, and improvement of pain with exercise. The patient or parents should be specifically asked about a family history of any of the spondyloarthropathies, psoriasis, and inflammatory bowel disease.

Ankylosing Spondylitis (AS)

AS is uncommon in children younger than 16 years of age. Onset is usually in young adulthood, again, primarily in males. Most patients will present with insidious, persistent chronic low back pain. Other features include enthesitis, peripheral arthritis, and less commonly extra-articular manifestations. Typical radiographic spinal changes of AS will not be present for years.

Reactive Arthritis/Reiter Syndrome

First described by Dr. Reiter in a German officer with bloody diarrhea, Reiter syndrome is a reactive arthritis, usually occurring after an enteric or genitourinary infection in young men (Chap 24). Because of Dr. Reiter's association with other Nazi physicians, many rheumatologists prefer to call this subtype simply reactive arthritis. The classical presentation is a triad of urethritis, arthritis, and uveitis, but most patients present with an acute arthritis alone. Women may present with subtle cervicitis. Arthritis is usually very abrupt, within a few days of the infection; a large weight bearing joint of the lower extremities is most often involved. The arthritis is usually mono or pauciarticular, and quite painful, lasting for weeks to months. Eye involvement is also abrupt and painful, in contrast to JIA uveitis which is usually painless and more indolent. Over time, patients will experience recurrent attacks of arthritis and may later develop mucocutaneous manifestations (mouth ulcers, rashes, nail changes) sacroiliitis or typical ankylosing spondylitis. Overall, clinically evident ankylosing spondylitis occurs in about 10% of cases.

Psoriatic Arthropathy

The arthropathy associated with psoriasis can be manifested in extremely varied ways; from peripheral asymmetric arthritis, a polyarthritis resembling RA, to spinal and sacroiliac disease, or even a combination of these manifestations. Most patients will have typical psoriasis skin lesions before developing arthritis (Chap. 19), but the psoriasis may appear at onset of the arthritis or, in a small percent, even years later. Psoriatic arthropathy is more common in adults, again with a male predominance, but does occur in children as well.

Enteropathic Arthropathy

Arthropathy occurs in about one-third of patients with inflammatory bowel disease and may be the

initial manifestation. Acute arthritis in peripheral joints usually coincides with active bowel inflammation and will subside once the gastrointestinal disease is controlled (Chap. 11). Ten percent of patients will eventually develop spinal disease, usually sacroiliitis and occasionally, ankylosing spondylitis. Other features include mouth ulcers, skin lesions (i.e., erythema nodosum, pyoderma gangrenosa), and uveitis. Interestingly, a high frequency of patients with other spondyloarthropathies have occult gastrointestinal inflammation demonstrated by endoscopic examination and biopsy.

Undifferentiated Arthropathy

Accurate classification of a spondyloarthropathy may not be possible for several years from onset of characteristic symptoms. It takes years before the classic radiographic findings of sacroilitis or spondylitis are present, especially in the younger patients. Patients with undifferentiated spondyloarthropathy will again be predominantly male, most will have HLA B27, and will not have RF or other auto antibodies. A subgroup of undifferentiated spondyloarthropathy was previously called seronegative enthesopathy or SEA syndrome; these patients were primarily young males with chronic enthesitis. Most of those individuals classified as undifferentiated arthropathy will over time have sufficient features to diagnose one of the spondyloarthropathies discussed above.

Laboratory and Radiographic Features

Determination of the presence or absence of HLA B27 can be helpful, particularly when combined with the patient's medical history and examination, family history, and radiographic evaluation. However, this antigen can be negative and is only used to support the clinical diagnosis. It is not a useful screening tool in asymptomatic individuals. In many patients, especially those with involvement of only a few joints, laboratory studies may be completely normal. Tests for rheumatoid factors and antinuclear antibodies will almost always be negative. Patients with significant inflammation may have a low grade anemia and elevation of acute phase reactants, such as CRP and the erythrocyte sedimentation rate.

Routine radiographs will be normal early on, except for soft tissue changes. For diagnosis of early disease, the most useful imaging procedure is an MRI examination. Other useful procedures include ultrasound and radionuclide scanning, particularly for evaluation of enthesitis. CT scanning is not useful for enthesitis, but can be quite useful for evaluation of sacroiliac disease. The most common radiographic changes are from enthesitis and from disease in the sacroiliac joints. Enthesitis is characterized radiographically first by bony erosion, then sclerosis and with longstanding disease, ankylosis of the adjacent bone. In sacroiliac disease, which can be unilateral, changes are similar and appear first on the iliac side of the joint. Before significant radiographic changes are present on plain films, MRI examination will show profound alterations in the sacroiliac joint, or in the case of enthesitis, alterations in involved bone, and attached connective tissues. Spondylitis occurs from a combination of arthritis and enthesitis, and begins in the lower spine first; it slowly progresses to involve the entire spine. Erosions develop at the vertebral corners, followed by formation of syndesmophytes and ultimately, leading to the bamboo spine appearance. A late feature is ankylosis.

Clinical Course and Prognosis

Most youngsters presenting with a spondyloarthropathy will do quite well and permanent disability is not common. Long term studies showing marked variation in progression to classic AS of rates of 10% to as high as 90%, mainly due to differences in classification criteria and length of follow-up. In a recent series of patients with childhood onset spondyloarthropathy, with at least 10 years disease duration, those with enteropathic or psoriatic arthropathy had remission rates of 50%–70%, whereas no patient with ankylosing spondylitis was in a remission; however, this was a very small series. In a study of 100 adults with typical ankylosing spondylitis, over 80% had daily pain, even after 20 years of disease, suggesting AS does not "burn out," as previously suggested. Similar findings were reported in a study of 328 patients with either AS or another spondyloarthropathy. In that series, factors associated with a more severe outcome

included presence of oligoarthritis, sausage digits, hip or lumbar spine disease, young age of symptom onset (<15 years), poor response to NSAID and persistently elevated erythrocyte sedimentation rate. Severe outcome was much more likely with hip involvement and/or three of the above factors.

Treatment

Similar to the treatment for children with JIA, the initial focus is on pain control, appropriate balance of rest and exercise, use of analgesics and a trial of NSAIDs. Exercises to preserve back flexibility, an appropriate exercise program, and inserts to protect heels and plantar fascia, can all be useful. For reactive arthritis, NSAIDs and pain relief are usually sufficient to control disease. Many rheumatologists will also treat an acute exacerbation of reactive arthritis with a course of doxycycline, as this has been shown to reduce the duration of the exacerbation. For more recalcitrant and persistent peripheral arthritis, other agents can be added and the dose and types of agents are similar to those used to treat RA and JIA. Medications include sulfasalazine, methotrexate, doxycycline, chronic NSAIDs, low dose prednisone, and potentially some of the newer biologic agents may control spondyloarthropathy as well. Injection of corticosteroids into involved joints and bursas may provide considerable and longstanding relief of symptoms. Vertebral compression fractures are a common, but often undiagnosed complication in adults with ankylosing spondylitis, as many of these patients have significant osteoporosis of the spine as a complication of the disease process.

RAYNAUD'S PHENOMENON

Raynaud's phenomenon refers to episodes of vasospasm precipitated by exposure to cold or emotional stress. In the full triphasic color response, the fingers turn white, then dusky blue, and with rewarming, turn bright red. Often only one or two digits will be involved and there will be a sharp line of demarcation on the involved digit. The patient may experience pain or numbness during an episode. The primary form occurs in individuals with no underlying medical disorders. Secondary Raynaud's phenomenon is most commonly associated with an underlying rheumatic disorder, but can also occur in individuals with carpal tunnel syndrome, vaso-occlusive arterial disorders, hyperviscosity states, and after exposure to environmental toxins or certain medications.

Raynaud's phenomenon is extremely common, occurring in 5%–10% of the general population, with three-fourths of cases occurring in women aged 15–40 years. Primary Raynaud's is more common and generally milder than secondary cases; overall 90% of cases are primary. In general, patients will show evidence of their underlying rheumatic disorder within a few years of the development of the symptoms of Raynaud's phenomenon. The presence of a positive ANA and abnormalities in the nail fold capillary loops (capillary drop-off, telangiectasias and focal areas of dilation) are predictive of the development of an underlying rheumatic disorder. Management consists of avoiding excessive cold exposure, appropriate warm clothing, and avoidance of tobacco products. More severe cases involving significant pain and/or damage to distal tissues may require management with vasodilating agents, including nifedipine and losartan. Treatment of secondary Raynaud's would also include management of the underlying medical disorder as well. Over 90% of patients with scleroderma have Raynaud's phenomenon and the incidence is about 10% in systemic lupus erythematosus (SLE), dermatomyositis, and adult RA.

SYSTEMIC LUPUS ERYTHEMATOSUS

SLE is an inflammatory disorder of unknown etiology, occurring predominantly in young women, with a male:female ratio of 1:10. The incidence of SLE is increased in Asian, Hispanic, and African American women. In the United States, the overall incidence is about 15–50 cases per 100,000 population. The hallmark of SLE is the production of multiple auto antibodies, vasculitis, and inflammation of multiple organ systems. The etiology is multifactorial; disease expression and long-term prognosis are quite unpredictable and quite variable. Diagnosis is based on exclusion of other rheumatic diseases and the presence of 4 out of 11 specific classification criteria, including rashes, presence of certain serologic markers, arthritis, nephritis, serositis, and neurologic or hematologic abnormalities (Table 12-6).

Clinical Features

SLE is characterized by the inappropriate production of autoantibodies to nuclear constituents which together with complement and other mediators can trigger an immune reaction in virtually any organ. Thus, patients with this disease can present to virtually any subspecialty, from the psychiatrist to the orthopedic surgeon. The disorder should be considered in any patient, especially a young woman, with unusual symptoms and evidence of inflammation. It is not uncommon for SLE to first present within the first few years after menarche, after institution of estrogen-containing oral contraceptives, or around pregnancy and delivery.

Among the most common symptoms of SLE are arthralgia and arthritis, fatigue, fever, headache, and weight loss. Cutaneous manifestations (Chap. 19) are frequent and include the classic butterfly malar eruption, generalized photosensitivity, alopecia, Raynaud's phenomenon, and cutaneous vasculitis (palpable purpura, livedo reticularis). Renal involvement occurs in 50%–70% of patients, ranging from minimal mesangial proliferation to diffuse proliferative glomerulonephritis on biopsy specimens. Inflammatory lesions can occur throughout the central nervous system, resulting in seizures, psychosis, stroke, and coma.

Laboratory Features

As in many other rheumatic diseases (including JIA), most SLE patients will have positive ANA. The ANA is a good screening test for SLE but lacks specificity. Antibodies to double-stranded DNA (anti-dsDNA) and various cytoplasmic antigens are much more sensitive and specific for a diagnosis of SLE. Active SLE often is accompanied by low

TABLE 12-6

DIAGNOSTIC CRITERIA FOR SLE

Criteria	Comment
Facial butterfly rash	Flat or raised malar erythema with or without edema. May develop vesicles, crusting, or ulcerations. Present in half of all cases. Nonspecific for SLE.
Discoid lupus	Scaly erythematous plaques predominating on face and scalp with or without scarring, atrophy, pigment changes, and telangiectasia. May be an isolated cutaneous disorder or part of a systemic disease. Other skin lesions that may be seen with SLE include urticaria, tender nodules on palms, fingertips, and soles, digit gangrene, and periungual erythema. See text.
Photosensitivity	Includes sun-exposure induced urticarial plaques on the skin.
Oral or nasopharyngeal ulceration	May result in epistaxis or perforation of the septum.
Nephritis or nephrotic syndrome	Renal involvement occurs in half of cases, involving persistent proteinuria, hematuria, or cellular casts (glomerular or tubular)
Joint swelling	Polyarthritis (two or more peripheral joints) similar to juvenile rheumatoid arthritis but without joint destruction. Present in nine of ten cases.
Pleuritis or pericarditis	Also may develop peritonitis, myocarditis, endocarditis (Libman-Sacks), or parenchymal lung disease. Cardiac tamponade is rare.
Psychosis or convulsions	Other CNS manifestations that may be seen include mononeuritis, cranial nerve neuropathy, chorea, myelopathy, aseptic meningitis, and cerebrovascular accidents.
Hemolytic anemia, leukopenia, lymphopenia, and/or thrombocytopenia	Coombs' test will be positive if hemolytic anemia is present. Splenomegaly is also seen.
Positive immunoserology	The LE cell is positive in 50% of SLE patients; not currently widely used. Other tests include anti-DNA antibody to native DNA in abnormal titer, anti-Sm antibody to Sm nuclear antigen, persistent false-positive serologic test for syphilis (with negative FTA test).
Antinuclear antibody	Fluorescence or equivalent assay

Established by the American Rheumatism Association or American College of Rheumatology in 1971 and revised in 1982. The presence of four or more of the criteria (serially or simultaneously) is associated with a positive pathologic diagnosis in nine of ten cases.

levels of the complement components C3 and C4. The combination of a depressed complement level and elevated anti-dsDNA is 100% specific for SLE. Similarly, anti-dsDNA titers and complement levels can be used to monitor disease activity and can often predict a disease flare.

Deficiencies of early complement components leading to lupus-like disease are suspected if the total hemolytic complement is quite low or persistently depressed. Hematologic features of SLE include leukopenia, lymphopenia, thrombocytopenia, and Coombs-positive hemolytic anemia.

Approximately one-third of SLE patients will have evidence of anti-phospholipid antibodies or another of the lupus anticoagulants.

Treatment

Treatment for SLE is based on the organ systems involved. All patients should be advised to use sunscreen and should be educated about the management of SLE. Arthritis and mucocutaneous disease are manageable with nonsteroidal drugs and hydroxychloroquine. Systemic corticosteroids are indicated for visceral involvement or severe hematologic disease and typically are begun at a dose of 2 mg/kg/day of prednisone (maximum 60–80 mg/day). The dosage of medication is titrated on the basis of the patient's symptoms and objective measures of disease activity (i.e., physical examination, urinary sediment, and levels of C3, C4, and DNA antibodies). Whenever possible, steroids should be converted to alternate-day dosing in an effort to minimize side effects. Severe SLE, such as progressive renal or pulmonary insufficiency, systemic vasculitis, and central nervous system (CNS) disease, may require treatment with large doses of intravenous pulse methylprednisolone (30 mg/kg, up to 1000 mg). Immunosuppressive therapy is added in children with severe uncontrolled disease or in whom the steroid dose cannot be reduced.

Significant renal involvement, such as diffuse proliferative glomerulonephritis, requires monthly intravenous cyclophosphamide, as corticosteroids alone are not sufficient to prevent end stage renal failure. Methotrexate and azathioprine are effective in managing nonrenal manifestations and can allow reduction of the corticosteroid dose. Autologous bone marrow transplantation has been used to control disease in severe SLE unresponsive to other therapies. Patients with SLE who have antiphospholipid antibodies or the lupus anticoagulant (about one-third of SLE cases) are prone to recurrent arterial and venous thromboses (stroke, thrombophlebitis) and miscarriage. These patients should be considered for treatment with low dose aspirin. SLE patients who have experienced a significant thrombotic event may require life-long treatment with anticoagulants.

Prognosis

The long-term outcome of SLE is variable and depends on the extent and severity of organ involvement. It is important to anticipate that over time, other organ sites will become affected. The prognosis of lupus has improved dramatically in the past 50 years and the 10 year survival is now greater than 90%. However, there is still considerable morbidity, both disease-related and from the complications of treatment; these complications include accelerated atherosclerosis, increased susceptibility to infection, and the musculoskeletal complications of prolonged corticosteroid use. The overall risk of corticosteroid induced avascular necrosis of the hips can exceed 25%. Death in SLE patients occurs primarily from infection, but can be a result of renal failure, pulmonary hemorrhage, severe CNS disease, and early myocardial infarction.

Other Lupus Syndromes

Discoid Lupus

Lupus can present with skin lesions alone (Chap. 19). These lesions typically occur in sun-exposed areas and are characterized by coin-shaped, scarring, skin lesions. Discoid skin lesions also occur in a third of patients with established SLE. Over time, 5%–10% of patients with discoid lupus will go on to develop SLE. Any patient with discoid lupus should be screened for SLE and monitored on a regular basis for signs and symptoms of SLE. Treatment of discoid lupus consists of sun avoidance, topical or intralesional corticosteroids and administration of hydroxychloroquine.

Drug-Induced Lupus

Drug induced lupus is seen in individuals taking any number of prescription drugs, most commonly antihypertensives (hydralazine, procainamide, and alpha methyldopa), so this disorder is more common in adults. Drug-induced lupus can be seen in children taking anticonvulsants, usually phenytoin and occasionally, phenobarbital. Rarely, a drug-induced lupus syndrome can occur with use of minocycline or after the hepatitis B immunization. The patient will develop vague constitutional symptoms, joint disease, rashes, mouth ulcers, and positive ANA. The adolescent may have pleuritis or pericarditis. Renal disease and positive anti-dsDNA are very unusual in drug-induced lupus. Most patients will have a positive ANA and usually have antihistone antibodies, but these antibodies can occur in SLE as well. The condition is self-limited and resolves when the medication is stopped. A short course of corticosteroids may be needed to control disease.

Mixed Connective Tissue Disease

Mixed connective tissue disease (MCTD) is one of the "overlap" syndromes with features of SLE, systemic sclerosis, myositis, and arthritis. It is defined by the presence of antibodies to the extractable nuclear antigen ribonucleoprotein (anti-RNP) and against U1-70 kd small nuclear ribonucleoprotein (snRNP). There is a marked female predominance and most cases occur in patients aged 15–25 years. The condition affects about three cases per 100,000 population. Classically, adolescents with MCTD present with Raynaud's phenomenon, puffy hands, and arthritis. They are less likely to have significant renal involvement than children with SLE. MCTD was initially thought to have a benign course and prognosis. However, recent long-term outcome studies have established pulmonary hypertension as the most common disease-related cause of death. The presence of anticardiolipin antibodies is a marker for development of pulmonary hypertension. Infections are also a major cause of death in MCTD. Over time, patients may ultimately evolve into a diagnosable rheumatic disorder, usually SLE or systemic sclerosis.

MCTD is a subset of conditions referred to as undifferentiated connective tissue disease. This term refers to patients with nonspecific rheumatic symptoms (e.g., Raynaud's, polyarthritis, positive ANA) who do not yet meet classification criteria for a definable rheumatic disease. Patients with rheumatic diseases can also have overlap syndromes where they have more than one rheumatic disease.

SCLERODERMA

Scleroderma encompasses a group of disorders falling into two main classes: systemic scleroderma and localized scleroderma. Systemic scleroderma (also called systemic sclerosis) is rare in children and adolescents. Most children with scleroderma have one of the localized forms, either linear scleroderma or morphea (isolated patches of sclerotic skin). A variant of systemic scleroderma, called CREST syndrome or limited scleroderma, is associated with calcinosis, Raynaud's phenomenon, esophageal dysmotility, sclerodactyly, and telangiectasias. Like most rheumatic diseases, the etiology of scleroderma is not known and this disorder also has a significant female predominance. Scleroderma is characterized by increased deposition of collagen in skin which manifests as progressive tightening of the skin.

The most severe form, diffuse scleroderma, involves internal organs–in particular, heart, lungs, and kidneys. Skin changes begin with edema, followed by induration, sclerosis, and eventually severe skin atrophy and contractures. The skin of the digits, hands, face, or arm is usually affected first; the disease then progresses proximally. Dysphagia results from thickening of the lower third of the esophagus. Hypertension, renal failure, pulmonary fibrosis, and cardiac involvement may also occur.

Systemic sclerosis is associated with Raynaud's phenomenon and can be relentlessly progressive. In most cases Raynaud's develops first and the individual will then develop scleroderma. The diagnosis is based on clinical suspicion and may be confirmed by a skin biopsy of affected sites. With the exception of biopsy, no single laboratory test is useful for the diagnosis. The ANA and RF may be positive, but are in lower titers than those found in patients with SLE. ANA patterns are usually nucleolar or centromere. Other auto antibodies seen in scleroderma include anti-SCL-70 in diffuse scleroderma and anticentromere antibodies in the CREST syndrome. Treatment of scleroderma is aimed at decreasing deposition of collagen and controlling associated disease manifestations, such as hypertension and digital necrosis. The long-term prognosis for children and adolescents with systemic sclerosis is not well established, but is probably similar to adult cases and depends greatly on the extent of systemic involvement. The major morbidity and mortality correlates with the degree of renal, cardiac, and/or pulmonary involvement. CREST tends to be more indolent than classic systemic sclerosis and is very unusual in youth.

The localized forms of scleroderma are not usually associated with systemic involvement, but some patients may have positive ANA. There are case reports of children with localized scleroderma developing typical systemic sclerosis as adults. Local involvement of skin and subcutaneous tissues can lead to flexion contractures and growth abnormalities. The natural history of localized scleroderma varies from total spontaneous remission to progression of lesions over several years. Treatment emphasizes good physical therapy to soften the skin and maintain range and function. Drugs are indicated for more severe or rapidly progressive disease. In several small series of patients with linear scleroderma, methotrexate has been shown to control disease extension and to soften involved skin.

DERMATOMYOSITIS

Clinical Features

Dermatomyositis is a rheumatic disorder characterized by chronic inflammation in skin, blood vessels and muscle. The etiology is not known and cases occasionally occur in clusters, suggesting an infectious trigger. The disorder occurs in 1:100,000 population with two distinct peaks–between ages 12and 17 and a larger peak in middle age.

The adolescent usually presents with painless, progressive proximal weakness over weeks to months. The distinctive dermatomyositis rash develops around the same time on sun exposed areas. Joint symptoms, fatigue, vague abdominal pain, mild dysphagia and low grade fever are also common. Some patients may have mild to moderate muscle pain as well; significant weight loss is not common. On physical examination, the child or teen will have the characteristic rash which consists of Gottron papules (reddish nodules on the knuckles), a psoriasiform eruption over the extensor surfaces of the elbows and knees, and a purplish discoloration of the eyelids (heliotrope rash). Photosensitive eruptions also occur on the face and can extend down the upper trunk in a V- or shawl-distribution. The facial rashes can be mistaken for the malar rash of SLE, but Gottron papules are not seen in SLE.

On muscle testing, the adolescent will have a positive Gowers' maneuver and diminished proximal muscle strength and normal reflexes. On laboratory testing, patients usually have a normal ESR, CRP, and CBC; occasionally, the platelet count can be mildly low. Muscle enzymes are moderately high and more than 70% of patients have positive ANA. Muscle biopsy reveals inflammation and inflammatory changes in capillaries. Other signs of vasculitis include nail-fold telangiectasias and ulcerative lesions of the skin and gastrointestinal tract. Diagnosis is made on the presence of four of five criteria: typical rash, muscle weakness, laboratory evidence of muscle involvement, typical biopsy findings, and characteristic abnormalities on electromyographic (EMG) testing. If weakness is documented, the rash is classic, and serum muscle enzyme concentrations are elevated, a diagnosis may be confirmed through characteristic changes in muscle seen on MRI. A third of adult patients with dermatomyositis have an occult malignancy; however malignancy is not seen in childhood dermatomyositis. Dermatomyositis, with its characteristic cutaneous findings, is usually a straightforward diagnosis. Polymyositis (idiopathic inflammatory muscle disease) can be confused with a variety of neurologic and myopathic processes including the muscular dystrophies, congenital neurodegenerative disorders, drug toxicities, and multiple sclerosis. Isolated polymyositis is uncommon in children, but can be seen in association with other rheumatic disorders such as SLE or systemic vasculitis.

Treatment of Dermatomyositis

Due to the seriousness of sequelae in untreated or inadequately treated patients, all children and adolescents with dermatomyositis should be referred to a specialist with experience in treating this condition. High-dose corticosteroid therapy is the mainstay of therapy for dermatomyositis, given either orally or as pulse methylprednisolone to control inflammation rapidly. Corticosteroids are continued in high doses until muscle strength improves and serum muscle enzyme levels normalize; then they are gradually tapered. It usually is not possible to convert to alternate-day dosing during periods of disease activity, and for unclear reasons, dermatomyositis patients can flare after a minor taper in the daily prednisone dose. Failure to respond to corticosteroids or the development of significant corticosteroid side effects calls for the addition of immunosuppressive therapy, usually methotrexate, given either orally or subcutaneously. Intravenous immune globulin (IVIG) has been shown in a randomized, placebo controlled trial to be efficacious as well. In refractory cases, cyclophosphamide, cyclosporine and other agents in combination with corticosteroids, have been tried. Hydroxychloroquine can be useful in treating the cutaneous disease, but has little effect on the muscle inflammation.

Prognosis

Untreated, the mortality rate for childhood dermatomyositis approaches 33% and historically, over two-thirds of untreated survivors had severe long term disability. Death is now uncommon (<1%), occurring in children or adolescents with fulminant disease or severe gastrointestinal disease with perforation. Patients can also die from infectious complications. More than 75% can be expected to have a monocyclic course lasting 2 years or less. Delay in diagnosis and lack of response to therapy is correlated with poorer outcome. Early complications include bowel perforation, infection, and respiratory compromise. Late complications are from the immobility and from treatment, such as corticosteroid induce osteoporosis. Calcinosis, a form of dystrophic calcification occurring in healing muscle, is seen in the majority of patients and is most severe in the most severely affected patients. Calcinosis can be quite difficult to treat and is associated with deformity, draining subcutaneous nodules, and secondary infection. Rarely,

dermatomyositis can overlap with scleroderma or other rheumatic disorders.

SYSTEMIC VASCULITIS

Vasculitis is the general term used to describe inflammation and damage to vessel wall endothelium. Damage to the vessel wall leads to increased vascular permeability, edema, further recruitment of inflammatory cells, release of an array of inflammatory mediators and local tissue destruction. Vasculitis has many causes, including a variety of infectious diseases, drugs, and toxins. The systemic vasculitides are a group of idiopathic disorders with distinct clinical manifestations and involvement of varying sizes of affected vessels. Vasculitis can occur in virtually any organ, and thus, the clinical signs and symptoms are extremely variable. In contrast to adults, the two most common vasculitis syndromes of childhood are Kawasaki disease (Chap. 9) and Henoch-Schönlein purpura (Chap. 16). Both conditions have an acute onset, a self-limited course, and overall good prognosis. Systemic vasculitis is quite rare in young children, but should be considered in older adolescents, particularly in a youngster with unexplained multi-system disease (especially rapidly progressive pulmonary and renal involvement), constitutional symptoms, and laboratory evidence of inflammation. Histologic examination of involved organs is essential to making an accurate diagnosis. The site of tissue for biopsy is determined clinically and the tissue biopsy must be obtained before starting corticosteroids. Accurate diagnosis, classification, and treatment are crucial to treating these rare and complex disorders, as many vasculitides can be fatal if not promptly recognized and treated.

Of equal importance is to identify diseases that can mimic vasculitis, such as drug reactions, infections (e.g., parvovirus, hepatitis, EBV), endocrine disorders, and gastrointestinal diseases. Although malignancies and cholesterol emboli are relatively common vasculitis mimics in adults, they are seldom the etiology of vasculitis mimics in children or adolescents.

Henoch Schönlein purpura (HSP) is the most common vasculitis of childhood and adolescence, with an incidence of about 15/100,000 children or teens; 75% of cases occur in children between ages 2 and 11, with a peak age of 5 years. HSP was first described in the nineteenth century. Other names include anaphylactoid purpura and allergic vasculitis. Histologic lesions show leukocytoclastic vasculitis and IgA deposition. Small vessels–capillaries, arterioles, and venules–are involved. Etiology is unknown, but cases have been shown after infection with several agents including EBV, adenovirus, enteric bacteria, and streptococcus. HSP is more common in the spring and fall months, and 75% of patients will report a preceding upper respiratory infection. Clinically, HSP typically presents with purpuric rash, abdominal pain, arthritis, and nephritis (Chap. 16). Other manifestations include intussusception (2%–3%), scrotal swelling, and renal involvement (20%–50%).

Long-term outcome depends on the extent of kidney involvement (Chap. 16). In general, renal involvement will be present within 2–3 months of onset. Progression to end-stage renal impairment is rare (<1%) and is more common in older children and adolescents. Treatment is primarily supportive. Intravenous fluids may be necessary for those with severe gastrointestinal symptoms. The role of corticosteroids is controversial. Corticosteroids will improve the rash, arthritis, and abdominal symptoms, as well as shorten the duration of hospitalization; however, it is unclear if they reduce the progression of renal disease. There are anecdotal reports of improvement of clinical symptoms after administration of intravenous immunoglobulin, cyclosporine, factor VIII, and plasmapheresis. An HSP-like rash, usually referred to as hypersensitivity vasculitis (leukocytoclastic vasculitis without the IgA deposition seen in HSP) can be seen in SLE, inflammatory bowel disease, RA, Wegener's granulomatosis, coagulopathies, and a variety of infections. Both HSP and hypersensitivity vasculitis predominantly affect small vessels.

Serum sickness occurs when a foreign protein (classically horse serum) is administered, resulting in circulating antigen-antibody complexes that fix to the walls of blood vessels and initiate an immune reaction and subsequent vasculitis. Serum sickness can occur after exposure to several drugs. Clinically, this is manifested as urticarial skin lesions and polyarthritis, often in association with fever. Commonly implicated drugs include antibiotics (e.g., cefaclor, sulfonamides, and penicillins) and anticonvulsants (e.g., phenytoin). Treatment is removal of the drug and supportive treatment. A short course of oral or parenteral corticosteroids can help ameliorate symptoms.

POLYARTERITIS NODOSA (PAN)/CUTANEOUS PAN

Classic polyarteritis nodosa (PAN) is a rare disorder (around 1:100,000), uncommon in youth and is typically seen in men in their 30s and 40s. PAN is a necrotizing vasculitis of medium sized vessels predominantly involving peripheral nerves, intestinal tract, kidneys, lungs, skin, and joints. Thirty percent of cases are associated with the presence of Hepatitis B surface antigen. Patients often present with hypertension and vague multisystemic symptoms. Laboratory evaluation will usually show signs of chronic inflammation, hematuria, proteinuria, a negative ANA, and presence of Antineutrophil cytoplasmic antibody (ANCA) in 20%–30% of cases. Untreated patients generally die within a few months of presentation, and it is imperative to consider this disorder in patients with suggestive clinical symptoms. Treatment usually requires large doses of corticosteroids and administration of cytotoxic agents, such as azathioprine or cyclophosphamide.

Cutaneous PAN is a less common entity, felt to be distinct from classic PAN by most rheumatologists and dermatologists. The skin lesions are the same as in PAN, but patients with cutaneous PAN will not have systemic involvement and the clinical course is much more favorable. Patients will present with painful nodules under the skin with secondary infarcts. Often, the patient will show livedo reticularis and painful edema of the muscles of the extremities. Low-grade fever, anemia, and acute phase reactants will be present. The patient will not have internal organ involvement. Most cases of cutaneous PAN in childhood are associated with Group A streptococcus infection and all adolescents suspected of having a vasculitis should be screened for streptococcal infection (by throat culture and ASO determination). Management consists of treatment of streptococcal disease or removal of an offending medication, as well as a course of corticosteroid. As the disease resolves, the corticosteroids can be tapered.

NONINFLAMMATORY MUSCULOSKELETAL CONDITIONS IN ADOLESCENCE

Osteoporosis

The past two decades have seen an explosion of research and new information in both the prevention and treatment of established bone loss. Approximately half of adult bone mass is acquired during adolescence, with bone mass increasing 8% each year during the adolescent growth spurt. Achievement of normal peak bone mass during childhood is quite important, as it may not be possible to correct this deficiency later in life. Conditions associated with decreased bone mass include chronic amenorrhea, eating disorders, renal, gastrointestinal and metabolic disorders, prolonged administration of corticosteroids or anticonvulsants and any of numerous disorders associated with limited mobility. JIA, RA, and spondyloarthropathy patients have diminished bone mass, even in the absence of corticosteroid use. Corticosteroids are frequently used in the treatment of the rheumatic diseases, and all patients on chronic corticosteroids should be considered at risk of osteoporosis. The risk and severity of corticosteroid induced osteoporosis is related both to the cumulative dose and to the duration of treatment. A careful balance between disease control and use of the lowest dose of corticosteroids is necessary. Osteomalacia refers to normal bone volume, but decreased mineralized bone matrix and is much less common than osteoporosis (normal bone mineral, but decreased bone volume). Osteomalacia is associated with renal disorders, vitamin D deficiency states, and inborn errors of vitamin D metabolism.

Evaluation and Screening for Osteopenia

A detailed history and physical examination will help identify those adolescents at risk of osteoporosis and the decision to perform screening studies is made on an individual basis. Unless severe, decreased bone density per se does not lead to musculoskeletal pain. Adolescents with osteoporotic vertebral stress fractures usually complain of chronic low grade back pain and progressive kyphosis, but can present occasionally with more acute severe pain. Many patients with significant osteoporosis are identified only after sustaining extremity or vertebral fractures and subsequent radiographs suggest low bone density. However, plain radiographs are not a useful screening tool, because the typical changes of osteopenia are not present until a third of the bone mass is lost. The study most frequently used currently to determine bone density is the dual energy x-ray absorptiometry (DEXA), because of its low radiation, wide availability and the presence of reference data in adults, adolescents and children. Quantitative CT measurements are precise, but are expensive, involve more irradiation, and there are limited data on healthy children and adolescents. Quantitative ultrasound of the calcaneus to determine bone density is not used as frequently. However, this procedure is relatively precise, uses no irradiation and is inexpensive.

By 1994 WHO criteria, an adult is said to have osteoporosis when the measurement of their bone density is more than 2.5 SD below the mean peak bone value of white women. There are several problems in trying to measure and interpret bone mass in children and adolescents. There is still insufficient bone density data based on large population studies in normal children. Age, body size, pubertal status, gender, and ethnic background are all variables with significant impact on the bone density of youths. Normative data on adults cannot be generalized to children and adolescents. In particular, a child or young teen's T-score is poorly predictive of the presence of osteoporosis, as a low T-score has a particularly high frequency of misinterpretation and false positive results. Accordingly, the WHO criteria define osteoporosis in children when the Z-score (SD based on age-matched controls) is below 2 SD.

Treatment

As part of routine health maintenance, all adolescents should be counseled about adequate calcium and vitamin D intake (Chap. 29), as well as the importance of sufficient regular physical exercise to maintain bone density. Any adolescent at risk of osteoporosis should be appropriately screened. The decision to treat will depend on the degree of osteoporosis, the etiology of the decreased bone mass, and the risk of fracture. Bone mass will increase significantly if the underlying condition can be identified and effectively treated. Indeed, in some instances, bone mass can eventually be restored to normal, without the need for pharmacologic agents. In steroid-induced osteoporosis, the corticosteroid dose should be reduced as much as clinically possible. If the steroid dose cannot be reduced, other anti-inflammatory agents should be added for disease control to allow a reduction in the daily steroid dose (steroid sparing effect), as discussed earlier in this chapter. Estrogen treatment may be indicated in females with estrogen deficiency states. Fluoride and calcitonin do not have sufficient effect on bone density to recommend their routine use, and there are virtually no data on their use in children and adolescents. Parathyroid hormone has been shown in animal studies and early clinical trials in humans to increase bone mass in osteoporotic individuals. However, this treatment is not yet FDA approved, nor has it been studied in children or adolescents. Currently, the bisphosphonates are the mainstay in the pharmacologic management of osteoporosis. There are commercially available agents—alendronate (Fosamax), risedronate (Actonel).

Although, the bisphosphonates have been studied and are effective in postmenopausal osteoporosis and in steroid induced osteoporosis in adults, there are very few studies on the use of these agents in children, adolescents, or young adults. The treatment recommendations for osteoporosis are in transition, and several large scale trials are underway to determine optimal doses and duration of therapy, as well as to determine the indications in younger patients.

CHRONIC PAIN SYNDROMES

A third of young patients presenting to a rheumatology clinic for consultation will not have a primary inflammatory disorder as a cause of their symptoms. Conditions include transient arthralgia or arthritis following an acute illness, overuse and orthopedic syndromes, somatization and mood disorders with arthralgia, and a variety of chronic pain syndromes. The chronic pain syndromes, also referred to as pain amplification syndromes are a heterogenous group of disorders characterized by diffuse pain, significant interruption of usual activities, absence of inflammation, and specific distinct clinical manifestations. It is important for clinicians to be aware of these disorders and to recognize the usual clinical presentations. Youngsters with these disorders are often put through a prolonged and unnecessary set of diagnostic studies and treatments. Chronic pain is extremely common and affects 10% of the general U.S. population.

Joint Hypermobility Syndrome

Up to 12% of school-aged children have hyperextensible joints; it is more common in younger children and girls. Joint laxity is also more prevalent among dancers, gymnasts, and instrumental musicians. Joint laxity leads to an increased incidence of arthralgia, transient joint effusions, dislocations, and diffuse pain syndromes such as fibromyalgia. Half of youngsters with joint hypermobility will consult a health care provider because of symptoms. Children and adolescents with hypermobility may also have mitral valve prolapse (Chap. 9). The diagnosis of hypermobility syndrome is based on the ability of the person to perform a series of five joint maneuvers (hyperextension of the knees and elbows, ability to touch the palms to the floor with the knees straight, dorsiflexion of the MCPs (metacarpal phalangeals) 90 degrees, and ability to touch the thumb to the forearm).

These children do not have skin laxity or other physical signs of the hereditary connective tissue disorders, such as Marfan's or Ehlers-Danlos syndromes (Chap. 21). However, joint laxity and increased pain do occur in those disorders as well. The management of hypermobility syndrome is conservative and includes curtailment of offending physical activities, physical therapy (strengthening, bracing, and pain control), and NSAIDs or analgesics as required. Hypermobility will improve or resolve with time.

Reflex Sympathetic Dystrophy (Complex Regional Pain Syndrome Type I)

Reflex sympathetic dystrophy (RSD) is an infrequent condition in adolescents: previous terms include reflex neurovascular dystrophy, causalgia, and Sudeck's atrophy. The term complex regional pain syndrome I is preferred, but most textbooks still refer to this condition as RSD. The adolescent will present with an extremely painful, swollen, mottled, cool extremity, usually after trauma; the trauma can be quite mild. The skin of the involved limb will be very dry or more commonly, will have increased sweating. Pain is extreme, with a burning or "pins and needles" sensation, and the individual will not use the extremity or tolerate even light touch. The condition can be confused with cellulites and inflammatory arthritis. Laboratory studies, including CBC and sedimentation rate are normal. Diagnosis is most often made clinically, but can be confirmed by bone scan or thermography. In longstanding cases of RSD the plain radiographs will show regional osteopenia. In adults, the condition is usually secondary to an underlying condition such as diabetes or degenerative cervical spine disease. In children, an underlying cause is not usually found, but occasionally a stress fracture or other orthopedic condition can trigger RSD.

Treatment is focused on pain control, prompt mobilization of the involved extremity and education of the patient as to the pathophysiology of the symptoms. NSAIDs or analgesics can be helpful. Narcotics should be used sparingly, if at all. Physical therapy, counseling, and biofeedback have

all been shown to be effective. There is a high incidence of psychosocial discord in the families of these children and adolescents which must be addressed as well. Most episodes will remit spontaneously, but can recur. Persistent and chronic disease can result in contractures and disability. In severe and refractory cases, referral to a pain specialist can be quite helpful.

Fibromyalgia

Fibromyalgia is quite common, particularly in older adolescent females, and occurs in about 3%–5% of adolescents. These patients have diffuse, longstanding chronic pain. Review of systems will usually reveal multiple complaints, including sleep disturbance, fatigue, mood disorders, generalized joint and muscle aching, back ache, abdominal pain and chronic headaches. Often, there is a lifelong history of vague chronic symptoms, sometimes starting with infantile colic. A positive family history of fibromyalgia or irritable bowel syndrome is also common. Physical examination will be completely normal, except for tender points across the back and anterior chest wall. The patient may occasionally have pain on joint examination, but should have no clinical signs of inflammation. Laboratory studies are normal, including serologic studies, acute phase reactants, radiographs, and routine blood tests. There is significant overlap of this condition with chronic fatigue syndrome, as well as with the mood and somatization disorders. School problems and other stresses are often present. Diagnostic criteria are listed in Table 12-7.

Management of these adolescents can be extremely challenging and at times, quite frustrating. The diagnosis of fibromyalgia is based on the typical history of chronic, stable diffuse pain persisting for at least 3 months, normal laboratory investigations, and the presence of specific tender points on physical examination. The focus is on pain control, patient education, normalization of sleep habits, stress reduction, and the use of nonnarcotic analgesics and physical therapy to control symptoms. An aerobic exercise program can be particularly effective. Fluoxetine, cognitive behavioral therapy, and aerobic exercise have been shown to

TABLE 12-7

DIAGNOSTIC CRITERIA FOR FIBROMYALGIA

A case must fulfill:
- All major criteria and four or more of the eight minor criteria

Major criteria:

1. Generalized aches or stiffness involving three or more anatomic sites for at least 3 months
2. At least six typical and reproducible tender points
3. Exclusion of any systemic condition that may cause similar symptoms

Minor criteria:

1. Generalized fatigue
2. Chronic headache
3. Sleep disturbance
4. Neuropsychiatric symptoms
5. Subjective joint swelling but no objective swelling
6. Numbness, tingling sensation
7. Irritable bowel syndrome
8. Modulation of symptoms by activity, weather, stress

Common bilateral tender points

1. Occiput, at the suboccipital muscle insertions
2. Low cervical, at the anterior aspects of the intertransverse spaces at C5-C7
3. Trapezius, at the midpoint of the upper border
4. Supraspinous, at origins, above the scapula spine near the medial border
5. Paraspinous, 3 cm lateral to the midline at the level of the mid scapula
6. Second costochondral junctions, maximum just lateral to the junctions on upper surfaces
7. Lateral pectoral, at the level of the fourth rib in the anterior axillary line
8. Lateral epicondyle, 2 cm to the epicondyles
9. Medial epicondyle, at the epicondyles
10. Gluteal, in upper outer quadrants of buttocks in anterior fold of muscle
11. Greater trochanter, posterior to the trochanteric prominence
12. Knees, at the medial fat pad proximal to the joint line

Source: From Komaroff AL, Goldenberg D. The chronic fatigue syndrome: Definition, current studies and lessons for fibromyalgia research. *J Rheumatol* 1989;16(Suppl 19):23.

Wolfe F. Fibromyalgia: The clinical syndrome. *Rheum Dis Clin North Am* 1989;15:1. with permission.

have significant effect in several separate controlled trials. Low-dose amitriptyline or nortriptyline given at night can improve sleep quality, as these agents have a mild sedative effect, without disturbing sleep rhythm. Management of concomitant mood disturbance (Chap. 36) is also quite important, as a third of patients will show clinical depression.

In the evaluation of these patients, an appropriate and limited workup is indicated, followed by a trial of conservative therapies. The parent, practitioner, and patient must come to an agreement as to what types of symptoms warrant further diagnostic evaluation and what therapies will be tried. Careful and consistent follow-up with a supportive health care provider can prevent a prolonged and unnecessary evaluation and has been shown to reduce the long term cost of treatment. Referral to a fibromyalgia support group, especially a group supervised by a health care provider, such as a social worker, can be tremendously helpful. In general, adolescents have a better prognosis than adults with fibromyalgia. In community based studies, most fibromyalgia patients will remain stable or improve over time. Predictive factors for a poorer outcome in fibromyalgia patients include lower socioeconomic status and the presence of a concomitant personality disorder.

Nonorganic Musculoskeletal Pain

Unexplained musculoskeletal pain is extremely common, and increases markedly with increasing age. Disorders include chronic fatigue syndrome, myofascial pain, fibromyalgia, nonspecific low back pain (discussed below), psychogenic rheumatism, and less commonly, conversion and factitious disorders. These conditions have considerable overlap. Nonorganic musculoskeletal pain can be one of the more challenging conditions to evaluate, as patients often have severe pain, prolonged symptoms, and seek evaluation from multiple health care providers. Parents become upset when no organic etiology can be determined as the cause of their youngster's pain. The term *psychogenic* is probably best avoided, as it can be perceived as pejorative, although it is important to discuss the role of psychological factors in pain expression when planning the diagnostic and therapeutic evaluation. Red flags for an organic cause include age under 10 years, the presence of systemic symptoms (fever and weight loss), inflammatory or nocturnal pain, neurologic signs or symptoms, and constant pain; the presence of any of these features requires further evaluation.

Malingering and/or factitious causes are not common in children, and can usually be ascertained by careful investigation. Symptom extension is quite common. In this entity the adolescent has persistent symptoms weeks after resolution of acute infection, when all the laboratory studies have normalized. Nonorganic musculoskeletal pain should be considered in the older child presenting with extended school absence, psychosocial stresses, bizarre, diffuse and/or vague symptoms with a normal laboratory and physical examination. Often the patient's reported disability and dysfunction is out of proportion to the physical examination. For these individuals, a limited diagnostic evaluation, careful observation and symptom control may be indicated as the first line of management. A trial of physical therapy, analgesics and/or NSAIDs is recommended and the adolescent should be scheduled for a reexamination in 4–8 weeks. The adolescent can be advised to keep a diary of symptoms, reassured in a sympathetic tone and transitioned back into school and to normal physical activity.

Chronic Back Pain

Back pain is a common symptom in adolescents, and its prevalence increases markedly with increasing age (Chap. 11). The incidence and prevalence in older adolescents is similar to adults. In adults, at any one time, 20%–40% will have experienced back pain (defined as any back pain lasting more than 24 hours) in the past month and adults have a lifetime 70%–90% probability of experiencing back pain. Over half of adolescents have experienced episodes of back pain, and 8%–30% have reported the presence of chronic back pain and pain usually in the lower lumbar area. Most of these adolescents will not seek medical evaluation. Of those

seeking evaluation, a specific cause will be found in only about half. A specific etiology is more often found in younger children, particularly in youngsters under age 10.

Adolescents presenting with nonorganic back pain have a higher incidence of psychosocial problems, disability claims, and pending litigation; similar findings have been seen in studies in adults with chronic back pain. In general, functional back pain is more common in patients with lower socioeconomic status, high stress, and in those patients with a higher incidence of self-reported physical or sexual abuse. Like other types of nonorganic musculoskeletal pain, nonorganic back pain can be one of the more challenging conditions to evaluate, as patients can have severe pain, prolonged symptoms, and seek evaluation from multiple health care providers.

All adolescents with back pain should have a careful history and physical examination, including family and social history. Red flags for an organic cause include age under 10 years, the presence of systemic symptoms such as fever and weight loss, pain interfering with sleep, inflammatory pain (worse in the morning with relief at the end of the day), neurologic signs or symptoms, involvement of the upper back, asymmetric back pain, and constant pain. Malingering and/or factitious causes are not common in children, and can usually be ascertained by careful investigation.

Treatment of chronic back pain should begin with patient education, an appropriate exercise regimen, control of pain, and stress reduction. Referral to physical therapy and various physical therapy modalities can be helpful as well.

PREOPERATIVE MEDICAL AND ANESTHETIC EVALUATION

Careful preoperative medical and anesthetic evaluation is necessary in all children (Table 12-8). Adolescents on systemic corticosteroid therapy need intravenous stress corticosteroid coverage and are at greater risk of infection. Involvement of the cervical spine, TMJs, and cricoarytenoid joints can make airway management difficult. C-spine stability

TABLE 12-8

PREOPERATIVE ASSESSMENT OF CHILDREN WITH RHEUMATIC DISEASES

All cases:
Anesthetic history, prior anesthetic difficulties
Careful attention to C-spine and jaw examination
Medication history
CBC

If indicated:
Cervical spine x-rays—any child with neck symptoms
   or limitation of motion (especially patients with
   polyarthritis)
Corticosteroid stress coverage for children on corticosteroids longer than 1 month in the past 6 months
Hold aspirin, consider holding other NSAIDs
   for 5–7 days
Hold methotrexate and other immune-suppressants
   for 1 week

should be assessed in any child or teen with C-spine arthritis. To evaluate adolescents for cervical spine disease or for preoperative assessment of the neck, the patient should have routine anteroposterior, open mouth, lateral, and extension-flexion radiographs of the cervical spine. Some rheumatologists advocate holding NSAIDs and methotrexate medication in the immediate perioperative period to reduce the risk of NSAID-induced bleeding and the potential inhibition of fibroblast function (and wound healing) from methotrexate. Any patient on chronic salicylates should stop these medications several days before the anticipated surgery.

Medications and other health problems should be reviewed, and consultations obtained with anesthesia, nursing, surgery, and other health care providers as indicated. Steps should be taken to reduce the patient's fear and anxiety. Anesthesia can be particularly challenging for the patient with severe JIA and polyarthritis. These individuals often have limited mouth opening, small mandibles, limited cervical spine extension and osteoporotic bone which lead to increased risks from anesthesia and endotracheal intubation. A careful preoperative examination of the neck should be performed on all those with JIA. Any

patient with neck pain or limited cervical spine movement should have cervical spine films (extension and flexion) obtained to look for subluxation or other abnormalities. Consideration should be given to fiberoptic intubation and consultation with the anesthesiologist to determine the most appropriate choices of anesthesia.

Children or adolescents on chronic corticosteroid medications (>10 mg daily for >30 days) should receive intravenous stress coverage during the surgery and until the patient is able to resume his/her usual oral steroid dose. Antibiotic prophylaxis for endocarditis is not necessary, unless the patient also has a heart defect (Chap. 9). Any NSAID medications may be stopped a few days before the surgery, and then restarted a few days later, due to the small risk of an effect on platelet function. Some rheumatologists recommend holding methotrexate or other immune suppressants the week of the surgery, because of the small potential for a delay in wound healing or increased risk of infection, though there are no firm data to confirm these risks. Omitting most rheumatic medications for a few days will have no long-term consequences on the underlying disease.

Suggested Readings

Bachrach LK. Bare-bones fact—children are not small adults. *N Engl J Med* 2004;351:924–926.

Brooks P. Use and Benefits of nonsteroidal anti-inflammatory drugs. *Am J Med* 1998;104:9S–13S.

Brik R, Keidar Z, Schapira D, Israel O. Bone mineral density and turnover in children with systemic juvenile chronic arthritis. *J Rheumatol* 1998;25:990–992.

Cabral DA, Malleson PN, Petty RE. Spondyloarthropathies of childhood. *Pediatr Clin North Am* 1995;42:1051–1070.

Cassidy JT, Petty RE. *Textbook of Pediatric Rheumatology.* 4th ed. Philadelphia, PA: W.B. Saunders, 2001.

Flatø B, Aasland A, Vinje O, Førre Ø. Outcome and predictive factors in juvenile rheumatoid arthritis and juvenile spondyloarthropathy. *J Rheumatol* 1998;25:366–375.

Gare RA. Epidemiology. *Baillieres Clin Rheumatol* 1998;12:191–208.

Gillette RD. A practical approach to the patient with back pain. *Am Fam Physician* 1996;53:670–678.

Gladman DD. Psoriatic arthritis. *Rheum Dis Clin North Am* 1998; 24:829–844.

Gran JT, Skomsvoll JF. The outcome of ankylosing spondylitis: A study of 100 patients. *Br J Rheumatol* 1997;36:766–771.

Greydanus DE: Rheumatoid disorders and other miscellaneous disorders. In: Hofmann AD, Greydanus DE, eds. *Adolescent Medicine.* 3d ed. Stamford, CT: Appleton & Lange, 1997; Chap. 20, pp. 432–453.

Grom AA, Passo M. Macrophage activation syndrome in systemic juvenile rheumatoid arthritis. *J Pediatr* 1996;129:630.

Hafner R, Truckenbrodt H, Spamer M. Rehabilitation in children with juvenile chronic arthritis. *Baillieres Clin Rheumatol* 1998;12:329–361.

Haldeman S. Diagnostic tests for the evaluation of back and neck pain. *Neurol Clin* 1996;14:103–117.

Hollinsworth P. Back pain in children. *Br J Rheumatol* 1996;35:1022–1028.

Ilowite NT. Current treatment of juvenile rheumatoid arthritis. *Pediatrics* 2002;109(1):109–115.

Isenberg DA, Miller JJ. *Adolescent Rheumatology.* London, UK: Martin Dunitz, 1999.

Jennette JC, Falk RJ. Small vessel vasculitis. *N Engl J Med* 1997;337:1512–1523.

Leboeuf-Yde C, Kyvik KO. At what age does low back pain become a common problem? *Spine* 1998;23: 228–234.

Miller M, ed. Pediatric Rheumatology. *Rheum Dis Clin North Am* 2002;3:1–10.

Moore MD. Rheumatic Diseases. In: Weinstein SL, ed. *The Pediatric Spine: Principles and Practice.* New York: Raven Press, 2000.

O'Dell JR: Therapeutic strategies for rheumatoid arthritis. *N Engl J Med* 2004;350:2591–2602.

Olivieri I, Barozzi L, Padula A. Enthesopathy: clinical manifestations, imaging and treatment. *Baillieres Clin Rheumatol* 1998;12:665–678.

Olsen NJ, Stein CM: New drugs for rheumatoid arthritis. *N Engl J Med* 2004;350:2167–2179.

Petty RE. Classification of childhood arthritis: a work in progress. *Baillieres Clin Rheumatol* 1998;12: 181–190.

Klippel JH, Crofford L, eds. *Primer on the Rheumatic Diseases.* 12th ed. Atlanta, GA: Arthritis Foundation, 2001.

Reveille JD. HLA-B27 and the seronegative spondyloarthropathies. *Amer J Med Sci* 1998;316:239–249.

Schaller JG. Juvenile rheumatoid arthritis. *Pediatr Rev* 1997;18:337–349.

Siegel DM, Janeway D, Baum J. Fibromyalgia syndrome in children and adolescents: clinical features at presentation and status at follow-up. *Pediatrics* 1998;101: 377–382.

Su CG. Extraintestinal manifestations of inflammatory bowel disease. *Gastroenterol Clin North Am.* 2002; 31(1):307–327.

Szer IS. Chronic arthritis in children. *Compr Ther* 1997; 23:124–129.

Urwin M, Symmons D, Allison T, Brammah T, Busby H, Roxby M, Simmons A, Williams G. Estimating the burden of musculoskeletal disorders in the community; the comparative prevalence of symptoms at different anatomical sites, and the relation to social deprivations. *Ann Rheum Dis* 1998;57:649–655.

Van der Linden S, Van der Heijde D. Ankylosing spondylitis—clinical features. *Rheum Dis Clin North Am* 1998; 24:663–676.

Wallace DJ. Lupus for the non-rheumatologist. *Bull Rheum Dis* 1999;48 (9):1–4.

APPENDIX: RESOURCES FOR FURTHER INFORMATION WEB SITES

www.arthritis.org—Arthritis Foundation—Also includes the American Juvenile Arthritis Organization. The Arthritis Foundation provides numerous excellent patient education materials. Local chapters coordinate summer camps and support groups for children with arthritis.

www.lupus.org—Lupus Foundation of America (LFA). A voluntary organization devoted to lupus, provides information to patients and research support for lupus.

www.niams.nih.gov—National Institute of Arthritis and Musculoskeletal and Skin Diseases. Has links to several related sites. Provides information to both patients and health professionals. A resource to locate ongoing investigational trials.

www.rheumatology.org—American College of Rheumatology—the professional organization of rheumatologists. The Web site provides materials and guidelines for health professionals.

13

NEUROLOGIC DISORDERS

Donald E. Greydanus and David H. Van Dyke

INTRODUCTION

Neurologic disorders are a common concern in the adolescent age group. Conditions reviewed in this chapter are seizure disorders, headaches, papilledema, vertigo and dizziness, Guillain-Barré syndrome, Bell's palsy, tic disorders, and cerebral palsy.

Suggested Readings

Behrman RE, Kliegman RM, Jenson HB, eds: The nervous system. In *Nelson Textbook of Pediatrics*. 17th ed. Philadelphia, PA: W.B. Saunders, 2004, Chap. 26, pp. 2048–2049.

Bradley WG, Daroff RB, Fenichel GM, Marsden CD, eds: *Neurology in Clinical Practice: Principles of Diagnosis and Management*, 3d ed. Available at: www.nicp.com

Greydanus DE: Neurologic disorders. In: Hofmann AD, Greydanus DE, eds: *Adolescent Medicine.* Stamford, CT: Appleton & Lange, 1997, Chap. 14, pp. 242–288.

Greydanus DE, Pratt HD, Van Dyke HD: Neurologic and neurodevelopmental dilemmas in the adolescent. *Adolesc Med* 13:413–686, 2002.

Swaiman KF, Ashwal S, eds.: Pediatric neurology: principles and practice. In: *The Epilepsy Foundation,* St Louis, MO: Mosby, 1999. Available at: www.epilepsyfoundation.org

SEIZURE DISORDERS

General: Epidemiology

A seizure is a discrete event with diverse manifestations; epilepsy (seizure disorder) defines a condition with recurring seizures. The annual incidence of a seizure disorder among 10–14 and 15–19-year-old adolescents is noted as 24.7 and 18.6 per 100,000, respectively. It affects 1% of the population and nearly one in four individuals with epilepsy are under the age of 18. The Mayo Clinic study from 1935 to 1967 recorded an incidence of newly diagnosed epilepsy as 36–48 per 100,000 per year in the 10–19 age group. (Hauser, 1975). Published prevalence rates range from 3 to 5 per 1000 adolescents. The disorder is therefore relatively common during the teenage years, either as a carryover from childhood or a new onset.

General: Etiology

A wide variety of underlying diseases may precipitate a seizure response (Table 13-1), but most cases are idiopathic, particularly in adolescents under 16 years. The probability of a causative space-occupying lesion increases with advancing age. Though idiopathic seizures gradually diminish in frequency, they still are commonly seen throughout the teenage years. Additional differential considerations

TABLE 13-1

EVALUATION OF SEIZURES IN ADOLESCENTS

Differential Diagnosis	Possible Precipitating Factors Idiopathic Seizures	Laboratory Evaluation*
Infectious: bacterial viral meningitis, encephalitis; systemic infection with fever, sepsis	1. Puberty[†]	1. CBC
	2. Menses	2. Urinalysis
	3. Trauma	3. Electrolytes
Congenital defects:	4. Fever	4. Glucose (fasting
AV malformations, porencephaly	5. Drugs (alcohol, phenothiazines,	& tolerance)
Trauma neoplasms: CNS primary, metastatic	tricyclic antidepressants, antihistamines, others)	5. BUN, creatinine
		6. Toxic drug screen:
Neurocutaneous syndromes:	6. Psychologic stress	urine, serum, gastric
Sturge-Weber, tuberous sclerosis, neurofibromatosis	7. Sleep/sleep deprivation	7. Lumbar puncture[‡]
	8. Hyperventilation	8. EEG
Metabolic: hypoglycemia,	(with absence types)	9. CT or MRI
hypoparathyroidism,	9. Photic stimuli (flashing or	10. Video EEG
hypocalcemia, hyponatremia,	flickering light, television)	11. Others: blood culture,
hypernatremia, hypomagnesemia,	10. Olfactory or tactile stimuli	liver function testes,
hypophosphatemia, inborn	11. Ingestion of certain foods	blood gases, serum
errors of metabolism	12. Reading	anticonvulsant level,
Vasculitis cerebrovascular accident:	13. Music	Wood's Lamp exam
ruptured aneurysm (congenital, mycotic), AV malformation, thrombocytopenia	14. Laughter	
Drug related: withdrawal from anticonvulsant drugs, withdrawal from CNS depressant addiction (including alcohol, cocaine), insulin overdose, phencyclidine overdose. Many drugs are reported (eg, antidepressants, antihistamines, various antibiotics, and sympathomimetics).		
Hypertensive encephalopathy: primary, renal, coarctation		
Others: collagen vascular diseases (SLE), porphyrias, liver disease, renal failure, Gaucher's disease, juvenile Huntington's disease, mitochondrial encephalomyopathy, shuddering attacks, pseudoseizures, syncope		

*Perform those tests indicated by clinical judgment and clinical signs.

[†]The role of puberty in precipitating seizures remains controversial.

[‡]Perform lumbar puncture only with great caution if cerebral bleed or increased pressure from other cause suspected. CT may be safer as first procedure. Never delay antibiotics for a lumbar puncture.

include conditions that may mimic a seizure disorder, such as hysteria (pseudoseizure), hyperventilation, vertigo, vasomotor syncope, migraine headaches, narcolepsy, night terrors, nightmares, chorea, Gilles de la Tourette syndrome, tardive dyskinesia, oculogyric crisis, or dystonia following phenothiazine ingestion. Evaluation of adolescents who present with new seizures can reveal an etiology due to head trauma, pseudoseizures, central nervous system infections, drug abuse, cancer or cancer treatment effects, cerebrovascular accidents, and idiopathic factors. Some seizures can occur as a complication of syncope, drug abuse or withdrawal, sleep deprivation, and other factors. Consider syncope if fainting and decrease in vision developed before unconsciousness and the face appeared pale, due to reduced blood pressure. Some primary generalized epilepsies present in adolescence, such as juvenile myoclonic epilepsy and juvenile absence epilepsy.

General Evaluation

Historical, physical, and laboratory evaluations are directed toward distinguishing between differential concerns (including partial vs. generalized seizures and epileptic syndromes) and detecting possible precipitating factors (Table 13-1). Particular historical points of note are prenatal and perinatal events, development, family history, and past or present injuries. It should be kept in mind that trivial head trauma is common in the life of children and the significance must be judiciously weighed. A careful description of the seizure itself and associated events will assist in classification and provide insight into precipitating factors. It is important to carefully evaluate the description of the aura, onset and duration of the seizure, as well as type of eye or limb movements, degree of consciousness (reactions to voice or pain), and presence/absence of incontinence. Classification of the seizure type requires identification of the ictal period as partial or generalized. Seizure classification is still mainly accomplished through a careful history. A careful assessment of medical and psychologic factors is necessary to identify pseudoseizures.

General Physical Examination

A careful physical examination is important and includes blood pressure evaluation (lying and standing for consideration of orthostatic hypotension), a thorough neurologic assessment, and auscultation for bruits (skull, orbits, and neck). Dermatologic clues can be important for identification of neurocutaneous syndromes. Body and extremity asymmetry may suggest chronic neurologic abnormality.

Laboratory Studies: EEG

The 16-channel electroencephalogram (EEG) should be performed while the patient is awake and, if possible, asleep or sleep deprived as well as during photic and hyperventilatory stimuli. The EEG, however, is only adjunctive or confirmatory to the diagnosis and may not be abnormal in every case. For example, complex partial seizures often have a normal EEG. In some situations, the EEG may become normalized as the child enters puberty. The patient should be treated, and not the EEG. Characteristic EEGs are especially noted with absence, Lennox-Gastaut, and infantile spasms.

Laboratory Studies: Other

Imaging techniques of value include ultrasound, computed tomography (CT), and magnetic resonance imaging (MRI). The MRI is better than CT for evaluation of the posterior fossa, temporal lobe, brain stem, and spinal cord. MRI is currently the imaging procedure of choice for evaluating youth with seizures of probable focal onset. Brain mapping remains experimental, technically challenging, and of little proven value. Positron-emission tomography (PET)–glucose metabolism with EEG correlation and single-photon-emission computed tomography (SPECT)–blood flow are also experimental studies.

Trauma and Seizures

An impact seizure is one that develops within seconds of head trauma and it alone does not increase the risk of overt epilepsy; thus use of anticonvulsant medication is not usually necessary. Early posttraumatic epilepsy (PTE) is noted within 7 days of the head trauma and may result from acute damage to the central nervous system. Later PTE develops over 7 days after the head injury. Risk factors for PTE include a depressed skull fracture, cerebral edema, subdural hematoma, focal signs, development of greater than 24 hours of post-trauma amnesia, and others. Post-traumic seizures are acutely controlled with intravenous phenytoin (10–20 mg/kg, given slowly). Approximately 25% of those who develop seizures during the first week after head trauma and 75% after the first week will continue with seizures and require ongoing anticonvulsant medication. Neuropsychologic testing is recommended for youth who develop posttraumatic brain injury.

Classification of Seizure Disorders

Classification of seizures has often been confusing, and periodic changes in terminology have added to this confusion. Current classification by the World Health Organization and International League Against Epilepsy (ILAE) use four basic seizure categories: primary generalized epilepsies, partial epilepsies, secondary generalized epilepsies, and unclassified epilepsies (Table 13-2). The international classification of seizures refers to episodes of bilateral onset (generalized) and local onset (partial types): simple (no loss of consciousness), complex (loss of consciousness), and secondarily generalized. Epilepsies have also been referred to as generalized (primary vs. secondary) and localized (primary vs. secondary). The terms generalized and idiopathic are now used interchangeably by many clinicians, as are the terms aura and simple partial seizure. Seizure classification systems also include situations that develop epileptic patterns secondary to specific events, such as change in body temperature, withdrawal of certain drugs, stress, changes in hormonal levels, and others. (See Committee, Epilepsia,1989.)

Absence, pure tonic-clonic, absence with tonic-clonic, clonic-tonic, juvenile myoclonic, complex-partial (mainly temporal-lobe epilepsy), and rolandic seizures are the most common seizure patterns in adolescents. The majority of patients experience only one pattern, though mixed patterns of two or more types (e.g., absence with tonic-clonic)

TABLE 13-2

CLASSIFICATION OF SEIZURE TYPES

Partial seizures	Simple partial
	Complex partial
	Progresses to unconsciousness
	Starts with unconsciousness
	Partial seizures secondarily
	generalized
	Simple partial develops
	into a generalized seizure
	Complex partial develops
	into a generalized seizure
	Simple partial develops
	into a complex partial,
	which develops into a
	generalized seizure
Generalized	Absence seizure
seizures	Atypical absence seizure
	Myoclonic seizure vs.
	myoclonic jerks
	Clonic seizure
	Tonic seizure
	Tonic-clonic seizure
	Atonic (astatic) seizure
Unclassified seizure	
disorders	
Others	

Source: Commission on Classification and Terminology of the International League Against Epilepsy: Proposal for revised classification of epilepsies and epileptic syndromes. *Epilepsia* 30:389–399, 1989. Reprinted by permission of the International League Against Epilepsy.

are common. The latter cases are more difficult to control.

These types generally have a good to excellent prognosis, and the majority are well controlled with proper use of antiseizure medications. The appropriate medication(s) is carefully titrated to each patient. The first line of anticonvulsants for partial seizures are carbamazepine and phenytoin, while second line medications include phenobarbital, valproate, gabapentin, and lamotrigine. Third line drugs include felbamate, benzodiazepines, and primidone. First line of anticonvulsants for generalized seizures include valproate and phenytoin, while the second line is the benzodiazepines. The third line of anticonvulsants include PHT, phenobarbital, lamotrigine, and acetazolamide.

The classification given can be used for seizures in older children and adolescents. Newer and more comprehensive classifications are helpful as they emphasize the importance of detailed seizure descriptions (see Engel, 2001).

Simple Partial Seizures (Focal Epilepsies)

General

Partial seizures include simple partial, complex partial, and partial seizures that become secondarily generalized seizures. Partial seizures include only part of the cerebral cortex, at least initially. Simple partial seizures usually consist of a brief period of tonic and clonic movements beginning in a single body part and extending progressively to other muscle groups on the ipsilateral side. Variations are noted with motor signs, sensory symptoms, autonomic symptomatology (sweating, flushing, pupillary dilatation, piloerection, pallor), hallucinatory symptoms (lights flashing, tingling, déjà vu), and mixed or compound forms.

A simple partial seizure can be confused with a migraine headache prodrome. Also, consciousness is not impaired in a simple partial seizure, though speech dysfunction or sensory symptomatology may occur. If consciousness is impaired, the seizure is classified as a complex partial seizure. Seizures that start locally suggest a structural etiology while seizures with a generalized onset suggest a more general etiology. If psychologic or psychic symptoms develop, it usually is classified as a complex partial seizure. Previous trauma or CNS infection with residual scarring is often causally implicated; tumor, focal bleeding, or one of the neurodermatoses also must be considered in the differential diagnosis. Treatment is usually with phenytoin or carbamazepine with phenobarbital as an alternative.

Rolandic Epilepsy

A special form of simple partial epilepsy seen in children and youth is rolandic epilepsy, also called benign epilepsy with rolandic spikes (BERS) or benign childhood epilepsy with centrotemporal spikes. It usually begins between ages 5 and 9, often disappearing between ages 14 and 20. One fourth of children with epilepsy may have BERS, in which the seizure comes from the rolandic or central sulcus. It is an autosomal dominant disorder, usually easily controlled with a single anticonvulsant drug. It may begin with a single tonic-clonic episode with focal onset, often at night. It may involve involuntary muscle contraction of one side of the face, arm, leg, or pharynx. Speech dysfunction can occur during the seizure. The EEG is characteristic, with rolandic (central) spikes. It is a self-limiting disorder. Antiseizure medications are not usually needed for brief, infrequent seizures. Teenagers who are treated with medications are usually very well controlled with either phenytoin or carbamazepine. Phenobarbital and primidone are also effective. Studies are currently underway evaluating the effectiveness of gabapentin and oxcarbazepine in BERS.

Complex Partial Seizure

General

Impairment of consciousness with a simple partial seizure reclassifies the pattern as a complex partial seizure. The temporal or frontal lobes are usually involved. Consequent to a temporal lobe focus, seizure pattern manifestations vary. An increased frequency of anovulatory menstrual cycles, decreased levels of unbound testosterone with hyposexuality in males, and low fertility rates are all described in patients with complex partial seizure disorders.

Temporal Lobe Seizure

In the temporal lobe seizure pattern (previously called psychomotor epilepsy) four stages are commonly seen: prodrome, aura, ictus, and postictal state. The prodrome is marked by irritability, confusion, headache, appetite changes, and pallor; it can develop from hours to days before the aura. The aura itself is manifested in a few minutes of sensory disturbances (taste, smell, and vision), psychologic aberrations (fear, rage, anxiety, depression, inappropriate laughter, mental confusion, and hallucinations), abdominal discomfort, and lacrimation, among other symptoms. A sense of familiarity can develop (déjà vu if visual, *déjà entendu* if auditory) and a sudden sense of unfamiliarity can also occur–*jamais vu*. The development of amnesia or early impairment of consciousness may interfere with the adolescent's aura awareness.

Ictus quickly follows, with both motor and psychic components. Motor phenomena vary from simple staring (ictal staring) to repetitive purposeless movements or complex automatisms (aimless walking, lip smacking, picking at clothes, picking at other objects, and pulling at body parts), as well as aphasia, numbness, a choking sensation, headache, and gastrointestinal disturbances. Psychic components are similar to those experienced during the aura. The seizure (ictus) phase lasts from one to several minutes or longer and gradually abates, giving way to the postictal state, with lethargy, confusion, hunger, and headache being the most common symptoms. Amnesia is often but not invariably present. There may be many episodes each day, or attacks may only occur at widely spaced intervals.

Diagnosis

Diagnosis can be difficult and requires a high index of suspicion, particularly in adolescents having bizarre or disturbed behavior. Misdiagnosis in ascribing a psychiatric cause is common. An EEG with an additional nasopharyngeal lead may demonstrate a temporal lobe focus, though this is not always the case as the tracing can be normal during the seizure-free state. Sphenoidal electrode tracings and intracranial (invasive) recordings may be helpful. Neuropsychologic abnormalities can be seen while MRI may note hippocampal defects. Monitoring with simultaneous EEG and video can be very helpful and avoid invasive monitoring.

Management

Response to antiseizure medication (phenytoin, valproate carbamazepine, phenobarbital, or primidone) is diagnostic as well as therapeutic. Currently, carbamazepine is considered by many clinicians to be the first drug of choice. The addition of clorazepate, valproate, or acetazolamide may be beneficial. Carbamazepine and valproic acid (valproate) are used for psychiatric disorders with aggression outbursts. Other types of complex partial seizures are described, for example, temporal lobe syncope (impaired consciousness, drop attack, and automatism), frontal lobe epilepsy, occipital lobe epilepsy, and somatosensory epilepsy (parietal lobe epilepsy). Phenytoin and carbamazepine are the drugs of choice for frontal lobe and parietal lobe epilepsies. Newer agents are very useful and include topiramate and oxcarbazepine.

Generalized Seizure Disorders

General

The primary generalized seizure disorder is one of the most common types seen in teenagers and is noted in 6% of first degree relatives (vs. 1% of controls). Various types are noted. There can be the clonic seizure, the tonic seizure, or the generalized tonic-clonic seizure GTC). It begins with a brief aura (flashing lights, peculiar taste, buzzing or ringing ears, feelings of depression, or premonitory anxiety) and rapidly progresses into generalized bilateral tonic (stiffening), clonic, or tonic-clonic movements, jerky respirations, tongue biting, and incontinence (fecal, urinary), with complete or partial loss of consciousness. The convulsions usually abate within 5 minutes or less and are followed by postictal somnolence lasting from a few minutes to several hours. Amnesia for the event is common. Some develop seizures during morning waking or evening relaxation. A variation is the atonic or astatic seizure with loss of muscle tone, ranging from loss of facial tone to drop attacks. The frequency of generalized seizures varies from several times a day to once or twice a year. Progression to status epilepticus is an infrequent complication. EEG abnormalities are usually present, but their nature varies. Treatment employs valproate as the initial drug of choice with carbamazepine, phenytoin, and phenobarbital as alternatives. Recent research suggests that carbamazepine is as effective as valproate and has fewer long-term side effects.

Absence Seizures

General

The typical absence seizures (petit mal epilepsies) are also classified as primary generalized seizure disorders. The typical absence seizure disorder often develops between the ages of 4 and 8 years and disappears by mid-adolescence. In 30% there is development into a generalized type of epilepsy, during adolescence or adulthood. A typical attack consists of a brief moment (15–30 seconds or less) of staring or lapse of consciousness without any prodrome, aura, or postictal state. Clonic movements or automatism is uncommon but may be seen on occasion. The brief disruption in consciousness noted in the absence seizure can be similar to that noted with a complex partial seizure. As the child matures, there may not be a full consciousness loss, as noted when he or she was younger. Typical absence seizures tend to occur with greater frequency than other types, sometimes as often as 100 or more times a day. Hyperventilation is a frequent precipitant and can be used diagnostically if 3 minutes of hyperventilation induces an absence seizure. Daydreams in some may be a subclinical manifestation of seizure activity. There is typically no postictal state. The EEG characteristically demonstrates a 3-per-second (range 2.5–4) spike and wave pattern and is a diagnostic finding. Treatment includes valproic acid or ethosuximide with clonazepam as an alternative. The prognosis is generally good, though some patients will develop other forms of generalized epilepsy in association with mild clonic elements, atonia, tonic elements, automatisms, and even autonomic components. Complex seizures may be very resistant to antiseizure medications.

Juvenile absence epilepsy is a form of absence seizure disorder that can develop around puberty. A generalized tonic-clonic or GTC form of epilepsy can be seen before or after the onset of the juvenile absence epilepsy. There is usually a greater than 3-per-second pattern on the EEG. A typical absence epilepsy can also be seen, with more pronounced tonal changes and/or less abrupt onset or cessation of symptoms.

Myoclonic Seizures

This seizure pattern can affect the entire person or produce isolated limb jerks. Myoclonic seizures are complex phenomena with various etiologies. Neuronal ceroid lipofuscinosis is a rare form of myoclonic seizure disorder with visual and cognitive deterioration requiring a skin biopsy and ERG (electroretinogram) to establish the diagnosis. Gaucher's disease can have hepatosplenomegaly and worsening intellectual functioning along with myoclonic seizure patterns. A bone marrow is diagnostic. A benign form of myoclonic seizure is the juvenile form (see next section).

Others: Generalized epileptic patterns can be seen secondary to trauma (see trauma section), anoxia, infection (as meningoencephalitis), congenital anomalies, neurocutaneous syndromes, and unknown factors (cryptogenic forms).

EPILEPTIC SYNDROMES

See Table 13-3.

Juvenile Myoclonic Seizure (Juvenile Myoclonic Seizure of Janz)

Juvenile myoclonic seizures, also called benign myoclonic seizure in late childhood and adolescence (ages 12–18) or impulsive petit mal of Janz, is a type of primary generalized seizure. It represents about 12% of all childhood epilepsy and has been mapped to the short arm of chromosome 6. It usually begins with myoclonic jerks of flexor muscles

TABLE 13-3

EPILEPSY SYNDROMES

Rolandic epilepsy (benign child epilepsy with centro-temporal spikes)
Juvenile myoclonic epilepsy of Janz
Juvenile absence epilepsy
Lennox-Gastaut syndrome
Epilepsy with GTC seizures on awakening
Others

in the neck and shoulder, along with clonic-tonic-clonic seizures–often soon after awakening. GTC seizures can develop 2 years after the myoclonus develops and both seizure patterns are worsened with drug/alcohol use, stress, and sleep deprivation. Some patients develop absence episodes also. Characteristic EEG patterns are described (4–6 Hz or multispike and wave pattern) and an excellent response to valproate is typical. Clonazepam can be used as an alternative. Other antiseizure medications can worsen the absence and myoclonus aspects of this syndrome. The vast majority will resume seizures within 5 years of drug cessation. As many as three agents may ultimately be required.

Rolandic Epilepsy

See Simple Partial Seizure section.

Juvenile Absence Epilepsy

See Absence section.

Lennox-Gastaut Syndrome

These mentally retarded youth have an epileptic encephalopathy and present with various seizure patterns called minor motor types. Various forms are seen, including akinetic, myoclonic, atypical absence, tonic, and others. Status epilepticus can develop, as well as drop attacks while awake and tonic seizures while asleep. The mental retardation is usually progressive. The EEG is described as a slow spike-wave pattern. Diverse etiologies are proposed and control of these seizures is often very difficult. Valproate has been used to control much of the seizure activity, along with phenytoin for control of sleep-induced tonic patterns. Clonazepam (Klonopin), a benzodiazepine, has also been used with some success. Felbamate (a dicarbamate) may be a better anticonvulsant for control of seizures in the Lennox-Gastaut syndrome; however, it has some significant potential side effects, including aplastic anemia and liver failure. Lamotrigine has shown some promise in the control of seizures in this syndrome without these side effects.

Special Considerations in Medication Treatment

Table 13-4 provides data relevant to the use of the more commonly employed anticonvulsant drugs. All have significant side effects requiring periodic monitoring and careful titration up to therapeutic doses. The precise dosage and combination of drugs required for control is a highly individualized matter. In addition, an increased dosage may be needed at certain times, such as during menstruation or infections. Monotherapy is attempted and it should be noted that plasma drug concentrations are suggestive of but not definitive for optimal drug dosages. Always treat the patient and not the plasma drug level.

When it is evident that more than one agent is required for control, a new drug should not be started until full therapeutic dosages of preceding ones have been achieved and the patient stabilized. A new drug also should be introduced gradually with careful titration and attention to drug interactions (Table 13-4), whereas old drugs deemed ineffective should be tapered rather than abruptly discontinued. Up to three agents ultimately may be required for the maximal possible control, which may take months or even years to achieve.

Historically, common practice was to initiate medication after a single seizure. Presently, this has been a matter of some debate. There is an increasing opinion to wait for the second or even third seizure. An isolated tonic-clonic seizure episode can be noted in an individual with a subsequent normal evaluation and no further seizure activity. Factors increasing the risk of recurrence include an abnormal EEG(s), abnormal neurologic examination, and a local or focal onset to the seizure. Epileptic activity secondary to syncope (as vasovagal reactions, orthostatic hypotension, hypoglycemia, anemia, or arrhythmias) do not usually require antiseizure medications, but attention to the cause of the syncope may be necessary. Such seizure activity can include violent myoclonic jerks, clonic movements and/or eye rolling with head extension, nuchal rigidity, and flexion of elbows with clenched fists.

TABLE 13-4

ANTICONVULSANT MEDICATIONS

Drug, Indication,* and Dose	Therapeutic Serum Levels and Drug Interactions	Side Effects and Comments
Phenobarbital G, T, SP: 2–5 mg/kg/day 150–250 mg/day SP: 100–250 mg/day	15–40 mcg/mL Increased by phenytoin, primidone, and valproic acid; decreases clonazepam effects; decreased plasma level of carbamazepine, propranolol, coumadin, others.	Drowsiness, lethargy (tend to improve with continued administration), stupor, coma (with levels over 60 mcg/mL), fever, nystagmus, and ataxia. Less commonly seen: osteomalacia with chronic use, hepatic dysfunction, leukopenia, lymphadenopathy, maculopapular or bullous rash, Stevens-Johnson syndrome. Behavioral and cognitive effects noted, as well as depression and teratogenicity.
Phenytoin (Dilantin) G, T, SP: 4–8 mg/kg/day 250–400 mg/day	10–20 mcg/mL Increased by valproic acid, cimetidine, chloramphenicol, isoniazid, others; decreased by phenobarbital, primidone, carbamazepine; decreased efficacy of oral contraceptives.	Gingival hyperplasia (can prevent with good oral hygiene), hypertrichosis, nystagmus (with levels over 25–30 µg/mL), ataxia, dysarthria, diplopia, choreoathetosis, lethargy, stupor, excitement, peripheral neuropathy, hepatic dysfunction, lymphadenopathy, hypocalcemia, osteomalacia, rickets, hyperglycemia, folic acid deficiency. Idiosyncratic reactions may occur (usually within first 1–4 weeks), including exfoliative dermatitis and other rashes, a lupuslike reaction, Stevens-Johnson syndrome. Overdose results in acute cerebellar symptoms, delirium, and coma. Can interfere with cognitive functions, contributing to academic dysfunction. Also, teratogenicity.
Ethosuximide (Zarontin) P: 15–40 mg/kg/day 750–1500 mg/day	40–100 mcg/mL Increased by valproate	Nausea, vomiting, lethargy, anorexia, hiccups, irritability, GI irritation, headaches, abdominal pain, skin rash, leukopenia, eosinophilia, ataxia, nystagmus, urticaria, bone marrow depression, lupuslike syndrome, dyskinesis, emotional reaction, including psychotic reactions.

(Continued)

TABLE 13-4

ANTICONVULSANT MEDICATIONS (*CONTINUED*)

Drug, Indication,* and Dose	Therapeutic Serum Levels and Drug Interactions	Side Effects and Comments
Carbamazepine (Tegretol) G, T SP: 10–25 mg/kg/day 400–1200 mg/day	4–12 mcg/mL Decreased by phenytoin, primidone, phenobarbital. Measure serum carbamazepine level and its active metabolite. Carbamazepine–10, 11 epoxide– also has toxic side effects	Fatigue, malaise, dizziness, anorexia, lethargy, nausea, vomiting, diplopia, nystagmus, ataxia, hepatic dysfunction, bone marrow depression, cardiac arrhythmias, inappropriate ADH secretion, leukopenia, skin rashes, eosinophilic myocarditis, Stevens-Johnson syndrome. Emotional liability and impaired task performance noted.
Primidone (Mysoline) G, T, SP: 10–20 mg/kg/day 500–1500 mg/day	5–12 mcg/mL Increased by carbamazepine	Lethargy, dizziness, vertigo, nausea, vomiting, ataxia, nystagmus, diplopia, megaloblastic anemia (folic acid deficiency), behavioral changes, bone marrow depression, edema, lupuslike syndrome. Tolerance develops if previously on phenobarbital. Often used as adjunct to phenytoin and carbamazepine.
Acetazolamide (Diamox) P, G: 8–30 mg/kg/day	10–14 mcg/mL	Sedation, teratogenicity, paresthesias, transient increased thirst, increased urination, hyperventilation.
Clonazepam (Klonopin) JM, A 0.03–0.3 mg/kg/day	20–80 mcg/mL Decreased by phenytoin and phenobarbital. Increased sedative effects with alcohol, antihistamines, psychotropic drugs, others.	Behavioral disturbances, ataxia, drooling, sedation
Clorazepate dipotassium (Tranxene) Complex partial, G 0.7–1.0 mg/kg/day	1–2 mcg/mL Increases sedative effects with alcohol, barbiturates, psychotropic drugs, others.	Sedation, ataxia, behavioral difficulties, drooling
Valproic acid or valproate (Depakene, Depakote) P, JM, G: 15–60 mg/kg/day 1000–3000 mg/day	40–150 µg/mL Increased by ethosuximide; decreased by carbamazepine; avoid with clonazepam; increases phenobarbital, diazepam effect, and phenytoin toxicity	Nausea, emesis, abdominal cramps, diarrhea, lethargy, transient alopecia, abnormal clotting, reduced platelets and platelet aggregation, pancreatitis, hepatic dysfunction, hair loss, encephalopathy, terato-genicity weight changes, increased

(Continued)

TABLE 13-4

ANTICONVULSANT MEDICATIONS (*CONTINUED*)

Drug, Indication,* and Dose	Therapeutic Serum Levels and Drug Interactions	Side Effects and Comments
		salivation, skin rashes, insomnia, headache. Take with meals to reduce GI side effects. Minimal cognitive impairment noted.
Felbamate (Felbatol) G, SP, P, JM 15–60 mg/kg/day 1200–3600 mg/day	Not established	Increasing aplastic anemia and acute hepatic failure reports have limited the use of this drug. Used alone or with other drugs for partial and secondarily generalized epilepsy and with other drugs for the complex epilepsy seen in the Lennox-Gastaut syndrome.
Gabapentin (Neurontin) G, SP, P 900–2400 mg/day	Not established	Usually well-tolerated. Side effects are often mild and transient: lethargy, ataxia, dizziness, and nystagmus. Does not induce or inhibit hepatic enzymes and does not interfere with other anticonvulsants. Used with other medications to control refractory partial and secondarily generalized epilepsy.
Lamotrigine (Lamictal) G, SP, P 100–500 mg/day	Not established	Used with other medications for complex partial and generalized epilepsy. Side effects include lethargy, headache, dizziness, blurred vision, rash, ataxia, diplopia, nausea and vomiting. Rash seen in 10% within 2 weeks of drug initiation and disappears when the drug is stopped. Stevens-Johnson syndrome noted in a few. Interference with valproate is seen.
Clonazepam (Clonopin) P, JM, Other minor motor seizures: 0.03–0.2 mg/kg/day 1.5–20 mg/day	13–72 ng/mL Decreased effect with phenobarbital and phenytoin; avoid with valproate	Lethargy, irritability, belligerence, aggression, hyperactivity, antisocial patterns, weight gain, ataxia, dysarthria. Tolerance can develop if given with valproic acid, as may be needed in petit mal. Behavioral disorders can occur.

(*Continued*)

TABLE 13-4

ANTICONVULSANT MEDICATIONS (*CONTINUED*)

Drug, Indication,* and Dose	Therapeutic Serum Levels and Drug Interactions	Side Effects and Comments
Topiramate (Topamax) G, T, SP, P, JM 1–3 mg/ kg/day, increasing weekly to 5–9 mg/kg/day at maximum	Not established	Reduce dose 50% with impaired renal function, cognitive slowing, behavioral change, word finding difficulty, may precipitate glaucoma
Oxcarbazepine (Trileptal) 8–10 mg/kg/day (maximum initial dose 600 mg/day). Increase 8–10 mg/kg/day as tolerated at 3–7 day intervals.	Carbamazepine—10, 11 epoxide levels can be measured	May produce dizziness, hyponatremia, double vision. Requires less hematologic evaluation than carbamazepine. Will occasionally give rash with carbamazepine sensitivity

*G, generalized seizures; T, temporal lobe seizures; SP, simple partial; P, petit mal seizure or absence seizure; JM, juvenile myoclonic seizures.

The decision to stop medication is equally debatable. An adolescent with idiopathic disease and only a single seizure or with a childhood onset who is wholly controlled by medication is probably a candidate for discontinuance after treatment for 2–4 years. Gradual tapering of the medication over 3–18 months is important to prevent recurrences. On the other hand, epilepsy with an adolescent onset and requiring 3 years or longer to control or seizures stemming from an identifiable organic disorder tend to persist and often return when medication is stopped. Under these circumstances, treatment for life is usually indicated. Most patients with generalized tonic-clonic and juvenile myoclonic epilepsy resume seizures within 5 years of medication cessation. The majority of those with pure absence seizures, unless complicated by tonic-clonic epilepsy, remain free of seizures. The decision to stop these medications after a seizure-free period is a controversial one. Careful consultation with a qualified neurologist is suggested in such cases. More research is needed to determine which youths can safely be removed from their medications.

Drug Interactions and Side Effects

Gabapentin does not interact with other drugs while lamotrigine interacts only with valproate; less drug interference is noted with the benzodiazepines. Also, estrogen lowers the seizure threshold while progesterone seems to offer some protection for the seizure threshold. Some adolescent females do develop increased seizure activity at the end of a menstrual cycle.

Unpleasant side effects of medications may lower compliance. For example gingival hyperplasia or the development of coarse facies is noted with phenytoin. Gastrointestinal symptoms, rash, weight gain, hair change or loss, impotence, and other side effects can be noted with carbamazepine and valproate. Menstrual dysfunction, polycystic ovaries syndrome, and hyperandrogenism are also noted with valproate.

Low self-esteem, severe parent-child conflicts, and family dysfunction are often noted in youths who do not take medication as recommended. Also noted is the failure of physicians to substitute medications with less upsetting side effects for medications having side effects that are intolerable to the youth. Behavior and cognitive dysfunction are often ascribed to anticonvulsant medications, as phenobarbital and phenytoin. However, the literature is not in agreement and some medications, such as carbamazepine, have been reported to improve such areas as reaction time and attention span. The causes of such dysfunction are complex and can involve the youth's reaction to chronic illness as well as adolescence in general, drug side effects, family stability, and others. Barbiturates and phenytoin are especially associated with cognitive difficulties. There is literature to suggest an association between the use of phenobarbital and the development of depression with or without suicidal behavior in some patients. Careful monitoring is necessary and many clinicians do not use phenobarbital if there is a personal or family history of depression. Phenobarbital should be stopped and another anticonvulsant used if depressive symptomology develops. See the Psychologic and Social Aspects section.

Summary

Approximately 30% percent of epileptics are not wholly controlled by a single anticonvulsant drug and the addition of a multidrug regimen results in another 10% with good seizure control. Thus, 20% of those with seizure disorders will not be well controlled with medication. Factors contributing to incomplete control include mixed or complex seizure disorders, underlying diseases, or metabolic processes that are difficult to manage in and of themselves (for example, cerebral edema, tumors, severe congenital or acquired brain damage, and pubertal changes). Other issues that should be considered are poor compliance with the recommended regimen, the use of an inappropriate drug, subtherapeutic dosage, drug interferences or interactions when two or more agents are combined, malabsorption, the development of physiologic drug tolerance, and incorrect diagnosis. The contribution of placing refractory patients on a ketogenic diet remains under current evaluation.

Status Epilepticus

Status epilepticus, a state of continuous (over 20 minutes) or rapidly sequential seizures (usually tonic-clonic type) without a return of consciousness, may occur with the precipitant removal of anticonvulsant medication (particularly phenobarbital), infection, metabolic dysfunction, alcohol or other substance abuse, cerebral edema, and trauma, among other causes. Although a favorable outcome with appropriate management is usually the expected course, death from exhaustion, anoxia, brain damage (infarction), and cardiovascular collapse is possible. Professional evaluation and treatment for this true medical emergency is critical; more patients with seizure disorder die from treatment complications than from the seizure itself.

Surgery

Epilepsy surgery is considered for a limited number of individuals who have intractable seizures resistant to medical treatment (Engel, 1996). A very thorough evaluation and medical treatment program is necessary before considering surgery. The evaluation includes extensive EEG monitoring (including use of invasive electrodes), PET scanning, magnetic resonance spectroscopy, psychometrical-neuropsychologic evaluation, CT/MRI evaluation, amobarbital injection into the carotid artery (Wada test) to assess language and memory location connections, and other measures. A defined abnormal focus for excision is critical for potential postsurgical improvement. Such extensive procedures as hemispherectomy and callosotomy remain controversial. Vagus nerve stimulation is a new nonpharmacologic treatment for adults and adolescents over age 12. Seizure reductions (mechanism not known) occur in 19%–53% of patients.

Psychologic and Social Aspects

General

Attention to the psychosocial dimension of the adolescent with epilepsy is also critical to successful management in ensuring optimal development progress and minimizing compliance problems. Youths with epilepsy, as with other chronic illnesses, should receive comprehensive education concerning their disorder. It is not unusual to find epileptic youths with limited knowledge of their own disorder. Exposure to flickering lights (video games, driving through a forest with flickering sunlight, and others) may increase seizures in some due to the influence of photic stimulation; special filtered glasses may help. The tendency of teenagers to become sleep-deprived may worsen their seizure patterns. Drug and alcohol use/abuse increases the risk for worsened seizures secondary to lowering of the seizure threshold. There is increased metabolism of sex steroid hormones due to antiseizure medications, with stimulation of sex hormone binding globulin (SHBG). The reduction in serum levels of unbound testosterone and result-ant reduced sex drive is noted in some males after years of epilepsy, especially temporal lobe epilepsy.

Specific concerns of an epileptic youth include driving, participation in sports, success in school, vocation, genetic counseling, and childbearing.

Driving

Well-controlled adolescents are usually eligible for a driver's license if seizure-free for 1 year (2 in some states) even if they are receiving medication. The actual length of required seizure-free time varies from state to state: 3 months to 2 years, with an average of 1 year. In some states, the physician must report a person of driving age with epilepsy to the state motor vehicle office. However, it may not be advisable to stop medication just at a time when driv-ing is important to the teenager. License restriction can lead to reduced self-esteem, limited socialization, limited job employment, and reduced compliance with motor vehicle regulations.

Sports

Youths with good seizure control can participate in most sports (including contact sports) if adequate supervision and medical support are provided (see Chap. 32). Careful analysis by the physician, youth, parent(s), and coach(s) is recommended in each case. Participation in sports can be a very positive aspect to the youth's life. In discussions with youths and parents, it is best to review the consequences of seizure activity during the desired event. In some cases, no real harm will occur. However, because potential seizure activity during certain activities can be harmful, these activities are restricted–i.e., high diving, rope climbing, competitive underwater swimming, and gymnastics with parallel bars. Sports with increased risk of head injury, such as football and hockey, are discouraged by some clini-cians. However, there is no conclusive evidence to suggest that physical activity per se causes or wors-ens seizures.

Contraception

Adolescent females should be counseled to avoid pregnancy, as it may exacerbate seizures as well as raise a host of other problems, including requiring a higher dose of antiseizure medications and a higher rate of limited compliance with medication usage. An effective contraceptive method(s) should be pro-vided if the patient is sexually active, and the clini-cian can provide information regarding barrier methods, injectable types (Depo-Provera, Norplant) (see Chap. 25 on contraception). Antiseizure drugs (especially phenobarbital, primidone, phenytoin, carbamazepine, ethosuximide, topiramate, and tiagabine) induce the hepatic microsomal enzyme system. Thus, they interfere with such drugs as oral contraceptives, steroids, and theophylline. Many anecdotal reports exist of pregnancy in individuals on antiseizure drugs and oral contraceptives, pre-sumably due to the antiseizure medication-induced increased metabolism of oral contraceptives. Breakthrough bleeding may be an indication of this and an increase in contraceptive steroids may be necessary to lower the pregnancy risk. Some anti-convulsant medications do not interfere with oral contraceptives, such as valproic acid, felbamate, gabapentin, and lamotrigine.

Pregnancy

If an unplanned pregnancy does occur, possible ter-atogenic effects of the seizure medications should be evaluated and taken into consideration when counsel-ing the youth. Some clinicians treat epileptic adoles-cents with folate in addition to the antiepileptic medication to reduce the potential incidence of neural tube defects as a complication of anticonvulsant medication usage. The dosage of folate is 1 mg/day up to 4 mg/ day if there is a family history of tube defects or of sickle cell disease. However, the fetus has more risk from seizure activity, which the pregnant epileptic may develop, than from the teratogenic risks of the antiseizure medications. An increased dose of medication is often necessary during pregnancy, as serum levels of antiseizure medications may drop; lower doses are usually necessary after delivery. Most adolescents, both male and female, will be also concerned for the possible genetic transmission of epilepsy to future offspring. Unless there is a strong family history of seizure disorders, they should be appropriately reassured.

Teratogenicity

Teratogenicity develops mainly in the first 8 weeks of pregnancy and it must also be considered in older adolescents and young adults taking antiseizure drugs who are contemplating becoming pregnant. A two- to three-times higher rate of birth defects is noted in offspring of parents (both mother and father) taking antiseizure medications. Tridione should not be given to adolescent females at risk of pregnancy because of the very high rate of stillbirths and congenital anomalies reported with this medication. Phenytoin and valproate are also linked with birth defects, the latter with spina bifida. If valproate is given during pregnancy, alpha-fetoprotein levels are monitored during the pregnancy because of the increased risk for spina bifida. Carbamazepine usage in pregnancy has been linked to neural tube abnormalities. The safety of gabapentin and lamotrigine during pregnancy has not been determined.

Vocational Counseling

Concerns about education and vocational success may also arise. Limited academic success can be secondary to various difficulties adjusting to a chronic illness, unhealthy family reactions to a chronically ill adolescent, coexisting learning difficulties, potentially negative effects of antiseizure medications on attention span, inadequate seizure control, and other factors. Reality dictates that certain vocations will be closed to the epileptic individual. It certainly would be ill advised for teenagers with uncertain control to contemplate any job that places them or others at physical risk should they have a seizure (operating certain types of machines, working at high altitudes in the construction business, and so on). Even those with full control will encounter difficulty in enlisting in the armed forces or obtaining acceptance into police or fire departments.

Psychiatric Issues

Psychiatric difficulties can occur in some adolescents with epilepsy, whether induced by the effects of status epilepticus, complications of medications (as ethosuximide), rapid withdrawal of antiseizure medications, problems induced by chronic illness, or other nonepilepsy-related factors in the development of mental illness in adolescents. Finally the presence of pseudoseizures can be a cause of poor response to the recommended treatment regimen. This refers to seizure activity of nonepileptic origin, and can occur with or without coexisting seizures. EEGs taken at the same time or with video recordings may be helpful to establish the correct diagnosis. A normal or nonepileptic EEG pattern can be seen, if coexisting seizures that produce abnormal EEGs are not present.

Bibliography

Chang BS, Lowenstein DH: Epilepsy. *N Engl J Med* 349:1257–1266, 2003.

Commission on Classification and Terminology of the International League Against Epilepsy: Proposal for revised classification of epilepsies and epileptic syndromes. *Epilepsia* 30:389–399, 1989.

Engel J Jr: A proposed diagnostic scheme for people with epileptic seizures and epilepsy: Report of the ILAE Task Force on Classification and Terminology. *Epilepsia* 37(Suppl 1):S26–S40, 1996; 42:796–803, 2001.

Greydanus DE, Van Dyke D: Epilepsy in the adolescent: The Sacred Disease and the Clinician's Sacred Duty. *Int Pediatr* 20(2):6–8, 2005.

Hauser WA, Kurland LT: The epidemiology of epilepsy in Rochester, Minnesota, 1935 through 1967. *Epilepsia* 16:1–16, 1975.

LaRoche SM, Helmers SL: The new antiepileptic drugs. *JAMA* 291:605–614, 615–620, 2004.

Liebenson MH, Rosman NP: Seizures in adolescents. *Adolesc Med* 2: 629–648, 1991.

Loring DW, Meador KJ: Cognitive and behavioral effects of epilepsy treatment. *Epilepsia* 42(Suppl 8):24–32, 2001.

Nordli DR Jr.: Special needs of the adolescent with epilepsy. *Epilepsia* 42(Suppl 8):10–17, 2001.

Paolicchi JM: Epilepsy in adolescents: Diagnosis and treatment. *Adolesc Med* 13:443–459, 2002.

Parmet S, Lynm C, Glass RM: Epilepsy. *JAMA Patient Page* 291:654, 2004.

Rimsza ME, Greydanus DE, Braverman PK: Contraception. *AAP Pediatric Update* 24:1–10, 2004.

Westbrook LE, Silver EJ, Coupey SM, et al: Social characteristics of adolescents with idiopathic epilepsy: A comparison to chronically ill and non-chronically ill peers. *J Epilepsy* 4:87–94, 1991.

HEADACHE

Epidemiology

Headache is one of the most common of adolescent complaints. During surveys, approximately 75% of females and 50% of males report a headache over the past 30 days of the survey; this includes 10% of the females and 5% of the males reporting four or more headaches or headache complexes a month. At least 25% of adolescents will seek medical attention for headache at least once during their adolescent years.

Classification

Headaches can be classified as to whether they reflect (1) spasm of the external musculature of the head, face, and neck with or without involvement of the external vasculature (tension headaches), (2) alteration of the intracranial vasculature (migraine headaches), or (3) an intracranial lesion. Although many conditions can cause headache (Table 13-5), most cases in adolescents are of the tension type. Migraine is also commonly encountered, but intracranial pathology is relatively rare.

History

Specific points to be noted in evaluation include the duration and frequency of acute episodes, a description of the pain, the degree of disability experienced, any associated symptomatology (weight loss, visual impairment, fever, vomiting, recent personality changes, neurologic deficits), possible precipitants, and a detailed neurologic as well as general examination. It is helpful for the teenager to keep a 30-day or more written record with descriptions of his/her headaches. A thorough psychosocial history is often critical in identifying specific headache types, particularly the psychogenic headache. It is unusual for sinusitis to be the cause of chronic headaches. Refractive errors may lead to dull, frontal headaches but rarely to severe, unremitting headaches. Both migraine and tension headaches are often readily diagnosed on the basis of the history and physical examination alone. These are often classic symptoms with no physical findings of note. Such headache types can exist together or in combination with other types. Headaches present for over 4 months without physical examination findings usually reflect a nonorganic etiology.

Laboratory Studies

Table 13-6 cites various laboratory procedures that may be useful in further evaluation, though how many to employ and in what sequence is a matter of judgment based on data already obtained. Neuroimaging procedures are considered for those with a history of headaches with seizures, papilledema, vision difficulties, and other neurologic abnormalities. Also consider such procedures for those with headaches that are worsening, which awaken the teenager from sleep or occur in early morning, and are associated with considerable psychologic changes (as new mental status aberrations). MRI and CT scans have replaced skull films

TABLE 13-5

DIFFERENTIAL DIAGNOSIS OF HEADACHES

CNS disorders

Infections: meningitis, encephalitis, brain abscess

Subarachnoid or subdural hemorrhage: trauma, spontaneous rupture of aneurysm or arteriovenous fistula, thromboembolism

Cerebral edema: pseudotumor cerebri, benign intracranial

Hypertension: complication of radiation treatment for a brain tumor

Brain tumor

Hydrocephalus

Subdural hematoma

Vascular disorders

Migraine headaches

As a component of tension headaches

Primary hypertension or hypertension secondary to renal disease, pheochromocytoma, carcinoid tumors; more typically seen in hypertensive crisis

Disorders of the eyes, ears, nose, and throat

Eye disorders: eye strain, optic neuritis, glaucoma

Pain, which is actually referred otalgia (secondary to disorders of the teeth, nasopharynx, temporomandibular joint)

Sinusitis

Otitis (acute or chronic)

Hay fever

Systemic and metabolic disorders

Endocrine dysfunction (hypoglycemia, diabetes mellitus, and hyperthyroidism)

Collagen vascular disorders

Acute and chronic infections other than CNS, particularly with fever and toxicity

Dialysis patients

Musculoskeletal disorders

Tension headaches

Cervical spine disorders

Systemic lupus erythematosus

Cervicogenic headache (cervical spine dysfunction)

Food- and drug-related disorders

Caffeine withdrawal (coffee, tea, cola beverages, and cocoa)

Ergotamine withdrawal (in relation to migraine treatment)

Use/abuse of alcohol, cocaine, marijuana, and other drugs.

Nicotine use or withdrawal (cigarettes)

Monosodium glutamate ingestion in susceptible persons

Nitrate and nitrite food preservatives

Foods that exacerbate migraine (see text)

Chronic use of large amounts of analgesics (as acetaminophen)

Carbon monoxide poisoning

Side effects of various medications, including antihypertensives, antidepressants, psychotropics

Psychiatric disorders

Psychosis

Depressions

Conversion disorder

Miscellaneous

Exercise

Trauma (as postconcussion)

Excessive video game use

Lack of sleep

Temporal arteritis

Trigeminal neuralgia

Sick building syndrome

Effect of toxins, such as lead

Electrolyte imbalance

Complication of lumbar puncture

Malingering

Migraine with CSF pleocytosis

---

in the evaluation of chronic headaches. The MRI is a better procedure than the head CT to identify some brain tumors and arteriovenous malformations. If a seizure disorder is suspected, EEG monitoring is necessary.

Migraine Headache

Epidemiology

Migraine affects 3%–15% of the population. It predominates in females (with a male to female

TABLE 13-6

CLINICAL AND LABORATORY EVALUATION OF HEADACHES

History	Location, description, duration, frequency, time of day or night, relation to time of year, effect on daily activity, sleep patterns, diet history, menstrual history, precipitating events or warning symptoms, disrupts sleep or interrupts activity, how relieved, associated symptoms and signs, other health and mental health issues, including use of drugs, alcohol, cigarettes, oral contraceptives, family history, psychosocial history, response to medication trials.
Physical examination	Particular attention to blood pressure, eyes (including fundi and visual acuity), ears (including Weber and Rinne tests and auditory acuity), nose, sinuses, TMJ, auscultation of skull and orbits, throat, cardiovascular system, neurologic system
Laboratory Tests[*]	Routine: complete blood count and urinalysis
	Erythrocyte sedimentation rate
	Blood values: glucose (fasting or tolerance test); if urinalysis is abnormal: urea nitrogen and creatinine
	Roentgenograms: cervical spine, sinuses, ear and mastoid, temporomandibular joint
	Other imaging procedures: head CT or MRI; except for evaluation of the cervical spine, the CT may be the better initial choice
	Lumbar puncture[†]
	EEG
	Visual fields, intraocular pressure
	Specialized neurologic and neuroendocrine procedures
	Therapeutic trial with selected medications in migraine suspects
	Psychologic or psychiatric evaluation
	Others: based on the specific situation

[*]To be preformed according to clinical judgment as suggested by prior findings and clinical course. A careful history (including family history) and examination remain the mainstay of headache evaluation. The yield of imaging studies is low in patients who have no history or physical findings suggestive of a space-occupying lesion inside the skull (ie, brain tumor, arteriovenous malformation, aneurysm, meningoencephalitis, or pseudotumor cerebri).

[†]Lumbar puncture is only useful for suspected infection or pseudotumor cerebri.

ratio of 1:3.5) and has a strong association with a positive family history (60% to 90%). In approximately one third of all cases migraine begins in childhood. The incidence gradually increases at the time of puberty, peaks during late adolescence, and thereafter declines. Childhood-onset migraine commonly abates during puberty, but initiation at the time of adolescence often presages the continuation of attacks into adulthood.

Etiology

Current research suggests that vasoconstriction-reactive vasodilatation is resultant but not the initial migraine mechanism. A migraine headache appears to be an electrochemical event involving activation of the trigeminovascular system with release of neuropeptides, as substance P, neurokinin A, and CGRP. Migraine prodromes have a hypothalamic origin while a cortical neuronal basis underlies the migraine aura and cognitive changes. Neurogenic inflammation involving the sensory C-fiber is identified as central to the pain of migraine headaches. Migraines start centrally, affecting blood vessels secondarily; the trigeminal vascular system is involved with pain production and blood vessel changes. Studies note that 5-HT (5-hydroxytryptamine) or serotonin may be released from platelets at the beginning of a migraine episode; free 5-HT levels increase at first and then decrease in later stages of the attack. 5-HT acts on different receptors and, depending on the type and amount of receptors found in different blood vessels, vasodilatation or vasoconstriction may occur. There are at least four classes of 5-HT receptors: 5-HT(1-4) beneficial medications used to treat acute migraine episodes interact at the 5-HT-1 receptor while medications helpful for prophylaxis of migraines interact at the 5-HT-2 receptor sites. Patients with migraine headaches (migraineurs) may also be at risk for the development of a number of comorbidities, including panic disorder, other anxiety disorders, depression, epilepsy, and stroke.

Classic pathophysiologic mechanisms implicate the intracranial vasculature, with an initial vasoconstrictive phase lasting several minutes to half an hour (the aura) followed by an extended period of vasodilation (the headache). Vasoconstriction may affect any part of the brain or brainstem; the precise vessels involved determining whether the aura is predominantly one of nausea and emesis (medulla), fever, edema, and irritability (hypothalamus), sensory changes relating to light, taste, sound, or motor function (cortex), or a combination of these. Spreading cerebral hypoperfusion during a migraine headache has been documented by blood-flow measurements with PET and oxygen-15-labeled water. This decrease in cerebral blood flow may begin in the occipital area and slowly spread throughout the brain in a pattern called cortical spreading depression. Vasodilation manifested in the typical headache appears closely related to the increased accumulation in the perivascular region of various pain sensitizers such as serotonin, catecholamines, histamine, bradykinin, angiotensin, and prostaglandins. Increased vessel permeability to these substances also may play a role.

There is a strong familial factor in many individuals with migraines. Also, a wide variety of precipitating events has been implicated in the vulnerable individual. These include fatigue, stress, menses, ovulation, flickering and/or very bright lights, barometric or humidity changes, head trauma, missed meals, changes in sleep patterns (too much, too little), hypertension, allergens, strong odors, exercise, coitus, and various ingestants or drugs such as oral contraceptives, chocolate, caffeine, alcohol (especially red wine), reserpine, vasodilator drugs, tyramine, nitrate preservatives, citrus fruits, sharp cheeses, and monosodium glutamate. Migraines are noted in increased incidence in individuals with primary and familial lipoproteinemias. A caffeine withdrawal syndrome has been identified in adults, with resultant headaches, drowsiness, fatigue, and/or depression. Individuals consuming two or more caffeinated beverages per day are at risk.

Symptomatology

A wide variety of manifestations and symptoms have been described (see following section), but the most common complaints among adolescents are of recurrent, unilateral, or bilateral, pounding headache associated with photophobia, pallor, nausea, vomiting, and anorexia. Diarrhea, constipation, diuresis, edema, fever, and blood pressure changes also have been described. Twenty-five percent of patients with migraine headaches experience an antecedent aura variably consisting of sensory phenomena (flashing lights, peculiar smell or taste, ringing or buzzing in ears), autonomic signs (pallor, syncope, hyperhidrosis, nausea, vomiting), psychic manifestations (apprehension, anxiety, mood changes), or motor abnormalities (from localized weakness to hemiparesis). Some patients develop migraine attacks in relation to menstrual periods and abatement of migraines may develop during pregnancy. Migraines can occur anytime and there may be prolonged periods in which there are no headaches. Patients with migraine headaches have an increased association with epilepsy and/or epileptiform EEGs. Also, migraine headaches can precipitate seizures. Differentiation of migraines and seizures can be difficult. Impaired consciousness is associated with epilepsy and not usually with migraines, while fortification scotoma is noted with some migraines but not epilepsy. The prodrome of migraines leads to headaches, while headache can develop after impaired consciousness and secondary GTCS in epilepsy.

Migraine with Aura (Classic Migraine)

Recent studies note that 4% of the population has this type of migraine headache over a period of a year and 6% report it at some time in their lives. Migraine with aura (formerly called classic migraine) presents with an abrupt, sharply defined aura lasting 10–30 minutes followed by a 4–6-hour unilateral, pounding headache with nausea, emesis, and anorexia. The aura may have various components: visual, sensory, speech, or motor. The visual aura involves the patient seeing lights, spots, or other phenomena. Syncope, confusion, and even coma can be part of auras in rare situations. It tends to occur two to four times per month at any time of the day and can last up to 72 hours. It can be worsened with physical activity and associated with hypersensitivity to light (photophobia) and sound (phonophobia). It can be misdiagnosed as a simple partial seizure of an occipital or parietal basis if the migraine has an aura with scotoma or lights, followed by unilateral neurodysfunction. Migraine with transient changes in consciousness or neurologic alterations is termed complicated migraine by some. Temporal lobe epilepsy may be confused with classic migraine if there is a visual aura or amnesia. Also, the prodrome of classic migraine is usually minutes in duration, versus seconds for simple partial seizure.

Migraine without Aura (Common Migraine)

The common migraine is now classified as migraine without aura. Recent studies suggest that 6% of the population have this type over a 1-year period and 9% at some time in their lives. The headaches are the same as with the classic form except that the aura is absent or less well defined and merges into the vasodilatory phase. The headache itself lasts 4–72 hours and, though usually unilateral, is bilateral one-third of the time. Withdrawal from caffeine, changes in sleep patterns (for example, excessive sleep on weekends), and stress appear to be significant precipitants. Although any of the factors discussed in the overview may be implicated, "let-down" migraine is a variant sometimes seen with the relief of stress such as during weekends, post-exams, vacations, or holidays. The frequency of attacks varies from daily episodes to ones separated by wide time intervals. The headache secondary to an alcoholic intoxication episode or hangover may be similar to a migraine complex. Hyperthyroidism and the effects of the flu syndrome can also produce similar headaches.

Rare and Unusual Forms of Migraine or Migraine-Like Headaches

Cluster migraine usually affects older males between 30 and 60 years and accounts for 4%–5% of all adult vascular headaches. There is an abrupt onset of unilateral headache with severe facial pain (retro-orbital), flushing, nasal discharge, lacrimation, conjunctival injection, and hyperhidrosis and occasional ptosis of the affected side. One out of five patients also demonstrates an ipsilateral Horner syndrome. Episodes tend to be nocturnal, last $\frac{1}{2}$–$1\frac{1}{2}$ hours, and recur in clusters over a period of 8–12 weeks, with subsequent remission for months to years. There is not usually a positive family history for cluster migraine complex and there is no progression to overt migraine headaches. Treatment of these headache complexes is often difficult and involves oxygen inhalation, ergotamine, intranasal drops of an anesthetic (numbing the sphenopalatine ganglion), steroids, lithium carbonate, indomethacin, and even surgery (dividing the nervus intermedius with limited ablation of the trigeminal nerve).

In unusual situations, migraine patients have been reported to have recurrent episodes of abdominal pain referred to as migraine equivalents. Ophthalmoplegic migraine consists of a typical headache and oculomotor paralysis lasting 3–5 days. Spontaneous clearing is the general rule, but permanent nerve injury has been noted. Temporary loss of vision in the affected eye due to transient retinal artery spasm or amaurosis fugax has been described in migraine patients. It usually clears without sequelae, unless there are other causes. Hemiplegic migraine is similar to ophthalmoplegic migraine but with hemiplegia, aphasia, or hemisensory deficits replacing eye signs. The differential diagnosis in either case includes intracranial tumor, cerebrovascular accident, other space-occupying lesions, multiple sclerosis, and encephalomyelitis, among others. All laboratory evaluation in either ophthalmoplegic or hemiplegic migraine, including cerebrospinal fluid, is negative. Research has linked familial hemiplegic migraine to a locus on chromosome 19. Cerebral infarction has been identified in rare situations.

Basilar artery migraine is primarily noted in females and appears to be closely related to menses. It is characterized by a 20–40-minute aura, with evidence of cranial nerve dysfunction, including loss of vision, emesis, vertigo, ataxia, dysarthria, paresthesias, weakness, tinnitus, and alteration of consciousness followed by a throbbing headache in the occipital region. This rare headache complex is also called the Bickerstaff syndrome. A seizure syndrome called childhood epilepsy with occipital paroxysms can be associated with migraine-like headaches. It is often noted during childhood but can be seen in adolescents with seizures characterized by daytime, visual hallucinations and a postictal headache; the EEG reveals abnormalities over the occipital area if the eyes are closed.

Acute Management of Migraines

General

Migraine may occur in conjunction with other disorders such as sinus, dental, or ear infections, or with tension headaches; attention should first be directed at isolating any such coexisting condition(s). A careful search of the patient's history for possible factors triggering the migraine itself (see overview) may suggest modifications in the patient's lifestyle, habits, food, or medications that may help to decrease the frequency of attacks. If the migraine complex precipitates seizure-like activity, antiepilepsy medications may be indicated. Headaches that improve on weekends or in different milieu may improve with careful attention to underlying stress factors. Caffeine may suppress migraines to some extent, but a tachyphylaxis phenomenon usually develops. The most effective treatment for migraine headaches is based upon

directing attention to the underlying pathophysiologic factors characteristic of migraines–the overproduction, excessive release, and recycling of the neurotransmitters serotonin and substance P. Psychogenic-type migraines are often very recalcitrant to pharmacotherapy and these patients usually do better with some form of behaviorallyoriented therapy. Migraine patients often do best with proper sleep habits, including the development of consistent sleep-awake cycles; moderation of caffeine use and reduction of stress is important, as well. Medication should be taken as early as possible and narcotics are to be avoided.

Analgesics

Nonsteroidal anti-inflammatory drugs (NSAIDs) are advocated by some as the first choice of medications for those with mild to moderate migraine headaches (Table 13-7). NSAIDs inhibit neurogenic inflammation in the trigeminovascular system, limit vascular vasoconstriction, and interfere with the neurotransmission of serotonin. Side effects can include dyspepsia and, rarely, gastrointestinal hemorrhage. Commonly used combination drugs include Midrin and Fiorinal (Table 13-7); they have not been shown to be better than plain analgesics. Fiorinal is approved by the FDA for tension headaches and Midrin is listed by the FDA as possibly effective for migraine headaches. It should be remembered that studies have noted that the chronic use of analgesics, as defined by their use more than once per week, can exacerbate headaches (analgesic rebound headaches) and thus, chronic use should be avoided. Narcotics and opiate medications should be avoided completely in adolescents.

Ergotamine

If NSAIDs are not helpful, specific drug treatment for an acute episode usually relies on ergotamine tartrate or triptan medications, such as sumatriptan (Imitrex) and others—see Table 13-8. Ergotamine is a 5-HT agonist and has vasoconstrictive properties; dihydroergotamine (DHE) has a high affinity for 5-HT-1D receptors and blocks release of substance P from the trigeminal nerve. It is effective in 50% in aborting an attack if given early in the cycle,

TABLE 13-7

DRUGS IN TREATING ACUTE MIGRAINE HEADACHES

Drug	Dosage
Ergotamine tartrate	
Cafergot tablets (1 mg ergotamine tartrate plus 100 mg caffeine; available as suppository in 2 mg dose)	Do not give more than 6 mg per 24 h or 10 mg/week; 1–2 tab p.o. stat, then 1 tab q 30 min if necessary; maximum dose, 6 tabs per 24 h, 10 tabs/week
Cafergot P-B suppositories (2 mg ergotamine tartrate, 100 mg caffeine, 0.25 mg Bellafoline, 60 mg pentobarbital sodium; available as p.o. tablet in different dose)	1 suppository stat, then 1 suppository in 1 h if necessary; maximum dose, 2 suppositories per 24 h, 5 suppositories per week
Migraine suppositories (1.0 mg Ergotamine tartrate, 100 mg caffeine, 0.1 mg belladonna alkaloids, 130 mg phenacetin; also available as p.o. tablets)	1–2 suppositories stat, then 1–2 suppositories q 15–30 min if necessary; maximum dose, 6 suppositories per 24 h, 12 suppositories per week
Ergotamine tartrate medihaler	1 inhalation stat, then 1 inhalation q 5 min if necessary;
Others: Migral, Ergostat,	maximum dose, 6 inhalations per 24 h
DHE 45 (dihydroergotamine	1 mL IM stat, then 1 mL q 60 min if necessary,
Mesylate injection)	maximum dose, 3 mL per 24 h (DHE)
Triptans	See Table 13-8
Analgesics	
Weak analgesics	
Acetaminophen (Tylenol)	15 mg/kg orally; 650 mg p.o. q 4 h
Fioricet (50 mg butalbital, 325 mg acetamin- ophen, 40 mg caffeine; as tablets	1–2 tabs q 4–6 h; maximum dose, 6 tabs per 24 h
Midrin (65 mg isometheptene mucate, 100 mg dichloralphenazone, 325 mg acetaminophen)	1–2 capsules q 4 h; maximum dose, 5 caps/24 h
Nonsteroidal anti-inflammatory drugs (NSAIDS)	
Naproxen sodium	250–500 mg b.i.d. for immediate release
(Aleve, NaProsyn)	375–00 mg b.i.d. for delayed release
Ibuprofen (200–800 mg p.o.)	200–800 mg t.i.d. to q.i.d.
(Motrin, Advil)	
Ketorolac (Toradol)	15–30 mg IV/IM q 6 h or 10 mg
Others	p.o. q 4–6 h; not over 5 days
Antinauseants	
Promethazine hydrochloride (Phenergan; available as tablet, suppository, or injectable)	12.5–25 mg p.o. or rectally q 4–6 h; adjust IM dose as needed. Demerol and Phenergan are often used together for relief of severe episodes.
Trimethobenzamide (Tigan; available as capsule, suppository, or injectable)	250 mg capsule b.i.d. or q.i.d.; 200 mg (2 mL) IM t.i.d. or q.i.d.
Hydroxyzine pamoate (Vistaril; available as capsules; injectable)	25 mg q.i.d. p.o. or IM (hydroxyzine)

(Continued)

TABLE 13-7

DRUGS IN TREATING ACUTE MIGRAINE HEADACHES (*CONTINUED*)

Drug	Dosage
Sedatives, Tranquilizers	
Chloral hydrate	250 mg t.i.d.-q.i.d. p.o.; maximum dose, 2 g per 24 h
Diazepam (Valium; also available as injectable	(Chloral Hydrate)
Chlorpromazine (Thorazine; also available as injectable)	2–10 mg b.i.d.-q.i.d. p.o. (Diazepam)
	50 mg p.o. or IM stat, then 50 mg q 30–60 min if necessary; maximum dose 300 mg first 4 h,
	1000 mg per 24 h (Chlorpromazine); ergotamine tartrate may be added
	Perphenazine and prochlorperazine also used for control of severe nausea and emesis.
Steroids, Prednisone	30–60 mg per 24 h × 3–5 days; taper to discontinue over 1 week

preferably at the first signs of an aura. Responsiveness to a clinical trial is also diagnostic in that other forms of headache are not alleviated. Ergotamine can be given in various forms: oral, intramuscular, sublingual, rectal, and inhalation. Ergotamine can be given with caffeine (Cafergot for example) for moderate episodes; the addition of caffeine increases ergotamine absorption and possibly its vasoconstrictor properties. Intramuscular or intravenous ergotamine (DHE-45) is used for severe migraine attacks.

Ergotamine, however, should not be prescribed for patients with prolonged auras (it will intensify the vasoconstrictive effects), those who are pregnant, and those who have peripheral vascular occlusive disease, hypertension, or other conditions that could be exacerbated by increased vascular resistance. Side effects include nausea, vomiting, muscle aches, paresthesias, habituation (in relation to use for headaches), rebound vascular headaches, ischemia of coronary or cerebral vessels, thrombophlebitis, abdominal pain, diarrhea, muscle cramps, and chronic ergotism (peripheral circulatory insufficiency, fatigue, depression, persistent nausea, and vomiting). Ergotism can be potentiated by concurrent use of dopamine, erythromycin, beta-adrenergic blockers, and troleandomycin. Failure of a response to ergotamine may be due to taking it too late in the migraine cycle, malabsorption, the coexistence of tension headaches, misdiagnosis, and, in some patients, individual idiosyncratic resistance.

TABLE 13-8

TRIPTAN MEDICATIONS FOR TREATMENT OF MIGRAINE HEADACHES

Sumatriptan (Imitrex):
25–50 mg orally; can be repeated after 2 h; maximum daily dose for adults is 200 mg.
Intranasal dose: 20 mg, repeated after 2 h if necessary
Subcutaneous dose: 6 mg, repeated after 1 h if necessary

Zolmitriptan (Zomig or Zomig ZMT [orally disintegrating pill]):
2.5 or 5.0 mg orally; can be repeated after 2 h; maximum daily dose for adults is 10 mg.
Intranasal dose: 5 mg, repeated after 2 h if necessary

Rizatriptan (Maxalt, Maxalt-MLT [orally disintegrating pill])
Oral dose: 5 or 10 mg to be repeated after 2 h if necessary; maximum dose is 30 mg

Naratriptan (Amerge): oral: 2.5 mg that can be repeated after 4 h if necessary;

Almotriptan (Axert): oral: 12.5 mg that can be repeated after 2 h if necessary

Frovatriptan (Frova): oral: 2.5 mg that can be repeated after 2 h if necessary (maximum daily dose: 7.5 mg)

Eletriptan (Relpax): oral: 20 or 40 mg that can be repeated after 2 h if necessary (maximum daily dose: 80 mg)

Sumatriptan (Imitrex) is a serotonin (5-HT) agonist used for oral and parenteral (SQ) treatment of migraine headaches. It constricts large intracranial blood vessels and decreases inflammation around sensory nerves. Oral sumatriptan is given in a 25 mg dose, with a range up to 100 mg, while the subcutaneous dose is 6 mg, repeated in 1 hour if necessary. It can also be given intranasally (20 mg), which can be repeated after 2 hours. The success rate increases only 10% with an oral dose beyond 25 mg while the risk for side effects then increases; these include nausea, emesis, skin tingling/burning, tachycardia, and a feeling of heaviness or pressure in the chest. The oral form appears to be less frequently effective than the parenteral but is worth trying first. The prepared vials contain 6 mg, which is appropriate for most teenagers. Parenteral sumatriptan (6 mg SQ) can also be used by some adult patients to treat themselves. Sumatriptan is not given with ergot medication, methysergide, monoamine oxidase inhibitor drugs, specific 5-HT-reuptake inhibitors, or lithium carbonate. It is used for those with occasional severe migraines and is usually coupled with a prophylactic agent. It is not used to prevent migraines. Other triptans are listed in Table 13-8.

Other Agents: Management of Acute Migraine Episode

Various combinations of analgesics, antiemetics, and sedatives or tranquilizers (Table 13-7) have been used to replace ergotamine or sumatriptan entirely when it is ineffective or when side effects require discontinuance or as a supplement when only partially effective. In the latter instance, ergotamine, combined with an analgesic and an antinauseant, may be helpful. Decreased gastric motility occurs during an acute migraine attack, and thus there can be decreased absorption of aspirin or other oral drugs. Metoclopramide (Reglan) may increase the drug enhancement by improving gastric motility. One method is to give 10 mg Reglan followed by 1 g aspirin 10 minutes later. However, caution is suggested when using metoclopramide, due to its infrequent, but well-known dystonia side effect.

Narcotic drugs, such as meperidine, have been used in emergency situations where other antimigraine medications have been ineffective or contraindicated. Intravenous dopamine antagonists have been used in emergency situations; these include chlorpromazine (0.1 mg/kg of body weight), prochlorperazine (10 mg dose), and metoclopramide (10 mg dose). These medications, including perphenazine, have been used in adults and some adolescents to control severe nausea and emesis; however, their use has been restricted in adolescents by some clinicians because of severe side effects, including the rare, but irreversible tardive dyskinesia. Prednisone has produced dramatic results in severe, persistent cases; however, its use is limited due to well-known side effects of steroids. Unremitting cases have been treated with some success by means of a deep sleep regimen using intravenous sedative and tranquilizer combinations.

Prophylaxis of Migraine Headaches

General

Patients with frequent episodes of migraine headaches (two to three or more per month) warrant a preventive regimen, with particular attention paid to precipitating causes, such as sleep deprivation, certain foods, irregular meals, stress, others. In addition to being given prophylactic medication, the patient should be instructed in alternative pain control techniques (operant conditioning, self-hypnosis, behavior modification, biofeedback techniques, guided imagery, meditation, body relaxation exercises). For example, double-blinded, crossover studies have demonstrated that 70% or more of persons with migraines may experience significant relief from biofeedback.

Specific Medications

A wide variety of agents have been employed in medical prophylaxis (Table 13-9). Regular use of NSAIDS is helpful to some adolescents to reduce the frequency of migraine attacks. Propranolol is commonly given to adolescents and adults with frequent migraines and is the only beta-blocker approved by the U.S. Food and Drug Administration for migraine prophylaxis. It modulates serotonergic neurons. It comes in a long-acting form, beginning

TABLE 13-9

DRUGS IN MIGRAINE PREVENTION

Drug	Comment
Propranolol hydrochloride (Inderal) Beta-adrenergic agonist	Dose, 80 mg/day initially, up to 160–240 mg/day. Most are helped with 80–120 mg/day dose. There are many side effects, including rebound headaches on withdrawal, if maximum dose not effective with 4–6 weeks, withdraw slowly over 2 weeks. Can see fatigue, hypotension, nausea. Start with a limited dose and work up slowly to reduce the side effects. Do not use in conjunction with ergotamine or in patients with sinus bradycardia, bronchial asthma, or congestive heart failure. The sustained-release Inderal LA (60–300 mg/day) can be taken once daily; side effects include weight gain, paresthesias, violent dreams. Other proposed β-blockers include timolol (20 mg/day) atenolol (40–100 mg/day), nadolol (80–240 mg/day), and metoprolol (200 mg/day).
Antidepressants Can block 5-HT reuptake and down-regulate 5-HT-2 receptors and some: 5-HT-2 receptor antagonist	Useful if depression underlies migraine. - Literature often lists amitriptyline as the antidepressant of choice; other (eg, imipramine or nortriptyline) can also be effective. Dose of amitriptyline is 25–50 mg h.s., up to 125–150 mg h.s. Selective serotonin reuptake inhibitors (fluoxetine {Prozac}, sertraline {Zoloft}, others) also effective in some.
Calcium-entry blockers Inhibit 5-HT release	Currently available agents: Verapamil (280–320 mg/day), nifedipine (30 mg/day), nimodipine (120 mg/day), others (as diltiazem). Side effects include constipation and rarely, hypotension as well as cardiac arrhythmias.
Acetazolamide (Diamox)	Useful for some menses-related migraines with few side effects. Given as 250 mg b.i.d. before, during and shortly after menstrual period.
Anticonvulsants (Valproic acid)	May be beneficial if EEG abnormal. Can see hair loss, weight gain, hepatic dysfunction, neurologic tube defect. Dose: 800–1000 mg per day. Others used include carbamazepine, topiramate, lamotrigine, and gabapentin.
Weak analgesics Aspirin (1300 mg/day) Naproxen sodium (1100 mg/day) Mefenamic acid (500–1500 mg/day) Ketoprofen (150 mg/day) Tolfenamic acid (300 mg/day) Other NSAIDS	Side-effects include gastritis, dyspepsia, GI bleeding, diarrhea, fluid retention.
Steroids	Prednisone: 30–60 mg/day or q.i.d.

(Continued)

DRUGS IN MIGRAINE PREVENTION (CONTINUED)

Drug	Comment
Cyproheptadine hydrochloride (Periactin) 5-HT-2- receptor antagonist	Dose, 4–8 mg t.i.d. Serotonin and histamine antagonist sometimes effective alone or with other medications. Side effects include lethargy, inappropriate appetite, weight gain; often need higher doses for benefit than the youth can tolerate.
Methysergide maleate (Sansert) 5-HT-2 receptor antagonist	Dose, 2–6 mg/day. Serotonin antagonist with many side effects, including nausea, vomiting, peripheral circulatory insufficiency, edema, depression, angina, and fibrosis of retroperitoneal, pulmonary, and cardiac regions. A respite for 2 months of every 6 months is recommended to reduce incidence of fibrosis. Not used often in the adolescent age group.

with doses of 60 mg, which may be useful to improve compliance. The usual dose is 2 mg/kg/day and side effects (as well as relative contraindications) include sedation, exacerbation of asthma, decline in athletic prowess, and impotence.

Calcium-channel blockers (such as verapamil [e.g., Calan] and nicardipine [Cardene]) have been used with success by some with severe migraines, especially for those with exercise-induced headache exacerbations. These medications come in regular and sustained released forms; regular forms are used twice daily and the usual dosage of verapamil is 1–2 mg/kg/day. Acetazolamide (Diamox) has been noted to be useful for catamenial exacerbation of headaches in females with predictable menstrual cycles. A usual dose of 250 mg b.i.d. is given 2–3 days before menses, during the flow and 1–2 days afterwards. It is well-tolerated by most women and only a limited number of side effects are reported. Angiotensin II receptor blockers (candesartan) may be effective in some as well.

Antidepressant medications (e.g., amitriptyline, imipramine, fluoxetine) have also been helpful in individuals in whom depression or anxiety is a precipitating factor; these medications can also be helpful in the prophylaxis of migraines in those not depressed due to effects on serotonin metabolism. They have also been used in some patients who could not tolerate the side effects of beta-blockers. See Chap. 42

(Psychopharmacology) for a review of antidepressant medication side effects. Anticonvulsants (especially valproic acid, gabapentin, and topiramate) have been helpful in selected cases. Cyproheptadine has been useful in younger children, but most adolescents do not tolerate the high doses needed to stop headaches. The side effects of all these medications must be carefully monitored.

Tension Headaches

General

Sustained contraction or spasm of the muscles about the head and neck with or without vascular involvement classically identifies the tension headache or tension-type headache. It is an exceptionally common complaint among adolescents, often reported once or twice a week. The etiology is unclear, though emotional tension and stress appear to be involved. They are classically described as having a tendency to be more common in the afternoon or evening (versus the morning) and to be more common in the beginning of the school year or on school days (versus the weekend). They can last several hours to days. Symptomatology varies greatly, but the pain is frequently described as a dull, constant ache over the entire head or as a sensation of tightness (bandlike, viselike) about the forehead,

head, and neck. Bitemporal or occipital locations are often noted. Other common features are positive family history, insidious onset, bilateral involvement, increase in discomfort as the day progresses, and onset or exacerbation with exposure to stress or anxiety. Tenderness of neck or scalp muscles may be present as well. An aura is notably absent, as are autonomic signs, and the pain is less likely to be pounding or unilateral, differentiating tension from migraine etiologies.

On the other hand, a middle ground exists where it may be difficult to differentiate common migraine from tension headaches, and, to further confuse matters, the two may coexist. Recent research has suggested that excess muscle contraction is noted in migraine headaches and does not differentiate tension from migraine headaches. Electromyogram studies of both headache complexes are nonspecific. The term primary headache has been suggested to serve as a disorder, which is a continuum between tension and migraine headaches, in which the term tension headache refers to a mild pain complex while more severe pain reflects a migraine with or without aura.

Diagnosis

Diagnosis can usually be made on clinical grounds alone. Deficits in visual acuity and chronic sinusitis should not be difficult to rule out, in that the pain and discomfort from these conditions usually are limited to the periorbital or sinus areas, with associated visual difficulties in one instance and tenderness to pressure or percussion over the frontal region in the other. Headaches due to intracranial lesions tend to be much more severe, well defined, and accompanied by neurologic deficits. Further evaluation (Table 13-7) may be indicated when signs and symptoms are more ambiguous or severe than commonly encountered.

Management

Treatment of tension headaches employs weak or mild analgesics alone or in combination with other agents (acetaminophen, aspirin, phenacetin, Fiorinal, and Midrin; see Table 13-8), though increasing favor is being given to body relaxation techniques and physical therapy, as well helping the patient to deal with stress more effectively as an alternative to drug-mediated solutions. Reassurance is also an important measure, as many adolescents believe their symptoms to be much more serious than they are. Improvement of underlying precipitating factors is often beneficial. Behavioral intervention may be indicated in cases where psychogenic factors are clearly involved. Antidepressant medications have proved useful in some cases.

Other Headache Complexes

General

The history and physical examination alone usually distinguish headaches other than those due to migraine and tension (Table 13-6) and give direction for further evaluation (Table 13-6). For example, a history of headaches that worsen in the spring or fall may reflect recurrent sinusitis exacerbated by allergies. Caffeine withdrawal is postulated as a cause of some postoperative headaches in adults. Referred pain headaches have many causes, including strabismus, glaucoma, poorly corrected refractive errors, temporomandibular dysfunction (TMJ), dental abscess, and so forth. Analgesic rebound headaches may develop after frequent use of analgesics, often only resolving after a period off the pain medication(s) and caffeine.

Psychogenic headaches are associated with psychiatric disorders and tend to be chronic as well as unresponsive to analgesic medications. The description of these pain complexes can be vivid or vague and they may have dramatic negative effects on the academic or social aspects of the affected teenager. There is often a positive family history for headaches, depression, and/or alcoholism. If depression, anxiety, or other behavioral issues are present, there usually is other evidence of these disorders, in addition to the chronic headaches. The psychogenic aspect behind these headaches may not be obvious and a psychiatric/psychologic diagnosis may not be clear without a thorough evaluation. Headaches that last beyond 7–10 days (especially those lasting weeks to months) fit into this category. Psychogenic headaches often do not respond to analgesic or other migraine medications and require psychiatric/behavioral consultation and therapy.

Cerebrovascular Accident

General

A cerebrovascular accident due to a ruptured congenital aneurysm or arteriovenous malformation can be a particularly serious cause of severe headache in adolescence and constitutes a medical emergency. Rheumatic heart disease, migraine headaches, and previously high estrogen oral contraceptives have been implicated in some studies. The onset tends to be sudden and commonly is occipital, with associated nuchal rigidity, confusion, lethargy, irritability, emesis, pyrexia, and, in 15%, convulsions. There may be a history of antecedent trauma and/or use of anticoagulants. Various neurologic deficits can be found if intracerebral hemorrhage occurs, including aphasia, hemiplegia, vision limitations, and others. A frequent location for aneurysmal hemorrhage is the anterior cerebral artery (proximal part), which produces third cranial nerve damage (pupillary dilatation, ptosis, and lateral eye deviation).

Laboratory Studies

CT of the head is now considered the diagnostic procedure of initial choice and should be performed on an emergent basis; however, the CT can be normal during the early stages of a bleed and thus a negative exam does not rule out a subarachnoid hemorrhage. The finding of blood in the cerebrospinal fluid is diagnostic, but a lumbar puncture should only be done with the greatest of caution because of the danger of brainstem herniation; thus it is done in suspicious cases after a negative CT scan. Further definition as to the site and nature of the causal defect may be obtained through angiography. The occipital location of the headache, infrequent nausea or emesis, presence of nuchal rigidity, and lack of a migraine history help to differentiate subarachnoid hemorrhage from a migraine without aura.

Management

Treatment includes bed rest, analgesics, oxygen, antifibrinolytics (Amicar), anticonvulsants, or surgery. Calcium antagonists (nimodipine and nicardipine) are also currently being used for their selective cerebrovascular effects (vasoconstriction) in cases of subarachnoid hemorrhage. If the patient survives the initial insult, the severity of the pain usually abates in 2–7 days, but full resolution may take several months. Additional neurosurgical evaluation is indicated in assessing the risk of a recurrence and what further intervention is required.

Traction Headaches

Traction headaches are noted with increased intracranial pressure because of hydrocephalus, brain abscess, or brain tumor. Traction headaches tend to occur during the night or upon awakening; this matinal or early morning symptom may be due to interference with cerebrospinal fluid drainage by the space-occupying lesion. The family history tends to be negative for brain tumors, except for the youth with a meningioma. Pain tends to be severe, dull, and consistent in manifestations. Pain and vomiting without nausea or diarrhea, often in the early morning, may be a particular clue; however, it may occur anytime, though usually not in association with meals. Brain tumor (Chap. 18) headaches vary in location, depending on the tumor's site. Papilledema is also present when the lesion is supratentorial but may be absent if it is infratentorial (for example, of the cerebellum or brainstem). In most instances, additional localizing neurologic signs are noted; particular attention should be given to examination of cranial nerves, visual fields, and cerebellar function. Posterior fossa tumors cause ataxia, brain stem gliomas lead to cranial nerve(s), and gait disturbances, while tumors of the cerebral hemispheres result in seizures. Some tumor patients may have headache with major emotional or behavioral changes but minimal neurologic signs. The evaluation of a brain tumor includes head CT, MRI, EEG, evoked responses, angiography, and usually as part of the follow-up, a lumbar puncture. It should be remembered that traction headaches can also be seen after a lumbar puncture removes cerebrospinal fluid. In general, if the CT or MRI is negative as part of the headache evaluation, no other studies are needed. Angiography (with a contrast MRI or arteriogram) is used to distinguish types or masses and/or if a tumor is suspected but the MRI is not definitive.

Others

Post-trauma headaches can occur after mild to severe trauma, can be of various types and duration, and usually start shortly after the accident (within minutes) to a few weeks. Associated symptomatology includes dizziness, vertigo, irritability, sleep difficulties, depression, and anxiety. Some develop a chronic headache pattern that may share many features with migraine without aura. Treatment involves analgesics, antidepressants, and counseling. Subdural hematoma may present only with a history of head trauma and headache. A whiplash injury can result from trauma. Pain and findings on examination can be focused on the occipital and cervical neck areas.

A psychiatric etiology for sudden alteration in personality or mood should be one of exclusion following careful investigation for an underlying organic cause(s). Evaluation for a substance abuse disorder should be part of the evaluation. Seizures in a youth with a history of recurrent, worsening headaches suggests the possibility of a brain neoplasm or vascular malformation. A head CT and/or MRI would be indicated. Migraine with cerebrospinal fluid (CSF) pleocytosis refers to an unusual migraine complex in which white blood cells are noted in the CSF. Current theories suggest that the headache may be precipitated by an upper respiratory tract or influenza-like infection, or that meningeal inflammatory response can be the result of a severe migraine headache. The sick building syndrome refers to a variety of symptoms noted in some individuals who spend a lot of time in modern office buildings. Headache, lethargy, and concentration difficulties are some of the complaints raised. The etiology is unclear, but lack of fresh air with a build-up of building contaminants is suggested, but not proven.

Suggested Readings

Akhhar N, Murray M, Rothner AD: Status migrainous in children and adolescents. *Sem Pediatr Neurol* 8:27–33, 2001.

Cutrer FM, Silberstein SD, Mathew NT, et al.: Antiepileptic drugs in migraine, cluster headache, and mood disorders. *Headache* 41(Suppl 1):S1–S10, 2001.

Lewis DW: Migraine headaches in the adolescent. *Adolesc Med* 13:413–432, 2002.

Lipton RB, Pan J, et al.: Is migraine a progressive brain disease? *JAMA* 291:493–494, 2004.

Mathew NT: Antiepileptic drugs in migraine prevention. *Headache* 41(Suppl 1):S18–S24, 2001.

Pakalnis A: Nonmigraine headaches in adolescents. *Adolesc Med* 13:433–442, 2002.

Rothner AD: Headaches in children and adolescents: Update. *Sem Ped Neurol* 8:2–6, 7–12, 2001.

Silberstein SD: Shared mechanisms and comorbidities in neurologic and psychiatric disorders. *Headache* 41(Suppl 1):S11–S17, 2001.

Zolmitriptan (Zomig) nasal spray for migraine. *Med Lett* 46:7–8, 2004.

PAPILLEDEMA

Benign Intracranial Hypertension

General

Headache (usually persistent), visual disturbances including diplopia (often due to sixth cranial nerve palsy), emesis (with or without nausea), neck stiffness, syncopal attacks (not universal) along with papilledema, and increased spinal fluid pressure comprise benign intracranial hypertension, or pseudotumor cerebri. This term generally refers to an idiopathic decrease in CSF reabsorption by the arachnoid granulations. These symptoms can develop gradually over several days, and there are no other signs of neurologic disorder. In many respects this is a diagnosis of exclusion; other causes of papilledema–primarily space-occupying lesions–must be thoroughly ruled out (Table 13-5), including hydrocephalus (primary or secondary), brain tumor, encephalopathies, CNS infections, and so forth. CSF pressure may exceed 180 mm H_2O and at times reaches 450 mm H_2O. In benign intracranial hypertension, head CT and MRI are normal, except for the possible demonstration of ventricular system compression. Thorough ophthalmologic evaluation is essential, including repeated funduscopic examinations, fundus photographs, intraocular pressure monitoring, repeat visual fields, and others.

Some cases of benign intracranial hypertension are idiopathic. Others may be seen in association with a wide variety of disorders, including young obese women, often with various menstrual disorders. Table 13-10 lists causes or associations of benign intracranial hypertension. A familial pattern is reported in rare situations. In most cases, however, a cause and effect relationship is unclear. The recent addition or withdrawal of certain medications is often an important clue in the development of benign intracranial hypertension.

Management

Treatment includes repeated lumbar punctures with the removal of up to 50 mL of spinal fluid each time to reduce pressure, oral steroids (dexamethasone), and attention to any coexisting related factors as noted above. Hyperosmolar medications, such as glycerin or mannitol, are also used. Acetazolamide (Diamox) is also used; it is a carbonic anhydrase inhibitor that decreases intracranial pressure by decreasing the production of cerebrospinal fluid.

TABLE 13-10

CAUSES/ASSOCIATIONS OF PAPILLEDEMA

Idiopathic[*]	Polyarteritis nodosa
Excess or deficiency of Vitamin A[*]	Iron deficiency anemia
Obesity, often in young women with menstrual dysfunction (hirsutism, galactorrhea, amenorrhea)[*]	Infectious mononucleosis
	Aplastic anemia
Recent menarche (often in obese teenagers)[*]	Polycythemia
Various drugs[*]	Galactorrhea
Thyroid medications, nalidixic acid, oral contraceptives	Hypophosphatasia
	Neurocysticercosis
Steroids (addition or withdrawal), tetracycline, minocycline, lithium	Galactokinase deficiency
	Obstructive nephropathy
Carbonate, tretinoin human chorionic gonadotropin hormone,	Sydenham's chorea
	Infections
Ciprofloxacin, danazol, amiodarone	Cerebral malaria
Hypoparathyroidism	Yersinia pseudotuberculosis
Pituitary hyperplasia	Lyme disease
Post-pituitary surgery	Typhoid fever
Eosinophilic granuloma	Mycoplasma pneumoniae infection
Post-transplantation surgery (heart, renal, bone marrow)	Aseptic meningitis
	Brucellosis
Congenital adrenal hyperplasia	Juvenile retinitis pigmentosa
Addison's disease	Behcet's disease
Head injury	Amaurosis fugax (transient vision loss in one eye due to transient loss of blood flow to the involved eye)
Pregnancy	
Lateral sinus thrombosis (lateral transverse sinus)	Hyperostosis
Mastoiditis	Bell's palsy
Pulmonary disease (carbon dioxide retention)	Others
Right heart failure	
Thoracic tumor (superior vena cava obstruction)	
SLE	

[*]Common causes of pseudotumor cerebri.

Some advocate a weight loss program with small amounts of dexamethasone for the young, obese adolescent. Rarely, surgical decompression may be required, whether optic nerve sheath incision or lumboperitoneal shunting. The prognosis generally is good, but it may take up to 3 months for headaches, papilledema, and other symptoms to improve and up to 12 months for headaches to disappear altogether. Ten percent of all patients experience a recurrence, and a few may have permanent visual impairment due to optic nerve atrophy.

PSEUDOPAPILLEDEMA

Not all instances of blurred optic discs reflect true papilledema. Some cases simply reflect a localized process of the optic nerve head and do not signify increased intracranial pressure. Table 13-11 provides differential points.

Suggested Readings

Albert DM, Jakobiec FA, eds: *Principles and Practice of Ophthalmology.* 2d ed. Philadelphia, PA: W.B. Saunders, 2000, pp. 4769–4770.

Behrman RE, Kliegman RM, Jenson HB, eds: *Nelson Textbook of Pediatrics.* 17th ed. Philadelphia, PA: W.B. Saunders, 2004, Chap. 596, pp. 2048–2049.

Evans RW, Dulli D: Pseudo-pseudotumor cerebri. *Headache* 41:416–418, 2001.

Haslam RHA: Pseudotumor cerebri. In: Behrman RE, Kliegman RM, Jenson HB, eds: *Nelson Textbook of Pediatrics.* 17th ed. Philadelphia, PA: W.B. Saunders, 2004, Chap. 596, pp. 2048–2049.

Kesler A, Fattal-Valevsk A: Idiopathic intracranial hypertension in the pediatric population. *J Child Neurol* 17:745–748, 2002.

Kosmorsky G: Pseudotumor cerebri. *Neurosurg Clin N Amer* 12:775–797, 2001.

CONSCIOUSNESS DISORDERS

Vertigo and Dizziness

Etiology

Vertigo (peripheral or central) is defined as the sensation of feeling oneself spinning in the environment or, alternatively, that the environment is spinning about oneself. The feeling of motion is integral to the diagnosis. Dizziness is defined as light-headedness

TABLE 13-11

PARTIAL DIFFERENTIAL FEATURES OF PAPILLEDEMA AND PSEUDOPAPILLEDEMA

	Papilledema	*Pseudopapilledema*
Definition	Noninflammatory swelling and edema of optic nerve heads with elevation of optic disks due to increased intra cranial pressure.	Indistinct disk margin due to localized cause; generally a benign finding
Disk appearance	Disk elevated; may be hyperemic; margins obliterated	Disk generally not elevated beyond its margins; margins only blurred
Retinal vessels	Dilated and tortuous with deflection and compression of all vessels over disk edge	Usually no abnormality
Retinal pathology	Peripapillary hemorrhages, exudates, and edema may be seen	Often none
Visual fields	Progressively enlarging blind spot	May have enlarged blind spot but not progressive

or giddiness but without the perception of motion. The latter is a common complaint among adolescents, whereas vertigo is rare. The conditions producing dizziness are usually relatively benign, often being related to standing up too quickly (orthostatic hypotension), hyperventilation, or a prodrome of vasovagal syncope. More significant but less common causes include peripheral vestibular disorders, peripheral neuropathy, visual disorders, hypertension, anemia, cerebral hypoxia due to cardiovascular disease, or carotid sinus hypersensitivity, and other neurologic or emotional disorders. Vertigo may also be due to a variety of conditions, generally of a more serious nature (Table 13-12), and sometimes coexistent with dizziness.

Diagnosis

The history is directed at differentiating between these two symptoms and elucidating possible underlying causes, including trauma, tinnitus, unilateral hearing loss, and other evidences of ear disease. Dizziness, turning, and rolling over in bed suggests vertigo. Physical examination is directed to the eyes, ears, heart, and neurologic system. Upright and supine blood pressures are taken to rule out orthostatic hypotension. A lateral jerk nystagmus is often noted with vertigo but not with dizziness. A head-hanging maneuver can be performed to check for positional nystagmus (Table 13-13). Check for a cholesteatoma or for vesicles associated with herpes zoster oticus (Ramsay Hunt syndrome); the latter may present with vertigo, ear vesicles, facial weakness, and deafness.

Laboratory Studies

The Weber and Rinne tests, audiometry, Barony response, caloric testing, electronystagmography (ENG), EEG, electrocardiogram (ECG), visual-evoked response (VER), brainstem auditory evoked response (BAER), somatosensory evoked response (SER), and other procedures as indicated also facilitate diagnosis. The CSF examination is used to evaluate for viral infections or multiple sclerosis. The MRI can identify an acoustic neuroma, other brain tumors, and the plaques of multiple

TABLE 13-12

DIFFERENTIAL DIAGNOSIS OF VERTIGO

Disorders of the ear
  Ceruminosis
  Otitis media
  Deafness
  Labyrinthine disease: benign paroxysmal positional
    vertigo
  Labyrinthitis (vestibular neuronitis)
  Meniere's disease
Head trauma (labyrinthine concussion)
Motion sickness
Otosclerosis
Other ENT disorders
  Herpes zoster oticus (Ramsay Hunt syndrome)
  Cholesteatoma
  Perilymph fistula
  Aminoglycoside ototoxicity
CNS disorders
  Acoustic neuroma
  Vertiginous seizure disorder
  Migraine headache (vertebrobasillar)
  Space-occupying lesions
    Subarachnoid hemorrhage (spontaneous; traumatic)
    Posterior fossa tumor
  Transient ischemic attacks (TIAs) including
    brainstem ischemia
    Vertebrobasilar TIA
  CNS infections:
    Meningitis
    Encephalitis
    Abscess
  Multiple sclerosis
Syncope (see Table 13-14)
Miscellaneous disorders
  Drug toxicity (licit, illicit):
    Aminoglycosides
    Aspirin
    Phenothiazides
    Alcohol
    Phenytoin
    Other CNS depressants
  Metabolic disorders
    Diabetes mellitus
    Hypoglycemia
    Hypothyroidism
    Hyperthyroidism
  Temporomandibular joint syndrome

drop of 20 mm Hg or more, as measured in the standing position, after a supine position (not sitting) for 5–10 minutes. Although many predisposing factors have been identified, a lag in the adjustment of carotid sinus sensitivity in relation to pubertal growth with its rapidly rising center of gravity and expanding blood volume may be a uniquely adolescent phenomenon. Other common associations are prolonged motionless standing, anemia, pregnancy, alcohol or other CNS depressants, tricyclic antidepressants, abuse of diuretics, weight loss (as in an eating disorder), and the administration of some antihypertensive agents or phenothiazines. More serious related conditions are rare in adolescents and, if present, give other indications and are not cited here. Treatment is by reassurance, instructions to rise more slowly from the lying or sitting state, and attention to underlying pathologic conditions. Vulnerable adolescents who must stand for long periods may attenuate their problem by isometric exercises of the legs and thighs.

Hyperventilation

This common phenomenon consists of deep breathing, usually in response to behavioral factors. As the cerebral hypoperfusion continues, numbness of the lips and fingertips develops, along with faintness, blurred vision, and hypocalcemic-induced spasms of facial as well as carpopedal muscles. Electrolyte abnormalities and acid-base imbalances are classic features of the prolonged breathing of hyperventilation. The EEG reveals diffuse slowing during the rapid breathing cycles and no abnormality in between episodes. Breathing into a paper bag or other means to breathe exhaled air usually aborts an acute episode. Attention to underlying emotional factors is necessary for youth presenting with recurrent episodes.

Postmicturition Syndrome

The postmicturition syndrome is occasionally seen among males who consume large amounts of alcohol, fall asleep, rise to urinate, and then faint. This appears to be due to the effects of vasodilation from alcohol and the warmth of the bed in combination with a sudden reflex reduction in the peripheral vascular resistance following bladder emptying. It is also noted in older adults who are on multiple medications and who develop orthostatic hypotension.

Situational Syncope

In addition to postmicturition syndrome, other examples of situational syncope include syncope secondary to severe stool straining (defecation syndrome), severe coughing (cough syncope), swallowing very hot or cold objects (swallow syncope), and exercise syncope (seen in weight lifting). Increased intrathoracic pressure may play a role in some of these types. Swallow syncope may be related to glossopharyngeal neuralgia. Cessation of the syncopal-provoking factor usually improves the syncopal episodes.

Voluntary Syncope

Voluntary syncope is sometimes induced by adolescents seeking an altered mental state. This is another example of situation syncope, and may be accomplished by the sequence of squatting, hyperventilating, standing up rapidly, and performing a Valsalva maneuver. Syncope also may be induced by having someone compress the chest with a sustained bear hug squeeze from behind.

Suggested Readings

Feinberg AN, Lane-Davies A: Syncope in the adolescent. *Adolesc Med* 13:553–567, 2002.

Hannon DW, Knilans TK: Syncope in children and adolescents. *Curr Probl Pediatr* 23(9):358–384, 1993.

Hotson JR, Baloh RW: Acute vestibular syndrome. *New Engl J Med* 339:680–685, 1998.

Soteriades ES, Evans JC, Larson MG, et al: Incidence and prognosis of syncope. *N Engl J Med* 347:878–885, 2002.

Walsh CA: Syncope and sudden death in the adolescent. *Adolesc Med* 12:105–132, 2001.

GUILLAIN-BARRÉ SYNDROME

Etiology

Guillain-Barré syndrome is an inflammatory, demyelinating polyneuropathy, which is characterized by an acute inflammation of the peripheral nerves and is manifested by a symmetric and rapidly ascending paralysis with a variable sensory loss. It has an incidence of 0.6–1.9 per 100,000 in the general population, with a slight predominance in females. The etiology is unknown, but hypersensitivity reactions (to peripheral nerve myelin), toxins, vaccines (as swine flu vaccine), and various viral and bacterial (Mycoplasma) infections have all been implicated at times in attempts to explain the immune attack on peripheral myelin of nerves. In about two thirds of cases the onset occurs 10–21 days after an upper viral respiratory or gastrointestinal tract infection. Cytomegalovirus (CMV) and Ebstein-Barr virus (EBV) are implicated in over 20% of episodes in youths; others include the hepatitis viruses, enteroviruses, *Campylobacter jejuni*, and others. Additional precipitants include pregnancy, lymphoma, and surgery. Identified immune reactions include increased IgG and oligoclonal levels in the CSF, increased antibodies against myelin in the serum and deposition of IgG, IgM, and IgA in Guillain-Barré lesions.

Symptomatology

An initial peripheral neuritis of the lower extremities with tender muscles and reduced deep tendon reflexes (or areflexia) is soon followed by flaccid paralysis. Involvement quickly progresses in an ascending fashion over several hours or days (or even weeks) to affect the abdominal, thoracic, and upper extremity musculature to variable degrees. Motor symptoms tend to occur more than sensory. Paresthesias, myalgias, mild meningeal signs, bulbar symptoms, sensory loss, and cranial nerve palsies may be evident as well. Autonomic dysfunction may develop, as evidenced by varying blood pressures and arrhythmias. Difficulty swallowing and handling secretions may develop, as well as total quadriplegia. Respiratory failure, due to involvement of the diaphragm and accessory muscles of respiration, can develop. Bladder or bowel dysfunction as well as optic nerve disease are usually not noted. The peak of symptoms is usually 3–4 weeks and the average hospitalization is over 30 days.

Laboratory Studies

The CSF characteristically reveals normal pressure, normal glucose, elevated protein (after the first 7 days), and an absence of pleocytosis (under 10 mononuclear leukocytes/square mm). This is called the albuminocytologic dissociation with increased protein but no increase of abnormal cells. Electrophysiologic studies (electromyographic [EMG], nerve studies) demonstrate an acquired demyelinating neuropathy with conduction delay. Electron microscopic studies reveal the presence of macrophages consuming myelin.

Differential Diagnosis

The differential diagnosis includes any condition that also manifests an acute peripheral neuritis or generalized muscular weakness (polyneuropathy). See Table 13-15. A Guillain-Barré syndrome-like disorder is noted in some adults with HIV infection. Diphtheria toxin can cause a GBS-like disorder, with prominent ocular and bulbar symptomatology. A number of lab studies are often done, including evaluating for EBV, CMV, Mycoplasma, and Campylobacter infections.

A number of variants are described, including the Fisher syndrome with areflexia, ataxia, and ophthalmoplegia. Another variant starts with extraocular muscle weakness or paralysis. Adults can develop a related disorder called CIDP (chronic inflammatory demyelinating polyneuropathy). This can have a subacute onset with increased sensory dysfunction and a worsened prognosis.

Prognosis

The prognosis generally is favorable, with symptoms often beginning to reverse after a few days or several weeks; full recovery, however, may take from 2 to 18 months. Adolescents tend to do better than adults, especially if symptoms gradually develop. Complications include pneumonia, paralysis of the muscles of respiration, inappropriate antidiuretic hormone secretion, and, in 1%–2%, death from respiratory failure and/or severe autonomic dysfunction. Motor disability can occur in

TABLE 13-15

**GUILLAIN-BARRÉ SYNDROME:
DIFFERENTIAL DIAGNOSIS**

Poliomyelitis (unimmunized individuals)
Multiple sclerosis
Hereditary sensory motor neuropathies
(as Charcot-Marie-tooth disease)
Toxic neuropathies (multiple drugs and toxins)
Glue sniffing   Thallium
Lead   Gold
Arsenic   Others
Conversion disorder
Polyarteritis nodosa
Wegener's granulomatosis
Other collagen vascular disorders
Lyme disease
Acute intermittent porphyria
Metabolic muscle diseases
Acute transverse myelopathy
Spinal cord tumor
Tethered cord
Myasthenia gravis
Acute cerebellar ataxia
Tic paralysis
Behçet's disease
Botulism
Cerebrovascular accident
Hypokalemic periodic paralysis
Diphtheria
Others

Table 13-15 is a partial list.

25%, including chronic muscle weakness and joint contractures. CIDP may be part of a recurrence or relapse picture in adults.

Management

Treatment is nonspecific, including ventilatory support, high quality nursing care, and physiotherapy to help prevent joint contractures. Steroids have been used but are without a clearly proven beneficial role. Plasma exchange therapy (plasmapheresis) and IV gamma globulin (IgG) therapy have been helpful by some reports. Plasmapheresis

has been noted to be of value for those within 7 days of acute symptoms to help reduce the incidence of the need for a ventilator or improve respiratory failure. Azathioprine has been studied but not shown to be of therapeutic value for the Guillain-Barré syndrome.

Suggested Readings

Joseph SA, Tsao C-Y: Guillain-Barré syndrome. *Adolesc Med* 13:487–494, 2002.

Haber P, DeStefano F, Angulo FJ et al.: Guillain-Barré syndrome following influenza vaccination. *JAMA* 292:2478–2481, 2004.

Hadden RD, Karch H, Hartung HP, et al.: Preceding infections, immune factors, and outcome in Guillain-Barré syndrome. *Neurology* 56:758–765, 2001.

Ropper AH: The Guillain-Barré syndrome. *N Engl J Med* 326(17):1130–1136, 1992.

BELL'S PALSY

Etiology

Bell's palsy is marked by the acute onset of facial weakness due to inflammation and compression of the seventh cranial nerve as it passes through the temporal bone. A positive family history is noted in some and an incidence of 23/100,000 is observed in adults and there is a female to male ratio of 2:1 and 10% of patients are teenagers. Neural dysfunction is thought to be due to nerve compression by neural edema within the narrow confines of the osseous facial nerve canal. The canal is narrowest in its labyrinthine segment and constriction appears to be most severe at this site. The most common result is spasm of the orbicularis oculi muscle with possible progression to the other muscles involved with facial expression. Disruption of the facial nerve at the stylomastoid foramen results in paralysis of all the muscles of facial expression on one side. Lesions of the nerves that are located in the facial canal above the junction with the chorda tympani but below the geniculate ganglion lead to both muscle paralysis and loss of taste over the anterior two thirds of the tongue. If a facial nerve is compressed or severed in the auditory canal, hearing loss usually occurs as well, due to involvement of the eighth cranial nerve. Intrapontine lesions that paralyze the face often also affect the abducens nucleus and the corticospinal and sensory tracts. Hypesthesia of the trigeminal nerve can develop also.

Though no clear etiology has been identified, diabetes mellitus does appear to be a risk factor for Bell's palsy. Also, acute otitis media, herpes simplex virus, and herpes zoster have been implicated; however, these associations are usually inconsistent. Recent reports note the spirochete of Lyme disease (*Borrelia burgdorferi*) can cause Bell's palsy with CSF pleocytosis. Research is looking at a link with intranasal vaccines. Other specific agents may also be identified. Current theory implicates an inflammatory response to a viral infection of the CNS. Bell's palsy can complicate the course of various disorders, including mastoiditis, diabetes mellitus, hyperthyroidism, pseudotumor cerebri, SLE, head trauma, and various CNS disorders.

Symptomatology

The appearance of weakness takes place rapidly over several hours and is usually without other symptoms or signs other than possible ear pain on the affected side. Progression to maximum paralysis usually develops in 2–5 days. Characteristic findings include the loss of the nasolabial fold, a drooping mouth corner, an inability to shut the eyelid, and a pulling of the mouth to the normal side on smiling or grimacing. Decreased tear formation, loss of taste over the anterior two thirds of the tongue, hyperacusis, and other auditory symptoms may also be evident, depending on the precise location and extent of the inflammation. The nerve damage is assessed by the physical examination and by electrophysiologic studies. Most patients recover spontaneously within a few weeks or months, but 10%–20% sustain permanent injury–5% severe. Recurrent cases of Bell's palsy can be seen. Imaging studies (MRI) can be done for Bell's palsy, which presents with atypical features: severe pain, involvement of more than 1 cranial nerve, mixed sensory-motor symptoms, slowly progressive symptoms, features that last over 2 months, and others.

Differential Diagnosis

The differential diagnosis includes any other lesion that may cause facial nerve palsy; these include brain tumor, skull fracture, meningitis, sarcoidosis, radiation therapy effects, parotid gland tumors, facial or trigeminal nerve neuroma, and other tumors (adenocarcinoma, lymphoma, melanoma, malignant paraganglioma, and so forth). Lyme disease is identified by many clinicians as a major etiologic agent in endemic areas. The Melkersson syndrome is a rare idiopathic condition marked by recurrent episodes of seventh nerve weakness and edema of the lips. Facial nerve paralysis may also be caused by nerve compression due to hemorrhage into the parotid gland or by sarcoid granulomatous infiltration and enlargement of the parotid gland (Heerfordt syndrome or uveoparotid fever).

Management

Treatment is first directed at protecting the cornea on the involved side by periodic irrigation with methylcellulose eyedrops and keeping the eye patched or taped shut. Steroids are used by some clinicians at the first signs of disease in an attempt to reduce the degree of nerve swelling and avoid permanent damage; however, there is no established proof of efficacy for this approach that often involves using prednisone, 40 mg/day for 3 days, and then tapered over 1 week. If some cases of Bell's palsy are linked to a viral etiology in children or adolescents, the use of steroids is questioned by some clinicians. If Lyme disease is noted, appropriate antibiotic therapy is necessary, as ceftriaxone, doxycycline, or ampicillin. Surgical decompression of the nerve itself has been tried when suggested by deteriorating electropotentials as measured by electromyography; however, this method also has not been proven to be effective.

Suggested Readings

Couch RB: Nasal vaccination, Escherichia coli enterotoxin, and Bell's palsy. *N Engl J Med* 350:860–861, 2004.
Peitersen E: Natural history of Bell's palsy. *Acta Otolaryngol Suppl (Stockh)* 492:122–124, 1992.

Shapiro ED, Gerber MA: Lyme disease and facial nerve palsy. *Arch Pediatr Adolesc Med* 151:1183, 1997.

Sarnat HB: Bell's palsy. In: Behrman RE, Kliegman RM, Henson HB, eds: *Nelson Textbook of Pediatrics.* 17th ed. Philadelphia, PA: Elsevier, 2004, Chap. 608. pp. 2081–2082.

Salman MS, MacGregor DL: Should children with Bell's palsy be treated with corticosteroids? A systematic review. *J Child Neurol* 26:565, 2001.

Tong JT: Blepharospasm and Bell Palsy In: Rudolph CD, Rudoplh AM, eds: *Rudolph's Pediatrics.* 21st ed. New York: McGraw-Hill, 2003, Chap. 26.4.6, p. 2366.

TIC DISORDERS

General

Tics (habit spasms) are sudden, brief, purposeless, involuntary, highly stereotyped movements that must be differentiated clinically from chorea, myoclonus, athetosis, dystonia, hemiballism, and tremor (Table 13-16). Tic disorders are divided into three basic groups: transient tic disorder, chronic motor tic disorder, and the Gilles de la Tourette syndrome.

Transient Tic Disorder

The transient tic disorder is described in 4%–20% of children (including young teenagers). One or more motor movements can develop that lasts at least 1 month but disappear spontaneously within 1 year, usually within several weeks. Voluntary suppression of the tics can occur for minutes to hours and the spasms may be stress related. The tics may be eye blinking, facial grimacing, shoulder shrugging, or others. Vocal tics are not present and in unusual cases, more than one motor tic is noted. There is a 2–3:1 male:female ratio and there is often a positive family history for tics. Specific treatment, except for reassurance, is not usually recommended. Observation for tic progression should be encouraged.

Chronic Motor Tic Disorder

Chronic motor tic disorder or chronic tic disorder involves more than three muscle groups at any one time, which are voluntarily suppressible for minutes to hours and are characterized by a persistent intensity for weeks to months. The overall disorder lasts

TABLE 13-16

DEFINITIONS OF VARIOUS INVOLUNTARY MUSCLE MOVEMENTS

Type	Definition
Athetosis	Slow, sinuous, writhing, involuntary movement that most frequently involves distal extremities; frequently increased by voluntary movements
Ballismus	Wild, flinging, coarse, irregular, involuntary movements beginning in proximal limb muscles.
Chorea	Rapid, irregular, nonrepetitive, sudden movement that may involve any muscle or muscle group; these movements generally interfere with voluntary movements.
Dystonia	Slow, twisting, involuntary movements associated with changes in muscle tone; movements generally involve trunk and proximal extremity muscles.
Myoclonus	Involuntary rapid, shocklike muscular contractions that are generally nonrepetitive; can be increased by voluntary actions.
Spasm	A slow and prolonged involuntary contraction of a muscle or group of muscles.
Tic	Involuntary, repetitive movement of related groups of muscles; movements do not interfere with voluntary muscle movements.
Tremor	Involuntary movement that may be a slow or rapid vibration of the involved body part; tremors may get worse with movement (intentional tremor) or may occur only at rest.

Source: Used with permission from S Kuperman, Tic disorders in children and adolescents. In: *Behavioral Pediatrics.* DE Greydanus and ML Wolraich, eds, New York: Springer-Verlag, 1992, Chap. 33, p. 452.

at least 1 year according to classification criteria. It is noted in approximately 1.6% of the population and it may be related to Tourette syndrome. A positive family history may be noted and the etiology is linked to a CNS dopamine metabolism dysfunction. Treatment with pharmacologic agents as haloperidol may be helpful. See below, under Tourette syndrome.

Gilles de la Tourette Syndrome

Epidemiology

The most severe of the complex tic disorders is the Gilles de la Tourette syndrome, which occurs in 5/10,000 and is 10 times more common in children as opposed to adults. There is a 3–4:1 male:female ratio. The onset is usually between 2 and 15 years (up to age 21 by definition) and the typical age of onset is usually stated as 7 years. Tourette's symptoms are present for at least 1 year before the criteria for Tourette syndrome are met. There is often a positive family history for tics (Tourette syndrome and/or chronic tic disorder) and research suggests that it is inherited as a highly penetrant, sex-influenced, autosomal dominant trait. Frequently, there is also a positive family history for attention-deficit/hyperactivity disorder (ADHD), learning disorders, obsessive-compulsive disorder (OCD), sleep disturbances, and nonspecific EEG changes.

Etiology

Theories vary and currently include dysfunction in CNS circuits linking such areas as the frontal lobe, thalamus, striatum, and globus palludum. A recent theory involves possible complications of infection with Group A beta-hemolytic streptococci and links with PANDAS (pediatric autoimmune neuropsychiatric disorders associated with streptococci).

Symptomatology

In this unusual neuropsychiatric disorder, which is etiologically linked to dopamine, and serotonin dysfunction, there is a combination of multiple, simple, or complex motor tics (involving the head, neck, trunk, and upper or lower extremities) with vocal tics (coughing, grunting, shouting, crying, barking, throat clearing, sniffing, and others). Complex vocal tics include echolalia (repeating words), palilalia (repeating the last sound), and the classic coprolalia (swearing). Common motor tics include eye blinking, lip smacking, shoulder shrugging, head tossing, grimacing, and so forth.

Motor tics usually begin before vocal tics, and the presenting symptom is a single tic in 50% and multiple tics in 50%. The most common motor tics involve the head and neck, while the trunk is involved in 50%, and the lower extremity in 40%. The presenting tic is the eye tic in 37% versus the head tic in 16%; a vocal tic is the presenting symptom in 18%. Coprolalia is the presenting feature in 0.1%, but eventually is noted in about one-third of patients, usually starting at age 13–14. Complex motor tics can occur, such as skipping, jumping, squatting, and hitting oneself or others. In 3% of Tourette's patients, sensory tics are present, in which an unpleasant sensation develops about a joint(s) or muscle group(s), which is relieved by a tic. There is a complex pattern of changing symptomatology that seems to occur independent of treatment. The adolescent can usually voluntarily suppress the tic temporarily until a feeling of unpleasantness becomes overwhelming and is only relieved by expression of the tic itself.

ADHD is noted in 30%–50% of patients with Tourette syndrome and usually develops first. Teenagers with Tourette syndrome have an increased incidence of other learning disorders (with or without ADHD), enuresis, OCD, oppositional defiant disorder, difficulties with anger and discipline, exhibitionism, and other behavioral disorders. Studies differ on the exact risk for OCD (33%–60+%) and various ritualistic behaviors can develop, including handwashing, touching, repetitive thoughts (aggressive, sexual), and others. Youth with Tourette syndrome often have various soft neurologic signs on examination, nonspecific EEG changes, and abnormal neuropsychologic findings; the precise influence of ADHD on these abnormalities is unclear.

Management

Comprehensive behavioral treatment must be provided for the youth and his/her family. The patient, family, and others (e.g., school personnel) must be educated about this very difficult disorder. Comorbid disorders (ADHD, OCD, other anxiety disorders, mood disorders, and oppositional defiant disorder) must also be comprehensively managed. Psychologic treatment, such as behavioral therapy, may be helpful.

Psychopharmacologic therapy includes the use of dopamine receptor antagonists (haloperidol, pimozide or *atypical antipsychotics* as risperidone or ziprasidone), alpha-2-receptor agonists (clonidine or guanfacine), and possibly stimulant medications (as methylphenidate). Coexistent OCD may be improved with selective serotonin reuptake inhibitors (SSRIs, e.g., fluoxetine [Prozac], sertraline [Zoloft], or paroxetine [Paxil]). Also helpful for OCD are the tricyclic antidepressants (e.g., imipramine Tofranil and amitryptiline Elavil) and the antidepressant, bupropion (Wellburtin). The use of psychostimulant drugs (e.g., methylphenidate Ritalin) to treat coexist attention-deficit/hyperactivity disorder can occasionally precipitate Tourette syndrome and in 33%, can worsen the tics in a youth with known Tourette syndrome. Its use for tic disorders is controversial, but it is used by some clinicians as a last medication resort if other medications are not helping to control the symptoms (especially if clonidine is not beneficial) and/or to treat severe sedative effects of haloperidol or pimozide.

Medications (e.g., haloperidol, respiradone, clonidine, pimozide) may suppress Tourette's symptoms but do not cure the disorder. Youth placed on neuroleptic medications often develop significant side effects as noted in Table 13-17. The incidence of

TABLE 13-17

MEDICATIONS FOR TOURETTE SYNDROME

Medications & Dose	Side Effects
Haloperidol (Haldol): Start with 0.5 mg HS; adjust q 5 days, average dose: 5 mg/day, maximum: 2–5 mg b.i.d. or t.i.d. (higher only with great caution)	Sedation, weight gain, decreased cognitive performance, irritability; anticholinergic symptoms; gynecomastia; lactation; acute dystonia; akinesia; akathisia; extrapyramidal symptoms, including tardive dyskinesia; others
Risperidone (Risperidol): *Atypical antipsychotic*; start with 0.25–0.5 mg at bedtime; raise weekly by 0.25 or 0.5 mg if necessary; range of effective daily dose: 0.5–4.0 mg given at bedtime or twice daily	There are reduced extrapyramidal side effects with atypical antipsychotics; main side effects of risperidone are weight gain and sedation
Pimozide (Orap) start: 2 mg/day; increase q 1 week; average dose: 2–12 mg/day; give in divided doses	Same as haloperidol; can also see a prolonged Q-T-c interval; get baseline and periodic electrocardiogram
Clonidine (Clonidine; Catapress) Initial dose: 0.05 mg/day; daily dose: 0.25 mg/day; give b.i.d. or t.i.d.; Range: 0.1 mg–0.4 mg/day	Sedation; orthostatic hypotension; dry mouth, headaches, irritability; sleep disturbances; less common: decreased glucose tolerance and worsening of preexisting cardiac arrhythmias; get baseline ECG and baseline glucose.
Guanfacine (Tenex); daily dosage range is 0.5–4 mg	Similar side effects to clonidine, including headaches, dizziness, and lethargy, may induce more agitation and headaches than clonidine.

extrapyramidal side effects is much lower with the atypical antipsychotics, such as risperidone, and the efficacy for Tourette's disorders similar to haloperidol or pimozide. Approximately 25% of patients on haloperidol (Haldol) note a 70% reduction in Tourette's symptoms at a low enough dose to avoid serious side effects. Approximately 50% note improvement but only at a dose that causes significant side effects while 25% are treatment failures, either because haloperidol is not effective or only effective at too high a dose, resulting in unacceptable side effects. Pimozide (Orap) can lead to 70%–80% improvement in Tourette's symptoms and often with less side effects, compared to haloperidol. Major side effects of risperidone are weight gain and sedation.

Prognosis

The prognosis for Tourette syndrome is varied, with spontaneous remissions in late adolescence described in 10%–20% of the patients and in others at least an improvement in the symptoms is noted. Very careful titration of the medication(s) is necessary, seeking to use the lowest dose that reduces the Tourette symptomatology to acceptable levels. Genetic counseling is important, since there is an increased risk for Tourette syndrome and chronic tic disorder in family members. For example, if a parent has Tourette syndrome, there is a 50% transmission to the son and a 35% transmission to the daughter. This transmission can be Tourette's, chronic tic disorder, OCD. Approximately 10% of those with Tourette's are socially impaired.

Suggested Readings

Tic Disorders. In: *Diagnostic and Statistical Manual of Mental Disorders DSM-IV* 4th ed. Washington DC: American Psychiatric Association, 1994, pp. 100–105.

Greydanus DE, Sloane MA, Rappley MA: Psychopharmacology of ADHD in adolescents. *Adolesc Med* 13:599–624, 2002.

Greydanus DE, Pratt HD: Attention-deficit/hyperactivity disorder in children and adolescents: Interventions for a complex costly clinical conundrum. *Pediatric Clin North Am* 50:1049–1092, 2003

Kuperman S: Tic disorders in children and adolescents. In: Greydanus DE, ML Wolraich, eds: *Behavioral Pediatrics.* New York: Springer-Verlag, 1992, Chap. 33, pp. 451–463.

Kuperman S: Tic disorders in the adolescent. *Adolesc Med* 13:537–551, 2002.

Varley CK, Smith CJ: Anxiety disorders in the child and teen. *Pediatr Clin North Am* 50:1107–1138, 2003.

CEREBRAL PALSY

General

Cerebral palsy is an umbrella term covering a group of nonprogressive, but often changing, motor impairment syndromes secondary to lesions or anomalies of the brain arising in the early stages of its development. Over 100,000 individuals under age 18 are diagnosed with cerebral palsy, which has an estimated incidence of 4 per 1000 live births. Table 13-18 reviews current classification criteria. Usually it has been diagnosed in early childhood and primarily poses therapeutic rather than diagnostic problems in the adolescent, with all the considerations raised by a chronic illness of any type. Mild degrees of cerebral palsy, however, may be missed until adolescence, when limb size disparity is magnified by pubertal growth, earlier clumsiness' is not outgrown, or the increased demands for coordination and athletic competence bring formerly modest, compensated deficits to greater light.

TABLE 13-18

CRITERIA FOR CEREBRAL PALSY CLASSIFICATION

A. Extremities involved
  1. Monoplegia
  2. Hemiplegia
  3. Diplegia
  4. Quadriplegia

B. Type of neurologic dysfunction
  1. Spastic type
  2. Hypotonic type
  3. Dystonic type
  4. Athetotic type
  5. Combinations

Symptomatology

Cerebral palsy is characterized by increased deep tendon reflexes, positive Babinski's signs, clonus, and spastic diplegia, together with a tendency toward contracture of involved muscle groups. Puberty tends to increase the disproportion between affected and non-affected extremities consequent to the former's restricted growth. Approximately 33% have epilepsy (50% with hemiplegia) and progressive scoliosis may develop in early adolescence. A number will have visual-motor disabilities, learning or cognitive disabilities, speech problems, scoliosis, extrapyramidal abnormalities, and epilepsy. The risk of these disabilities increases with the increased severity of the cerebral palsy. Approximately 30% are classified with mental retardation.

Management

Treatment is rehabilitative and behavioral. Muscle relaxers are used, such as diazepam, baclofen, and dantrolene. Scopolamine patches may help with the chronic problem of drooling. Botulinum toxin (Botox) is used in cases of chronic spasm. Careful titration of antiseizure medications is necessary for youths with epilepsy.

Suggested Readings

Bottos M, Feliciangeli A, Sciuto LS, et al.: Functional status of adults with cerebral palsy and implications for treating children. *Dev Med Child Neurol* 431:516–528, 2001.

Johnston MC: Cerebral palsy. In: Behrman RE, Kliegman RM, Henson HB, eds: *Nelson Textbook of Pediatrics.* 17th ed. Philadephia, PA: Elsevier Science-Saunders, 2004, Chap. 591.1, pp. 2024–2025.

Krach LE: Pharmacotherapy of spasticity: oral medications and intrathecal beclofen. *J Child Neurol* 16:31–6, 2001.

Wollack JB, Nichter CA: Cerebral palsy. In: Rudolph CD, Rudolph AM, eds: *Rudolph's Pediatrics.* 21st ed. New York: MCGraw-Hill Medical Publishing, 2003, Chap. 25.5.1, pp. 2197–2202.

C H A P T E R

14

SLEEP DISORDERS IN THE ADOLESCENT

John N. Schuen

INTRODUCTION

Knowledge of sleep disorders has grown tremendously over the last decade, shedding light on previously under-diagnosed disorders that have plagued the adolescent population for centuries. With newly established pediatric clinical guidelines, primary care providers, sleep specialists, and the media have begun to spread the word about sleep disorders in young people. Pediatric sleep centers have arisen around the country to help uncover sleep disorders and guide management. Entirely new disorders are being identified and novel approaches to well-known adolescent sleep problems are being uncovered. Current principles of sleep disorder management are reviewed in this chapter. Standard abbreviations used in discussing sleep disorders are listed in Box 14-1.

SLEEP IN THE ADOLESCENT POPULATION

Significance of the Problem

The National Sleep Foundation (NSF) recently commissioned a study looking into adolescent sleep behavior.[1] Although our adolescents require between 8.8 and 9.5 hours of sleep, the vast majority

is getting far less.[2] Wolfson and Carskadon[3] reported that, during the school week, the mean hours of sleep in adolescents, 19 years of age or younger, was significantly less than 8 hours. In the same report, more than 25% of adolescents slept 6.5 hours or less. Sleep deprivation in an American adolescent is no surprise, considering contributing factors such as

BOX 14-1

ABBREVIATIONS USED IN SLEEP DISORDERS

PSG	Polysomnography/polysomnogram
EOG	Electro-oculogram
EtCO$_2$	End-tidal carbon dioxide
PS	Primary snoring
UARS	Upper airway resistance syndrome
OSAS	Obstructive sleep apnea syndrome
OH	Obstructive hypoventilation
SRBD	Sleep-related breathing disorders
RDI	Respiratory distress index
OI	Obstructive index
AHI	Apnea + hypopnea index
PAP	Positive airway pressure
CPAP	Continuous positive airway pressure
BiPAP	Bi-level positive airway pressure
PLMD	Periodic limb movement disease

academic demands, extracurricular activities, social demands, after school jobs, and early high school start times. Daytime sleepiness represents an inconvenience when a term paper is due the next day; however, when an adolescent falls asleep driving on a highway, the outcome may be deadly. In 1994, the National Highway Transportation Safety Administration (NHTSA) reported that more than 50% of all drowsy-driving motor vehicle accidents were caused by drivers under the age of 25 years.[4] A more recent report notes that 44% of drivers under the age of 21 years say that they experienced falling asleep while driving in the last 6 months.[5] Yet, the 2003 NHTSA report also noted that adolescents were significantly less likely to take action (e.g., napping on roadside, getting off the road, or getting out of the car to stretch) that would increase wakefulness than older adults. Therefore, young and relatively inexperienced drivers pose a tremendous risk for the rest of drivers on the road when sleep deprivation occurs.

Normal Sleep

Understanding normal adolescent sleep serves as an important foundation for care providers to assess appropriate sleep duration and habits. The NSF report noted key features of adolescent physiologic and social change, which are detailed in Table 14-1.[1] Given that these features are so common, providers need to proactively educate preadolescents and families on common sleep-related problems. Also, the first ever percentile curves with standard deviation were published from Switzerland for infants, children, and adolescents.[6]

Sleep stages occur throughout the life span and can be identified even in the neonatal period. Humans enter sleep via nonrapid eye movement (NREM)

TABLE 14-1

KEY FEATURES OF ADOLESCENT SLEEP ADAPTED FROM THE NATIONAL SLEEP FOUNDATION REPORT

Physiologic features

- Adolescents require at least as much sleep as they did as preadolescents (8.5–9.5 h per night).
- Daytime sleepiness increases. Even in the presence of normal amounts of sleep, adolescents are sleepier than prepubescent young people.
- Adolescent sleep patterns undergo a phase delay that is physiologic. Sleep-related phase delay represents an internal tendency to fall asleep and awaken later in the day.

Behavioral and psychosocial features

- Many U.S. adolescents do not get enough sleep, especially during the week.
- Adolescents have irregular sleep patterns, in particular, their weekend sleep schedules are very different from their weekday schedules, to some extent as a direct consequence of weekday sleep loss.
- Irregular sleep schedules—including significant discrepancies between weekdays and weekends—can contribute to a shift in sleep phase, trouble falling asleep or awakening, and fragmental (poor quality) sleep.

Consequences of poor sleep quantity and/or quality in adolescents

- Increased risk of unintentional injuries and death
- Low grades and poor school performance
- Negative moods
- Inability to stay focused
- Impulsivity
- Difficulty completing tasks
- Aggressive behaviors
- Increased likelihood of stimulant use

Source: National Sleep Foundation: Adolescent Sleep Needs and Patterns: A Research Report and Resource Guide. Washington, DC, National Sleep Foundation, 2000.

sleep, which is composed of light and deep sleep stages. Stage 1 and Stage 2 make up the first category, while Stage 3 and Stage 4 represent slow-wave or delta sleep. Rapid eye movement (REM) sleep is characterized by loss of muscle tone and a significant variability in the regulation of bodily functions, such as temperature, blood pressure, respiratory rate, and heart rate. In the adolescent, REM sleep occurs approximately every 60–90 minutes throughout the sleep cycle. Therefore, the average adolescent experiences 4–6 sleep cycles in a night's sleep. Although we briefly awake between sleep cycles, these micro-arousals are so brief that we do not recall them and this is considered normal. The architecture of sleep also changes slowly but significantly throughout the second decade of life. As compared with toddlers and older children, adolescents have significantly less slow-wave sleep (Stages 3 and 4). Slow-wave sleep is restorative in nature, and approximately 40% decline occurs between 10 and 20 years of age, resulting in a modestly less efficient night's sleep in the adolescent. There is also a gradual decrease in the amount of REM sleep.[7] These changes represent subtle changes in sleep pattern and efficiency that contribute to longer sleep duration and needs than the general population normally expects.

SLEEP DISORDERS

Overview

It is no surprise that the most common sleep complaint in adolescence is excessive daytime sleepiness. By far, the overwhelming majority of these cases represent insufficient or inadequate sleep from a variety of external causes and pressures. Mercer and coworkers reported, via a questionnaire given to high school freshmen, that 63% of the adolescents in the study (especially females) wanted more sleep on school nights.[8] Table 14-2 provides a list of common reasons for why young people may find themselves sleepy. When parents or young people seek their medical provider for assistance, many will have a chaotic sleep pattern that is readily evident by history. If questions remain after history and physical examination, a

TABLE 14-2

ETIOLOGY OF EXCESSIVE DAYTIME SLEEPINESS IN THE ADOLESCENT

Common causes

Inadequate amounts of sleep

Poor sleep hygiene

Obstructive sleep apnea syndrome

Delayed sleep phase syndrome

Use of caffeine or other drugs/alcohol

Withdrawal from or use of illegal drugs/alcohol

Uncommon causes

Insomnia

Psychiatric illnesses

Narcolepsy

Kleine-Levin syndrome

Periodic limb movement disease restless leg syndrome

Movement disorders (e.g., paroxysmal nocturnal dystonia)

Parasomnias (e.g., pavor nocturnus and somnambulism)

number of tools are available to the clinician to uncover sleep-related problems.

A sleep diary, available from a variety of commercial sources, represents a preprinted age appropriate method of recording sleep and wakefulness. It provides patients an efficient way to record their sleep and wakefulness cycles over a 24-hour period each day for typically 1–3 weeks. When kept accurately, by either the adolescent or a parent (and sometimes both), a sleep diary frequently identifies trends and problems in the sleep-wake cycle.

Actigraphy represents another tool of the sleep physician that identifies motion over extended periods of time (i.e., days to weeks). Now utilized in clinical medicine for over a decade, actigraphy has become a well validated tool for the adolescent population.[9] Actigraphs are worn on the wrist or ankle and have measures in size and weight similar to a wrist watch. Motion is automatically recorded over a specific, modifiable time interval (e.g., motion per minute of time), and then downloaded to a proprietary software program to graphically illustrate motion over time. In more sophisticated devices, light may be recorded and even specific event markers are available. The basic actigraph tracks motion and may be used to determine wakefulness (motion) and sleep (no or very little motion). Actigraph records help to uncover sleep-wake cycles over many days, and understand sleepiness in an adolescent when sleep diaries are not completed, or in the presence of a normal polysomnogram (PSG).[10] When combined with a sleep diary, they are even more powerful in elucidating sleep-wake cycles in the patient.

Like every test, actigraphy has limitations. Actigraphy may overestimate sleep time in individuals with insomnia, due to prolonged periods of quiet wakefulness typically spent in bed. Actigraphy may underestimate sleep in people who have movement disorders, because regular movement of the extremity (e.g., periodic limb movement disorder) gives the false impression of wakefulness.[11] In many cases, this diagnostic tool can dramatically improve the clinician's picture of circadian cycle of the adolescent.

When daytime symptoms put the adolescent at risk for obstructive sleep apnea syndrome (OSAS) or fail to be explained by sleep diaries or by history and physical examination, a sleep study—PSG—is often diagnostic. The PSG monitors a patient's night sleep in a sleep laboratory for a minimum of 6 hours in the presence of an experienced sleep technician. Pediatric sleep laboratories are designed specifically for infants, children, and adolescents and their special developmental as well as ergonomic needs. A sleep study measures EEG (brain waves), EOG (eye movements), electromyographic (EMG) (chin and tibial movements), electrocardiogram (ECG) (lead two), heart rate trend, oronasal airflow, nasal pressure, oxyhemoglobin saturations, end-tidal carbon dioxide ($EtCO_2$) level, movements of the chest and abdomen, and a video record of the study. Pediatric standards for child and adolescent sleep studies were originally published in 1996 by the American Thoracic Society,[12] and normal PSG values were originally published by Carole Marcus and colleagues in 1992.[13] Additional studies, such as expanded seizure montages to identify epileptiform activity or multiple sleep latency testing to diagnose narcolepsy, also expand the capabilities of the basic nocturnal PSG.

Poor Sleep Hygiene

The most common sleep problem plaguing our youth today is poor sleep hygiene. The reasons for poor sleep hygiene are numerous but all result in significant consequences of poor quality and/or quantity of sleep as mentioned in Table 14-1. Environmental causes include hot or cold bedrooms, loud noise, excessive light, video games, television, radio, or CD players that continue throughout the night disrupting sleep. Other common causes include irregular sleep times, eating within 2 hours of bedtime, and strenuous activity or stimulants. Caffeine, the most common worldwide stimulant available, is known to disrupt sleep even when consumed in small quantities in the morning. When consumed in the afternoon or evening, caffeine causes significant insomnia, frequent awakenings, and disrupted sleep architecture at any age. History, actigraphy, and sometimes even sleep studies provide clues that identify poor sleep hygiene. Changing environment and behavior early in life is important because adolescents will frequently continue either positive or poor sleep hygiene into adulthood leading to a lifetime of alertness or sleepiness.

Delayed Sleep Phase Disorder

Some adolescents experience a pathologic shift toward later and later bedtimes, which is felt to be, at least in part, a circadian rhythm disturbance. A delayed sleep phase syndrome (DSPS) occurs when the individual falls asleep at progressively later bedtimes (and subsequent later rise times) every night. By definition, this problem persists over at least a 6 month period.[14] Weekends, holidays, and vacations may potentiate the problem, but sleepiness occurs when the weekdays require waking up at an earlier time than the young adult is accustomed to. Sleep onset can be significantly delayed to 3:00 a.m. or later and if the patient is allowed, the rise time occurs in the afternoon. When the patient is forced to conform to the typical early morning high school start times, it becomes difficult or impossible to arouse the adolescent. Daytime sleepiness is the typical consequence and is perpetuated by "napping." Although, experts have uncovered that most adolescents have some modest phase delay as a normal physiologic change through adolescence, it is important to rule out behavioral etiologies such as school avoidance. Ferber notes that there are several distinguishing features between DSPS and overt school avoidance, or school refusal syndrome.[15] In the sleep laboratory, the PSG is normal and usually the adolescent does not have difficulty waking up as long as the wake time is later in the morning.

Multiple therapies are frequently employed simultaneously to keep a person with DSPS awake and alert during the daytime. Chronotherapy is a therapeutic intervention used to reset the circadian clock and get the adolescent back to a more academically appropriate bedtime.[16] Bedtime is systematically delayed by 3 hour increments each day until the desired bedtime is reached and the 24 hour day is then established. Once desirable sleep-wake times are achieved, strict sleep hygiene is required to maintain ongoing success. This includes regular bedtimes, avoidance of naps, a quiet sleep-promoting environment, regular daytime physical activity, and bright light in the morning. Successful light therapy as the only intervention for DSPS was demonstrated by Rosenthal and colleagues in 1990 using 2500 lux for 2 hours from 7 to 9 a.m.[17] In general, bright light from 2500 to 10,000 lux for 1–2 hours per day represents therapeutic light exposure that will shift circadian sleep and core body temperature rhythms.[18] Exogenous melatonin has emerged as another beneficial therapy for circadian rhythm disturbances.

Narcolepsy

Narcolepsy represents the intrusion of REM sleep at inappropriate times while awake. The classic diagnostic pentad of narcolepsy is noted in Table 14-3.[19] The prevalence of narcolepsy in the general population is 0.03% to 0.16%, which is similar to cystic fibrosis.[19] Although narcolepsy often begins in adolescence or early adulthood, diagnosis may be delayed for years due to the subtle onset and indolent progression of this disorder. Only a tiny percentage of adolescent patients have all the characteristics of narcolepsy (Table 14-3). Since

TABLE 14-3

FEATURES OF NARCOLEPSY

Excessive daytime sleepiness
Cataplexy
Hypnagogic hallucinations
Sleep paralysis
REM onset sleep

excessive daytime sleepiness is a frequent complaint in the teenage population, this disease may be attributed to sleep deprivation or poor sleep hygiene for many months or years, thereby delaying accurate diagnosis. Morrish and colleagues reported a median delay of 10.5 years in their report on narcolepsy from the United Kingdom.[20]

Clinical presentation of narcolepsy varies from quite subtle to distinctly abnormal. The sudden onset of sleep usually occurs during sedentary activity, but may occur during quiet mealtimes, standing, or even as a spectator in an auditorium. A transient loss of facial or limb muscle tone without a change in consciousness, called cataplexy, is present in majority of narcoleptic adults; however, this occurs rarely in adolescence and children. Strong emotions or unsettling events (e.g., suddenly scared) may trigger a cataplectic attack, which results in brief decrease or loss of striated muscle tone. Sleep paralysis is described as an inability to move one's body for a short period of time (typically less than 1 minute), just as the individual with narcolepsy is falling asleep or awakening from sleep. Hypnagogic hallucinations represent vivid visual, auditory, or even tactile dream-like states that occur as the individual makes the transition between the awake and sleep state. Although surreal to the individual who experiences the hallucination, they often appear in "real" environmental settings, such as the bedroom.

Narcolepsy is often found in families, though the inheritance pattern is unclear. Researchers in 1983 observed an association between narcolepsy and two specific serologically defined HLA class II antigens, DR2 and DQ1.[21] Another study determined that HLA DQB1*0602 of chromosome 6 was the most closely associated HLA marker for narcolepsy and that it is a specific marker for cataplexy in those with narcolepsy.[22] Another identified gene was DQA*0102.[23] However, these genetic markers have been found in people who express no clinical symptoms of excessive daytime sleepiness or narcolepsy. Since the presence of these HLA types results in significant risk of having narcolepsy, an autoimmune pathogenesis is a possibility. Therefore, these markers increase a person's likelihood of having narcolepsy, but are not diagnostic for the disease.

Understanding the pathophysiology of narcolepsy has progressed significantly in the last decade. In 1999, canine narcolepsy research uncovered a hypocretin receptor 2 gene deficiency;[24] which was also noted in orexin-deficient knock-out narcoleptic mice.[25] In humans with cataplexy, hypocretin-1 deficiency was noted in the cerebrospinal fluid (CSF) as compared to controls,[26] and also found to be absent in cataplectic patients with HLA DQB1*0602 markers.[27] Hypocretin, a neuropeptide neurotransmitter, is released broadly from the lateral hypothalamus to central nervous system centers that maintain wakefulness and suppress REM sleep. This cellular and molecular understanding will help to shape future medical therapies in the treatment of narcolepsy.

Diagnosis typically depends upon the above history and a sleep study during the night as well as a multiple sleep latency test (MSLT) the following day. The nighttime sleep study establishes a patient's sleep quality and eliminates other causes of excessive daytime sleepiness (e.g., obstructive sleep apnea and periodic limb movement disorder). The night following the PSG, an MSLT is performed in the sleep laboratory where the patient is asked to take a series of 4–5 naps. A PSG diagnosis of narcolepsy is based upon a normal overnight PSG with at least two sleep-onsets REM periods and a shortened sleep latency (i.e., time to sleep onset of less than 5 minutes).[23] Although rare in adolescence, excessive daytime sleepiness and witnessed cataplexy also meet diagnostic criteria.[23] Other considerations in the differential of excessive daytime sleepiness include anemia, hypothyroidism, mononucleosis, drugs of abuse, Lyme disease, and seizure disorders.[28] Marcus described a case series of secondary narcolepsy patients who met criteria for narcolepsy, but revealed central nervous system tumors on MRI as the root cause for their symptoms.[29] Rosen also described a number of patients with excessive daytime sleepiness and narcolepsy in his retrospective review of young people with central nervous system tumors.[30]

Medical treatment involves use of stimulants such as methylphenidate, dextroamphetamine, or rarely pemoline for the treatment of excessive daytime sleepiness, sleep paralysis, as well as hypnogogic hallucinations. An antidepressant, such as imipramine or other tricyclic antidepressants, are prescribed for cataplexy. The first medication, the Federal Drug Administration (FDA) approved for narcolepsy, modafinil, is chemically distinct from currently available stimulants. Modafinil is thought to induce neurotransmitter output to the posterior hypothalamus known to promote wakefulness. This drug was shown to be effective in adults during MSLT and is well tolerated.[31] Although not FDA approved for young people under the age of 14 years, Ivanenko and colleagues reported in a small number of patients that modafinil use, for up to 18 months in the pediatric populations, was well tolerated and effective in treating narcolepsy and idiopathic hypersomnia.[32]

Nonpharmacologic treatments play a significant role in narcolepsy and can help minimize the need for medication for months or years. Strict adherence to regular bedtimes with adequate sleep duration help minimize daytime sleepiness. Differences between weekday and weekend bedtimes should not vary by more than 1–2 hours. The school should encourage brief daytime naps, usually around noon for 20 minutes or less, and again in the late afternoon as well. For the adolescent, arranging physical activity in the midst of expected periods of sleepiness may be helpful in reducing or avoiding medication. Employing these therapies with medications can significantly boost the level of alertness of the narcoleptic teen in order to allow the young person to achieve academic success and to safely drive automobiles.

Kleine-Levin Syndrome

Kleine-Levin syndrome represents another hypersomnolence disorder. Also referred to as recurrent hypersomnia, the clinical pattern typically begins in adolescence with extended periods of sleep as long as 18–20 hours per day.[33] Hyperphagia and distinct personality changes such as confusion, withdrawal, or loss of sexual inhibitions occur concomitantly. This constellation of symptoms is self-limited and usually lasts for several weeks with normal degrees of wakefulness, sleep behaviors, and personality between episodes. The hypersomnolence occurs in a cycle phase, and returns regularly over a period of weeks or months. This syndrome is more commonly described in males and may appear following a viral illness or a significant head injury. Significant stress may trigger a bout of hypersomnolence as well. Sleep studies note the increased total sleep time (REM or dreaming sleep and deep, NREM sleep) and short REM latency. Although some researchers believe that the underlying etiology is secondary to intermittent hypothalamic instability, Mayer et al. studied five patients and could not find cortisol, thyroid stimulating hormone (TSH), or follicle stimulating hormone (FSH) alterations.[34] This syndrome commonly fades away by adulthood.

Post-Traumatic Hypersomnolence

Excessive daytime sleepiness and long sleep duration may follow significant trauma to the central nervous system. Characterized in detail by Guilleminault and colleagues, post-traumatic hypersomnolence lasts for 6–18 months.[35] Symptoms of long sleep duration and excessive daytime sleepiness are most noticeable in the first few weeks following the traumatic event. PSG is unremarkable and an MSLT reveals short sleep latency (less than 10 minutes) with less than two sleep onset REM periods (SOREMPs). Other diagnoses to consider include depression, encephalopathy, seizure disorder or secondary narcolepsy. Treatment with stimulants is controversial, given that this disorder resolves within a relatively short period of time and efficacy of stimulants is unclear.

Parasomnias

Parasomnias can appear in adolescence and represents disorders of arousal, partial arousal, and sleep stage transitions. Sleep talking, nightmares, nocturnal enuresis, sleep terrors, and somnambulism (sleep walking) occur less often in adolescents than in young children. Nightmares usually occur during REM sleep, are often remembered, and may be precipitated by drug withdrawal (especially alcohol) or underlying psychologic problems or stress. Somnambulism requires safeguarding the house from injury. Locking doors that lead to lower levels, the outdoors, and into pool areas is the key safeguard to avoid injury. Placing barriers in front of plate glass windows or other potential dangers in the home is another preventative strategy for wandering young people. Alarming the bedroom door may alert other family members that the sleepwalker is on the move. Finally, medication therapy is an uncommon therapy, but is discussed under in the sleep terror section.

Sleep terrors (night terrors or *Pavor Nocturnus*) usually reflect a benign condition and rarely represent underlying significant psychopathology.[36] Sleep terrors are distinct from nightmares, usually occurring in NREM sleep. They typically begin with loud vocalizations (i.e., crying and screaming) and increased autonomic reactions (i.e., tachycardia, tachypnea, and diaphoresis) with a typical duration of less than 30 minutes. Patients virtually never recall events from the prior night. Night terrors tend to occur at regular times each night. A familial tendency is also noted with night terrors. Age range is typically 4–12 years, but will occasionally persist, or become worse, during adolescence and adulthood. In most cases, night terrors disappear within several months or a year and therefore do not require treatment. DiMario and Emery report that approximately 36% of children with sleep terrors persist with this sleep disorder into adolescence.[37] Although alternative diagnoses are extremely uncommon, the differential diagnosis includes nocturnal panic attacks, confusional arousals, and complex partial seizures.[38]

Management includes both behavioral and medication options. Since night terrors occur about the same time each night, one behavioral intervention awakens the patient up 15–30 minutes prior to an episode. This awakening results in a change in sleep stage that often stops or reduces the number of night terrors. Another variation of this technique involves awakening the patient 15–30 minutes after falling asleep at the beginning of the night. Neither of these therapies have undergone scientific scrutiny. Stress reduction therapy also reduces the frequency and severity of sleep terrors. If behavioral interventions fail to stop night terrors or somnambulism, then treatment may include an antidepressant medication (such as imipramine), and benzodiazepines (such as clonazepam). These medications may decrease Stage 2 sleep or modulate the change between NREM and REM sleep, where sleep terrors typically begin in children. Selective serotonergic reuptake inhibitors, such as sertraline, have been used anecdotally with some efficacy, although none of these medications have been FDA approved for this indication. Duration of medical therapy is initially 3–6 months; then, a medication holiday is suggested to reevaluate the continued presence of sleep terrors or other parasomnias.

Sleep Disordered Breathing

Sleep disordered breathing diagnosed in a pediatric sleep laboratory spans the continuum of dynamic, intermittent upper airway obstruction; this range is from (minimal) primary snoring (PS) with no gas exchange abnormalities, to upper airway resistance syndrome (UARS), to obstructive hypoventilation (OH), and to obstructive sleep apnea (complete obstruction, OSA).[39] Research over the last decade regarding the snoring adolescent has dramatically changed our perceptions of pathologic conditions.

Epidemiologic studies around the globe seek to clarify the magnitude of and the risk factors for this problem. Snoring has been studied in a variety of population with a prevalence of approximately 10% with considerable variability.[40–43] Snoring still represents the most common indication for referral to a pediatric sleep laboratory.[40] The incidence of OSAS and OH has been reported to be roughly 2% with an equivalent male to female ratio.[41] Population estimates of UARS and OH are not available, due to the lack of a diagnostic "gold standard." In a recent large epidemiology study by Redline and colleagues, risk factors for OSA included family history, obesity, African American race, sinus disease, and "persistent wheeze."[42] Prematurity also increases the risk for the broad continuum of sleep disordered breathing in ages 8–11 years, and the significance in adolescent years is yet unclear.[43]

The pathophysiology and medical sequelae sleep-related breathing disorders are well characterized. Sleep-disordered breathing results from abnormally elevated upper airway resistance due to a combination of one or more of the following: abnormal neuromuscular control, shape of the upper airway, or anatomic abnormalities (Table 14-4). In an obstructive event, the upper airway briefly halts the normal passage of gas in and out of the chest, though the respiratory muscles continue to attempt to breathe. The end-result of these obstructive events is intermittent, but recurrent hypoxemia and hypercarbia to varying degrees (Fig. 14-1). Even a partial obstruction causes tremendous, transient negative

TABLE 14-4

ASSORTED FEATURES LEADING TO INCREASED RISK FOR SLEEP DISORDERED BREATHING

Nasal:	Rhinitis, Choanal atresia, nasal stenosis, pharyngeal flap surgery, adenoid hypertrophy, nasal polyps
Pharyngeal:	Infiltrative disorders (e.g., mucopolysaccharidoses), airway narrowing (obesity), cleft palate repair, tonsil enlargement, micrognathia, retrognathia
Laryngeal:	Laryngeal Web, subglottic stenosis, vocal cord paralysis, laryngomalacia, laryngeal masses, inflammation of upper airway (e.g., gastroesophageal reflux)
Neurologic:	Cerebral palsy, Arnold-Chiari malformation
Pharmacologic:	Sedation, anesthesia
Other:	Allergy or atopy, cigarette smoke, sleep deprivation

Source: Carroll J: Obstructive sleep-disordered breathing in children: new controversies, new directions. Clin Chest Med 24:261–282, 2003.

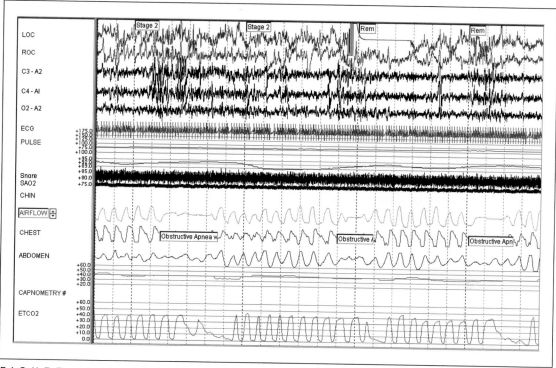

FIGURE 14-1

MULTIPLE OBSTRUCTIVE EVENTS DURING SLEEP IN A YOUNG PERSON WITH OBSTRUCTIVE SLEEP APNEA SYNDROME.

Note absence of airflow during continued respiratory effort associated mild oxyhemoglobin desaturations (nadir of 89%). Normal end-tidal CO_2 ($EtCO_2$) peaks throughout this example. Poor $EtCO_2$ waveform during obstructive events reflects little or no airflow. Paradoxical inward rib cage motion represent increased work of breathing that occurs throughout this portion of sleep preceding, during and following obstructions.

intrathoracic pressures (Fig. 14-2).[44] Sleep architecture is spared in all but the most severe cases of OSAS, which is why children are generally alert during the day. OSAS has been associated with impaired growth, right and left ventricular hypertrophy,[45] gastroesophageal reflux,[46] aspiration of upper airway secretions into the lower airway tract,[47] neurologic abnormalities (seizures and increased intracranial pressure), abnormal blood pressure variability,[48] and surgical complications (e.g., respiratory compromise). Reuveni and coworkers found that young people with OSAS resulted in a 226% increase in health care utilization at all ages over those who did not have sleep disordered breathing.[49]

Our understanding of the neurocognitive sequelae of untreated sleep apnea has expanded significantly. Excessive daytime sleepiness in the adolescent population is an uncommon feature, but presents as the most common symptom in adult obstructive sleep apnea. More commonly, the adolescent with OSAS or OH may exhibit behavioral difficulties, suboptimal academic performance, and psychiatric diagnoses (like ADHD) at approximately three times the risk of the population at large.[50] No large, prospective studies document any specific connection between ADHD and OSAS. However, Chervin, in two different publications, noted a significantly higher incidence of behavioral problems, hyperactivity and attention difficulties in young people with sleep-disordered breathing.[51,52]

The history and physical examination provides a basic screen for further investigation, but surprisingly, is limited as an evaluation tool. The American Academy of Pediatrics (AAP) now recommends that every adolescent well visit should incorporate sleep screening questions regarding snoring.[53]

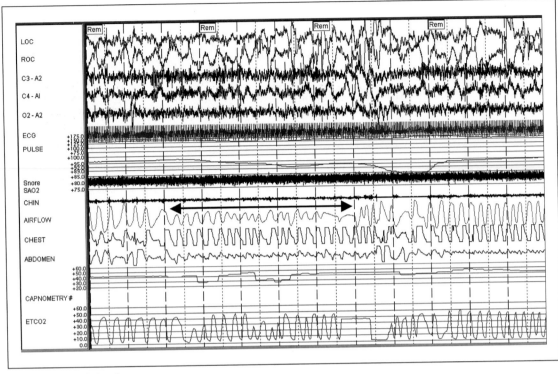

FIGURE 14-2

EXAMPLE OF OBSTRUCTIVE HYPOPNEA (PARTIAL OBSTRUCTIVE EVENT) IN 13-YEAR-OLD FEMALE WITH SNORING AND DIFFICULTY BREATHING.
Double head arrows span the event that is followed by oxyhemoglobin desaturation to 85%. Normal $EtCO_2$ throughout tracing. Diagnosed with obstructive sleep apnea syndrome.

Other important questions include duration of sleep, quality of sleep, and level of alertness during the day. The young adult who reports any of the following on a regular basis requires further evaluation: snoring, apnea, struggling to breathe during sleep, cyanosis, nocturnal enuresis, paradoxic inward rib cage motion, and choking or gagging during sleep. Although snoring during an upper respiratory infection may be expected, persistence of seasonal trends may signal allergic rhinitis. If the family is unsure, a sleep diary usually clarifies symptoms and trends. A trial of antihistamines, prior to ordering a sleep study, helps reduce unnecessary referrals to the sleep laboratory. McColley and colleagues identified an increased prevalence of allergies from control, as determined by radioallergosorbent test (RAST) testing, in habitual snorers presenting for PSG.[54] A suggested algorithm for the work-up of

snoring in the adolescent is presented in Fig. 14-3 from the AAP consensus paper.[56]

There is no good alternative to the sleep study. An audio and video recording by home camcorder is not equivalent to a formal sleep study. Home videotapes of the adolescent's sleep may indicate the presence of significant OSAS, but is likely to miss mild OSAS, does not measure gas exchange, and will never accurately diagnose OH or UARS. Pulse oximetry is helpful if oxyhemoglobin desaturation is demonstrated, but cannot rule out significant OSA if normal. Unattended home sleep studies have been shown to be unreliable due to significant loss of data compromising accuracy.[55] Therefore, the laboratory-based sleep study still represents the best means for accurate diagnosis of and estimation of severity of OSAS.

Pediatric definitions of these disorders have been established for PS, OSAS, and OH, but are not

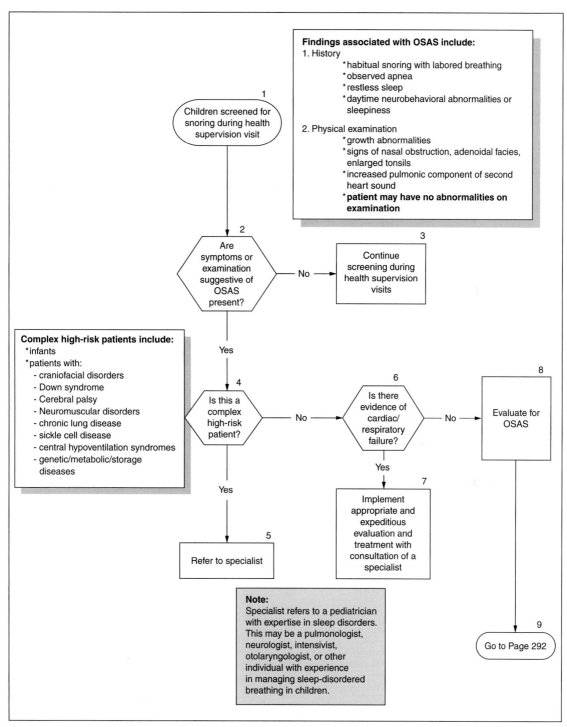

FIGURE 14-3

DIAGNOSIS AND TREATMENT OF THE SNORING YOUNG PERSON.

Source: Guilleminault C, Relayo R, Leger D, et al.: Recognition of sleep disordered breathing in children. Pediatrics 98:1235–1239, 1996.

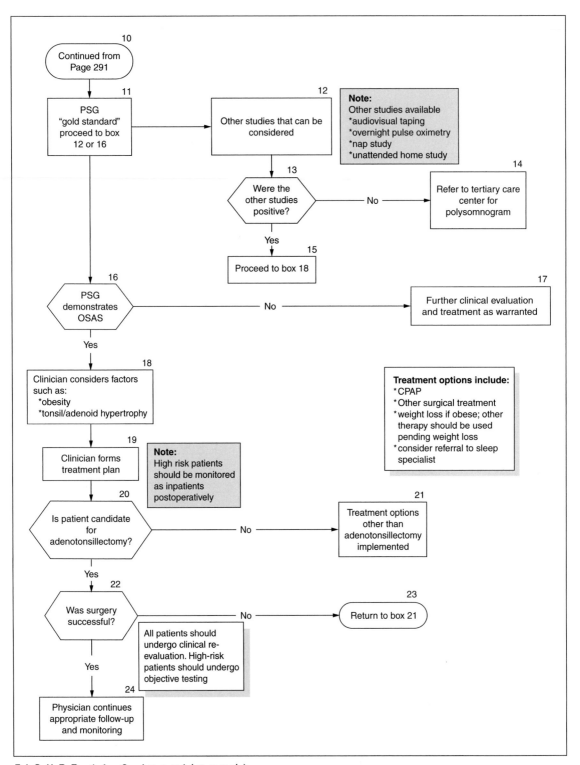

FIGURE 14-3 (continued)

validated in large multicenter population studies. Specifically, multiple definitions of OH have been published, further confusing the current diagnostic picture. There is no pediatric definition for UARS adopted by the American Thoracic Society or American Academy of Sleep Medicine and clinicians typically use the findings of Guilleminault as a reference.[56]

Although the clinical significance of OSA is clearly pathologic, the concept of PS has undergone significant revision. Until 1998, OSA and OH were considered pathologic conditions and PS was considered a "benign" condition. In 1998, Gozal reported that elementary school age children with snoring experienced significantly worse academic performance than nonsnoring peers.[57] Those who underwent adenotonsillectomy significantly improved their school performance. More recently, Kennedy and colleagues found significant neurocognitive impairment (e.g., average global IQ scores, sustained attentions scores, and mean memory index) in a group of children diagnosed with snoring on PSG.[58] Emerging literature on snoring suggests the need to reevaluate the approach to a snoring child. It is important to rule out other medical problems, such as allergic rhinitis and sinusitis, while considering behavioral as well as neurocognitive evaluation in adolescents who perform poorly in school or exhibit significant behavioral abnormalities.

Medical and surgical options are available for the treatment of sleep-disordered breathing. Adenotonsillectomy is indicated as the clear therapy of choice for OSAS, UARS, OH, and PS. Sleep study results will help guide the preoperative work-up and postoperative care. Young adults with severe sleep-related obstructive disease should undergo a 12-lead ECG, and hemoglobin/hematocrit testing to verify right ventricular hypertrophy or polycythemia, respectively. An elevated serum bicarbonate level for possible chronic respiratory acidosis can be seen in more severe cases. High-risk surgical candidates (Table 14-5) should spend the first night after surgery in a monitored bed, to allow prompt intervention in the event of respiratory compromise or failure.[59]

For most patients, outpatient adenotonsillectomy has become the standard. Adenotonsillectomy is typically curative in a high percentage of patients with

TABLE 14-5

RISK FACTORS FOR RESPIRATORY COMPROMISE FOLLOWING ADENOTONSILLECTOMY

Children or adolescents with the following
complicating medical conditions
Neuromuscular disorders
Pulmonary hypertension
Dwarfism
Craniofacial abnormalities
Marked obesity
Hypotonia and related syndromes (e.g., Down
syndrome and Prader-Willi syndrome)
Severe OSAS
Obstructive index >10
Apnea-hypopnea index >15
Oxyhemoglobin saturation nadir ≤75%
Age less than 3 years

Source: Modified from Lipton A, Gozal D: Treatment of obstructive sleep apnea in children: do we really know how? Sleep Med Rev 7:61–80, 2003.

mild to moderate OSAS who do not have other complicating factors.[60] Adenotonsillectomy also results in significant neurocognitive improvement in those with OSAS.[61] For those who have severe sleep-related obstructive disease or who fail to resolve their daytime or nighttime symptoms after adenotonsillectomy, a follow-up PSG is indicated in 6–8 weeks after surgical intervention. Uvulopalatopharyngoplasty (UPPP) is an option more common in the adult population. This operation provides short-term relief of upper airway obstruction, but may not be as helpful months and years after surgery.[62] A small retrospective study involving children and adolescents revealed that UPPP was effective in improving AHI and gas exchange in postsurgical PSGs.[63] Long-term studies are indicated to better understand the best utilization of this procedure. For the rare patient who is refractory to the aforementioned surgical and available medical therapies, tracheostomy is a definitive therapy.

Medical options exist for those who prefer to avoid surgery or are not surgical candidates. Treatment of other contributing factors and/or the use of noninvasive nocturnal assisted ventilation should be considered. For example, obesity is a risk factor for OSAS, which persists after adenotonsillectomy. Weight management with a multidisciplinary team, including a dietician, will reduce obstructive index in many individuals; however, follow-up sleep studies are critical in reevaluation of sleep-disordered breathing. Some researchers recommend weight loss even before surgical intervention if the family is motivated, closely monitored, and properly supported with an experienced weight management team. Rapid palatal expansion is a new nonsurgical option and marks the first validated dental option proven to resolve significant OSA.[64] Supplemental oxygen has also been studied in children and found to be generally safe and effective in increasing the mean and nadir oxyhemoglobin saturation, but it did not significantly change sleep architecture or obstructive index.[65] Marcus and colleagues did note several children who experienced a significant increase in $EtCO_2$ with supplemental oxygen and had to discontinue its use. Therefore, when considering supplemental oxygen as a therapy for OSAS, a PSG should be done first to determine safety. For the individual with OSA and allergic rhinitis, fluticasone nasal spray has shown to significantly reduce the number of obstructions in mild disease.[66] Lastly, montelukast has been shown, in a recent abstract, to provide significant improvement in the obstructive index in young people with mild OSA with no history of allergic rhinitis or atopy.[67] This new and promising therapy requires further validation but, if true, suggests that inflammation plays a role in sleep-disordered breathing.

Another medical alternative is a positive airway pressure (PAP) device. PAPs have become an effective alternative therapy for sleep-related breathing disorders.[68] Noninvasive nocturnal assisted ventilation with continuous positive airway pressure (CPAP) or bi-level positive airway pressure (BiPAP) devices are effective means of maintaining a patent airway and normal gas exchange during sleep. A retrospective study involving nine academic sleep laboratories, concluded that CPAP is generally safe and effective in children and adolescents, although a wide variation in indications and practices were noted.[69] Pediatric experience with the auto PAP device has recently been published and noted to be safe.[70] However, the study involved a monitored setting and,

currently, cannot be recommended for independent use. In our pediatric sleep center's experience, a PAP device is provided for the home so that the adolescent may acclimate to the apparatus. Then, once the person can wear the device through the night, a sleep study with BiPAP or CPAP titration fine tunes the pressure to overcome obstructions without very high pressures causing frequent arousals. A multidisciplinary team approach with behavioral assessment and frequent office visits are indicated to enhance compliance with this therapy.[71]

Identification, diagnosis, and treatment of sleep disorders in adolescents have progressed significantly with innovative diagnostic and treatment options. Still, readily available inexpensive means of diagnosing these disorders remains elusive. The pediatric sleep community also needs to focus on establishing and validating sleep disordered breathing PSG criteria that are universally applicable in every pediatric laboratory. The media and schools need to provide sleep awareness and education in multiple formats to reach a diverse population.

References

1. National Sleep Foundation: Adolescent Sleep Needs and Patterns: A Research Report and Resource Guide. Washington, DC, National Sleep Foundation, 2000.
2. Carskadon M, Harvey K, Duke P, et al.: Pubertal changes in daytime sleepiness. Sleep 2:453–460, 1980.
3. Wolfson A, Carskadon M: Sleep schedules and daytime functioning in adolescents. Child Dev 69:875–887, 1998.
4. National Highway Traffic Safety Administration: U.S. Department of Transportation. Crashes and fatalities related to driver drowsiness/fatigue. Research Notes, 1994.
5. National Highway Traffic Safety Administration: U.S. Department of Transportation. National Survey of Distracted and Drowsy Driving Attitudes and Behavior: 2002. Vol. 1: Findings. Washington, DC, The Gallup Organization, 2003.
6. Iglowstein I, Jenni O, Molinari L, et al.: Sleep duration from infancy to adolescence: Reference values and generational trends. Pediatrics 111:302–307, 2003.

7. Dahl RE: The development and disorders of sleep. Adv Pediatr 45:73–90, 1998.

8. Mercer PW, Merritt SL, Cowell JM: Differences in reported sleep need among adolescents. J Adol Health 23:259–263, 1998.

9. Littner M, Kushida C, Anderson W, et al.: Practice parameters for the role of actigraphy in the study of sleep and circadian rhythms: an update for 2002. Sleep 26:337–341, 2003.

10. Gracia J, Rosen G, Mahowald M: Circadian rhythms and circadian rhythm disorders in children and adolescents. Semin Pediatr Neurol 8:229–240, 2001.

11. Ancoli-Israel S, Cole R, Alessi C, et al.: The role of actigraphy in the study of sleep and circadian rhythms. Sleep 26:342–392, 2003.

12. ATS Consensus Statement: Standards and indications for cardiopulmonary sleep studies in children. Am J Respir Crit Care Med 153:866–878, 1996.

13. Marcus CL, Omlin KJ, Basinki DJ, et al.: Normal polysomnographic values for children and adolescents. Am Rev Respir Dis 146:1235–1239, 1992.

14. International Classification of Sleep Disorders: Diagnostic and Coding Manual. Delayed sleep phase disorder. Rochester, MN, American Academy of Sleep Medicine, 2001, pp. 128–133.

15. Ferber R: Circadian rhythm sleep disorders in childhood. In Ferber R, Kryger M (eds), Principles and Practice of Sleep Medicine in the Child, Philadelphia, PA, W. B. Saunders, 1995, Chap. 10, pp. 91–98.

16. Czeisler CA, Richardson GS, Coleman RM, et al.: Chronotherapy: resetting the circadian clocks of patients with delayed sleep phase insomnia. Sleep 4:1–21, 1981.

17. Rosenthal N, Joseph-Vanderpool J, Levendosky A, et al.: Phase-shifting effects of bright morning light as treatment for delayed sleep phase syndrome. Sleep 13:354–361, 1990.

18. Baker S, Zee P: Circadian disorders of the sleep-wake cycle. In Kryer M, Roth T, Dement W (eds), Principles and Practice of Sleep Medicine, 3d ed., Philadelphia, PA, W. B. Saunders, 2000, p. 610.

19. Guilleminault C, Anagnos A: Narcolepsy. In: Kryer M, Roth T, Dement W (eds), Principles and Practice of Sleep Medicine, 3d ed., Philadelphia, PA, W. B. Saunders, 2000, pp. 677–686.

20. Morrish E, King M, Smith I: Factors associated with a delay in the diagnosis of narcolepsy. Sleep Med 5:37–41, 2004.

21. Honda Y, Asake A, Tanaka Y, et al.: Discrimination of narcolepsy by using genetic markers and HLA. Sleep Res 12:254, 1983.

22. Mignot E, Hayduk R, Black J, et al.: HLA DQB1*0602 is associated with cataplexy in 509 narcoleptic patients. Sleep 20(11):1012–1020, 1997.

23. International Classification of Sleep Disorders: Diagnostic and Coding Manual. Narcolepsy. American Association of Sleep Medicine, Rochester, MN, 2001, pp. 38–43.

24. Lin L, Faraco J, Kadotani H, et al.: The sleep disorder canine narcolepsy is caused by a mutation in the hypocretin (orexin) receptor 2 gene. Cell 98:365–376, 1999.

25. Chemelli R, Willie J, Sinton C: Narcolepsy in orexin knockout mice: molecular genetics of sleep regulation. Cell 98:437–451, 1999.

26. Nishino S, Ripley B, Overeem S, et al.: Hypocretin (orexin) deficiency in human narcolepsy. Lancet 355: 39–40, 2000.

27. Krahn L, Pankratx S, Oliver L, et al.: Hypocretin (Orexin) levels in cerebrospinal fluid of patients with narcolepsy: relationship to cataplexy and HLA DQB1*0602 status. Sleep 25:733–736, 2002.

28. Brown LW, Billiard M. Narcolepsy, Kleine-Levin Syndrome, and Other Causes of Sleepiness in Children. In Ferber R, Kryger M (eds), Principles and Practice of Sleep Medicine in the Child, Philadelphia, PA, W. B. Saunders Co, 1995, Chap. 14, pp. 125–134.

29. Marcus C, Trescher W, Halbower A, et al.: Secondary narcolepsy in children with brain tumors. Sleep 25:435–439, 2002.

30. Rosen G, Bendel A, Neglia J, et al.: Sleep in children with neoplasms of the central nervous system: case review of 14 children. Pediatrics 112:e46–e54, 2002.

31. Fry JM: Treatment modalities for narcolepsy. Neurology 50(Suppl 1):S43–S48, 1998.

32. Ivanenko A, Tauman R, Gozal D: Modafinil in the treatment of excessive daytime sleepiness in children. Sleep Med 4:579–582, 2003.

33. International Classification of Sleep Disorders: Diagnostic and Coding Manual. Recurrent Hypersomnia. Rochester, MN, American Association of Sleep Medicine, 2001, pp. 43–46.

34. Mayer G, Leonhard E, Krieg J, et al.: Endocrinological and polysomnographic findings in Kleine-Levin syndrome: no evidence for hypothalamic and circadian dysfunction. Sleep 21(3): 278–284, 1998.

35. Guilleminault C, Faull K, Miles L, et al.: Posttraumatic excessive daytime sleepiness: A review of 20 patients. Neurology 33:1584–1589, 1983.

36. Kales J, Kales A, Soldatos C: Night terrors: clinical characteristics and personality patterns. Arch Gen Psychiatry 37:1413–1417, 1980.

37. DiMario F, Emergy E: The natural history of night terrors. Clin Pediatr 26:505–511, 1987.

38. Mahowald M. NREM Arousal Parasomnias. In Kryer M, Roth T, Dement W (eds), Principles and Practice of Sleep Medicine, 3d ed., Philadelphia, PA, W. B. Saunders, 2000, pp. 696–700.

39. Carroll J: Obstructive sleep-disordered breathing in children: new controversies, new directions. Clin Chest Med 24:261–282, 2003.

40. Brouillette R, Hanson D, David R, et al.: A diagnostic approach to suspected obstructive sleep apnea in children. J Pediatr 105:10–14, 1984.

41. Marcus C: Sleep-disordered breathing in children. Am J Respir Crit Care Med 164: 16–30, 2001.

42. Redline S, Tishler P, Schluchter M, et al.: Risk factors for disordered breathing in children: associations with obesity race, and respiratory problems. Am J Respir Crit Care Med 159:1527–1532, 1999.

43. Rosen C, Larkin E, Kirchner H, et al.: Prevalence and risk factors for sleep-disordered breathing in 8 to 11 year-old children: association with race and prematurity. J Pediatr 142:383–389, 2003.

44. Guilleminault C, Korobkin R, Winkle R, et al.: Children and nocturnal snoring: evaluation of the effects of sleep related respiratory resistive load and daytime functioning. Eur J Pediatr 139:165–168, 1982.

45. Amin R, Kimball T, Bean J, et al.: Left ventricular hypertrophy and abnormal ventricular geometry in children and adolescents with obstructive sleep apnea. Am J Respir Crit Care Med 165:1395–1399, 2002.

46. Buts JP, Barudi C, Moulin D, et al.: Prevalence and treatment of silent gastroesophageal reflux in children with recurrent respiratory disorders. Eur J Pediatr 145:396, 1986.

47. Konno A, Hoshino T, Togawa K: Influence of upper airway obstruction by enlarged tonsils and adenoids upon recurrent infection of the lower airway in childhood. Laryngoscope 90:1709, 1980.

48. Raouf S, Carroll J, Jeffries J, et al: Twenty-four-hour ambulatory blood pressure in children with sleep-disordered breathing. Am J Respir Crit Care Med 169:950–956, 2004.

49. Reuveni H, Simon T, Tal A, et al.: Health care services utilization in children with obstructive sleep apnea syndrome. Pediatrics 110:68–72, 2002.

50. Schechter M: American Academy of Pediatrics, Section of Pediatric Pulmonology, Subcommittee on Obstructive Sleep Apnea Syndrome. Technical report: diagnosis and management of childhood obstructive sleep apnea syndrome. Pediatrics 109:e69, 2002.

51. Chervin R, Dillon J, Archbold K, et al.: Conduct problems and symptoms of sleep disorders in children. J Am Acad Chld Adolesc Psychiatry 42:201–208, 2003.

52. Chervin R, Archbold K, Dillon J: Inattention, hyperactivity, and symptoms of sleep-disordered breathing. Pediatrics 109:449–456, 2002.

53. American Academy of Pediatrics, Section of Pediatric Pulmonology, Subcommittee of Obstructive Sleep Apnea syndrome. Clinical practice guideline: diagnosis and management of childhood obstructive sleep apnea syndrome. Pediatrics 109:704–712, 2002.

54. McColley S, Carroll JL, Curtis S, et al.: High prevalence of allergic sensitization in children with habitual snoring and obstructive sleep apnea. Chest 111: 170–173, 1997.

55. Golpe R, Jimenez A, Carpizo R: Home sleep studies in the assessment of sleep apnea/hypopnea syndrome. Chest 122:1156–1161, 2002.

56. Guilleminault C, Relayo R, Leger D, et al.: Recognition of sleep disordered breathing in children. Pediatrics 98:1235–1239, 1996.

57. Gozal D: Sleep-disordered breathing and school performance in children. Pediatrics 102: 616–620, 1998.

58. Kennedy J, Blunden S, Hirte C: Reduced neurocognition in children who snore. Pediatr Pulmonol 37: 330–337, 2004.

59. McColley S, April M, Carroll J, et al.: Respiratory compromise after adenotonsillectomy in children with obstructive sleep apnea. Arch Otolaryngol Head Neck Surg 118:940–943, 1992.

60. Lipton A, Gozal D: Treatment of obstructive sleep apnea in children: do we really know how? Sleep Med Rev 7:61–80, 2003.

61. Friedman B, Hendeles-Amitai A, Kozminsky E, et al.: Adenotonsillectomy improves neurocognitive function in children with obstructive sleep apnea syndrome. Sleep 26: 999–1005, 2003.

62. Janson C, Gislason T, Bengtsson H, et al.: Long-term follow-up of patients with obstructive sleep apnea treated with uvulopalatopharyngoplasty. Arch Otolaryngol Head Neck Surg 123: 257–262, 1997.

63. Wiet GJ, Bower C, Seibert R, et al.: Surgical correction of obstructive sleep apnea in the complicated pediatric patient. Intnatl J Pediatr Otolaryngol 41:133–143, 1997.

64. Pirelli P, Saponara M, Guilleminault C: Rapid maxillary expansion in children with obstructive sleep apnea syndrome. Sleep 27:761–766, 2004.

65. Marcus CL, Carroll JL, Bamford OS, et al.: Supplemental oxygen during sleep in children with sleep-disordered breathing. Am J Respir Crit Care Med 152:1297–1301, 1995.

66. Brouillette R, Manoukian J, Ducharme F, et al.: Efficacy of fluticasone nasal spray for pediatric obstructive sleep apnea. J pediatr 138:838–844, 2001.

67. Goldhart A, Gozal D: Leukotriene modifier therapy for mild sleep disordered breathing in children. Sleep 27(abstract):A101, 2004.

68. Guilleminault C, Nino-Murcia G, Heldt G, et al.: Alternative treatment to tracheostomy in obstructive sleep apnea syndrome: nasal continuous positive airway pressure in young children. Pediatrics 78: 797–801, 1986.

69. Marcus Cl, Davidson-Ward SL, Mallory GB, et al.: Use of nasal continuous positive airway pressure as treatment of childhood obstructive sleep apnea. J Pediatr 127:88–94, 1995.

70. Palombini L, Pelayo R, Guilleminault C: Efficacy of automated continuous positive airway pressure in children with sleep-related breathing disorders in an attended setting. Pediatrics 113:e412–e417, 2004.

71. Koontz K, Slifer K, Cataldo M, et al.: Improving pediatric compliance with positive airway pressure therapy: the impact of behavioral intervention. Sleep 26:1010–1015, 2003.

15

ENDOCRINE DISORDERS

Martin B. Draznin

DIABETES MELLITUS

Classification of Diabetes

Diabetes mellitus is a symptom complex due to deficiency of insulin or its action on tissues. There are numerous etiologies, mainly type 1 and type 2 diabetes; however, diabetes secondary to another illness and the uncommon genetically determined maturity onset diabetes of youth (MODY) emerge as the other most important etiologies in adolescents. Type 1 diabetes is further subdivided into type 1a, the form due to autoimmune destruction of beta cells, and type 1b, the form due to other causes for loss of beta cell function. This chapter mainly addresses type 1 diabetes, and then type 2 diabetes to a lesser extent.

In type 1a diabetes mellitus, there is usually a progressive loss of beta cell mass and function for varying times, until insulin deficiency manifests with asymptomatic glucose intolerance followed by frank diabetes. Approximately one-third of those with type 1 diabetes are diagnosed at presentation with ketoacidosis, while one-third have symptoms of polyuria and polydipsia with or without significant weight loss, and the remaining one-third are noted with routine screening of blood glucose or by urine analysis.

True type 2 diabetes mellitus is diagnosed more frequently in adolescents today than in past decades, in part due to the alarming increase in obesity in the population at large, including young children. In type 2 diabetes the symptoms are predominately polydipsia and polyuria; ketoacidosis, however, may be present in as many as 25% of newly diagnosed type 2 patients, as there is a phenomenon of "glucose toxicity" whereby prolonged hyperglycemia inhibits release of insulin. Some adolescents are found to have type 2 diabetes on screening laboratory evaluation when their primary care providers investigate an overweight condition or find physical signs suggesting presence of the metabolic syndrome.

The occasionally confusing overlap of symptoms and laboratory findings between the two main types of diabetes found in youth has recently been reviewed. The presence of antibodies to insulin and to islet cell components, in addition to an insulin or C-peptide level that is quite low, support the diagnosis of type 1 diabetes. A very high insulin or C-peptide level during hyperglycemia makes the diagnosis of type 2 more likely. Illnesses leading to destruction of the pancreas, such as cystic fibrosis, or to significant resistance to insulin action, such as Cushing syndrome or during treatment with atypical antipsychotic medicines, can give rise to secondary forms of diabetes. The term MODY should be reserved to refer to a group of distinct hereditary single gene disorders of islet cell function, and not to refer to true type 2 diabetes with insulin resistance and eventual deficiency that occurs in youth.

Prevalence of Diabetes

The prevalence of type 1 diabetes is estimated at 1 million in the United States with 25% of cases occurring in children and adolescents, or as many as one in 500 under the age of 20. The alarming increase in type 2 diabetes in youth seen in some urban academic centers comprises from 30% to more than 50% of new diabetes cases. The overall burden of diabetes in the country is estimated to be 17 million diagnosed cases and a third as many undiagnosed. Very few cases of type 1 diabetes would remain undiagnosed for long due to the typical symptoms. Of concern is that type 2 diabetes may have the same long preclinical course of tissue damage in youth that has been well documented in older patients before it is diagnosed and adequately treated.

Diagnosis of Diabetes

Symptoms at the onset of type 1 diabetes can be dramatic or subtle; the classic triad of polydipsia, polyuria, and polyphagia may not be noticed at first, or may be attributed to other things. Table 15-1 lists the diagnostic criteria for diabetes developed by the American Diabetes Association. Weight loss is often seen, and anorexia may replace the more adaptive polyphagia as ketosis ensues. The time course of symptoms before the diagnosis is made can be weeks to months if the adolescent does not seem to be acutely ill. Once vomiting occurs, there is a chance that misdiagnosis of gastroenteritis may be entertained. Kussmaul breathing, a later symptom

T A B L E   1 5 - 1

DIAGNOSTIC CRITERIA FOR DIABETES MELLITUS

Symptoms, such as polyuria, polydipsia, and unexplained weight loss, with nonfasting plasma glucose of ≥200 mg/dL, *or*

Fasting plasma glucose ≥126 mg/dL, *or*

Two hour plasma glucose level of ≥200 mg/dL on a standardized oral glucose tolerance test using 1.75 mg/kg (no more than 75 g) oral glucose

Source: Modified with permission by the American Diabetes Association.

that is true hyperpnea not just rapid respiration, may be misinterpreted as a pulmonary problem. Surprisingly, even in families where diabetes has been diagnosed in another member, the symptoms may not be noted until they are quite severe before attention is sought. Candida vaginitis, or persistent cutaneous infections, such as furuncles, may be a presenting complaint; this is due to the high glucose concentrations in body fluids and poor antibacterial activity of white blood cells during exposure to high levels of glucose.

Conditions Associated with Diabetes

Associated autoimmune endocrinopathies, such as Hashimoto thyroiditis and Addison's disease, are seen more frequently in persons with type 1 diabetes; thus, annual screening for thyroid insufficiency is recommended in those with type 1 diabetes. Additionally, pernicious anemia and celiac disease are important autoimmune nonendocrine disorders reported to occur more frequently in type 1 diabetes patients than in the general population. In type 2 diabetes obesity is a frequent feature, and further findings associated with insulin resistance include pseudoacanthosis nigricans, hypertension, and signs of hyperandrogenism in females.

Initial Therapy of Diabetes

In diabetic ketoacidosis (DKA), the lack of insulin leads to hyperglycemia, lipolysis, proteolysis, dehydration, metabolic acidosis, and total body potassium and phosphate depletion. Therapy designed to reverse and repair these perturbations is outlined in Table 15-2. Key elements of any plan to correct such a severe disorder of metabolic function include: assessment of the nature and degree of metabolic derangement, a scheme to deliver the corrective fluids and insulin that can quickly be modified as the patient's condition may change rapidly, and a scheme to monitor outcomes using appropriate variables to assess progress.

The plan used in our institution was designed to limit the rate of fluid administration to minimize the risk of cerebral edema, to replace potassium loss in part with potassium phosphate to minimize hyperchloremia, and to use the "two bag" intravenous

TABLE 15-2

MANAGEMENT OF DIABETIC KETOACIDOSIS

Assessment prior to starting treatment

Blood glucose >300 unless previously taking insulin

Arterial pH <7.3 or venous pH <7.25 or serum bicarbonate <15

Electrolytes, BUN, creatinine, anion gap

Precipitating cause assessed if possible

Assess extent of dehydration, tissue wasting

Assess peripheral circulatory adequacy, capillary refill time

Mental status

Kussmaul respirations, acetone odor of breath

Correction of dehydration and electrolyte imbalance

Assume 10%–15% dehydration; deliver repair fluid over 36–48 h

Reserve resuscitative bolus for patients in or near circulatory compromise infuse physiologic saline (0.9%)
10–20 mL/kg over first hour if needed

Limit total rate of fluid infusion to ≤ twice maintenance level whether that is 4 L/m^2 surface area, or as
calculated by weight, this total to include any resuscitative fluids given at start of therapy

Use 0.45% saline, containing 20 meq/L K Phos and 20 meq/L KCl

Have a second bag of IV fluid containing 0.45% saline, 20 meq/L K Phos, 20 meq/L KCl, and 10% dextrose at the
bedside

Adjust total rate of glucose infusion by infusing each of the two bags of fluid at the desired rate, i.e., 50:50 to yield
5%, 25:75 to yield 7.5%, and 0:100 to yield 10% glucose. This "two bag" scheme minimizes delay between the
decision to adjust fluid and the actual adjustment

Bicarbonate may be used if pH very low, such as 7.0 arterial, *never* by push, always by infusion over at least 1 h

Insulin infusion

Whichever system is employed by the particular unit, to yield initial rate of 0.1 unit/kg/h. Bolus dosing of insulin is
not needed

Adjust rate of insulin downward only if blood glucose drops and increased rate of glucose infusion cannot maintain
it between 100 and 200.

Maintain insulin drip until clearance of ketones from urine/normalization of imbalance of electrolytes and acidosis

Monitoring of progress

Hourly vital signs with neurologic assessment

Electrolytes, BUN, Cr every 2 h at first, then less often once stable

If corrected sodium level trends down, give less free water

Capillary blood glucose (or from central line) hourly

Intake and output and daily weight

Resolution and transition

Continue insulin by IV until significant overlap with insulin given subcutaneously

Use IV fluid only until patient stable and able to take oral liquids, may take much longer or shorter to resolve than
anticipated

Initial injected insulin dose

Discuss with patient which system he or she will be using

Mixed-split least complex, least flexible, basal bolus most work, most flexible

Adolescent dose higher 1–1.5 units/kg/day but may need to start lower

(Continued)

TABLE 15-2

MANAGEMENT OF DIABETIC KETOACIDOSIS (*CONTINUED*)

Mixed split 2/3 insulin in A.M., 4/9:2/9 of day's dose NPH to short-acting insulin

　　1/9 of day's dose as short acting at dinner

　　2/9 of dose as NPH at bedtime

"Basal-bolus" 50:50 basal and rapid acting insulin, start basal at the usual time even if IV drip not quite finished,

　　e.g., if acidosis nearly clear by bedtime of the first night.

Calculate bolus dose by rule of 1800 if using analog short acting for meals

Begin diabetes survival skill education

When patient well enough to participate

Topics are: blood glucose monitoring, insulin administration, ketosis recognition and treatment, hypoglycemia

　　recognition and treatment, and contacting a team member daily for help with adjustments or for problems

Meal plan started

Nutrition consultation, or make rough calculation based on age or weight

　　1000 kcal plus 100 kcal/year of age vs. 100 kcal/kg for first 10 kg

　　and 50 kcal/kg for next 10 kg, and 25 kcal/kg for rest

Carbohydrate content stability for mixed split, carbohydrate counting for basal bolus system

Limit fat: ≤30% of calories with ≤10 from saturated fat, carbohydrate 50%–60% of calories

solution method to speed adjustments as well as minimize waste when changing from glucose-free to glucose-containing fluids. Transition from the acute repair phase to the replacement phase takes place by 24–36 hours in most adolescents. The adolescent and family begin their learning of diabetes self-care skills as soon as they are able. Diabetes educators and nursing staff help them choose a treatment program that seems best suited to their perceived needs. Physician input in this phase is mostly to support the education. Many more questions arise, in rapid order, than can be dealt with during the hospital stay; and feelings of fear, anger, guilt, and loss must be acknowledged and legitimized as the family begins to deal with them.

Advances in Diabetes Care

Intensification of Care

The movement to intensify type 1 diabetes management to minimize long-term complications was validated by the Diabetes Control and Complications Trial and subsequent publications. Such research has indicated the continuing benefit of tight blood sugar control (i.e., target hemoglobin A1c level

≤7%) even years after the initial trial was concluded. Proponents of this system of care hold that youth with diabetes would also benefit from working with a multidisciplinary team to give them the skills, knowledge, and support needed to achieve the goals of better metabolic control. Publications show that there is benefit for patients with type 2 diabetes from improved metabolic control; this suggests that youth with type 2 diabetes may benefit from the same intensity of support as for type 1 diabetes, even though they perform fewer self-management tasks per day. Recommendations for standards of care by the American Diabetes Association, the American Association for Clinical Endocrinology, and others are readily available. There is a substantial lay literature for self-education for support of the patient with diabetes as well.

Insulin Therapy

Advances in the treatment of type 1 diabetes have allowed clinicians to continue to strive for the goal of near normal blood glucose levels without increasing the risk of severe hypoglycemia (Table 15-3). Human insulin analogs of recombinant DNA origin, such as lispro or aspart, have a much more rapid

T A B L E   1 5 - 3

TYPES OF INSULIN REGIMENS

Insulin Regimen	Advantages	Disadvantages
Mixed short (regular or analog) and intermediate acting insulin given at breakfast and evening meal	Smallest number of injections No injection at school except for correction of hyperglycemia Requires only 4 capillary blood glucose tests a day to regulate	Must mix insulin accurately Inflexible time schedule required for best outcome Snacks mandatory to match long peak of intermediate insulin More overnight hypoglycemia
"Mixed-Split" As above, but split the evening dose, give intermediate insulin at bedtime, short acting with evening meal	Less overnight hypoglycemia No injection at school except for correction of hyperglycemia Requires only 4 capillary blood glucose tests a day	More injections needed Still needs accurate mixing Still has inflexible timing Still requires snacks
Bedtime intermediate insulin with regular insulin at meals (European style)	Smooth coverage Said to be good for athletes Same number of tests will allow regulation	More shots, lunch time shot mandatory, regularly requires 30–45 min wait between injection and eating, analog insulins do not cover long enough between meals
Premixed insulin, i.e., 70:30, 75:25, NPH with regular or with an analog given twice a day	Fewer shots No need to mix insulin Still need to test four times a day	Least flexible system Least amount of adaptability to changing daily needs, does not foster independence from team Have to have short-acting insulin for corrections Most patients can master mixed-split and do better than this system allows
"Basal-Bolus" with Glargine or Detemir long-acting insulin and analog insulin for meals. Ultralente is now much less used for basal	Very flexible, meal times can vary, can skip meals Less hypoglycemia overnight or with sports Snacks not mandatory	Must have insulin shot at lunch More testing needed to master system Carbohydrate counting needed for accurate dosing Must cover snacks having carbohydrate content
Continuous subcutaneous insulin infusion "pump"	Most flexible system No shots Adjustments in "basal" rates to match varying needs day and night Temporary basal rates available	Expense of pump, infusion sets Just as difficult to master as "basal-bolus" system Not magic Occasional pump failure or dislodgement of infusion set require insulin injection

onset of action and shorter duration than regular human insulin (Table 15-4). This makes these insulins well-suited for coverage of meals and snacks; they are injected by syringe, by pen, or through an insulin pump infusion set 15 minutes before eating as compared to regular insulin, which ideally should be injected 30–45 minutes before eating (Table 15-5). Few patients would inject insulin that much in advance on an every meal basis; and, this schedule made meals away from home fraught with worry or even danger, if there was a prolonged delay in availability of food after the insulin was given.

Pen injector devices improve portability of insulin, allow increased precision and accuracy of dosing, and are easier to use than syringes with vials of insulin. The basal insulin analog, glargine, may provide 24 hours of essentially "peakless" coverage for non-food-related insulin requirements,

minimizing the risk of hypoglycemia overnight; rapid acting insulin analogs are used at meals to cover ingested carbohydrates. There are other insulin products in development designed to provide basal coverage, as well as inhaled insulin or insulin in other forms to cover meals and snacks. Insulin pumps and their delivery sets have been made dramatically more adjustable, reliable, and comfortable; they have many customizable features to fit the insulin dosing to the life of the patient, instead of the patient "living around" the insulin concentration curve.

Blood Glucose Monitoring

Updated techniques and equipment make it easier to monitor the outcome of diabetes care (Table 15-6). Capillary blood glucose monitoring, using ever smaller amounts of blood, and using sites other

TABLE 15-4

TYPES OF INSULIN

Type of insulin	Onset	Peak	Duration	Use	Advantages	Disadvantages
Regular	45 min	2 h	6 h	Meal coverage, hyperglycemia	Inexpensive, No Rx needed	Slower onset, longer duration than optimal for meals
Lispro	15 min	45 min	4 h	Meal coverage, hyperglycemia	Less hypoglycemia	Expensive, Rx only
Aspart	15 min	45 min	4 h	Meal coverage, hyperglycemia	Less hypoglycemia	Expensive, Rx only
Lente	2 h	6 h	12 h	Basal twice a day, lunch coverage	Inexpensive, No Rx needed	"Compromise" inflexible, can not premix, must suspend correctly
NPH	2 h	6 h	12 h	Basal twice a day, lunch coverage	Inexpensive, No Rx needed, can premix	"Compromise" inflexible, must suspend correctly
Ultralente			12–24 h	Basal once or twice daily	Can mix with short acting	Must suspend correctly, significant peak effects
Glargine			24 h	Basal once a day	Smooth basal	Expensive, stings, can not mix
Detemir			24 h	Basal once a day	Smooth basal	Not yet available in the United States

TABLE 15-5

DELIVERY OF INSULIN

System of Delivery	Advantages	Disadvantages
Syringes and vials	Inexpensive	Skill, need to have vial of insulin as well as syringe, disposal of syringe
Pen injectors and pen needles	More precise for small doses, easier to set dose	May be harder for small hands, disposal of cartridge or pen
Jet injectors	No needles	Special adaptors needed to load, expensive, sterilization needed, seem to be more painful
Pumps	Most flexible, near physiologic way to administer insulin, less a privacy issue to "dial up" a dose than to inject in public	Most complex system to learn, costly, infusion set and pump failure issues
Inhaled	No injection	Only short-acting form available, accuracy and long-term safety questions
Other; such as (a) Implantable "artificial pancreas"	Optimal insulin dosing and delivery to optimal tissue	Major surgery needed, in development, an unknown quantity at present
(b) Islet cell or stem cell transplant	No shots	Toxicity of antirejection regimen, need for more cells than are available at present, long-term efficacy and safety unknown

than finger tips when the blood glucose is not likely to be rapidly changing, has continually been upgraded. Monitors have memories to store readings covering months at a time, and most meters can be downloaded into computers to give graphic displays to assist in analysis of treatment strategies. Some interact directly with insulin pumps, while others allow storage of insulin dose and carbohydrate ingestion records. Continuous monitoring of subcutaneous tissue glucose levels can be made available for selected patients with troublesome glucose curves; in this system, the recording unit must be downloaded into a computer after up to 3 days of readings have been made. Thus, it is not a method to protect against overnight hypoglycemia; rather it serves as an analytical tool. There is a watch sized device worn on the arm that can give up to 12 hours of continuous recording and real time readings with a low blood glucose alarm capacity.

Both these sophisticated devices have practical limitations in their application, but can be of benefit in selected cases. The companies that make them are working to improve their function and utility.

Glycated hemoglobin, representing a retrospective report of average blood glucose, is at present the most predictive index of risk for long-term complications of diabetes of any type. A device providing rapid analysis from finger stick specimens has allowed this measurement to be reviewed at the time of the office visit. The glycohemoglobin is compared to the stated report of how management has been going, the glucose meter is downloaded, and any paper logbook that has been kept can be reviewed; such feedback can be a powerful educational tool. Changes in the treatment plan, thus, can be made face to face during the visit to enhance understanding rather than by letter or telephone notification.

TABLE 15-6

VARIABLES MONITORED IN DIABETES MANAGEMENT

Monitored Variable	Characteristics
Urine glucose	Time delay from blood glucose, easy to do, not used in modern care
Urine ketones	Easy to do, needed for "sick day" routine, may not be done often enough, hard to do in infants, incontinent patients
	Done by patient as needed and during office visit
Timed urine for excessive protein, microalbuminuria	Signs of nephropathy, microalbuminuria may be transient
	Done associated with office visit
Blood glucose	Need finger poke (or other site), need strips and monitor, get current status, harder to do, more likely to be omitted, painful technique
	Done by patient as needed and at office visit
Blood beta hydroxybutyrate	Can find ketosis when urine sample unavailable
	Need special monitor and strip that may not be readily available
	Done by patient, usually not needed with adolescents
Intensive blood glucose monitoring, pre- and 2 h postinjection of short-acting meal coverage insulin, and at bedtime	Most helpful in "basal bolus" injection system, or with pump.
	Most difficult to accomplish
	Done by patient
Continuous glucose monitoring system	Inserted glucose electrode monitors for up to 3 days. Expensive device, must calibrate with capillary blood glucose readings, need to download for analysis, newer version will have real time reading, positional loss of signal
	Done by patient after learning how to use in office visit, analysis done by physician or team member
GlucoWatch	Pads on skin allow sampling for up to 13 h per set, alarms for low can be helpful, real time reading can be useful
	Pads can be quite irritating, need to calibrate, will not operate if wet
	Positional loss of signal may occur
	Done by patient after learning how to use in office, download analyzed by physician or office staff, real time alarms, and so forth, by patient
Hemoglobin A1c	"Averages" over past 3 months, most highly correlated to risk for long-term complications
	Usually done with office visit
Thyroid hormone, TSH	Annual screen for Hashimoto Thyroiditis in type 1 patients
	Usually done with office visit
Lipid panel	Annual screen for diabetes related dyslipidemia
	Usually done with office visit
Screen for other autoimmune endocrine or nonendocrine disorders	Addison's disease, celiac disease in type 1 patients reportedly increased
	Usually done with office visit

An Example of a Diabetes Clinic Visit

A typical interdisciplinary diabetes clinic visit is now reviewed. The adolescent, on arrival, goes to the laboratory to have glycohemoglobin measured at each three-monthly visit. Free thyroxine level, thyroid-stimulating hormone (TSH), lipid panel, and renal function screening are recommended to be done yearly for patients with type 1 diabetes. The recent reports of increased incidence of celiac disease in type 1 diabetes patients suggest that screening for this too may become standard care. The patient and family fill out a questionnaire about their system of diabetes management and the overall health of the youth since the last visit. This questionnaire elicits the insulin dosing and meal plan used, the estimated blood glucose ranges, problems with hyperglycemia and hypoglycemia, illnesses with and without ketosis, and whether a "sick day" regimen had to be employed. It is also important to know the time of the last visit to the primary care physician if diabetes care is provided by a diabetes specialty clinic. In general, primary care for all nondiabetes matters is best provided at the "medical home."

Recommendations for influenza and pneumococcal vaccination, dental care to prevent gingivitis, and ophthalmologic screening are followed by asking when these were last done. Other information reviewed includes patient requests for prescription refills and any questions or concerns the adolescent and family bring with them. The clinic nurse brings the patient to the examining room to obtain vital signs and measurements, to download the meter(s) and insulin pump if appropriate, and print out the reports. The accuracy of the blood glucose monitor(s) is checked, prescription forms for supplies are filled out for physician signature, and a work or school absence form is given as needed. Samples of needed supplies may be given; different glucose monitors are often tried on a sample basis. A certified diabetes educator addresses questions, suggests appropriate changes in the management plan, reminds families of seasonal changes, and continues to provide ongoing education for diabetes self-care knowledge and skills. Performance of the care and decision making about the care are assessed for appropriateness for developmental level of the youth and for accuracy. A nutritionist reviews the meal planning, answers questions, makes adjustments in the meal plan for growth or weight control, and also delivers ongoing education. If psychologic support or social work support are requested or otherwise deemed necessary, a referral can be made.

The clinician reviews the information with the family and performs the physical examination. Changes in injection sites, such as lipohypertophy from infrequent rotation of sites, a screen of the retina through the handheld ophthalmoscope, thyroid palpation, and other diabetes related or associated findings are sought. Discussion about the treatment plan is continued. This would include review of all suggested changes in the care plan, setting a time to call or fax in readings of blood sugars between visits to help with adjusting insulin dosing, starting of new insulin dosing regimens, scheduling for insulin pump education, and other matters. Results of the laboratory studies are transmitted directly to the family as well as to the primary care physician with recommended treatment, suggestions for referral to other specialty providers, and so forth. Letters of support for the patient to do the care plan at school or at work may be required; information regarding travel is sometimes needed. Specialized material is prepared in the form of handouts for the family to use in adjusting the management, and handling "sick days" and other matters.

Care of Type 2 Diabetes

In the case of the adolescent with type 2 diabetes, the self-care skill set will not be as extensive until insulin production is lost and insulin administration started. Glucose monitoring should still be done at least in the morning. Meal planning is critical and adherence to the recommended intake is urged, as weight control or weight loss is the most widely recommended initial step in care. Increased physical activity should also be advocated since it helps to improve insulin sensitivity as well as weight loss.

Use of Metformin can significantly lower glycated hemoglobin if other aspects of care are accurate. Metformin is given with meals, starting with 500 mg at the evening meal; a second dose can be added at breakfast if needed. The dose(s) can be increased as needed to control blood glucose.

It is preferable to adjust upward from a lower dose to allow for adaptation to side effects; most adolescents will tolerate the dose they need if it is gradually introduced. An extended release form of Metformin is also available and is usually taken with the evening meal. Insulin may be required if Metformin, meal planning, and exercise do not suffice to keep glycohemoglobin in the target range.

There are several ways in which insulin can be administered. For example, intermediate acting insulin (NPH or Lente) can be given twice a day, or fast acting analog insulin can be given in addition to the intermediate insulin or instead of it. Another approach is to give the insulin glargine once a day with doses of rapidly acting analog insulin for meal coverage. Once insulin treatment is started, it is important to remember the underlying insulin resistance, and thus, Metformin or other treatment to sensitize the tissues to insulin is continued. Laboratory screening for autoimmune disorders is less pertinent in type 2 diabetes; however, lipid levels and renal function assessment are still needed. At present, the other insulin sensitizers and agents that are available to minimize glucose excursion or absorption are used less often in adolescents with diabetes than in adults with diabetes.

The Family as Team Concept of Diabetes Care

The parent or guardian is encouraged to participate in the visit. At our institution, we believe that knowledge of and responsibility for this particular aspect of adolescent health care must be shared by the family. Issues of privacy, autonomy, and other matters, such as sexuality and drinking or drug experimentation, often require the adolescent to be seen alone, Such issues can be handled in another setting, such as during a sub session of the diabetes visit (Chaps. 2 and 3). The daunting difficulty, emotional drain, and high volume of the care skills needed for avoidance of problems with the diabetes demand that the adolescent have knowledgeable adult partners.

Occasionally it becomes an overwhelming burden for the youth to accurately perform all the required care without respite, requiring someone else to give an injection, to help with calculating a correction, and other aspects of care. Thus, the parent or guardian is routinely included during the information sharing and adjustment of the care plan. Diplomatic handling of this "full team" visit is advisable. Since the adolescent has increasing responsibility for self-care based on ability to perform the skills, and to make gradually more independent judgment about adjustments of care, at no time should the providers be perceived by family members or the adolescent to be "diabetes cops" or persons who are agents of the parent trying to control the adolescent. The providers should instead acknowledge that they work *for* the adolescent with diabetes and *with* the adults who also help in the care, as opposed to working *for* the adults and *on* the adolescent.

The goals and outcome of the treatment should be adopted by the youth and the family, and not merely represent something that the physician wants them to do. For example, there is a risk that constant physician praise of correct procedures and successful outcomes, or criticism of perceived failures, may lead to distortions of the information shared with the team by the adolescent in a mistaken attempt to "make the doctor like me more." Also, a seemingly negative or judgmental approach to the patient's treatment, monitoring, and outcomes will often fail to help the patient make appropriate adjustments. Reminding the adolescent of whose health is at risk, for whom the care plan is designed, who is the "employer" (patient), and who is the "employee" (provider), should be done in a matter of fact style. When the adolescent believes that the provider is working for him or her and is supportive even when there are problems with the adherence to care, or in lack of success with the care, the clinician will be able to hear more accurately what has been going on, what is needed, and what the adolescent can be realistically expected to achieve in self-care.

Diabetes Care is Really Done Between the Office Visits

Support of the family performance of the care plan should continue between office visits. Calls for help with adjustment should be handled by providers, knowledgeable in the system of care that is being employed. When problems occur, awareness of the multiple possible causes is needed; the adolescent is then given tips and information on how to investigate the problem, to find and apply the correct remedy, and is invited to get back in touch with the clinician if further help is needed. Some problems are easier to identify, such as a mistake in the dose of insulin, a malfunctioning pump, or a missed dose of insulin would usually be known to the patient at the time of the call; corrective measures can then be suggested. Sick day plans, how to treat hypoglycemia, alternative insulin delivery if a pump is malfunctioning, and similar support should be available to the patient by calling or paging the provider. The use of preprinted instruction sheets for various changes in care, handling of problems, and other matters is beneficial.

This part of the care that is between the office visits can be the least convenient, most time consuming, and most vexing; however, it is also the most valuable for successful self-care to be learned and followed by an adolescent with diabetes. It is the safety net that lends credence to the care plan made at the visit. It will also demonstrate to these adolescents that they indeed can find and fix problems successfully. Most families will master the needed adjustments for all but the most arcane of situations in the first 2 years after diagnosis, if a supportive team member can always be contacted in a timely manner. The immediacy of the problem means that the lesson will be more completely learned. By comparison, attempting to teach everything that will ever be needed at the time of the diagnosis is not feasible.

Difficult to Manage Blood Glucose Levels

There are some families for whom this system of care does not seem to work. Blood glucose levels are not in the recommended range and no obvious explanation exists. Many possible reasons for lack of success must be thought of and eliminated by careful, supportive history taking, physical evaluation, and when indicated, laboratory investigation (Table 15-7). Remediation for the various causes of difficulty in management can then be focused on the cause with more chance for success.

TABLE 15-7

DIFFICULT TO MANAGE BLOOD GLUCOSE

Psychosocial problems typical of adolescence, developmental issues
  Errors of management and/or excess catecholamine release
Psychosocial problems unique to the patient and family
Errors of management not due to stress
  Glucose monitor malfunction, test strip malfunction
  Inappropriate dose calculation (by team or by teen)
  Use of wrong insulin for a particular purpose (e.g., large dose of lispro instead of glargine at bedtime)
  Fatigue leading to error of interpretation, calculation
  Deliberate mismanagement for secondary gain
  Insulin not kept at proper temperature or kept too long
  Pump malfunction ignored by patient who does not like shots
  Omission of BG testing, dosing insulin by "how it feels"
Intercurrent illness such as infections, trauma, or surgical stress
Addison's or Cushing's disease complicating diabetes
Pregnancy
Alcohol or other drug abuse
Use of medicines that affect blood glucose such as decongestants, steroids, and so forth
Inaccurate following of meal plan, overeating
Over treatment of hypoglycemia, or eating for symptoms of hypoglycemia at normal BG
Withholding of insulin to lose weight
Missing injections due to fatigue, embarrassment, denial
High progesterone phase of menstrual cycle or oral contraceptives not recognizing pattern of high readings relating to cycle
Large growth spurt
Injection site abnormalities due to lack of rotation of site
Insulin resistance due to chronic poor control
Change in exercise or sleep amount or schedule without change of insulin regimen

The Sick Day Plan

The days when many of the patients were admitted with recurrent episodes of DKA are long in the past; thanks to improved techniques of blood glucose and urinary ketone monitoring, as well as to development of aggressive but safe sick day routines. It is advised to give the full base dose of insulin during acute illness, regardless of appetite. Withholding insulin during an acute illness may lead to ketoacidosis. Should ketones be present, it is advised to give frequent supplemental injections of rapid acting analog insulin based on the concentration of urinary ketones, frequent monitoring of blood glucose levels, adjustment of oral intake to maintain hydration, and keeping blood glucose levels from falling too low as a consequence of the extra insulin If the amount of oral fluid that can be taken is insufficient to maintain the blood glucose in a safe range, or if repeated vomiting renders oral fluid and glucose support impossible, intravenous fluid therapy is required. Thus, a definite time over which to allow this system to work or fail has to be agreed on at the start and the next phase, office or emergency department intravenous care, entered rapidly.

How to fit in Fitness, Exercise, and Sports

The benefits of exercise, fitness, and participation in competitive sports should not be denied to youth with diabetes of either type. In type 1 diabetes, there are concerns regarding possible interference by exercise with blood glucose level control; in type 2 diabetes, this is usually not as much of an issue. There are several publications available to assist in the assessment of a youth with diabetes for participation in sports. Some detail the effect of many types of exercise on carbohydrate metabolism, while others stress the individualization of the planning. The information needed to adjust the diabetes regimen for participation in exercise (including organized fitness programs or a sport) is gathered and assessed by the athlete and the diabetes care team; in this process, adjustments to the daily care are suggested and tested. Fine-tuning of the program is then continued throughout the season.

This is not to state that it is an easy process or that the provider will have many ready-to-use plans; rather, this must be true teamwork, involving an exploration of needed adaptations to allow safe and successful sports participation. In many instances, what makes diabetes management for athletes most gratifying is the chance to help them utilize their strong desire to do well in their sport that is also consistent with good diabetes care. It is their drive to succeed and their self-discipline that leads to success in sport that can best be applied to the diabetes care as well.

Driving, Drinking, Drugs, Dating

Adolescents with diabetes will need to master the same set of developmental and life skills as their peers and at the appropriate developmental stages. The teaching of diabetes self-management, therefore, must take these activities into account. Driving is a privilege, not a right; thus, keeping a safe level of blood glucose to allow full alertness is mandatory, and this should not be a negotiable issue. In some cases, the use of driving as a metaphor for diabetes care can be a helpful didactic tool. For example, the clinician can note that one does not drive off without looking out the windshield; one should not go about one's daily routine, including driving, without checking blood glucose to see where one is headed. Unless driver license applications require that diabetes is mentioned and physician clearance obtained, this information must be offered by the team in anticipation of driver training. Important points the clinician can stress include having knowledge of the blood glucose before turning on the ignition, keeping a source of rapidly available carbohydrate at hand when driving to treat low blood sugars, and having a method of diabetes identification (such as medical identity card, necklace, or bracelet), in case of being stopped by authorities or needing medical attention while driving.

Youth should be taught that it is too dangerous for them to use alcohol; not only is alcohol consumption illegal for adolescents (Chap 34), it may predispose diabetic adolescents to severe hypoglycemia by interfering with hepatic glycogenolysis/gluconeogenesis. Further, the youth with diabetes, who volunteers to remain sober and be a designated driver, could still be at unacceptable risk in the event of severe hypoglycemia; in this situation, there may only be inebriated, and thus, unwitting, uncaring, or incompetent helpers available in such an emergency. The abuse of so-called street drugs may also be an important issue (Chap. 34). Their use, in addition to being illegal, may have other devastating long-term consequences. For example, drug experimentation or abuse is very dangerous if it masks the symptoms of hypoglycemia or interferes with the cognitive and physical ability to take correct action when diabetes care is not working correctly.

Issues of adolescent sexuality are reviewed in Chap. 22, and briefly considered here. A key health issue for the adolescent female with diabetes concerns the serious risk to her own health from an unplanned pregnancy, as well as the risk of significant damage to the fetus from high maternal blood glucose levels. Abstinence, if practiced, is the most efficacious system for birth control and avoidance of sexually transmitted diseases (STDs). When abstinence is not practiced, contraceptive and anti-STD methods are recommended (Chaps. 24 and 25). However, when a pregnancy is planned and desired, preconception blood glucose control should be very tight. A perinatologist or other experts in the care of diabetes in pregnancy should supervise diabetes care during the pregnancy to prevent, or at least minimize, the potential damage to mother and child that unhealthy maternal glucose levels present.

Complications of Diabetes Mellitus

Acute Complications and Problems

Acute complications of diabetes include DKA, hyperosmolar nonketotic coma, and severe hypoglycemia. DKA is a very dangerous metabolic derangement with up to 2% fatality, while hyperosmolar non ketotic coma in youth with type 2 diabetes, can also cause fatalities. Severe hypoglycemia from use of insulin has risks for serious injury, central nervous system damage, or death. Cerebral edema, as a complication of DKA treatment, is

mentioned separately because its risk may be minimized by careful fluid administration. Deaths from DKA can also be due to vascular collapse, acidosis, and electrolyte imbalance. Poorly controlled type 1 diabetes may subject the patient to episodes of recurrent ketoacidosis with the attendant risks of morbidity or mortality, loss of school time, and further disruption of the patient's life; less poorly controlled diabetes is much more subtle, but ultimately leads to increased risk for complications as a young adult.

On the other hand, repeated episodes of severe hypoglycemia may cause memory impairment and poor school performance; they can also subject these youth to increased risk of injury or death if episodes occur while driving, performing vigorous or dangerous sporting activities, or even when just being off alone with no one to assist them if severe hypoglycemia develops. There can be a gradual loss of hypoglycemia awareness with longer duration of the diabetes. There is also a lowering of the threshold for symptoms of hypoglycemia with lowering of the average blood glucose level. A frank discussion of the limits of safe blood sugar control should be done. To overly frighten the adolescent about hypoglycemia will defeat attempts at control of high readings; however, pushing tight control to a level of obsession with low averages, leading to severe lows, is not appropriate either. It is a healthy balance that the clinician and adolescent should seek.

A major area of emotional risk with lasting impact is the imposition of arbitrary changes in many aspects of the adolescent's daily life. The basic level of so-called intensive therapy for type 1 diabetes consists of three or more injections of insulin a day, four capillary blood glucose checks a day, and mindfulness of the amount of carbohydrate ingested at meals. It requires a rigid schedule of meals and snacks to match the arbitrary and non-physiologic insulin concentrations noted with subcutaneous insulin injections. Advanced intensive management involves a shift to so-called "basal-bolus" dosing of insulin, employing both very long-acting and very short-acting analog insulins by injection or very short-acting insulin via an insulin pump; this requires a more intensive schedule of blood glucose monitoring, and much more knowledge about carbohydrate counting.

The basal-bolus systems can allow more flexibility of meal times, sleeping in on the weekend, spontaneity (e.g., going out for a pizza with friends after the game), and less risk of hypoglycemia.

No part of the day is spared the effect of diabetes. Sleep is not seen as a safe haven if severe hypoglycemia may occur; sports participation can be frustrating or dangerous in that exercise may elevate blood sugar so high that ketoacidosis occurs, or, plunge it so low that hypoglycemia and unconsciousness occur. Timing of the capillary blood glucose checks, injections, meals, and required snacks often subjects the youth to loss of privacy; performance of self-care usually requires negotiations with the school or workplace as to what can be done when and where. Others responsible for the safety of these youth may not always respond appropriately to medical needs, leading to anxiety, anger, frustration, and poor control.

Even though outward manifestations of diabetes are not present, these youth may feel that they are different from their peers and the stigmatization can be felt to be severe, regardless of what those around them actually are thinking. Loss of autonomy and the need to ask for advice about matters previously mastered (such as eating, play, sports, others) may be a very painful experience for many youth. The impact of emotional illness on adequacy of diabetes self-care cannot be too strongly stated. Inaccuracy of self-management, for whatever reason, leads to elevated or chaotic blood glucose levels and increased risk of acute and chronic complications. Type 2 diabetes is less likely to lead to severe acute complications, once the diagnosis had been made; however, nonketotic hyperosmolar coma is still a risk if careful blood sugar control is not maintained. Blood glucose testing during acute illness, and not skipping doses of medication or insulin should be stressed.

Medications for type 2 diabetes can be associated with problematic symptoms or cause illness. Metformin acts by diminishing postprandial release of glucose from the liver. It is known to cause intestinal cramps, and more severe gastrointestinal disturbances, such as diarrhea, in a significant fraction of patients, when initially started. In the face of renal insufficiency, metformin therapy may predispose to lactic acidosis. The thiazolidinedione insulin sensitizers, which act on muscle, have been linked to fatal hepatic failure, in the case of the first generation Rezulin; edema and worsening congestive heart failure have been noted with second generation forms, especially when dosed with insulin. These effects are not as well studied in youth as in adults, and may be less common in youth; nevertheless, the thiazolidinedione agents are not yet Federal Drug Administration (FDA) approved for use in patients younger than 16.

Chronic Complications

Chronic complications of diabetes accrue during the entire time that blood glucose is elevated, and may not manifest during childhood or youth. However, with the recent trend of very early onset diabetes in children younger than 5, the long-term exposure to high blood glucose will put more adolescents with diabetes at risk of earlier onset of long-term complications than widely recognized. Thus, renal damage, manifesting as proteinuria and hypertension, must be sought and treated aggressively to preserve renal function. Screening for high blood pressure is done at each office visit (Chaps. 9 and 16). Urine screening for microalbuminuria or quantitative urine testing for proteinuria and microalbuminuria, once reserved until five or more years after onset, may need to be started sooner (Chap. 16). Yearly dilated pupil examination is recommended in adolescents as well as in children having had 5 years of diabetes before adolescence. Since effective therapy for some aspects of nonproliferative retinopathy is available, and early changes in the retina may serve as a cue to improve self-management, screening should not be left until late in the diabetes development.

Peripheral neuropathy can lead to painful legs and feet, disordered gait, absence of protective pain sensations, and ultimately, diabetic foot complications; such neuropathy is also unusual until quite a few years of poor blood sugar control. Upper extremity neuropathy may also occur. Autonomic neuropathy, which may manifest as cardiac, gastrointestinal, or erectile dysfunction symptoms, may be a problem; it is not clear how early it may manifest, as symptoms may be subtle and nonspecific at first. Skin manifestations of diabetes are also variable in timing of onset; unfortunately, they have no specific therapy. In the case of type 2 diabetes, obesity comes associated with a negative image and the admonitions to lose weight, exercise more, take medications accurately, and take insulin if needed; the latter can be a burden, just as noted in the more intensively treated type 1 patients.

Treatment of Complications

Acute problems with diabetes care, such as hypoglycemia, hyperglycemia, and ketoacidosis, can be readily treated with immediate benefit. Long-term complications require specific ameliorative or palliative interventions. Proteinuria due to diabetes, persistent microalbuminuria, or elevated blood pressure require therapy with angiotensin converting enzyme (ACE) inhibitors or angiotensin receptor blockers (ARBs); this is important in order to preserve renal function (Chap. 16). The clinician, if prescribing these medications, should develop familiarity with them, especially with their dosing, side effects, and strict warnings needed to avoid pregnancy if using ACE inhibitors. The clinician may prefer a nephrology consultant's input in this regard. Infections are more frequent in patients with poor blood sugar control. They require accurate diagnosis, aggressive treatment, and, at the same time, intensification of blood glucose control. Problems with nonproliferative retinopathy, such as macular edema, may be serious enough to require a laser certified retina expert; the unusual development of cataract formation requires appropriate ophthalmologic evaluation and treatment.

Neurologic complications are not common in young adolescents or in those with a shorter duration of diabetes; however, their presence may require highly specialized consultation and management. Autonomic neuropathy, an unusual development in diabetic youth, can be dangerous, frightening, and hard to manage; it can manifest as gastroparesis, orthostatic hypotension, erectile dysfunction, or other symptoms. The psychologic

burden of a chronic illness must be considered a complication as well. Adolescents with diabetes and their families may need help to assess their most effective learning styles as well as coping skills; arrangements should be made to obtain therapy for specific emotional or psychologic concerns that may arise.

Other Assistance in Care

It is often worthwhile to counsel the family and youth to seek out community resources, such as support groups for youth with chronic conditions, such as diabetes. Many states have summer diabetes camps for children and youth. Peer to peer networking, support, and information sharing available from these resources cannot credibly be provided by the clinician, or the rest of the diabetes team; they are not adolescents living with diabetes. Use of the Internet to learn about diabetes is a mixed benefit. Several excellent sites can be accessed to assist in learning about self-care, advocacy, current research breakthroughs, how to network with others to minimize feelings of separateness, and other benefits. However, there is no effective peer review of Internet postings. While many Web sites that are devoted to diabetes are of great help, others may cause undue feelings of guilt or worry, give false hopes for treatments that do not work, or blame diabetes on factors that probably had nothing to do with it.

New Developments

Human insulin analogs with altered properties have been in service since insulin lispro was introduced in the 1990s. Both of the currently available rapid acting insulin analogs, lispro and aspart, demonstrate an improved match of their course of action to the shape of the concentration curve of glucose absorbed from meals, when given properly; also, they offer less worry of delayed hypoglycemia. The long-acting insulin glargine seems to provide for basal, or non-food-related needs for insulin over 24 hours, with a minimal peak of action in most, though not all, patients. The insulin, glargine, also seems less associated with hypoglycemia occurring overnight or after exercise;

however, it is not completely free of those problems in all patients. A newer long-acting analog, insulin Detemir, is in final phases of clinical trials. It is possible that, in addition to a long peakless action curve, it may exhibit other improved properties, such as miscibility with a short-acting analog without altering the time curve of either insulin.

Work continues in several commercial venues to develop a true closed loop artificial pancreas system, in which very frequent readings of instantaneous blood glucose levels would be used to control the release of insulin into subcutaneous tissue, the peritoneal cavity, or the portal vein. The transplantation of beta islet cells is still undergoing research and development. While the Edmonton protocol dramatically increased the yield of long-functioning beta cells and the years of freedom from insulin injections in some of their adult subjects, knowledge of immunosuppressive regimes is not yet at a stage where islet cell transplantation can be confidently recommended to adolescents, due to concerns about the risks of long-term toxicity.

Some Clinical Scenarios in Diabetes

14-Year-Old Girl

She reports having very high readings of blood sugar in the morning, sometimes with urine ketones at trace to small concentrations. Questions to ask include: What is the insulin regimen: three injections, basal bolus with injections, or an insulin pump? What are the blood glucose readings at bedtime? Is there a bedtime snack? How well has she slept overnight when the readings have been high the next morning? How well rested does sleep leave her feeling the next morning? Does the blood sugar run high all morning or can it be controlled by an adjustment at the breakfast dose?

These questions are designed to explore a number of issues. Is this adolescent "running out of insulin" overnight, which is known as the Dawn phenomenon, or could she be experiencing the Somogyi phenomenon? In the Dawn phenomenon, normal release of growth hormone leads to early morning insulin resistance. In the Somogyi

phenomenon, overnight hypoglycemia leads to rebound hyperglycemia and insulin resistance. The appropriate time to test blood glucose to differentiate between these two phenomena is during the night, usually at midnight and 2 A.M. It may be that the bedtime snack is too large, the bedtime dose of basal insulin too small, the coverage of the bedtime snack with short-acting insulin too low, or a serious hypoglycemic excursion is occurring followed by a rebound. In order to resolve this problem, there should be monitoring of the overnight readings, if using an insulin pump, to check how well it functions overnight; also, assess whether the bedtime insulin dose injection site is rotated and if the site is in normal skin, rather than in an area of scarring or lipohypertrophy.

16-Year-Old Male Adolescent Athlete

He has had episodes of very severe hypoglycemia over night on days when there is basketball practice, but not on the weekends. Questions for the clinician to ask include: Does he check his blood glucose before and after practice? Does he take any carbohydrate during the practice? When is the practice in relation to insulin doses, meals, and snacks? What is the bedtime glucose reading after exercise as opposed to on nights without exercise? and is any carbohydrate taken after exercise?

These inquires seek to look at the complex effects that exercise has on diabetes control. Initial hormone mediated release of glucose from glycogen stores in the liver and lactic acid from muscle (to be used in hepatic gluconeogenesis) may elevate blood glucose in diabetes. At the same time, the markedly increased flow of blood to exercising muscles increases uptake of insulin by the muscle allowing it to be used more rapidly; also, increased blood flow to the skin of exercising limbs may increase uptake of insulin from the injection site. Utilization of the stored carbohydrates sets the stage for later "preferential" glucose uptake and glycogen storage by liver and muscle after exercise, regardless of blood glucose concentration, since muscle and liver cells have glucose transporters while the brain depends solely upon glucose absorption via diffusion; hence, there is a need for a higher blood glucose concentration to obtain glucose. As noted by the metaphor of driving, the empty reserve tank will be filled before the main tank; thus, extra carbohydrate must be provided during and often after exercise. Research suggests that appropriate amounts of carbohydrate use are needed for periods of different types of exercise. Specific monitoring and record keeping are needed to sort out the magnitude of these different effects.

An Adolescent Who Takes the Wrong Insulin

He calls, sounding quite panicky, and says he has given himself a large dose of a rapid acting insulin analog in place of his usual bedtime glargine dose. Questions that the clinician should ask include: what is his blood sugar now, what is the ratio of grams of carbohydrate per unit of short-acting insulin, and can he eat enough carbohydrate over the next few hours to match the amount of short-acting insulin just taken?

The clinical concern is that glargine is a clear appearing form of insulin, as are the short-acting analogs. This makes it easier, due to fatigue or distraction, to give the wrong insulin, unless a pen device is always used for the short-acting insulin analog and a syringe for glargine. This mistake is very frightening to the patient, who will have heard about, and may have already experienced hypoglycemic coma and seizure; however, when it is identified so quickly after the injection, almost all patients will be able to treat it successfully at home. Calm support is needed. The ratio of insulin to carbohydrate is used to calculate the amount of carbohydrate that must be ingested to match the excess insulin. Since the size of the injection is often much larger than the usual amount of rapid acting analog used for meals, this large volume may yield a mass action effect that may be helpful in slowing down absorption. Thus, the carbohydrate to cover the insulin can be taken over several hours. It is important to advise retesting of blood glucose levels every hour or if the symptoms of hypoglycemia occur. Occasionally, intravenous administration of glucose might be needed, requiring support in a hospital emergency department or by trained emergency transport medics; however, eating a large amount of extra carbohydrate is usually not a problem for the adolescent.

Suggested Readings

American Diabetes Association. Type 2 diabetes in children and adolescents: Consensus conference report. Diabetes Care 2000;23:381–389.

American Diabetes Association Clinical Practice Recommendations 2004, Diabetes Care 2004;27(Suppl 1): Diagnosis and classification S5–S10, Standards of medical care S15–S35, Nutrition principles S36–S46, Physical activity/exercise S58–S62, Insulin administration S106–S110, Influenza and pneumococcal immunization S111, Diabetes care in the school and day care setting S122–S18, Diabetes care at diabetes camps S129–S131.

Bricker LA, Draznin MB, Hare JD, Greydanus DE. Diabetes in adolescent patients: Diagnostic dilemmas. Ind J Pediatr 2001;68:457–465.

Brink SJ. Complications of pediatric and adolescent type 1 diabetes mellitus. Curr Diab Rep 2001;1:47–55.

Brink S, Miller M., Moltz KC. Education and multidisciplinary team care concepts for pediatric and adolescent diabetes mellitus. J Pediatr Endocrinol Metab 2002;15:1113–1130.

Cameron FJ. The impact of diabetes on health-related quality of life in children and adolescents. Pediatr Diabetes 2003;4:132–136.

Ciechanowski PS, Katon WJ, Russo JE, Hirsch IB. The relationship of depressive symptoms to symptom reporting, self-care and glucose control in diabetes. Gen Hosp Psychiatry 2003;25:246–252.

Draznin MB. Type 1 diabetes and sports participation: Strategies for training and competing safely. Phys Sportsmed 2000;28:49–56.

Kamboj M. Diabetes on the college campus. Pediatr Clin North Am 2005;52:279–305.

Kent SC, Legra RS. Polycystic ovary syndrome in adolescents. Adolesc Med 2002;13:73–88.

Rowell HA, Evans BJ, Quarry-Horn JL, Kerrigan JR. Type 2 diabetes mellitus in adolescents. Adolesc Med 2002; 13:1–12.

Weissberg-Benchell J, Antisdel-Lomaglio J, Seshadri R. Insulin pump therapy: A meta-analysis. Diabetes Care 2003;26:1079–1087.

Winter WE. Molecular and biochemical analysis of the MODY syndromes. Pediatr Diabetes 2000;1:88–117.

HYPOGLYCEMIA

The true incidence of hypoglycemia is probably much less than is suspected by the lay public. In evaluating an adolescent with possible hypoglycemia, the distinction needed is whether there is a symptomatic fall of blood glucose following a meal (suggesting a condition that can be managed with nutritional manipulation), or whether there is hypoglycemia due to an endocrine condition, such as hormone deficiency or even an insulinoma. The history of the episodes, and of any documentation of reliably measured low blood glucose readings at the time of the symptoms, will often separate postprandial syndrome from postprandial hypoglycemia, and that from true fasting hypoglycemia. Usually the serious conditions lead to fasting hypoglycemia, while postprandial symptoms and hypoglycemia associate with the nutritional or so-called reactive form of hypoglycemia. The gold standard for assessing presence or absence of hormonal and metabolic abnormality remains the critical sample of blood levels of glucose, insulin, growth hormone, cortisol, alanine, and other metabolic intermediates obtained when low blood glucose is found. It may be necessary to precipitate this event with a prolonged supervised fast, as an opportunity to get the appropriate blood sample during a spontaneous event may not be readily available.

Suggested Readings

Cryer PE. Glucose homeostasis and hypoglycemia. In Larsen PR, Kronenberg HM, Melmed S, Polonsky KS (eds.), *Williams Textbook of Endocrinology*, 10th ed. Philadelphia, PA:W.B. Saunders, 2002, pp. 1585–1618.

Haymond MW, Sunehag A. Controlling the sugar bowl: Regulation of glucose homeostasis in children. Endocrinol Metab Clin North Am 1999; 28:663–694.

THYROID DISORDERS

Hypothyroidism

Most cases of hypothyroidism acquired during adolescence will be due to Hashimoto thyroiditis, an autoimmune disorder with a strong familial tendency and human leukocyte antigens (HLA) linkages that are strong within, but not usually across ethnic groups. In addition, approximately one infant in every 3000 is born with congenital hypothyroidism every year. Since congenital hypothyroidism is usually permanent, a youth who omits treatment may present with symptoms similar to those of acquired hypothyroidism. Other less common causes of hypothyroidism in the United States include iodine deficiency, rarely iodine excess, ingestion of soy products that contain organic goitrogens in sufficient amount to interfere with thyroid function, complication of taking lithium for mental disorders, and following radiation therapy for tumors in which the field of radiation includes the thyroid bed.

Growth failure is a strong indicator of hypothyroidism in younger children. Hypothyroidism should be ruled out, if an adolescent is in the early to middle phases of the growth spurt and the growth rate falls. Otherwise, once the growth spurt has ended, the signs and symptoms of hypothyroidism are much as those in adults. Features that suggest acquired hypothyroidism include cold intolerance, diminished activity, increased sleeping, fatigue, dry skin, constipation, dry brittle hair, menometrorrhagia, waxy skin with pallor, facial features appearing immature for age, weight gain, and myxedema. Tall, "pink," active obese adolescents rarely have hypothyroidism! School performance may not be particularly worsened in acquired hypothyroidism.

Physical findings of hypothyroidism may include short stature, pale skin with myxedematous swelling (in severe cases this may manifest as pseudohypertrophy of calf muscles), puffy facies, immature appearing facial features, dry skin, cool extremities, "hung up" deep tendon reflexes, a firm goiter with an irregular nodular surface, a Delphian lymph node just superior to the thyroid isthmus, diminished heart sounds in the presence of a pericardial effusion, and increased weight.

Laboratory investigation reveals diminished level of free thyroxine and elevation of TSH. There may be elevated liver enzymes and cholesterol levels as well as microcytic or macrocytic anemia.

Antibodies to thyroglobulin and to the thyroid peroxidase enzyme are diagnostic of autoimmune thyroid disease and are usually found in hypothyroidism caused by Hashimoto thyroiditis. An ECG may show diminished precordial voltages due to the presence of pericardial effusion.

The treatment for hypothyroidism is with levothyroxine, at a dose calculated based on approximately 1.66 µg of thyroxine per kilogram body weight. The therapeutic goal is relief of symptoms, normalization of signs, and normalization of both free thyroxine and TSH levels. Loss of excessive weight is not assured upon normalization of laboratory values; even the increase in activity to prior normal levels may not be enough to allow for loss of the excess weight that had been gained. Thus, dietary control to reduce weight is needed in some patients. With treatment, the myxedema and puffiness diminishes and the youth will feel much more energetic and, in most ways, better. An increased level of energy may be misinterpreted by teachers as attention deficit disorder. There is no proven benefit of treatment with premixed thyroxine and triiodothyronine products, since the peripheral tissues deiodinase thyroxine on taking it up from the circulation and generate enough of the active hormone triiodothyronine from that process. There is also no indication for the use of desiccated thyroid preparations in adolescents.

Occasionally, pseudotumor cerebri may complicate the initiation of thyroid replacement. Thus, a careful retina examination is needed before treatment so it can be compared later to rule out pseudotumor cerebri, if severe headaches develop during the early part of treatment. If this condition does develop, stop the thyroid hormone replacement for a few days to a week, and then gradually reintroduce it, starting with a lower dose and working gradually to full replacement over several weeks. This method should prevent recurrence of the pseudotumor cerebri.

Fortunately, the cardiac decompensation reported in elderly hypothyroid patients rapidly restored to normal levels is not usually an issue in youth with normal hearts. Adolescent females who had developed hypothyroid-induced menorrhagia, metrorrhagia, or the combination of the two, will resume normal menses as the thyroid condition stabilizes. Hashimoto thyroiditis is frequently found to be associated with preexisting type 1 diabetes; 25% of females and 8% of males with type 1 diabetes are expected to develop hypothyroidism due to Hashimoto thyroiditis. However, diabetes is diagnosed only slightly more frequently in cases of preexisting thyroiditis patients than in the general public.

Hyperthyroidism

Graves' Disease

Graves' disease is less common in children and youth than in adults, comprising 5% of all cases; the majority of which occur in adolescents under age 20. There is also a thyrotoxic phase of Hashimoto thyroiditis in some individuals, called "Hashitoxicosis." Since both Graves' disease and Hashimoto thyroiditis are autoimmune in nature, it is possible that some of these individuals may have had both entities at once. Hashitoxicosis is described as resolving to a hypothyroid state, while Graves' disease continues on; acute thyroiditis may have a thyrotoxic phase. Thyrotoxicosis factitia, defined as the taking of thyroid hormone for secondary gain, is a rare disorder that may occur in adolescents.

Symptoms of thyrotoxicosis include nervousness, weight loss, shakiness, emotional lability, sleep dysfunction, exercise intolerance, heat intolerance, and increased appetite. Some adolescents manage to gain weight when hyperthyroid. Other associated symptoms include amenorrhea, moist skin, and tachycardia with or without palpitations. Ophthalmologic findings include eyes that are protruding, irritated, or even just dry; there may be diplopia on upward gaze, on gaze away from the midline, or even at rest in the rare case of severe exophthalmos.

Signs of Graves' disease may include a goiter, which is usually smooth and rubbery in consistency; there can also be increased heart rate and pulse pressure, increased skin moisture, stare, lid lag, fidgeting, extreme emotional instability, apparent thought disorder, bounding pulse to palpation, and a bruit over the thyroid gland with or without a palpable thrill. In comparison to adults, exophthalmos is much less frequent in adolescents and is usually less severe.

Laboratory testing will reveal an elevation of free thyroxine and a depressed level of TSH, while positive antithyroid antibodies are found in many cases; a positive test for thyroid-stimulating immunoglobulin is also helpful.

Treatment for Graves' disease in children and youth is usually initiated with antithyroid medications, and propylthiouracil (PTU), or methimazole are used in the United States (Table 15-8). Beta adrenergic blocking agents may be needed to control severe cardiovascular and neurologic symptoms. A recommended starting dose of PTU is 7–10 mg/kg/day divided into three doses. Methimazole, being 10 times more potent than PTU, is often effective at 10–20 mg twice a day; however, it often seems to require a higher dose at initiation of therapy than for maintenance. Some youth will need three times a day dosing of methimazole for initial control of excessive thyroid hormone levels

In the past, pediatric endocrinologists were trained to treat Graves' disease with suppressive doses of antithyroid medications until the TSH level became elevated and then continue suppression of thyroid activity with the antithyroid agent, with addition of thyroxine to yield normal TSH and thyroxine levels simultaneously. The rationale for this combined therapy was that thyroid rest for 2–4 years would lead to an improved chance for a prolonged drug free remission. A retrospective survey of a large group of children and adolescents with Graves' disease from one clinic instead suggested that two physical findings at presentation of the disease had good predictive value; these two findings were the size of the goiter and the weight of the patient compared to the median for age. A large goiter and weight more than 0.5 SD below the median for age were poor prognostic indicators. Adult endocrinologists often "titrate" monotherapy with a single antithyroid drug, frequently adjusting the dose to maintain the euthyroid state.

The side effects of antithyroid medications include rash, a lupus-like syndrome, myalgia, arthralgia, arthritis, and leukopenia. More severe reactions include agranulocytosis and autoimmune hepatitis. These thionamide drugs have a strong bitter metallic taste, making good adherence to the dosing schedule hard for some patients. In children and youth, the permanent therapies of thyroidectomy and radioiodine ablation, have been reserved

TABLE 15-8

THERAPY FOR GRAVES' DISEASE

Mode of Therapy	Advantages	Disadvantages
Antithyroid drugs	Reversible in event of spontaneous remission	Side effects common, unpleasant
		Complications uncommon, severe
		Bitter disagreeable taste and inconvenience increase likelihood of poor adherence
		Long duration of therapy
Surgical ablation of thyroid	No medical toxicity or side effects	Scar, pain, exposure to general anesthesia universal
		Risk of hypoparathyroidism or vocal cord paralysis small but measurable
		Can not operate when very thyrotoxic, risk of thyroid storm
		Permanent hypothyroidism is goal, meaning lifelong replacement therapy needed
Radioiodine ablation of thyroid	Very easy to do	Patient and parental worries about radiation long-term risk
		Permanent hypothyroidism is goal, meaning lifelong replacement therapy needed

in the past for cases of severe toxicity from antithyroid medications, or failure of the medical therapy to control hyperthyroidism; in contrast, radioiodine ablation is often the first line treatment in adults.

The preferred surgery, near-total thyroidectomy, requires the services of a highly skilled surgeon who has had significant experience with this procedure, as the potential complications include damage to recurrent laryngeal nerve(s) and/or the parathyroid glands. In a small number of cases, vocal cord paralysis or permanent hypoparathyroidism are reported. Excellent metabolic control must be achieved prior to induction of anesthesia for this operation to minimize the risk for intraoperative thyroid storm. For years, radioiodine ablation has been considered best reserved for adults and older adolescents, due to uncertainty about the long-term risk for neoplasia. However, reports from centers with large numbers of patients treated in adolescence and childhood with radioiodine ablation, suggest that this procedure is as safe in adolescents as in the elderly and may be preferable to the small but real risks of surgery. Once the adolescent has been rendered hypothyroid (the preferred outcome) by surgery or radioiodine therapy, addition of thyroxine replacement will control the TSH level and maintain a euthyroid state.

Euthyroid Goiter

The most common cause of euthyroid goiter in adolescents is Hashimoto thyroiditis, perhaps affecting one or more adolescent females per hundred. Unless the gland enlargement causes pressure symptoms, or is large, it may be missed. Treatment can be offered with thyroxine if the TSH is elevated, to minimize further growth of the goiter; however, lymphocytic infiltration is not affected by this treatment. Other causes are much less seen in the United States.

Thyroid Neoplasia

Thyroid tumors in youth are considerably less common than in adults. Benign lesions include a nodular form of Hashimoto thyroiditis, thyroid cysts, adenomas, ectopic thyroid masses, or a thyroglossal duct cyst; the latter is a remnant of an embryologic connection of the thyroid gland to the pharynx. Malignant neoplasms include papillary carcinoma, follicular carcinoma, mixed papillary-follicular carcinoma, medullary carcinoma, and anaplastic (undifferentiated) thyroid carcinoma. Radiation to the neck or mediastinum in childhood may be a predisposing factor for thyroid carcinoma (papillary or follicular) development. Metastatic lesions, especially lymphomas, may be found in the thyroid. Ultra-sonography, radionuclide scanning, and, in appropriate cases, fine needle aspiration, may all be employed to assess a palpable nodule and plan the further evaluation and treatment needed.

Suggested Readings

Foley TP. Acquired hypothyroidism in infants, children, and adolescents. In: Braverman LE, Utiger RD (eds.), *Werner and Ingbar's The Thyroid: A Fundamental and Clinical Text*, 8th ed. Baltimore, MD: Lippincott Williams & Wilkins, 2000, pp. 993–988.

Generic Levothyroxine. Med Lett 2004;46:77–78.

Hanna CE, LaFranchi SH. Adolescent thyroid disorders. Adolesc Med 2002; 13:13–36.

Rivkees SA. Hypothyroidism and hyperthyroidism in children. In: Pescovitz OH, Eugster EA (eds.), *Pediatric Endocrinology: Mechanisms Manifestations and Management*, Baltimore, MD: Lippincott Williams & Wilkins, 2004, pp. 508–521.

Rivkees SA, Cornelius EA. Influence of iodine-131 dose on the outcome of hyperthyroidism in children. Pediatrics 2003;111:745–749.

Siegmund W, Spieker K, Weike AI, et al. Replacement therapy with levothyroxine plus triiodothyronine (bioavailable molar ratio 14:1) is not superior to thyroxine alone to improve well-being and cognitive performance in hypothyroidism. Clin Endocrinol 2004;60:750–757.

Zimmerman D. Thyroid tumors in children. In: Lifshitz F (ed.), *Pediatric Endocrinology*, 4th ed. New York: Marcel Dekker, 2003, pp. 407–420.

GROWTH DISORDERS

Short Stature

Short stature of medical significance is usually present before the onset of puberty; however, a departure from the growth curve during the time of expected increased rate of growth should indicate the need for evaluation. Many short male adolescents are also delayed in onset of puberty and have so-called constitutional delay of growth and development; this is a physiologic and often familial growth pattern. Another group of normally short adolescents will be found to have familial short stature. In many academic endocrine clinics, the incidence of endocrine disorders among patients referred for short stature is approximately 15%.

Plotting of growth measurements on standardized growth charts is the most important method for initial analysis of the child's growth. Charts from the Centers for Disease Control that are currently available were published in 2000 and should be used. A free-ware utility program for personal digital assistant (PDA) users can be used to calculate percentiles or standard deviation scores for the height, weight, and body mass index. If there are two sets of properly performed and accurately recorded measurements separated by sufficient time, the rate of growth can be calculated and assessed as well. There are also standard growth charts for syndromes associated with short stature, which allow comparison with expected measurements for the appropriate cohort of children and youth; examples include growth charts for Turner syndrome and Down syndrome.

It is important to note that omission of measurements; inaccurate measurements due to improper technique or equipment, or misplotting of the measurements on the growth chart can lead to difficulties in use of growth as an index of health. Such problems make evaluation of a growth disorder difficult. In addition, the rate of growth is more powerful in making a determination of whether there is a problem than is the presence of a single measurement that is lower on the chart than expected. In fact, normal stature with a slowing growth rate is more troublesome than short stature with a normal or accelerating growth rate. While the Tanner-Davies growth charts from the late 1980s are no longer current, the concept of tempo of growth is still important. It is important to compare the patient to the proper cohort of youth. Thus, the timing of entry into puberty, the rate of growth, the current pubertal status, and the history of timing of the growth spurt,

and important pubertal milestones in family members are important data to have in hand, when making a determination whether there is a growth disorder or a pattern of growth that is normal for that child but not typical of his/her age peers.

In addition to Tanner staging, bone age x-rays can be used to determine where the individual should be placed on the continuum of growth curves. The Greulich and Pyle atlas of bone age films is based on an old study, and the population sampled was not representative of all ethnic or socioeconomic groups; however, given these caveats, it still can serve to help in evaluating the pattern of growth. Contained in the atlas are the Bailey-Pinneau tables of predicted height, which are based on bone age, and separate children into cohorts by their apparent tempo of growth. They can be used to help assess the growth of the adolescent and make predictions for future growth; however, the statistical error inherent in this prediction is several inches, as is the prediction of adult height based on the height of the parents.

Among causes of short stature, genetic or familial short stature and constitutional delay of growth and puberty, are the most common. In fact, most short children and adolescents are healthy and do not have a disorder of growth. Key characteristics of familial short stature are a normal degree of pubertal maturation, a normal bone age for chronological age, and, most important, a normal rate of growth. The final height in adulthood agrees with that predicted by heights of the parents, and of older siblings who have finished growth.

In constitutional delay, the bone age, and pubertal stage lag behind the chronological age by up to several years. In addition to the concerns about height, the delay of onset of puberty compared to peers causes much anxiety for some. The rate of growth will be normal for the appropriate stage of puberty and for the appropriate cohort, late developing youth. While the age peers are undergoing their growth spurt, youth with delayed puberty may still be in the prepubertal, slowing phase of growth; this will accentuate the differences and exacerbate the concerns. The diagnosis of constitutional delay can only be made certain by eliminating other causes. It is often helpful to track growth, pubertal progression and the advance of the bone age over 6 or more months to minimize the number of healthy youth who otherwise would undergo extensive and unnecessary testing.

Screening laboratory indices of health include complete blood count (CBC), differential count, erythrocyte sedimentation rate, urinalysis, and multiple so-called "panel" blood chemistry tests to assess renal, osseous, and hepatic status. These can be done at the start of the evaluation or the testing can be reserved for those youth whose growth rate at the return visit seems too slow. Testing for celiac disease has been advocated by some consultants.

Free thyroxine and TSH levels, insulin-like growth factor 1 (IGF-1) and its major binding protein (IGFBP-3), have been used in screening as well. IGF-1 and IGFBP-3 are growth hormone (GH) dependent and the levels in the circulation fluctuate less throughout the day than that of GH. Thus, this can be a good test to represent GH adequacy whereas random levels of GH are not helpful, due to the infrequent, pulsatile releases of GH. It is also important to remember that there are other causes for a low level of IGF-1, such as malnutrition; thus, it is suggestive of but not diagnostic for growth hormone deficiency (GHD). IGF-1 levels must also be interpreted in relation to the pubertal stage of the patient, as there is a large difference between the levels measured during the growth spurt and those of prepubertal youth.

The prevalence of GHD is thought to be from 1:10,000 to as many as 1:4000. It may be isolated or associated with deficiency of other pituitary hormones. The etiology may be idiopathic, genetic, secondary to tumor, trauma, radiation, vascular accident, or from developmental anomalies involving the hypothalamus and pituitary. The onset of growth abnormality can occur at any age from birth to adolescence, depending on the cause. Appropriate continuing care for a youth previously diagnosed with GHD includes periodic measurements and bone age films to assess adequacy of growth response, surveillance for the uncommon side effects and complications associated with GH treatment, and adjustment of the dose of GH to optimize outcome. When linear growth is finished, testing to find those individuals who have continuing growth deficiency, as determined by adult criteria, is recommended, as a significant percentage of children

and youth who needed treatment with GH to grow normally are able to release enough GH to maintain normal health; however, those who need continued replacement need to be found.

Excessively Tall Stature

Excessively tall stature may indicate a syndrome, such as Marfan syndrome or Klinefelter syndrome; true pituitary giants are very rarely encountered. The subjective decision by the family that height is excessive often brings the youth to the clinician for evaluation. In the absence of a disorder of growth associated with a syndrome or pathologic tall stature (such as caused by pituitary giantism), treatment is less a medically driven necessity than one mediated by psychologic issues. Considerations of appropriateness of care in normal tall stature that is subjectively excessive take on ethical and cultural dimensions; this is especially noted in the case of a tall normal girl desiring to be shorter than her predicted stature requesting high dose estrogen to prematurely fuse her epiphyses.

Suggested Readings

Allen DB. Growth hormone treatment. In: Lifshitz F (ed.), *Pediatric Endocrinology*, 4th ed. New York: Marcel Dekker, 2003, pp. 87–112.

Bayley N, Pinneau SR. Tables for predicting adult height from skeletal age: Revised for use with the Gruelich-Pyle hand standard. J Pediatr 1952;40:563–571.

Gruelich WW, Pyle SI. *Radiographic Atlas of Skeletal Development of the Hand and Wrist*, 2d ed. Stanford, CA: Stanford University Press, 1959.

Lifshitz F, Botero D. Worrisome growth. In: Lifshitz F (ed.), *Pediatric Endocrinology*, 4th ed. New York: Marcel Dekker, 2003, pp. 1–46.

National Center for Health Statistics in collaboration with the National Center for Chronic Disease Prevention and Health Promotion. CDC Growth Charts United States, 2000. Available at: http://www.cdc.gov/growthcharts

STAT Growth-BP™ Ver 2.50. Growth 2 PDA freeware available from Statcoder.com.

Tanner JM, Davies PSW. Clinical longitudinal standards for height and weight velocity for North American children. J Pediatr 1985;107:317–329.

Obesity

Obesity is rarely due solely to a disorder of hormone synthesis and release (Chaps. 29 and 31). The critical information needed to assess the likelihood that obesity is secondary to thyroid hormone deficiency or glucocorticoid excess, for example, requires thorough history taking. This includes careful attention to the growth records of family members as well as that of the youth who presents for evaluation. Glucocorticoid excess, whether from Cushing's disease, Cushing syndrome of adrenal origin, or due to high doses of glucocorticoids, is associated with poor linear growth in children. By contrast, the child or youth with exogenous obesity usually appears healthy, unless the obesity is so severe as to impair movement or sleep. There is usually excellent linear growth in exogenous obesity.

Weight loss requires expenditure of more calories than are taken in. This is difficult to accomplish, at any age. The normal approach to weight loss should be advised for the youth whose abnormal weight was induced by a hormone disorder, once the disorder is under effective treatment. Hormone regulation alone may not have any effect on the excess weight. For example, some youth with Graves' disease are quite upset to discover that they gain excessive weight on resolution of the hypermetabolic state with successful treatment, mimicking hypothyroidism. Thus, they should be warned in advance not to let their weight increase rapidly.

Suggested Readings

Dietz WH. Overweight in childhood and adolescence. N Engl J Med 2004;350:855–857.

Greydanus DE, Bhave S. Obesity and adolescents: Time for increased physical activity. Ind Pediatr 2004;41: 545–550.

DISORDERS OF PUBERTAL ONSET

Delayed Puberty

Delayed puberty is part and parcel of constitutional delay of growth and puberty or of a syndrome, such as Turner syndrome. However, in cases of delayed puberty where there is normal linear growth and absence of signs suggesting syndromes or symptoms suggesting chronic illness, other conditions should be investigated. A statistically based and helpful definition of delay is absence of breast development by age 13 in girls, or absence of testicular enlargement in boys by age 14. While many normal youth will start puberty at or later than these limits, it is appropriate to consider starting the investigation at these ages.

Causes of pubertal delay, roughly in order of prevalence, include constitutional delay, undernutrition (due to poor dietary intake or to excessively high levels of exercise output), stimulant medication for attention deficit disorder (with or without hyperactivity), eating disorder, chronic illness or syndrome (associated with delayed growth and development, as Turner syndrome, see Chap. 21), recently acquired interference with pubertal onset or progression from disorders of the hypothalamus and/or pituitary (such as tumor, trauma, or infiltrative disease), damage to gonads from therapy for another illness, isolated disorders of sexual development and puberty (such as the hypogonadotropic hypogonadism of Kallmann syndrome), and isolated gonadal dysgenesis, as in some cases of mosaic Turner syndrome, or in Klinefelter syndrome (see Chap. 21).

The initial screening evaluation of delayed puberty includes a careful family history, including growth and timing of pubertal development of the parents and siblings. The physical examination should verify absence of pubertal signs. It is possible that the early signs are not known to the concerned parent and are indeed present, making the rest of the evaluation less problematic. Also, as part of the physical assessment, a careful search is needed for features of syndromes, and Tanner staging needed for any pubertal signs that are found. A bone age x-ray is the initial recommended laboratory study during the screening process. Measurement of luteinizing hormone (LH), follicle stimulating hormone (FSH), and sex steroid hormone levels would start the focused investigation. The investigation should be done in a stepwise and focused manner; specific diagnostic tools may be available only from research groups.

The two main divisions in pathologically delayed puberty are hypogonadotropic hypogonadism (secondary) and hypergonadotropic hypogonadism (primary). A tall, anosmic, hypogonadal male with low LH and FSH is most likely to have Kallmann Syndrome. Klinefelter syndrome should be considered in a tall hypogonadal young man, with high LH and FSH levels, gynecomastia, school or learning difficulties, and small firm testes. Turner syndrome (ovarian dysgenesis) occurs in 1 of every 2000 female births (Chap. 21). Rarely, other disorders can be found, such as mutations of steroidogenic enzymes interfering with sex steroid production, or processing, and sex steroid receptor mutations.

Treatment of delayed puberty should be tailored to the underlying condition, the current needs of the adolescent for continued development of secondary sexual characteristics, and long-term considerations. Provision of sex steroid hormone replacement is appropriate either for delayed normal puberty or for when the hypogonadal state is permanent. In pituitary or hypothalamic disorders, the provision of gonadotropin replacement would be deferred until there is a desire to attempt to develop fertility; it is not needed for development of secondary sexual characteristics and accrual of bone mineral density.

Suggested Readings

Achermann JC. Delayed puberty. In: Pescovitz OH, Eugster EA (eds.), *Pediatric Endocrinology: Mechanisms Manifestations and Management*. Baltimore, MD: Lippincott Williams & Wilkins, 2004, pp. 334– 348.

Cedars MI. Polycystic ovary syndrome: What is it and how should we treat it? J Pediatr 2004; 144:4–5.

Herman-Giddens ME, Kaplowitz PB, Wasserman R. Navigating the recent articles on girls' puberty in *Pediatrics*: What do we know and where do we go from here? Pediatrics 2004;113:911–917.

Lee PA. Puberty and its disorders. In: Lifshitz F (ed.), *Pediatric Endocrinology*, 4th ed. New York: Marcel Dekker, 2003, pp. 211–238.

Midyett LK, Moore WV, Jacobson JD. Are pubertal changes in girls before age 8 benign? Pediatrics 2003;111:47–51.

Reiter EO, Lee PA. Delayed puberty. Adolesc Med 2002;13:101–118.

Stepanian M, Cohn DE. Gynecologic malignancies in adolescents. Adolesc Med 2004;15:555–570.

Premature Thelarche and Premature Adrenarche

Premature thelarche refers to early breast development in female children, most commonly starting within the first 2 years of life; pubarche and menarche do not develop as a result of this condition that has a prevalence of 2%. Various causes are noted, including hereditary factors, increased sensitivity to estrogen, increased estrogen (adrenal gland-induced), increased dietary estrogen, transient estrogen-secreting follicular cysts of the ovaries, oral contraceptive ingestion, application of estrogen cream to the nipples, and transient partial activation of pubertal axis with increased FSH. A careful evaluation will distinguish this condition from precocious puberty. Laboratory studies are normal, though the serum estradiol may be mildly elevated. Management is exclusion of precocious puberty, reassurance, and periodic observation. Breast development may regress after a few years and only rarely progresses; menarche is usually normal.

Premature adrenarche (premature pubarche) refers to the development of sexual hair in girls before 8 years and in males before 9 years, without other signs of puberty. It usually occurs in later childhood, before the timing of normal puberty, often between 6 and 8 or 9 years of age. There may be other features, such as increase in adrenal androgens, penile enlargement, body odor, perspiration, and acne. The growth rate and bone are normal, or slightly increased. A careful evaluation should rule out precious puberty and atypical precocious adrenarche (with increased growth, severe acne, and other pubertal signs). Management for premature adrenarche is reassurance and periodic observation. Perhaps half of these females are at increased risk for hyperandrogenism and polycystic ovary syndrome.

Precocious Puberty

This disorder is, by definition, puberty developing before a child is of an age at which it is normal; therefore, it occurs before ages associated with adolescence. A child previously diagnosed and under therapy will have a very different experience of starting puberty than peers starting with their cohort do at the usual time. In addition to the usual dramatic physiologic and psychologic changes noted with puberty in general, there is the inappropriateness of the early pubertal onset, with attendant psychologic risks from stigmatization. There are reports of early experimentation with sexual behavior or other high-risk behaviors in children with precocious puberty, and there may be a risk for sexual exploitation as well.

The medical attention and treatment may also have a negative effect on self-image in spite of the best efforts of the family and physician to reassure the child. Short adult stature is a serious concern in precocious puberty if effective therapy was not instituted early enough; this is because the bone age, during precocious puberty, often advances beyond the advance in so-called height age, with premature fusion of epiphyses. In the less common forms of precocity, such as McCune Albright syndrome, associated problems, such as fibrous dysplasia of bone, need to be addressed.

Ambiguous Genitalia/Intersex

A small but important group of adolescents are born with nontypical genital development, leading to difficulties with making the correct sex assignment at birth. There is much current interest and controversy about what, if any, procedures should be done for these children to alter the appearance of their genitalia. Other concerns include when and by whose decision such changes should be done. An expert panel to study those aspects of these disorders and to possibly redefine what procedures should be done at which ages for such an individual has been assembled in recent years.

A youth who has genital ambiguity, for whatever reason, needs expert advice and support. Humans predominately think of themselves as male or female; there is apparently no middle or mixed gender identity, although other aspects of human sexuality, such as gender role, may be more complex. The development of gender identity has been shown by studies in the past decades to involve much more than having "normal" appearing external genitalia. There are significant genetic and hormonally directed differences between male and female, presumably from early in embryogenesis. Thus, provision of expert, sensitive assessment and guidance ideally should have been made available to the family at the birth of the child; hopefully, by adolescence, many issues ideally should have been addressed. Where this has not been available and where remaining concerns or problems persist, expert help ideally should be sought. Unfortunately, there is not yet a broad consensus about whose expertise, whose experiences, and which studies to rely on in some conditions to give the most favorable outcome for the adolescent with genital ambiguity who needs help.

Suggested Readings

Berenbaum SA. Management of children with intersex conditions: Psychological and methodological perspectives. Gr Genet Horn 2003;19:1–6.

Blizzard RM. Intersex issues: A series of continuing conundrums. Pediatrics 2002;110:616–621.

Gallagher MP, Oberfeld SE. Disorders of sexual differentiation. In: Pescovitz OH, Eugster EA (eds.), *Pediatric Endocrinology: Mechanisms Manifestations and Management*. Baltimore, MD: Lippincott Williams & Wilkins, 2004, pp. 243–254.

Wisniewski AB, Migeon CJ. Gender identity/role differentiation in adolescents affected by syndrome of abnormal sex differentiation. Adolesc Med 2002;13: 119–128.

ADRENAL DYSFUNCTION

Adrenal Insufficiency

Congenital adrenal hyperplasia (CAH) of the salt-wasting or simple virilizing varieties will have been diagnosed at birth or early in childhood. What is needed in adolescence is continuation of proper provision of glucocorticoid and mineralocorticoid replacement therapy. The goal of treatment is to minimize the effects of continuing adrenal androgen excess without stunting growth or inducing Cushing syndrome. Provision of extra cortisol is mandatory during significant acute illnesses to mimic the normal adrenal stress response. Surveillance is needed in males for growth of adrenal rest tissue in the testes, made worse in case of poor adherence to the treatment plan. Innovative ideas, such as employing additional therapeutic agents to improve the control of adrenal androgen effects, or performing laparoscopic adrenalectomy to remove the source of the androgens have been discussed with much interest; however, at present, these are seen as issues for further research and refinement rather than current established therapy.

The more common nonclassical form of CAH may manifest as premature adrenarche in childhood, as signs of excess androgen in pubertal girls, or with little or no sign or symptom in adolescent males. As the nonclassical form of CAH is thought to predispose to a polycystic ovarian phenotype, careful investigation and treatment are needed. The most common cause of all forms of CAH is a defect in the gene for the steroid 21 hydroxylase enzyme leading to diminished cortisol synthesis, elevation of adrenocorticotropic hormone (ACTH) level, and increased generation of adrenal androgens. Unlike the salt-wasting or simple virilizing forms of CAH, there is no genital ambiguity and there is less risk for adrenal insufficiency in the nonclassical form. Thus, treatment should be designed to avoid androgen excess in girls, but with care to minimize side effects of the glucocorticoid. It is often recommended that the patient be considered to be at risk for adrenal suppression once undergoing treatment; thus, stress dosing of cortisol, including injection therapy by the family, is taught.

Addison's disease, due to autoimmune destruction of adrenal cortical cells, may be as prevalent as 0.1% in youth with type 1 diabetes; it can arise in the absence of diabetes or in association with other autoimmune endocrine disorders. However, it may also be due to HIV/AIDS or tuberculosis. Manifestations of Addison's disease include weakness, weight loss, abdominal pain, hypoglycemia, an unusual bronze appearing hyperpigmentation of the skin, and mental status changes. Laboratory findings include hypoglycemia, hyponatremia, metabolic acidosis, elevated ACTH, and low cortisol levels. The adolescent with Addison's disease can present in

"adrenal crisis"; this can mimic a surgical condition of the abdomen, placing the patient at extreme risk for circulatory collapse during surgery if not discovered prior to induction of anesthesia. Treatment with replacement cortisol and mineralocorticoid is easier to adjust than in CAH; symptom relief and control of ACTH level can be accomplished with lower doses than those needed to suppress adrenal androgens in CAH, minimizing the risk of inducing Cushing syndrome. For the crisis situation, intravenous infusion of 10% dextrose in 0.9% saline with 100 mg/L of soluble cortisol is recommended as the resuscitative fluid of choice. It directly addresses all areas of concern, such as cortisol deficiency, volume depletion, sodium deficiency, and hypoglycemia.

Adrenal Excess

Cushing's disease from pituitary ACTH excess, and Cushing syndrome from adrenal cortisol excess or from high dose exogenous glucocorticoids, manifest with metabolic derangement, increased weight, proximal muscle wasting, striae, and other signs and symptoms. In growing children, there is attenuation or cessation of linear growth; nearly full-grown adolescents may not exhibit growth failure and will present more as adults do. The specific cause of cortisol and other adrenal hormone excess should be found and treated. In Cushing's disease, adrenal androgens are often secreted in excess leading to varying degrees of virilization. In adolescents, these may be less dramatic than in prepubertal children.

Suggested Readings

Shulman DI, Root AW. Hyperadrenocorticism. In: Pescovitz OH, Eugster EA (eds.), *Pediatric Endocrinology: Mechanisms, Manifestations and Management*. Baltimore, MD: Lippincott Williams & Wilkins, 2004, pp. 582–591.

Speiser PW. Congenital adrenal hyperplasia. In: Pescovitz OH, Eugster EA (eds.), *Pediatric Endocrinology: Mechanisms, Manifestations and Management*. Baltimore, MD: Lippincott Williams & Wilkins, 2004, pp. 601–613.

Ten S, New, Laclaren N. Clinical review: Addison's disease. J Clin Endocrinol Metab 2001;86:263–315.

Witchel SF. Hyperandrogenism in adolescents. Adolesc Med 2002; 13: 89–100.

DISORDERS OF CALCIUM METABOLISM

Hypocalcemia

Hypocalcemia diagnosed during adolescence in the United States is often due to hypoparathyroidism or a type of pseudohypoparathyroidism that did not present with phenotypic abnormalities in infancy or early childhood. Symptoms include muscle tetany, muscle cramps and pain, seizures of varying type, and severity; however, symptomatology may be subtle. One youth seen at our institution presented to an Emergency Department with eyelid ptosis. While undergoing an MRI to investigate the cause of his ptosis, he became anxious and hyperventilated, leading to severe carpopedal spasm and the diagnosis of hypocalcemia due to hypoparathyroidism. An adolescent girl had absence seizures in class. The consulting neurologist made the diagnosis of hypocalcemia due to pseudohypoparathyroidism. She has no signs of Albright's hereditary osteodystrophy and is of normal height and intelligence suggesting type Ib or type II pseudohypoparathyroidism.

Transient parathyroid depression presumably due to edema following thyroidectomy is more common than permanent loss of function from severe damage to or removal of all four glands with the thyroid. Less likely in adolescents in the United States, is severe dietary deficiency of vitamin D, calcium, or hypomagnesemia, leading to inability to release parathyroid hormone (PTH). Laboratory testing reveals low total and ionized calcium, elevated phosphorus, low 1, 25-dihydroxy vitamin D level. PTH will be abnormally low if deficient, or elevated in pseudohypoparathyroidism.

The initial treatment is with calcium and calcitriol, 1,25-dihydroxy vitamin D. Not all patients will need calcium supplementation if their diets are calcium sufficient. Monitoring the levels of ionized calcium, phosphorus, and urine calcium to creatinine ratio or quantitative urinary calcium over 24 hours must be done to adjust therapy to minimize symptoms while avoiding nephrocalcinosis and loss of renal function.

Hypercalcemia

Hypercalcemia can be due to primary hyperparathyroidism, or immobilization after an injury or during a debilitating illness, both leading to bone resorption. It may also be due to a complication in the course of malignancies, either with bony destruction from metastases or marrow replacement, or from elevated levels of parathyroid hormone related peptide released by the tumor cells. Symptoms of hypercalcemia include abdominal pain, loss of appetite, weakness or fatigue, polydipsia, and polyuria due to loss of renal ability to concentrate urine. Acute management should provide hydration with 0.9% saline to protect renal function coupled with a calciuretic diuretic to diminish the calcium burden. Glucocorticoids may act to interfere with absorption of calcium from the gut; bisphosphonates can interfere with mobilization of calcium from bone. Definitive therapy for the underlying condition is needed for ultimate resolution.

Suggested Readings

Greydanus DE, Bricker LA. Parathyroid disorders in the adolescent. Asian J Paediatr Pract 2005;23: 123–129.

Perheentupa J. Hypoparathyroidism and mineral homeostasis. In: Lifshitz F (ed.), *Pediatric Endocrinology*, 4th ed. New York: Marcel Dekker, 2003, pp. 421–468.

Rivkees SA, Carpenter TO. Hyperparathyroidism in children. In: Lifshitz F (ed.), *Pediatric Endocrinology*, 4th ed. New York: Marcel Dekker, 2003; pp. 469– 468.

DIABETES INSIPIDUS

Diabetes insipidus (DI) can occur following significant head trauma leading to transection of the pituitary stalk, as a consequence of surgery in the area of the hypothalamus and pituitary, and as a result of infiltrative disease or to a neoplasm in the region of hypothalamus and pituitary. Classically, the symptoms of acquired DI occur suddenly, with massively increased urine output and thirst requiring large volumes of water. Cold water is said to be the preferred drink. An overnight water deprivation test will result in hemoconcentration while the urine stays dilute. Provision of antidiuretic hormone in the form of desmopressin restores ability of the kidneys to concentrate urine. In cases of "idiopathic" DI, it is necessary to follow closely the

MRI as small or slow growing lesions capable of causing DI may not be detected for months to several years after onset of symptoms.

Suggested Reading

Robertson GL. Diabetes insipidus. In: Pescovitz OH, Eugster EA(eds.), *Pediatric Endocrinology: Mechanisms Manifestations and Management.*, Baltimore, MD: Lippincott Williams & Wilkins, 2004, pp. 94–99.

16

GENITOURINARY AND RENAL DISORDERS

Donald E. Greydanus, Alfonso D. Torres,
and Julian H. Wan

URINARY TRACT INFECTIONS

Sites of Infection

Lower Urinary Tract Epidemiology

Bacterial urinary tract infections (UTI) are common bacterial infections affecting humans throughout life. This is particularly true for females who may develop UTIs from infancy through old age. Cystitis is three to five times more common in females than in males and most often occurs as a primary infection in an otherwise healthy individual. The incidence of first time infection decreases during the first decade of life, but then gradually increases with age, particularly in females. This is probably due to several gender-specific factors listed in Table 16-1. Studies note that at least 5% of females aged 5–18 will have a UTI and more than 20% of all females will experience at least one episode of acute cystitis during their reproductive years. In some series, as many as 30% of these will have recurrent infections. Recurrence is unusual in young adult males. The incidence of UTIs in males tends to be higher at the extremes of life, during the first year of life and after age 55 due to prostatic hypertrophy.

Etiology

The uropathogens most frequently associated with cystitis in adolescents include *Escherichia coli* and coagulase negative staphylococci, though other enteric bacteria may cause urinary infections, particularly in males. Urine bacterial colony counts are usually $\geq 10^5$ colony forming units (CFU)/mL for acute cystitis or pyelonephritis. They can be lower, between 10^2 and 10^5 for bouts of symptomatic urethritis, particularly in boys. A negative routine urine culture, particularly in a sexually active individual, should suggest the possibility of urethral infection with *Chlamydia trachomatis*, *Neisseria gonorrhoeae*, *Trichomonas vaginalis*, or herpes simplex virus (Chap. 24). The presence of concomitant cervicitis, vaginitis, or pelvic pain increases the likelihood of simultaneous urethral infection with *Candida albicans* or one or more of these organisms in females.

As can be seen in Table 16-1, the pathogenic factors determining the risk of primary and recurrent infections are complex and multiple. Virulence factors may enhance the pathogenicity of certain serotypes of bacteria within the urinary tract. Certain pili on the outer surface of the bacteria (type

TABLE 16-1

FACTORS CONTRIBUTING TO THE RISK OF UTI

Females
Anatomic short urethra
Poor perineal hygiene
Coital irritation, change of coital patterns, new sexual partner (honeymoon cystitis)
Vulvovaginitis
Vaginal or rectal colonization with pathogenic bacterial serogroups (viz. *E. coli*)
Pregnancy (abnormal ureteral peristalsis)
Bladder contamination secondary to douching
Vaginal foreign body
Diaphragm and/or spermicide use (controversial for disease)
Males
Urethral strictures (extremely rare in girls who have not had prior surgery, trauma, or radiation)
Posterior urethral valves
Phimosis
Meatal stenosis
Sexual practices exposing the urethra to fecal flora
Males or females
Urologic abnormality with stasis and/or obstruction (dysfunctional bladder [neurogenic or other], ectopic ureter, nephrolithiasis, and so forth)
Vesicoureteral reflux
Urethral instrumentation (catheters, foreign bodies, and masturbatory)
Urethral trauma
Other foci of infection (direct extension from kidney, prostate, vagina, or hematogenous spread from distant site)
Lowered host resistance to infection (including due to HIV infection)
Multiple antibiotic usage and development of resistant organisms
Infrequent or incomplete voiding
Voluntary urinary retention
Chronic illnesses such as diabetes

II P-fimbriated *E. coli*) have been shown to increase adherence to urothelial cell membranes and are more frequently associated with invasive UTIs. Other bacterial factors may increase adhesion, tissue invasiveness, or provide protection from host defense systems. The clinical significance of many of these factors is currently under investigation. It may be possible to use immunization to augment host resistance or to introduce benign competitive bacteria. Host factors that appear to contribute to the risk of UTI include structural, functional, and biochemical characteristics.

Structural factors include the relatively short urethra of the female, the intact prepuce in the male, and underlying structural abnormalities of the upper or lower urinary drainage system. *Functional factors* include various types of voiding dysfunction, which may lead to incomplete or infrequent bladder emptying. Urine biochemical factors, which have been purported to contribute to host resistance to UTI, include urine pH, osmolality, urea concentration, and the presence of urinary Tamm-Horsfall glycoprotein. In addition, phenotypic expression on urothelial cells of cell surface receptors capable of binding to *p*-fimbriae appears to increase the risk of urinary infection in certain individuals. Finally, 20% of females with bacteriuria will have vesicoureteral reflux (VUR) and over 10% of the children of these females will become bacteriuric themselves. There is also a strong tendency for VUR to be clustered in families. Siblings of a child with VUR have about a 30% chance of having VUR themselves, and should be studied.

Symptomatology

Clinical symptoms of upper and lower urinary tract sites of infection overlap considerably (Table 16-2). Dysuria and other associated symptoms of lower urinary tract irritation and/or inflammation frequently accompany infection of the lower genitourinary system.

TABLE 16-2

SYMPTOMS OF UTI

Dysuria
Urinary frequency
Nocturia
Hesitancy
Urgency
Low abdominal pain (including suprapubic pain)
Low-grade temperature elevation
Hematuria (gross or microscopic)

In this clinical setting, several anatomical sources for these symptoms must be considered. In some cases of pyelonephritis, clinical findings are indistinguishable from those of cystitis. UTI symptoms may also occur with the acute urethral syndrome and urethritis. However, as opposed to the abrupt onset usually associated with cystitis, symptoms of urethritis tend to develop more gradually. Dysuria may also occur in patients with vaginitis. In this setting, urinary frequency and urgency are uncommon, and evidence for vulvovaginal inflammation is noted with the history and physical examination.

Upper Urinary Tract Etiology

Contributing factors are similar to those for cystitis, though there is a much higher association with urogenital structural abnormalities. In upper UTIs, *E. coli* is the most frequently cultured bacterial isolate; however, other organisms, including gram-positive cocci and drug-resistant enteric pathogens, also may occur, particularly in those individuals with chronic or recurrent disease. Any pattern of unexplained recurrent pyelonephritis should prompt the clinician to consider an occult abnormality of the urinary tract.

Symptomatology

Characteristic findings in patients with acute pyelonephritis are symptoms of acute cystitis and a positive urine culture, together with some combination of fever, chills, costovertebral tenderness, elevated white blood cell (WBC) count, and elevated erythrocyte sedimentation rate. As mentioned above, however, the clinical presentation is often less clear, with only a low-grade fever, simple backache, or variable abdominal pain.

Asymptomatic (or covert) bacteriuria occurs in all age groups, predominantly in females. The term is best reserved for those patients with no evidence of urinary voiding symptoms and who have no history of antecedent UTI, since patients with previous urinary infections and bacteriuria may have radiographic evidence of renal parenchymal scarring and/or VUR. It is a diagnosis of exclusion and refers to patients with typically normal blood pressure, normal upper urinary tract, normal bladder function, and no VUR.

As many as 3%–5% of asymptomatic adolescent females will be found to have $>10^5$ CFU/mL of the same bacterial organism on repeated urine cultures. The significance of asymptomatic bacteriuria in the individual with a normal genitourinary tract is unclear. Although half of these patients will completely resolve spontaneously, a significant proportion will have intermittent recurrences of bacteriuria over the ensuing years, such that only a small proportion remain bacteria-free. While short courses of appropriate antibiotics can eradicate the bacteriuria, it recurs in the vast majority of patients. Follow-up studies of adolescents and young adults who had asymptomatic bacteriuria occurring during childhood, suggest that progressive renal injury does not occur in those patients whose urinary tracts were normal at the time of initial evaluation. However, during pregnancy, there is an increased risk of bacteriuria recurrence (both symptomatic and asymptomatic) in those patients having had asymptomatic bacteriuria during childhood. Furthermore, during pregnancy, those patients who were bacteriuric as children and not treated with long-term urinary antibiotic suppression had less renal adaptation to pregnancy compared to treated patients.

Although still somewhat controversial, the routine treatment of asymptomatic bacteriuria in the nonpregnant female does not appear to be warranted, and runs the risk of altering the urinary flora from probably low-virulence organisms to those with higher pathogenic potential. The exceptions to this approach are the affected sexually active females who appear to have a higher incidence of postcoital cystitis, and those who become pregnant, in whom there is a greater likelihood of the occurrence of pyelonephritis. In the latter instance, there may be an increased risk of miscarriage and infection to the fetus as well. Antibiotic treatment and subsequent urinary antibiotic prophylaxis in this setting may be justified.

Laboratory Studies: UTI

The evaluation of adolescents suspected of having a UTI can be challenging. The clinician has the responsibility to identify the causative organism so that rational therapy may be implemented. Effort has to be made to localize the site of the infection.

This task is not easy because of the overlapping of symptoms often observed, and the lack of specificity of the available laboratory studies. It is necessary to recognize the existence of contributing factors that modify the clinical management of the individual patient and finally consider potential long-term consequences of a UTI in a particular adolescent.

Laboratory data supporting the diagnosis of a UTI include those listed in Table 16-3. Urine dipsticks often include tests of leukocyte esterase and nitrite for WBCs and gram-negative bacteria, respectively. However, negative results in the symptomatic patient should be interpreted carefully, since gram-positive and nonbacterial infections can be missed. In addition, specificity data for the leukocyte esterase and nitrate tests indicate a significant rate of false negative results. A pelvic examination may also be necessary to differentiate UTI from vulvovaginitis due to *C. albicans* or *T. vaginalis* (Chap. 24). Also, frequency and urgency can occur as the result of viral cystitis and even as a reaction to carbonated beverages, caffeine, and chocolate.

Conventionally, a colony count of $>10^5$ CFU/mL of a single bacterial species on a clean voided specimen defines the causative organism. However, adolescents with symptoms of cystitis or pyelonephritis, may have colony counts as low as 5×10^4/mL. As previously discussed, counts as low as 10^2 may be significant in the setting of urethritis or when urine specimens are obtained by catheterization or suprapubic aspiration. A single positive culture from a voided specimen correlates with true infection in 80%, and with false positives in 20%. Two positive cultures in which the same organism is recovered increase the probability of infection to 95%. Mixed cultures, even of significant colony counts, usually indicate specimen contamination. Storing the urine on ice or in a 4°C refrigerator until it is cultured will substantially reduce the incidence of overgrowth contamination.

More than 60% of patients with a UTI, if cultured, will have significant bacteriuria with $>10^5$ CFU/mL; however less than 30% will not fulfill this criteria, as noted in the acute urethral syndrome. Some of these patients will have a true UTI with a CFU of 10^2 per mL and others, when sexually active, may have urethral infection caused by sexually transmitted organisms. Cultures for the identification of these pathogens are important. Only 70% of youth with bacteriuria have infections localized to the bladder and 30% will have infections localized to both the bladder and the upper urinary tracts as well.

E. coli is the most common cause of isolated episodes of acute cystitis, being implicated 80%–90% of the time. Chronic or recurrent infection, however, may be due to any of a wide variety of organisms in addition to *E. coli*, including those listed in Table 16-4. *S. saprophyticus* is the etiologic agent in more than 15% of the cases. Recurrent infection may occur with the same (relapse) or a different (reinfection) organism; occasionally, two or more pathogenic strains are present simultaneously, particularly after multiple antibiotic administration. A relapse usually is due to incomplete treatment possibly complicated by urolithiasis or an underlying structural abnormality. A pelvic examination may be necessary to rule out pelvic inflammatory disease.

T A B L E   1 6 - 3
LAB DATA SUGGESTING UTI

Pyuria of more than 10 white blood cells per high power microscope field of spun urine sediment
Positive gram stain with one or more bacteria per high power field of uncentrifuged urine
Positive urine culture with antibiotic sensitivities identifying the causal organism (most important)

T A B L E   1 6 - 4
ETIOLOGIC AGENTS IN UTIS

Escherichia coli (80%–90%)
Staphylococcus saprophyticus (15%)
Klebsiella
Enterobacter
Enterococcus
Pseudomonas
Proteus
Staphylococcus aureus
Streptococcus fecalis
Serratia sp.

A single isolated episode of cystitis in adolescent females does not necessarily require investigation for an anatomic cause, particularly if external precipitants are identified. The occurrence of two to three episodes of cystitis in a female within a span of 12–24 months, however, is an indication for further evaluation, starting with renal ultrasonography. In males, however, a single episode is sufficient to warrant a full evaluation because of the greater likelihood that a urogenital abnormality is responsible. Ultrasound provides an initial evaluation for upper tract structural abnormalities (e.g., hydronephrosis and renal cysts) and can usually identify renal calculi, as well. Computed tomography (CT) scans and intravenous urography may be required if calculi are suspected, but remain unidentified by sonography. Finally, voiding cystourethrography (isotope or contrast) is used to detect VUR and bladder and urethral abnormalities.

In cases of suspected overt or subclinical pyelonephritis, the technetium ^{99}m-dimercaptosuccinic acid (DMSA) renal scan has proved to be very sensitive for the detection of infectious foci in the renal parenchyma; reduced uptake of the radionuclide is noted in the kidney in areas of acute pyelonephritis with this study. The DMSA renal scan can also demonstrate residual renal scarring as the result of previous kidney infections. In perplexing situations, a CT or ultrasound study can help identify an abscess.

Management: UTI

Asymptomatic female adolescents with a history of recurrent, noncomplicated UTIs, when well known to the clinician and appropriate follow-up is assured, may be treated with a short course of antibiotics without obtaining a urine culture. In most cases of acute, uncomplicated cystitis in females, the UTI can be effectively treated with a 3-day course of an oral antibiotic, such as trimethoprim-sulfamethoxazole, trimethoprim, or a fluoroquinolone (Table 16-5). While single-dose antibiotic treatment regimens have been studied with a variety of antibiotics, relapse appears to occur with greater frequency. Increasing prevalence rates of common uropathogens resistant to amoxicillin and sulfonamides make these selections

TABLE 16-5

ANTIBIOTIC TREATMENT OF SIMPLE UTI

Trimethoprim-sulfamethoxazole double strength (160 mg/800 mg): twice daily for 3 days
Trimethoprim: 100 mg twice daily for 3 days
Nitrofurantoin: 50–100 mg four times daily for 7 days
Ciprofloxacin: 250 mg twice daily for 3 days*
Levofloxacin 250 mg once a day for 3 days*

*Used off label for prepubertal patients.

less appropriate unless specific sensitivities have been obtained. In addition, ampicillin and cephalosporins may alter fecal and periurethral flora such that the emergence of multidrug resistance occurs more frequently. The course is extended by 7 days in the presence of complicating factors, such as pregnancy, diabetes, a history of UTI recurrence, or use of a diaphragm. Cystitis in the male is treated for 7–10 days.

Clinically, mild cases of pyelonephritis can be effectively treated with oral antibiotics for 7–10 days on an ambulatory basis. Commonly used antibiotics include trimethoprim-sulfamethoxazole, fluoroquinolones, or third-generation cephalosporins. Those with more severe illness, possible urosepsis, pregnancy, or inability to sustain oral intake warrant hospitalization and parenteral therapy. Broad-spectrum intravenous antibiotic coverage is generally provided, commonly using ceftriaxone or ampicillin in combination with an aminoglycoside, until specific sensitivities are available; nafcillin can be substituted for ampicillin. Once the patient has had a clinical response with complete defervescence, oral antibiotics may be substituted to complete a 10–14-day total course of therapy.

In patients with cystitis/urethritis syndromes as the result of sexually transmitted bacteria or nonbacterial infection, the selection of an agent should be obviously based on the specific organism isolated. Females who have recurrent episodes of cystitis despite the absence of any genitourinary abnormality may benefit from antibiotic prophylaxis for 4–6 months (Table 16-6). When coitus appears to be a major contributing cause, 50–100 mg of nitrofurantoin, $\frac{1}{2}$ tablet (or 1 tablet) of

TABLE 16-6

AGENTS COMMONLY USED FOR URINARY BACTERIAL PROPHYLAXIS

Medication	Prophylactic Oral Dose
Nitrofurantoin	50–100 mg at night
Trimethoprim-sulfamethoxazole	100 mg at night
(80 mg/400 mg)	Half tablet at night

trimethoprim-sulfamethoxazole (double-strength), or 250 mg of ciprofloxacin taken immediately after coitus, may be effective. Improved hygiene and post-coital voiding also help to reduce the frequency of postcoital UTI. Initial suppressive treatment should be tried for 2–6 weeks. If the use of a diaphragm and spermicide appear to be contributing factors, alternative forms of birth control should be considered.

Suggested Readings

Bent S, Nallamothu BK, Simel D, et al.: Does this woman have an acute uncomplicated urinary tract infection? *JAMA* 287:2701–2710, 2002.

Bonny AE, Brouhard BH: Urinary tract infections among adolescents. *Adolesc Med* 16:149–161, 2005.

Fihn SD: Acute uncomplicated urinary tract infection in women. *N Engl J Med* 349:259–266, 2003.

Gupta K, Hooton TM, Roberts PL, et al.: Patient-initiated treatment of uncomplicated recurrent urinary tract infections in young women. *Ann Intern Med* 135:9–16, 2001.

Holroyd-Leduc JM, Staus SE: Management of urinary incontinence in women. Scientific review. *JAMA* 291:986–995, 2004.

Hooton TM: Recurent urinary tract infection in women. *Int J Antimicrob Agents* 17: 259–268, 2001.

Kennedy T: Urinary tract infection. In: Rudolph CD, Rudolph AM (eds.), *Rudolph's Pediatrics*. New York: McGraw-Hill, Chap. 21.6, pp. 1667–1669, 2003.

Roberts JA: Management of urinary tract infections in the adolescent male. *Adolesc Med* 7: 1–8, 1996.

Ronald A: The etiology of urinary tract infection: Traditional and emerging pathogens. *Am J Med* 113 (Suppl 1A):14S–19S, 2002.

Scholes D, Hooton TM, Roberts PL, et al.: Risk factors for recurrent urinary tract infection in young women. *J Infect Dis* 182:1177–1182, 2000.

Weir M, Brien J: Adolescent urinary tract infections. *Adolesc Med* 11:293–313, 2000.

DISEASES OF THE KIDNEY

Introduction

Clinical symptoms of an underlying acute or chronic renal parenchymal disorder, when present, usually relate to the dominant physiologic disturbance. For instance, patients with chronic reflux nephropathy and moderately severe hypertension may complain of blood pressure-related headaches or visual disturbances. By contrast, patients with acute nephritis may experience flank pain while those with the severe anemia characteristic of medullary cystic disease may be most concerned about their fatigue and diminished mental performance. In many patients, the clinical course of the kidney disease is silent until the process is sufficiently advanced so as to produce findings such as diminished growth, edema, uremia, oliguria, hypertension, or colic from urolithiasis. Therefore, many of those cases with initially silent clinical courses may only be discovered at the time of routine health screening examinations.

Many serious renal disorders which present in childhood may, for the adolescent, progress to become the problems of chronic or even end-stage renal disease, dialysis, and transplantation. Other disorders do not appear until the teenage years, with diagnostic and early treatment issues as the principal clinical concerns. The importance of chronic renal insufficiency in adolescents is reflected in the finding that between 25% and 27% of chronic renal failure in pediatric patients is reported in children between 13 and 17 years. This section will primarily focus on those renal disorders that may arise and require evaluation during the teenage years.

Proteinuria

General: Etiology

Clinically asymptomatic proteinuria is a frequent finding in adolescents and young adults. The vast majority of patients with asymptomatic proteinuria will be found to have orthostatic (postural) or intermittent proteinuria. Orthostatic proteinuria has a good prognosis and intermittent proteinuria is carefully followed up to ensure it does not become persistent. Also, proteinuria is a common hallmark of many renal diseases; unless it is sufficiently severe as to cause nephrotic syndrome, clinical findings may be scant. The situation may become more clouded since fever, strenuous exercise, dehydration, extreme cold, and, possibly, emotional stress, often increase the rate of protein excretion both in normal individuals and patients with kidney disease-associated proteinuria. False-positive dipstick results for urine protein should be considered in all asymptomatic patients with unexplained proteinuria. Common causes of false-positive results are listed in Table 16-7. Also note that urine proteins other than albumin are not readily detected by standard dipstick testing. Thus, gamma globulins, Bence Jones proteins, hemoglobin, lysozyme, and others may produce negative results. Detection of nonalbumin urinary proteins can be routinely accomplished using sulfosalicylic acid. A positive dipstick for proteinuria is an indication for quantification of proteinuria.

Quantification of Proteinuria

The traditional method for quantification of proteinuria has been the 24-hour urine collection, expressed as g/L or g/24 hour. Normal values range between 30 and 150 mg/24/hours in adults and

TABLE 16-7

CAUSES OF FALSE-POSITIVE URINE PROTEIN BY DIPSTICK

Highly buffered urine from alkaline medications or storage
Leaving dipstick in urine too long thereby washing out buffer
Contamination of urine by quaternary ammonium cleaning compounds
Treatment with phenazopyridine (in some dipstick brands)
Urine pH >7.0

around 100 mg/m^2/day in children. A more practical alternative is the measurement of the protein to creatinine ratio expressed as gram of protein per gram of creatinine in a randomly collected urine sample. It has an excellent correlation with the 24-hour urine collection. Normal values are <0.2 after 5 years of age.

Orthostatic Proteinuria

Orthostatic proteinuria is a condition most generally described as the presence of abnormally high rates of protein excretion occurring in the upright position only. When unassociated with any other urinary abnormality (i.e., hematuria), long-term follow-up studies have demonstrated that the risk of underlying significant renal disease is not increased for the normal population. Since the majority of adolescents evaluated for protein in the urine will be found to have intermittent or orthostatic proteinuria, the clinician's first task is to screen out those patients with a benign diagnosis. Normal males excrete 20–26 mg/kg/day of creatinine while normal females excrete 14–22 mg/kg/day. The upper limit of normal protein excretion is approximately 100 mg/m^2/24 hours (150–200 mg/24 hours). The diagnosis of orthostatic proteinuria is based on first-morning recumbent urine protein testing by dipstick that is negative or trace, increased values during daytime activity, and less than 1000 mg protein/24 hours (some authors suggest an upper limit of 2000 mg/24 hours).

A number of different algorithms for the diagnosis of orthostatic proteinuria have been proposed. A useful approach is described below which can be applied to the adolescent found to have proteinuria and no historical or physical finding suggestive of underlying renal or urologic disease; this method allows one to demonstrate the orthostatic component of the proteinuria:

A 24-hour "split" urine collection is recommended. The test requires two clean containers, usually provided by the laboratory performing the test. On the day of the test, the first voided urine specimen is discarded and the time is noted. All the urines voided the rest of the day are collected in one container and labeled "daytime urine collection." Before retiring to bed, the teen should rest, reclining for 1–2 hours.

Just before going to bed the teen should urinate, place the urine in the daytime urine collection container, note the time, and the teen retires to bed for the night. The following morning, the teen should urinate, if possible by the bedside. The urine is collected in the second container and labeled "nighttime urine collection." Both containers are taken to the laboratory for determination of volume, protein, and creatinine content; also, the ratio of protein to grams of creatine excretion in each container is established. The normal urine protein to urine creatinine excretion ratio is <0.2; an elevated protein excretion during the daytime in the presence of normal protein excretion during the night establish the presence of orthostatic or postural proteinuria.

The general consensus among nephrologists is that orthostatic proteinuria has a good prognosis and that renal biopsy is not necessary; it seems prudent to follow these patients at yearly or every 2-year intervals. Indications for a renal biopsy are listed in Table 16-8. Rapid deterioration of renal function requires an emergency renal biopsy to exclude or confirm crescentic glomerulonephritis. Isolated microscopic hematurias in which all other studies are normal require follow-up, but the need for prompt renal biopsy is less clear. Few contraindications for renal biopsy exist and include uncontrolled bleeding diathesis, uncontrolled hypertension, uncooperative patient, renal neoplasm, and renal

infection multiple cyst; a solitary kidney is a relative contraindication.

Other Proteinuria: Etiology

Persistent, pathologic proteinuria can be the result of acute or chronic glomerular diseases, tubulointerstitial diseases, or overflow proteinuria, due to abnormal production of low molecular weight proteins. Proteinuria frequently occurs in association with pregnancy and chronic congestive heart failure. Chronic renal scarring can result from structural abnormalities or pyelonephritis. Reflux nephropathy frequently presents as persistent proteinuria, and is a progressive renal disease; it is characterized by VUR, renal scarring, hypertension, and elevated creatinine. Virtually any form of acute or chronic nephritis (e.g., acute or chronic glomerulonephritis, cystic kidney diseases, focal sclerosis, IgA nephropathy, hereditary nephritis, cystic kidney diseases) may also present in a similar fashion; however, other hallmarks of renal disease are frequently present, such as hypertension, hematuria, abnormal anion gap, metabolic acidosis, or azotemia.

Laboratory Studies

Adolescents with persistent proteinuria, particularly associated with one or more of renal factors listed above, should be considered for referral to a subspecialist for further evaluation and possible renal biopsy. Although many tests for underlying renal disease may be performed by the primary care physician, tests beyond quantitative protein excretion measurements and basic renal function studies are oftentimes best done in the context of a formal nephrology evaluation. Once the proteinuria has been characterized as a nonorthostatic, persistent proteinuria (see above) and appropriate measures taken, serial quantitative changes of protein excretion may be approximated without the need of repeated 24-hour urine collections. The technique for this estimate uses a random daytime specimen of urine in which protein and creatinine concentrations are measured. The protein concentration divided by the creatinine concentration (in the same units, e.g., mg/dL, g/L) multiplied by the factor 0.63, gives the result in grams of protein excreted/m²/24 hours. This method of long-term

TABLE 16-8

INDICATIONS FOR RENAL BIOPSY

Nephrotic syndrome

Acute renal failure in whom the etiology is not clear

Rapid deterioration of renal function

Persistent mild proteinuria and persistent microscopic hematuria

Persistent, non-orthostatic proteinuria

Unexplained chronic renal failure

Renal transplant dysfunction

Isolated microscopic hematuria in whom all other studies are normal

reevaluation is an attractive alternative to the often-dreaded task of 24-hour urine collections by adolescents attending school or working.

Urinalysis is an important aspect in the evaluation of any patient with proteinuria; unfortunately, the microscopic evaluation of the urinary sediment is becoming an infrequent exercise for many physicians. A simple estimation of renal function can be obtained by measuring blood urea nitrogen (BUN), creatinine, electrolytes, and CO_2 in serum. Adolescents with nonorthostatic proteinuria require renal ultrasound evaluation to detect structural abnormalities, such as number of renal units, cystic diseases, renal asymmetry, or hydronephrosis. These basic studies can be performed by the primary care physician; however, adolescents with nonorthostatic proteinuria, need to be referred to a nephrologist for further evaluation and management.

Diabetic Nephropathy

Even the presence of low-grade proteinuria in an adolescent with diabetes mellitus should prompt a consideration for diabetic nephropathy. Diabetic nephropathy may begin during adolescence, since overt renal injury may be evident as early as 15 years following its onset. Progressive renal function impairment and hypertension are frequent manifestations of diabetic nephropathy. Microalbuminuria (30–300 mg of albumin per 24 hours or >20 μg of albumin per minute) can develop as early as 5 years post diabetes onset; in 5–10 more years, overt albuminuria (over 300 mg albumin per 24 hours) is seen in those who develop nephropathy. Hypertension usually develops during this time also. Renal functional impairment, heavy proteinuria, and, ultimately, renal failure, often occur over the next 10–15 years in affected individuals. If overt proteinuria does not develop after 20–25 years of insulin-dependent diabetes mellitus (IDDM), the risk of nephropathy decreases. Current clinical data indicate that the development of nephropathy can be delayed with excellent glycemic control (see Endocrine Disorders Chap. 15). Data also suggest that angiotensin-converting-enzyme inhibitors, angiotensin II receptor blockers, and the simultaneous use of both classes of

medications may slow the progression of the renal disease in diabetic nephropathy.

Nephrotic Syndrome

Etiology

The extreme clinical form of proteinuria manifests as the nephrotic syndrome, a generic term describing the concomitant presence of features listed in Table 16-9. In recent years, important developments have occurred in the understanding of the etiology in some diseases associated with the nephrotic syndrome. At present, it is recognized that multiple factors are associated with the etiology of the nephrotic syndrome and this chapter can only briefly review basic concepts of its etiology. In children, the nephrotic syndrome has been most frequently associated with the minimal change (*nil lesion*) nephrotic syndrome. However, during the second decade of life, prevalence of the nephrotic syndrome is increasingly associated with various forms of glomerulonephritis, including those listed in Table 16-10. The concurrent findings of hypertension and microscopic hematuria in adolescents with new-onset nephrotic syndrome are unusual in minimal change disease. Such findings should raise the clinical index of suspicion for the presence of an underlying glomerulonephritis or focal sclerosis as the cause. Secondary causes of the nephrotic syndrome are listed in Table 16-11. Those of viral origin include hepatitis B, which can lead to membranous nephropathy, and hepatitis C which can lead to mesangiocapillary glomerulonephritis and polyarteritis nodosa. HIV-infected adolescents can

T A B L E   1 6 - 9

FEATURES OF NEPHROTIC SYNDROME

Edema

Hypoalbuminemia

Massive proteinuria (>3.5 g/1.73 m^2/day. In children 50 mg/kg/day or >40 mg/m^2/h)

Hyperlipidemia

TABLE 16-10
PRIMARY CAUSES OF NEPHROTIC SYNDROME

Minimal change disease
Focal and segmental glomerulosclerosis
Immune complexes glomerulonephritis:
    Acute proliferative (postinfectious) glomerulonephritis
    Membranoproliferative glomerulonephritis
        (mesangiocapillary glomerulonephritis)
    Membranous nephropathy
    IgA nephropathy
Crescentic glomerulonephritis
Collapsing glomerulopathy (collapsing focal segmental
    glomerulosclerosis)

develop focal segmental glomerulosclerosis (FSGS) and IgA nephropathy.

Focal Segmental Glomerulosclerosis

Primary FSGS is of particular concern to the physician caring for adolescents. It is the most common cause of glomerular disease resulting in end-stage renal disease in this age group, particularly in African American adolescent males. It is now recognized that the prevalence of primary FSGS in nephrotic black patients is two to four times that of the Caucasian population. The incidence of FSGS in children and in adults is increasing in all ethnic groups.

TABLE 16-11
SECONDARY CAUSES OF NEPHROTIC SYNDROME

Medications
Infections
Multisystem diseases:
    Systemic lupus erythematosus
    Henoch-Schönlein purpura nephritis
    Other vasculitis
Neoplastic diseases
Metabolic disorders (as diabetes mellitus)
Hereditofamilial disorders (as Alport's).

Primary FSGS is characterized by proteinuria, frequently associated with the nephrotic syndrome; hematuria and hypertension occur more often than in minimal changes disease (MCD). Renal biopsy reveals a histologic pattern of injury with segmental glomerular scarring, obliteration and hyalinosis of the glomerular capillaries, and adhesions to the Bowman's capsule. There is interstitial fibrosis and tubular atrophy; similar histologic findings are also observed in secondary forms of FSGS. Clinically steroid resistance is common. Persistent proteinuria more than 3.5 g/day, despite therapy, predicts progression to end-stage renal disease in 5–10 years in >50% of patients. Poor prognosis is also predicted by the severity of the interstitial fibrosis and creatinine levels >1.3 mg/dL at diagnosis. The etiology of primary FSGS remains unclear. Circulating factors produced by lymphocytes have been implicated, but none has been identified. In recent years, mutations in several genes related to proteins in slit diaphragm in podocytes have been identified and associated with familiar and sporadic cases of steroid resistant nephrotic syndrome with progression to ESRD.

The management of patients with FSGS requires the expertise of an experienced nephrologist. In general, up to 40% of patients with primary FSGS respond to prolonged (up to 6 months) use of steroids; it is therefore justified to start treatment with prednisone in adolescents with this disease. Many adolescents however, are overweight, and the use of steroids requires careful consideration of their side effects. Other forms of treatment will be considered in patients with steroid resistant nephrotic syndrome, patients that relapse and in those with genetically determined forms of the disease that do not respond to immune suppression.

Membranoproliferative Glomerulonephritis

Membranoproliferative glomerulonephritis (MPGN), also known as mesangiocapillary glomerulonephritis, is characterized by histologic findings of diffuse proliferative lesions and widening of capillary loops, often with appearance of double contour. By electron microscopic examination, three types of MPGN have been described. Type I is defined as the presence of immune complexes in the subendothelial space and in the mesangium. Type II MPGN is also known as dense deposits disease; it is characterized by the presence of extremely osmophilic dense deposits in the capillary wall. Type III is a variant of type I, with electron dense aggregates diffusely present in subendothelial and subepithelial areas of the membrane. MPGN type I is the most common form of the disease; it may be primary or secondary. Type I and type III usually presents in older children, adolescents, and young adults; it affects males and females with equal frequency and is responsible for 5%–20% causes of the nephrotic syndrome in Europe and North America. The general impression is that the incidence of MPGN is declining in these parts of the world. The presence of persistent circulating immuno-complexes, as seen in chronic bacterial, viral or parasitic diseases, immunologic diseases (autoimmune), neoplasias, and paraproteinemias, play an important role in the development of MPGN type I. MPGN type II is idiopathic in the majority of cases, but abnormalities in factor H are described in rare familial forms of the disease; it is also seen in association with partial lipodystrophy.

The clinical presentation of MPGN may assume several forms: nephrotic syndrome in about 30% of cases, as persistent microscopic hematuria and proteinuria in 35% of cases, as a chronic progressive glomerulonephritis in 20% of cases, or as a rapid progressive glomerulonephritis in 10% of cases. Laboratory abnormalities include depletion of complement C3, total hemolytic complement (CH50), and in some cases, C4. At least three mechanisms have been implicated as responsible for the hypocomplementemia in MPGN: circulating immune complexes activating the classical pathway, NF (an autoantibody directed against complement proteins), and excessive breakdown of C3 by C3 convertase of the alternative pathway.

The clinical course of MPGN is generally progressive and prognosis for renal survival is poor, particularly in adults with MPGN type II. The prognosis is better in younger individuals and in type I. Indicators of poor renal prognosis include: hypertension, impaired renal function, nephrotic syndrome, more than 20% of crescents present, sclerosis, mesangial deposits, and tubulointerstitial disease.

Less strong association is seen with macroscopic hematuria and male sex; no correlation is seen with serum complement levels. There is no specific therapy for primary MPGN. Children with MPGN type I and III were treated by the Cincinnati group with steroids at 2 mg/kg/day, up to 80 mg every other day for up to 2 years; there was dose reduction according to clinical response. They reported improvement in renal survival. Similar improvement was also reported by the International Study of Kidney Disease in Children with alternated day use of steroids. Treatment of secondary forms of MPGN should be directed to the cause, as for example, interferon for hepatitis C and steroids as well as cyclophosphamide for SLE. Nonspecific treatment, including normalization of blood pressure and the use of angiotensin-converting enzyme (ACE) inhibitors to decrease proteinuria, are also indicated.

Membranous Nephropathy

Membranous nephropathy is a chronic glomerular disease in which immune deposits of IgG and complement develop mainly in the subepithelial space of the glomerular capillary wall, inducing morphologic and functional changes. Morphologically, there is increasing thickening of the glomerular basement membrane; with silver methenamine staining, there are "spikes" surrounding the intramembranous deposits. Membranous nephropathy is the most common cause of the nephrotic syndrome in the Caucasian adult population; it is responsible for 20%–25% of cases of idiopathic nephrotic syndrome in this age group. In the young the incidence of membranous nephropathy is not well established, but is uncommon. In contrast to adults in whom primary membranous nephropathy is more frequent (23%), the secondary forms of the disease predominate in the young (35%). (Table 16-12) The nephrotic syndrome is the most common presentation of the disease, but in 7%, nonnephrotic range proteinuria and/or abnormal urinary sediment may be the presenting findings.

Diagnosis of membranous nephropathy: There are no specific clinical or laboratory findings that permit the diagnosis of membranous nephropathy. Histopathologic diagnosis is established by renal

TABLE 16-12

CAUSES OF SECONDARY MEMBRANOUS NEPHROPATHY

Infections
Hepatitis B
Congenital syphilis
Malaria
Parasitic infections

Medications and toxins
O-penicillamine
Gold
Mercury
NSAIDs

Autoimmune diseases
Systemic lupus erythematosus
Autoimmune enteropathy
Rheumatoid arthritis
Crohn's disease
Hashimoto's thyroiditis
Graves' disease

Neoplasms
Ovarian tumor
Neuroblastoma
Gonadoblastoma
Lungs
Stomach
Melanoma
Bladder

biopsy, with special staining techniques (silver-methenamine, PAS), immunofluorescence, and electron microscopy. Plasma C3 is usually normal; terminal complement component C5b-9 is reported to be elevated in urine. Because secondary forms of the disease are more common in the young, a report of the renal biopsy read as membranous nephropathy means it becomes necessary to exclude secondary causes of the disease before starting the patient on potentially toxic immunosuppressive medication. This possibility is particularly relevant in the elderly individual in whom the risk of neoplasia is high. There is no specific treatment for membranous nephropathy; additionally, spontaneous remission of membranous nephropathy may occur in up to 40% of the nephrotic syndrome in the young. A period of nonspecific treatment with

ACE inhibitors, close supervision of renal function, and monitoring of severity of proteinuria, is a reasonable approach for the adolescent with membranous nephropathy. Immunosuppression is indicated if there is deterioration of renal function or if the proteinuria is >10 g a day.

Certainly, several other forms of the nephrotic syndrome occur in the adolescent, as noted in Tables 16-11 and 16-12. In addition to the underlying disease causing the nephrotic syndrome, the severe hypoproteinemia and the nature of the protein loss also cause potential clinical problems. For example, there is the increased independent risk of *serious bacterial infections* (particularly with *Streptococcus pneumoniae, Hemophilus influenzae*, and gram-negative enteric organisms); sepsis, peritonitis, and cellulitis are among the most frequent sites of infection. This increased risk is multifactorial, but to a large part, it is the result of the urinary loss of bacterial opsonins in the proteinuric state. Thus, this is a problem generic to the nephrotic syndrome itself. Thromboembolism may also occur, largely the result of dysfunction of the coagulation regulatory systems. Again, this is largely the result of the loss of regulatory proteins into the urine.

Collapsing Focal Segmental Glomerulosclerosis is characterized by collapsing of glomerular capillaries, hypertrophy as well as hyperplasia of podocytes, and interstitial nephritis; the etiology is unknown, but has been associated with viral infections and drug toxicity. This disorder has been described in African American and Caucasian children, adolescents, and adults. It predominantly affects African American males 18 to 28 years of age. Though it is more common in patients with a history of HIV infection and intravenous heroin addiction, there is no history of high risk behavior or serologic evidence of HIV infection in 20% of these patients. Clinically this disorder is manifested by severe nephritic syndrome, resistance to steroids, and rapid advance to end stage renal disease (ESRD). Unfortunately, there is no known effective therapy.

Management

Current strategies for the treatment of nephrotic syndrome in these various disorders are continuously evolving and undergoing considerable reassessment. Most specific treatments require the use of high-dose corticosteroids and, frequently, systemic immuno-suppressive agents. The potential short and long-term side effects of these agents are considerable. Where eradication or medical control of the underlying disease is not possible, symptomatic treatment is often used. These treatments most often use a combination of modest dietary sodium restriction in conjunction with diuretics to control the degree of edema, while taking care not to compromise the plasma volume. New strategies for the symptomatic medical control of nephrotic edema and the long-term management of intractable proteinuria are currently under investigation. Treatment of associated infections is always important.

Hematuria

Etiology

Gross or microscopic hematuria in an adolescent is a common occurrence. Evaluation of the possibility of red blood cell (RBC) products in the urine requires both dipstick and microscopic analyses. Most dip and read urine stick products are very sensitive, with detection ranges as low as the equivalent of 2–5 RBCs per high power field on microanalysis. Red or red-brown discolored urine or clear urine testing positive for blood on dipstick may indicate the presence of hemoglobinuria or myoglobinuria, rather than hematuria. The absence of RBCs on micro-analysis should suggest either of the two former diagnoses, though the possibilities of RBC lysis in a very hypotonic urine (specific gravity <1.007) or a false positive result should also be considered. False positives may occur in the presence of oxidizing contaminants, such as hypochlorite disinfecting solutions and high urinary bacterial contents with release of bacterial peroxidases. False negative results occur in the presence of high urinary ascorbic acid concentrations. Non-RBC products that may give the urine a reddish, smoky, or dark appearance should also be considered when the dipstick fails to be positive for blood. Urate crystals, berries, beets, vegetable dyes, as well as alcaptonuria, tyrosinosis, porphyrin compounds, and bile may all cause facti-tious hematuria.

The presence of ≥ RBCs/high power field on a spun urine specimen is considered abnormal in most laboratories. However, borderline RBC counts should be reaffirmed on at least two additional uri-nalyses, since as many as 80% of cases of micro-scopic hematuria detected on an initial urinalysis will be transient. Transient hematuria may be encountered in association with various conditions, as noted in Table 16-13. Vigorous exercise or a period of strenuous training can cause hematuria that may be accompanied by proteinuria as well as casts; it typically clears within 24 hours.

Diagnosis

Persistent or recurrent hematuria warrants a thorough investigation for an underlying cause. The initial evaluation should include a carefully focused history, family history, and physical examination, all of which can contribute significantly to the diagnostic evaluation. Table 16-14 describes general compo-nents of the initial clinical evaluation that often prove useful. The diagnostic studies appropriate to the ado-lescent with hematuria will largely depend on the suspected site and etiology of the bleeding.

Laboratory Studies

Localization of the site of urinary bleeding is often useful in the initial diagnostic evaluation. Hematuria originating in the kidney is often characterized by brown or cola-colored urine. The concomitant pres-ence of >2+ protein by dipstick, or RBC casts, WBC casts, deformed (dysmorphic) RBC, or renal tubular

TABLE 16-13

CONDITIONS ASSOCIATED WITH TRANSIENT HEMATURIA

Infections (generalized, urinary, prostatic,
  and vulvovaginal)
Genitourinary foreign bodies
Coagulation defects
Sickle cell trait or anemia
Posttrauma (both recognized and unrecognized, as
  may occur in contact sports)

TABLE 16-14

COMMON COMPONENTS OF THE CLINICAL EVALUATION OF HEMATURIA

History of:	Suggests:
Dysuria, fever	Upper or lower UTI
Headache, rash, arthralgias, *others*	Systemic infection, vasculitis, collagen vascular diseases, Henoch-Schönlein nephritis
Sinusitis, cough, headache, epistaxis	Wegener's granulomatosis
Flank pain	Renal calculus, acute urinary obstruction, subacute pyelonephritis, cystic diseases
Intermittent gross hematuria	IgA and IgG nephritis; urethritis, foreign body, hypercalciuria, neoplasm (rare)
Antecedent viral illness	Postinfectious nephritis, IgA nephropathy, other nephritis
Cola-colored urine, edema, hypertension	Glomerulonephritis
Bloody diarrhea	Hemolytic-uremic syndrome (serotoxin-producing *E. coli* and others)
Family history of:	
Microhematuria	Thin basal membrane disease, hereditary nephritis, hypercalciuria
Hearing loss	Hereditary nephritis
Renal failure	Hereditary nephritis, cystic kidney disease
Anemia	Sickle cell disease or trait
Physical findings of:	
Hypertension	Acute or chronic glomerulonephritis
Edema, ascites	Glomerulonephritis, membranous nephropathy, focal sclerosis
Bruising	Coagulopathy, collagen vascular disease
Heart murmur, fever	Subacute bacterial endocarditis
Purpura	Systemic infection, Henoch-Schönlein nephritis
Flank mass	Polycystic kidney disease, obstructive uropathy, renal tumor, multicystic dysplastic kidney

epithelial cells in urine sediment, increases the likelihood of bleeding from the renal parenchyma, especially from glomerular causes. Lower urinary tract bleeding is more often characterized by terminal hematuria, passage of blood clots, and/or normal RBC morphology on microanalysis.

If the cause of the hematuria is not evident from historical and physical findings, the initial empirical evaluation should begin with a urine microanalysis, from which it is determined whether the bleeding is more likely glomerular or extraglomerular (i.e., nonparenchymal). As noted above, the presence of no RBCs and/or pigmented urine casts should raise the possibility of pigmenturia from hemoglobin or myoglobin. Intravascular coagulation, mechanical RBC damage (e.g., artificial heart valves), hemolytic anemia (e.g., G6PD deficiency, mismatched blood transfusion), as well as muscle injuries (crush, electrical, posttraumatic compartment syndrome), myositis, and rhabdomyolysis should be considered in the appropriate settings.

A microanalysis showing a dysmorphic RBC subpopulation or RBC casts is indicative of glomerular or renal parenchymal bleeding. In this case, a serum C3 is often useful to distinguish hypocomplementemic from normocomplementemic causes of renal parenchymal bleeding (Table 16-15). In contrast, the absence of urinary casts and the presence of

TABLE 16-15

CAUSES OF NORMOCOMPLEMENTEMIC AND HYPOCOMPLEMENTEMIC RENAL PARENCHYMAL BLEEDING

Normocomplementemia	Hypocomplementemia
Normocomplementemic nephritis	Poststreptococcal nephritis
IgA nephropathy	Lupus nephritis
Henoch-Schönlein purpura	Membranoproliferative nephritis
nephritis	Nephritis with chronic infection
Hereditary nephritis	Hepatitis B (early)
Nephritis of vasculitis	Malaria
Rapidly progressive nephritis	Infected ventriculo-atrial shunts
Chronic nephritis (idiopathic)	
Wegener's granulomatosis	
Nonnephritic glomerular bleeding	
Vasomotor nephropathy	
Hemolytic-uremic syndrome	
Renal dysplasia/cystic diseases	
Renal vein thrombosis	
Renal artery embolism/thrombosis	
Renal trauma	

morphologically normal RBCs on microanalysis should suggest extraparenchymal bleeding. Causes of this form of urinary bleeding include those listed in Table 16-16.

Ultrasound of the kidneys and bladder is a useful and noninvasive tool in the initial evaluation of suspected renal structural abnormalities. Hypercalciuria

TABLE 16-16

CAUSES OF EXTRAPARENCHYMAL URINARY BLEEDING

Urinary infection
Hypercalciuria ± urolithiasis
Abdominal or flank trauma
Urinary tract structural malformations
Medical/nonmedical instrumentation of the lower
 urinary tract
Hemoglobinopathies
Medications
Tumors
Hemorrhagic diatheses

also appears to be increasingly associated with hematuria and the subsequent risk of urolithiasis. A random daytime urine specimen, in which the ratio of the calcium concentration divided by the creatinine concentration (both expressed in the same units) is greater than 0.21, suggests the presence of hypercalciuria (see below). In the setting of a history or family history suggestive of renal parenchymal disease, or the identification of physical or laboratory findings compatible with underlying glomerulonephritis or renal dysfunction, the decisions as to the most appropriate subsequent evaluation and/or treatment including the possible need for renal biopsy should be made in conjunction with a specialist in nephrology.

Glomerulonephritis

General

Acute poststreptococcal glomerulonephritis (PSGN), Henoch-Schönlein purpura (HSP), and hemolytic-uremic syndrome (HUS) are three forms of glomerulonephritis occurring in adolescence and young adulthood that deserve special mention.

Poststreptococcal glomerulonephritis

General

PSGN is the most commonly encountered form of postinfectious nephritis in children and younger adolescents. This inflammatory renal disorder results from immune complex formation and localization within the glomerulus associated with specific M-serotype nephritogenic Group A as well as Group C streptococcal infections. Most commonly, the sites of infection are the upper respiratory tract (pharyngitis, otitis, sinusitis) and the skin. The appearance of respiratory tract-associated PSGN is typically 7–14 days after onset of the infection, while onset of pyoderma-associated nephritis may take as long as 3 weeks. Late treatment (>36 hours after onset of infection) or treatment at the time of appearance of the nephritis does not appear to modify the course of the renal disease. The typical clinical findings of PSGN include the triad of sudden onset of gross hematuria, volume overload (often manifesting as edema or cardiopulmonary congestion), and hypertension. However, many patients may be discovered to have asymptomatic disease, especially during periods of epidemic streptococcal disease.

PSGN: Laboratory Studies

The diagnosis of PSGN relies on the demonstration of the causative organism, though prior empiric therapy may preclude this option. Serologic tests for evidence of a preceding streptococcal infection are often useful; however, both chronic asymptomatic streptococcal carriage as well as elevated streptococcal-associated antibody levels are frequently present in unaffected individuals. Most patients with suspected PSGN are screened with the streptozyme test, which screens for antibodies to several streptococcal antigens. A positive test should be confirmed with specific titers. Approximately 70% of those patients with pharyngitis-associated PSGN will have increased titers of antistreptolysin-O (ASO), though the rise of the ASO titer in pyoderma-associated PSGN is less common. The combination of ASO, antihyaluronidase, and antideoxyribonuclease B (anti-DNAase B) titers should provide evidence of a recent streptococcal infection in almost all patients.

Decreased serum C3 levels are detected in approximately 90% of the cases. Therefore, adolescents with acute glomerulonephritis, who have normal C3 values at the time of onset, should have consideration for other forms of nephritis. In addition, the serum C3 levels almost invariably return to normal within 6–8 weeks of onset of the nephritis. Thus, serial complement measurements are necessary to document the diagnosis. Since other forms of chronic glomerulonephritis may clinically exacerbate in association with an acute viral illness, variation from the typical clinical presentation and course should prompt a more thorough evaluation. Also, other acute bacterial and viral illnesses may be associated with a similar clinical presentation of acute nephritis.

Prognosis

Current data indicate that the vast majority of patients with PSGN can fully recover if morbidity can be avoided that is associated with the clinical presentation (e.g., hypertensive encephalopathy, congestive heart failure, mineral imbalance associated with acute renal failure, and serious infection). This favorable prognosis excludes that very small percentage of patients with PSGN manifesting as the clinical syndrome of acute oliguric renal failure associated with crescentic glomerulonephritis.

Henoch-Schönlein Purpura (HSP)

HSP is a common vasculitic syndrome most often characterized by involvement of joints (arthritis), gastrointestinal tract (abdominal pain, diarrhea), and skin (purpuric/petechial rash primarily involving lower extremities, buttocks, and distal upper extremities). It can also involve the scrotum and mimic torsion of the testicle. Glomerulonephritis occurs in 20%–30% of the patients, though severe nephritis (nephrotic-range proteinuria, hypertension, and azotemia) occurs less than 10% of the time. Renal manifestations of HSP include isolated gross or microscopic hematuria, proteinuria, and occasionally, the nephrotic syndrome.

Hemolytic Uremic Syndrome (HUS)

General

HUS is not truly a glomerulonephritis. Rather, it results from a small vessel vasculopathy leading to glomerular capillary thromboses. It is a common cause of acute renal failure in children. It has an average age of onset of 3 years (2–6 years), though it can also affect younger and older individuals. In the United States, it often follows a diarrheal illness due to exotoxin (verotoxin)-producing *E. coli* (especially 0157-H7) and other infectious agents, including *Salmonella typhi, Shigella*, or *Campylobacter*. HUS with diarrhea is identified as D+HUS; hematochezia is often present. Atypical forms of HUS are usually diarrhea negative or D-HUS and have been associated with such infectious disease agents as *Streptococcus pneumonia* as well as HIV; other associations include cancer chemotherapy, immunosuppressive drugs (e.g., cyclosporine), pregnancy (including preeclampsia and during the postpartum period), malignant hypertension, and scleroderma. D-HUS has also been reported in families with an autosomal recessive or dominant pattern of inheritance.

Diagnosis

The three cardinal features of this HUS are microangiopathic hemolytic anemia, thrombocytopenia, and azotemia. These may be frequently associated with hypertension, petechiae, seizures, and/or encephalopathy. The initial renal findings in HUS include variably diminished renal function (which may be seen as oliguric renal failure), proteinuria, and hematuria. Adolescents presenting with features of HUS, in whom central nervous system and hemorrhagic findings predominate, should also be considered to have thrombotic thrombocytopenic purpura (TTP); TTP is a distinct entity from HUS.

Prognosis

With aggressive and early treatment of fluid and electrolyte imbalances (especially potassium imbalance), control of elevated blood pressure, and institution of early dialysis when required, the prognosis associated with the epidemic (D+HUS) form is good; with excellent management, the mortality is less than 5% in young children, though in some patients there may be long-term persistent residual renal dysfunction, hypertension, neurologic sequelae, or colonic strictures. The severity of the HUS is worse in the atypical cases (D-HUS), particularly in the familial and recurrent forms of the disease, and in patients with TTP; management includes plasma exchange and plasmapheresis therapy. The short and long-term prognosis in these patients is less favorable, and they should be managed in collaboration with a nephrologist.

Suggested Readings

Abitbol CL, Lawrence B. Friedman LB, Zilleruelo G: Renal manifestations of sexually transmitted diseases: STD's and the kidney. *Adolesc Med* 16:45–65, 2005.

Andrioli SP: Acute renal failure. *Urr Opin Pediatr* 17:713–717, 2002.

Balow JE, Austin HA: Maintenance therapy for lupus nephritis—something old, something new. *N Engl J Med* 350:1044–1046, 2004.

Blowey DL: Nephrotoxicity of over-the-counter analgesics, natural medicines and illicit drugs. *Adolesc Med* 16:31–43, 2005

Boulware IE, Jaar BG, Tarver-Carr ME, et al.: Screening for proteinuria in US adults. A cost-effective analysis. *JAMA* 290:3101–3114, 2003.

Boydstun II: Acute renal failure in adolescents. *Adolesc Med* 16:1–9, 2005.

Boydstun II: Chronic kidney disease in adolescents. *Adolesc Med* 16:185–199, 2005.

Colberg JW: Urologic abnormalities of the genitourinary tract. In: Rudolph CD, Rudolph AM (eds.), *Rudolph's Pediatrics.* New York: McGraw-Hill, Chap. 21.16, pp. 1735–17434, 2003.

DeWiler RK, Hogan SL, Falk RJ, et al.: Collapsing glomerulopathy (CG): A distinct clinical and pathologic entity. *J Am Soc Nephrol* 3:310, 1992.

Eddy AA: Glomerular disorders. In: Rudolph CD, Rudolph AM (eds.), *Rudolph's Pediatrics.* New York: McGraw-Hill, Chap. 21.8, pp. 1677–1699, 2003.

Ellis EN: Diabetes mellitus and the kidney in adolescents. *Adolesc Med* 16:173–184, 2005.

Gordon C, Stapleton FB: Hematuria in adolescents. *Adolesc Med* 16:229–239, 2005.

Hannu Jalanko: Pathogenesis of proteinuria: Lessons learned from nephrin and podocin *Pediatr Nephrol* 18:487–491, 2003.

Hogg RJ: Adolescents with proteinuria and/or the nephritic syndrome. *Adolesc Med* 16:163–172, 2005.

Kaplan BS, Meyers KE, Schulman SL: The pathogenesis and treatment of hemolytic uremic syndrome. *J Am Soc Nephrol* 9:1126–1133, 1998.

Keaney CM, Springate JE: Cancer and the kidney. *Adolesc Med* 16:121–148, 2005.

Lau KK, Wyatt RJ: Glomerulonephritis. *Adolesc Med* 16:67–85, 2005.

McDonald SP, Craig JC: Long-term survival of children with end-stage renal disease. *N Engl J Med* 350:2654–2662, 2004.

Milliner DS: Pediatric renal-replacement therapy-coming of age. *N Engl J Med* 350:2637–2639, 2004.

Nathan DM, Writing Team for the Diabetes Control and Complications Trial/Epidemiology of Diabetes Interventions and Complications Research Group: Sustained effect of intensive treatment of type 1 diabetes mellitus on development and progression of diabetic nephropathy. The epidemiology of diabetes interventions and complications (EDIC) study. *JAMA* 290:2159–2167, 2003.

Orth SR, Ritz E: The nephrotic syndrome. *N Engl J Med* 338:1202–1211, 1998.

Patel DR, Torres AD, Greydanus DE: Kidneys and sports. *Adolesc Med* 16:111–119, 2005.

Smith JM, McDonald RA: Renal transplantation in adolescents. *Adolesc Med* 16:201–214, 2005.

Wilson PD: Polycystic kidney disease. *N Engl J Med* 350:151–164, 2004.

HYPERTENSION

The Seventh Joint National Committee Report (JNC7) defines hypertension in adults as a systolic blood pressure of 140 mmHg and a diastolic blood pressure of 90 mmHg (see Chap. 9). This report cautions about the characterization of an individual as hypertensive only in base of numeric values of blood pressure, and consider this definition inadequate because it fails to take in consideration risk factors, comorbidities, and end-organ damage (EOD) in order to assess the prognosis and to guide therapy.

Currently in the United States, the diagnosis of hypertension in children and adolescents is based on recent research (see Fourth Report, Pediatrics, 2004). Hypertension is defined as an average systolic blood pressure (SBP) and/or diastolic blood pressure (DBP) ≥95th percentile for gender, age, and height on ≥3 occasions. Prehypertension in children is defined as average SBP or DBP levels that are ≥90th percentile but <95th percentile. Adolescents with blood pressure levels ≥120/80 mm Hg should be considered prehypertensive, and preventive life style modifications should be recommended. A patient who is hypertensive at the physician's office or clinic, but normotensive outside a clinical setting, has "white-coat hypertension;" ambulatory blood pressure monitoring is often necessary for this condition.

As in the adults, there is a correlation between the severity of hypertension and evidence of organ damage, if appropriate markers are utilized, such as left ventricular hypertrophy (LVH), retinopathy, microalbuminuria, and others. The existence of comorbidity issues, such as diabetes, renal disease, cardiovascular disease, and positive family history, are important considerations in the decision to intervene therapeutically. Common causes of hypertension in adolescents are indicated in Table 16-17.

Evaluation of the Hypertensive Adolescent

As a general rule, the severity of hypertension is directly related to secondary causes of hypertension and inversely related to the patient age. Most pediatric patients below 10 years of age have secondary causes of hypertension, whereas most adolescents have primary hypertension. Adolescents with mild to moderate hypertension and a positive family history of primary hypertension have themselves primary hypertension. These patients require basic laboratory and imaging screening test, common to all hypertensive patients; this includes a CBC, electrolytes, BUN, creatinine, and urinalysis. Serum uric acid elevation is a frequent finding in patients with primary hypertension and should be measured as well as a fasting lipid profile. Echocardiographic examination is also indicated.

Patients with symptomatic severe hypertension, regardless of their age, need to rapidly be treated in order to bring their blood pressure down to safer

TABLE 16-17
CAUSES OF HYPERTENSION IN ADOLESCENTS

Primary (essential) hypertension
White coat hypertension
Secondary causes of hypertension

Renal
Renal parenchymal diseases: acute and chronic
  glomerular diseases, chronic interstitial disease,
  polycystic kidney disease, reflux nephropathy,
  obstructive uropathy
Renovascular disease: renovascular hypertension
  due to renal artery muscular dysplasia
Extramural compression of renal artery:
  neurofibromatosis

Endocrine
Congenital adrenal hyperplasia, adrenal adenoma,
  bilateral adrenal hyperplasia, and Cushing syndrome
Pheochromocytoma of the medulla of the adrenal
  glands, extra adrenal chromaffin cell tumor
Hyperthyroidism, hypothyroidism

Medications and illicit drugs
Glucocorticoids, mineralocorticoids, cyclosporin,
  erythropoietin, sympathomimetics, contraceptives,
  nonsteroidal anti-inflammatory medications,
  monoamine oxydase inhibitors, licorice, herbal
  remedies, heavy metals cocaine alcohol, and so forth

Exogenous obesity
Insulin resistance, sleep apnea

Spinal cord injury
Paraplegia, quadriplegia
Peripheral neuropathy: Guillain-Barré syndrome

Mendelian forms of hypertension
Apparent mineralocorticoid excess (AME)
Glucocorticoid-remediable hyperaldosteronism (GRH)
Liddle syndrome
Gordon syndrome

inhibitors or diuretics. The history, physical examination, basic laboratory data, and renal ultrasound results guides the clinical decision for more specific testing needed for the evaluation of secondary forms of hypertension in these adolescents (Table 16-18).

Management of Hypertension in Adolescents

Nonpharmacologic intervention is the first step in the management of adolescents with mild to moderate hypertension. This requires a lifelong-lasting commitment in lifestyle that includes modifications in diet, exercise, avoidance and treatment of obesity, and cigarette smoking avoidance or cessation. Adolescents with mild to moderate hypertension will

TABLE 16-18
TESTS FOR EVALUATION OF SECONDARY HYPERTENSION IN ADOLESCENTS

Renal parenchymal
Proteinuria, hematuria, RBC casts, complement C3,
  C4, ASO titers, ANA, anti-double-strand DNA,
  ANCA titers, renal biopsy

Reflux nephropathy
Proteinuria, urine culture, VCUG, DMSA renal scan

Renal artery stenosis
Plasma rennin activity, captopril renogram, spiral
  computed tomographic angiography, magnetic
  resonance angiography

Endocrine causes
Pheochromocytoma: plasma metanephrines,
  clonidine suppression tests. Localization of tumor
  by CT, MRI, metaiodobenzylguanidine (MIBG)
Primary aldosteronism: serum potassium, serum
  aldosterone/plasma renin ratio, CT MRI of adrenal
  glands
Cushing syndrome morning serum cortisol after
  dexamethasone suppression
Hyperthyroidism/hypothyroidism, total and free
  thyroxin TSH

Medications/drug abuse
History of prescribed and not prescribed
  medications, herbal remedies. Drug screening

levels to prevent further target organ damage; this should be done even before a definitive diagnosis is established. An effort should be made to obtain laboratory tests that may be altered by administration of medications, such as plasma catecholamines with Labetalol, or plasma rennin levels with ACE

benefit from regular, moderate aerobic exercise. An increase in fruits and vegetables, as part of normal nutrition, is associated with demonstrable decrease in systolic and diastolic blood pressure; reduction in salt intake to less than 100 mmol (less than 3 g of Na) a day causes reduction of blood pressure. Weight reduction in obese individuals decreases systolic and diastolic blood pressure. Aerobic exercise of moderate intensity three to five times a week is associated with moderated reduction in blood pressure. The effect of resistance exercise in blood pressure is less clear. These changes in lifestyle are the foundation for risk reduction of hypertension-related cardiovascular events later in life.

Those with more severe hypertension need to be evaluated and treated. The decision regarding participation in organized sports needs to be individualized. Pharmacologic treatment of hypertension is indicated in adolescents with primary hypertension and evidence of end-organ damage, with blood pressure consistently over the 99th percentile, in those that do not respond to or are unable to comply with life style modifications, and in patients with secondary forms of hypertension. Current recommendations in the literature regarding the use of antihypertensive medications in children and adolescents are unsatisfactory to help guide clinicians in the management of hypertensive adolescents. For example, doses of antihypertensive medications are extrapolations of doses in adults or based on studies with limited number of patients and different causes of hypertension; fortunately, better studies are now been conducted in these age groups.

Pharmacologic treatment needs to be individualized; some of the factors to keep in mind include the effects of medication on electrolytes disturbances, glucose and lipid metabolism, and renal as well as cardiovascular function. Medication can also interfere with physical and intellectual activities, and interact with other medications. Additional factors to consider include preexisting conditions, patient compliance with taking medications, and medication cost. Adolescents with hypertension requiring pharmacologic intervention should be under the supervision of consultants in nephrology or cardiology who are familiar with hypertension in adolescents.

Table 16-19 lists the most commonly used drugs for the management of hypertension in children, adolescents, and adults.

Pregnancy in adolescents deserves special consideration in view of the high risk of the development of hypertension in pregnant teens with the potential for complications threatening the well-being of the mother and the infant. Severe hypertension in the mother increases the risk for hypertensive encephalopathy, intracranial bleeding, and renal insufficiency. In the fetus, the risk of premature delivery increases, with all its consequences. Small-for-gestational age infants are born with decreased number of nephrons and are at risk of developing hypertension. The evaluation of the hypertensive mother is complicated. Common radiologic or nuclear scans are contraindicated. The use of angiotensin converting enzyme inhibitors, and angiotensin II receptor antagonists are teratogenic and are contraindicated in pregnancy. These patients are better served when followed by a team that includes an obstetrician, perinatologist, and a nephrologist.

Suggested Readings

Chobanian AV, Bakris GL, Black HR, et al.: The Seventh Report of the Joint National Committee on Prevention, Detection Evaluation, and Treatment of High Blood Pressure: The JNC 7 Report. *JAMA* 289:2560–2572, 2003.

Flynn J: Hypertension in the adolescent. *Adolesc Med* 16:11–29, 2005.

Fourth Report on the Diagnosis, Evaluation, and Treatment of High Blood Pressure in Children and Adolescents. *Pediatrics* 114(Suppl):S555–S576, 2004.

Goodfriend TL, Colhoun DA: Resistant hypertension, obesity, sleep apnea, and aldosterone theory and therapy. *Hypertension* 43:518–524, 2004.

Initial therapy of hypertension. *Med Lett* 46:53–55, 2004.

Luckstead EF: Cardiovascular disorders in the college student. *Pediatr Clin North Am* 52:243–278, 2005.

Vogt BA, Davis DI: Treatment of hypertension. In: Avner ED, Harmon WE, Niaudet P (eds.), *Pediatric Nephrology.* 5th ed. Philadelphia, PA: Lippincott Williams & Wilkins, Chap. 62, pp. 1199–1866, 2004.

TABLE 16-19

ANTIHYPERTENSIVE MEDICATIONS: FOR CHRONIC HYPERTENSION—CHILDREN/ADOLESCENTS

Class	Drug	Starting Dose	Interval	Max Dose	Adults
ACE inhibitors	Captopril	0.5–1.0 mg/kg predose	tid	6 mg/kg/day	12.5–450 mg PO (tid)
	Enalapril	0.2 mg/kg/per dose	bid	1 mg/kg/day	2.5–40 mg/day PO (qd or bid)
	Lisinopril	0.2 mg/kg/day	qd	1 mg/kg/day	5–40 mg/day PO (qd)
Angiotensin II receptor antagonists	Losartan	?		?	25–100 mg/day (qd)
					25–100 mg/day PO (qd)
	Candesartan	?		?	8–32 mg/day pL (qd)
	Irbesartan	?		?	150–300 mg/day PO (qd)
	Telmisartan	?		?	40–80 mg/day PO (qd)
α and β antagonists	Labetalol	2–3 mg/kg/day	bid	10–12 mg/kg/day up to 2.4 g	200–2400 mg/day (bid)
B antagonists	Atenolol	0.5–1 mg/kg/day	qd	2 mg/kg/day	25–100 mg/day PO (q do or bid)
	Metoprolol	1–2 mg/kg/day	bid	6 mg/kg/day up to 450 mg/day	100–450 mg/day PO (qd or bid)
	Propranolol	0.5–8 mg/kg/day	bid	16 mg/kg/day	80–480 mg/day PO (bid)
Calcium channel blockers	Amlodipine	0.1–0.3 mg/kg/day	qd or bid	0.6 mg/kg/day up to 20 mg/day	2.5–20 mg/day PO (qd)
	Isradipine	0.05–0.15 mg/kg/day	tid or qid	0.8 mg/kg/day up to 20 mg/day	2.5–20 mg PO (qd)
	Extended release nifedipine	0.25–0.5 mg/kg/day	qd or bid	3 mg/kg/day up to 180 mg/day	30–180 mg/day PO (qd)

(Continued)

ANTIHYPERTENSIVE MEDICATIONS: FOR CHRONIC HYPERTENSION—CHILDREN/ADOLESCENTS (CONTINUED)

Class	Drug	Starting dose	Interval	Max dose	Adults
CNS α_2 agonists	Clonidine	0.05–0.3 mg PO	bid or tid	0.3 mg	Same as children
	Clonidine (Patch)	TTS-1	Once a week		Same as children
		TTS-2	Once a week		Same as children
		TTS-3	Once a week		Same as children
	Methyldopa	10 mg/kg/dose	bid		65 mg/kg/day up to 3 grams/day
Diuretics	Chlorothiazide	10–20 mg/kg/day	bid	40 mg/kg/day	125–500 mg/day PO (bid)
	Furosemide	0.5–2.0 mg/kg/day	bid or qid	10–15 mg/kg/day	Same as children
	Hydrochlorothiazide	1 mg/kg/dose	bid	4 mg/kg/day	25–200 mg/day PO (qd or bid)
	Metolazone	0.2–0.4 mg/kg/PO			2.5–200 mg/day PO (qd or bid)
	Spironolactone	3.3 mg/kg/day	bid		25–200 mg/day PO (qd or bid)
Vasodilators	Hydralazine	0.25 mg/kg/PO	tid–qid	7.5 mg/kg/day up to 200 mg/day	Seldom used
	Minoxidil	0.1–0.2 mg/kg/ PO	bid–tid	1 mg/kg/day up to 50 mg/day	20–100 mg/day PO (bid)

NEPHROLITHIASIS

Etiology

Nephrolithiasis should be considered in a patient presenting with unexplained acute abdominal or flank pain with hematuria. Crystals form in the urine as the result of some combination of two major factors: the increased (supersaturated) concentration of a potential stone-forming salt within the urine (due to increased excretion of a substance or decreased water excretion) and alterations of crystal inhibiting factors (Table 16-20). The relative contribution of each of these factors to clinical stone disease varies with the condition. Crystals mixed with urinary protein adhere most often to renal papillae where the aggregates increase in size to form a definitive stone. The stone may vary in size from only a few millimeters to a large staghorn calculus filling the entire pelvis. The smallest stones tend to pass out in the urine unnoticed; slightly larger ones may appear as sand in the urine; still larger ones may induce ureteral obstruction and/or colic. Any stone that causes obstruction also predisposes the urinary tract to infection. Other general factors contributing to stone formation include those listed in Table 16-20.

Disorders associated with renal stones are listed in Table 16-21. After early childhood in

TABLE 16-20

FACTORS LEADING TO STONE FORMATION

Increased concentration of certain salts
Changes in crystal inhibiting factors
Urinary stasis
Urinary pH that diminishes crystal solubility
Deficiencies of endogenous urinary stone-inhibiting
  substances:
a. Including the urinary proteins:
  Nephrocalcin
  Uropontine
  Tamm-Horsfall mucoprotein
b. Concentrations of citrate, pyrophosphate, sodium,
  and magnesium
Disorders that increase the concentration or amount
  of stone-forming substances in the urine

TABLE 16-21

DISORDERS ASSOCIATED WITH RENAL STONES

Urologic obstruction
Urinary tract infections (with stasis)
Medullary sponge kidney
Renal tubular acidosis
Alkaptonuria
Primary hyperoxaluria
Cystinuria
Gout
Xanthinuria
Hypercalciuric states
1. Hypercalciuria with hypercalcemia
   a. Hyperparathyroidism
   b. Sarcoidosis
   c. Cushing syndrome, steroid administration
   d. Neoplasm
   e. Immobilization
   f. Hypervitaminosis D
   g. Hyperthyroidism
   h. Milk-alkali syndrome (increased intake of
      antacids with sodium bicarbonate)
   i. Adrenal insufficiency
2. Hypercalciuria with normal serum calcium
   a. Idiopathic
   b. Immobilization (casting, prolonged bed rest,
      paraplegia-quadriplegia)
   c. Steroid administration
   d. Some endocrine disorders
   e. Distal renal tubular acidosis
Normocalciuria with normal serum calcium and
  calcium stones
Others
a. Ethylene glycol ingestion
b. Large amount of ascorbic acid ingestion
c. Rhubarb
d. Furosemide administration

the United States, the most common constituent of renal stones is calcium, most often as one of the calcium phosphate or calcium oxalate crystalline forms. However, other chemical compositions occur in children and adolescents in a variety of clinical settings. Aspects of the more common forms are outlined in Table 16-22. Bladder dysfunction

T A B L E   1 6 - 2 2

CHARACTERISTICS OF COMMON FORMS OF UROLITHIASIS

Type	Description	Initial Treatment
Calcium stones	Calcium oxalate stones are radiopaque and may be due to hyperoxaluria (excess dietary intake of oxalate-containing foods, excessive intake of vitamin C, oxalosis, and others). Calcium phosphate stones also are radiopaque and due to abnormal calcium metabolism. Together, calcium oxalate and phosphate stones are the most commonly encountered (50%–70%) of all types of stones. Many also contain hydroxyapatite and some uric acid.	Eliminate excess calcium intake; increase fluid intake (2500 mL per 24 h); administer thiazide diuretics, potassium citrate, sodium phosphate, cellulose phosphate, and/or magnesium gluconate; treat underlying disorders of secondary hypercalcemia; An effective prophylactic regimen can significantly reduce the need for specific stone removal procedures.
Cystine stones	Weakly radiopaque, milky glass appearance; most common cause of stone formation in young children and is autosomal recessive inheritance; accounts for 2%–5% of stones overall (including adults). Urine turns purple in the presence of cyanide-nitroprusside. Typically flat, hexagonal crystals seen in urine.	Low methionine diet, increase water intake (3–4 L/day); alkalinize urine with divided dose sodium bicarbonate or sodium citrate; chemolysis with α-mercaptopropionyl-glycine or treatment with D-penicillamine.
Uric acid stones	Slightly radiopaque to radiolucent; occur in hyperuricemic states (gout, neoplastic disease, diuretic treatment, diabetic ketoacidosis, renal failure, rapid weight loss, sickle cell anemia, lead poisoning, psoriasis, sarcoidosis, hyperparathyroidism, or hypoparathyroidism). Also can form with normal serum and uric acid levels. Accounts for 5%–10% of stones overall.	Treat uric acid levels over 9 mg/mL with or without symptoms (probenecid; allopurinol) alkalinize urine with potassium citrate and restrict dietary protein; increase fluid intake.
Triple phosphate stones (struvite or infection-related stones)	Radiopaque; consist of calcium phosphate and magnesium-ammonium phosphate. Form in urine with pH over 6.5; often seen with ureteropelvic obstruction and urinary tract infections where gram-negative, urease-generating bacteria produce alkaline urine and promote stone formation with precipitation of phosphate salts. Bacteria include *Proteus*, *Pseudomonas*, *Klebsiella*, *Providencia*, *Serratia*, and rarely, *Staphylococci*. Also seen with urinary tract infection vesicoureteral reflux, neurogenic bladder, posterior urethral valves. May become exceptionally large filing renal pelvis (staghorn calculus). Accounts for 15% of stones overall.	Remove stone by ESWL or newer endoscopy techniques; treat infection with antibiotics (acute and prophylactic), thiazide diuretics to decrease the urine calcium excretion.

(particularly neurogenic bladder), chronic UTIs, and exogenous steroids are among the more common contributory factors seen in adolescents; however, a significant number of cases are idiopathic. While calcium oxalate stones are usually less than 2 cm, others (struvite, uric acid, and cystine stones) can fill the renal collection system (staghorn calculi). Most ureteral stones less than 0.5 cm pass spontaneously while larger stones usually do so less frequently.

Symptomatology

The presence of nephrolithiasis should be suspected in instances of acute or recurrent colicky abdominal (or flank) pain, hematuria, pyuria, recurrent UTIs, or where there is a history of passing sand. Flank pain suggests renal pelvic obstruction while groin pain with radiation to the scrotum or labia suggests distal ureteral colic or obstruction. The obstruction may have long-term consequences if it remains silent for a significant period of time. A dietary history may reveal increased intake of calcium (milk, cheese, ice cream, antacids) or oxalate (tea, oranges, cranberry juice, spinach, rhubarb). Injudicious vitamin intake also may also contribute to stone formation since vitamin D promotes gastrointestinal calcium absorption and vitamin C promotes oxalate formation.

Endogenous causes of calcium oxalate stones include primary hyperparathyroidism, idiopathic hypercalciuria, low urine citrate concentrations, hyperoxaluria, and hyperuricosuria. Renal tubular acidosis or other forms of chronic urinary alkalization may promote calcium phosphate stone formation, while low urine pH and hyperuricosuria promote uric acid stone formation. Infection with bacteria that excrete urease leads to struvite stones while cystinuria leads to cystine stones.

Laboratory Studies

Ideally, the medical evaluation of renal calculi is guided by the type of stone. When available for chemical analysis, infrared spectroscopy is the preferred method. Polarization microscopy and x-ray diffraction can also be used. Stones frequently may be obtained by passing all urine through a cloth sieve or one of the proprietary urine filters generally available.

Laboratory studies that contribute to the evaluation of stone disease include those listed in Table 16-23. Radiologic studies often prove useful in the diagnostic evaluation of stones. Kidney and bladder sonography is a noninvasive technique that has an excellent level of sensitivity in the detection of renal calculi, though plain films of the abdomen are better in localization of ureteral stones. Spiral noncontrast CT scan is now the preferred modality of imaging. It will show nearly all types of stones and also can detect hydronephrosis. Even stones that are normally radiolucent on plain x-ray are visible on CT. Only stones that are aggregations of drugs are not visible on CT. Protease inhibitors such as indinavir sulfate used to treat HIV positive patients may develop stones formed from the drug. These stones are not visible on CT, and should be kept in mind when assessing patients on these medications. Intravenous urography is less commonly utilized

TABLE 16-23

POTENTIAL LABORATORY STUDIES IN THE EVALUATION OF STONE FORMATION

Urinalysis

Urine culture

Urine pH

24-h urine collection (for total calcium, uric acid, citrate, magnesium, oxalate, amino acids, and creatinine)

Blood tests:

Serum calcium

Phosphorus

Alkaline phosphatase

Uric acid

Electrolytes

Urea nitrogen

Creatinine

Parathyroid hormone

Magnesium

Albumin

Total protein

because it is more invasive. It still has a role in helping to define the anatomy more completely, particularly in cases where duplication, ureterocele, or ureteropelvic junction (UPJ) obstruction may be suspected.

Stone density on plain x-ray may often give a clue to the composition of the stone. Calcium stones are densely radiopaque; cystine stones are more softly radiopaque and generally larger and smoother than calcium stones. Uric acid and xanthine stones are radiolucent, while struvite stones are of mixed radiographic appearance. The list of possible studies below should be used as a menu from which is selected those blood and urine tests of the greatest likely benefit in any given clinical setting.

Management

Some basic principles of therapy for stone disease are useful, though the treatment of urolithiasis also is based partly on the composition of the stone and partly on the underlying cause (Tables 16-21 and 16-22). In addition, the pain of renal colic may be sufficiently severe as to require narcotic analgesia. In the past, surgical removal was often necessary in many instances, but modern minimally invasive methods have limited open surgery to only the largest of staghorn calculi. Stones that are reasonably small (i.e., 5 mm or less in diameter) have a 90% chance of passing spontaneously with only analgesics and hydration. For other patients whose stones have become impacted and they have become septic, cystoscopy with stenting or percutaneous nephrostomy can relieve the obstruction.

Three methods predominate stone treatment today: extracorporeal shockwave lithotripsy (ESWL), ureteroscopy with laser or electrohydraulic lithotripsy (URS), and percutaneous nephrolithopaxy with ultrasonic, electrohydraulic, or laser lithotripsy (PCN). ESWL has largely supplanted the need for open surgical procedures to remove stones from the kidney or upper ureter. Focused shock waves disintegrate the stones into smaller more easily passed fragments. Advances in fiberoptics have created ureteroscopes, which can be passed retrograde all the way to the renal pelvis. Allied with small laser fibers (3 Fr) these new scopes allow successful treatment of stones, which

would otherwise be unreachable by ESWL. Finally, for large, awkwardly positioned, or very hard stones in the kidney, PCN treatment is the preferred method. Combination treatments are also commonly done. A large stone can be debulked using PCN and small fragments disintegrated by ESWL.

Preventive measures for stone disease should be a priority in many patients. Wherever possible, the underlying cause should be corrected. Increased water intake with consequently decreased urinary stone salt concentrations is often helpful. Patients with paraplegia, quadriplegia, or a neurogenic bladder from some other cause, as well as those who may be immobilized for prolonged periods, are at risk and should be closely monitored. Treatment measures include the avoidance of excessive protein intake. The role of dietary calcium restriction in many forms of calcium stone disease may actually be counterproductive and should be approached with caution, particularly in growing adolescents. However, diminution of sodium intake may have a net beneficial effect on calcium stone formation. Alkalinization of the urine using oral alkali can control the recurring and potentially obstructive stones of cystinuric patients.

Suggested Readings

Coe FL, Favus, Asplin MJ, Asplin JR: Nephrolithiasis. In: Brenner BM (ed.), *Brenner and Rector's: The Kidney,* 7th ed. Philadelphia, PA: W.B. Saunders, Chap. 39, pp. 1819–1886, 2004.

Langman CB: Nephrolithiasis. In: Rudolph CD, Rudolph AM (eds.), *Rudolph's Pediatrics.* New York: McGraw-Hill, Chap. 21.12, pp. 1715–1716, 2003.

Srivastava T, Alon US: Urolithiasis in adolescent children. *Adolesc Med* 16:87–109, 2005.

Idiopathic Hypercalciuria

General

The most common cause of calcium containing stones is idiopathic hypercalciuria. Rather than a single entity, this category represents several pathophysiologic entities. Research in adults and children has demonstrated that idiopathic hypercalciuria may be associated with a variety of symptoms before the first renal stone appears. These include asymptomatic microscopic or gross hematuria, urinary frequency, dysuria, enuresis (nocturnal or diurnal), and colicky abdominal pain. The idiopathic hypercalciuria syndromes are invariably associated with normocalcemia (Table 16-21). Although the pathophysiologic basis for each of the hypercalciuria syndromes is incompletely understood, current data suggest that some form of 1,25-dihydroxy vitamin D dysregulation may occur. At the intestinal level, increased vitamin D-induced calcium absorption can result in the so-called absorptive form of hypercalciuria. In circumstances where the kidney produces more 1α hydroxylase activity than is needed for calcium homeostasis, calcium mobilization, and consequent renal excretion can occur, thus producing the primary renal form of hypercalciuria. Other factors, including sodium intake, also appear to impact on the degree of hypercalciuria. Hypercalciuria has been generally defined by a calcium excretion rate of >4 mg/kg/day. Alternatively, a random calcium: creatinine ratio (in the same units: mg to mg) of >0.2 (if 5 years or older) on a late morning random specimen suggests hypercalciuria. This should be confirmed with a 24-hour urine collection wherever possible. A similar ratio on a random first morning urine specimen after an overnight fast suggests the absorptive form.

Management

The treatment of idiopathic hypercalciuria remains controversial. Although dietary calcium restriction and/or thiazide diuretic therapy may decrease calcium excretion, these are not without possible risks. Also, dietary calcium restriction does not actually decrease the formation of calcium oxalate stones and it aggravates bone mineral loss; this is especially worrisome in children (with unknown long-term effects) and also women who will eventually become menopausal and face osteoporosis. Furthermore, thiazide treatment may be associated with disturbances of cholesterol balance. Although these patients have an increased risk of subsequent stone formation, the presence of microscopic hematuria or occasional gross hematuria should not prompt immediate and aggressive treatment. A more rational approach to the

management of hypercalcemia with nephrolithiasis includes increased water intake, sodium and protein restriction, the addition of potassium citrate to inhibit calcium oxalate crystallization, and the administration of thiazide diuretics or other agents to promote tubular calcium reabsorption. Patients with recurring flank pain, dysuria, or frequently recurring episodes of gross hematuria are candidates for treatment.

ENURESIS

Epidemiology and Etiology

The prevalence of enuresis is approximately 3%–4% at age 12; it falls to 1% or less by age 19 whether intervention has occurred or not. Sixty percent of the cases have been present from early childhood without interruption. The remainder of these cases are secondary, appearing after at least 3–6 months of total urinary continence. Nocturnal enuresis occurs more frequently in males while females constitute the greater proportion of those with diurnal enuresis.

It is worthwhile enquiring about symptoms of enuresis, since the embarrassed adolescent may not volunteer such information if not directly asked. Most cases of primary nocturnal enuresis are idiopathic, but various familial, constitutional, and social factors (Table 16-24) play contributory roles. A positive family history of enuresis increases the risk of enuresis in the offspring; if both parents had nocturnal enuresis, 70%–75% of their children will be affected. This figure decreases to 45% with one affected

TABLE 16-24

FACTORS ASSOCIATED WITH PRIMARY, NOCTURNAL ENURESIS

Heredity
Low socioeconomic status
Institutionalization
Deep sleep
Deficiency of a nocturnal surge of ADH
Functional reduction of bladder capacity
Unstable bladder
Chronic illness

parent as compared to a 15% incidence if neither parent had enuresis. Pure primary nocturnal enuresis undoubtedly results from several causes. Among those proposed etiologies are genetic factors, decreased nocturnal antidiuretic hormone (ADH) secretion, unstable bladder syndrome and a maturational lag in nocturnal bladder control (Table 16-25). Studies evaluating enuresis as a sleep disorder have yielded conflicting results.

Table 16-25 lists other causes of enuresis. When contemplating evaluation, treatment, and prognosis, it is important to distinguish those adolescents with pure, asymptomatic nocturnal enuresis from those with accompanying voiding symptoms, UTIs, or daytime enuresis. Anterior displacement of the posterior labial frenulum, often seen in obese females, may cause urethrovaginal reflux with urine leakage after urination. Nocturnal enuresis present from birth may be associated with the so-called "unstable bladder." This describes a group of patients who experience insuppressible detrusor contractions and have not yet acquired the ability to voluntarily suppress the infantile voiding reflex. When possible, the patient forcefully contracts the external sphincter, sometimes with external pressure as well through a squatting posture. The high intravesical pressures generated can lead to dilatation of the bladder and urethra and increased risk of UTI.

TABLE 16-25

MISCELLANEOUS CAUSES OF ENURESIS

Unstable bladder
Hinman-Allen syndrome
Obstructive lesions of the urethra or bladder
Urinary tract infection
Diabetes mellitus
Diabetes insipidus
Psychogenic water intoxication
Sickle cell disease (trait and anemia)
Renal disorders (such as tubulointerstitial disease)
Food allergies
Lumbosacral disorders (including acquired spinal
   dysraphic states)
Mental retardation and other developmental disorders
Anterior displacement of the posterior labial frenulum

At the extreme of the continence disturbances is the Hinman-Allen syndrome, also termed the non-neurogenic neurogenic bladder. In addition to both diurnal and nocturnal enuresis, these patients often have histories of encopresis, constipation, and UTIs; on radiographic evaluation of the urinary tract, they are often found to have large, trabeculated bladders, incomplete bladder emptying and VUR.

Laboratory Studies

Adolescents with primary nocturnal enuresis typically have a normal physical examination, normal urinalysis, and negative urine cultures. Further medical evaluation of these youth is unnecessary. Secondary or diurnal enuresis is only slightly more likely to have an underlying organic cause. A renal sonogram, voiding cystourethrogram, and cystometric study are usually reserved for patients with a history of UTI and symptoms suggestive of an occult neurologic problem. Patients with Hinman-Allen syndrome or those with suspected neurogenic abnormalities should undergo thorough neurologic evaluation. A psychiatric evaluation is also advisable for these patients.

Management

Treatment (Table 16-26) of idiopathic nocturnal enuresis produces variable results; whether therapy or time is the critical factor is unknown in light of the high rate of spontaneous resolution. Daytime enuresis is often managed with a combination of pharmacologic and behavior modification therapy (Table 16-26).

Pharmacologic Methods

There are three commonly prescribed drugs used to treat nocturnal enuresis: desmopressin acetate (DDAVP), imipramine, and oxybutynin. DDAVP is a synthetic analogue of ADH. Available both as an oral pill or nasal spray, it has become widely used because of its efficacy and safety. The initial dose is one pill (0.2 mg) or one nasal spray (10 µg) each night about 20–30 minutes before bed. The dosage

TABLE 16-26

METHODS OF ENURESIS TREATMENT

Tincture of time
Pharmacologic
    Imipramine (25–125 mg PO at night)
    Oxybutynin (5 mg PO at night to 5 mg PO three
    times daily)
    DDAVP (0.2–0.6 mg PO or 10–40 µg intranasal at
    night)
Behavior modification
    Operant conditioning devices—wetting alarm
    Scheduled voiding program
    Counseling or psychotherapy
    Hypnosis
    Acupuncture
    Diet manipulations

can be adjusted upward to a maximal dose of three pills or four puffs as needed. If the initial dose is not effective after 2–3 weeks, the dosage is increased to two pills and sprays for another 2–3 weeks. This is repeated to a maximum of three pills or four puffs if necessary. The pills can be chewed if the patient cannot swallow them whole, without any loss of efficacy. Once a successful dose has been found, it should be used for at least 3–6 months before attempting to wean the patient off. The chief benefit of DDAVP is its ease of use; it can be used discreetly, and has few side effects. There have been reports of hyponatremia in patients with underlying liver and kidney disease, but these have been rare. Also, nose bleeds and headaches have been reported with the nasal form. It must be used in conjunction with aggressive fluid restriction.

Typically, patients are asked to hold all fluid intakes starting $1\frac{1}{2}$–2 hours before bed. This includes fruit, vegetables, bowls of cereal, ice cream, and other snacks. One must be quite explicit about this point. It is surprising what some adolescents and parents assume to be acceptable foods and liquids on a fluid restriction. Some families prefer to restrict the use of the medication to just special occasions such as sleepovers, campouts, or other social events. If this is the pattern of use, always have the family

try the drug out first at home to see if the child or adolescent responds and at what dose. Not everyone is a responder; however about half of the patients who do respond will develop intermittent or complete return to nocturnal enuresis 1 year after stopping the medication.

Patients who do not respond to DDAVP or to alarm devices can be offered imipramine (Tofranil). This was the drug of choice in the treatment of nocturnal enuresis prior to the development of DDAVP. It is a tricyclic antidepressant and has weak alpha adrenergic and anticholinergic effects on the bladder. It also can affect the sleep cycle of the brain. About 50% of patients will respond. The typical dosage is 25 mg PO taken 20–30 minutes before bed; this can be gradually raised to 50 mg and 75 mg depending on the size, age, and weight of the adolescent.

Caution is necessary when prescribing imipramine because it can have severe side effects, such as blurring of vision and alteration of concentration. It must be kept in a childproof container and secured. Overdose can result in fatal arrhythmias. If effective, the drug is continued for 3–6 months before gradually weaning off. Side effects of imipramine include restlessness, anxiety, poor concentration, weight loss, syncope, and constipation, though these tend to be less pronounced with a single bedtime dose than with divided doses during the day.

Oxybutynin may be given as a single 5 mg PO nighttime dose or as frequently as three times daily for daytime enuresis associated with an unstable bladder. It is an anticholinergic and helps to suppress uninhibited bladder activity. Patients should be alerted to the common side effects of anticholinergic medications, including dry mouth, constipation, and flushing. It is important to avoid overheating on hot days. If successful, it is used for 3–6 months before attempting to wean off. For patients who are not responsive to medications individually, combination therapy using two drugs and/or devices together can sometimes be effective.

Nonpharmacologic Methods

Pharmacologic treatment of enuresis is often combined with one of several behavior modification programs (Table 16-26) in order to improve bladder capacity and control. A number of operant conditioning devices are available; the wetting alarm is prototypical. A cotton absorbent pad equipped with a sensor is placed in the patient's underwear or pajama bottom. This is linked to an alarm module, which attaches to the shirt or top. When the sensor becomes wet, the alarm sounds and/or vibrates, and it is hoped that the patient wakes sufficiently to finish urinating in the bathroom. There are many models and manufacturers (Palco Wet Stop, Nytone Enuresis Alarm, and Malem Bedwetting Alarm among many). The older style models which have a complete rubber pad or sheet are no longer as popular because of their bulk, expense, and the observation that the patient has to be quite wet before the alarm is triggered.

The chief benefit of the alarm is that when they work, and the patient responds, the effect usually endures and has a low recidivism rate. About three fourths of those who initially respond will still be dry 1 year after the alarm is stopped. Unfortunately many patients with enuresis are heavy sleepers and may not respond at all. They cannot be used discreetly and can also wake up siblings and other family members. Alarms take time to use and the family and child or adolescent has to be patient and adjust its placement. Finally, not all insurance plans and third party payers will cover them.

Bladder retention exercises have been employed with success on occasion in the past, but are no longer a preferred method. The patient would be instructed to try to hold his or her urine for increasingly longer periods of time after experiencing the urge to void. This method unfortunately rarely works because it depends on the conscious mind to engage physical tricks (i.e., crossing one's legs) or mental tricks (i.e., thinking of calm thoughts) to help hold the bladder longer. These tricks are not available to the unconscious sleeping patient. It is now felt that a scheduled voiding program which asks the patient to try to void on a regular basis throughout the day, regardless if there is a sense of fullness or urgency, is a more useful form of conditioning.

Fluid restriction in the evening and rousing the patient to void when the last family member goes to bed, so-called "night waking," may be helpful adjunctive measures but generally are futile in themselves. Counseling or psychotherapy can be tried, but have been minimally successful in ameliorating enuresis per se; however, they may help manage emotional distress or coexistent emotional problems. It is not common for simple nocturnal enuresis to be the result of an occult psychologic problem; however, psychologic problems can develop from misguided draconian measures. Reassurance that enuresis does not adversely affect sexual function is an important component of counseling for enuretic teenagers. Hypnosis, diet manipulations, acupuncture, and other therapies have been reported to help some patients as well, but lack evidence of long-term efficacy. Finally commercial programs that offer money back guarantees have not been shown to be any more effective than the techniques described above and which are readily available to any practitioner.

Suggested Readings

Austin PF, Ritchey ML: Dysfunctional voiding. *Pediatr Rev* 21:336–341, 2000.

Elder JS: Voiding dysfunction. In: Behrman RE, Kliegman RM, Jenson HB (eds.), *Nelson Textbook of Pediatrics,* 17th ed. Philadephia, PA: W.B. Saunders, Chap. 535, pp. 1808–1812, 2004.

Evans JHC: Evidence-based management of nocturnal enuresis. *Br Med J* 323:1167–1169, 2001.

Fergusson DM, Horwood LJ: Nocturnal enuresis and behavioral problems in adolescence: A 15-year longitudinal study. *Pediatrics* 94:662–668, 1994.

Fritz G, Rockney R, Work Group on Quality Issues: Summary of the practice parameter for the assessment and treatment of children and adolescents with enuresis. *J Am Acad Child Adolesc Psychiatry* 3(1):123–125, 2004.

Ghoniem GM, Sakr MA: Bladder dysfunction syndromes. *Adolesc Med* 7:35–46, 1996.

Glazener CM, Evans JH, Peto RE. Tricyclic and related drugs for nocturnal enuresis in children. *Cochrane Database Syst Rev* 3:CD002117, 2003.

Greydanus DE, Torres AD, O'Donnell DM, et al.: Enuresis: Current concepts. *Ind J Pediatr* 66:425–438, 1999.

Palmer LS, Franco I, Rotario P, et al.: Biofeedback therapy expedites the resolution of reflux in older children. *J Urol* 168:1699–1703, 2002.

Pennesi M, Pitter M, Bordugo A, Minisini S, Peratoner L. Behavioral therapy for primary nocturnal enuresis. *J Urol* 171(1):408–410, 2004.

Schulman S, Stokes A, Salzman PM: The efficacy and safety of oral desmopressin in children with primary nocturnal enuresis. *J Urol* 166:2427–2431, 2001.

Sher PK, Reinberg Y: Successful treatment of giggle incontinence with methylphenidate. *J Urol* 156:656–658, 1996.

SCROTAL DISORDERS

Table 16-27 provides a list of various scrotal disorders in adolescent males; the more common conditions are described in this section. Sexually transmitted disorders are reviewed in Chap. 24.

Hydrocele

Etiology

A hydrocele is a collection of peritoneal fluid within the tunica vaginalis or processus vaginalis. There are two common forms: communicating and noncommunicating. Among adolescents, the most common form is the communicating or patent processus vaginalis. The path through which the testicle made its descent into the scrotum has not sealed completely. It remains open or patent and the fluid that normally bathes the peritoneal structures can trickle down into the scrotum. Fluid flows freely between the peritoneum and tunica vaginalis. Often it increases in size during the day and with activity and can become smaller at night. Noncommunicating hydroceles are uncommon in adolescents; typically they are found in the elderly. In these hydroceles, there is no open passageway, but rather something has irritated the inner lining of the tunica vaginalis causing it to secrete more fluid. Recurrent trauma, injury, or irritation, have been identified as causes, though many cases are idiopathic. The communicating hydrocele and indirect inguinal hernia are essentially the same condition with the difference being in the former, there is only fluid passing

TABLE 16-27

CAUSES OF SCROTAL PAIN AND/OR SWELLING

Testicular torsion (acute or intermittent)
Torsion of appendix testis (hydatid or Morgagni)
Torsion of appendix epididymis
Orchitis
Epididymitis
Acute idiopathic scrotal edema
Henoch-Schönlein purpura (with spermatic cord vasculitis)
Hernia (strangulated)
Hydrocele
Varicocele
Spermatocele
Hematocele
Testicular tumor
Paratesticular tumor
Generalized edema
Scrotal cellulitis
Fat necrosis
Spermatic venous thrombosis
Fournier syndrome: acute scrotal gangrene
Epididymal cyst
Adrenal rest
Splenogonadal fusion
Fibroma (tunica albuginea)
Trauma: hematoma

down; in the latter, there is a solid structure, such as a tongue of omentum or a loop of bowel.

Symptomatology

A hydrocele typically presents as a nontender, firm or tense, often intermittent scrotal swelling which transilluminates. The testis on the affected side may or may not be palpable. In very fair patients, it may have a bluish cast or tint because the blue wavelength of light is the shortest and is least absorbed.

Diagnosis

Diagnosis is by clinical signs and Table 16-28 provides a differential diagnosis list for a hydrocele.

TABLE 16-28

**DIFFERENTIAL DIAGNOSIS FOR A SWOLLEN
SCROTUM**

Hydrocele
Hernia
Varicocele
Trauma-induced hematocele
Testicular torsion
Testicular tumor
Epididymitis

Occasionally, acute hydroceles may appear as the result of scrotal trauma, epididymitis, testicular tumor, or torsion. Scrotal ultrasound should be performed if a tumor is suspected.

Management

Aspiration is contraindicated due to the risk of introducing infection or of bowel perforation if a hernia is present. Communicating hydroceles are usually repaired electively as an outpatient. Noncommunicating hydroceles can be treated by open surgery or aspiration and sclerotherapy. Open surgery is done directly through a scrotal incision unlike communicating hydroceles, which are operated on through an inguinal approach. The dilated tunica vaginalis tissue is resected and the edges oversewn. Aspiration and sclerotherapy is usually not advisable in this age group because the inflammatory reaction of the sclerosing agent can affect the testicle, epididymis, and vas deferens and lead to subfertility or infertility.

Hernia

Indirect hernias are more common than direct hernias in teenagers. The indirect hernias are palpated with an index finger in the external inguinal ring; the hernia may become more prominent with a Valsalva maneuver. If the bowel is in the scrotum, the testes and epididymis can be palpated separately from the bowel and bowel sounds are frequently present on scrotal auscultation. Direct hernias occur most frequently in adult males as the result of strenuous activity; a defect at the external inguinal ring can be palpated, especially with Valsalva maneuver. Femoral hernias can occur in females and the defect palpated in the femoral canal.

Surgical repair is indicated for identified hernias. Swelling of a hernia with pain and/or overlying erythema suggests bowel incarceration, prompting emergency surgery to prevent bowel ischemia, necrosis, and perforation. An asymptomatic hernia may be repaired electively. Laparoscopic methods and techniques involving placement of synthetic meshes, umbrellas, and other devices have been used in some adults; however, for the vast majority of adolescents, open surgical repair by any of the commonly used techniques is preferable. They are durable, time tested, and do not involve placement of a foreign object.

Varicocele

Etiology

Varicoceles are found in 15%–20% of older adolescents and young adults. They result from the tortuous dilation of pampiniform plexus veins in the scrotum. A primary varicocele is usually left-sided. It is believed that the greater length of the left spermatic vein, its connection with the left renal vein and not the inferior vena cava, and its fewer number of valves to block retrograde flow, make it more susceptible to varicoceles formation. Bilateral varicoceles can occur. Right-sided varicoceles are usually secondary to mechanical venous obstruction in the lower abdomen or pelvic region, as may occur with a retroperitoneal or kidney tumor. Solitary, right-sided varicoceles should be imaged promptly by CT or Doppler ultrasound for this reason. Varicoceles have been associated with infertility, and up to 30%–40% of men who present to an infertility clinic will be found to have varicoceles. It is believed that the extra pooling of blood increases the temperature in the scrotum, thereby affecting testicular function and development.

Symptomatology

Examination of the standing patient reveals dilated, wormlike cords (*bag of worms*) running the scrotal length. Varicoceles can be graded on a scale from 1 to 3. Grade 1 varicoceles are usually not prominent visually but can be palpated and become more prominent with Valsalva maneuvers. Grade 2 varicoceles are more visible and can be readily palpated without the Valsalva maneuver. Grade 3 varicocele is most easily seen and the large tortuous veins can be readily defined without palpation or the Valsalva maneuver. A primary varicocele disappears in the recumbent position and increases with the Valsalva maneuver; a secondary varicocele (usually right-sided) does not disappear when the patient lies down. This is an important distinction, as a secondary lesion requires a vigorous search for causal pathology, whereas the primary form requires no such investigation.

Management

There are three major reasons why varicoceles are repaired. First, if the varicocele is quite large and uncomfortable, it may warrant repair. It should be noted that not all groin and scrotal discomfort is due to the varicocele; also, the patient and family should bear in mind that even successful repair of the varicoceles may not necessarily lead to complete discomfort relief. Second, if there is a legal reason for repairing the varicoceles. Certain occupations require the applicant to be free of hernias and varicoceles. Typically these are jobs that require repetitive heavy exertion and labor. Third, if there is concern of future subfertility or infertility, treatment may be warranted. Because most of these adolescent patients are not in a position where there is an active desire to start a family, the concern is to prevent the development of future problems. If the testicle on the left side is markedly smaller (greater than 0.5 cm in its length) than the right one, surgery may be recommended. If the testicle is similar in size and volume, regular annual assessment is advisable. Surgical ligation is usually carried out as an outpatient and with the aid of an operating microscope, which decreases the risk of postoperative hydrocele because fewer lymphatics are disrupted.

Spermatocele

A spermatocele is a small, usually nontender cyst that develops as an extrusion from epididymal tubules and is superior-posterior to and distinct from the testis. It transilluminates and contains milky, sperm-filled fluid. They are often bilateral and even multiple. There is no effect on fertility or sexual function. Evaluation should rule out a testicular tumor or other cause of a scrotal mass (Tables 16-27 and 16-28). Surgical excision may be performed if discomfort or pain develops.

Hematocele

A hematocele is a hematoma of the scrotum. It usually develops after scrotal injury, inducing scrotal swelling and pain. Ultrasound can be helpful in diagnosing the lesion. Treatment includes scrotal elevation, ice packs, and analgesics. Occasionally surgical drainage is necessary. Large hematoceles associated with trauma or accidents should be evaluated by scrotal ultrasound. Subtle testicular ruptures can be missed. If not repaired, the rupture renders the testicle infertile.

Testicular Torsion

Symptomatology

Acute torsion is usually unilateral and only rarely bilateral; however, if one side is affected, the adolescent is at risk for a similar episode occurring on the opposite side at a future time. The patient with torsion classically experiences the sudden (occasionally gradual) onset of acute scrotal pain, accompanied by scrotal swelling and discoloration. Sometimes the onset is spontaneous; it can also be associated with exercise or trauma. Inguinal canal or lower abdominal pain can also occur. Previous episodes with spontaneous resolution have been described. Nausea and vomiting are present in 25% of the cases; there are no urinary voiding symptoms. Physical examination reveals a very tender, swollen testicle lying in a transverse position high in the scrotal sac; the equally tender epididymis is in an anteroposterior rather than its usual posterolateral position. Elevation of the testicle does not relieve the pain (negative Prehn's sign) and it does not transilluminate. The cremasteric reflex is usually absent. Scrotal edema and less frequently, a reactive hydrocele can develop.

Laboratory Studies

The urinalysis is normal. A testicular blood flow scan with technetium-99m shows reduced perfusion, but is usually not done because it takes too long to be available on an emergent basis. Scrotal Doppler ultrasound may also be a useful adjunct in the demonstration of the presence or absence of vascular pulsations and the determination of testicular viability. The diagnosis is a clinical one and in the face of a strong history as well as clinical findings, one should not wait to do an imaging study, but operate to relieve the torsion. As noted with cases of suspected appendicitis, there will be a percentage of false positive explorations, but this reduces the chances of missing a true torsion.

Management

The most frequent challenge is to distinguish acute testicular torsion from epididymal orchitis. Inflammation of epididymitis and orchitis is noted in about one-third of cases presenting with scrotal pain and tenderness. Differentiation of these diagnoses is urgent, and any case of suspected torsion should be viewed as a potential surgical emergency. Initial venous flow obstruction and thrombosis ultimately lead to arterial flow obstruction. It is essential that the torsion be reduced and normal blood flow returned as quickly as possible. Irreversible infarction occurs in 5–6 hours and Leydig cell necrosis in 10–12 hours, though testicular survival times up to 24 hours have been reported in 10%–20% of the cases with minimal flow. Manual detorsion after premedication may be tried, but immediate surgical exploration is still needed even if pain is relieved. When the testis can be salvaged, reduction of the torsion should be followed by fixation so that there will be no recurrence. Since the contralateral testicle is also vulnerable to torsion, it too should be explored and fixed. Intermittent testicular torsion has been described in some patients who have symptoms consistent with torsion, but which have resolved by the time the patient presents to the emergency department. After several episodes, elective bilateral scrotal pexy is often offered to prevent future occurrences.

Other Torsions

The appendix testis or appendix epididymis may also develop torsion and account for up to 25% of the cases of acute testicular pain and swelling. The sudden or gradual onset of pain is usually localized to the testicular upper pole with minimal nausea or emesis. The twisted appendix forms a pea-size swelling which may be visible in the fair skinned; a finding called the blue-dot sign. The appendix testis torsion usually resolves in less than 14 days, but persistent or severe pain may prompt surgical incision. Clinical signs may be indistinguishable from torsion of the entire testis or they may be somewhat milder. If differentiation can be made, surgical intervention is not necessary and there is no damage to testicular function. If in doubt, surgical exploration is the treatment of choice.

Acute Epididymitis

Etiology

Inflammation of the epididymis can be precipitated by many factors, including those listed in Table 16-29. It is unusual in the absence of sexual activity or a urologic abnormality. Chlamydial or

TABLE 16-29

CAUSES OF EPIDIDYMAL INFLAMMATION

Urethritis
Urinary tract infection
Prostatitis
Testicular tumor
Urologic surgery or instrumentation
Respiratory tract infection
Genitourinary tuberculosis
Mumps
Other viral infections
Bacterial infections capable of hematogenous spread

gonococcal urethritis and idiopathic causes account for most cases (40%–60%) in adolescents. Coliforms, *Pseudomonas*, and gram-positive cocci occur in youths who have engaged in anal coitus. Idiopathic epididymitis may be the result of trauma or exercise-induced reflux of sterile urine through the vas deferens, with resultant chemical irritation. In some instances, inflammation involves the testicle as well, producing epididymal orchitis.

Symptomatology

Epididymitis is characterized by the gradual or sudden onset of epididymal pain, tenderness, and local swelling, including scrotal swelling. As mentioned, it is usually observed in sexually active patients. Inflammation of the epididymitis may be mild or severe. In contrast to torsion, elevation of the testicle and epididymis does relieve pain (positive Prehn's sign) and an intact cremasteric reflex is usually found; however, neither is specific for acute epididymitis. Nausea is not usually found with acute epididymitis. Urethritis, symptoms simulating cystitis (such as urinary frequency and dysuria), fever, pyuria, bacteriuria, and positive urethral cultures are variable findings. Oligo- or azoospermia can result from acute epididymitis, especially when due to *C. trachomatis*. Other possible complications include epididymal abscess, infarction, and atrophy. Testicular atrophy can increase testicular cancer risk.

Laboratory Studies

A urethral culture may identify *N. gonorrhoeae* or *C. trachomatis* (Chap. 24). A first voided urine cultured for sexually transmitted infectious agents can be tested for leukocyte esterase as well. Epididymal aspirates can be also obtained for culture. A scrotal scan with technetium-99m reveals increased or normal vascularity in contrast to decreased vascularity in torsion. Doppler ultrasound may also distinguish acute epididymitis from testicular torsion.

Management

Persistence of inflammation for more than 14 days should prompt reevaluation. Testicular tumors have been misdiagnosed as simple epididymitis. Table 16-30 outlines a treatment approach. Surgical exploration is indicated if testicular torsion has not been ruled out promptly by clinical and laboratory findings.

Orchitis

Symptoms of orchitis can range from mild to severe testicular swelling and pain. More severe cases may also display chills, fever, and nausea. Causes of orchitis include mumps, varicella, coxsackievirus, influenza, and Epstein-Barr viruses as well as *Mycobacterium tuberculosis*, and, occasionally, bacterial organisms. Thirty percent of pubertal males with mumps develop orchitis that is usually unilateral. Treatment includes bed rest, analgesics, and scrotal support. Sterility is unusual, though testicular atrophy may occur in as many as 60% of cases following mumps.

Testicular Neoplasms

Epidemiology

Testicular neoplasm represents 1% of all cancer in males (see Chap. 18). The published incidence of

TABLE 16-30

TREATMENT OF EPIDIDYMITIS

1. Bed rest with cold compresses
2. Scrotal elevation (by means of a towel placed between the legs and an athletic supporter)
3. Analgesics
4. Antibiotics for suspected sexually transmitted organisms
   a. Ceftriaxone (250 mg IM once) in combination with:
   b. Doxycycline (100 mg bid for 10 days)
   c. Alternatives:
      i. Erythromycin base (1 g orally qid for 10 days)
      ii. Erythromycin ethylsuccinate (800 mg orally qid for 10 days)
      iii. Ofloxacin (300 mg orally bid for 10 days)
5. Anti-inflammatory drugs (oxyphenbutazone, steroids) for severe disease

testicular tumors is 1.0 to 2.0 per 100,000 males in the 15–19-year age group, and, 6 per 100,000 in 15–24-year age group. Patients with ectopic or undescended testes are at 10- to 40-fold greater risk for testicular tumors than the population at large; other predisposing factors are unknown. Although less common than leukemia, bone tumors, and tumors of the central nervous system, testicular neoplasm occurs with sufficient frequency to mandate examination of the testes in all routine physical examinations and to educate the adolescent to palpate his gonads himself on a regular basis. Testicular tumor is the most common solid neoplasm in the 15–39-year old male; establishing self-examination habits early in adolescence will allow an early diagnosis and maximal cure rate.

Classification. Adolescents are vulnerable to both prepubertal and postpubertal types of testicular tumors. The postpubertal or adult types are seminoma, embryonal cell, choriocarcinoma, teratoma, yolk sac, and mixed forms. Affected patients are treated like adults with testicular tumor. Prepubertal testicular tumors differ in their makeup and composition. Germ cell tumors comprise 95% of postpubertal testicle tumors, but only 75% of prepubertal tumors. Seminoma, the most common adult testicle tumor is quite rare in prepubertal patients. Yolk sac, teratoma, paratesticular rhabdomyosarcoma, and gonadal stromal tumors (Leydig and Sertoli cell tumors) predominate prepubertal tumors. Yolk sac and teratoma are the most common, comprising 80% of all prepubertal testicle tumors.

Symptomatology

A firm, painless testicular mass or a nodule palpated within the testes is the most common presenting finding and should raise a high index of suspicion. The mass does not transilluminate. Pain is uncommon, occurring only in approximately 10% of the time, and only if necrosis or hemorrhage has occurred. Patients may not admit to having a mass but will voice vague reports of testicular size change, or an uncomfortable scrotal sensation. A reactive hydrocele can sometimes occur but should not be confused with a true tumor. A hydrocele transilluminates and does not a have a hard rocky feeling on palpation,

which is characteristic of a testicle tumor. Scrotal ultrasound is very useful in distinguishing between these two diagnoses. Epididymitis can swell the epididymis and testicle but should be associated with a positive urine analysis and culture.

Evaluation

The full evaluation and treatment of testicular tumors is a complex subject and beyond the scope of this chapter. Several points are worth noting for the primary care clinician. Radical orchiectomy should be performed to obtain a definitive tissue diagnosis. If the patient has gone through puberty, he should be evaluated and treated like an adult testicle tumor patient. Serum markers should be drawn before treatment is started. Yolk sac tumors produce α-fetoprotein (AFP) with a half-life of 5 days, and a postoperative persistence or elevation of AFP suggests residual tumor. Postpubertal choriocarcinoma and the spermocytic variant of seminoma have elevated levels of the other tumor marker, β-hCG. The most common sites of metastases are the lungs and retroperitoneal lymph nodes. Chest x-ray and CT scan of the abdomen are needed to complete the evaluation for metastasis.

Management

Treatment includes radical orchiectomy of the affected testicle, retroperitoneal lymph node dissection, chemotherapy, and radiotherapy. The prognosis depends on the tumor type and the clinical staging. Among prepubertal patients, the best outcome occurs with teratomas. Unlike adult teratomas, prepubertal teratomas have a benign course with no reported metastases. All three germinal layers (endoderm, ectoderm, and mesoderm) should be present and sometimes, because of characteristic appearance on ultrasound, it is possible to suggest the pathology preoperatively. Because of its benign nature in prepubertal patients, a testis sparing approach is often used. After complete exposure and vascular control, the tumor is shelled out and the diagnosis confirmed by frozen section pathology. Seminomas have the best outlook in postpubertal patients; it is highly radiosensitive and responds well to platinum-based chemotherapy with better than a 90%5-year survival rate, even if the tumor is metastatic.

The testicle is a potential sanctuary for leukemic cells because the blood-testis barrier may protect tumor cells from chemotherapy. Acute lymphocytic leukemia is the most common type of leukemia to infiltrate the testicles, occurring in up to 25% of patients. In patients with a history of leukemia and development of a testicular mass, testicular biopsies should be done. Testicular metastasis is not just a local occurrence, but may be a warning of occult residual disease occurring systemically.

Paratesticular rhabdomyosarcoma, though extratesticular, is usually discussed along with the testicular tumors. Up to 10% of intrascrotal tumors in prepubertal boys are rhabdomyosarcomas. They are the most common spermatic cord tumors in adults and children. There is no consistent tumor marker. There are two histologic types described: favorable and unfavorable. Nearly 90% of paratesticular rhabdomyosarcomas are of the embryonal (favorable) subtype. CT scanning is used to rule out retroperitoneal metastases, but may not be as accurate in peripubertal patients. After radical orchiectomy, chemotherapy is recommended with patients with positive retroperitoneal lymph nodes also receiving external beam radiation. Retroperitoneal lymph node dissection is currently recommended in postpubertal patients, even if the CT scan is negative due to the high rate of false negative scans. This is of particular concern for the adolescent as there is a risk of postoperative retrograde ejaculation; because of the effects of chemotherapy, pretreatment sperm banking is recommended.

Suggested Readings

Adelman WP, Joffe A: Genitourinary issues in the male college student: A case-base approach. *Pediatr Clin North Am* 52:199–216, 2005.

Belman AB: The adolescent varicocele. *Pediatrics* 114:1669–1670, 2004.

Davenport M: ABCs of general surgery in children: Acute problems of the scrotum. *Br Med J* 312:435–437, 1996.

Dyment PG, (ed.): Symposium on male reproductive health. State of the art reviews: *Adolesc Med* 7:1–162, 1996.

Jayanthi VR: Adolescent urology. *Adolesc Med* 15:521–534, 2004.

Joffe A, Blythe MJ, (eds.): Genitorinary—Handbook of Adolescent Medicine. *Adolesc Med* 14:387–393, 2003.

Klein EA, Kay R, (eds.): Symposium on testis cancer in adults and children. *Urol Clin North Am* 20(1):1–192, 1993.

Monga M, Sofikitis N, Hellstrom WJG: Benign scrotal masses in the adolescent male: Varicoceles, spermatoceles, and hydroceles. *Adolesc Med* 7:131–140, 1996.

Monga M, Hellstrom WJG: Testicular trauma. *Adolesc Med* 7:141–148, 1996.

Perez-Brayfield MB, Baseman A, Andrew J. Kirsch AJ: Adolescent urology. *Adolesc Med* 16:215–227, 2005.

Process of Care Consensus Panel. Position paper. The process of care model for evaluation and treatment of erectile dysfunction. *Int J Impot Res* 11:59–74, 1999.

Rabinowitz R, Hulbert WO: Acute scrotal swelling. *Urol Clin North Am* 22(1):101–106, 1995.

Skoog SJ, Roberts KP, Goldstein M, et al.: The adolescent varicocele: What's new with an old problem in young patients? *Pediatrics* 100:112–121, 1997.

Thomas R: Testicular tumors. State of the art reviews. *Adolesc Med* 7:149–156, 1996.

Wan J, Bloom DA: Genitourinary problems in adolescent males. *Adolesc Med* 14:717–732, 2003.

Workowski KA, Levine WC: Sexually transmitted diseases treatment guidelines, 2002. *MMWR* 51/RR-6:1–72, 2002.

PROSTATITIS

Etiology

Prostate infections are uncommon in adolescents. When they occur, they are usually as complications of some other urogenital infection. Contributing factors include urethritis, UTIs, sepsis, and urethral instrumentation. *E. coli* is the most commonly implicated organism, but *N. gonorrhoeae* follows as a close second. The prostate may be the reservoir for the gonococcus in asymptomatic male carriers; this condition may be accompanied by prostatic enlargement. A number of other cases are caused by *Staphylococcus* or *Streptococcus* and recent data suggest the possible contribution of *Clamydia trachomatis, Pseudomonas aeruginosa, Salmonella, Bacteroides fragilis, Clostridium perfringens*, and others.

Symptomatology

Acute prostatitis is characterized by a number of features, as reviewed in Table 16-31. Rectal examination reveals a large, tender, boggy prostate. Vigorous examination or massage should be avoided in acute prostatic infection in order to avoid precipitating hematogenous spread of the causative infection. Recurrent prostate infection is common and most often due to residual bacteria, this tissue being relatively resistant to penetration by antibiotics. Recurrent UTIs and prostatic abscess may occur as well.

Laboratory Studies

Differentiation between prostatitis and cystitis is made by comparing bacterial colony counts of prostatic fluid (ejaculate) and urine; prostatic infection is indicated by a 10-fold higher count. Evaluation of prostatic secretions reveals inflammatory cells, including numerous WBCs and lipid-filled macrophages. Cultures should be obtained from both the urine and prostatic secretions.

Management

Antibiotics useful for the treatment of prostatitis include ampicillin, tetracycline, cephalosporins, or sulfonamides for at least 10–14 days in acute cases, and for up to 28 days in chronic cases. A 6–12-week course has been used in some chronic cases. Trimethoprim-sulfamethoxazole is the preferred drug if causative organisms are sensitive, as it appears to penetrate prostatic tissues in higher concentrations than other antimicrobial agents. Ofloxacin is a suitable

TABLE 16-31

SYMPTOMATOLOGY OF PROSTATITIS

Fever
Dysuria
Urinary frequency
Painful erection or ejaculation
Painful defecation
Constipation
Perineal discomfort
Sometimes, lower abdominal or lower back pain

alternative treatment at 300 mg orally, twice a day for 6 weeks; ciprofloxacin is also used as an alternative. Highly febrile and toxic patients should be hospitalized and treated intravenously. The combination of ampicillin with an aminoglycoside can be used as a regimen pending culture results. Chronic disease is particularly difficult to eradicate and has a high recurrence rate; weekly massage as an adjunctive measure to antibiotics may be helpful. Other forms of prostatitis include nonbacterial prostatitis and prostatodynia (symptoms present with no laboratory evidence for infection). This more frequently occurs in older adult males; treatment is uncertain as the etiology is unknown. Nonbacterial prostatitis, which is related to infection with *C. trachomatis* or *U. urealyticum*, is often treated with oral doxycycline (100 mg twice a day) for 3–4 weeks.

Suggested Readings

Krowchuk DP: Nongonococcal urethritis: Diagnosis, management and complications. *Adolesc Med* 7:63–83, 1996.

Krieger JN: Prostatitis, epididymitis, and orchitis. In: Mandell GL, Bennett JE, Dolin R (eds.), *Principles and Practice of Infectious Diseases.* 4th ed. New York: Churchill Livingstone, Chap. 91, pp. 1098–1103, 1995.

MISCELLANEOUS DISORDERS

Hematospermia

This is a condition in which blood is noted in the ejaculate. It is usually benign and most often resolves spontaneously. The physical examination is normal, though small tears in the frenulum or in the meatus should be excluded before this diagnosis of hematospermia is made. Patients with malignant melanoma can develop melanospermia, in which melanin can stain the ejaculate black. Evaluation of patients with hematospermia for sexually transmitted infections is recommended. No specific treatment is known for hematospermia.

Urethrorrhagia

This is recurrent blood spotting of the underwear in adolescent males. It is a common and chronic condition; it rarely occurs as the result of a urethral diverticulum. Blood spotting in females suggests a urethral prolapse, which should be visible on examination of the introitus

Balanoposthitis

Inflammation of the penile prepuce (*posthitis*), penile glans (*balanitis*), or both (*balanoposthitis*) may be due to phimosis, masturbation injury, urethritis, or, on occasion, paraphimosis (inability to replace the retracted prepuce). Differentiation from a sexually transmitted disease is necessary. If complete foreskin retraction is difficult, the adolescent should carefully retract his foreskin during cleaning to loosen the narrowing at the distal foreskin area. Treatment involves oral antibiotics and antibiotic compresses, while in severe cases, incision of the prepuce and surgical drainage is necessary. Circumcision is usually recommended after paraphimosis occurs or if severe phimosis is noted.

Hypospadias

Though commonly thought of as referring to a low urethral meatus, hypospadias usually has three consistent findings. First, the urethral opening is low, being off of the glans. The most common location is at the junction of the penis shaft and glans. Second, the foreskin is incomplete, being present on the dorsum but absent ventrally. Third, there is usually a ventral curvature of the penis, which is termed chordee. These three findings can vary in severity but are typically found in patients with hypospadias. This constellation of findings occurs in 3–5 per 500 male births. It is a congenital abnormality that should have been recognized and dealt with by surgery in childhood. Repairs utilize the foreskin and thus, circumcision should be avoided if there is a question of chordee or hypospadias at birth. Teenagers with previously corrected hypospadias need careful follow-up to ensure proper growth of the urethral meatus and the absence of urethral obstruction.

Historically, evidence supported a possible association of hypospadias with diethylstilbestrol (DES) exposure in utero. Other recognized correlates are epididymal cysts, reduced sperm density, and bilateral testicular hypoplasia. Thus, in the past, the presence of hypospadias led to inquiries about DES exposure, which in turn led to evaluation of possible infertility and counseling at an appropriate time. Since DES use in pregnancy stopped in 1971, DES complications are no longer seen in children or teenagers. Boys born by in vitro fertilization and other reproductive technologies, such as intracytoplasmic sperm injection, appear to have a higher than normal incidence of hypospadias.

Suggested Readings

Keating MA, Duckett JU: Recent advances in the repair of hypospadias. *Surg Ann* 22:405, 1990.

Silver RI, Rodriguez R, Chang TS, Gearhart JP: In vitro fertilization is associated with an increased risk of hypospadias. *J Urol* 161(6):1954–1957, 1999.

Simpson JL, Lamb DJ: Genetic effects of intracytoplasmic sperm injection. *Semin Reprod Med* 19:239–249, 2001.

BENIGN PENILE SKIN LESIONS

A number of benign lesions can be encountered on the penis and need to be distinguished from human papillomavirus lesions (condyloma acuminata—see Chap. 19 and 24). Dermoid cysts and mucosal subcutaneous cysts are usually noted along the median penile raphe while benign pink pearly papules are noted along the penile corona. Dermoid cysts may also occur along the scrotal raphe.

Buried Penis

A large pubic fat pad in an obese youth may partially cover the penis, giving it a false impression of being smaller than its actual length: the so-called "buried" penis. The teenager is often too embarrassed to mention it, but compressing the fat pad will reveal the true penile size. In an unusual situation, there may be abnormal development of tissue at the penile base that must be surgically released for the actual penile size to be seen.

Trauma

Renal trauma was previously discussed in the hematuria section. Bladder rupture can be spontaneous, but is more likely seen when a teenager with a full bladder is in a motor vehicle accident. Urethral injury can occur with catheterization or instrumentation; accidental causes also include pelvic fractures and straddle injuries. The recent popularity of the new extreme sports, such as trick skateboarding and rollerblading, has seen increased number of straddle injuries when riders fail to successfully ride their boards down guard rails or pipes. Urethral injuries are best evaluated by careful retrograde urethrography before any catheterization is attempted. In the proper setting, bloody spotting or dripping from the urethra, independent of voiding, should raise the suspicion of urethral injury. Penile injury can also occur from zipper entrapment, vacuum cleaners (and other attempts at aided masturbation), or other such activity.

Priapism

Low Flow Priapism

Priapism is the involuntary and prolonged erection of the corpora cavernosa. There are two broad groups of causes: low blood flow and high blood flow. The majority of patients have low blood flow priapism. Decreased venous outflow leads to increased intracavernosal pressure and subsequent decreased arterial inflow. This leads to stasis of blood, hypoxia, and acidosis. The glans penis and spongiosum are characteristically flaccid. Recurrent and extended bouts of low flow priapism can lead to corporal fibrosis and impotence. The most common low flow situation occurs in patients with sickle cell disease. Priapism can occur as an isolated event or as part of a diffuse sickle crisis. Management is like that for a sickle crisis: oxygenation, diluting hemoglobin S, alkalinization, and pain control. When conservative management fails, irrigation with an α-adrenergic agent, such as phenylephrine, and shunting can be considered. Shunting refers to the surgical creation of a temporary connection between the corporal body and the corpus spongiosum.

Leukemia is another low flow cause of pediatric priapism. Although chronic granulocytic leukemia accounts for only a small percentage of pediatric leukemia, about 50% of leukemic priapism occurs in these patients. Leukemic cells can sludge within the corporal bodies. Treatment is directed at lowering the WBC count, while shunts are used in refractory cases. Other uncommon causes of low flow priapism include blunt perineal trauma, spinal cord injury, and medications. Priapism has been associated with the medications listed in Table 16-32. For example, commonly prescribed antidepressants (such as trazodone or sertraline) and antipsychotics (such as chlorpromazine) have been implicated in priapism. Prompt recognition and halting the medication is the crucial step in these cases. Irrigation and shunting may help, but often the priapism persists until the offending drug completely clears.

High Flow Priapism

This is caused by unrestrained arterial inflow. The problem does not involve venous occlusion; thus, there is no hypoxia or acidosis. Almost all cases of high flow priapism are due to penile or perineal trauma. An injury to the cavernosal artery results in a cavernosus-to-corporal body fistula. The key diagnostic observation is the finding of well-oxygenated red blood on corporal aspiration. In contrast to the flaccidity found in low flow priapism, the glans and spongiosum in high flow priapism are engorged with blood and are quite firm. Treatment is by angiographic occlusion of the fistula. There is also a rare, poorly understood, idiopathic high flow variant that is usually managed by oral α-adrenergic blockers.

T A B L E   1 6 - 3 2

MEDICATIONS ASSOCIATED WITH PRIAPISM

Buspirone	Papaverine
Clozapine	Phenothiazines
Cocaine	Phenytoin
Fluphenazine	Prazosin
Hydralazine	Tamoxifen
Labetalol	Testosterone
Mesoridazine	Thioridazine
Molindone	Thiothixene
Nifedipine	Trazodone

Suggested Readings

Emir L, Tekgul S, Karabulut A, Oskay K, Erol D: Management of posttraumatic arterial priapism in children: Presentation of a case and review of the literature. *Int Urol Nephrol* 34(2): 237–240, 2002.

Molitierno JA Jr, Carson CC III: Urologic manifestations of hematologic disease sickle cell, leukemia, and thromboembolic disease. *Urol Clin North Am* 30(1): 49–61, 2003.

Thomas A, Woodard C, Rovner ES, Wein AJ: Urologic complications of nonurologic medications. *Urol Clin North Am* 30(1): 123–131, 2003.

OTHER SEXUAL DYSFUNCTIONS

Many drugs cause interference with sexual functioning, resulting in loss of libido, erection or ejaculatory dysfunction, and/or orgasmic dysfunction. The most commonly implicated drugs are antihypertensives, antidepressants, and antipsychotic drugs.

Suggested Reading

Greydanus DE, Pratt HD, Baxter T: Sexual dysfunction and the primary care physician. *Adolesc Med* 7:9–26, 1996.

17

ADOLESCENT HEMATOLOGY

Roshni Kulkarni, Renuka Gera, and Ajovi B. Scott-Emuakpor

HEMATOLOGIC DISORDERS IN THE ADOLESCENT

Hematologic disorders in the adolescent pose unique challenges to the physician. While the manifestations of some inherited disorders continue into adolescence, diagnosis of others may be delayed until adolescence. Many acquired disorders similar to those seen in adults also affect adolescents. This chapter views hematologic disorders in the adolescent.

HEMOSTATIC DISORDERS

The dynamic process of hemostasis reflects a delicate balance between bleeding and thrombosis. Appropriate diagnosis, management, and education of such disorders may prevent future morbidity in adulthood. For instance, in an adolescent with menorrhagia, a diagnosis of von Willebrand's disease (VWD) may result in appropriate treatment, and thereby improve quality of life and prevent unnecessary obstetric procedures. Similarly, early detection of thrombophilic disorders may lead to appropriate treatment and initiation of preventive strategies. Adolescence can be a demanding period for the parents as well as the health team. Issues with compliance, control, anger, independence, rebellion,

sexuality, peer pressure, and financial requirements pose distinctive challenges.

Congenital Coagulation Disorders

Hemophilia A (F [factor] VIII deficiency) and B (F IX deficiency) and VWD represent approximately 80%–85% of the inherited bleeding disorders. Deficiencies of fibrinogen, prothrombin, F–V, VII, X, XI, XIII, and combined V and VIII account for 15% of congenital bleeding disorders. Screening tests to assess the degree of hemorrhage and the adequacy of hemostasis are given in Fig. 17-1. Hemophilia is seen in all ethnic groups, shows no racial predilection and occurs in 1:5000 males whereas VWD is more common and occurs in 1%–3% of the U.S. population. The *F VIII* and *F IX* genes are located at the tip of the long arm of the X chromosome and the gene for VWD is located on chromosome 12. Based on the plasma levels of F VIII or F IX (normal levels are 50%–150%) that correlate with severity and predict bleeding risk, hemophilia is classified as mild (>5%), moderate (1%–5%), and severe (<1%). Approximately two thirds of persons with hemophilia have severe disease, 15% have moderate disease and 20% have mild disease.

Hemophilia A and B are clinically indistinguishable and specific factor assays are the only

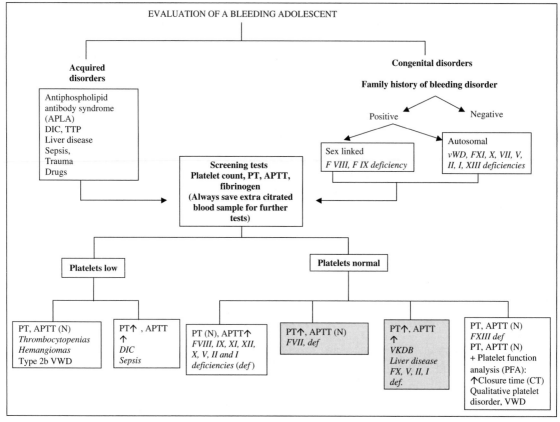

FIGURE 17-1

SCREENING TESTS ASSESS THE DEGREE OF HEMORRHAGE AND THE ADEQUACY OF HEMOSTASIS
IN A BLEEDING ADOLESCENT.

way to differentiate between them and confirm the diagnosis. Both should be differentiated from VWD. The latter is characterized by either a quantitative (types 1 and 3) or a qualitative (type 2 and subtypes 2a, 2b, 2m, and 2n) defect of the von Willebrand's factor (VWF). Table 17-1 gives the details about the characteristics and differences between the hemophilias and VWD.

Individuals with severe hemophilia and type 3 VWD bleed spontaneously and are diagnosed in early childhood. Patients with mild hemophilia and types 1 and 2 VWD often remain undiagnosed until adolescence or adulthood and may experience bleeding with severe trauma or surgery. An adolescent girl with VWD may present with menorrhagia as the first sign of a bleeding disorder. Both adolescent boys and girls may present with

prolonged bleeding following dental extraction. Occasionally, diagnosis is made on screening tests done prior to a surgical procedure.

The goal of treatment of hemophilia and VWD is to raise factor levels to approximately 30% or more for minor bleeds (such as hematomas or joint bleeds) and 100% for major bleeds (such as intracranial hemorrhage or surgery). This is accomplished by administration of appropriate factor (F VIII, F IX, or VWF) concentrates; 1 unit (U)/kg raises F VIII levels by 2%, F IX levels by 1.5%, and VWF (Ristocetin cofactor activity) levels by 1.5%, respectively. Recombinant factor concentrates are recommended. If unavailable, pathogen-safe-plasma-derived concentrates can be used. Concentrates can be administered either as bolus or continuous infusion. For mild hemophilia A and

TABLE 17-1

CHARACTERISTICS AND DIFFERENCES BETWEEN HEMOPHILIAS AND VON WILLEBRAND'S DISEASE

	Hemophilia A	*Hemophilia B*	*von Willebrand's Disease*
Incidence	1:5,000	1:30,000	1%–3% of U.S. population
Abnormality	Factor (F) VIII deficiency. Normal levels: 50%–150%	F IX deficiency. Normal levels: 50%–150%	VWF abnormality
Inheritance	X-linked, affects males. Gene at the tip of X-chromosome.	X-linked, affects males	Autosomal dominant (gene on chromosome 12). Affects males and females
Site of production	Unknown	Liver, vitamin K dependent protein	Megakaryocytes and endothelial cells
Function of protein	Cofactor; forms "tenase" complex with FIX and activate FX	Clotting protein (zymogen). Activated by F XI or VIIa and forms a "tenase" complex with FVIII and activates FX	Platelet adhesion, protection of F VIII
Classification (Normal plasma levels of FVIII and IX = 50–150%)	Mild (>5%) Moderate (1%–5%) Severe (<1%)	Mild (>5%) Moderate (1%–5%) Severe (<1%)	Types 1 Type 2 (2A, 2B, 2M, 2N) Type 3
Clinical manifestations	Positive family history (30% new mutation). Hemarthroses, hematomas, intracranial hemorrhage, hematuria, gastrointestinal hemorrhage, and so forth	Positive family history (30% new mutation). Milder disease, though identical hemorrhage sites as hemophilia A	Positive family history Mucocutaneous (epistaxis, menorrhagia, postdental bleeding). Type 3 may present as hemophilia A
PFA/Bleeding time	Normal	Normal	May be prolonged
PT	Normal	Normal	Normal
APTT	Prolonged	Prolonged	Prolonged or normal
F VIII assay	Decreased or absent	Normal	↓ or Normal
F IX assay	Normal	Decreased or absent	Normal
VWF: antigen	Normal	Normal	Decreased or absent (type 3)
VWF R: Co	Normal	Normal	Decreased or abnormal
VWF multimers	Normal	Normal	Normal or abnormal
Specific treatment	Recombinant (r) F VIII (preferred), virally safe plasma derived concentrates	Recombinant F IX, virally safe plasma derived concentrates	DDAVP (intranasal or intravenous) VWF concentrates (plasma derived)
Inhibitor patients	rFVIIa, FEIBA	rFVIIa	Rare
Adjunct treatment	Antifibrinolytics	Antifibrinolytics	Oral contraceptives, antifibrinolytics

VWD the synthetic vasopressin analog desmo-pressin acetate (1-deamino-[8-D-arginine]-vaso-pressin, [DDAVP]) increases plasma concentrations of coagulation F VIII and VWF two- to sixfold through endogenous release and is the treatment of choice. Antifibrinolytics such as Epsilon Amino Caproic acid (Amicar) or tranexamic acid can be used as adjunct hemostatic therapy for mucosal bleeds (epistaxis, dental extraction, oral bleeds etc.). Amicar is available in the tablet (500 mg), elixir (250 mg/ml or intravenous forms (250 mg/ml). The oral dose is 100–200 mg/kg (maximum 10 grams) followed by 50–100 mg/kg every 6 hours. The dose for tranexamic acid is 25 mg/kg every 6–8 hours. It is available only in the intravenous or capsule (500 mg) form. Antifibrinolytics are often used for a period of 7–10 days following dental extraction and tranexamic acid has been used to prevent blood loss in menorrhagia.

Prophylactic administration of concentrates (F VIII 25–40 U/kg every other day, F IX 25–40 U/kg twice weekly because of longer half-life of F IX) is aimed at preventing debilitating effects of joint dis-ease and often begun at 1–2 years of age and con-tinued throughout life. Adolescents should be encouraged to self-infuse regularly and prior to any planned strenuous activity. Because of the complica-tions of central venous catheters (infections, throm-bosis, and mechanical), use of a peripheral vein is encouraged.

Inhibitory antibodies to F VIII and F IX should be suspected if a patient fails to respond to an appro-priate dose of clotting factor concentrate. They fur-ther exacerbate bleeding episodes and hemophilic arthropathy.

Adolescents with bleeding disorders should be encouraged to attend the regional hemophilia treat-ment centers (HTC) where, besides education, patients are trained to self-infuse, calculate dosage, maintain treatment logs and call the center for seri-ous bleeding episodes. Soucie et al. (2000) reported a lower mortality rate among patients who received care at HTC than those who did not (28.1% vs. 38.3%, respectively). Table 17-2 lists the issues that physician caring for adolescents with bleeding disorders should be aware of. A brief description is given below.

TABLE 17-2

ISSUES IN ADOLESCENTS WITH BLEEDING DISORDERS

- Bleeding issues
  - Joint bleeds, hemophilic arthropathy
  - Menorrhagia in VWD and carriers
  - Inhibitors
  - Hepatitis C
  - Compliance with therapy
- Sports, exercise, physical therapy.
- Dental issues, nutrition, transition to adult physician
- Insurance
- Education
  - Academic achievement
  - Support groups, NHF, HTC
  - Importance of medic alert badges
- Sexuality
  - Bleeding during sexilio, psoas bleeds
  - Guilt of passing gene
  - Sexually transmitted disease
  - Pregnancy
- Travel
  - Letter
  - Self-infusion
  - Medication

Joint Disease

In severe hemophilia, debilitating effects of joint disease commence in childhood and often continue in the adolescent and young adult. Chronic joint disease with decreased joint range of motion severely impairs ability to participate in sports. This may result in denial, refusal to attend school, and/or depression. Compliance with prophylaxis drops during adolescence and there is a positive correlation between school absenteeism and bleed-ing episodes. Children with more school absences have lower scores in mathematics, reading, and total achievement, even after adjusting for IQ and level of education of parents. The quality of life is often compromised. More recently, Soucie et al. (2004) in a study of 4343 males aged 2–19 with hemophilia reported limitation of joint range of motion positively correlated with older age, non-Caucasian race, and increased body mass index.

Human Immune-Deficiency Virus, Hepatitis C Virus, and Other Blood Borne Pathogens

While the currently available concentrates are made using recombinant technology or donor screened and pathogen safe plasma, during the early 1980s over 50% of hemophiliacs treated with plasma derived concentrates became infected with human immune-deficiency virus (HIV) and/or hepatitis C virus (HCV). Although many of these individuals with HIV died, some survivors are currently in their late adolescence. HCV is often asymptomatic but may lead to chronic hepatitis, cirrhosis or liver cancer. Current treatment includes a combination of pegylated interferon and ribavirin, though HIV/HCV coinfection results in poor response to therapy. Adolescents with bleeding disorders should be immunized against hepatitis A and B. Constant vigilance against potential emerging pathogens that may be blood borne, such as parvovirus, variant Creutzfeldt-Jakob disease and newer viruses, should be maintained.

Sports and Exercise

Adolescents with hemophilia should be encouraged to participate in sports activities that promote not only "joint health" by muscle building and strengthening but also psychologic well-being and acceptance by peers. Sports activities have been divided into three categories. Category 1 activities such as swimming, golf, and running are safe; category 2 activities include weight lifting, bowling, and bicycling where the psychologic, social, and physical benefits outweighs the risks; category 3 sports such as boxing, skateboarding, and football should be avoided.

Adolescents should be encouraged to wear medic alert tags (necklace or wrist or ankle bracelet) that may be life saving, allowing early and appropriate treatment in the event of an accident, as well as join support groups such as the local HTC and the National Hemophilia Foundation (NHF). The goal of the NHF's national prevention program (available at www.hemophilia.org) is to prevent or reduce complications of bleeding disorders by "doing the 5," namely: (1) annual comprehensive check ups, (2) vaccination for hepatitis A and B, (3) early treatment of joint bleeds, (4) exercise for joint health, and (5) regular testing for blood borne pathogens.

Adolescence, Sexuality, and Bleeding Disorders

Menorrhagia in an adolescent may be the first indication of a bleeding disorder(s) (VWD, platelet function defect, thrombocytopenia, and deficiency of F V, XI, XIII, VII, II, and carriers of hemophilia). Approximately 11%–33% of adolescents admitted for menorrhagia have been reported to have an underlying bleeding disorder. Menorrhagia may be problematic and may lead to increased school absenteeism and participation in activities. The American College of Obstetrics and Gynecology (ACOG) in a committee opinion recommended that adolescent girls with menorrhagia should be screened for a bleeding disorder. Intranasal DDAVP, antifibrinolytics or oral contraceptives are often prescribed for adolescents with VWD or symptomatic carries of hemophilia A to control excess bleeding. More recently a levonorgestrel-releasing intrauterine contraceptive device (Mirena) has been used to control menorrhagia.

Sexual activity may pose a risk not only for bleeding but also for transmission of pathogens. While the currently available concentrates are pathogen safe, reducing sexual transmission through changing behavior remains challenging. Reluctance to disclose serostatus may lead to unprotected sex, though there appears to be no correlation between disclosure and condom use. The guilt of passing an abnormal gene may lead to anger and antisocial behaviors.

Travel and other Issues

Travel for an adolescent reflects independence. For individuals with a bleeding disorder it is important to be educated about their disorder and have a letter that specifies the diagnosis and management in case of an emergency. Furthermore, they should be taught to self-infuse, travel with a supply of factor concentrate, wear medic alert bracelet/necklace, and avoid risky behavior during their travels.

Transition to adult physician may sometimes be anxiety provoking and a team approach may be helpful. Guidelines for transition at every stage, from infancy to adulthood, are available at the NHF (MASAC document #147, available at *www.hemophilia.org*).

Bibliography

ACOG Committee on Gynecologic Practice. Committee opinion: Number 263, December 2001. von Willebrand's disease in gynecologic practice. *Obstet Gynecol* 98:1185, 2001.

Bevan JA, Maloney KW, Hillery CA, et al. Bleeding disorders: A common cause of menorrhagia in adolescents. *J Pediatr* 138:856, 2001.

Bolton M, Pasi KJ. Haemophilias A and B. *Lancet* 36:1801, 2003.

Geary MK, King G, Forsberg AD, et al. Issues of disclosure and condom use in adolescents with hemophilia and HIV. Hemophilia Behavioral Evaluative Intervention Project Staff. *Pediatr AIDS HIV Infect* 7:418, 1996.

Hord JD. Anemia and coagulation disorders in adolescents. *Adolesc Med* 3:359, 1999.

Montgomery RR, Gill JC, Scott JP. Hemophilia and von Willebrand disease. In: Nathan DG, Orkin SH (eds.), *Nathan and Oski's Hematology of Infancy and Childhood*, 6th ed. Philadelphia, PA: W.B. Saunders, 2003, p. 1547.

National Hemophilia Foundation Medical and Scientific Advisory Council (MASAC). *Treatment Recommendations. Medical Advisory No. 151.* New York: National Hemophilia Foundation; Nov. 2003. Available at *www.hemophilia.org* (as document #151)

National Hemophilia Foundation Medical and Scientific Advisory Committee (MASAC). *MASAC Recommendation Regarding the Use of Recombinant Clotting Factor Replacement Therapies.* New York: National Hemophilia Foundation; Nov. 2000. Available at *www.hemophilia.org* (as document #106)

National Hemophilia Foundation Medical and Scientific Advisory Council (MASAC). *MASAC Recommendation Concerning Prophylaxis (Prophylactic Administration of Clotting Factor Concentrate to Prevent Bleeding).* New York: National Hemophilia Foundation, June 2001. Available at *www.hemophilia.org* (as document #117)

Soucie JM, Nuss R, Evatt B, et al. Mortality among males with hemophilia: Relations with source of medical care. *Blood* 96:437, 2000.

Soucie JM, Cianfrini C, Janco RL, et al. Joint range-of-motion limitations among young males with hemophilia: Prevalence and risk factors. *Blood* 103:2467, 2004.

Wilde JT. HIV and HCV coinfection in haemophilia. *Haemophilia* 10:1, 2004.

THROMBOTIC DISORDERS AND THROMBOPHILIA

Thrombotic disorders in adolescents are being recognized with increased frequency and may be inherited or acquired as a result of blood vessel or a coagulation factor abnormality. They can be venous or arterial and are frequently associated with risk factors such as infections, cancer, or pregnancy (Table 17-3). Arterial thrombi are generally considered as platelet thrombi, though they may sometimes have a venous origin and enter the systemic

TABLE 17-3

RISK FACTORS FOR THROMBOSIS IN ADOLESCENTS

Venous
Thrombophilias
Infections
Obesity
Venous stasis and immobility
Pregnancy/oral contraceptives
Medical conditions: cancer, sickle cell disease, inflammatory bowel disease, systemic lupus erythematosus
Indwelling venous catheters
Arterial
Thrombophilias
Smoking
Diabetes, hyperlipidemia, hypertension
Strong family history
Vessel wall abnormality, trauma, malignancy, Kawasaki disease, Takayasu's arteritis

circulation through a shunt or a defect in the cardiac septum. The incidence of symptomatic venous thromboembolic events (VTE) in the Canadian Thrombophilia Registry is 0.07/10,000 children and 5.3/10,000 hospital admissions. It shows a bimodal peak with greatest risk for children below 1 year and during adolescence (Chan et al., 2003). The term thrombophilia indicates an inherited or acquired disorder of the hemostasis that predisposes to clot formation. Inherited disorders include mutations (prothrombin G20210A, F V Leiden, MTHFR C677T, plasminogen activator inhibitor polymorphism (PAI-1 4G/4G), or abnormalities of clotting factors such as elevated F VIII, F VII, dysfibrinogenemias, F XII, and naturally occurring anticoagulants (protein C & S, antithrombin III, plasminogen) as well as elevation of lipoprotein(a). The most common inherited thrombophilic disorder in the Caucasian population is F V Leiden and the acquired disorder is antiphospholipid antibodies. Levy et al. (2003) reported a 54% incidence of thromboembolic event (TE) in pediatric patients with systemic lupus erythematosus; the median age of the first TE was 15.1 years. Adolescents, without an underlying medical condition, who present with a thrombotic episode, should be screened for thrombophilia. A strong family history of thrombosis at a young age may suggest an inherited thrombophilia. Selected patients may require lifelong anticoagulation. The clinical features, diagnosis, and treatment of arterial and venous thromboses are listed in Table 17-4.

References

Chan AK, Deveber G, Monagle P, et al. Venous thrombosis in children. *J Thromb Haemost* 1:1443, 2003.

Levy DM, Massicotte MP, Harvey E, Hebert D, Silverman ED. Thromboembolism in paediatric lupus patients. *Lupus* 12:741, 2003.

PLATELET DISORDERS

Immune thrombocytopenic purpura (ITP) is characterized by immune mediated destruction of platelets by reticuloendothelial cells resulting in peripheral blood thrombocytopenia. It is classified on the basis of duration as acute (<6 months) or chronic, or on the basis of age (childhood versus adult). Acute ITP is more commonly seen in children following a viral infection and is self-limited; 80% achieve remission. Chronic ITP on the contrary is often seen in adults (predominantly females) and is associated with complications and a frequent need for splenectomy. ITP in adolescents shares features of both childhood and adults. Bruising and petechiae occur when the platelet counts fall below 20,000/mm^3. Lowe and Buchanan reviewed 126 patients aged 10–18 years with ITP; 57% had chronic ITP, 27% acute ITP, and 15% the cause was unknown. Chronic ITP was associated with slight female predominance; higher platelet counts at diagnosis and a need for splenectomy in 38% of the cases.

Treatment of ITP remains controversial and ranges from observation only to the use of steroids, intravenous immune globulin, and anti-D immune globulin (WinRho). Splenectomy is a treatment option in refractory cases. Immune-suppressive drugs or chemotherapy drugs are used in cases unresponsive to splenectomy.

Other causes of thrombocytopenia in the adolescents include thrombotic thrombocytopenic purpura (TTP), a microangiopathic hemolytic anemia that shares many clinical features with hemolytic uremic syndrome (HUS). In some cases of familial or acquired TTP, severe deficiency or inhibitory antibodies against VWF cleaving metalloprotease termed ADAMTS-13 (a disintegrin and metalloprotease with thrombospondin domain) results in production of unusually large VWF multimers. These bind to platelets resulting in thrombocytopenia. In TTP platelet rich thrombi are seen predominantly in the brain, and to a lesser extent in the heart, pancreas, adrenals, and kidneys. In HUS, the thrombi are largely confined to the kidney and it is frequently associated with a toxin produced by 0157:H7 strain of *Escherichia coli* or *Shigella* infection. Treatment is primarily supportive with plasma exchange, corticosteroids, and platelet transfusions.

Disseminated intravascular coagulation, sepsis, and massive transfusions as may occur following trauma as well as (heparin induced thrombocytopenia)

TABLE 17-4

CLINICAL MANIFESTATIONS OF ARTERIAL AND VENOUS THROMBOSES

	Arterial	Venous

Location and manifestation	Carotid and/or vertebral arteries or intracerebral arteries: ischemic stroke
	Peripheral arteries, usually in the leg: ischemia/gangrene
	Coronary arteries: myocardial infarction
	Mesenteric arteries
	Retinal arteries causing loss of vision
	Placenta arterial thrombosis leading to:
	  Placental insufficiency
	  Miscarriage
	  Eclampsia and preeclampsia
	  Abruptio placentae
	  Intrauterine growth retardation
		Pulmonary embolism (PE): dyspnea, tachypnea, sudden death
		Cerebral sinus (brain)
		Renal vein thrombosis:
		Retinal veins: vision changes
		Deep vein thrombosis (DVT):
		  pain swelling fever
		Mesenteric vein: abdominal pain
		Veins in bones, (hip or jaw) causing osteonecrosis
		Paget-Schroetter syndrome: axillary vein thrombosis
		Placenta venous thrombosis: same as arterial

Diagnosis	Magnetic resonance imaging (MRI), MR arteriogram Contrast angiography Echocardiogram	Serial compression ultrasound with color Doppler (duplex scanning) MRI, MR venogram (MRV) Spiral CT scan of lungs for PE Ventilation perfusion VQ scan for PE CT scans Contrast venography or angiography
Treatment	Thrombolytic therapy (tissue plasminogen activator [tPA]) Antiplatelet agents, anticoagulants Surgical embolectomy	Systemic anticoagulants: Unfractionated heparin, low molecular weight heparin, direct thrombin inhibitors, anti-Xa inhibitors Oral anticoagulants Inferior vena cava filters

are rare causes of thrombocytopenia in an adolescent. Treatment involves treatment of the underlying cause and supportive therapy.

Platelet function disorders may be congenital or acquired and present with mucocutaneous hemorrhage. Bernard-Soulier syndrome, Glanzmann thrombasthenia, and storage pool defects are examples of congenital disorders. Many drugs inhibit platelet function; the most common among them is aspirin. It inhibits cyclooxygenase thereby causing impaired thromboxane synthesis. It is therefore used as an adjunct to anticoagulant therapy.

Suggested Readings

Lowe EJ, Buchanan GR. Idiopathic thrombocytopenic purpura diagnosed during the second decade of life. *J Pediatr* 141:253, 2002.

Moake JL. Thrombotic microangiopathies. *N Engl J Med* 347:589, 2002.

ANEMIAS

Anemia is defined as a reduction in the number of red blood cells (RBCs) or hemoglobin concentration. In the adolescent, anemia may either be due to failure to reach normal developmental levels of hemoglobin or a result of inherited or acquired disease processes. The effect of the reduction in oxygen carrying capacity due to decreased hemoglobin may be as subtle as diminished performance or overt exhaustion. As adolescents transition from childhood to adulthood, hematopoiesis responds to meet the increased demand placed by the growth spurt and the hemoglobin levels increase. Thus, the knowledge of normal growth and development and its impact on erythropoiesis is critical in evaluating an adolescent with anemia.

During adolescence, as the body mass increases, the red cell mass increases several-fold to maintain a normal hematocrit. In adolescent males, under the influence of testosterone the hematocrit increases by 1% with each successive increase in sexual maturity rating. This rise is not seen in adolescent girls because of menstrual losses that average 40 mL (20 mg iron) per menstrual period. Mean hemoglobin, hematocrit, and mean corpuscular volume (MCV) values at various stages of adolescence are given in Table 17-5.

While these values can detect most patients with anemia, they fail to identify adolescents with cardiorespiratory insufficiency and those with high affinity hemoglobins who usually have higher than normal hemoglobin levels secondary to hypoxia.. Furthermore, anemia in adolescents may signal an underlying nutritional deficiency or an inherited condition such as Fanconi's anemia; rarely, it may be the first sign of malignancy.

Anemias can be classified into two broad categories, namely, those caused by increased destruction or decreased production of RBCs. The reticulocyte count accurately reflects the process and is very helpful in making this distinction. It is increased in anemias secondary to RBC destruction and is reduced in those caused by decreased RBC production. The factors responsible for red cell production or destruction also influence red cell size. Based on the RBC size, (normal size is 7–8 μm) anemias are classified as normocytic, microcytic (smaller than normal RBC), and macrocytic (larger than normal RBC). Therefore, a simplified classification of anemia that incorporates these variables is more practical and is given in Table 17-6. Macrocytic anemias are very rare in adolescents. Strict vegetarian/vegan/macrobiotics diet may result in vitamin B_{12} deficiency. Adolescent girls on oral contraceptives may also develop macrocytic anemia due to folate deficiency. A brief evaluation and management of adolescents with common types of anemia is discussed below.

Iron Deficiency Anemia

Iron deficiency is the most common cause of anemia in adolescence. Due to the increased growth velocity and expansion of red cell mass, the iron requirement

TABLE 17-5

NORMAL VALUES FOR HEMOGLOBIN, HEMATOCRIT, AND MCV FOR ADOLESCENTS

Age (years)	Hemoglobin (g/dl)		Hematocrit (%)		MCV (μ^3)	
	Mean	Lower Limit	Mean	Lower Limit	Mean	Lower Limit
12–14						
Female	13.5	12	41	36	85	78
Male	14	12.5	43	37	84	77
15–17						
Female	14	12	41	36	87	79
Male	15	13	46	38	86	78

TABLE 17-6

CLASSIFICATION OF ANEMIAS

Microcytic Hypochromic	
Decreased Production	*Increased Destruction*
Iron deficiency	Thalassemia
Lead poisoning	
Chronic inflammation	
Sideroblastic anemia	
Normocytic Normochromic	
Decreased Production	*Increased Destruction*
Aplastic anemia	Autoimmune hemolytic anemia
Bone marrow replacement	Microangiopathic anemia
Drugs	Congenital hemolytic anemia
Infections	• Red cell membrane defects
	a. Hereditary spherocytosis
	b. Hereditary elliptocytosis
	• Red cell enzyme defects
	a. G-6PD deficiency
	• Hemoglobinopathies
Macrocytic Anemia	
With Megaloblastic Bone Marrow	*Without Megaloblastic Bone Marrow*
B_{12} deficiency	Aplastic anemia
Folic acid deficiency	Fanconi's anemia
	Hypothyroidism
	Down syndrome
	Liver disease
	Dyserythropoietic anemia
	Valproic acid
	Bone marrow replacement

during adolescence is high. Failure to meet the increased demands results in an iron deficient state. Poor dietary habits, common in this age group further accentuates the iron deficiency.

Only 27.7% of adolescent girls and 83.1% adolescent boys (ages 12–19) in the United States meet the criteria for use of the recommended daily allowance (RDA) for iron intake. In developed countries, the prevalence of iron deficiency in adolescents aged 12–15 years is 14% among girls and 3.7% among boys. The prevalence of iron deficiency in the United States as estimated by the National Health and Nutrition Examination Survey (NHANES) 1999–2000 was 9% for females aged 12–15 years and 11% for those aged 16–19 years. Approximately 2% of the girls aged 12–19 years had iron deficiency anemia, whereas 5% boys aged 12–15 had iron deficiency without any evidence of anemia.

Iron deficiency without anemia is common in adolescence. During the initial stages of iron deficiency, low serum ferritin levels characterize depletion of iron stores. With further iron depletion the serum iron falls, total iron binding capacity (TIBC) increases, and the soluble transferrin receptor (sTfR) levels increase. The ratio of sTfR to the log of ferritin (sTfR/Log Ferritin index) appears to be a sensitive index of iron deficiency before erythropoiesis is affected. It can differentiate between iron deficiency anemia and anemia of chronic disease. Values of >1.5 suggest iron deficiency and <1.5 suggest anemia of chronic disease. Hypochromic microcytic anemia suggests late stages of iron deficiency. Anemia of chronic illness may present with hypochromic microcytic RBCs, however, unlike iron deficiency anemia, both TIBC and sTfR are low and ferritin levels are elevated. Common causes of iron deficiency are shown in Table 17-7.

Treatment of Iron Deficiency

Due to a high prevalence of iron deficiency in 12–18-year-old females, nutritional counseling, as well as baseline hemoglobin and hematocrit determination should be an integral part of routine health maintenance visits. Girls with previous history of iron deficiency, heavy menstrual losses, or low iron intake should be screened annually. Due to

TABLE 17-7

CAUSES OF IRON DEFICIENCY IN THE ADOLESCENT

Decreased iron intake
Nutritional deficiency:
Reliance on unhealthy or junk food

Blood loss
Metromenorrhagia
Inflammatory bowel disease
Peptic ulcer disease
NSAID-induced gastritis
Epistaxis

Decreased iron absorption
Intestinal malabsorption
Antacid abuse

TABLE 17-8

CAUSES OF POOR RESPONSE TO ORAL IRON THERAPY IN ADOLESCENTS

Noncompliance
Ongoing blood loss
High gastric pH antacids
Inhibitors or iron absorption
    Chronic inflammation
    Neoplasia
Incorrect diagnosis

increased iron requirements, pregnant adolescents are at risk for developing iron deficiency. Routine screening is not recommended for adolescent boys because of the lower risk of anemia. However, boys with previous history of anemia or with other chronic illnesses are candidates for routine screening. Hemoglobin increase of 1 g/dl after a 4-week trial of 60–120 mg oral iron daily supports iron deficiency in a patient with mild anemia and eliminates the need for more specific tests for iron deficiency. Iron supplementation should be continued for 2–3 months after hemoglobin normalizes and hemoglobin levels should be rechecked at 6 months after correction. Ferrous iron sulfate is an inexpensive and effective treatment for iron deficiency. A single 325 mg ferrous sulfate tablet (65 mg of elemental iron) given at night is well tolerated and may be adequate to treat mild to moderate iron deficiency. Gastrointestinal discomfort and bloating are the distressing side effects. Ferrous gluconate is better tolerated than ferrous sulfate. Newer polysaccharide iron complexes have fewer unpleasant gastrointestinal side effects and could be used to treat patients who fail to tolerate other iron preparations. The causes of poor response to oral iron are listed in Table 17-8. Patients with severe anemia or those who fail to respond to oral iron need further evaluation.

Suggested Readings

Iron Deficiency—United States, 1999–2000, Morbidity and Mortality Weekly Report, Center for Disease Control and Prevention, 51:897, 2002.

Orkin SH, Brugnara C, Nathan DG. A Diagnostic Approach to the Anemia Patient. In Nathan DG, Oski SH, Ginsburg D, Look AT, eds. *Nathan and Oski's Hematology of Infancy and Childhood*. 6th ed. Philadelphia, PA: W.B. Saunders; 2003 p. 417.

Rasmussen SA, Fernhoff PM, Scanlon KS. Vitamin B$_{12}$ deficiency in children and adolescents. *J Pediatr* 138:10, 2001.

Samuelson G, Bratterby LE, Berggren K, et al. Recommendations to prevent and control iron deficiency in the United States. Morbidity and Mortality: Dietary iron intake and iron status in adolescents. *Acta Paediatr* 85:1033, 1996.

APLASTIC ANEMIA

Aplastic anemia is defined as peripheral pancytopenia due to decreased productions of hematopoietic progenitors in the bone marrow. Although the majority of cases of aplastic anemia in this age group are due to acquired disease processes, sometimes inherited conditions such as Fanconi's anemia may present as aplastic anemia in this age group. In some cases, a combination of both acquired and inherited factors may be responsible for bone marrow failure. Drugs or chemicals are often implicated as a common cause of aplastic anemias. The list of drugs associated with bone marrow failure is long. The categories of drugs often associated with bone marrow failure are chemotherapy, chloramphenicol, nonsteroidal anti-inflammatory, antihistaminics, and heavy metals such as gold, arsenic, and mercury. In the majority of cases, however, there is no identifiable cause. The peak age of presentation of idiopathic aplastic anemia is 15–25 years. Allogeneic bone marrow transplantation (BMT) for patients with HLA-identical siblings is the first-line therapy and long-term survival of approximately 90% can be expected with state-of-the-art therapy (Strob, 2002). Unfortunately 75% of the patients do not have suitable matched donors and are candidates for immunosuppression with a combination of antithymocyte globulin (ATG) and cyclosporine and/or other agents to reduce T-cell activity. Occasionally aplastic anemia may be the first sign of Fanconi's anemia. Short stature and unexplained macrocytosis may be the only signs of Fanconi's anemia in some patients until aplastic anemia develops. Hence, chromosome breakage studies for Fanconi's anemia should be considered in any adolescent who presents with aplastic anemia

Suggested Readings

Georges GE, Storb R. Stem cell transplantation for aplastic anemia. *Int J Hematol* 75:141, 2002.

Young NS. Immunosuppressive treatment of acquired aplastic anemia and immune-mediated bone marrow failure syndromes. *Int J Hematol* 75:129, 2002.

HEMOLYTIC ANEMIA

Shortened red cell survival, reticulocytosis, and hyperbilirubinemia are the hallmark of the hemolytic anemias. Most patients with congenital hemolytic anemia due to red cell enzyme defects, hemoglobinopathies, thalassemia, and red cell membrane defect present in early childhood. Autoimmune hemolytic anemia may present throughout childhood. An adolescent presenting with new onset anemia, reticulocytosis, and jaundice (with and without splenomegaly) should be evaluated with a direct Coombs test. A positive Coombs test establishes the diagnosis of autoimmune hemolytic anemia. Individuals with a negative Coombs test require further evaluation for other causes such as hereditary spherocytosis (HS), red cell enzyme deficiency, and hemoglobinopathies. HS, a very important cause of hemolysis, occurs in all racial and ethnic groups. The inheritance is autosomal dominant. The clinical presentation may vary from classical triad of anemia, jaundice, and splenomegaly, to mild anemia, jaundice, or reticulocytosis. Patients with mild or atypical HS may present later in life. While patients with severe HS often undergo splenectomy by age 9, the role of splenectomy for the treatment of mild-to-moderate hereditary spherocytosis remains controversial and different models for decision making are proposed. The patients with milder features of HS who escape splenectomy will continue to have mild anemia, jaundice, and cholelithiasis through their adolescence years. Similarly, patients with milder form of red cell enzyme defect may go undiagnosed until adolescence. A high index of suspicion will direct the practitioner to the right diagnosis.

Suggested Reading

Marchetti M, Quaglini S, Barosi G. Prophylactic splenectomy and cholecystectomy in mild hereditary spherocytosis: Analyzing the decision in different clinical scenarios. *J Intern Med* 244:217, 1998.

HEMOGLOBINOPATHIES

Hemoglobinopathies are autosomal disorders of globin chain synthesis. Thalassemia is caused by reduced production of alpha or beta chain, sickle cell disease, methemoglobinemia, or unstable hemoglobins due to abnormal beta chain synthesis. Normal human hemoglobin, an oxygen carrying protein in the red cells, is made up of four polypeptide chains (globins) wrapped around a heme (iron) core. The Greek characters, alpha, beta, gamma, delta, and epsilon designate the polypeptide chains. Four genes located on the short arm of chromosome 16 control the alpha chains. The genes for the beta, delta, and gamma chains are located on the short arm of chromosome 11. Hemoglobin contains soluble globin tetramers composed of two alpha and two nonalpha chains. Excess alpha and nonalpha chains are insoluble and are removed and any excess accumulation results in shortened red cell life span. There are three types of hemoglobins in the normal adult. Hemoglobin A_1 (HbA$_1$) (adult) consists of two alpha (α) and two beta (β) chains and is the major hemoglobin (97%). Hemoglobin A_2 (HbA$_2$) consists of two α and two delta (δ) chains and the relative amount in blood is approximately <3.5 %) and hemoglobin F (HbF) (fetal) is composed of two α and two gamma(γ) chains (Table 17-1). HbF is the predominant hemoglobin of the normal fetus, and is gradually replaced postnatally by HbA$_1$ by the age of 6–9 months. The relative proportions of these three hemoglobins on hemoglobin electrophoresis changes with underlying

hemoglobinopathies. Hemoglobin electrophoresis is part of routine new born screening in the United States. This practice has resulted in early diagnosis of hemoglobinopathies. Some children with unusual hemoglobinopathy or those who miss newborn screening may not be diagnosed until their adolescence.

Thalassemias

Thalassemia is a genetic defect (deletion or mutation) that results in reduced, defective or absent synthesis of α or β chains. The α-thalassemias are secondary to a deficiency in the production of α-chain and β-thalassemias are due to a deficiency of synthesis of β-chain. There are two genes that regulate production of the β-chains; either one or both may be affected. When one gene is affected (β^+/β, β/β^0), it results in mild anemia and is often clinically referred to as thalassemia minor or trait. When both genes are affected, it may result in variable degrees of anemia. Thalassemia major (Cooley's anemia or β^0 thalassemias [β^0/β^0, β^+/β^0]) is associated with severe anemias whereas thalassemia intermedia or β^+ thalassemias (β^+/β^+) are associated with moderately severe anemias. There are four genes that regulate the α-chain production. The α-thalassemias, are classified based on the loss of gene(s) as silent carrier state (one gene loss), mild α-thalassemias (two genes loss), hemoglobin H disease (three genes loss), and Hydrops fetalis (four genes loss). There are other minor thalassemias such as δ-thalassemia and $\delta\beta$-thalassemia that are rare. Because of their rarity in the adolescent population, they will not be discussed further. The reader is referred to several excellent reviews on the thalassemias available in the literature.

Clinical Presentations in the Adolescent

The thalassemias are one of the most common inherited human diseases and they are found commonly in persons of African, Mediterranean, and Southeast Asian heritage. Clinically, the thalassemia minors are associated with mild anemia as well as microcytosis and hypochromia, while the thalassemia majors are associated with severe

LABORATORY TESTS FOR THE DIAGNOSIS OF HEMOGLOBINOPATHIES

Defect	Anemia	RBC Count/ RDW	Reticulocyte Count	Serum Bilirubin	Serum Iron	TIBC	Ferritin	HbA$_2$	HbF	Iron Therapy
Iron deficiency	Mild → severe	RBC count↓ RDW↑	Low	Normal	Low	High	Low	Normal	Normal	Improved anemia
β-Thalassemia traits	Mild	RBC count↑ RDW (N)	Variable	Variable	Normal	Normal	Normal	High (mild >3.5%)	Variable	No change
β-Thalassemia major	Severe	RBC count↑ RDW (N)	High	High	High	Low	High	High (marked)	Very high >90%	Contraindicated
α-Thalassemia trait	None → mild	RBC count↑ RDW (N)	Variable	Variable	Normal	Normal	Normal	Normal	Normal	No change
Hemoglobin H disease	Moderate → severe	RBC count↑ RDW (N)	High	High	Normal → high	Normal → low	Normal → high	Normal*	Normal	Contraindicated

*In absence of alpha chain, β-tetramers (HbH), and γ-tetramers (Hb Barts) are formed.
Abbreviations: TIBC = total iron binding capacity, RBC = red blood cells, RDW = red cell distribution width.

anemia, microcytosis, and hypochromia. In the severe varieties, besides decreased levels of cellular hemoglobin, unbalanced excess globin chains results in membrane damage and early destruction of the red cell leading to ineffective erythropoiesis. Presence of inclusion bodies leads to further destruction of mature cells in either the spleen or bone marrow.

Severe iron deficiency can mask a diagnosis of thalassemia traits in an adolescent and should be corrected prior to obtaining a hemoglobin electrophoresis. The healthcare provider should be able to distinguish β-thalassemia from iron deficiency, employing the guidelines provided in Table 17-9. Homozygous α-thalassemia due to deletion of all four genes results in hydrops fetalis and is seldom seen later on in life. However, hemoglobin H disease due to deletion of three out of four alpha genes results in moderately severe anemia and may be seen in adolescence.

The clinical features of thalassemia are dependent on the severity. Table 17-10 lists the more common clinical findings in severe thalassemias. The majority of these patients have iron overload that results from a combination of repeated blood transfusions and abnormal iron absorptions. There is growth impairment, puberty is usually delayed, and, on rare occasions, completely absent. The transfusional and absorptive iron overload may cause deposition of iron in various organs resulting in cardiomyopathy, endocrinopathies, and hepatic dysfunction. Heart failure, cirrhosis, and hepatic failure are late complications of iron overload.

Management

In Africa and in the Middle East, where thalassemia major (Cooley's anemia) is a major problem, adolescents were rarely found with this disease because death occurred in infancy. In the last decade, advances in red cell transfusions coupled with iron chelation therapy, and recently bone marrow transplantation, have transformed this disease from a chronic illness to one that permits a near normal survival. For patients who do not have a BMT donor or the resources to undergo a bone marrow transplant, the management is essentially based on a program of careful and regular blood transfusions (chronic transfusion therapy) followed by chelation with an iron binding agent, desferrioxamine

T A B L E 1 7 - 1 0

CLINICAL FEATURES OF THALASSEMIA MAJOR

Clinical Presentation	Underlying Pathology
Pallor, exercise intolerance, generalized malaise	Anemia
Thalassemic facies (gnathopathy), sternum and skull (hair-on-end appearance on x-ray), osteoporosis	Bone marrow hyperplasia
Scleral icterus	Hemolysis
Leg ulcers	Peripheral vascular insufficiency
Abdominal pains, organomegaly	Cholelithiasis, extramedullary hematopoiesis
Heart failure, liver failure, arthritis, gonadal failure, diabetes mellitus, hypothyroidism, hypoparathyroidism, skin pigmentation	Iron overload (transfusional and absorptive)

(Desferal) to prevent iron mediated damage to organs. Deferiprone or L1 is an oral chelating agent currently licensed in Europe and India and is used alone or in combination with Desferal. It is associated with side effects such as agranulocytosis, zinc deficiency, and gastrointestinal disturbances. Supplemental therapies include oral vitamin C to increase iron excretion, splenectomy to reduce transfusion requirements, and endocrine replacement therapy (insulin for diabetes, bisphosphonates, calcium, and vitamin D for osteoporosis). Compliance with chelation is critical and would result in decreased morbidity and mortality. Adherence to rigid chelation program during adolescence is a real challenge. Transplantation using HLA-identical bone marrow or umbilical cord cells have been used, mostly in Europe, as a cure for this disease with some success.

Suggested Readings

Cao H, Stamatoyannopoulos G, Jung M. Induction of human gamma globin gene expression by histone deacetylase/inhibitors. *Blood* 103:701, 2004.

Lawson SE, Roberts IA, Amrolia P, et al. Bone marrow transplantation for beta-thalassaemia major: The UK/ experience in two paediatric centres. *Br J Haematol* 120:289–295, 2003.

Lo L, Singer ST. Thalassemia: Current approach to an old disease. *Pediatr Clin North Am* 49:1165, 2002.

Piomelli S. Management of Cooley's anaemia. *Baillieres Clin Haematol* 6:287, 1993.

Thein SL. Beta-thalassaemia prototype of a single gene disorder with multiple phenotypes. *Int J Hematol* 76(Suppl 2): 96, 2002.

SICKLE CELL DISEASE AND OTHER HEMOGLOBINOPATHIES

The sickle cell hemoglobinopathies are defects resulting from a single gene mutation, more specifically, a single base substitution. Those of clinical significance are β-globin defects, that result in abnormal beta chain synthesis. Sickle cell anemia, a hemoglobinopathy that causes significant morbidity and mortality, is caused by a single amino acid substitution, here, the acidic amino acid glutamic acid is replaced by the neutral valine at the sixth position of the β-globin chain. The gene for β chain is located in chromosome 11 and it is inherited in simple Mendelian fashion.

Since the discovery of the sickle cell defect, referred to as HbS, several other globin chain abnormalities have been discovered and they have been designated by alphabets (e.g., HbC, HbE, and HbG). Of all of these abnormalities, HbS is the most significant and problematic clinically.

Sickle Cell Disease

This condition is characterized by formation of sickle-shaped red blood cells (SRBC) under conditions of low oxygen content of the tissues. SRBCs have a shortened life span, leading to anemia. The repeated sickling of RBC creates rather rigid cells (irreversible sickle cells) with greatly diminished ability to deform, causing entrapment in small capillaries. The resulting vaso-occlusion leads to ischemia and infarct and, ultimately, severe pain and end-organ damage. The various types of sickle cell diseases, genotypes, and modes of inheritance are shown in Table 17-11. The prevalence rate is 1 in 375 African Americans, 1 out of every 1000 Spanish Americans and 1 out of every 70 West Africans, making it one of the most common genetic disorders in the United States and in the world.

The common sickle cell disease variants are shown in Table 17-12. All of these variants do not have specific characteristics that distinguish them clinically from HbSS. These variants are usually a result of compound heterozygosity of another β-globin abnormality inherited with the β-sickle gene. A high proportion of the milder sickle cell disease forms fall into this variant category.

The frequency of HbS trait (carrier) is about 8% in African Americans, 0.5%–3% in Spanish Americans, and about 25% among West Africans. The frequency of HbC is about 2.5% among African Americans and about 20% among West Africans. HbSC disease is the second most common sickle cell disease variant and accounts for nearly 20% of sickle cell disease. HbS/β-thalassemia has clinical features that are dependent on the severity

TABLE 17-11

SICKLE CELL DISEASES, GENOTYPES, AND MODES OF INHERITANCE

Condition	Genotype	Zygosity
Sickle cell anemia	HbSS	Homozygote
Sickle cell disease	HbS/HbC	Compound heterozygote
Sickle β-thalassemia	HbS/β-Thal	Compound heterozygote*
Sickle-cell disease	HbS/HbE	Compound heterozygote†

*Sickle β-thalassemia is quite complex. The sickle cell gene could be in combination with β^0 (no chain production) or β^+ (reduced β chain production)

†Massive immigration of southeast Asians to the United States has led to the increased recognition of HbS/HbE compound heterozygotes.

of the thalassemia component. The more severe type is in combination with the β^0 gene and the milder type is associated with the $\beta+$ gene. In general, the HbS/β-thalassemia variant is the third most common form of sickle cell disease.

A third variant is HbS and $\delta\beta^0$-thalassemia in a compound heterozygous state. On a hemoglobin electrophoresis, the pattern of this variant is similar to that of HbSS, but HbF levels may be as high as 20%–25%. There are several subtypes of hereditary persistence of fetal hemoglobin (HPFH), each of which may interact with *HbS* gene to produce a variety of sickle cell diseases. The pancellular type, in which HbF is distributed evenly throughout the red cells, is found in 0.1% of the African American population and is responsible for the most common form of this variety of sickle cell disease. HbSD disease and HbSO Arab disease are very rare varieties of sickle cell disease.

Clinical Manifestation in Adolescents

The hallmark of sickle cell disease is vasoocclusion and practically every organ in the body is involved. In the lungs, it results in acute chest syndrome, a medical emergency often caused by fat/bone marrow embolus and infections with *Chlamydia, Mycoplasma,* or a viral infection. Vaso-occlusive crises in the bones, results in infarcts, abnormalities of the vertebrae (fish mouth), osteopenia, avascular necrosis ultimately leading to growth disturbances, and joint replacement. In the genitourinary system it causes priapism and renal disease (e.g., nephrotic syndrome), and in the central nervous system it causes stroke. Aplastic crises are also a common occurrence and may be associated with parvovirus infections.

The adolescent with sickle cell disease is particularly vulnerable to the features listed in Table 17-13.

TABLE 17-12

SICKLE SYNDROMES

Syndrome	HbA₁ ($\alpha_2\beta_2$)%	HbS ($\alpha_2\beta_2^S$)%	HbF ($\alpha_2\gamma_2$)%	HbA₂ ($\alpha_2\delta_2$)%	HbC ($\alpha_2\beta_2^C$)%
Normal	95–98	0	<<2	<<3.5	0
HbSS (homozygous HbS)	0	75–95	2–25	<<3.5	0
Sickle/β^0 thalassemia	0	80–90	2–15	3–7.5	0
Sickle/HbC (HbSC disease)	0	35–55	1–5		45–55
Sickle/β^+ thalassemia	5–30	65–90	2–10	3–6	0
Sickle/HPFH	0	65–70	20–30	1–3.5	0
Sickle/$\delta\beta$ thalassemia	0	60–80	15–25	1–3.5	0
Sickle cell trait (carrier)	45–60	35–45	<<2	<<3.5	0

TABLE 17-13

MAJOR CLINICAL FEATURES OF SICKLE CELL DISEASE AT VARIOUS AGES

	Infancy	Childhood	Adolescent
A. Impairment of circulation	Pain, hand and foot syndrome	Pain, stroke, arthralgia, hematuria, hyposthenuria	Chronic pain, stroke, autosplenectomy, renal insufficiency, avascular necrosis
B. Red blood cell destruction (hemolysis)	Pallor, jaundice, lethargy	Pallor, jaundice, lethargy, splenomegaly, cardiomegaly, shortness of breath	Exercise intolerance pallor, jaundice, gall stones, chronic lung disease, chronic transfusion, and iron overload
C. Stagnation of blood in organs	Sequestration	Sequestration	Priapism, hepatomegaly, chronic leg ulcers
Combination of A, B, and C	Fever, pneumonia, osteomyelitis, susceptibility to infections (*Pneumococcus* and *Haemophilus influenzae*)	Fever, pneumonia, osteomyelitis, susceptibility to infections (*Pneumococcus* and *H. influenzae*)	Fever, osteomyelitis (*Salmonella* sp.), acute chest syndrome, pulmonary hypertension, retinopathy delayed sexual maturation, pregnancy complications, depression, pain intolerance, narcotic dependence, increased school absenteeism

The difficulties related to their chronic illness pose tremendous challenges to the adolescent with sickle cell disease. They must cope with their personal and sexual identity, their sense of self-worth, and their role in society. Pregnancy poses a risk for the mother and the fetus and is complicated by an increase in the severity of painful crises, acute chest syndrome, exaggerated anemia, toxemia, and death. Fetal complications secondary to placental infarctions include prematurity, abortion intrauterine growth retardation. Chronic transfusion therapy during pregnancy may prevent some of these complications.

Management

Most adolescents with sickle cell disease will have periods of freedom from serious medical symptoms; it is not unusual for these patients to start experiencing an increase in the number of crises resulting in high morbidity. The other unique problems seen in adolescence include delayed sexual development, avascular necrosis, cholelithiasis, priapism, proteinuria, and airway disease. The additional issues during adolescence relate to drug use, birth control methods, and academic performance. Therefore, the management of adolescents with sickle cell disease should involve periodic comprehensive evaluation, including assessment by the nutritionist, social worker, psychologist, and the medical team. The frequency is individualized and depends on the clinical severity of the disease presentation. Laboratory studies during each comprehensive evaluation will include a complete blood count (CBC) with differential, a reticulocytes count, and a comprehensive chemistry. Ferritin levels are of value for patients on "chronic transfusion therapy" or those who have need for multiple blood transfusions.

Usually by adolescence the spleen in patients with sickle cell disease is nonfunctional (autosplenectomy). The dysfunction of the immune system resulting from this leads to high risk for overwhelming infections with encapsulated organisms (e.g., *Pneumococcus* and *Haemophilus influenzae*). Adolescents with sickle cell disease, especially those with SC disease and HbS/β-thalassemia variants may sometimes present with large spleens and continue to remain at risk for acute splenic sequestration and may present with precipitous drop in hemoglobin concentration that may be life threatening. Acute splenic sequestration is treated with blood transfusion. To avoid recurrence the patient also needs elective splenectomy.

Stroke contributes one of the most devastating problems in adolescents with sickle cell disease. Fortunately, screening by transcranial Doppler (TCD) has led to early detection of those at risk, enabling the early institution of preventive measures, such as chronic transfusion therapy.

Common bone disorders in sickle cell disease are osteomyelitis, bone infarction from vasoocclusion and aseptic necrosis of the weight-bearing joints. All of these conditions have to be managed symptomatically. Ophthalmologic problems that are encountered in sickle cell disease include occlusion of small retinal vessels with neovascularization, retinal detachment, and central retinal artery occlusion. These eye problems must be treated energetically. Also, about 5% of patients with sickle cell disease will develop chronic renal failure. Consequently, routine monitoring of kidney function and cautious use of nephrotoxic drugs is very important.

Pulmonary function tests performed annually on adolescents with sickle cell disease will help with early diagnosis and institution of measures to prevent chronic lung disease. A majority of males with sickle cell disease would have experienced priapism of varying severity by the time they reach adulthood. Patients with persistent priapism may be candidates for chronic transfusion therapy as well as other therapeutic measures such as use of epinephrine in order to prevent impotence.

Blood transfusion is an important aspect of management of sickle cell related complications. However because of the risk of alloimmunization and iron overload, the transfusion should be used with caution. The indications for blood transfusion include stroke, acute chest syndrome, heart failure, multiorgan failure, splenic sequestration, and aplastic crises and before surgical procedures. The goals of transfusion therapy are to increase oxygen carrying capacity while at the same time decrease the percentage of sickle hemoglobin. However, caution should be exercised not to increase the hemoglobin to >11 g/dL, as it may increase blood viscosity. Straight transfusions are indicated when the hemoglobin is <8–9 g/dL and exchange transfusions are preferred when the hemoglobin concentrations are high. Besides exposure to transfusion transmitted pathogens and transfusion reactions, adolescents who have received numerous blood transfusions are at risk for iron overload that may lead to endocrine failure, cirrhosis of the liver, and cardiomyopathy. Desferal chelation is effective in decreasing iron overload. However, it is very tedious and requires compliance on the part of the adolescent. Oral iron chelators may be effective, but toxicity has to be taken into consideration. It may be combined with intermittent intravenous Desferal.

Treatment of pain in adolescents with sickle cell disease is one of the most challenging issues. Most pain arises from tissue ischemia secondary to vasoocclusion and is unpredictable. Pain management teams may be helpful in optimizing treatment options. Patient controlled analgesia (PCA), non-steroidal anti-inflammatory drugs (NSAIDs), and hydroxyurea can be used as adjunct therapies to narcotics. In addition, a comprehensive team strategy approach helps in removing misconceptions and concerns about opiate addiction or dependence.

Other therapies: The use of hydroxyurea (15–20 mg/kg) is now very widespread in the treatment of adolescents. Besides increasing hemoglobin F that inhibits sickle cell polymerization, hydroxyurea increases red cell deformability, alters adhesive receptors on reticulocytes, and decreases white cell counts (white cells are less deformable and more adhesive). Careful monitoring is required;

hydroxyurea should not be used during pregnancy. There are several reviews of hydroxyurea efficacy. Other therapies include Butyrates and Decitabines, which have been shown to increase circulating HbF. There are other agents being studied including Niprisan (nix—0699), a naturally occurring product discovered in West Africa, nitric oxide, clotrimazole, and magnesium. Bone marrow/stem cell/umbilical cord blood cell transplantation, while curative, is indicated in severe cases with a poor quality of life.

Suggested Readings

Claster S, Vinchinsky EP. Managing sickle cell disease. *Br Med J* 327:1151–1155, 2003.

Covas DT, De Lucena Angulo I, Vianna Bonini Palma P, et al. Effects of hydroxyurea on the membrane of erythrocytes and platelets in sickle cell anemia. *Haematologica* 89:273, 2004.

Hadar RW, Vinchinsky EP. Major changes in sickle-cell disease. *Adv Pediatr* 47:249–272, 2000.

Locatelli F, Rocha V, Reed W, Eurocord Transplant Group, et al. Related umbilical cord blood transplantation in patients with thalassemia and sickle-cell disease. *Blood* 101:2137, 2003.

Scott-Emuakpor AB. Genetic aspects of sickle-cell disease. In: Scott RB (ed.), *International Aspects of Sickle Cell Disease.* Washington, DC: Howard University Center for Sickle Cell Disease, 1979, pp. 11–19.

Vinchinsky, EP. New therapies in sickle-cell disease. *Lancet* 360:629–631, 2002.

18

MALIGNANT DISEASES IN ADOLESCENTS

W. Archie Bleyer and Karen H. Albritton

INTRODUCTION

Among 15–24-year olds in the United States, accidents and homicides are the most frequent as causes of death. Cancer and intentional self-harm (suicide) are the next two most common causes of death and the two most frequent causes of death due to disease. In the age group, cancer kills far more females than suicide and overall is the second most common cause of death. It is estimated that 4374 U.S. adolescents between 15 and 19 years of age were diagnosed with invasive cancer in the year 2000.

This chapter reviews the incidence and mortality burden of cancer in the adolescents, the unique distribution of cancer types, general diagnostic and treatment principles, and the concerning lack of improvement in survival and quality of survival. The emphasis is on issues that make management of this population of oncology patients unique and challenging, and the goal is to heighten awareness of a relatively neglected group of patients and improve their recognition, management, and out come. Because of common standard age groupings for analytical purposes, much of the data are ascertained for 15–19-year-olds, who are therefore the focus of the chapter, but many of the principles are applicable to the

12–15 year olds-and the next older group of patients, especially to those 20–30 years of age.

EPIDEMIOLOGY

Incidence and Incidence Trends

In the most recent National Cancer Institute Surveillance, Epidemiology, and End Results data (1997–2001), the incidence of invasive cancer in persons of 15–19 years of age in the United States was 200 new cases per million persons per year. Based on the year 2000 United States census and incidence rates, the number of persons diagnosed yearly with cancer in the United States between 15 and 20 years of age exceeds 4000, the highest of all 5-year age groups younger than age 20, 1.9 times the number in 5–9-year-olds, and 1.7 times that in 10–14-year olds (Table 18-1).

The incidence of cancer has been increasing during the past quarter century in most, if not all, age groups. In 15–19-year olds, the overall incidence increased an average of 0.5% per year from 1975 to 2001 (Fig. 18-1) (Ries et al., 2004). All of the younger age groups in the United States have also shown similar increases during this 26 year interval (Fig. 18-1). In the first half of the interval, the

TABLE 18-1

INCIDENCE OF INVASIVE CANCER IN CHILDREN AND ADOLESCENTS, UNITED STATES,
BY 5-YEAR AGE INTERVALS

| | Age at diagnosis (years) | | | |
	0–4	5–9	10–14	15–19
United States population, year 2000 census	19,175,798	20,549,505	20,528,072	20,219,890
Average annual increase in invasive cancer, 1975–2001*	0.8%	0.4%	0.9%	0.5%
Estimated incidence of invasive cancer, year 2000, per million*	204	114	129	200
Estimated number of persons diagnosed with invasive cancer, year 2000	3,912	2,343	2,648	4,044

*Data from United States National Cancer Institute Surveillance, Epidemiology, and End Results program.

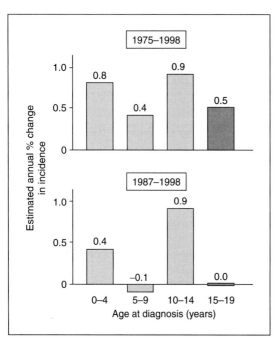

FIGURE 18-1

CHANGE IN INCIDENCE FROM 1975 TO 1998 (UPPER
PANEL) AND FROM 1987 TO 1998 (LOWER PANEL)
AS A FUNCTION OF 5-YEAR AGE INTERVALS.
The lower panel represents the trends during the last
11 years of the 23-year interval represented in the upper
panel.
Source: Data from the United States National Cancer Institute
Surveillance, Epidemiology, and End Results program. Modified
from Bleyer 2002.

cancer incidence in 15–19-year olds increased out
of proportion to other age groups (at an estimated
annual increase of 1.6% per year) but this trend has
gradually waned from 1987 to 2001, whereas it
slowed down but did not abate in younger children
(Fig. 18-1). Testicular and ovarian germ cell
tumors, gonadal carcinomas, osteosarcoma, and
non-Hodgkin's lymphoma (NHL) have shown the
greatest increases in incidence rates over this time
interval in the 15–19 age group. After 1986, none
of the common types of cancer in 15–19-year olds
underwent a statistically significant increase or
reduction in incidence.

Because cancer in 15–19-year olds occurs at the
interface of pediatric and adult oncology, with overlapping age-specific classes of cancer (Fig. 18-2),
the types of cancer in this age group have a unique
distribution (Fig. 18-3). The cancers that predominate in adults, such as carcinomas of the breast and
aerodigestive and genitourinary tracts, are particularly rare among adolescents. Similarly, most of the
malignancies common in children younger than 5
years are virtually absent in adolescents, including
the embryonal malignancies of Wilms' tumor, neuroblastoma, medulloblastoma, ependymoma, hepatoblastoma, and retinoblastoma (Table 18-2). What
are seen is a mix of "pediatric" cancers (cancers
that account for a large portion of the cancers
treated by pediatric oncologists; Fig. 18-3, shaded
portions) and some "adult" cancers rarely seen

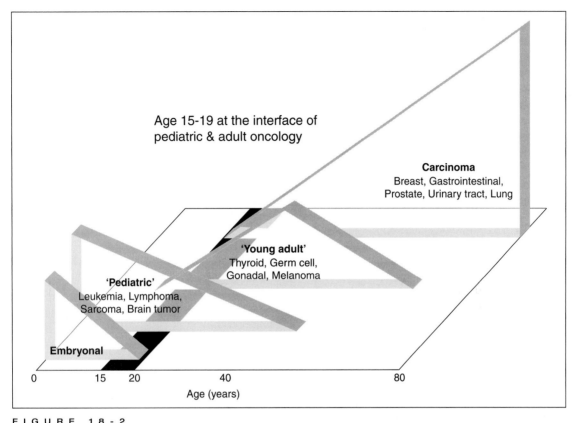

Age 15-19 at the interface of pediatric & adult oncology

Carcinoma
Breast, Gastrointestinal,
Prostate, Urinary tract, Lung

'Young adult'
Thyroid, Germ cell,
Gonadal, Melanoma

'Pediatric'
Leukemia, Lymphoma,
Sarcoma, Brain tumor

Embryonal

0   15   20   40   80

Age (years)

F I G U R E   1 8 - 2

DISTRIBUTION OF TYPES OF CANCER IN ADOLESCENTS, 15–19 YEARS OF AGE, COMPARED WITH OTHER AGE GROUPS. RB-RETINOBLASTOMA, NB-NEUROBLASTOMA, RMS-RHABDOMYOSARCOMA.

before age 15 (Fig 18-3, clear portions). The most common cancers among 15–19-year olds in the United States are Hodgkin's disease (19%), germ cell tumors (14%), central nervous system (CNS) tumors (10%), NHL (7%), thyroid cancer (7%), malignant melanoma (7%), and acute lymphoblastic leukemia (ALL) (6%) (Fig. 18-3, Table 18-2).

Nosologic systems used to classify malignancies depend on age. For example, the International Classification of Diseases (ICD) system is based primarily on organ site and applies to adults with cancer. Children with cancer are generally classified according to the International Classification of Childhood Cancer (ICCC), which is based on histology. Given the mix of cancers, neither histology nor topography provides a completely accurate basis on which to classify the cancers of adolescents. However, with minor modification,

the childhood cancer system is probably more applicable to the cancers of adolescents. One group has recommended that colorectal, salivary, and lung carcinomas be named and enumerated independently from other carcinomas within the group of carcinoma and other epithelial tumors. Breast cancer should also probably be enumerated in this way.

The bone sarcomas-osteosarcoma and Ewing sarcoma-peak in incidence between 15 and 19 years of age, and several hypotheses have been made relating this to growth spurts and hormonal milieu. The types of soft tissue sarcoma that occur in 15–19-year olds are also distinct from those in younger patients. Specifically, rhabdomyosarcoma predominates among the sarcomas of childhood, accounting for more than 60% of the soft tissue sarcomas in children younger than 5 years.

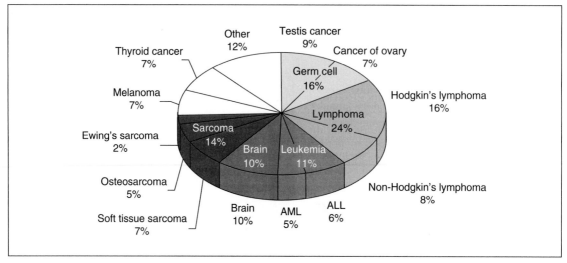

FIGURE   18-3

TYPES OF CANCER IN ADOLESCENTS, 15–19 YEARS OF AGE. THE SHADED SECTIONS INDICATE TUMOR
TYPES COMMONLY FOUND IN CHILDREN AND YOUNGER ADOLESCENTS.
Source: Data from the United States National Cancer Institute Surveillance, Epidemiology, and End Results program, 1986–1995.
AML-Acute myeloid leukemia. ALL-Acute lymphoblastic leukemia. NHL-Non-Hodgkin's lymphoma. Modified from Bleyer 2002.

In 15–19-year olds, rhabdomyosarcoma accounts for only 25% of the soft-tissue sarcomas. Non-rhabdomyosarcomatous soft-tissue sarcomas, including synovial sarcoma, liposarcoma, malignant fibrous histiocytoma, and malignant peripheral nerve sheath tumors in which are rare before age 15, rise in incidence and account for the rest.

The distribution of leukemias and lymphomas in older adolescents also differs from that in young children. ALL has a peak incidence between age 2 and 3 and accounts for 30% of all cancers in children less than age 15 but only 6% of all cancers in adolescents aged 15–19 years. This makes acute myelogenous leukemia (AML), an uncommon disease throughout childhood and adolescence, nearly as common as ALL in 15–19-year olds. The incidence of chronic myelogenous leukemia (CML) increases steadily with age from infancy but is not as common as either ALL or AML in 15–29-year olds. Juvenile myelomonocytic leukemia is uncommon in all four 5-year age groups before age 20 but especially rare in the 15–19 group. In adolescents, NHL is more common than ALL. The incidence of NHL increases

steadily with age, but the subtype distribution changes, from a predominance of lymphoblastic and Burkitt's lymphomas during early childhood to a predominance of diffuse large-cell lymphoma during adolescence and early adulthood. The incidence of Hodgkin's disease rises dramatically during adolescence and peaks between 20 and 29 years of age.

Ethnic and racial differences in incidences are particularly apparent between African American and non-Hispanic Caucasian older adolescents (Smith MA, 1999). For example, among 15–19-year olds in the United States, the overall incidence of cancer is 50% higher among Caucasians than among African Americans. The incidences of specific cancers such as melanoma and Ewing's sarcoma are strikingly higher in Caucasians than African Americans in all age groups. ALL, germ cell tumors, and thyroid cancer are at least twice as common among Caucasians as among African Americans in all age groups. Among the common cancers in this age group, only soft-tissue sarcomas, considered as a group, are more common among African Americans than among Caucasians.

TABLE 18-2

AGE-SPECIFIC CANCER INCIDENCE RATES PER MILLION BY CANCER TYPE AND AGE GROUP, 1975–1998

	Age at diagnosis (years)			
	0–4	*5–9*	*10–14*	*15–19*
All cancer	193.7	107.9	116.5	197.1 (100.0%)
Tumor group (ICCC category†)				
Lymphomas & reticuloendothelial neoplasms	6.9	13.3	24.3	51.7 (26.2%)
Hodgkin's disease	0.5	4.2	13.3	36.8 (18.7%)
Non-Hodgkin's lymphoma	5.7	8.9	10.6	14.6 (7.4%)
Carcinomas	1.6	2.9	10.7	41.3 (21.0%)
Germ-cell, trophoblastic,	6.1	2.2	6.1	27.3 (13.9%)
Leukemia	67.6	34.8	24.0	22.6 (11.5%)
Acute lymphoblastic leukemia	55.3	28.4	16.0	11.7 (5.9%)
Acute myeloid leukemia	5.2	3.4	4.2	6.0 (3.0%)
Central nervous system tumors	32.7	30.3	23.9	19.2 (9.7%)
Astrocytoma	13.4	15.3	14.0	12.1 (6.1%)
Other gliomas	4.8	5.8	4.1	3.4 (1.7%)
Malignant bone tumors	1.2	5.0	13.1	15.0 (7.6%)
Osteosarcoma	0.5	2.4	7.5	8.3 (4.2%)
Ewing's sarcoma	0.6	2.3	4.3	4.8 (2.4%)
Soft-tissue sarcomas	10.2	8.5	10.3	15.0 (7.6%)
Fibrosa, other fibromatous neoplasms	1.8	1.5	3.5	5.5 (2.8%)
Rhabdomyosarcoma, embryonal sarcoma	6.5	4.8	3.1	3.5 (1.8%)
Renal tumors	19.2	6.1	1.3	1.2 (0.6%)
Sympathetic nervous system tumors	29.7	3.2	1.1	1.1 (0.6%)
Hepatic tumors	4.5	0.6	0.6	0.9 (0.5%)

Source: Modified from Bleyer 2002; data from United States National Cancer Institute Surveillance, Epidemiology, and End Results program.
*Percent of all 15–19-year-old patients with cancer.
†International Classification of Childhood Cancer.

Although the incidence of cancer is 20% higher in boys than girls younger than 15 years, the overall incidence is essentially equal among males and females of 15–19 years. However, individual tumor types have unequal sex distributions in the older adolescent populations (Smith MA, 1999). The most striking difference is in the incidence of thyroid carcinoma; adolescent females are 10 times more likely to develop this disease than males. The next greatest sex-related difference in 15- to 19-year-olds is the incidence of ALL; males are more than twice as likely as females to be affected. Adolescent females are 50% more likely to develop melanoma and about 15% more likely to have Hodgkin's disease. Compared with females, males are nearly twice as likely to be diagnosed with NHL or Ewing's sarcoma, 50% more likely to develop osteosarcoma, and 20%–30% more likely to have a brain tumor. Internationally, the incidence of melanoma varies the most among members of this age group. Rates in adolescents (and adults) living in Australia are up to five times higher than elsewhere worldwide.

Mortality Rates and Burden

From 1994 to 1998, the cancer mortality rate in the United States was 38 deaths per million in 15–19-year olds, 41% higher than the rate of 27 per million in all quintiles below age 15. The mortality rate is a function of the survival and incidence rates. In the 5–9 and 10–14-year age groups, the lower incidence rate accounts for the lower mortality rate. However, the 0–4-year age group has a similar incidence to older adolescents but a lower mortality rate, implying that older adolescents have not fared as well as younger children with cancer.

The improvement in mortality (as measured by the average annual percentage change in the mortality rates) waned between 1975 and 1998 in all age groups under 20 years of age (Fig. 18-4). The magnitude of the change is least apparent in the adolescents, particularly in older adolescents, most notably during the last half of the interval, 1987–2001 (Fig. 18-4). Since the 15–19-year-old age group had the smallest increment in the incidence among all the age groups below 20 years they should have had the greatest reduction in mortality rate if all age groups had the same improvement in survival. Yet, they had the least reduction in mortality; and as shown in Fig. 18-5, they have had the least improvement in survival. In sum, in the last quarter of the twentieth century, adolescents in the United States, compared to younger children, have had a higher incidence of cancer, a higher mortality rate, and the least improvement in survival and mortality rates.

More than 80% of the cancer mortality burden in the United States for 15–19-year olds is caused by four malignancy groups: sarcomas, leukemia and lymphomas, CNS tumors, and germ cell tumors. The leukemias/lymphomas are the primary contributors to the cancer mortality burden for 15–19-year olds. Although thyroid carcinoma and melanoma are among the more common cancers in this age group, they contribute little to the

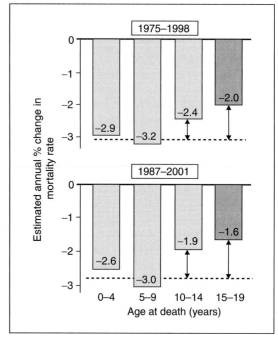

FIGURE 18-4

CHANGE IN UNITED STATES CANCER MORTALITY RATES FROM 1975 TO 1998 (UPPER PANEL) AND FROM 1987 TO 1998 (LOWER PANEL) AS A FUNCTION OF 5-YEAR AGE INTERVALS. THE LOWER PANEL REPRESENTS THE TRENDS DURING THE LAST 11 YEARS OF THE 23-YEAR INTERVAL REPRESENTED IN THE UPPER PANEL. Source: Data from the United States National Cancer Institute Surveillance, Epidemiology, and End Results program. Modified from Bleyer 2002.

overall cancer mortality burden in this group because of their high survival rates. The former has all but disappeared and the latter rarely occurs in the current era.

Etiology

As in younger patients, little is known about the causes of cancer in adolescents. Very few cancers in this age group have been attributed to environmental or inherited factors. Two notable exceptions are clear cell adenocarcinoma of the vagina or cervix in adolescent females (most cases of which were caused by diethylstilbestrol taken prenatally by the patients' mothers to prevent spontaneous

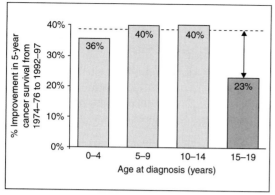

FIGURE 18 - 5

IMPROVEMENT IN THE 5-YEAR SURVIVAL RATE FROM INVASIVE CANCER FROM 1974–1976 TO 1992–1997 AS A FUNCTION OF 5-YEAR AGE INTERVALS. THE HORIZONTAL DASHED LINE REPRESENTS THE INCREASE AMONG PATIENTS LESS THAN 15 YEARS OF AGE AT DIAGNOSIS.

The increase among 15–19-year olds, 23%, is 57% of the improvement in younger patients.

Source: Data from the United States National Cancer Institute Surveillance, Epidemiology, and End Results program.

abortion) and radiation-induced cancer in adolescence after an exposure during early childhood.

Skin cancer, lymphoma, sarcoma, and hepatic cancers occur at higher frequencies among persons with some inherited conditions such as neurofibromatosis, ataxia telangiectasia, Li-Fraumeni syndrome, xeroderma pigmentosum, Fanconi pancytopenia, hereditary dysplastic nevus syndrome, nevoid basal cell carcinoma syndrome, multiple endocrine neoplasia syndromes, and Turner syndrome. In the aggregate, however, these cancers account for only a small proportion of the cancers that occur during adolescence. If the primary care physician recognizes major cancer genetic syndromes, he should make a referral for genetic counseling and testing, and follow recommended screening guidelines.

The cumulative exposure to potential environmental carcinogens is directly proportional to age. Therefore, the occurrence of tobacco-, sunlight-, or diet-related cancers would be expected to be higher in older adolescents than in younger children. However, these environmental carcinogens, which are known to induce cancer in older adults, have

not been demonstrated to cause cancer with significant frequency in adolescents. It appears to take considerably longer than one or two decades in most persons for these environmentally related cancers to become manifest. An exception to this general rule is the frequency of melanoma in Australian teenagers, a finding that suggests that solar exposure may be able to induce skin cancer before the end of the second decade of life, at least among the population of Australia. This possibility is strengthened by the observation that the location where the greatest increase in melanoma has occurred is the trunk and extremities of females, and more so the legs than arms, which is consistent relative to the increased sun exposure by adolescents during the past couple of decades, and particularly among females who have taken to wearing less clothes, leading to melanoma in previously unexposed areas of the body.

DIAGNOSIS

Prevention and Screening

Unlike the detailed guidelines for cancer screening in adults provided by the American Medical Association and other organized groups, there are no guidelines for prevention and screening of pediatric or adolescent cancers. Given the relative rarity of malignancy, it is unlikely that any screening test will ever be cost-effective in children or adolescents. However there are elements of the history and physical examination that can be adapted to screen for common cancers, and there are teaching points that can be stressed during the counseling portion of the visit (Table 18-3).

Adolescents should be taught to adopt lifestyles that will help prevent cancer later in life. Avoidance of tobacco and ultraviolet exposure (sunburns and tanning parlors) are obvious examples. Whether they should be taught self-testicular or self-breast examinations is controversial, since there is no high-level evidence that cancer mortality is decreased by introducing these practices in adolescents. Overzealous workup of minor abnormalities found on breast, skin, or testicular examinations can result in unnecessary anxiety or diagnostic procedures

TABLE 18-3

CANCER-RELATED HISTORY, PHYSICAL EXAMINATION, AND COUNSELING FOR ADOLESCENTS

History	Physical Examination	Counseling
Unexplained weight loss	Thyroid gland nodule or enlargement	Sun avoidance
Fevers/night sweats	Lymphadenopathy (especially supra-	Tobacco avoidance
Headaches (with vomiting)	clavicular, axillary)	Breast and testicle self-examination
Soft tissue, lymph node,	Testicular mass	Skin examination
or bony mass	Abnormal pigmented skin lesion	
	Soft tissue or bony mass	
	Bruising	

with attendant morbidity. It also might be considered difficult to bring up and teach these topics at this age. Countering this perception, however, is the finding from a preliminary assessment of teaching testicular self-examinations to high school and college students that showed that anxiety was no greater in students who were exposed to presentations on testicular cancer and testicular self-examination than in those who did not receive this training (Friman et al., 1986). There is consensus that self-examination is important for individuals with testicular or breast cancer risk factors, such as undescended testes or families with known BRCA mutations. Overall, self-examination of the skin and breasts can be introduced, as can the importance of awareness of symptoms of testicular cancer in young men. Health counseling may include guidance about smoking cessation, diet, physical activity, and a beginning discussion of benefits and risks of undergoing various screening tests as they age into adulthood. Lastly, efforts should be made to educate teenagers about the treatment and cure rates of cancer in children and young adults in order to dispel the fatalistic perception that arises from knowing older individuals (grandparents and others) who have died from cancer.

Symptoms and Signs

Physicians who see adolescents should be cognizant of the cancers common in this age group, and the most common presentations (Table 18-4). The healthcare professional who is aware of cancer as a diagnostic possibility, and particularly the prominence of sarcomas, thyroid cancer, testicular cancer, and melanoma in this age group, can consider these possibilities when taking the history and performing the physical examination.

Because the kinds of cancer during adolescence are unique to the age group, the signs and symptoms of cancer in adolescents differ from those of both cancers of children and the carcinomas of adults. Symptoms are more likely to be those caused by solid tumors or their metastases (masses, localized bone pain, and lymph nodes) than those systemic symptoms (fever, weight loss, diffuse bone pain, and fatigue) seen in younger children who are more likely to have disseminated disease due to hematologic or hematogenously spread cancers.

Because of medical, psychologic, economical, and social factors, older adolescents are at higher risk for a delay in diagnosis, and can present with quite advanced disease. In a study of the interval between symptom onset and diagnosis in 2665 children participating in Pediatric Oncology Group therapeutic protocols between 1982 and 1988, a multivariate analysis showed that for all solid tumors except Hodgkin's disease, as age increased, lag time increased (Pollock et al., 1991). The reasons for delay in seeking medical care and obtaining a diagnosis are multiple (Table 18-5). It is unknown how much such delays might compromise outcome.

Compared to the diagnosis of cancer in children, the diagnosis of cancer in adolescents is facilitated by the older patient's ability to describe and localize the symptoms and signs caused by the

COMMON CANCERS IN ADOLESCENTS: PRESENTATION, TREATMENT, SURVIVAL, AND LATE EFFECTS

Cancer	Common Signs and Symptoms	Treatment Modalities and Average Duration	Possible Long-Term Issues	Survival for Adolescents (%) (Smith, 1999)
Acute lymphoblastic leukemia	Fatigue, fever, bone pain, bruising	IV and PO and intrathecal chemotherapy for 2–3 years	Neurocognitive changes, avascular necrosis, congestive heart failure	51
Acute myeloid leukemia	Fatigue, fever, bruising	IV chemotherapy, +/– bone marrow transplant; 6–9 months	Infertility, thyroid dysfunction, osteoporosis, secondary malignancy (leukemia)	42
Non-Hodgkin's lymphoma	Lymphadenopathy, weight loss, fever	IV chemotherapy, radiation; 4–24 months	Pulmonary dysfunction, congestive heart failure, secondary cancer (leukemia), infertility, avascular necrosis	69
Hodgkin's disease	Lymphadenopathy, weight loss, fever, night sweats	IV chemotherapy, radiation; 2–7 months	Secondary cancers (breast, thyroid), pulmonary dysfunction, congestive heart failure, thyroid dysfunction, infertility	90
Sarcoma	Bone pain, mass	Chemotherapy, surgery, +/– radiation; 30–50 weeks	Limb dysfunction, secondary malignancy, cardiac dysfunction, hearing loss	45–63
Testicular cancer	Testicular mass	Orchiectomy, +/– retroperitoneal lymph, node dissection, chemotherapy; 9–18 weeks	Infertility, pulmonary dysfunction, renal dysfunction, hearing loss, gonadal dysfunction	90
Thyroid cancer	Thyroid mass/nodule	Surgery +/–I[131]	Hypothyroidism	99
Brain tumors	Headaches, vomiting, neurologic dysfunction	Surgery +/– radiation, +/– chemotherapy; 2 weeks–2 years	Neurocognitive dysfunction, motor dysfunction, visual damage, secondary cancers, pituitary or hypothalamic hormone failure	75
Melanoma	Changing skin, lesion (pigmented, asymmetric)	Surgical resection, chemotherapy, and/ or biologic therapy for disseminated; 2 weeks–1 year	Disfiguration from resection, depression or weight loss from interferon	92

TABLE 18-5
POTENTIAL REASONS FOR DELAY IN DIAGNOSIS OF ADOLESCENTS WITH MALIGNANT DISEASE

- Adolescents have a strong sense of immortality and invincibility. Out of denial, they may delay seeing a physician for symptoms. Even when seen, they may give poor historical information, especially to a physician untrained to "read between the lines" of an adolescent's history.
- Older adolescents have one of the lowest rates of primary care use of any age group and are therefore often not receiving routine medical care (see Chap. 2). Without a primary physician who knows the patient's baseline health status, the symptoms of cancer can be missed.
- Young adults are the most underinsured age group, falling in the gap between parental coverage and programs designed to provide universal health insurance to children (such as Medicaid) and the coverage supplied by a full time secure job (Mills R and Bhandari S, 2003). There is evidence that in the United States the diagnosis of cancer in 15–19-year-olds is significantly delayed in those who are under- or uninsured than in those with private insurance (Bleyer et al., 2005).
- Physicians may be poorly trained or unwilling to care for adolescents.
- Adolescents and young adults are not supposed to have cancer. Clinical suspicion is low, and symptoms are often attributed to physical exertion, fatigue, and stress.
- Adolescents are often too embarrassed to bring the problem to anyone's attention.
- Other factors include pressures to remain in school or in the workplace if the patient is employed.

malignancy and the greater ease with which biopsies can be obtained. Knowing the most common sites and histology of malignancies in the age group assists the radiologist and pathologist in evaluating symptoms and selecting the most appropriate imaging and biopsy procedures. Noninvasive imaging without the need for sedation, endoscopy, and minimally invasive surgery are all available for patients in this age group.

TREATMENT

Treatment Location and Specialist

As is true of the care of adolescents in other specialties, there are no rules that govern whether an adolescent is seen and treated by a pediatric oncologist or an adult oncologist. Several studies have shown that although children under age 10 are almost always seen by a pediatric oncologist at a pediatric center, the percent drops off between age 10 and 15, and the minority (approximately one-third) of 15–19-year olds are seen by pediatric specialists or centers. Research is being done only now to ascertain the reasons for this practice pattern.

The only survey of medical oncologists on the subject had a poor response rate (29%) and concluded that medical oncologists believe that they appropriately treated adolescents as adults (Brady, 1993).

It is unclear if there is a single right answer to where and by whom the adolescent with cancer should be treated. A 1997 American Academy of Pediatrics consensus statement considered referral to a board-eligible or board-certified pediatric hematologist-oncologist and pediatric subspecialty consultants as the standard of care for all pediatric and adolescent cancer patients (American Academy of Pediatrics, 1997). A wider consensus panel that included adult oncologists, the American Federation of Clinical Oncologic Societies, also concluded that "payors must provide ready access to pediatric oncologists, recognizing that childhood cancers are biologically distinct" and that the "likelihood of successful outcome in children is enhanced when treatment is provided by pediatric cancer specialists" (American Federation of Clinical Oncologic Societies. Consensus statement on access to quality cancer care. J Pediatr Hematol Oncol 1998; 20: 279–281). However, neither of these statements defines an age cutoff for the recommendation.

The answer to which specialist is most appropriate certainly varies from case to case. Patients at any age who have a "pediatric" tumor, such as rhabdomyosarcoma, Ewing's sarcoma, and osteosarcoma, will probably benefit from the expertise of a pediatric oncologist, at least in the form of consultation. Children under the age of 18 and their parents may benefit from the social and supportive culture of a pediatric hospital regardless of the diagnosis. Individuals between the ages of 16 and 24 may have varying levels of maturity and independence, and choice of physician and setting for their care should be individually determined. Pediatric oncologists may be less adept at a nonpaternalistic relationship with the patient (and potentially his or her spouse) and less inclined to consider issues such as sexuality, body image, fertility, and so forth. Adult oncologists are more permissive of dose delays and adjustments and may be less willing to be aggressive with dosing that can be tolerated by the younger patient. Adolescent patients are more verbal about their desire to receive treatment close to home, in order to maintain a normal social life, whereas younger children are more easily uprooted and transported by parents to centers at a distance. This may deprive adolescents the advantages of a tertiary care center including expertise, experience, and clinical trial availability.

In the end, the decision should be based in large part on which setting will provide the patient with the best outcome. If these are equivalent, "social" or "supportive" factors should weigh into the decision. However, increasing data suggest a disparity of objective survival outcomes. For those malignancies that have been treated by both pediatric and adult oncologists, with approaches typical of their respective disciplines, comparisons have shown that the pediatric therapy has been more effective. ALL, Ewing's sarcoma, osteosarcoma, and rhabdomyosarcoma have been found to have better survival rates when treated with the pediatric treatment approach (Stock, 2000; Paulussen, 2003; Mitchell, 2004; Ferrari, 2003). At the University of Texas M.D. Anderson Cancer Center and the Dana Farber Cancer Institute, the more rigorous pediatric regimen for ALL was adopted successfully years ago. Subsequently, the M.D. Anderson Cancer Center is integrating the more intensive AML regimen used by pediatric oncologists into the adult therapy program for AML. The use of childhood cancer regimens for the treatment of older adolescents with sarcomas appears "rational and feasible" without excessive dose delays or modifications (Verrill, 1997).

Treatment Modalities

A treatment regimen for the adolescent with cancer will include one or more elements of surgery, radiation, and chemotherapy (Table 18-3).

Surgery

In general, surgery is more readily performed in an adolescent compared to a child, and anesthesia is easier to administer. Compared to adults, adolescents are generally healthier, which also helps. The main disadvantage relative to children is that the fully-grown patient generally has fewer compensatory mechanisms to overcome deficits and disabilities rendered by surgical resection of large tumors. For example, an amputation in a toddler is compensated for within a short interval and many do so well that they prefer no prosthesis; an adolescent may struggle for years and may never accommodate. The increasing prevalence of obesity in the adolescent population has created more challenges for anesthesia and surgery.

Radiation Therapy

Adolescents are generally spared the adverse effects of ionizing radiation to vulnerable developing tissues. This is particularly true for the central nervous system (CNS), the cardiovascular system, connective tissue, and the musculoskeletal system, each of which may be irradiated to higher doses and/or larger volumes with less long-term morbidity in the older adolescent than the young child. Accommodating school or work schedules for the daily routines of radiotherapy, as well as the increasing prevalence of obesity has complicated radiotherapy planning and delivery in adolescents.

Chemotherapy

As is true at any age, choice of chemotherapy depends on the type and stage of the tumor. In general, however, the therapeutic management of cancers in adolescents differs from that in adults because of physiologic, psychologic, and psychosocial differences. Adolescents tolerate more intensive chemotherapeutic regimens than most adult patients since they have fewer coexisting morbidities and better renal, hepatic, and cardiac function. This should encourage those treating patients in this age group to push the limits of dose intensification.

On the other hand, adherence to therapy regimens is much more problematic in teenagers than in either younger or older patients. Compliance with oral chemotherapy is particularly unreliable in the adolescent cancer patient (Kyngas, 2000).

In general, the acute and chronic toxicities of chemotherapeutic agents are similar in children and adolescents. Exceptions are that older patients in this age range may experience a greater degree of anticipatory vomiting and have a somewhat less rapid recovery from myeloablative agents.

Issues for the Primary Care Provider

While on therapy, the adolescent with cancer receives most medical care from the oncologic specialist. However, several scenarios commonly involve the primary care provider. Because of the myelosuppression of chemotherapy, fever in the face of neutropenia (an absolute neutrophil count less than 500 cells/mm^3, calculated by multiplying the percentage of neutrophils [segmented neutrophils and bands] by the total white cell count) is common. Several guidelines, both pediatric and adult, have been published on the management of febrile neutropenia that are easily applicable to adolescents (Orudjev, 2002). The primary care provider, if comfortable, may manage uncomplicated cases locally with specialty support, guidelines (Table 18-6), and feedback.

Another role the primary care provider may play is as supplier of appropriate immunizations (American Academy of Pediatrics, 2003). In general, adolescents should be up-to-date if they have received their Td and MMR boosters, and are immune to varicella by infection or immunization.

Boosters can be deferred during therapy (as they may not be effective in the immunocompromised host anyway), and no live vaccines should be given. It is useful to check immunization titers prior to and after the completion of chemotherapy, as reimmunization or boosters may be required after the end of therapy. Those living in the household of a cancer patient should not receive the oral polio vaccine, as live virus can be excreted in the feces, but should receive the varicella vaccine. If adolescents with cancer have a negative varicella titer and are exposed to chicken pox or zoster, they should receive varicella zoster immune globulin (1 vial per 10 kg body weight) within 72 hours of exposure. Any suspected case of varicella zoster infection (recognizing that cases in immunocompromised patients may present atypically and subtly) should be treated promptly with intravenous acyclovir. Other restrictions due to therapy and immunosuppression depend on the patient and intensity of treatment. The treating oncologist can provide specifics for an individual patient.

In general, adolescents with cancer should be encouraged to continue schooling and a reasonable activity schedule to maintain a sense of normalcy, self-esteem, and continue social development. Consistency of rules and household activities are important too, as many adolescents report feeling that parents are overprotective after a cancer diagnosis. Safe measures to minimize the risk of infection include avoiding crowded environments, frequent hand washing, proper dental and mouth hygiene, and avoidance of constipation. Diet or food preparation rarely needs to be altered (although fresh fruit and vegetables should be washed well, peeled, or cooked). Pets are valuable and allowable, with the exception of reptiles and amphibians, which may carry salmonella, and exemption from the chore of cleaning up pet waste. Immunosuppressed adolescents should not garden or play in dirt, or be in proximity to construction work that may expose them to fungal spores.

Lastly, the management of some symptoms related to cancer therapy may be accomplished by the primary care physician. The cytopenias that result from chemotherapy may benefit from transfusions. Individual oncologists may have their own recommendations for thresholds for transfusions, and should be consulted for each case. In general,

TABLE 18-6

MAN AGEMENT OF FEVER AND NEUTROPENIA

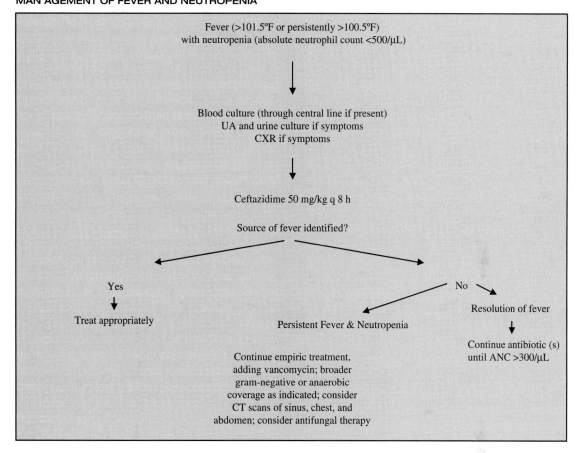

Fever (>101.5°F or persistently >100.5°F)
with neutropenia (absolute neutrophil count <500/μL)

Blood culture (through central line if present)
UA and urine culture if symptoms
CXR if symptoms

Ceftazidime 50 mg/kg q 8 h

Source of fever identified?

Yes

Treat appropriately

No

Resolution of fever

Persistent Fever & Neutropenia

Continue antibiotic (s)
until ANC >300/μL

Continue empiric treatment,
adding vancomycin; broader
gram-negative or anaerobic
coverage as indicated; consider
CT scans of sinus, chest, and
abdomen; consider antifungal therapy

adolescents tolerate anemia well unless symptomatic, and do not need a red cell transfusion unless their hemoglobin approaches 7 g/dL. Likewise, the stable, afebrile, nonbleeding patient will tolerate platelet counts down to 10,000/μL (Schiffer C, 2001). All transfused blood products should be leukocyte depleted and irradiated. Patients are usually given a battery of agents by their oncologist to combat the nausea associated with therapy. Particularly useful agents in adolescents for acute nausea appear to be dexamethasone, lorazepam, and oral cannaboids.

Psychosocial and Supportive Care

The greatest challenge and difference between the management of an adolescent patient and a younger

one is in their psychosocial and supportive care. Adolescents have special needs that are not only unique to their age group but also broader in scope and more personally intense than those at any other time in life. The primary goal of the adolescent is autonomy, separating from parents and family, and succeeding at independent decision making. The diagnosis and treatment of cancer reverses this trajectory and brings the adolescent, by circumstance and/or choice, back to a dependent role with parents and authority figures. Older adolescent patients may have developed some autonomy from the nuclear family but may have not yet developed a network of adult support relationships. Because of these complex issues, decision making during cancer therapy is different and more challenging for the patient, family, and physician of an adolescent than for either younger or older patients. The older adolescent patient may wish to make his or her own decisions, but his or her understanding of the illness may be incomplete or flawed. To achieve and maintain a good trusting relationship with the adolescent, the physician must balance open and considerate communication with the patient and endorsement of parental discretion and authority.

Honing social and interpersonal skills is an important developmental milestone during adolescence. Cancer treatment for these patients must accommodate this important developmental process. Treatment may have to be scheduled around sentinel events like final examinations, school performances, college and job interviews, and the senior prom. Other challenges include the time away from school, work, and community that therapy requires, and the financial hardships that occur at an age when economic independence from family is an objective. There may be guilt if not attending to these responsibilities, or stress and fatigue if trying to keep up a semblance of normal activity.

Yet boundaries must be set, so that treatment effectiveness is not compromised to keep a "social calendar." Certainly, cancer therapy causes practical problems in social arenas. Adolescent patients who are developmentally dependent on peer group approval often feel isolated by their experience; the cancer patient's issues are illness and death, while their peers are consumed by lipstick and homework.

Adolescents are particularly disdainful of hospital admissions, and compliance is often threatened. Efforts should be made to allow the adolescent to personalize their room environment and, as medically appropriate, allow many visitors. There is a growing trend to try to transform a section of the hospital to an environment particularly appealing to adolescent cancer patients; in the United Kingdom there are already several designated adolescent cancer units. The important features seem to include age appropriate recreation (television, video games, pool tables, lounges, and so forth), relaxed visitation and dress rules, and proximity to other patients of the same age. This combats the strong sense of loneliness and isolation of which adolescents with cancer often complain.

In adolescents with cancer, compelled to be isolated from peers and society by having a disease that makes them different and having to be treated separately is often devastating. All adolescents agonize over their personal appearance and hate to be singled out or to appear different. Many of the adverse effects of therapy can be overwhelming to an adolescent's self-image, which is often tenuous under the best of circumstances. Weight gain, alopecia, acne, stunted growth, and mutilating surgery to the face and extremities are examples of adverse consequences that can be damaging to an adolescent's self-image. In particular, hair loss is cited over and over as a huge blow to the adolescent, especially the female, with cancer.

For young adults, this is a period when sexuality, intimacy, and reproduction are central. A young adult is supposed to attract a mate and reproduce. But the young adult with cancer may feel or look unattractive, may be uninterested in or unable to have sex, and may be infertile. A feeling of impotence can pervade. Relationships will be tested by the strain of the cancer diagnosis and its therapy. Patients may wonder whether the partner stays in the relationship out of guilt or sympathy. Some significant others may feel ignored by medical staff because they are not formally family members. After treatment, commitment to the relationship in the face of fear of relapse or infertility can be difficult for both parties. Those contemplating having children often worry about passing on a genetic predisposition to cancer.

A wide range of financial situations is seen in the older adolescent population. Some patients are still happily dependent on their parents. Some are just striking out on their own but without a long-standing job or savings, may have to return to dependence on parents or get public assistance. Others are trying to begin a career but long work absences threaten their job security or growth. Older adolescent and young adult patients incur high medical bills at a time in life when they may least be able to afford them. Future insurability is certainly a stressful issue for all these patients.

Medical professionals caring for adolescents and young adults may be used to the psychosocial problems more common in either younger children or older adults. Extra effort, including patient and family support groups specifically geared to this age bracket, should be made to uncover and address these needs to increase compliance, reduce stress, and improve the quality of life during cancer therapy.

Psychologic and/or psychiatric support is often needed and prescription of antidepressants for situational depression may be beneficial.

OUTCOME

Survival

In the two decades from the mid 1970s to the mid 1990s, the proportion of 5-year survivors among children with cancer in North America has increased nearly 40%. Advances in the treatment of leukemias, lymphomas, sarcomas, brain tumors, germ cell neoplasms, and cancer of the kidney account for much of the improvement. Unfortunately, older adolescents with cancer have not fared as well. Table 18-7 shows the 5-year survival rates for all cancers and for different cancer types for each of the 5-year age intervals up to 19 years of age during 1985–1997. For all patients 15–19 years of age, the 5-year survival rate for the recent reporting period was 78%, which was slightly higher than that for each of the

TABLE 18-7

5-YEAR SURVIVAL RATES DURING 1985–1997 BY CANCER TYPE AND COMPARISON OF 15–19-YEAR OLDS WITH AGE GROUPS LESS THAN 15 YEARS

	Age at diagnosis (years)			
	0–4	*5–9*	*10–14*	*15–19*
All cancer	74.2	74.1	73.6	77.7
Cancer with a worse outcome in 15–19-year-olds than in <15-year-olds as a group				
Tumor group (ICCC category)*				
Lymphomas & reticuloendothelial neoplasms				
Hodgkin's disease	†	90.8	93.2	91.8
Non-Hodgkin's lymphoma	72.7	78.2	75.0	69.8
Leukemia	76.4	76.0	59.2	47.0
Acute lymphoblastic leukemia	83.9	82.3	68.7	54.3
Acute myeloid leukemia	38.8	47.3	41.4	38.3
Malignant bone tumors	†	70.9	66.2	62.9
Osteosarcoma	†	65.5	68.5	63.1
Ewing's sarcoma	†	74.4	56.6	54.8
Soft tissue sarcomas	76.2	74.4	70.6	64.7
Rhabdomyosarcoma, embryonal sarcoma	78.3	68.3	51.7	46.0
Renal tumors	91.1	88.7	88.0	75.6
Cancer with a comparable outcome in 15–19-year-olds and <15-year-olds as a group				
Central nervous system tumors	59.0	67.0	73.1	75.9
Astrocytoma	80.3	74.7	75.6	74.4
Other gliomas	56.7	43.4	68.2	75.1
Germ cell, trophoblastic	86.2	81.1	85.5	90.3
Carcinomas	73.7	91.9	90.5	89.1

Source: Modified from Bleyer 2002; data from United States National Cancer Institute Surveillance, Epidemiology, and End Results program.
*International Classification of Childhood Cancer.
†Statistic could not be calculated.

5-year intervals younger than 15 years of age. Whereas the 5-year-survival between 1975 and 1998 improved 36%–40% among children younger than 15 years old, the corresponding increment was only 23% in 15–19-year olds (Fig. 18-5). If this trend continued until 2000, the 5-year survival rate reached 80% in 15–19-year olds and 85% in younger patients, reversing the 10% advantage in the 5-year survival rate for older adolescents diagnosed in 1975 to a disadvantage of 5% for these patients in 2000.

AML, ALL, the bone sarcomas (osteosarcoma and Ewing's sarcoma) and the soft-tissue sarcomas (rhabdomyosarcoma and other soft-tissue sarcomas), NHL, and renal tumors have shown less improvement in survival in older adolescents than the gains seen in children (Fig. 18-6). Brain tumors in 15–19-year olds have outcomes equal or better (5-year survival = 76%) than in younger patients, but it is the histologic type and stage of brain tumors seen during late adolescence that drive the more favorable prognosis, not age independently. Older adolescents with thyroid carcinoma, melanoma, and germ cell tumors have fared as well as younger patients with the corresponding malignancy, with a survival that is so high (>95%) that a relative difference cannot be feasibly demonstrated.

Reasons for this lack of progress include issues specific to this age group. Some are inherent in the disease or the patient (differences in biology or intolerance of therapy), some are inherent in the system (treatment by physicians less familiar with the disease, delay in recognition of malignancy (Pollack, 1991), lack of availability, and participation in clinical trials), and some are influenced by the psychosocial milieu of the patient (lack of medical insurance and financial resources, delays in seeking medical attention with symptoms of cancer, poor compliance with treatment, and unwillingness to participate in clinical trials).

There is evidence that in the United States the diagnosis of cancer in 15–19-year-olds is significantly delayed in those who are under- or uninsured than in those with private insurance (Bleyer et al., 2005).

More than 90% of children less than 15 years of age with cancer are managed at institutions that are members of an NCI-sponsored clinical trials organization, and 65% are entered on clinical trials.

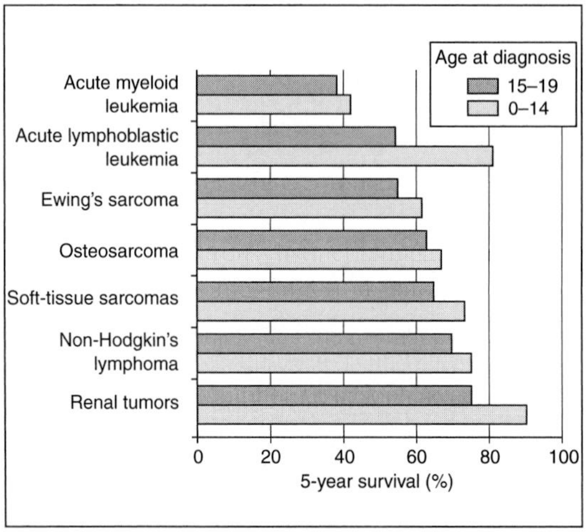

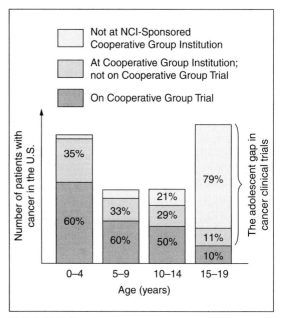

FIGURE   18 - 6

5-YEAR SURVIVAL RATES FROM 1974–1976 TO 1992–1997, BY TYPES OF TUMOR.
Source: Data from the United States National Cancer Institute Surveillance, Epidemiology, and End Results program. Modified from Bleyer 2002.

FIGURE   18 - 7

THE "ADOLESCENT GAP" IN CANCER CLINICAL TRIALS. MODIFIED FROM BLEYER 2002.

In contrast, about 20% of 15–19-year olds with cancer are seen at one of these institutions, and only about 10% of the patients are entered onto a clinical trial (Fig. 18-7) (Bleyer, 1996, 1997, 2002). This gap has been observed throughout the United States and spares no geographic region or ethnic group. This dramatic deficit in clinical trial participation in older adolescents may help explain a lower than expected level of progress in older adolescents and young adults. There is evidence that children who participate in clinical trials have a more favorable outcome than those who do not (Murphy, 1995).

Quality of Survival

The quality of life is generally poor for the cancer patient during the period of active therapy. The acute and delayed toxic effects of cancer therapy are undeniably among the worst toxic effects associated with the treatment of any chronic disease. Acute nausea, vomiting, mucositis, alopecia, weight gain or excessive weight loss, acne, bleeding and infection are to be expected. During treatment, delayed complications may be of less concern to patients in this age group (whose vision of the future is myopic) than to older adults and parents of younger children, but after therapy has been completed, such complications can be surprisingly disheartening, fearful, and can have terrible consequences. Examples include second malignancies, depression, infertility, avascular necrosis, cognitive dysfunction, or cardiac failure.

Remarkably little has been published on the quality of life of survivors of cancer during adolescence. Most of the reports are on adolescent survivors of childhood cancer, instead of survivors of cancer during adolescence, and may not be appropriate to extrapolate. In one study, 41 adolescents who were evaluated at a mean age of 17 had completed treatment for cancer at 2–8 years of age. Of these, one quarter had poor global functioning or was considered counterphobic and hypochondriacal (Fritz and Williams, 1988). About one-half of the survivors had body image problems, and many had subtle concerns about sexuality, attractiveness to the opposite sex, and reproductive capacity,

which may not be different than the general population at this age. Depression was found to be no more common (8%) than in the general age-matched population (7%), and self-concept scores were higher than the normative values. Another study also reported higher risk-taking behavior among survivors of Hodgkin's disease that occurred during childhood or adolescence (Wasserman, 1987).

Many adolescent and young adult cancer survivors cite fertility as a primary concern that impacts the quality of their life. Yet most do not recall an adequate discussion of the risks of infertility or methods to decrease the risks with their physician at the initiation of therapy (Duffy, 2005). The provider must consider the estimated risk of infertility, the patient's maturity, and the need to initiate therapy immediately in framing the conversation about infertility and the options of germ cell preservation. Rates of infertility are very hard to predict for an individual and depend on gender, age, radiation dose and schedule, and chemotherapeutic agent and dose.

Because of a decreasing pool of ovarian follicles, rates of amenorrhea and infertility are positively associated with increasing age of the female patient at the time of treatment, so that the rates in adolescents and between the lower rates. Although permanent failure may not occur, there may be more subtle changes, including decreased libido and premature menopause (with resultant increase in risk of osteoporosis, heart disease, and so forth), which only prolonged follow-up of many cancer survivors will quantify. Even if ovulation does return after the end of therapy, the patient should be counseled about the risk of premature ovarian failure, as it may narrow the window of fertility. There are no established techniques to preserve fertility for women undergoing chemotherapy but experimental approaches are being studied at specialized centers.

Rates of infertility appear higher in male survivors than female. Thankfully, fertility preservation options are more feasible and successful. Sperm cryopreservation should be discussed with all sexually mature males, usually collected via masturbation but epididymal aspiration and testicular wedge biopsy are also possible options. After both radiation and chemotherapy, spermatogenesis may return after years of apparent azoospermia and adolescents should be counseled regarding this possibility.

Other late effects are specific to the therapies received (Table 18-4). The patient should be educated by their oncologist about the possibility of these and the primary care physician and oncologist should coordinate monitoring for them. This task is aided by a comprehensive document prepared by the Children's Oncology Group and available on their Web site www.survivorshipguidelines.org. The follow-up for adolescent cancer patients is made difficult not only by their sense of invincibility (especially after surviving cancer), and their mediocre compliance, but, if they have received care in a pediatric system, their inevitable transition to adult services.

CONCLUSIONS

Adolescents with cancer are unique and have special needs in virtually every aspect of cancer management, be it detection, diagnosis, treatment, or follow-up. The array of types of cancer that affect this age group does not occur at any other age, and several types of cancer peak in incidence during this age interval. About one-third of the cancers are adult types of malignancies and approximately one-half of the types of cancer are pediatric in nature in that they are common among childhood cancers. Cancer is nearly twofold more common in adolescents 15–19 years of age than in 5–14-year-olds. Diagnosis is often delayed and many adolescents present with metastases or disseminated disease.

Their epidemiologic, medical, physical, psychologic, and social needs remain largely unmet despite their age juxtaposition with younger patients whose outcomes have so much improved. There is evidence of a lower degree of reduction in cancer mortality in the United States and Canada in adolescents than in younger or older persons. In the United States, only about 10% of 15–19-year olds with cancer are entered onto clinical trials, in contrast to 60%–65% of younger patients providing at least a partial explanation for the relative lack of progress.

Cancer during adolescence and early adulthood has been relatively neglected as an independent topic and merits enhanced national research programs and resources. Improvements in the overall survival, quality of care, and quality of survival of adolescents with cancer will require surmounting the challenges unique to this group of patients.

Bibliography

Albritton K, Bleyer A: The management of cancer in the older adolescent. Europ J Ca 39:2548–2599, 2003.

American Academy of Pediatrics. Immunocompromised Children. In: Pickering LK, ed. Red Book: 2003 Report of the Committee on Infectious Diseases. 26th ed. Elk Grove Village, IL: American Academy of Pediatrics; 2003:69–81. Available at: http://aapredbook.aappublications.org/cgi/content/full/2003/1/1.6.3.

American Academy of Pediatrics Section on Hematology/ Oncology: Guidelines for the Pediatric Cancer Center and role of such centers in diagnosis and treatment. Pediatrics 99:139–141, 1997.

American Federation of Clinical Oncologic Societies. Consensus statement on access to quality cancer care. J Pediatr Hematol Oncol 20:279–281, 1998.

Bleyer A, Albritton K: Special considerations for the young adult and adolescent. In Kufe DW, Pollack RE, Weichselbaum RR, Bast RC, Holland JF, Frei E (eds), Cancer Medicine, 6th ed, BC Decker, Hamilton, Ontario, BC, pp. 2414–2422, 2003.

Bleyer A: Older adolescents with cancer in North America: Deficits in outcome and research. Pediatr Clin North Am 49:1027–1042, 2002.

Bleyer A, Ulrich C, Martin S, Munsell M, Lange G, Taylor S: Status of health insurance predicts time from symptom onset to cancer diagnosis in young adults. Proc Am Soc Clin Oncol 23(16S):547s, 2005.

Bleyer WA, Montello M, Budd T, et al.: Cancer incidence, mortality, and survival: Young adults are lagging further behind. Proc Am Soc Clin Oncol 21:389a, 2002.

Bleyer WA, Tejeda H, Murphy SM, et al.: National cancer clinical trials: Children have equal access, adolescents do not. J Adol Health 21:366–373, 1997.

Bleyer WA: The adolescent gap in cancer treatment. J Registry Management 23:114–115, 1996.

Brady AM, Harvey C: The practice patterns of adult oncologists' care of pediatric oncology patients. Cancer 71(10 Suppl):3237–3240, 1993.

Corpron CA, Black CT, Singletary SE et al.: Breast cancer in adolescent females. J Pediatr Surg 30:322–324, 1995.

Duffy CM, Allen SM, Clark MA: Discussions regarding reproductive health for young women with breast cancer undergoing chemotherapy. J Clin Oncol 23(4): 766–773, 2005.

Dunsmore J, Quine S: Information, support and decision making needs and preferences of adolescents with cancer: Implications for health professionals. J Psychosoc Oncol 13:39–56, 1995.

Ferrari A, Dileo P, Casanova M, et al.: Rhabdomyosarcoma in adults. A retrospective analysis of 171 patients treated at a single institution. Cancer 98(3):571–580, 2003.

Franks LM, Bollen A, Seeger RC, et al.: Neuroblastoma in adults and adolescents: An indolent course with poor survival. Cancer 79:2028–2035, 1997.

Friman PC, Finney JW, Glasscock SG, et al.: Testicular self-examination: Validation of a training strategy for early cancer detection. J Appl Behav Anal 19: 87–92, 1986.

Fritz GK, Williams JR: Issues of adolescent development for survivors of childhood cancer. J Am Acad Child Adolesc Psychiatr 27:712–715, 1988.

Golden E, Beach B, Hastings C: The pediatrician and medical care of the child with cancer. Pediatr Clin North Am 49:1319–1338, 2002.

Kyngas HA, Kroll T, Duffy ME: Compliance in adolescents with chronic disease: A review. J Adol Med 26:379–388, 2000.

Lewis IJ: Cancer in adolescence. Br Med Bull 52:887–897, 1996.

Manne S, Miller D: Social support, social conflict, and adjustment among adolescent with cancer. J Pediatr Psychol 23:121–130, 1998.

Mills R and Bhandari S: Health Insurance Coverage in the United States: Current Population Reports, US Census Bureau 60–223, *http://www.census.gov/prod/ 2003pubs/ p60-223.pdf*, 2003.

Mitchell AE, Scarcella DL, Rigutto GL, et al.: Cancer in adolescents and young adults: Treatment and outcome in Victoria. Med J Aust 180:59–62, 2004.

Murphy SB: The National Impact of Clinical Cooperative Group Trials for Pediatric Cancer. Med Pediatr Oncol 24:279–280, 1995.

Novakovic B, Fears TR, Wexler LH, et al.: Experience of cancer in children and adolescents. Cancer Nurs 19:54–59, 1996.

Oeffinger KC, Mertens AC, Hudson MM, et al.: Health care of young adult survivors of childhood cancer: A report from the Childhood Cancer Survivor Study. Am Fam Med 2:61–70, 2004.

Orudjev E, Lange BJ: Evolving concepts of management of febrile neutropenia in children with cancer. Med Pediatr Oncol 39:77–85, 2002.

Paulussen S, Ahrens S, Juergens HF: Cure rates in Ewing tumor patients aged over 15 years are better in pediatric oncology units. Results of GPOH CESS/EICESS studies. Proc Amer Soc Clin Oncol 22:816, 2003.

Pollock BH, Krischer JP, Vietti TJ: Interval between symptom onset and diagnosis of pediatric solid tumors. J Pediatr 119:725–732, 1991.

Rait DS, Ostroff J, Smith K, et al.: Lives in balance: perceived family functioning and the psychosocial adjustment of adolescent cancer survivers. Fam Process 4:383–397, 1992.

Reaman GB, Bonfiglio J, Krailo M, et al.: Cancer in adolescents and young adults. Cancer 71 (Suppl): 3206–3209, 1993.

Ries LAG, Eisner MP, Kosary CL, et al. (eds): SEER Cancer Statistics Rev, 1975–2001, National Cancer Institute, Bethesda, MD. 2004. *http://seer.cancer.gov/ csr/1975_2001.*

Schiffer C, Anderson K, Bennett C, et al.: Platelet transfusion for patients with cancer: Clinical practice guidelines of The American Society of Clinical Oncology. J Clin Oncol 19:1519–1538, 2001.

Smith MA, Gurney JG, Ries LA: Cancer in adolescents 15–19 years old. In: Ries LAG, Smith MA, Gurney JG, Linet M, Tamra T, Young JL, Bunin GR (eds): Cancer incidence and survival among children and adolescents: United States SEER Program 1975–1997, National Cancer Institute, SEER Program. NIH Pub No. 99-4649, Bethesda, MD, 1999.

Stock W, Sather H, Dodge RK, et al. Outcome of adolescents and young adults with ALL: a comparison of Children's Cancer Group (CCG) and Cancer and Leukemia Group B (CALGB) regimens. Blood 96(11):467a, 2000.

Thomson AB, Critchley HO, Wallace WH: Fertility and progeny. Eur J Cancer 38:1634–1644, 2002.

Verrill MW, Judson IR, Fisher C, et al.: The use of paediatric chemotherapy protocols at full dose is both a rational and feasible treatment strategy in adults with Ewing's family tumours. Ann Oncol 8:1099–1105, 1997.

Wasserman AL, Thompson EI, Wilimas JA, et al.: The psychological status of survivors of childhood/adolescent Hodgin's disease. Am J Dis Child 14:141:626–631, 1987.

Whyte F, Smith L: A literature review of adolescence and cancer. Eur J Cancer Care 6:137–146, 1997.

Wiest MD, Finney JD: Training in early cancer detection and anxiety in adolescent males: A preliminary report. Dev Behav Pediatr 17:98–99, 1996.

Wites RE: Therapies for cancer in children—past successes, future challenges. N Engl J Med 2003; 348: 747–749.

19

DISORDERS OF THE SKIN

Daniel P. Krowchuk

INTRODUCTION

The management of skin conditions is an important component of adolescent health care. According to the National Ambulatory Medical Care Survey, an ongoing survey of office-based physician practice, in 2002 there were an estimated 37.5 million visits made by adolescents 12–19 years of age to general or family physicians, pediatricians, or internal medicine physicians. In 11% of visits, a diagnosis of a dermatologic disorder was made. Among the most commonly encountered conditions were acne, warts, and skin infections. This chapter reviews the identification and management of these and other dermatologic diseases that affect adolescents. Given limitations of space, the chapter is not all inclusive; it addresses those disorders most likely to be encountered by clinicians. Representative photographs of selected disorders are presented; for additional images, readers are referred to an online atlas (e.g., Dermatlas, available at *http://dermatlas.med.jhmi. edu/derm/*) or a standard text.

ACNE VULGARIS

Acne vulgaris is the most common skin disease treated by physicians. It is a disorder of the pilosebaceous follicle, a structure composed of a follicle, sebaceous gland, and rudimentary or vellus hair.

The concentration of pilosebaceous follicles is highest on the face, chest, and back, thus explaining the appearance of acne lesions in these areas.

Etiology

Although the exact cause of acne is not known, several factors contribute.

Androgens

Androgens play an integral role in acne. At age 8 or 9, prior to the appearance of secondary sexual characteristics, the adrenal glands begin to produce increasing amounts of the androgen dehydroepiandrosterone sulfate (DHEAS). Rising levels of DHEAS cause sebaceous glands to enlarge and produce more sebum. Sebum secretion peaks during adolescence and begins to decline after age 20; rates of sebum secretion correlate with acne severity. Despite the importance of androgens in causing acne, most patients have normal hormone levels, though some females have elevations of free testosterone and DHEAS, and reductions of sex hormone binding globulin.

Bacteria

Propionibacterium acnes is an anaerobic, gram-positive diphtheroid that colonizes pilosebaceous follicles. The organism uses sebum as a nutrient and its numbers correlate with the concentration of triglycerides in sebum. Although a normal skin inhabitant, *P. acnes* is more abundant in patients who have acne than in those who are unaffected. *P. acnes* produces chemoattractant factors that cause polymorphonuclear neutrophils (PMNs) to enter pilosebaceous follicles. As PMNs ingest *P. acnes*, enzymes are released that damage the follicle wall, resulting in dispersion of follicular contents into the surrounding tissue. In addition, within the follicle, *P. acnes* hydrolyzes triglycerides to free fatty acids, a factor that may contribute to the inflammatory process and increase follicular obstruction.

Abnormal Keratinization

Pilosebaceous follicles are lined with squamous epithelium that is continuous with the skin surface. In persons who have acne, epithelial cells lining the follicle are not shed properly resulting in a collection of cells and sebum within the follicle. This process, called comedogenesis, is central to the development of acne lesions.

Genetics

Although familial trends are well recognized in patients who have acne, an exact pattern of inheritance has not been defined and it is not possible to predict the severity of disease in an individual patient based on family history.

Clinical Manifestations

Initially, obstruction within the follicle is microscopic and cannot be perceived clinically; such lesions are termed microcomedones. As comedones enlarge, they become apparent as open comedones (blackheads) or closed comedones (whiteheads). Open comedones represent follicles with widely dilated orifices. Closed comedones are small white or skin-colored papules without surrounding erythema. They represent follicles that have become dilated with cellular and lipid debris but possess only microscopic openings to the skin surface. Patients who have inflammatory acne exhibit erythematous

papules (<5 mm), pustules, or nodules (≥5 mm). After inflammatory lesions resolve, erythematous or hyperpigmented macules may remain for as long as 12 months and are often mistaken for true scars. Some patients, particularly those with nodules, develop scars as inflammatory lesions resolve. On the face, acne scars have the appearance of pits, while on the trunk they look like small hypopigmented spots. True cysts, compressible nodules that lack overlying inflammation, also may be observed in patients who have acne.

Management

Adolescents and their families should be advised about the causes of acne and possible exacerbating factors (including the use of oil-based skin care products, picking at or traumatizing lesions, wearing athletic gear that applies pressure to the skin); myths about acne (e.g., the role of diet and the need for vigorous washing of the skin) should be dispelled. They should be counseled that a realistic goal of treatment is to reduce the number and severity of lesions and to prevent scarring, and that 6–8 weeks may be required for medications to work. Although there is no standardized treatment plan for acne, rational guidelines exist based on the types and extent of lesions present, and the severity of disease (Table 19-1). The severity of facial acne may be graded as mild (one fourth or less of the face involved, no nodules, no scarring), moderate (one half of the face involved, few nodules), or severe (three fourths of the face involved, many nodules, scars may be present). Medications used to treat acne may be separated into topical and systemic preparations.

Topical Therapies

Benzoyl Peroxide

Benzoyl peroxide (BP) has an antibacterial effect and is useful in controlling inflammatory acne. It may also decrease the formation of free fatty acids, thereby improving obstructive (comedonal) disease. These two actions make it a useful first-line drug in the management of patients who have mild inflammatory or mixed (i.e., inflammatory and comedonal) acne. BP also prevents the emergence of antibiotic

TABLE 19-1

MANAGEMENT OPTIONS FOR FACIAL ACNE

Acne Severity	Lesion Type	Initial Treatment	If No Response
Mild	Comedonal	BP or topical retinoid*	If BP used initially, substitute with or add topical retinoid* once daily
	Inflammatory	BP (or topical combination preparation†)	Increase BP application to twice daily, or substitute combination product† or oral antibiotic‡
	Mixed (i.e., comedones and inflammatory lesions)	BP (or topical combination product†) alone or with topical retinoid* Azelaic acid as monotherapy	If BP used initially, add topical retinoid* once daily (for comedonal component) and/or substitute topical combination product† or oral antibiotic‡ (for inflammatory component)
Moderate	Comedonal	Topical retinoid*	Increase strength of topical retinoid*
	Inflammatory	Topical combination product† (or oral antibiotic‡,§)	If topical combination product† used, add or substitute oral antibiotic‡,§ and add topical retinoid*
	Mixed (i.e., comedones and inflammatory lesions)	Topical combination product† (or oral antibiotic‡,§) and topical retinoid* Azelaic acid as monotherapy	Increase strength of topical retinoid* (for comedonal component) If combination product† used alone, substitute oral antibiotic‡,§ (for inflammatory component) and add topical retinoid*
Severe	Comedonal	Topical retinoid* once daily	Increase strength of topical retinoid* or refer to dermatologist
	Inflammatory	Oral antibiotic‡,§ and topical retinoid*	Consider alternate antibiotic‡,§ or refer to dermatologist
	Mixed (i.e., comedones and inflammatory lesions)	Oral antibiotic‡,§ and topical retinoid*	Consider increasing strength of topical retinoid* (for comedonal component) and/or beginning alternate antibiotic‡,§ (for inflammatory component), or refer to dermatologist

* For example, tretinoin cream 0.025%, Retin-A gel micro 0.04% and 0.1%; Differin; or Avita.

† For example, clindamycin or erythromycin combined with BP (clindamycin and erythromycin used alone are not favored due to potential antibiotic resistance).

‡ For example, tetracycline (or possibly erythromycin) 250–500 mg twice daily.

§ Some experts advise the use BP in patients treated with oral antibiotics to prevent the emergence of antibiotic resistant *P. acnes*.

resistance among *P. acnes*; therefore, it may be used adjunctively for patients receiving long-term antibiotic therapy. BP is available with or without a prescription in concentrations ranging from 2.5% to 10% and in a variety of vehicles, including creams, lotions, washes, or gels. The application of a product containing a 5% concentration once or twice daily is adequate for most patients. As with all topical acne medications, patients should be advised to apply a thin coat of medication to the affected area (a pea-sized amount should be sufficient to cover the face). To treat larger areas, such as the chest or back, a BP wash may be employed, though it may be somewhat less effective than a form that is left on the skin. Common adverse effects include drying, erythema, and burning. These may be lessened or prevented by using a water-based gel or an emollient vehicle. BP also may bleach bedding and clothing.

Topical Antibiotics

Topical antibiotics reduce concentrations of *P. acnes* and inflammatory mediators. As a result, they are useful in treating mild to moderate inflammatory acne that is limited to the face. Topical clindamycin and erythromycin are used most commonly, though concerns about bacterial resistance may limit their efficacy when used as single agents. Products that combine BP 5% and clindamycin or erythromycin prevent this resistance and are more effective than either drug alone. For this reason, they are preferred by many clinicians. Sodium sulfacetamide, with or without sulfur, also is available.

Topical Retinoids

Topical retinoids are indicated for patients who have numerous comedones. These agents normalize the keratinization process within follicles, reducing obstruction and the risk for follicular rupture. A topical retinoid also is recommended in those who have moderate to severe inflammatory acne, even in the absence of clinical evidence of obstructive lesions. Tretinoin (Retin-A and others) is available in creams (0.025%, 0.05%, 0.1%), gels (0.01%, 0.025%), and a liquid (0.05%). The vehicle has an impact on efficacy; creams are less potent (and less irritating) than gels (which are of greatest benefit for patients who have oily skin). Newer formulations (e.g., Retin-A Micro Gel 0.04%, 0.1%, and Avita) appear to be as effective but less irritating than traditional varieties. Tretinoin is also available in generic form.

Other retinoids are also available. Adapalene (Differin) has been shown to be as effective as tretinoin but less irritating. It is available as a 0.1% gel, cream, solution, or as pads. Tazarotene (Tazorac) is formulated in 0.05% and 0.1% gels and creams. Although proven effective in clinical studies,

tazarotene is more expensive and may be more irritating than other retinoids. For these reasons, it is not widely prescribed for the treatment of acne.

Many adolescents who use retinoids experience irritation, redness, or dryness, though this may be avoided or minimized by initiating therapy with a low strength preparation (e.g., tretinoin cream 0.025% or adapalene) and advising use every third night progressing as tolerated to nightly application over 2–3 weeks. Other adverse effects include an apparent temporary worsening of acne 2–3 weeks after beginning treatment and increased sensitivity to sunlight caused by skin irritation. Since BP inactivates topical retinoids, the two drugs should not be applied simultaneously. Rather, BP or a combination product (BP with an antibiotic) may be applied in the morning and the retinoid at night. Although there have been no reports of malformations occurring in infants born to women who used tretinoin during pregnancy, it and adapalene are classified as pregnancy category C and, therefore, should not be used during pregnancy. Tazarotene is classified as category X and is contraindicated in pregnancy. For those who cannot tolerate topical retinoids, products containing salicylic acid may be beneficial.

Azelaic Acid

Azelaic acid 20% (Azelex) is both antibacterial and anticomedonal. It is applied twice daily and appears to be well tolerated, although some patients experience pruritus, burning, stinging, tingling, or erythema. Azelaic acid is an alternative for patients who have mild to moderate inflammatory and comedonal acne, or those who cannot tolerate tretinoin.

Systemic Therapies

Oral Antibiotics

Oral antibiotics possess greater efficacy than topical preparations and, for this reason, are prescribed for patients who have severe or extensive inflammatory acne. They exert their anti-inflammatory effect by decreasing bacterial colonization and inhibiting neutrophil chemotaxis; however, they also reduce the concentration of free fatty acids in sebum. Although many antibiotics are used to treat acne, tetracycline and erythromycin are most often prescribed initially. For those who fail to respond to or cannot tolerate tetracycline or erythromycin, doxycycline or minocycline often are effective (Table 19-2). As with other acne therapies, 6–8 weeks often are required before oral antibiotics produce a significant clinical effect. Once the appearance of new lesions has ceased or been satisfactorily reduced, the dose may be tapered or eventually withdrawn in favor of topical agents.

An area of concern related to the use of systemic or topical antibiotics is the emergence of resistant forms of *P. acnes*. Over the past three decades, in some geographic areas the percent of patients carrying antibiotic-resistant organisms has risen from 20% to 60%. Resistance to erythromycin is observed most often and cross resistance to clindamycin and other macrolide antibiotics is frequent. Among tetracyclines, resistance to tetracycline is more common than to doxycycline and rare to minocycline. With this

issue in mind, some clinicians do not prescribe oral erythromycin for acne or use it only for previously untreated patients who are unlikely to harbor resistant organisms. Similarly, the use of topical erythromycin or clindamycin as monotherapy (i.e., not combined with BP) may be ineffective due to bacterial resistance. Adding BP to the treatment program decreases bacterial resistance and is recommended for patients who are receiving long-term antibiotic therapy.

Isotretinoin

Isotretinoin (13-cis retinoic acid, Accutane, and others) is an oral analog of vitamin A that is highly effective for the treatment of severe, scarring acne. It typically is prescribed at a dose of 0.5–1.0 mg/kg/day for a course of 16–20 weeks. Despite its efficacy, oral isotretinoin therapy may be associated with important adverse reactions, the most serious of which is

TABLE 19-2

SOME ORAL ANTIBIOTICS USED IN THE TREATMENT OF ACNE

Antibiotic	Dose	Selected Adverse Effects
Tetracycline	250–500 mg bid	Must be taken on empty stomach
		Should not be used during pregnancy or in those <8 years of age
		Gastrointestinal upset
		Esophageal ulceration
		Photosensitivity
		Pseudotumor cerebri
		Onycholysis
Erythromycin	250–500 mg bid	Gastrointestinal upset
		Potential *P. acnes* resistance
Doxycycline	50–100 mg bid	Analogous to tetracycline
		More likely than tetracycline to cause photosensitivity
Minocycline	50–100 mg bid	Analogous to tetracycline
		Dizziness
		Pigmentation of skin, teeth, mucosa (uncommon)
		Autoimmune syndromes: serum-sickness-like reaction, hypersensitivity syndrome, lupus-like syndrome, hepatitis (all rare)

teratogenicity. Presently, all isotretinoin prescriptions require that a qualification sticker be affixed. To obtain these, physicians must have read educational materials provided by the manufacturer and signed a letter of understanding regarding the use of the drug and its potential adverse effects. However, it is anticipated that the Food and Drug Administration (FDA) will soon implement a strengthened risk minimalization action plan that will include a registry of prescribers, patients, and dispensing pharmacies. Reports to the FDA have raised concern that isotretinoin use may predispose patients to depression or suicide. Although an association has not been clearly demonstrated, clinicians caring for patients who are receiving isotretinoin should remain alert to the presence or development of mental health disorders, including depression and suicidal ideation.

Hormonal Therapy

Combined oral contraceptives (OCs), those containing an estrogen and progestin, may improve acne by reducing free testosterone and ovarian androgen production. Despite this, these agents are not viewed as a primary therapy for acne but as an adjunct to standard medications.

Follow-Up

A follow-up visit typically is scheduled 2 months following initiation of therapy to assess compliance, determine the patient's impression of response to treatment, discuss any adverse effects, and make an objective assessment of the effect of therapy. Based on this information, adjustments to the treatment program can be made.

DERMATITIS

Atopic Dermatitis

In adolescents, atopic dermatitis usually represents a continuation of disease that began during infancy or childhood. Its cause is unknown but likely is multifactorial; genetics, the environment, a defective skin barrier, and altered immunologic responses all appear to play a role.

Clinical Manifestations

The manifestations of atopic dermatitis vary with the patient's age and racial background. Adolescents exhibit flexural involvement (e.g., antecubital and popliteal fossae) but may develop lesions on the hands, neck, and face. Lesions often appear as dry, sometimes scaling patches, but erosions may occur. Those who have lightly pigmented skin exhibit lesions that are erythematous and tend to be flat. In persons of color, erythema is less obvious, the eruption often is papular, and postinflammatory hypo- or hyperpigmentation may be present. Generally the skin is dry, a factor that is exacerbated by decreased environmental humidity during colder months. However, flares also may occur during warmer months as a result of becoming overheated. In response to chronic scratching, the skin may become thickened with accentuated skin creases (i.e., lichenification).

Since individuals who have atopic dermatitis frequently are colonized with *Staphylococcus aureus*, scratching may lead to secondary infection characterized by increasing erythema and erosions. Individuals who have atopic dermatitis also are prone to viral infections, including herpes simplex virus (HSV) infection (i.e., eczema herpeticum) and molluscum contagiosum.

The diagnosis of atopic dermatitis is made clinically. The essential criteria include pruritus, typical morphology and distribution of the rash, a chronic relapsing course, and a personal or family history of atopy.

Management

The management of atopic dermatitis rests upon daily skin care (designed to prevent disease flares) (Table 19-3) and treatment of exacerbations (Table 19-4). Daily measures are intended to hydrate the skin (since most patients have dry skin that contributes to itching and scratching) and control pruritus (primarily through the avoidance of precipitants).

TABLE 19-3

DAILY MEASURES TO MANAGE ATOPIC DERMATITIS

Control Pruritus	*Hydrate the Skin*
• Apply an emollient once or twice daily as needed to control dry skin (one application should take place immediately after emerging from a bath or shower). Lotions work well for most individuals. Ointments are the best moisturizers but, because of their greasy feel, may not be well tolerated.	• Apply an emollient once or twice daily as needed.
• Use a mild, unscented soap or soap substitute for bathing.	• Limit the frequency of bathing. Bathing too often can dry the skin and remove natural moisturizing factors.
• Use a mild detergent for laundering clothes.	• Consider the use of a room vaporizer or humidifier during cold weather months.
• To the extent possible, wear cotton clothing next to the skin. Avoid bathing in very hot water.	

Although food allergies play a role in a minority of children, this is less likely in adolescents. The role of inhalants (pollen, mold, and dust mites) is controversial.

During disease flares, the keys to management are to reduce inflammation (through the application of a topical corticosteroid or noncorticosteroid immuno-modulator), control pruritus (by using a sedating antihistamine at bedtime), and treat secondary infection, if present (Table 19-4). As an exacerbation improves, topical corticosteroids may be withdrawn or tapered in strength, and the antihistamine discontinued.

Contact Dermatitis

Contact dermatitis occurs when an antigen penetrates the epidermis and sensitizes T lymphocytes. For potent antigens, such as urushiol (present in poison ivy, oak, and sumac), sensitization takes 7–10 days; weaker agents may require multiple exposures over many weeks. Once sensitization

TABLE 19-4

TREATING FLARES OF ATOPIC DERMATITIS

Reduce inflammation
- Apply a topical corticosteroid twice daily as needed.
  - Face or anatomically occluded area: Use a low-potency preparation (e.g., hydrocortisone cream 1% or 2.5%).
  - Extremities: Use a mid-potency preparation (e.g., triamcinolone cream 0.1%).
  - Hands or feet: Use a mid-potency preparation. However, a more potent agent (e.g., fluocinonide 0.05% cream or ointment may be required).
- Apply a topical immunomodulator (e.g., tacrolimus). These agents are effective but expensive. They are most useful in the management of facial dermatitis (where potent topical corticosteroids cannot be used) or adjunctively (with topical corticosteroids) in the management of recalcitrant dermatitis.

Control pruritus: Use a bedtime dose of a sedating antihistamine.

Control infection: If there is evidence of secondary bacterial infection (e.g., crusting or oozing) consider an oral anti-staphylococcal antibiotic (e.g., cephalexin).

occurs, reexposure to the antigen will induce an eruption within 12–24 hours.

Potent antigens such as urushiol typically cause an acute dermatitis manifested by vesicles, bullae, erythematous papules, and edema. Lesions may appear in a linear array or be distributed in a patchy fashion. The rapidity of onset and severity of the rash depend on an individual's sensitivity to the antigen and the amount of antigen in contact with the skin. Thus, a concentrated application of the resin produces vesicles while a less intense exposure results in fine erythematous papules. New lesions continue to appear over several days and, if untreated, the rash may persist for 3–4 weeks.

In contrast, weaker antigens produce erythema, scaling, and lichenification (i.e., a subacute dermatitis). Antigens commonly responsible include nickel (present in jewelry, belt buckles, or clothing snaps); potassium dichromate (present in some shoes); neomycin, thimerosal, or formaldehyde (used in topical medications); or Balsam of Peru or other fragrances (used in perfumes or soaps). The key to recognizing contact dermatitis is the observation that the eruption is limited to certain areas (Table 19-5).

If the contact dermatitis is mild, a mid-potency topical corticosteroid (e.g., triamcinolone 0.1%) may be applied. However, when more than 10%–15% of the body surface is involved, the disease is severe, or areas such as the face or perineum are significantly affected, oral prednisone is recommended, tapering the dose over 12–21 days. Sedating oral antihistamines offer relief from itching.

TABLE 19-5

RECOGNIZING CONTACT DERMATITIS

Location of Lesions	Agent Likely Responsible
Linear lesions on exposed areas	Poison ivy, oak, sumac
Ear, neck, wrist, umbilicus	Nickel in jewelry
Below umbilicus	Nickel in clothing snap or belt buckle
Eyelid	Rubber in eye shadow applicator
	Colophony (pine resin) in mascara
	Acrylates in artificial nails, nail repair kits
Face	Preservatives or perfumes in cosmetics
	Rubber in make-up applicator or removal sponge
	Cocoamidylpropyl betaine in shampoo
	Acrylates in artificial nails, nail repair kits, eyeglass frames
	Nickel in eyeglass frames
Dorsal feet	Potassium dichromate used in shoe leather

2% ketoconazole cream or 1% hydrocortisone cream.

Seborrheic Dermatitis

Seborrheic dermatitis is a disorder of uncertain cause, though it may be related to an inflammatory response to the yeast *Pityrosporum ovale*. In adolescents, it presents as scaling of the scalp, eyebrows, or eyelashes, or as erythematous scaling patches in the nasolabial folds, postauricular creases, or presternal regions. Scalp involvement is treated with an antiseborrheic shampoo (e.g., one containing zinc pyrithione, selenium sulfide, ketoconazole, or tar). If signs of inflammation are present, a mid-potency corticosteroid solution may be applied to the scalp as needed at bedtime. Skin lesions respond to the application of

Dyshidrotic Eczema

Dyshidrotic eczema likely represents a variant of atopic dermatitis. It is not, as the name suggests, related to dysfunction of the eccrine apparatus. The condition affects the hands and feet, particularly the palms, soles, and lateral aspects of the digits, with deep-seated, intensely pruritic vesicles (Fig. 19-1). Conditions to be differentiated from dyshidrotic eczema include contact dermatitis, fungal infection, and an id reaction. Treatment involves the application of a mid- to high-potency corticosteroid twice daily during flares. If erosions are severe, wet-to-dry dressings may be employed to promote drying.

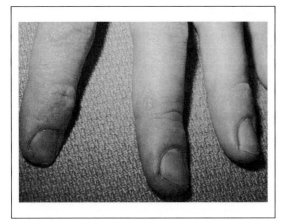

FIGURE 19-1

DYSHIDROTIC ECZEMA IS CHARACTERIZED BY TINY VESICLES TYPICALLY LOCATED ON THE LATERAL ASPECTS OF THE DIGITS.

Pityriasis Alba

Pityriasis alba, commonly observed in patients who have atopic dermatitis, likely represents an area of mild inflammation that has disturbed the normal process of pigmentation. It is characterized by hypopigmented macules that may have a fine scale. Lesions are round or oval and occur most commonly on the face, though the neck, upper trunk, and proximal extremities may be affected. The borders of lesions are ill-defined with a gradual transition from normal to abnormal pigmentation. In less pigmented individuals, pityriasis alba often is noted following sun exposure; the normal skin becomes darker but affected areas do not, accentuating contrast between the two. The differential diagnosis includes tinea corporis, tinea versicolor, vitiligo, and psoriasis. Treatment is with an appropriate topical corticosteroid (e.g., hydrocortisone 1% or 2.5% for facial lesions) for 2–3 weeks to reduce inflammation. The patient should be counseled that repigmentation may take as long as 1 year.

DRUG REACTIONS

Exanthematous Drug Eruptions

Exanthematous eruptions are responsible for an estimated 50% of drug-induced rashes. They likely are immunologically mediated and typically appear 7–14 days after beginning a new medication, but may occur several days after discontinuing a drug. On rechallenge, the rash appears more rapidly. The eruption begins as erythematous macules that may become slightly elevated. Initially, the trunk and upper extremities are involved but the rash subsequently spreads more widely. Aminopenicillins, cephalosporins, sulfonamides, and anticonvulsants are common offending agents. Whenever possible, the agent believed to be responsible should be withdrawn. A topical corticosteroid and oral antihistamine may be used to control pruritus pending resolution of the eruption.

Urticarial Drug Eruptions

Urticarial eruptions account for approximately 25% of drug eruptions. These reactions are IgE-mediated, and their onset generally is sudden, usually occurring hours or days after drug exposure (prior sensitization to the drug results in a more rapid onset of the eruption). Individual lesions (i.e., wheals) are transient, but the entire process may last for 4–6 weeks. Urticaria may be accompanied by angioedema (i.e., edema of the subcutaneous and submucosal tissues resulting in swelling of the face, particularly the lips and eyes, or other areas) or, rarely, anaphylaxis. Antibiotics (e.g., penicillins, aminopenicillins, cephalosporins, and sulfonamides), nonsteroidal anti-inflammatory agents, and radiocontrast media are the agents most likely to cause this type of reaction. Treatment involves removing the suspected offending agent and administration of an antihistamine.

Fixed Drug Eruptions

Unlike other drug eruptions, fixed drug eruptions are localized in their distribution. Lesions are discrete, erythematous, or violaceous plaques that often are single or few in number and generally are asymptomatic. They commonly involve the lips, genitalia, hands, and feet. As the lesions resolve, they leave hyperpigmentation (Fig. 19-2). If the responsible drug is administered again, the rash will appear in the identical location. On initial exposure, the eruption begins within 1–2 weeks; on reexposure, it appears within 24 hours. Nonsteroidal anti-inflammatory agents, sulfonamides, barbiturates, tetracyclines, and

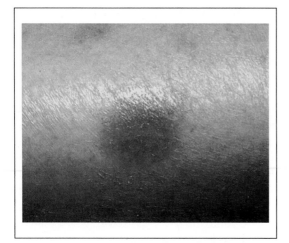

FIGURE 19-2

A HYPERPIGMENTED MACULE OFTEN OCCURS
DURING THE RESOLUTION OF A FIXED DRUG
ERUPTION.

carbamazepine most often are implicated. If a fixed drug eruption is diagnosed, future use of the drug should be avoided. The eruption may be treated with a topical corticosteroid and the patient advised that several months will be required for hyperpigmentation to resolve.

Hypersensitivity Syndrome

Hypersensitivity syndrome, also known as Drug Reaction with Eosinophilia and Systemic Symptoms (DRESS) is a severe reaction that likely results from defects in drug metabolism. It begins 2–6 weeks after initiating a drug. Patients develop fever and a morbilliform eruption; facial edema commonly is present. Lymphadenopathy and arthralgias may occur. Hepatitis may be fulminant; other complications include myocarditis, pneumonitis, and nephritis. Performance of a complete blood count reveals eosinophilia and, frequently, the presence of atypical lymphocytes. The agents most often implicated in the hypersensitivity syndrome are anticonvulsants (e.g., phenobarbital, phenytoin, carbamazepine, and lamotrigine), antibiotics (e.g., sulfonamides and minocycline), and allopurinol. Early withdrawal of the agent suspected is essential; systemic corticosteroids are employed in severe cases.

Other Drug Eruptions

Photosensitivity reactions, including phototoxic and photoallergic eruptions, are discussed in the section Photosensitivity Diseases (Drug Photosensitivity). Stevens-Johnson syndrome and toxic epidermal necrolysis are addressed in the section Hypersensitivity Disorders.

HAIR LOSS

Alopecia Areata

Alopecia areata is a disease of unknown cause, though autoimmune mechanisms are believed to be responsible. Affected individuals develop well-circumscribed round or oval patches of complete or nearly complete hair loss. The scalp is normal in appearance without scale, erythema, or scarring. At the periphery of lesions, short hairs (a few mm in length) that are broader distally than proximally (i.e., exclamation point hairs) may be seen. One or multiple patches of alopecia may be present. If all scalp hair is lost, the condition is termed alopecia totalis; alopecia universalis describes the loss of all body hair. Individuals who have alopecia areata often exhibit tiny punctate depressions in the nail surface (i.e., nail pits). Although alopecia areata may occur in association with other autoimmune diseases (e.g., Hashimoto thyroiditis and vitiligo) routine laboratory testing is not indicated.

The course of alopecia areata is unpredictable. Even without therapy the majority of patients regrow hair within a year, though nearly one third of these will experience a recurrence. When hair regrows, it often initially is white or hypopigmented. Individuals in whom alopecia areata appears in a bandlike distribution around the scalp (i.e., ophiasis) are at risk of losing all scalp hair and have a poor prognosis.

A wide variety of therapeutic techniques have been employed in alopecia areata with variable results. Initial treatment often involves intralesional or potent topical corticosteroids or topical minoxidil. Application of anthralin, tacrolimus or imiquimod, or contact sensitization (e.g., with squaric acid dibutyl ester or other agents) may be employed. For patients who have widespread hair loss, use of a wig may be beneficial. Most patients who have alopecia areata will benefit from consultation with a dermatologist. Support and information may be obtained from the National Alopecia Areata Foundation (available at *http://www.naaf.org/*).

Trichotillomania

Repetitive twirling, twisting, rubbing, or pulling the hair on the scalp or elsewhere may cause it to break, a condition called trichotillomania. Individuals who have scalp involvement exhibit well-defined but irregularly-shaped patches of alopecia. The hair loss is incomplete; within patches of relative alopecia are hairs of differing lengths (Fig. 19-3). The scalp usually appears normal, though petechiae or hemorrhagic crusts may be seen if the hair has been pulled out.

In most adolescents, trichotillomania represents a habit but in a minority it may be a reaction to stress or evidence of a more severe psychologic problem. Treatment focuses on behavioral modification: positive reinforcement is provided, and patients are encouraged to substitute another activity when tempted to manipulate their hair and to employ

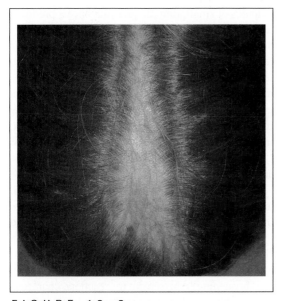

FIGURE   19 - 3

TRICHOTILLOMANIA IS A PATCH OF ALOPECIA WITHIN WHICH HAIRS ARE BROKEN AT DIFFERENT LENGTHS.

relaxation techniques. For those with severe or recalcitrant disease, referral to a mental health professional or institution of a selective serotonin reuptake inhibitor is indicated.

Telogen Effluvium

Telogen effluvium is characterized by diffuse but rarely complete hair loss. Normally, 90%–95% of hair follicles on the scalp are in the anagen (or growing) phase, which lasts for approximately 3 years. The remainder are in the telogen (or resting) state, which lasts for 3–6 months and is followed by shedding of hairs. As a result, it is normal to lose 50–100 hairs from the scalp daily. In telogen effluvium, a stressful event causes many of the follicles in the anagen phase to be converted to the telogen stage. Inciting factors include febrile illnesses, drug reactions, and the delivery of a baby. Hair loss begins 2–4 months after the inciting event. Telogen effluvium is self-limited; within 5–6 months hair regrowth is complete. The diagnosis may be confirmed by pulling out a few hairs and examining their roots. Anagen hairs have a large pigmented bulb; telogen hairs have smaller bulbs that lack pigment. In telogen effluvium, this examination demonstrates a larger than anticipated number of hairs in the telogen phase. Patients who have telogen effluvium should be reassured; no treatment is necessary.

Androgenetic Alopecia

Androgenetic alopecia (AGA) is believed to result from the effects of androgens on genetically susceptible hair follicles. Under the influence of dihydrotestosterone, genes are activated that reduce the length of the hair growth cycle and the size of the follicle. As a result, shorter and finer hairs are produced. In men, temporal and eventually frontal hairline recession is observed. Women typically have diffuse hair loss that is most noticeable at the vertex. For women with marked temporal recession or other signs of androgen excess, hormonal evaluation is indicated. The initial treatment of AGA in men is with minoxidil 5% applied topically or finasteride orally. In women, topical minoxidil often is employed.

HYPERSENSITIVITY REACTIONS

Urticaria

Urticaria is a common hypersensitivity reaction characterized by the release of mediators, principally histamine, from cutaneous mast cells. The lesions result from localized vasodilation (causing erythema) and transudation of fluid from capillaries and small blood vessels (causing swelling). Individual lesions (i.e., wheals) are transient, lasting a few hours and never longer than 24 hours. They are erythematous papules and plaques that may be round or oval, or form rings or arcs. Occasionally, the centers of lesions will appear dusky mimicking purpura or erythema multiforme (EM). Pruritus is a common feature. Approximately one half of patients have associated angioedema, a process analogous to urticaria that occurs in the submucosa, deep dermis, and subcutaneous tissue. It appears as poorly defined areas of swelling with little or no erythema often located around the eyes or lips.

Urticaria may be separated into acute (lasting <6 weeks) and chronic (lasting ≥6 weeks) forms. Acute urticaria has many causes but the agents most often responsible include drugs (e.g., antibiotics and nonsteroidal anti-inflammatory agents), foods (e.g., nuts, shellfish, strawberries, and peanuts), infections (e.g., *Streptococcus pyogenes*, many viruses, and parasites), and arthropod bites and stings. Less common causes are contactants (e.g., latex), systemic diseases (e.g., collagen vascular diseases and inflammatory bowel disease), occult infections (e.g., sinusitis and dental abscesses), blood products, and physical agents (e.g., heat, cold, pressure, light, vibration, and water). Cholinergic urticaria is a distinctive form manifested by the appearance of 2–3-mm papules surrounded by large erythematous flares. These flares are very pruritic and follow the onset of sweating. Given the wide variety of inciting agents, identifying the cause of urticaria often is difficult, particularly for patients who have chronic urticaria.

The disorders that may be confused with urticaria are EM and urticarial vasculitis. Although the lesions of EM are annular, unlike those of urticaria they remain fixed in location for 7 days or more; are concentrated on the distal extremities and face; do not assume unusual shapes such as large plaques or arcs; and develop a central change, such as a violaceous discoloration, vesicle, or crust. If urticarial appearing wheals persist longer than 24 hours, urticarial vasculitis should be suspected and a skin biopsy performed.

The first step in treatment is to remove, treat, or avoid an identified cause. A first-generation (e.g., sedating) antihistamine will reduce pruritus and hive formation. If drowsiness occurs or control of symptoms is incomplete, a second-generation (e.g., nonsedating) agent may be substituted or added. Systemic corticosteroids generally are not required.

Erythema Multiforme (EM)

EM is a cutaneous hypersensitivity reaction that traditionally has been separated into two types, minor and major, depending on the extent and severity of lesions. However, at present, the minor form is simply called EM, while the major form is termed Stevens-Johnson Syndrome (SJS). EM often is caused by HSV types I or II infection; preceding herpes labialis is reported in one half of patients. In EM (unlike SJS) prodromal symptoms are absent. The rash is composed of erythematous macules or small, thin plaques that have a predilection for acral surfaces, including the palms, soles and face, with relative sparing of the trunk. Lesions remain fixed in location for up to 3 weeks before resolving. Over several days, a central violaceous discoloration, vesicle, or crust develops (i.e., a target lesion) (Fig. 19-4). Oral erosions that are few in number are observed in one half of patients; involvement of other mucosal sites is rare. EM typically resolves in 1–2 weeks and treatment is supportive.

EM must be differentiated from urticaria, SJS, and toxic epidermal necrolysis (TEN). In EM, unlike in urticaria, pruritus is less common, lesions are fixed in location (not evanescent), and unusual lesion shapes (e.g., arcs, plaques with serpiginous borders) are not seen. SJS and TEN are severe and potentially life-threatening hypersensitivity reactions characterized by blisters that rupture leaving large areas of denuded skin; target lesions are absent or few in number.

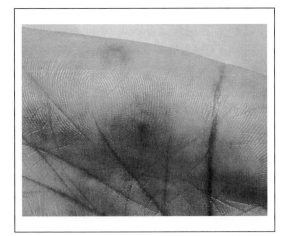

FIGURE 19-4

TARGET LESIONS ON THE HAND OF A PATIENT
WHO HAS ERYTHEMA MULTIFORME.
Source: Courtesy of Alan B. Fleischer, Jr. MD.

The treatment of EM is supportive. Acyclovir is of benefit in the prevention of recurrent episodes of EM triggered by HSV infection, but is not useful once lesions of EM are established. There is no evidence to support a role for corticosteroids in the treatment of EM (minor).

Stevens-Johnson Syndrome (SJS)/ Toxic Epidermal Necrolysis (TEN)

SJS (formerly called EM major) and TEN represent severe and potentially life-threatening hypersensitivity reactions to drugs (e.g., antibiotics, anticonvulsants, or nonsteroidal anti-inflammatory agents) or, less commonly, infectious agents (e.g., *Mycoplasma pneumoniae*). Both are characterized by large areas of epidermal necrosis. Although some controversy exists, many experts believe that SJS and TEN are the same disease, differing only in extent. In both disorders, patients experience prodromal symptoms, including fever, sore throat, rhinitis, cough, headache, vomiting, or diarrhea. Within 14 days, erythematous macules and patches appear on the trunk and extremities. Blisters form rapidly then rupture leaving large areas of denuded skin. In SJS there is epidermal loss of <10% of the body surface, while TEN is diagnosed when patients lose >30% of the

epidermal surface; those with 10%–30% involvement are said to have SJS/TEN overlap. Target lesions (seen in EM) are absent or few in number. Mucosal involvement is prominent with hemorrhagic crusting of the lips, oral ulcers, and purulent conjunctivitis. The mucosae of the trachea, bronchi, and gastrointestinal tract also may be involved.

Patients who have SJS or TEN ideally should be managed in a burn or intensive care unit with careful attention to fluid and electrolyte status, nutrition, skin and eye care, and the potential for secondary bacterial infection. If a precipitating drug is suspected, it should be withdrawn promptly. Intravenous immunoglobulin may be beneficial; the role of systemic corticosteroids is controversial. Long-term complications of SJS/TEN involve the eye, skin, and nails.

Erythema Nodosum

Erythema nodosum represents a hypersensitivity reaction to various infections, drugs, and other conditions. It is a form of panniculitis, an inflammation of the subcutaneous fat. It begins as painful, erythematous, warm nodules with indistinct borders most often located on the pretibial surfaces (Fig. 19-5). Over several days, the nodules evolve from red to brown-red or purple and later to yellow-green, as seen with bruises.

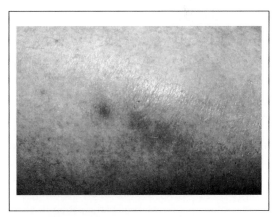

FIGURE 19-5

ERYTHEMA NODOSUM IS CHARACTERIZED BY
ERYTHEMATOUS OR VIOLACEOUS NODULES
TYPICALLY LOCATED OVER THE SHINS.
Source: Courtesy of Alan B. Fleischer, Jr. MD.

In most cases, no precipitant is identified in patients who have erythema nodosum. Among infectious precipitants, the most common is a preceding streptococcal infection. Others include infection with Epstein-Barr virus or *Yersinia enterocolitica*, tuberculosis, histoplasmosis, coccidioidomycosis, and leptospirosis. An association with inflammatory bowel disease, particularly Crohn disease, and sarcoidosis has been observed. Drugs most frequently incriminated include estrogen-containing oral contraceptives and sulfonamides. Chronic or recurrent episodes suggest systemic disorders, such as a collagen vascular disease, lymphoma, or inflammatory bowel disease.

The lesions of erythema nodosum initially may be confused with cellulitis, insect bites, or bruises. If necessary, a biopsy will assist in diagnosis, revealing inflammation in the subcutaneous fat, including around vessels. If a precipitating factor is identified, it should be managed appropriately. Most patients respond to relative rest and the use of an oral nonsteroidal anti-inflammatory agent; occasionally potassium iodide is employed. Typically, erythema nodosum resolves within a few days to 3 weeks.

INFECTIONS

Bacterial Infections

Impetigo

Crusted (nonbullous) impetigo: Crusted or nonbullous impetigo is caused primarily by *Staphylococcus aureus*, though *Streptococcus pyogenes* occasionally is implicated. It begins as tiny vesicles that rapidly rupture leaving a golden or honey-colored crust. Lesions may spread locally and any area of the body may be involved, though the region around the nares commonly is affected. Infection is spread by direct contact, including that which occurs as the result of participation in close contact sports (e.g., wrestling). When impetigo is widespread, therapy with an oral antibiotic active against *S. aureus* and *S. pyogenes* (e.g., cephalexin or dicloxacillin) is indicated. For localized disease, topical mupirocin is effective.

Bullous impetigo: Strains of *S. aureus* that produce exfoliative toxins A and B are responsible for bullous impetigo. The toxins cause superficial intraepidermal cleavage that results in the formation of flaccid bullae filled with cloudy fluid. Bullae rupture rapidly, leaving round or oval erosions that become crusted and are surrounded by a rim of scale, the remnant of the blister roof. If diagnostic uncertainty exists, culture of blister fluid will reveal the causative organism. Treatment is with an oral antistaphylococcal antibiotic (e.g., cephalexin or dicloxacillin).

Folliculitis

Staphylococcal folliculitis: Infections of the hair follicle unit are caused most frequently by *S. aureus*. Lesions are pustules centered around follicles and surrounded by a small rim of erythema. Commonly affected sites include the buttocks in those wearing occlusive clothing, areas that have been shaved (e.g., the beard area, axillae, legs, or groin), and areas of the skin that are rubbed by padding in athletes. If localized, folliculitis can be treated successfully with the use of an antibacterial soap and application of a topical antibiotic (e.g., clindamycin) or benzoyl peroxide. More widespread disease usually requires treatment with an oral antistaphylococcal antibiotic (e.g., cephalexin and dicloxacillin).

Gram-negative folliculitis: A folliculitis caused by gram-negative organisms (e.g., *Escherichia coli*, *Enterobacter* spp., or *Klebsiella* spp.) may occur in adolescents who have acne and are treated with systemic antibiotics. The key to suspecting the diagnosis is a sudden flare of inflammatory papules and pustules surrounding the nose and extending to the central face in an individual receiving an oral antibiotic. Treatment generally requires withdrawal of antibiotic therapy and initiation of isotretinoin.

Hot tub folliculitis: Hot tub or whirlpool folliculitis is caused by superficial infection with *Pseudomonas aeruginosa*. It is characterized by the appearance of erythematous macules, papules, or pustules 8–48 hours after immersion in a hot tub, or after using a swimming pool or water slide.

The lesions may occur on any part of the body immersed but typically are concentrated under swimsuits. Because the infection is superficial, normally no treatment is required. Hot tubs should be chlorinated and the pH maintained appropriately. Deeper inoculation of *Pseudomonas* may result from abrasion of the skin by rough surfaces in pools or hot tubs. Inflammation of the subcutaneous fat occurs producing tender nodules located on the palms or soles (the *Pseudomonas* "hot foot" syndrome).

Pitted Keratolysis

Pitted keratolysis is a superficial infection with *Micrococcus sedentarius* or *Corynebacterium* spp. These organisms produce proteolytic enzymes that digest the stratum corneum. The result is multiple small (a few mm in diameter), well-defined, superficial pits on the plantar surfaces of the feet (Fig. 19-6). Lesions occasionally are hyperpigmented and may coalesce to form large superficial erosions. Patients may complain of an unpleasant odor or excessive sweating, but many are unaware of the condition's

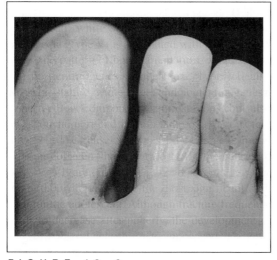

FIGURE 19-6

PITTED KERATOLYSIS: SUPERFICIAL PITS AND EROSIONS ON THE PLANTAR SURFACE OF THE TOES.

Source: Courtesy of Alan B. Fleischer, Jr. MD.

existence. If therapy is desired, a topical antibiotic (e.g., clindamycin or erythromycin) may be applied twice daily to control odor. Associated hyperhidrosis is treated with topical aluminum chloride in a 12% or 20% concentration (see Hyperhidrosis in the section Miscellaneous Conditions).

Erythrasma

Erythrasma, a superficial infection caused by *Corynebacterium minutissimum*, results in the appearance of reddish-brown patches located in flexural areas, such as the groin or axillae. The diagnosis may be confirmed by examining affected areas with a Wood lamp in a darkened room; in the presence of infection, a coral-red fluorescence will be observed. Localized forms may be treated topically (e.g., with clindamycin or erythromycin), while more widespread infection should be managed with oral therapy (e.g., with erythromycin for 5–7 days). Unlike tinea cruris with which it often is confused, the lesions of erythrasma do not have elevated borders and do not produce scale.

Arcanobacterium Haemolyticum–Induced Rash

Arcanobacterium haemolyticum is a gram-positive bacillus that causes pharyngitis and a rash similar to that caused by group A β-hemolytic streptococci. Infection usually occurs in adolescents or young adults. Fever, pharyngeal erythema and exudate, and lymphadenopathy are common. A rash is present in one half of patients; it typically is scarlatiniform, being composed of fine erythematous papules that first appear on the distal extensor surfaces of the extremities and then spread centrally to the trunk. Following resolution of the rash, desquamation may be observed. If infection is suspected clinically or confirmed by bacterial culture, treatment with erythromycin is indicated. Penicillin is not consistently effective.

Erythema Migrans

Erythema migrans is the earliest clinical manifestation of Lyme disease, being present in 80%–90% of those with documented infection. About 7–14 days following the bite of an infected tick, an erythematous papule or macule appears at the site of the bite. Without antibiotic treatment, the rash enlarges forming an erythematous patch, ring, or concentric rings. The lesions are flat or slightly elevated, persist for 1–2 weeks, and usually are asymptomatic, though local burning, pruritus, or pain may be present. Patients who have erythema migrans may experience fever, headache, malaise, myalgias, or arthralgias. Days to weeks after the onset of erythema migrans, dissemination of the organism may result in small secondary cutaneous lesions at sites distant from the bite. Treatment of erythema migrans is with doxycycline (for those 8 years and above) or amoxicillin (for all ages).

Toxic Shock Syndrome

Toxic shock syndrome (TSS) results from infection with certain toxin-producing strains of *S. aureus*. In the absence of protective immunity, the toxins, TSS toxin-1 and staphylococcal enterotoxins, induce the formation of cytokines that produce characteristic symptoms and signs. The rash of TSS is a diffuse sunburn-like erythema. Additional signs include hyperemia of the conjunctivae and other mucous membranes, fever, shock, and multisystem involvement (e.g., gastrointestinal, muscular, renal, hepatic, hematologic, and central nervous system).

When first described, 90% of cases of TSS occurred in association with menses, often in women using super-absorbent tampons. With the institution of preventive measures, the incidence of TSS has declined and, at present, approximately 50% of cases are associated with menses. Nonmenstrual TSS may occur following staphylococcal infection of the respiratory tract (e.g., bacterial tracheitis or sinusitis), sites of trauma, burns, or surgical wounds. Treatment is supportive; patients should receive a parenteral antistaphylococcal antibiotic.

Fungal Infections

Tinea Corporis

Tinea corporis represents a superficial infection caused by *Trichophyton tonsurans, Microsporum canis, T. mentagrophytes*, or other dermatophytes.

It occurs commonly in adolescents and often is seen in wrestlers or others involved in close contact sports. The typical lesion begins as a scaling papule or small plaque. As it enlarges, a ring is formed; the border generally is scaly and slightly elevated and, at times, may contain tiny vesicles or pustules. Lesions usually are solitary or few in number and round; however, multiple lesions occasionally are present and unusual shapes may be noted, including coalescent rings or lesions with incomplete borders. Tinea corporis usually is asymptomatic, though pruritus may be present. If necessary, the diagnosis may be confirmed by a potassium hydroxide preparation that reveals branching hyphae or a fungal culture. The conditions most frequently confused with tinea corporis are granuloma annulare, the herald patches of pityriasis rosea, and nummular eczema. Treatment consists of application of a topical antifungal agent, such as an imidazole (e.g., miconazole or clotrimazole), twice daily for 2–3 weeks or until the lesion resolves. If lesions are multiple or involvement extensive, oral therapy (e.g., with griseofulvin) may be indicated.

Tinea Pedis

Tinea pedis is the most common fungal infection of adolescents and adults. Several clinical patterns have been identified. The interdigital form, caused by *Trichophyton rubrum* or *Epidermophyton floccosum*, presents with pruritus, redness, scaling, fissuring, and maceration between the toes. *T. rubrum* may cause a more diffuse infection that involves much or all of the sole and sides of the feet (the "moccasin" type). Finally, in the vesicular form, caused by *T. mentagrophytes*, the patient develops vesicles or bullae located on the instep of the foot. The diagnosis usually is accomplished clinically, though it may be confirmed by the performance of a potassium hydroxide preparation or fungal culture. Conditions that may mimic tinea pedis include atopic dermatitis, dyshidrotic eczema, pitted keratolysis, contact dermatitis, or psoriasis. For mild infections, application of a topical imidazole (e.g., miconazole or clotrimazole), terbinafine, or naftifine will be effective. Patients who have the moccasin type require oral therapy (e.g., with griseofulvin or one of the newer oral antifungals) as do those who desire treatment of concomitant nail infection (nail infection typically is treated with terbinafine, itraconazole, or fluconazole, see Nail Disorders, later).

Tinea Cruris

Tinea cruris is the result of infection with *T. mentagrophytes* or *E. floccosum* and commonly occurs in adolescents and young adults. It produces well-defined patches with erythematous, slightly raised, scaling borders. Tinea cruris involves the proximal medial thighs and crural folds; it may be unilateral or bilateral and typically spares the penis and scrotum. The differential diagnosis includes candidiasis, intertrigo, erythrasma, and irritant or allergic contact dermatitis. Application of an imidazole antifungal agent (e.g., miconazole and clotrimazole) for 2–3 weeks is effective.

Tinea Versicolor

Tinea versicolor is caused by the yeast *Pityrosporum ovale* (*Malassezia furfur*). The organism is a normal component of the skin flora but when it converts to the mycelial form it may cause disease. Patients exhibit hyper- or hypopigmented macules and patches on the neck, chest, and back (Fig. 19-7). Lesions have well-defined borders, are round or oval, and have a fine scale. Often, individual macules coalesce to form large patches. Pruritus is variable.

The diagnosis is usually apparent clinically but may be confirmed by performing a potassium hydroxide preparation on scale obtained from a lesion. Spores and hyphae (spaghetti and meatballs) of *Pityrosporum ovale* will be observed. Wood light examination in a darkened room often reveals a yellow-orange to blue-white fluorescence. The differential diagnosis includes pityriasis rosea, postinflammatory hypopigmentation, and vitiligo.

Tinea versicolor usually is treated topically with selenium sulfide 2.5% lotion. Various regimens exist; in one commonly employed, the lotion is applied to all affected areas for 10 minutes once daily for 7 days. To prevent recurrences, patients should be advised to apply the medication for 8–12 hours once every 1–2 months for a period of 4–6 months.

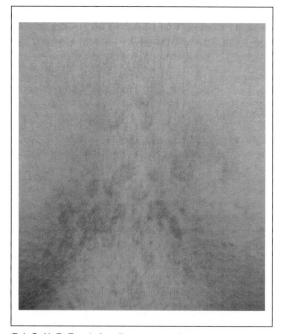

FIGURE 19-7

HYPERPIGMENTED SCALING MACULAE ON THE CHEST OF A PATIENT WHO HAS TINEA VERSICOLOR.

Adverse effects associated with selenium sulfide use include stinging (particularly with longer application times) and an unpleasant odor. An alternative topical treatment is ketoconazole shampoo applied for 5 minutes daily for 1–3 days. If infection is very localized, a topical imidazole may be employed. Oral ketoconazole (400 mg po once or 200 mg/day for 5 days), itraconazole (200 mg/day for 7 days), or fluconazole (400 mg po once) generally are reserved for patients who fail therapy with selenium sulfide. Although each of these agents eradicates the primary infection, prophylactic therapy with selenium sulfide lotion should be employed. Patients should be advised that several months are required for normalization of pigmentation.

Candidiasis

Cutaneous candidal infections are relatively uncommon in adolescents. When they occur, the crural region often is affected with confluent erythema that involves the skin creases. Satellite lesions (i.e., erythematous papules or pustules) may be observed. The penis and scrotum often are involved unlike in tinea cruris. Candidal infection also may involve the angles of the mouth, the axillae, the area beneath the breasts, or the nails (see Nail Disorders, later). Recurrent or persistent candidal infection should suggest the presence of an underlying disorder, such as diabetes mellitus, hypoparathyroidism, Addison disease, acquired immunodeficiency syndrome, or malignancy. Usually, infection can be treated effectively with the application of an anticandidal agent, such as nystatin or an imidazole antifungal agent (e.g., clotrimazole or miconazole).

Viral Infections

Warts

Warts are the result of infection with various types of human papillomavirus (HPV). HPV types often are related to a specific clinical presentation of the wart; for example, types 1, 2, and 4 cause common warts on the hands and plantar warts on the feet, while types 3 and 10 cause flat warts. Transmission of warts is believed to occur primarily by direct contact; however, autoinoculation and spread by fomites also may occur. Untreated warts generally persist a few months to several years; in children, two thirds disappear within 2 years. The clinical features of various wart types are summarized in Table 19-6.

The response of individual warts to any therapy is variable. A recent Cochrane analysis of pooled data found cure rates of 75% for both topical salicylic acid preparations and cryotherapy; two trials comparing the two modalities found no difference. Because most warts resolve spontaneously, no intervention is a reasonable choice for some patients. Commonly employed options for the treatment of warts are presented in Table 19-6.

Molluscum Contagiosum

Lesions of molluscum contagiosum, caused by a poxvirus, are translucent papules that upon initial examination may mimic vesicles. Typically lesions are one to a few mm in diameter, but occasionally reach 1 cm or more. Larger lesions may have a central umbilication. The number of lesions may vary from a few to hundreds. A dermatitis surrounding molluscum lesions is common. Typically, spread is by direct contact but autoinoculation occurs frequently. Individuals who have atopic dermatitis are prone to the development of widespread lesions in areas of active dermatitis.

Although no treatment is an option, the condition may last months to years, and patients frequently request therapy. If lesions are few in number, they can be treated with liquid nitrogen, removed with a curet, or the surface opened with a needle and the contents expressed. Imiquimod (alone or used in combination with a keratolytic), keratolytics, cantharidin, and podophyllin also have been used. Tretinoin also may be effective but irritation of surrounding normal skin may preclude its continued use.

Herpes Simplex Virus Infection

Cutaneous HSV infections, due to HSV type 1 or 2, typically produce grouped vesicles on an erythematous base. The vesicles become pustular then rupture forming erosions that crust. Several forms of infection may occur.

Herpes labialis: Herpes labialis is the most common form of recurrent HSV infection in adolescents. A prodrome of pain or tingling often precedes the appearance of vesicles, which are located on the lip and perioral skin. Vesicles rupture and crust, and healing takes place over 8–10 days. Recurrences often are precipitated by a febrile illness, trauma, menses, stress, or sun exposure. Treatment is supportive. Topical agents are of little value; topical acyclovir is ineffective and topical penciclovir reduces the duration of disease by only 1 day. Docosanol, an agent that blocks viral replication, is available without a prescription. In several trials, it was either ineffective or reduced the time of healing by only 18 hours. Oral antiviral agents are also of little value in treating recurrences, reducing the duration of disease by 1 day or less. When used suppressively, they are of benefit in reducing the frequency of recurrences.

CLINICAL FEATURES AND TREATMENT OPTIONS FOR WARTS

Wart Type	Clinical Features	Treatment Options	Comments
Common	Rough skin-colored papules May occur on any body site but common on the hands Tiny dark specks (thrombosed capillaries) may be seen through the surface	Keratolytic topically	Available in liquid, gel, pads, and bandages Use 17% concentration for common warts Leave product on for 24 h; soak wart in warm water, dry, and debride wart with coarse nail file or emery board; reapply medication
		Cryotherapy	Use keratolytic (as above) in interval between treatments to prevent wart regrowth
		Tape (e.g., duct tape)	Apply and leave in place for 6 days; remove tape and debride wart with emery board or coarse nail file; reapply tape
		Imiquimod 5%	Apply daily (use in conjunction with keratolytic [i.e., use one product in the morning and one at hs])
		Cantharidin	Applied in office. Induces blister formation; when blister heals, some or all of wart is lost. Not approved for use by the Food and Drug Administration
Plantar	Single or clustered Thrombosed capillaries are present	Each of the therapies listed for common warts may be used for plantar warts	If using a keratolytic, may select a product containing a concentration of salicylic acid greater than 17%
Flat	Small (few mm in diameter), skin-colored papules or thin plaques Surface is smooth, may coalesce to form plaques or appear in a linear array May spread extensively as a result of shaving	Each of the therapies listed for common warts may be used for flat warts Tretinoin	Apply daily
Genital	Skin-colored to hyperpigmented papules that may coalesce into plaques	Imiquimod 5%	Applied by patient q hs three times weekly for as long as 16 weeks
		Podofilox 0.5%	Applied by patient bid for 3 days then 4 days without therapy
		Cryotherapy	Applied by provider
		Podophyllin 10% or 25%	Applied by provider
		Trichloroacetic acid or bichloroacetic acid	Applied by provider

Herpes gladiatorum: Herpes gladiatorum occurs in wrestlers and others who participate in sports that involve close physical contact. Infection often is the result of inoculation from a competitor who has herpes labialis. Herpes gladiatorum may be treated with an oral antiviral agent, although the efficacy of this approach has not been established.

Genital herpes: Genital herpes (i.e., herpes progenitalis) typically is caused by HSV-2; 20% of cases are due to HSV-1. During primary infections, patients may exhibit systemic symptoms, including fever, genital pain, dysuria, and regional lymphadenopathy. Recurrent episodes often are asymptomatic. In males, clustered vesicles on an erythematous base appear on the glans or shaft of the penis. Women exhibit vulvar ulcers with surrounding erythema. Treatment of primary infections with an oral antiviral agent results in a 2-day reduction in symptoms, 4-day decrease in time to healing, and 7-day reduction of viral shedding. In recurrences, the impact of therapy is less (e.g., a 1-day decrease in symptoms and time to healing, and a 2-day decrease in viral shedding). For those with frequent recurrences (e.g., 6 or more in 1 year), suppressive oral antiviral therapy may be considered.

Herpes zoster: Herpes zoster, or shingles, is caused by reactivation of varicella-zoster virus (VZV) following primary infection (i.e., varicella). The rash often is preceded by several days of a stinging or burning sensation. Lesions begin as clustered erythematous papules that evolve over several days into vesicles. They appear in a dermatomal distribution and only rarely cross the midline. Lesions may not be continuous within a dermatome and, on occasion, more than one dermatome is affected. In a minority of patients, especially those who are immunocompromised, zoster may become generalized. Lesions that appear on the nose or around the eye may be associated with ophthalmic involvement (i.e., Ramsay-Hunt syndrome). VZV may be spread by direct contact with the lesions of zoster. Herpes zoster typically resolves without sequelae in 7–14 days. Persistent pain in the area previously affected (i.e., postherpetic neuralgia)

is unusual in immunocompetent adolescents and young adults.

Most patients who have zoster can be managed supportively with an analgesic and the application of a topical antibiotic to prevent secondary bacterial infection. Treatment with oral antiviral agents (e.g., acyclovir, famciclovir, or valacyclovir) reduces the duration of symptoms. However, such therapy generally is reserved for those who have extensive infection, ophthalmic involvement, or are immunocompromised.

Viral Exanthems

Several systemic viral infections have cutaneous manifestations. Although a complete discussion of these diseases is beyond the scope of this chapter, the dermatologic features of the most common viral exanthems that occur in adolescents are summarized in Table 19-7.

INFESTATIONS

Pediculosis

Pediculosis is caused by infestation with the head louse (*Pediculus humanus capitis*), crab louse (*Pthirus pubis*), or body louse (*Pediculus humanus humanus*). Infestation with head lice is spread by direct contact or fomites. It is most prevalent in childhood but adolescents may be affected. The primary symptom is pruritus that often is severe at night. Examination reveals nits attached to hairs, lice, or crusted erythematous papules at sites of feeding.

Pubic lice usually are acquired through sexual contact but may be spread by fomites, such as shared clothing or bedding. The lice usually cling to pubic hair, but may attach to other body hair or eyelashes. Symptoms include pruritus or a sense that something is crawling on the skin. Examination reveals nits, crusted papules, or the louse itself. Sometimes, bluish gray, faint purpuric spots (i.e., maculae ceruleae) may be seen at the sites of feeding by the louse.

Infestation with body lice is less common than other forms. The lice generally can be found in the

TABLE 19-7

FEATURES OF SELECTED VIRAL EXANTHEMS

Disease	Etiologic Agent	Clinical Features
Erythema infectiosum	Parvovirus B19	The rash begins as confluent erythema of the cheeks followed by a lacy, reticulated pink erythema of the extremities or trunk. The eruption fades after 3–5 days but may return for up to 4 months following exercise, overheating, or sun exposure.
Infectious mononucleosis	Epstein-Barr virus	Symmetrically distributed eruption composed of erythematous macules (i.e., morbilliform). The rash may occur spontaneously or following the administration of ampicillin or amoxicillin or, occasionally, penicillin or cephalosporins.
Measles	Measles virus	Characterized by fever, cough, coryza, conjunctivitis and an exanthem composed of erythematous macules and papules. The rash first appears on the lateral aspects of the neck and behind the ears. It then progresses to involve the face, trunk, and extremities. By the time the rash reaches the feet, the face is clearing. Koplik spots may be observed on the buccal mucosa.
Rubella	Rubella virus	Erythematous macules first appear on the face and then spread to the trunk and extremities. As the rash appears on the distal extremities it is resolving on the face and trunk. Patients may have associated fever, posterior cervical lymphadenopathy, or arthritis.
Varicella	Varicella-zoster virus	The lesions of varicella are erythematous macules or papules that rapidly develop a central vesicle. Vesicles then rupture forming a crust. Crops of new lesions appear for 3–4 days; they usually begin on the trunk and subsequently spread to the extremities and head. Vesicles that rapidly rupture to form ulcers may occur on mucosal surfaces.

seams of clothing. Infestation results in pruritic papules or pustules located on the trunk and in the perineum; hyperpigmented macules may be present at sites of healing lesions.

Treatment of head or pubic lice infestation consists of an application of permethrin 1% to the affected area for 10 minutes. Alternate therapies include a pyrethrin or lindane, though the latter is considered a second-line therapy and should be used with caution. Treatment should be repeated in 7–10 days to kill lice that have hatched since initial therapy. Clothing and bedding should be laundered. If the eyelashes are involved, petrolatum, applied several times daily for 7 days, may prove effective. The treatment of body louse infestation is analogous to that of head or pubic louse infestation, though particular attention should be given to laundering clothing where the lice reside.

Scabies

Scabies is an infestation with the mite, *Sarcoptes scabiei.* Female mites burrow into the stratum corneum where they deposit eggs. Symptoms and signs develop 2–3 weeks after infestation and are thought to be the result of sensitization to the mite and its products. Thus, an individual may be infested and transmit it to others without having symptoms.

A key feature of scabies is pruritus that is intense and often worse at night. Lesions are papules, vesicles, or pustules, many of which are excoriated. Burrows, linear or "S"-shaped tunnels, may be observed. In adolescents, lesions are most numerous on the hands, particularly in the webs of the fingers; on the wrists; in the axillae; at the belt line; on the areolae of women; and on the penis and scrotum in males.

Although the symptoms and findings on examination may suggest a diagnosis of scabies, an attempt to confirm the presence of infestation is prudent. A few nonexcoriated lesions are scraped with a scalpel blade coated with immersion oil. The material is transferred to a glass slide and a coverslip applied. The slide is then examined microscopically at low power for the presence of mites, eggs, or feces.

Scabies is treated with the application of 5% permethrin cream from the neck down for 8–14 hours. Since permethrin is not always ovicidal, a second application 7–10 days later is recommended. An alternative to permethrin 5% is lindane applied for 6–8 hours. Concerns about potential toxicity if it is used inappropriately or inadvertently ingested limit its use and, at present, it should be considered a second-line therapy. Lindane should not be used to treat pregnant women and is best avoided in infants and young children. Even if treatment is successful, pruritus may persist for several weeks.

All asymptomatic family members and close contacts should receive a single treatment at the time the index case is initially treated. Failure to do so may result in cycles of reinfestation. Clothing worn and bedding used by the family before treatment should be washed or stored in a plastic bag for 72 hours.

NAIL DISORDERS

Onychomycosis

Fungal infection of the nail, also known as onychomycosis or tinea unguium, is caused most often by *Trichophyton rubrum, T. mentagrophytes,* or *Epidermophyton floccosum.* Infection usually presents with thickening of the nail, and a yellow discoloration distally or laterally that indicates separation of the nail from the nail bed (distal and lateral subungual onychomycosis, respectively). Debris tends to accumulate beneath the nail plate. Occasionally only the surface of the nail is involved with white discoloration and a fine, powdery scale (i.e., superficial white onychomycosis).

Treatment of onychomycosis generally requires oral therapy. Terbinafine (250 mg/day for 3 months for toenail disease) and itraconazole (for toenail disease: 200 mg/day for 3 months, or 200 mg bid 1 week/month for 3–4 months) are approved for the treatment of onychomycosis; fluconazole is employed by some. Cure rates as high as 80% have been reported but recurrences are common, particularly with toenail disease. Clinicians prescribing these agents should be aware of potential drug interactions and adverse effects, and the need for laboratory monitoring. Griseofulvin also is approved for use but requires prolonged therapy and has a lower cure rate. Topical agents (e.g., ciclopirox [Penlac]) should be considered only for those who have superficial white onychomycosis or who cannot tolerate oral therapy.

Pseudomonas Infections

Pseudomonas infections of the nail produce a greenish blue discoloration of the nail bed. Paronychial pain and swelling occasionally are present. Since immersion in water is an important contributing factor, keeping the nails dry is important. Application of or soaking the nail in bleach three times daily may be effective in clearing the infection.

Candidal Infections

Infections with *Candida* spp. are seen most often in adolescents whose occupations require repeated immersion of the hands in water. The key to diagnosis is the observation of swelling and erythema of the skin at the base of the nail and lateral to it. The cuticle is absent and the nail itself may be discolored, thickened, and separated from the nail plate distally. Unlike acute bacterial paronychia, pain is uncommon. Treatment consists of removal of the source of continued wetness (to the extent possible) as well as application of a topical anticandidal agent to the infected nail and surrounding skin. If this treatment fails, oral therapy with itraconazole or fluconazole may be considered.

NEVI

Acquired Melanocytic (Nevocellular) Nevi

Acquired melanocytic nevi begin to appear during childhood and increase in number until the third decade after which they tend to disappear. Caucasians have greater numbers of nevi than more deeply pigmented individuals. Acquired melanocytic nevi typically are a few mm in diameter and may be separated into three clinical types: junctional nevi (brown and flat), compound nevi (brown but slightly elevated), and intradermal nevi (slightly pigmented or skin-colored and dome-shaped).

Acquired nevi do not require removal unless they develop changes suggestive of melanoma. Although malignant change is uncommon in adolescents, features that should prompt further evaluation include asymmetry, border irregularity, color variation within the lesion (particularly the appearance of pink, red, blue, or white colors), or those with a diameter of >6 mm. Evaluation is also indicated if a lesion is increasing in size, undergoes spontaneous bleeding or ulceration, develops satellite lesions, or becomes inexplicably painful or pruritic.

Atypical (Dysplastic) Nevi

Atypical (i.e., dysplastic) nevi are larger (5–12 mm) than common acquired nevi and are characterized by irregular and ill-defined borders (Fig. 19-8). Often their color is variegated, with shades of tan, dark brown, or pink. At times, lesions have a central elevated component making their appearance simulate that of a "sunny-side up" fried egg.

Atypical nevi begin in adolescence and continue to appear into adulthood. They occur sporadically or in a familial pattern. Persons who have atypical nevi are at increased risk of developing malignant melanoma; the risk varies with the number of nevi and the family history. For those who have a few

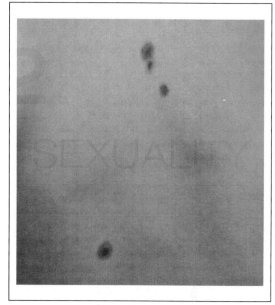

FIGURE 19-8

ATYPICAL NEVI ARE LARGE, ASYMMETRICAL, AND OFTEN HAVE A CENTRAL ELEVATED COMPONENT.

atypical nevi but no family history of melanoma, the lifetime risk of developing melanoma is only minimally elevated. However, for the individual with atypical nevi in whom there is a family history of melanoma in two or more first-degree relatives, the risk is very high. Adolescents who have atypical nevi should be referred to a dermatologist for periodic surveillance and removal of suspicious nevi.

Halo Nevi

Acquired nevi occasionally develop a hypopigmented ring around them and, over time, disappear. These halo nevi are believed to represent an immunologic response to melanocytes. They almost always are benign; further evaluation for possible malignant melanoma is warranted if the halo is irregular or incomplete, or if the central nevus is unusual in its appearance (e.g., has irregular borders and color variation).

Becker's Nevus

Becker's nevus typically appears at puberty and is more common in males. Its cause is unknown, although androgenic stimulation may play a role. Classically, Becker's nevus appears as a single large hyperpigmented patch overlying the shoulder. The borders are irregular, pigmentation within the affected area often is patchy rather than complete, and increased hair growth within the lesion nearly always is present. Becker's nevus is a benign lesion and no treatment is required.

PAPULOSQUAMOUS DISORDERS

Papulosquamous disorders are characterized by elevated lesions (e.g., papules or plaques) that form scale. In addition to the disorders discussed in this section, certain fungal infections (e.g., tinea corporis and tinea cruris) and seborrheic dermatitis produce papulosquamous lesions.

Pityriasis Rosea

Pityriasis rosea is a disorder of unknown cause believed, but not proven, to be viral in origin. It occurs most commonly in adolescents and young adults. Most cases occur sporadically but small epidemics have been reported.

In about one half of patients, pityriasis rosea begins with the appearance of a herald patch, a solitary erythematous patch or minimally elevated plaque that may be mistaken for tinea corporis. One to two weeks later, a generalized eruption begins. It is composed of oval lesions that are concentrated on the trunk and have their long axes parallel to lines of skin stress. On the patient's back, this arrangement creates the appearance of the branches of a fir tree. Individual lesions are minimally elevated and erythematous or hyperpigmented. Most are covered by a fine scale centrally and peripherally. At times, particularly in more deeply pigmented individuals, lesions may be more papular or hyperpigmented, or the eruption may be concentrated on the extremities and face, sparing the trunk (i.e., inverse pityriasis rosea). Occasionally, the lesions may be urticarial wheals or may become purpuric.

Typically, pityriasis rosea lasts 6–8 weeks but occasionally may persist longer. There is no specific therapy. Pruritus, present in one half of patients, may be managed with an emollient containing menthol or phenol, a topical nonsensitizing anesthetic (e.g., pramoxine), or an oral antihistamine. Judicious exposure to sunlight (avoiding burning) may hasten the resolution of the eruption and reduce pruritus.

The differential diagnosis of pityriasis rosea includes nummular eczema and psoriasis. Secondary syphilis may produce an eruption similar to pityriasis rosea, though patients usually are ill, have lymphadenopathy, and exhibit lesions on the palms and soles. Nevertheless, a serologic test for syphilis should be considered if the patient is sexually active.

Psoriasis

Psoriasis is an inherited disorder the onset of which occurs before 16 years of age in 25%–45% of patients. Lesions are well-defined erythematous papules or plaques covered with a silvery scale. Removing scale may cause pinpoint bleeding (i.e., Auspitz sign). The distribution is symmetrical, with plaques commonly appearing over the knees and elbows, sites of repeated trauma (Fig. 19-9). The eyebrows, ears, umbilicus, and gluteal cleft frequently are involved. Other findings include a thick, adherent scale on the scalp, nail involvement (punctate stippling or pitting, or discoloration and thickening), or scaling and fissuring of the palms and soles.

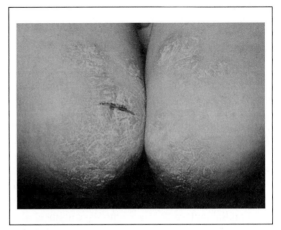

FIGURE 19-9

PSORIASIS: ERYTHEMATOUS, SCALING PLAQUES ON THE ELBOWS.

The Koebner phenomenon (i.e., the appearance of rash at sites of physical, thermal, or mechanical trauma) often is evident. Rarely, psoriasis may present with multiple individual and coalescent pustules.

The differential diagnosis of psoriasis includes uncommon disorders, such as pityriasis rubra pilaris, parapsoriasis, and lichen planus. Atopic dermatitis, pityriasis rosea, tinea corporis, and seborrheic dermatitis also may mimic psoriasis.

The course of psoriasis is unpredictable and consultation with a dermatologist is indicated for all but the mildest forms. Most patients who have plaque psoriasis will require combined therapy with a topical corticosteroid and calcipotriol (a vitamin D3 analog that normalizes epidermal proliferation and inhibits neutrophil and monocyte function). Topical coal tar preparations, anthralin, and tazarotene (a retinoid) also may be employed. Exposure to sunlight, with care taken not to burn the skin, often is beneficial. Patients who have severe, widespread, or recalcitrant disease may require phototherapy (ultraviolet [UV] B), photochemotherapy (UVA combined with psoralen), or systemic treatment with acitretin, methotrexate, or cyclosporin.

Lupus Erythematosus

Lupus erythematosus is a multisystem disease that is believed to be autoimmune in nature. Several variants of cutaneous disease exist, defined to some degree by the location of the inflammation within the skin. Acute cutaneous lupus, which often is associated with systemic disease, is characterized by the so-called butterfly rash, a slightly raised erythematous or violaceous thin plaque or patch with fine scale located over the malar areas and bridge of the nose. This rash tends to appear following sun exposure but is transient. Patients may also exhibit discoid lesions, round, well-demarcated, erythematous to violaceous plaques with telangiectases, an adherent scale, and areas of atrophy (Fig. 19-10). They appear most commonly on the face and scalp and in the ears and represent a form of chronic cutaneous lupus. Discoid lesions may result in scarring but most patients do not have systemic involvement. Other cutaneous lesions include transient erythematous annular lesions in sun-exposed areas (i.e., subacute

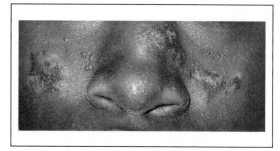

FIGURE 19-10
ERYTHEMATOUS, SCALING PLAQUES ARE TYPICAL OF DISCOID LUPUS ERYTHEMATOSUS.

cutaneous lupus erythematosus), red or purple nodules, scaling patches on the dorsa of the fingers (located between the interphalangeal joints, not overlying the joints as occurs in dermatomyositis), and scarring and nonscarring alopecia.

For patients who have mild, localized cutaneous disease, treatment may include sunscreens, topical or intralesional corticosteroids, or hydroxychloroquine. A discussion of the treatment of systemic disease is beyond the scope of this chapter; however, hydroxychloroquine, prednisone, or immunosuppressive agents often are employed.

PHOTOSENSITIVITY DISORDERS

Sun and Sun Protection

Sun exposure is linked to the development of skin cancer and skin aging (i.e., wrinkling and laxity of the skin, mottled hyperpigmentation, open comedones). Some 1.3 million Americans develop skin cancer each year. The majority of these are nonmelanoma skin cancers (e.g., basal cell and squamous cell carcinomas) that are associated with cumulative sun exposure. However, more than 54,000 persons develop malignant melanoma annually and 7600 of these die as a result of their disease. Melanoma risk appears to be linked, in part, to intermittent intense sun exposure, such as that which produces blistering sunburns. Other factors of importance include skin pigmentation (Caucasians have a 10-fold greater risk than African Americans), lower latitude of residence (owing to greater sun exposure in areas closer to the equator), family history of melanoma, and personal or family history of atypical nevi.

A key element of anticipatory guidance is to counsel adolescents about the risks of sun exposure and elements of sun protection; these are summarized in Table 19-8. The need for sun protection varies with skin type, specifically, the degree of skin pigmentation. Those with the greatest need for protection are fair-complexioned Caucasians who burn

TABLE 19-8

SUN PROTECTION STRATEGIES

- To the extent possible, minimize prolonged outdoor activities between the hours of 10:00 A.M. and 4:00 P.M.
- Wear protective clothing such as a wide-brimmed hat, long-sleeved shirt, and long pants. Several manufacturers offer lightweight clothing that has an SPF of 50 or more, even when wet (see *http://store.yahoo.com/coolibar/index.html http://radicoolcanada.com/products.asp?IID=1* or *http://tugasunwear.com*). For clothing such as T-shirts, consider using a laundry additive that will increase the SPF value (e.g., Sungard).
- Use a sunscreen regularly. Choose a product with an SPF of 15 or greater that provides UVA and UVB protection.
  - Consider a product that is not alcohol based (will not sting) and that is labeled nonacnegenic or noncomedogenic (will not block pores and make acne worse)
  - Apply liberally (using too little decreases the SPF value), ideally 30 min before beginning outdoor activities, even on cloudy days
  - Apply every 2 h, particularly if you are swimming or sweating
- To prevent cataracts and ocular melanoma, wear sunglasses labeled "maximum of 99% UV protection or blockage," "special purpose," "UV absorption up to 400 nm," or "meets ANSI UV requirements."

easily and do not tan; often these individuals have red hair and freckles. In contrast, deeply pigmented individuals who never burn are at little risk. Those with intermediate degrees of skin pigmentation may tan or burn and, therefore, require counseling about sun protection.

Sunscreens are an essential component of sun protection. They work by absorbing (i.e., chemical agents) or blocking (i.e., physical agents) ultraviolet (UV) radiation. Chemical sunscreens typically employ combinations of agents to provide the desired range of protection. Physical sunscreens contain microfine titanium dioxide or zinc oxide to provide both UVA and UVB protection. SPF values apply only to UVB protection; there is no agreed upon measure of UVA protection.

Adolescents can be advised to select a sunscreen that (1) has an SPF of at least 15 that offers both UVA and UVB protection, (2) is not alcohol-based (to avoid stinging, particularly when used around the eyes), and (3) that is labeled nonacnegenic or noncomedogenic (to avoid exacerbating acne). The product should be applied liberally; in an adolescent, approximately 1 oz of product is required to cover the entire body surface once. Most individuals use one quarter to one half the recommended amount, a factor that diminishes the effective SPF value by 50%–75%. Sunscreens should be applied frequently; a "waterproof" product provides protection through 80 minutes of immersion, "sweat-resistant" products can protect the skin after 30 minutes of heavy perspiration.

Artificial Tanning

Artificial tanning is popular among adolescents. However, epidemiologic evidence links the use of artificial tanning devices (which use fluorescent lights to produce UV radiation, 95% of which is UVA) to melanoma and nonmelanoma skin cancer. In addition, indoor tanning may cause burns and photoinduced drug reactions, and contribute to skin aging. Thus, for adolescents who desire a tan, the use of tanning beds should be discouraged and "sunless" alternatives discussed. The active ingredient in sunless tanning products is dihydroxyacetone (DHA). It reacts with basic amino acids in the stratum corneum to produce a darkening that begins within 1 hour of application, is maximal in 8–24 hours, and fades over 5–7 days. These products may be applied by the patient or by personnel in spas or salons. In addition, they may be sprayed on in sunless tanning booths. DHA is considered safe, though it should not be applied to the lips or near the eyes.

Sunburn

Sunburn represents a phototoxic reaction characterized by vasodilation, increased vascular permeability, and leukocyte migration to the site of injury. It appears within 4 hours of exposure and peaks by 6 and 24 hours. In addition to erythema and pain, individuals may develop vesicles or bullae. If extensive, sunburn may be associated with fever, headache, and fatigue. Sunburn may be treated with an oral nonsteroidal anti-inflammatory agent, cool compresses, or a topical corticosteroid. Application of aloe vera and vitamin E, though popular, has not been studied with respect to efficacy.

Drug Photosensitivity

Drug reactions to light have been divided into two types, toxic and allergic. Phototoxic reactions occur when UV radiation (typically UVA) activates an agent. Thus, with a sufficient dose of a drug and UVA, all individuals are potentially susceptible. A phototoxic reaction results in cellular damage through nonimmunologic mechanisms (e.g., free radical damage to cells). These reactions occur 2–6 hours after sun exposure and are characterized by erythema (that mimics sunburn) or, occasionally, bullae on sun-exposed surfaces. Nonsteroidal anti-inflammatory agents, tetracyclines (e.g., doxycycline), quinolones, phenothiazines, furocoumarins (responsible for phytophotodermatitis), and diuretics (e.g., furosemide, thiazide, and hydrochlorothiazide) are the agents most often implicated.

Most photoallergic reactions result from delayed hypersensitivity. After sensitization, within 24 hours of reexposure to the drug and sun, a pruritic, eczematous eruption appears on sun-exposed and partially covered skin. The agents responsible for photoallergic reactions include sunscreens (the most common cause), fragrances, topical antibacterial agents (e.g., chlorhexidine and hexachlorophene), and phenothiazines.

Treatment of drug photosensitivity reactions rests upon identification and removal of the offending agent. However, if the offending drug is considered therapeutically essential, photoprotection and nighttime dosing could be advised and may prevent further episodes. For established reactions, cool compresses, an oral antihistamine, and topical or systemic corticosteroids may be used.

SEXUALLY TRANSMITTED INFECTIONS

A number of sexually transmitted infections (STIs) have cutaneous manifestations that can serve as clues to diagnosis (Chap. 24). STIs that produce papules in the genital region, including scabies, pediculosis pubis, molluscum contagiosum, and genital warts, are discussed elsewhere in this chapter. Table 19-9 summarizes the clinical features, differential diagnosis, and treatment of STIs that cause genital ulcers. The cutaneous manifestations of syphilis, disseminated gonococcal infection (DGI), and Reiter disease will be discussed briefly here.

Syphilis

Syphilis is separated into primary, secondary, tertiary, and late stages. The cutaneous manifestations of primary and secondary syphilis will be discussed here. Primary syphilis is characterized by a chancre (Table 19-9) that usually is solitary. It begins as an erythematous macule that develops into an ulcer with an indurated border and a firm, rubbery base. Unless it becomes secondarily infected, a chancre is painless. Even without treatment, chancres resolve within 3–6 weeks. If untreated, 60%–90% of those who have primary syphilis will develop secondary syphilis. This stage begins 6–8 weeks following infection (3–6 weeks after appearance of the chancre). Patients who have secondary syphilis may exhibit a variety of cutaneous findings. An erythematous,

DIFFERENTIAL DIAGNOSIS OF GENITAL ULCERS CAUSED BY SEXUALLY TRANSMITTED INFECTIONS

Infection (cause)	Incubation Period	Primary Lesion(s)	Pain	Inguinal Lymphadenopathy	Diagnosis	Preferred Treatment[*]
Herpes simplex virus	3–14 days	Grouped vesicles on an erythematous base that rupture forming erosions Fever and malaise often occur in primary infection	Common, especially in primary infections	Common, especially in primary infections; usually bilateral	Tzanck smear, culture, direct fluorescent antibody, polymerase chain reaction (PCR)	Acyclovir, famciclovir, valacyclovir
Syphilis (Treponema pallidum)	9–90 days	Chancre: well-defined erythematous ulcer with a firm "rubbery" base	Uncommon unless secondarily infected	Common; usually nontender and non-suppurative. May be bilateral or unilateral	Darkfield examination, RPR, VDRL	Primary syphilis: benzathine penicillin G
Chancroid (Haemophilus ducreyi)	3–14 days	Small red papule that erodes to form a ragged ulcer with undermined edges	Common	Common; usually painful and unilateral; may be suppurative	Clinical (exclude HSV, syphilis); culture (not widely available); PCR	Azithromycin, ceftriaxone, ciprofloxacin, erythromycin
Lymphogranuloma venereum (Chlamydia trachomatis)—occurs rarely in the United States	3–30 days	Small red erosion that may be overlooked Fever, malaise, arthralgias, myalgias are common	Variable	Common; usually; unilateral nodes above and below the inguinal ligament create the "groove" sign	Clinical (exclusion of other causes); complement fixation	Doxycycline
Granuloma inguinale (Calymmatobacterium granulomatis)—occurs rarely in the United States	2–10 weeks	Red papule or nodule that ulcerates and forms "beefy-red" granulation tissue that is friable	Rare	Rare; pseudobubos (perilymphatic granulomas) may mimic lymphadenopathy	Tissue smear (Donovan bodies) or biopsy; organism difficult to culture	Doxycycline, trimethoprim sulfamethoxazole

[*]For specific dosing and treatment course see: Centers for Disease Control and Prevention. Sexually transmitted diseases treatment guidelines 2002. MMWR 2002;51(RR-6). Available at http://www.cdc.gov/std/treatment/TOC2002TG.htm (browsable version).

Source: Adapted from Clayton BD, Krowchuk DP. Skin findings and STDs. Contemp Pediatr 1997;14(9):119–137.

macular eruption is the earliest skin manifestation, appearing 9–10 weeks after initial infection. It begins on the trunk and extremities; with time, however, lesions become somewhat elevated, develop a copper-red color, and involve the palms and soles. Plaque-like lesions (resembling psoriasis) or rings (that mimic tinea corporis) also may be observed. Involvement of mucous membranes is common with the appearance of condylomata lata (macerated, skin-colored, or gray papules in the genital or perianal regions) or mucous patches (oval gray erosions in the oral cavity or on the genitalia). A patchy, "moth-eaten" alopecia also may occur. In the absence of treatment, the cutaneous lesions of secondary syphilis resolve in 2–10 weeks.

Disseminated Gonococcal Infection

DGI is an unusual complication of urethral or cervical infection with *Neisseria gonorrhoeae*. It is characterized by polyarthralgias, a rash, and constitutional symptoms, including fever. Joint pain usually results from an immune-mediated tenosynovitis, not septic arthritis. The fingers, toes, wrists, and ankles are symmetrically involved. The rash is composed of gray pustules on an erythematous base often located overlying joints. Petechiae, vesicles, macules, and papules also may be seen. Diagnosis of DGI may be confirmed by Gram stain or culture of material obtained from a pustule; however, testing of samples obtained from the cervix or urethra is more sensitive. Initial management includes hospitalization and administration of ceftriaxone or cefotaxime.

Reiter Syndrome

Reiter syndrome is defined by reactive arthritis, urethritis, ophthalmologic changes, and mucocutaneous lesions that are triggered by infections of the genital or gastrointestinal tracts. Among the genital pathogens, *Chlamydia trachomatis* most often is responsible, although *N. gonorrhoeae* and *Ureaplasma urealyticum* occasionally are implicated. The initial manifestation of Reiter syndrome, occurring 7–14 days after exposure to a genital tract pathogen, is urethritis. Within several days, the patient develops conjunctivitis, iritis, or uveitis. Three to four weeks later, there is the onset of a symmetrical oligoarthritis that involves the sacroiliac joints, knees, ankles, hands, or feet. One half of affected individuals manifest unique cutaneous eruptions, the most common of which is circinate balanitis. This rash begins as vesicles that rapidly evolve into crusted erosions or plaques with serpiginous borders located on the glans or shaft of the penis. Keratoderma blennorrhagicum occurs in a minority of patients. It is a psoriasis-like eruption composed of scaling papules and plaques usually located on the palms and soles, though nearly any body site, including the scalp and genitalia, may be involved.

MISCELLANEOUS DISORDERS

Acanthosis Nigricans

Acanthosis nigricans is a hyperpigmented velvety thickening of the skin. The most common sites of involvement are the nape and sides of the neck, the axillae, and the groin; the elbows and knuckles also may be affected. In adolescents, acanthosis nigricans usually is associated with obesity and insulin resistance. However, it also may occur in association with other endocrinologic disorders (e.g., diabetes mellitus, Addison disease, Cushing disease, hypothyroidism, hyperandrogenism, or hypogonadism [e.g., Prader-Willi syndrome]) or, rarely, malignancy. No effective therapy is available for the lesions, though tretinoin and keratolytics are advocated by some. Lesions may regress with treatment of the underlying cause.

Acne Keloidalis

Acne keloidalis is a disorder of unknown cause, though it is postulated that shaving or cutting tightly curled hairs causes them to turn back into the skin precipitating an inflammatory response. Lesions of acne keloidalis are papules or plaques located on the lower occipital scalp. Pustules may be present and a scarring alopecia may develop. Affected individuals are almost always African American. Patients should be advised to employ preventive measures, such as avoiding tight-fitting garments or head gear that may cause mechanical irritation, and not to use a razor in this area. Initial therapy of noninflamed lesions includes combining topical tretinoin and a potent topical corticosteroid. If pustules are present, a topical (e.g., clindamycin) or systemic antibiotic may be used. For persistent nodules or plaques, surgical or laser excision may be indicated.

Keratosis Pilaris

Keratosis pilaris is a common benign skin condition characterized by follicular papules distributed most commonly on the extensor surfaces of the upper arms, thighs, or face. Lesions possess a central plug of keratinaceous material and occasionally have surrounding erythema. The lesions are distinctive and readily diagnosed, though when present on the face they may be mistaken for acne. The cause of keratosis pilaris is unknown but it occurs most often in individuals who have atopic dermatitis or ichthyosis vulgaris. For patients who desire treatment, keratolytics, such as emollients containing ammonium lactate, urea, or lactic acid, can be applied once or twice daily. Once the desired effect (i.e., a reduction in the size or roughness of the papules) is achieved, the agent may be discontinued and reinstituted as necessary. Tretinoin also may prove effective, though it may be irritating. If there is evidence of inflammation surrounding the papules, an appropriate topical corticosteroid may be used in conjunction with the keratolytic agent. Patients should be counseled that treatments for keratosis pilaris rarely are completely successful.

Hidradenitis Suppurativa

Hidradenitis suppurativa results from obstruction of pilosebaceous follicles and secondary inflammation. Patients develop painful inflammatory nodules in the axillae and anogenital region. Sinus tracts, malodorous drainage, and keloidal scarring are chronic sequelae. Management of hidradenitis suppurativa is difficult

and consultation with a dermatologist is indicated. Topical (e.g., clindamycin) or systemic antibiotics often are used in a fashion analogous to that for acne management. Surgical excision or laser ablation of affected areas may be considered for patients who fail medical therapy.

Hyperhidrosis

Hyperhidrosis of the axillae, hands, or feet is a common complaint among adolescents. It is believed to result from increased neural impulses to the eccrine glands. Several options exist for management. For axillary hyperhidrosis that has failed standard antiperspirants, one may advise the use of agents containing higher concentrations of aluminum chloride (e.g., Certain Dri [12%] or DrySol [20%]). These products are applied nightly at bedtime under occlusion using plastic wrap inside a tight fitting shirt. The agent is washed off in the morning. Once an acceptable reduction in sweating is achieved (usually within several days), the frequency of application may be reduced to once or twice a week and, for some patients, occlusion may be discontinued. The primary adverse effect of this therapy is skin irritation that may be limited by not shaving immediately prior to an application. For those who fail this treatment, other options include injections of botulinum toxin A (injections generally need to be repeated one to three times a year) or surgical ablation of the axillary sweat glands. The treatment of hyperhidrosis of the palms or soles is analogous to that for axillary disease. First-line therapy is the application of 20% aluminum chloride (DrySol) at bedtime under occlusion with vinyl gloves. Other options include iontophoresis (see Drionic device available at *www.drionic.com*), botulinum toxin injections, or for severe, recalcitrant cases, surgical sympathectomy.

Piercing

Body piercing at sites other than the ear lobe has become increasingly prevalent among adolescents. As with tattooing, body piercing at sites other than the ear lobe is associated with an increased risk of involvement in health risk behaviors, including substance use and sexual activity. To avoid the development of an allergic contact dermatitis, patients should select jewelry that is composed of surgical stainless steel, niobium, or titanium. Healing times are related to the site pierced. Typical times to healing are 4–6 weeks for the tongue, 6–8 weeks for the earlobe or eyebrow, 2–12 months for ear cartilage, 3–6 months for the lip, and 4–12 months for the navel. After piercing, the area should be washed twice daily with an antibacterial soap until healed; isopropyl alcohol, hydrogen peroxide, and betadine should be avoided. The most common complication of piercing is local infection, usually with *Staphylococcus aureus*. Rarely, bacteremia, meningitis, or toxic shock syndrome have occurred. Infection with *Pseudomonas aeruginosa* that may result in deformities of the pinna is a recognized complication of ear cartilage piercing. Thus, patients who develop pain, erythema, or swelling following piercing of ear or other cartilage should have a bacterial culture performed and be treated presumptively with an antibiotic active against both *Pseudomonas* spp. and *S. aureus*. Information for patients, including assistance in deciding whether to have a body piercing, criteria for selecting a body artist, instructions for care of the piercing site, and healing times can be found at *http://www.vh. org/pediatric/patient/dermatology/ tattoo* (the Virtual Hospital of the Children's Hospital of Iowa).

Pseudofolliculitis Barbae

Pseudofolliculitis barbae is a chronic inflammatory condition that affects men with skin of color; it is analogous to acne keloidalis (discussed earlier). Shaving causes tightly curled hairs to penetrate the skin precipitating an inflammatory response. The condition is characterized by pustules or erythematous or hyperpigmented papules located in the beard area. Patients should be advised not shave too close, not shave against the direction of hair growth, and to dislodge any ingrown hairs with a toothpick or sterile needle. Alternately, they may avoid shaving and use a depilatory. Topical or systemic antibiotics, used in a fashion analogous to that for the management

of acne, may be of some benefit due to their anti-inflammatory properties.

Striae

Striae or "stretch marks" frequently appear during adolescence. Their cause is not known but they are believed to result from breaks in connective tissue at sites of increasing body size. Initially, the lesions may appear red or red-blue, but they become skin-colored and atrophic with time. In boys, the shoulders, thighs, and lumbosacral regions are involved, while in girls, common sites are the breasts, hips, and thighs. Although usually an isolated finding, striae may result from systemic corticosteroid therapy, Cushing disease (in this disorder, striae typically are larger and more widespread), or locally following the application of potent topical corticosteroids for prolonged periods. Patients may be counseled that the appearance of striae improves with time. No universally effective therapy exists. Topical tretinoin has been reported to improve the appearance and reduce the length and width of early striae, and pulsed dye laser therapy has been used in the management of erythematous striae.

Tattooing

Tattooing, one form of body modification, is common among adolescents. Reasons stated by adolescents for getting a tattoo include wanting to be part of a group or to express independence. However, tattoos also may be marks of gang membership. Often these tattoos are dots, crosses or spider webs located in the space between the thumb and index finger. Although tattooing has become more acceptable, studies suggest that adolescents who have tattoos are more likely to be involved in health risk behaviors, such as disordered eating, substance use and sexual activity.

Several potential complications of tattooing exist. Local infection may follow placement of a tattoo and usually is caused by *Staphylococcus aureus*. There is also a risk of transmission of hepatitis B and C, and concern also exists about the potential for transmission of human immunodeficiency virus infection, though this has not been documented. The tattoo may enhance local photosensitivity and use of a sunscreen is recommended. Allergic reactions to the dyes are well documented; red pigments, derived from mercury, are the most common offenders. The reaction may occur long after the tattoo is placed and may be precipitated by laser removal. The allergy usually is manifest as an eczematous eruption at the tattoo site; however, some patients develop generalized urticaria. Lastly, keloid formation or the development of granulomas within the tattoo may occur.

A common consequence of tattooing is eventual dissatisfaction with its presence. Q-switched (QS) laser treatment is the primary modality used for tattoo removal. The choice of laser is determined by the absorption spectra of the ink colors in the tattoo. Black pigments may be removed with the QS ruby, alexandrite, or neodymium (Nd):YAG (yttrium-alexandrite garnet) lasers; red, blue, and green with the QS ruby or alexandrite; and red, orange, or yellow with the QS Nd:YAG However, removal may be incompletely successful, is expensive and not covered by insurance, and requires multiple treatments. Patient information about tattooing (including a discussion of decision-making, advice about selecting a body artist, and instructions for caring for a tattoo) may be obtained by visiting *http://www.vh.org/pediatric/patient/ dermatology/tattoo* (the Virtual Hospital of the Children's Hospital of Iowa).

Vitiligo

Vitiligo is an uncommon disorder that affects approximately 2% of the general population. In one half of patients the disease begins before 20 years of age. The cause of vitiligo is unknown, but autoimmune, autocytotoxic, and neuronal dysfunction mechanisms have been suggested as reasons for melanocyte destruction. Patients who have vitiligo are more likely than those who are unaffected to have a family member with an autoimmune disorder and to develop such disorders (e.g., Hashimoto thyroiditis, Graves disease, alopecia areata, diabetes mellitus, Addison disease, and pernicious anemia).

The lesions of vitiligo are well-defined macules or patches that lack any pigment (i.e., are depigmented) and, therefore, the affected skin is white. Vitiligo may be separated into generalized and segmental forms.

Generalized vitiligo is the most common form. Lesions are located bilaterally and symmetrically, often appearing around body orifices. The most frequent sites of involvement are the face, backs of the hands and wrists, umbilicus, and genitalia. In contrast, segmental vitiligo is limited to one area of the skin (e.g., one arm).

Several options exist for treating vitiligo but none are satisfactory. For lightly pigmented individuals, use of sunscreen (SPF > 50) and protective clothing, and sun avoidance reduce the contrast between affected and unaffected areas. Others with limited involvement may choose a covering cosmetic. Potent topical corticosteroids result in the return of normal skin color in approximately 20% of treated patients, and 50% of those treated will have 75% or more repigmentation. A concern, however, is the potential for local skin atrophy following prolonged use of these agents. Topical tacrolimus is effective for the treatment of lesions located on the face. Treatment with psoralens and UVA light, UVB light, or autologous grafting of unaffected epidermis or cultured melanocytes generally are reserved for individuals with significant disease who fail other therapies. Regardless of the therapy selected, care must be taken to protect the depigmented skin from sunburn. Patients may benefit from referral to the National Vitiligo Foundation (available at *http://www.nvfi.org/*) which provides information about the disorder.

The prognosis for vitiligo is guarded. Generalized vitiligo tends to be a progressive disease and spontaneous remission is uncommon. Although segmental vitiligo also is progressive, patients typically do not progress to generalized disease.

Suggested Readings

Abbasi N, Shaw HM, Rigel DS, et al. Early diagnosis of cutaneous melanoma. *JAMA* 2004;292:2771–2776.

Carroll ST, Riffenburgh RH, Roberts TA, Myhre EB. Tattoos and body piercings as indicators of adolescent risk-taking behaviors. *Pediatrics* 2002;109:1021–1027.

Centers for Disease Control and Prevention. Sexually transmitted diseases treatment guidelines 2002. *MMWR* 2002;51(RR-6):1–84. Available at *http://www.cdc. gov/std/treatment/rr5106.pdf* (printable version).

Clayton BD, Krowchuk DP. Skin findings and STDs. *Contemp Pediatr* 1997;14:119–137.

Gibbs S, Harvey I, Sterling JC, Stark R. Local treatments for cutaneous warts. *Cochrane Database Syst Rev* 2004;(3):CD001781.

Gupta AK, Ryder JE, Johnson AM. Cumulative meta-analysis of systemic antifungal agents for the treatment of onychomycosis. *Br J Dermatol* 2004;150: 537–544.

Haider A, Shaw JC. Treatment of acne vulgaris. *JAMA* 2004;292:726–735.

Krowchuk DP. Managing adolescent acne: A guide for pediatricians. *Pediatr Rev* 2005;26:250–261.

Lee DJ, Eichefield LF. Atopic, contact, and seborrheic dermatitis in adolescents. *Adolesc Med* 2001;12: 269–283.

Martel S, Anderson JE. Decorating the "human canvas": Body art and your patients. *Contemp Pediatr* 2002; 19:86–102.

Truong A, Friedlander SF. Superficial fungal infections in adolescents. *Adolesc Med* 2001;12:213–227.

RESOURCES FOR CLINICIANS (ELECTRONIC ATLASES)

http://tray.dermatology.uiowa.edu/DermImag.htm

An atlas of general dermatology maintained by the Department of Dermatology at the University of Iowa. Images of conditions are listed alphabetically.

http://www.dermis.net/doia/mainmenu.asp?zugr=d &lang=d

Dermatologic Online Image Atlas maintained by the University of Erlangen, Germany. It contains over 2200 images of adult and pediatric dermatologic disorders. Conditions may be searched alphabetically or by body area. There is a quiz to test your knowledge.

http://dermatlas.med.jhmi.edu/derm/

Johns Hopkins University Dermatlas. Contains over 4700 images of pediatric dermatologic disorders. Each image is accompanied by a brief case history. One may search by diagnosis, disease category, or body site involved. There is a quiz to test your knowledge.

GENERAL RESOURCES

http://www.aap.org/topics/html

Health topics section of the American Academy of Pediatrics website. Offers brief audio programs for patients on acne and piercing. Also provides text information on acne.

http://www.aad.org/patient_intro.html

Public resources section of the American Academy of Dermatology website. Provides information for patients on common skin disorders that affect adolescents.

http://www.webmd.com

WebMD provides patient information on a number of dermatologic disorders. Patients may use the search engine on the home page. Because there is considerable product advertising, they should be advised to look for "WebMD Search Results" and find the "Topic Overview."

RESOURCES FOR SPECIFIC DISEASES

Acne: *http://www.skincarephysicians.com/acnenet/index. html*

Located at the website of the American Academy of Dermatology, this site provides information about acne, treatments, and frequently asked questions.

Alopecia areata: *http://www.naaf.org/*

The National Alopecia Areata Foundation provides information about the disease and ongoing research and lists products (e.g., head coverings and hair pieces) for patients.

Tattooing and Piercing: *http://www.vh.org/pediatric/ patient/dermatology/tattoo* Information on tattooing and piercing provided by the Virtual Hospital of the Children's Hospital of Iowa.

Website of the National Vitiligo Foundation. Provides patient information about vitiligo, a list of physicians who treat the condition, and research information: *http://www.nvfi.org/*

20

INFECTIOUS DISEASES OF INCREASED INCIDENCE IN THE ADOLESCENT

Russell W. Steele

Infections of skin and skin structure, bone and joints, and diseases related to outdoor exposure are relatively more common in adolescents because of their increased physical activity combined with their risk taking behavior. Other infections have an increased incidence for reasons that are not entirely clear; examples include *Mycoplasma pneumoniae* pulmonary infection, and Epstein-Barr virus (EBV) infectious mononucleosis syndrome.

SKIN AND SKIN STRUCTURE INFECTIONS: ABSCESSES

Among skin and skin structure infections, cutaneous abscesses should be distinguished from impetigo, cellulitis, and wound infections, where treatment is somewhat different.

Etiology

The organisms most frequently recovered from skin and soft-tissue abscesses are *Staphylococcus aureus* and group A β-hemolytic streptococci (GABHS). Anaerobes are present in approximately

25% of cutaneous abscesses in adolescents and another 25% are caused by mixed aerobes and anaerobes. Occasionally, *Enterobacteriaceae* such as *Escherichia coli* are responsible pathogens. An increasing prevalence of methicillin-resistant *S. aureus* strains are currently being observed as the etiology of community-acquired infection. These strains are more virulent than methicillin-sensitive *S. aureus* and require antibiotics other than semi-synthetic penicillins and cephalosporins for treatment. Abscesses in the perianal region are almost always associated with mixed infection, including numerous anaerobic bacteria and aerobic pathogens, mainly *S. aureus* and *E. coli*, though streptococci and other aerobes each account for approximately 10% of infections.

Treatment

All abscesses should be incised and drained. When there is a question as to whether a lesion is fluctuant, EMLA cream can be applied to the skin and an 18-gauge needle and syringe used to aspirate material or probe the abscess. An incision can then be made and a wick placed to ensure continued drainage.

This is all that is necessary for *S. aureus* and most other organisms. Group A streptococci require penicillin or an appropriate alternative oral antibiotic to sterilize the larger areas of cellulitis. Bacteremia from cutaneous abscesses is extremely rare but should be considered with extensive involvement, high fever, or in the immunocompromised host.

For the management of perianal abscesses, in contrast to infection in other anatomic areas, simple drainage may be inadequate. Fistulae must be identified, opened, and excised. Perianal abscesses therefore require surgical consultation. Suggested antibiotics are clindamycin and a third-generation cephalosporin (or as directed by Gram stain and culture), though they are only necessary for extensive involvement, systemic symptoms, and immunocompromised hosts.

Acute Necrotizing Fasciitis

Acute necrotizing fasciitis (ANF) is a life-threatening invasive soft-tissue bacterial infection characterized by a rapid widespread necrosis of fascia and subcutaneous tissue with relative sparing of the skin and underlying tissue. The disease is frequently accompanied by severe toxicity and its progression is often fatal unless promptly recognized and aggressively treated.

Clinical Manifestations

The initial diagnosis of ANF is a clinical one relying on the recognition of predisposing factors and a high index of suspicion. Severe local pain, out of proportion to the physical findings in a patient with systemic toxicity is the most frequently described presentation.

Etiology

The site of infection is an important predictor of etiologic pathogens. Abdominal and perineal infections tend to be polymicrobial while infections in the extremities tend to be monomicrobial, caused mainly by GABHS.

Epidemiology

Associated factors, reported mostly in adults, include diabetes mellitus, alcoholism, illicit intravenous drug abuse, peripheral vascular disease, malignancy, and immunosuppression. However, ANF usually occurs in otherwise healthy young individuals. In adolescents, varicella, surgery, and minor trauma are the most common initiating factors.

Diagnosis

Because rapid diagnosis and early therapeutic intervention are the keys to a good outcome, soft tissue and fascial exploration with biopsy plus extensive soft-tissue excision are recommended whenever the diagnosis is clinically suspected. Full thickness frozen section biopsy is of value only early in the evolution of infection because once the necrotizing process becomes extensive and all of the soft-tissue layers become involved, ANF is difficult to differentiate from other necrotizing processes. The incision must be sufficiently deep to include fascia and muscle of all tissue layers, since the location of the necrotizing process is of prime importance. Earlier blood culture data had been quite variable, but in more recent reports of streptococcal toxic shock syndrome (TSS) associated ANF, bacteremia has occurred in up to 60% of cases.

Radiographic imaging studies have offered limited information, particularly plain radiographs, which are usually normal. Soft-tissue gas may be present but not until the necrotizing process is well advanced. Computed tomography (CT) is superior for the detection of small amounts of gas and particularly useful for delineating subcutaneous and fascial edema, thus defining the extent of debridement required. Magnetic resonance imaging (MRI) is a more reliable method for determining the depth of soft-tissue involvement, delineating the extent of inflammation, and identifying fluid in tissues. The definitive diagnosis of ANF is achieved at surgery by direct visualization of the gray, ragged, stringy appearance of the fascia, associated with a thin, serosanguinous exudate and extensive undermining along the plane just superficial to the deep fascia.

Treatment

The initial and most important aspect of therapy in ANF is prompt surgical exploration with extensive and aggressive debridement of all necrotic tissue. Management should also include vigorous fluid resuscitation with correction of electrolyte imbalances and meticulous supportive care. Coagulopathy, respiratory insufficiency, and renal failure are seen frequently enough to warrant continuous monitoring for their development.

Parenteral antibiotics should be instituted at initial diagnosis. In cases in which a polymicrobial infection is suspected (i.e., perineal and abdominal ANF) the regimen should include a penicillinase-resistant penicillin for streptococcal and staphylococcal coverage, an aminoglycoside for gram-negative enteric bacilli, and either clindamycin or metronidazole for anaerobes. Antimicrobial therapy should always be modified once responsible pathogens and their antimicrobial susceptibilities are identified. In cases of trauma in water, coverage for marine vibrios should be provided. Penicillin, sulfas, erythromycin, tetracycline, and gentamicin are all effective.

Penicillin remains highly effective for the treatment of almost all GABHS infections. However, for ANF, where high concentrations of streptococcal bacteria are seen, efficacy of penicillin therapy appears diminished. This is explained by the fact that high concentrations of GABHS reach the stationary phase of bacterial growth quickly and penicillin is not effective at killing organisms that are not in the logarithmic phase of growth. Penicillin failure can also be explained by the recent observation that certain penicillin-binding proteins (PBPs) are not expressed by streptococci during the stationary phase.

In experimental models of fulminate streptococcal infection, clindamycin has proven more effective than penicillin, likely a consequence of its mechanism of action i.e., the inhibition of protein synthesis, independent of the size and stage of growth of the bacterial inoculum. Clindamycin also suppresses the production of bacterial toxins and facilitates the phagocytosis of GABHS by inhibiting M protein synthesis. Therefore, it appears reasonable to add clindamycin to those cases in which ANF due to GABHS is suspected.

Ceftriaxone has also been shown to provide more rapid killing of GABHS than penicillin in cases of severe infection. This is believed to be the result of the greater affinity of ceftriaxone for streptococcal penicillin-binding proteins.

TOXIC SHOCK SYNDROME

GABHS and *S. aureus* are causative agents of this syndrome. TSS is an illness seen in all age groups, though it is more commonly found in the clinical settings of antecedent fasciitis (GABHS), chickenpox (GABHS), or in young menstruating women (*S. aureus*). Shock is the result of exotoxins produced by these organisms.

Clinical Manifestations

With both GABHS and *S. aureus*, TSS is characterized by fever, hypotension, and multisystem organ failure. There may be watery diarrhea, vomiting, rash, conjunctival injection, and severe myalgias with *S. aureus*-mediated TSS but less commonly with *S. pyogenes*-mediated TSS. There may be no identifiable focus of infection, but many cases are associated with pneumonia, osteomyelitis, bacteremia, septic arthritis, and endocarditis.

Etiology

Most *S. aureus* strains causing TSS produce at least one of the staphylococcal enterotoxins. *S. pyogenes*-mediated TSS is caused by stains producing at least one of several different protein superantigenic exotoxins: streptococcal pyrogenic exotoxins A, B, or C; mitogenic factor; or streptococcal superantigen.

Epidemiology

S. aureus-mediated TSS is associated with tampon use in menstruating women, with a predilection for adolescents and young women who do not have antibody to causative toxins.

In adolescents, toxic-shock syndrome toxin-1 (TSST-1) producing strains of *S. aureus* may be part of the normal flora of the anterior nares and the vagina, producing protective antibody, and more than 90% of adults have antibodies to TSST-1. *S. aureus*-mediated TSS with TSST-1-producing strains occurs in individuals who do not have antibodies to TSST-1. Menses-related cases generally develop on the third or fourth day of menses.

The incidence of *S. pyogenes*-mediated TSS is lower in adolescents than young children primarily because of strong association with varicella. Adolescents at increased risk include those with diabetes mellitus, chronic cardiac or pulmonary disease, human immunodeficiency virus infection, and intravenous drug and alcohol abusers. The incubation period is not clearly defined but is reported as short as 14 hours in cases associated with subcutaneous inoculation of organisms after penetrating trauma.

Diagnostic Tests

S. aureus-mediated TSS remains a clinical diagnosis as fewer than 5% of patients have bacteremia, while blood cultures are positive for *S. pyogenes* in more than 50% of TSS patients. With both pathogens, cultures usually are positive from the site of infection and should be obtained as soon as the site is identified. If *S. aureus* is isolated in the laboratory, it is important to obtain antimicrobial susceptibilities because methicillin-resistant *S. aureus* strains are particularly associated with TSS.

S. pyogenes uniformly is susceptible to penicillins and cephalosporins. Antimicrobial susceptibility should be determined only for non-β-lactam antimicrobial agents, such as clindamycin and erythromycin, to which *S. pyogenes* may be resistant. A significant increase in antibody titers to antistreptolysin O, antideoxyribonuclease B, or other streptococcal extracellular products 4–6 weeks after infection may help confirm the diagnosis if culture results were negative. For both forms of TSS, laboratory studies may reflect multisystem organ involvement and disseminated intravascular coagulation.

Treatment

Management is similar for TSS caused by *S. aureus* and *S. pyogenes*. Aggressive fluid replacement and correction of respiratory or cardiac failure are immediate priorities. Because distinguishing between the two forms of TSS may not be possible, initial empiric antimicrobial therapy should include a β-lactamase-resistant antistaphylococcal antimicrobial agent and a protein synthesis-inhibiting antimicrobial drug, such as clindamycin. Both should be given parenterally at maximal doses for age. Clindamycin is more effective than penicillin for treating well-established *S. pyogenes* infections because this antibiotic inhibits protein synthesis resulting in suppression of synthesis of the *S. pyogenes* antiphagocytic M protein and bacterial toxins. Clindamycin should not be used alone as initial empiric therapy, because in the United States, 1%–2% of *S. pyogenes* strains are resistant to clindamycin. Because methicillin resistant *Staphylococcus aureus* (MRSA) now causes over half of community-acquired infections in many regions of the United States, vancomycin should be used routinely as initial empiric therapy. The total duration of therapy should be individualized and based in large part on the underlying infection, such as pneumonia, septic arthritis, and ANF.

Immune globulin intravenous (IGIV) may be considered as adjunctive therapy for either form of TSS. The mechanism of action of IGIV appears to be neutralization of circulating bacterial toxins. Various regimens of IGIV, ranging from 150 to 400 mg/kg/day for 5 days and a single dose of 1–2 g/kg, have been used, but the optimal regimen is unknown.

Isolation of the Hospitalized Patient

Standard precautions, as well as droplet and contact precautions, are recommended for all patients with *S. pyogenes*. Because person-to-person transmission of *S. aureus*-mediated TSS is uncommon, only standard precautions are needed.

HEMATOGENOUS OSTEOMYELITIS

Hematogenous osteomyelitis begins in the metaphysis of tubular long bones adjacent to the epiphyseal growth plate, therefore more common in growing children and adolescents. Thrombosis of the low velocity sinusoidal vessels due to trauma or embolization is considered the focus for bacterial seeding in this process. This avascular environment allows invading organisms to proliferate while avoiding the influx of phagocytes, the presence of serum antibody and complement, the interaction with tissue macrophages, and other host defense mechanisms. The proliferation of organisms, release of organism enzymes and by-products, and the fixed volume environment contribute to progressive bone necrosis.

Clinical Manifestations

The signs, symptoms, and pathologic progression vary by age. In adolescents focal symptoms are usually present, with very localized point tenderness, mild restriction of movement, and limp suggesting not only the diagnosis of osteomyelitis, but its location. Fever and malaise are also common symptoms.

Etiology

The bacterial etiology of hematogenous osteomyelitis demonstrates an age-specific pattern, but in adolescents *S. aureus* accounts for more than 90% of cases in otherwise healthy adolescents with no predisposing factors. Other epidemiologic factors, predisposing chronic diseases, and exposure history may suggest unusual pathogens (Table 20-1).

Epidemiology

Infectious agents are introduced into bone by (a) hematogenous infection from bacteremia, (b) local spread from contiguous foci such as cellulitis or

TABLE 20-1

SPECIFIC ETIOLOGIES OF OSTEOMYELITIS

Clinical Circumstances	Probable Etiology
Human bite	Anaerobes
Dog or cat bite	*Pasteurella multocida*
Puncture wound of foot	*Pseudomonas aeruginosa*
Sickle cell disease	*Salmonella* sp.
Rheumatoid arthritis	*Staphylococcus aureus* (from joint)
	Pasteurella multocida
Diabetes mellitus	Fungi
Uncommon etiologies	
Facial and cervical area; in the jaw; sinus drainage; lytic bone changes with "egg shell" areas of new bone	*Actinomyces* sp.
Vertebral body or long bone abscesses; systemic signs and symptoms	*Brucella*
Regional distribution; systemic findings; vertebral body, skull, long bone involvement	*Salmonella* *Coccidioides*
Skin lesion; pulmonary involvement; skull and vertebral bodies most common, but long bone involvement is reported	*Blastomyces*
Very distinct, slowly progressive bony lesions can occur	Cryptococcus
Exposure to cats, fever of unknown origin (FUO), liver granulomas, chronic adenitis	*Bartonella henselae* (cat scratch disease)

infected varicella lesions, and (c) direct inoculation following trauma, invasive procedures, or surgery. The incidence of osteomyelitis is greater in males (2.5 times more often than females) and approximately 40% of cases occur in patients less than 20 years of age. Tubular long bones are primarily involved, especially of the lower extremities.

Differential Diagnosis

Other etiologies of children with bone pain and fever include: septicemia, cellulitis, toxic synovitis, septic arthritis, thrombophlebitis, or in a sickle cell disease patient, a bone infarction.

Diagnosis

A technetium bone scan remains the procedure of choice for establishing a diagnosis of osteomyelitis and localizing disease. However, routine plain x-rays are initially obtained since they are readily available and may identify other etiologies of bone pain. The diagnosis of osteomyelitis on routine roentgenographs can be subtle to obvious depending on the duration of disease and are adequate for differentiating patients with trauma, including physical abuse. X-rays are also fairly sensitive for identifying leukemic infiltrates, which represent one important cause of bone pain.

Diagnosis of bone infection is enhanced with the use of technetium scanning, which can be completed in 1–2 hours. This study should be obtained for any patient who has obvious evidence of focal bone pathology, fever of undetermined etiology with bone tenderness on physical examination, and an elevated C reactive protein or sedimentation rate or suggestive findings on routine radiographs. The bone scan can also aid in directing aspirate procedures for diagnosis and culture. In situations where osteomyelitis is suspected on physical examination but the technetium bone scan is equivocal or nondiagnostic, secondary radionuclide imaging including MRI may be performed. In selected cases, including pelvic, vertebral, or small bone (hands/feet) osteomyelitis, the use of MRI or CT can be useful in establishing a diagnosis or directing surgical intervention.

The diagnosis of osteomyelitis is confirmed with isolation of organisms from bone, subperiosteal exudate, or contiguous joint fluid. Needle aspiration through normal skin over involved bone at a subperiosteal site or at the metaphyseal area combined with a potentially involved joint aspiration should be performed by an orthopedic surgeon. Aspirates of involved focal areas yield positive cultures in 80%–85% of cases that have not been pretreated with antibiotics. However, because early institution of antimicrobial therapy is so common, only 50% of suspected cases are culture positive. Blood cultures have been reported to be positive in as many as 50% of cases so should be obtained routinely prior to initiation of antimicrobial therapy.

NONHEMATOGENOUS OSTEOMYELITIS

Bone involvement arises through spread from a contiguous focus of infection or direct inoculation. The following are the more common types of nonhematogenous osteomyelitis in adolescents.

Pseudomonas Osteochondritis

The predilection of *Pseudomonas* to involve cartilaginous tissue and the relative amount of cartilage in children's tarsal-metatarsal region are the reasons for this infection being classified as an "osteochondritis." The classic history is a nail puncture through a tennis shoe. This entity is seen as early as 2 days postinjury but frequently requires up to 21 days to manifest clinically. The proper initial management of this trauma is vigorous irrigation and cleansing of the puncture wound in conjunction with tetanus prophylaxis. Upon diagnosis of *Pseudomonas* osteochondritis from wound, drainage culture, or surgical curettage culture, intravenous antibiotics should be initiated and guided by antibiotic sensitivity testing. The crucial factor for successful therapy is complete evacuation of all necrotic, infected bone and cartilage. If this is accomplished, only 7–10 days of parenteral antibiotics are necessary (depending on soft-tissue healing and appearance) for completion of therapy.

Pseudomonas osteochondritis of the vertebrae or pelvis should lead one to suspect intravenous drug abuse.

Patellar Osteochondritis

Patellar osteochondritis is seen in children 5–15 years of age when the patella has significant vascular integrity. Direct inoculation via a puncture wound yields symptoms within 1 week to 10 days. Constitutional symptoms are uncommon. *S. aureus* is the most common etiology. Roentgenographs may take 2–3 weeks to show bone sclerosis or destruction.

Contiguous Osteochondritis

Infection is most common in adolescents and adults. It is associated with nosocomial-infected burns or penetrating wounds. The clinical course characteristically includes 2 to 4 weeks of local pain, skin erosion, ulceration, or sinus drainage. Multiple organisms are common and draining sinus cultures correlate well with bone aspirate or biopsy cultures. *S. aureus*, streptococci, anaerobes, and nosocomial gram-negative enterics are the etiologic organisms; peripheral leukocyte count or erythrocyte sedimentation rates are usually normal.

Treatment of Osteomyelitis

The treatment of hematogenous osteomyelitis should be guided initially by Gram stain and subsequently by susceptibilities of organisms recovered from bone or joint aspirates. Empiric therapy on an age- and disease-related basis administered parenterally should be initiated once a diagnosis is confirmed and cultures have been obtained.

Parenteral antibiotics in acute bacterial hematogenous osteomyelitis are indicated initially because: physiologic and constitutional changes are not ideal for oral antibiotic absorption; there is propensity for dissemination and abscess formation (especially for *S. aureus*); and compliance must be assured during early treatment. Although the route of administration of antibiotics remains controversial, oral absorption is adequate for the continuation of therapy. Parenteral therapy should be continued until a clinical response is documented, usually 3–5 days. The duration of antibiotic therapy (parenteral and oral) should generally be 3 weeks and may have to extend longer depending on the site of infection and clinical response. The use of home intravenous antibiotics for selected cases can substitute for part of the initial therapy or for the entire course if oral continuation therapy is felt to be suboptimal for age, site, or severity (*Pseudomonas* osteochondritis following puncture wound of the foot and surgical debridement is an exception). Surgical drainage or debridement of subperiosteal abscesses or soft-tissue abscesses should be considered. Immobilization of an affected extremity is necessary for pain relief and to enhance healing.

Duration of Treatment

Most cases of hematogenous osteomyelitis are culture negative after 21 days of therapy. Exceptions are vertebral osteomyelitis which should be treated for 6 weeks and puncture wound osteochondritis caused by *Pseudomonas* which can be sterilized after 7–10 days of antimicrobial therapy in conjunction with adequate surgical debridement.

SEPTIC ARTHRITIS

Pathogenesis

With the production of joint fluid by the synovial membrane, the kinetics of capillary diffusion of fluid into the joint space and the effective blood flow of the joint space, the relatively high frequency of joint infections is not surprising. Bacteria can enter the joint space by direct inoculation (such as kneeling on a needle or trauma), contiguous extension (osteomyelitis), or via a hematogenous route. In adolescents, infection in the lower extremities accounts for over 80% of cases.

Clinical Manifestations

The diagnosis of septic arthritis is made earlier than in osteomyelitis due to the onset of constitutional symptoms within the first few days of the infection. Patients almost always have fever, focal findings in the joint (e.g., swelling, tenderness, heat, and limitation of motion), and placement of the joint in a neutral, nonstressed position. Resistance to movement or pain on internal rotation of the joint should be evaluated. An obvious portal of entry in septic arthritis is uncommon.

Diagnosis

The diagnosis of suspect joint infection by roentgenograms depends on finding evidence of capsular swelling. In the case of hip involvement, roentgenograms can be valuable; placement of the adolescent in the frog-leg position for an anteroposterior radiograph shows displacement of fat lines. Obliteration or lateral displacement of the gluteal fat lines or a raised position for Shenton's line with widening of the arc, are consistent with hip joint effusion under pressure. The presence of a significant joint effusion by hip ultrasound is adequate to dictate a joint aspiration. Radionuclide imaging or MRI may be a useful adjunct in a complex or uncharacteristic case for early diagnosis. The use of hip ultrasound followed by a technetium bone scan (or CT/MRI) in selected cases is a reasonable progression of tests based on usefulness, cost, and radiation exposure.

The confirmatory procedure for diagnosis is a joint aspiration with Gram stain, culture, and cytology-chemistry evaluation. Joint aspiration of knees (most common joint involved) should be a procedure for all primary care physicians; aspiration of hips or shoulders should be limited to an experienced orthopedist (under fluoroscopic control for hip aspirations). Joint fluid should be processed for Gram stain and aerobic and anaerobic cultures. The fluid should be analyzed for glucose concentration (compared to a concomitant blood glucose), leukocyte count, and differential ability to spontaneously clot, and mucin clot test. Joint fluid should be obtained in a heparinized syringe to assure leukocyte analysis. To perform the mucin clot test, glacial acetic acid is added to the joint fluid while stirring; normal fluid reacts with a white precipitate (rope) that clings to the stirring rod with a clear supernatant.

Etiologic diagnosis of septic arthritis can be aided by blood cultures; some series have reported up to 20%–30% of sterile joint fluids with concomitant positive blood cultures. Additional laboratory studies include a hemogram to screen for anemia (hemoglobinopathy), CRP or ESR (usually elevated in septic arthritis), serum or urine for bacterial antigen detection (only in partially treated cases with suspect group B streptococci, *Haemophilus influenzae*, pneumococcus, or meningococcus), and accessory cultures: wound, infected skin lesions (secondarily infected varicella lesions over the involved joint), cellulitis, or urethral-cervical-rectal cultures in sexually active adolescents (gonorrhea).

The differential diagnosis of arthritis includes joint fluid inflammation due to a variety of etiologies. More common in adolescents than other age groups are infections caused by parvovirus B19, rubella vaccine virus, mycoplasma, Reiter syndrome, and Lyme disease. Other etiologies of arthritis are serum sickness (drug, postinfectious), acute rheumatic fever, collagen vascular disease, anaphylactoid purpura, leukemia, pigmented villonodular synovitis, primary bone tumor, gout, hyperparathyroidism, agammaglobulinemia, Behçet syndrome, hepatitis, diabetes mellitus, peripheral nerve or spinal cord injury, leprosy, trauma (to include physical abuse), hemophilia, aseptic necrosis, osteochondritis, bursitis, sarcoidosis, inflammatory bowel disease, familial Mediterranean fever, Tietze syndrome, and reactive arthritis following *Shigella, Salmonella, Yersinia*, and *Campylobacter* enteric infections. The causative bacterium in most cases of septic arthritis in sexually active adolescents is *Neisseria gonorrhoeae*. In other adolescents, *S. aureus* remains the most frequent single pathogen.

Treatment of Septic Arthritis

The empiric choice of antimicrobial therapy in septic arthritis should be guided by the site of involvement, underlying disease, and Gram stain of joint fluid but should consider *S. aureus* in all cases and *N. gonorrhoeae* in sexually active adolescents. The penicillins, cephalosporins (first, second, and third generation), macrolides, and aminoglycosides, all attain effective concentrations in joint fluid, averaging 30%–40% of peak serum concentration. Intraarticular antibiotics therefore add no benefit. Larger joints may require open drainage. The duration of antibiotic therapy should be 3 weeks minimum with the first 3–5 days administered parenterally followed by oral continuation therapy as long as the following criteria are met: no gastrointestinal (GI) disorder to underlying disease that would diminish oral absorption, clinical response to parenteral antibiotics, and surgical management has been established; the organism is sensitive to a class of antibiotic in oral form and compliance can be guaranteed. Some experts administer a trial dosage of oral antibiotics during inpatient management.

To evaluate the effectiveness of antibiotic therapy in more difficult cases, serial joint aspirations can be performed. Although cultures may be positive for up to 5–7 days in nonsurgically drained joint fluid, a decrease in leukocyte density should be seen by 1–2 weeks of therapy. In studies using serial joint aspirations, by days 1 through 10 of antibiotic therapy those patients who subsequently recover had less than 5000 cells/mm^3 compared to those with recrudescent infection who had more than 60,000 cells/mm^3. The best predictor of outcome and complications is the duration of signs and symptoms prior to diagnosis and effective therapy.

MYCOPLASMA INFECTION

Clinical Manifestations

In adolescents, *Mycoplasma* infection presents most commonly as pneumonia, but also as acute bronchitis and upper respiratory tract infections, including pharyngitis. Associated signs and symptoms frequently include malaise, fever, and headache. In patients with pneumonia, cough is an early manifestation and persists for 3–4 weeks. The cough is nonproductive initially but later may become productive, particularly in adolescents. A maculopapular rash is occasionally seen. Radiographic abnormalities are most commonly bilateral, diffuse infiltrates. Approximately 20% of patients have a small pleural effusion. Focal abnormalities, such as consolidation and hilar adenopathy, may occur.

Other occasional manifestations include aseptic meningitis, encephalitis, cerebellar ataxia, transverse myelitis, and peripheral neuropathy. Myocarditis, pericarditis, polymorphous mucocutaneous eruptions (including Stevens-Johnson syndrome), hemolytic anemia, and arthritis have all been observed. More severe pulmonary disease is seen in patients with sickle cell disease, Down syndrome, immunodeficiencies, and chronic cardiorespiratory disease.

Etiology

M. pneumoniae are the smallest free-living pleomorphic microorganisms that lack a cell wall.

Epidemiology

M. pneumoniae disease, seen only in humans, is transmitted by respiratory droplets during close contact. The incubation period ranges from 1 to 4 weeks. There is a higher incidence of disease in adolescents and outbreaks have been reported in young adults and adolescents on military bases, colleges, and summer camps. Community-wide epidemics occur every 4–7 years. Because patients remain colonized for weeks after treatment is completed, familial spread may continue for many months. Immunity after infection is not long lasting.

Diagnostic Tests

Culture of *M. pneumoniae* is impractical because incubation in special enriched broth requires up to 21 days. A rapid test (bedside cold agglutinins) can be readily performed for early diagnosis. Two to five drops of blood are placed in a small (blue top) tube containing sodium citrate, which is then submerged in a cup containing ice and water for 30–60 seconds. Agglutination of red blood cells occurs when mycoplasma antibody titers are 1:64 or greater. Specificity of this test is virtually absolute, but unfortunately the sensitivity is only 50%.

Specific immunofluorescence and enzyme immunoassay methods are available commercially and both detect *M. pneumoniae*-specific immunoglobulin (Ig) M and IgG antibodies. The IgG antibody titer peaks at approximately 3–6 weeks and persists for 2–3 months after infection. IgM antibodies suggest recent infection, but persist in serum for several months and, in adolescents, may remain increased for years. However, an increased specific IgM against *M. pneumoniae* in an adolescent with pneumonia is acceptable for etiologic diagnosis. False-negative results also occur with these serologic assays.

Treatment

Bronchitis and upper respiratory tract illness are self-limited and do not require antimicrobial therapy. Macrolides, such as erythromycin, azithromycin, and clarithromycin, are the preferred antimicrobial agents for treatment of pneumonia. Tetracycline and doxycycline are equally effective.

Isolation of the Hospitalized Patient

Standard and droplet precautions are recommended for the duration of symptomatic illness. Prophylaxis of exposed contacts is not recommended with the exception of close household contacts with sickle cell disease.

EPSTEIN-BARR VIRUS INFECTIONS

EBV causes numerous distinct clinical entities, the most common being infectious mononucleosis. Others are the x-linked lymphoproliferative syndrome, posttransplantation lymphoproliferative disorder, Burkitt lymphoma, nasopharyngeal carcinoma, undifferentiated B-cell lymphomas of the central nervous system, aseptic meningitis, encephalitis, and Guillain-Barré syndrome.

Infectious Mononucleosis

Infectious mononucleosis in adolescents is characterized by fever, exudative pharyngitis, lymphadenopathy, splenomegaly, and atypical lymphocytosis.

The incubation period for infectious mononucleosis is 1–2 months. Many patients may be asymptomatic only showing evidence of infection by the development of EBV antigen-specific antibodies.

Etiology

EBV is a member of the herpes group of viruses that replicates in B-lymphocytes.

Epidemiology

EBV is species-specific for humans, transmitted primarily by close contact. The virus can be isolated from saliva and can infect white blood cells resulting in transmission through blood transfusions. The virus may be isolated from saliva for 3–6 months after symptomatic disease and intermittent excretion occurs lifelong. Outbreaks of infectious mononucleosis have frequently been reported among adolescents in educational institutions or among those housed in common dormitories.

Diagnosis

Nonspecific tests for heterophile antibody are usually positive in adolescents with typical manifestations of infectious mononucleosis during the first 2 weeks of illness, becoming negative after 4–6 months. In typical cases of infectious mononucleosis, no further testing needs to be done. Serologic testing for EBV-specific antibody is used to make the diagnosis in atypical cases. The best documentation for recent infection (less than 3 months) is IgM antiviral capsid antigen (VCA) antibody. Other serologic studies include IgG to VCA, which is present as early as IgM, but persists for longer than 3 months and in about 20% of individuals persists for life. Antibody to EBV nuclear antigen (EBNA) is present 2–6 months after onset of infection and persists for life.

Treatment

A short course of corticosteroids is recommended for patients with enlarged "kissing" tonsils which are judged to potentially cause airway obstruction. Some experts have also recommended steroids for prolonged illness (>28 days), massive splenomegaly, hepatitis, myocarditis, hemolytic anemia, and the hemophagocytic syndrome. The dosage of prednisone is 1 mg/kg/day, maximum 20 mg for 7–10 days. In patients with splenomegaly, contact sports must be discontinued.

Pertussis

It is now apparent that adolescents and young adults, usually parents or other household members are the contact sources for most pediatric cases of whooping cough. Illness in adolescents is often undetected because it is so mild, yet might be transmitted to young infant contacts resulting in severe disease. Although active whooping cough during childhood usually confers immunity for 15 years, protection from vaccine wanes by age 11–15, just 6 years after the last booster dose is given. Therefore, booster doses of pertussis vaccine during early adolescence is an important strategy for further reduction of disease.

Etiology

The genus *Bordetella* currently contains six species: *B. pertussis, B. parapertussis, B. hinzii, B. holmesii, B. bronchiseptica,* and *B. avium.* The first four have host species specificity for humans while *B. bronchiseptica* can infect dogs causing severe respiratory disease, occasionally associated with a high mortality in these animals, and *B. avium,* causing respiratory illness in turkeys and other birds. The live *B. bronchiseptica* vaccine used to immunize dogs has been shown to cause severe illness in young children exposed to recently vaccinated dogs and milder symptoms in adolescents exposed directly to the aerosolized vaccine.

CLINICAL MANIFESTATIONS

Illness is classically divided into three stages: catarrhal lasting approximately 2 weeks, paroxysmal lasting 4–6 weeks, and then a convalescent stage which can continue for as long as 2 months. Duration of each stage is somewhat dependent on the patient's age in that fully immunized adolescents and adults may exhibit only paroxysmal coughing for a few weeks. This infection is unique in that patients are generally afebrile and do not show an elevation in the erythrocyte sedimentation rate nor increase in other classic acute phase reactants. Most characteristic is a marked lymphocytosis of both T and B cells. Pertussis is one of the more common causes of a leukemoid reaction with leukocyte counts often exceeding 50,000 cells/mm^3. The classic chest radiographic finding is a "shaggy heart" produced by bilateral perihilar infiltrates, interstitial edema, and atelectasis. The presence of fever, neutrophilia, or consolidated pneumonia should suggest a secondary bacterial infection in the lungs and antibiotics should be selected to empirically cover pneumococcus and *S. aureus.*

Diagnosis

Cultures for *B. pertussis* or fluorescent stain of posterior nasopharyngeal secretions are equally sensitive for confirmation of diagnosis. Culture requires special media such as Regan-Lowe or Bordet-Gengou. Fluorescent stains are preferred because cultures may require incubation for as long as 2 weeks. Unfortunately the direct immunofluorescent assay has relative low specificity thereby yielding a high percent of false-positive results. Many experts therefore recommend culture when accurate epidemiologic information is being sought.

Treatment

Erythromycin is the drug of choice, recommended at a dosage of 40–50 mg/kg/day, orally, in four divided doses; maximum 2 g/day. Duration of therapy is 14 days. Recent studies have shown that azithromycin (10–12 mg/kg/day, orally, in one dose for 5 days; maximum 600 mg/day) and clarithromycin (15–20 mg/kg/day, orally, in two divided doses; maximum 1 g/day for 7 days) are equally effective.

ROCKY MOUNTAIN SPOTTED FEVER

Rocky Mountain spotted fever (RMSF) caused by *Rickettsia rickettsii*, is transmitted by tick bites. The organisms replicate within the endothelial cells of blood vessels, causing a generalized vasculitis and producing clinical findings.

Clinical Manifestations

The triad of high fever, severe headache, and a centrifugal petechial rash are the characteristic features of RMSF. The incubation period is 1–8 days. When early nonspecific symptoms appear following a tick bite, RMSF should be seriously considered and early treatment instituted. It is difficult to differentiate RMSF from the myriad other causes of febrile exanthems. Its diagnosis is also frequently overlooked in patients who do not present with the typical rash or in whom a history of tick bite cannot be elicited.

Diagnosis

Serologic tests for antibody to *R. rickettsii* are the usual method of diagnosis but do not become positive until 7–14 days after onset of illness.

Treatment

Treatment of RMSF should be instituted as soon as the diagnosis is suspected clinically. In addition to antibiotic therapy, careful supportive intensive care is often needed.

TULAREMIA

Clinical Manifestations

There are five clinical presentations of tularemia. Most common is the ulceroglandular syndrome, characterized by a painful ulcer at the site of the tick bites, associated with painful adenitis, which may drain spontaneously. The glandular syndrome is similar but without an ulcer. Less common disease presentations are: oculoglandular (severe conjunctivitis

and preauricular lymphadenopathy), oropharyngeal (severe exudate stomatitis, pharyngitis, or tonsillitis and cervical lymphadenopathy), typhoidal (high fever, hepatomegaly, and splenomegaly), intestinal (intestinal pain, vomiting, and diarrhea), and pneumonic (pneumonia). With all clinical forms there is an abrupt onset of fever, chills, myalgia, and headache.

Etiology

Francisella tularensis, the causative agent, is a gram-negative pleomorphic coccobacillus.

Epidemiology

In the United States, tick bites and skinning rabbits are major sources of human infection. Adolescents at risk are those with recreational exposure to ticks and to infected animals or their habitats, such as rabbit hunters and trappers. In the United States, ticks are the most important arthropod vectors, and most cases occur during summer months. Infection also may be acquired by ingestion of contaminated water or inadequately cooked meat, or inhalation of aerosolized organisms or contaminated particles.

Clinical Manifestations

The incubation period usually is 3–5 days, with a range of 1–21 days.

Diagnostic Tests

A single serum antibody titer of ≥1:128 determined by microagglutination (MA) or of ≥1:160 determined by tube agglutination (TA) supports a presumptive diagnosis. Confirmation by serologic testing requires a fourfold or greater titer change been two sera obtained at least 2 weeks apart, with one of the specimens having a minimum titer of ≥1:128 (MA) or ≥1:160 (TA). Low titer nonspecific cross-reactions can occur with antibodies to *Brucella* species and *Legionella* species. Culture of ulcer exudate is not recommended because of the potential for severe disease in laboratory personnel handling these specimens.

Treatment

Aminoglycosides: streptomycin, gentamicin sulfate, or amikacin are recommended for treatment with streptomycin preferred because of greater experience and because it can be given twice a day. Recommended duration of therapy is 10 days.

Control Measures

Protective clothing and frequent inspection for and removal of ticks from the skin and scalp offer the best prevention. Rubber gloves should be worn by hunters when skinning rabbits. Game meats should be cooked thoroughly.

PLAGUE

Clinical Manifestations

In the United States, plague is most commonly seen in adolescents presenting in the bubonic form, with acute onset of fever and painful swollen regional lymph nodes (buboes), most commonly in the inguinal region. Plague may also present with hypotension, acute respiratory distress, intravascular coagulopathy, pneumonia, or meningitis. Fever, chills, headache, and rapidly progressive weakness are characteristic in all forms. Occasionally, patients have only mild lymphadenitis or prominent GI tract symptoms.

Etiology

Plague is caused by *Yersinia pestis*, a pleomorphic, bipolar-staining, gram-negative coccobacillus.

Epidemiology

Rodents, carnivores, and their fleas are the reservoir of plague reported throughout the western United States with New Mexico reporting the highest number of cases. Bubonic plague usually is transmitted by bites of infected rodent fleas. Septicemic plague occurs most often as a complication of bubonic plague. Primary pneumonic plague is acquired by exposure to respiratory droplets from infected humans or animals. The incubation period is 2–6 days for bubonic plague and 2–4 days for primary pneumonic plague.

Diagnostic Tests

Y. pestis is readily identified in affected tissues, especially lymph nodes, spleen, and liver. A fluorescent antibody test is also available to confirm the presence of *Y. pestis* in direct smears or cultures from infected sites. A single positive serologic test result by passive hemagglutination assay or enzyme immunoassay is highly suggestive of disease and a fourfold increase in antibody titer between two serum specimens obtained 4 weeks to 3 months apart provides confirmation.

Treatment

Streptomycin, 30 mg/kg/day in two divided doses, given intramuscularly is the treatment of choice. Gentamicin is an equally effective agent. Drainage of abscessed buboes is necessary keeping in mind that material may be infectious during the first day or two after beginning antimicrobial therapy.

Isolation of the hospitalized patient

For bubonic plague, only standard precautions are necessary while droplet precautions are indicated for pneumonic disease.

Suggested Readings

Cohen JI: Epstein-Barr virus infection. *N Engl J Med.* 343:481–492, 2000.

Darenberg J, Ihendyane N, Sjolin J, et al.: Intravenous immunoglobulin G therapy in streptococcal toxic shock syndrome: A European randomized, double-blind, placebo-controlled trial. *Clin Infect Dis* 37:333–340, 2003.

Dennis DT, Chow CC: Plague. *Pediatr Infect Dis J* 23:69–71, 2004.

Floyed RL, Steele RW: Culture-negative osteomyelitis. *Pediatr Infect Dis J.* 22:731–735, 2003.

Jacobs RF, Cabe HC: Tularemia. *Adv Pediatr Infect Dis* 12:55–69, 1997.

Lee MC, Rios AM, Aten MF, et al.: Management and out-come of children with skin and soft tissue abscesses caused by community-acquired methicillin-resistant *Staphylococcus aureus*. *Pediatr Infect Dis J* 23: 123–127, 2004.

Quinonez JM, Steele RW. Necrotizing fasciitis. *Semin Pediatr Infect Dis* 8:207–214, 1997.

Smith JW, Piercy EA: Infectious arthritis. *Clin Infect Dis* 20:225–231, 1995.

Stevens DL: Dilemmas in the treatment of invasive *Streptococcus pyogenes* infections. *Clin Infect Dis* 37:341–343, 2003.

Taylor-Robinson D: Infections due to species of *Mycoplasma* and *Ureaplasma*: An update. *Clin Infect Dis* 23:671–684, 1996.

Thorner AR, Walker DH, Petri WA: Rocky mountain spotted fever. *Clin Infect Dis* 27:1353–1360, 1998.

21

GENETICS IN ADOLESCENT MEDICINE

Helga V. Toriello

INTRODUCTION

This chapter is composed of several parts, all dealing with aspects of genetics and adolescent medicine. The first section reviews principles of genetics and modes of inheritance while the next section reviews genetic counseling issues as they pertain to the adolescent. The final section describes several common syndromes and specific issues for management in adolescents with that particular syndrome.

MODES OF INHERITANCE

This section serves as a review of different modes of inheritance, including chromosomal, monogenetic, multifactorial, and nontraditional modes of inheritance.

Chromosomal Inheritance

Humans have 46 chromosomes, arranged in 23 pairs. Twenty-two of the pairs are called autosomes and numbered 1–22; the 23rd pair is the sex chromosomes with an XX complement present in a female and an XY complement present in a male. Chromosome anomalies can either be numeric or structural. Numeric anomalies pertain to a chromosome number of either more or less than 46. One common such anomaly is Down syndrome, in which the individual usually has 47 chromosomes, with trisomy for chromosome 21. Structural anomalies are those in which the chromosome number is normal, but detailed analysis demonstrates either a deletion or duplication of all or part of a particular chromosome.

Chromosome studies are indicated in any individual with a pattern of multiple malformations with an unknown diagnosis. However, it should be borne in mind that individuals with chromosome anomalies generally have involvement of several parts of the body, and include both major and minor anomalies. Second, most individuals with chromosome anomalies have growth deficiency of either prenatal or postnatal onset, as well as mental retardation. Therefore, an individual with one or two anomalies, but with normal growth and psychomotor development, is not a good candidate for chromosome analysis. Exceptions of course apply, particularly regarding sex chromosome anomalies and very small deletions or duplications, the detection of which may require special techniques. One example is the use of fluorescent *in situ* hybridization (FISH) to detect the deletion responsible for the velocardiofacial, or 22q deletion syndrome.

Monogenic Patterns of Inheritance

Monogenic traits are generally inherited in either a dominant or recessive mode, and can be autosomal or X-linked, depending on the nature of the chromosome on which the gene lies. Dominant conditions occur when a single mutant gene is sufficient to cause the condition. If an individual has a dominant trait, it is either inherited from a parent who also has the condition, inherited from a parent who may appear clinically unaffected but is mosaic for the trait, or a new mutation occurred in the egg or sperm of a parent. The genes responsible for autosomal dominant traits are on the autosomes (numbered chromosomes), whereas those responsible for X-linked dominant traits are on the X chromosome. In both cases the condition can be passed from one generation to the next, with the exception that male to male transmission virtually never occurs in an X-linked dominant trait (Figs. 21-1 and 21-2).

Features often found with autosomal dominantly inherited traits are incomplete penetrance and variable expressivity. An individual that has the mutant gene but no manifestations of the condition

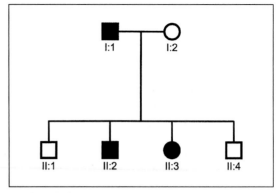

FIGURE 21-1

AUTOSOMAL DOMINANT INHERITANCE. IN THE PEDIGREE, SQUARES REPRESENT MALES, CIRCLES REPRESENT FEMALES. FILLED IN SYMBOLS INDICATE THAT THE INDIVIDUAL IS AFFECTED.

is said to exhibit lack of penetrance for the condition. In some cases this may be a function of age. For example, in Huntington disease, penetrance is close to 100% by age 70, but only approximately 50% at age 40.[1] In other cases penetrance is a function of

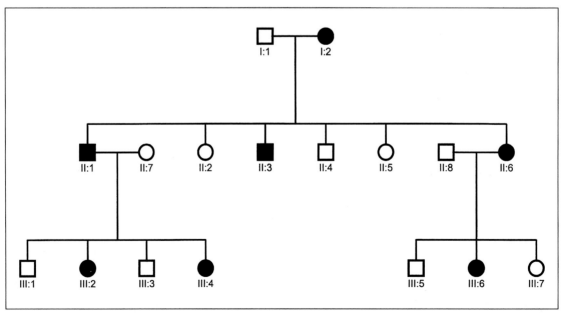

FIGURE 21-2

X-LINKED DOMINANT INHERITANCE. SEE FIG. 21-1 FOR EXPLANATION OF SYMBOLS.

the depth of investigation. An individual with a mutant gene may appear clinically unaffected, but on further evaluation found to have biochemical differences typical of the disorder. A trait that has variable expressivity can have manifestations that range from mild to severe, even within a family. For example, in a family in which neurofibromatosis occurs, some family members may have a severe expression of the condition, whereas others have milder expression. Finally, there are rare situations in which clinically unaffected parents will have more than one child affected with a trait inherited in an autosomal dominant fashion. Although incomplete penetrance in one of the parents could be the cause, another possible explanation is somatic mosaicism in one of the parents. This means that some of that parent's cells (including germ cells) have the mutation whereas other cells do not. Although rare, there have been instances of siblings with achondroplasia being born to unaffected parents. Somatic mosaicism is almost certainly the cause of this phenomenon. The above concepts can also apply to X-linked dominant traits.

Conditions that are inherited as autosomal recessive traits require that both alleles (an allele is one of the members of the pair of genes at a particular locus) of the gene pair be mutated. In that case each parent, who usually only has one copy of the mutated gene, is unaffected but said to be a carrier for the trait. There is usually no family history, other than siblings, of similarly affected individuals, unless the condition is a common one (e.g., hemochromatosis) (Fig. 21-3). When couples are consanguineous (related to each other), their chance of having a child with a condition inherited as an autosomal recessive trait is higher than that of the general population.

X-linked recessive traits are those that are carried by the mother and affect her sons, with each son having a 50% chance of being affected. Her daughters each have a 50% chance of being a carrier like the mother (Fig. 21-4). A male that has an X-linked recessive trait will have no affected children (unless by chance his partner is a carrier for the same condition), but his daughters will all be carriers. In many cases carrier mothers will have

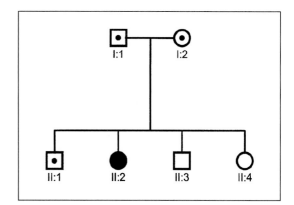

FIGURE 21-3

AUTOSOMAL RECESSIVE INHERITANCE. THE DOT WITHIN THE SYMBOL INDICATES CARRIER STATUS FOR THE TRAIT.

minor manifestations of the condition, such as Lowe syndrome (the features of which include cataract, mental retardation, vitamin D-resistant rickets, and aminoaciduria) in which mothers may have lens opacities.[2] In other cases inheritance is said to be X-linked with irregular dominance, in that the penetrance is reduced in females, but the expression is generally the same in males and

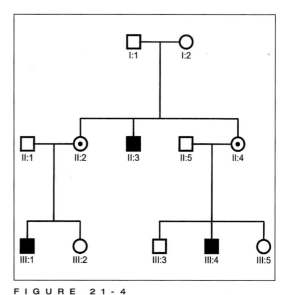

FIGURE 21-4

X-LINKED RECESSIVE INHERITANCE.

TABLE 21-1
GENETIC RISKS

Risk to Offspring If	Individual Affected	Sibling Affected
Autosomal dominant	50%	Not affected (provided penetrance 100%)
Autosomal recessive	Assuming partner unaffected, carrier frequency time $1/2$	Carrier frequency times $2/3$ times $1/4$
X-linked recessive	If affected is a male, 0% for male offspring and 100% for female offspring to be carriers. For female carriers, 50% for affected male and 50% for carrier female.	For female with affected male sibling, . risk depends on family history. If multiple affected family members, risk is $1/4$ for affected male and $1/4$ for carrier female. If no family history, risks less, but not 0%.

females.[3] These situations are fairly rare, however. See Table 21-1 for a summary of risks associated with each mode of monogenic inheritance.

Multifactorial Inheritance

Multifactorial inheritance is thought to result from a combination of genetic and environmental factors.[4–8] There may be several predisposing genes involved, or only one or two. The contribution from environmental factors may be significant, or rather small. However, there are several characteristics of multifactorial traits that must be kept in mind. First, the recurrence in relatives is greater than the frequency of the disorder in the general population, with the risk higher to close relatives than to more distant ones. For example, a sibling or child of an individual with cleft lip/palate has a 3%–4% chance of being similarly affected, whereas a cousin's risk would only be approximately twice that of the general population risk of 0.1%. Second, the chance of recurrence increases with each additional affected family member. If a child has cleft lip and neither parent is affected, the recurrence risk is 3%–4%. However, if one of the parents also has a cleft lip/palate, the risk increases to 10%. Third, the more severe the condition, the higher the risk to relatives. The chance of having a second affected child with a cleft is greater when the index case has a bilateral cleft lip and palate than when he/she has a unilateral cleft lip. Fourth, if there is a sex difference in the frequency of the condition (i.e., females affected more often than males), the risk to relatives is greater when the trait occurs in the sex less often affected.

Table 21-2 lists some of the risks associated with multifactorial conditions. This is not meant to be an exhaustive table, but to rather convey the general idea of risks for multifactorial traits. For example, if the patient's sister has an eating disorder, one would look up the risk to a first degree relative (the patient) because a sibling is affected. Similarly, if a pregnant patient with a cleft lip wants to know the chance of her child also being affected, one would look under cleft lip/palate, first degree relative (because the parent, the patient, is affected). However, if the pregnant patient herself does not have a cleft, but her sister has cleft lip/palate, one would look under the second degree relative column, because the baby's aunt is affected.

Nontraditional Modes of Inheritance

Some types of genetic patterns are not explained by the above-described modes of inheritance. These are uniparental disomy, genomic imprinting, mitochondrial inheritance, and trinucleotide repeat disorders.

Uniparental Disomy

In uniparental disomy, two copies of a given chromosome come from one parent, and none from the other.

TABLE 21-2

RECURRENCE RISKS, WHERE KNOWN, FOR MULTIFACTORIAL CONDITIONS

Risk of Relative Being Affected If Relative Has:	First Degree (Child, Sibling, Parent)	Two First Degrees	Second Degree (Half-sib, Grandparent, Aunt, Uncle)	Third Degree (Cousin, Great-aunt, Great-uncle, Great-grandparent)
Cleft lip/palate[1]	3%–4%	10%	0.6%	0.3%
Cleft palate[1]	2%	8%	~0.2%	~0.1%
Heart defect[1]	2%–3%	10%	~1%	Not increased
Spina bifida, anencephaly[1]	2%	10%	1%	0.5%
Scoliosis, idiopathic[4]	5%–7%		3%–4%	1%–2%
Talipes equinovarus[5]	2%–6%		0.6%	0.2%
Hip dysplasia[1]	6%	36%	1%	
Diabetes, insulin-dependent[1]	7%	16%		
Eating disorders[6]	14%			
Schizophrenia[1]	9%	15%	3%	1%–2%
Bipolar disorder[1]	13%–20%	20%–30%	5%	2%–3%
Inflammatory bowel disease	5%–8% for Crohn's disease, 2%–4% for ulcerative colitis[7]		2%–4%[8]	

This situation usually occurs when the conception had trisomy for that chromosome, with subsequent loss of a chromosome in one of the early cell divisions. If both of the remaining chromosomes are from the same parent, then uniparental disomy is present. For example, in .02% of cases, cystic fibrosis occurs because of uniparental disomy for chromosome 7.[9] In this case the pertinent chromosome 7 has the mutant allele for cystic fibrosis, and only one parent (whose chromosome 7 it is) is a carrier. However, 20%–30% of cases of Prader-Willi syndrome arise in this way.

Imprinting

It is often assumed that the influence of a gene is independent of the source, but that is not necessarily true. There are situations where modifications of genetic material occur depending on whether it is inherited from the mother or the father. The term that describes this phenomenon is genomic imprinting. For example, a deletion of a region of the paternally inherited chromosome 15 results in Prader-Willi syndrome; if a deletion of the same region occurs in the maternally inherited chromosome, Angelman syndrome is the result.

Mitochondrial Inheritance

Mitochondrial inheritance is characterized by transmission of the disorder from a mother to all of her children. However, only females transmit the condition, since the zygote contains mitochondria that are only maternally derived. We do know that the expression of mitochondrially inherited disorders varies widely, even within sibships. That occurs because not all of the mitochondria will have the gene mutation, and one child could have a greater proportion of mitochondrial mutations than another child.

Trinucleotide Repeat Disorders

In the past, anticipation was the term used to describe either an adult-onset condition appearing earlier in successive generations, or the presence of increasing severity with successive generations.[10] This phenomenon can now be explained by the disorder being caused by repeated trinucleotide sequences within the gene. Below a certain number of repeats, the gene is considered stable. A small increase in the number of repeats leads to instability of the gene, but with little, if any, effect on the phenotype. Above a critical level, the condition becomes clinically apparent. In some conditions, the expansion occurs during female meiosis, whereas in others during male meiosis. For example, if a man with Huntington disease (condition characterized by motor, cognitive, and psychiatric disturbances) has a repeat size of 43 (36 or more repeats is considered a mutant allele,[11] the expected age of onset is 44 years.[12] However, if his son or daughter inherits a further expanded allele of 50 repeats, the age of onset is predicted to be 27 years.[12]

GENETIC COUNSELING AND TESTING ISSUES IN ADOLESCENTS

Genetic counseling is defined by the American Society of Human Genetics as the communication process that deals with the human problems associated with the occurrence or risk of occurrence of a genetic disorder in a family. This process involves an attempt by one or more appropriately trained persons to help the individual or family to (1) comprehend the medical facts including the diagnosis, probable course of the disorder, and the available management, (2) appreciate the way heredity contributes to the disorder and the risk of recurrence in specified relatives, (3) understand the alternatives for dealing with the risk of recurrence, (4) choose a course of action which seems to them appropriate in view of their risk, their family goals, and their ethical and religious standards and act in accordance with that decision, and (5) make the best possible adjustment to the disorder in an affected family member and/or to the risk of recurrence of that disorder.[13] One component of this process includes obtaining a three-generation family history, and documenting age and cause of death (for those deceased); ethnic background; relevant health information for the patient, his or her parents, siblings, half siblings, aunts and uncles, cousins, and grandparents; and information about consanguinity.[14] Another component is the discussion of genetic testing options that might be available.

A genetic test is generally defined as a laboratory analysis to detect DNA, RNA, or chromosome abnormalities that cause or are likely to cause a specific disease or condition. There are various forms of genetic tests, including carrier tests (used to predict whether an individual carries a single copy of a mutant gene for a condition inherited as an autosomal or X-linked recessive trait, or carries a chromosome rearrangement that could be unbalanced in an offspring), prenatal diagnosis (used to detect a genetic condition in a fetus), preimplantation diagnosis (used to detect a genetic condition in an embryo conceived by in vitro fertilization), newborn screening (used to detect certain genetic disorders for which early diagnosis and treatment are available), diagnostic/confirmatory testing (used to identify or confirm a genetic condition in an individual), and presymptomatic/predictive testing (used to determine the probability that an asymptomatic individual will develop a certain genetic disorder). As discussed by Wertz et al.,[15] genetic testing of minors falls into four general categories. These are:

1. Testing that offers immediate medical benefits for the minor (e.g., diagnosis, prevention, and early treatment).
2. Testing for which there are no medical benefits, but testing is of benefit to the minor in terms of making reproductive decisions.
3. Testing offers no benefits of either type, but parents or the minor request it.
4. Testing is done solely for the benefit of another family member.

Hoffman and Wulfsberg[16] expanded on the above list, and identified seven categories of genetic testing in minors. These are:

1. Testing is of immediate benefit to the individual, and includes newborn screening, confirmatory or diagnostic testing in a symptomatic individual, or presymptomatic testing for a condition that has a treatment that is available and beneficial.
2. Reproductive testing for adolescents, and which is carrier rather than diagnostic testing.
3. Testing is for the benefit of other family members who may be making reproductive decisions, and where it may be necessary to test both affected and unaffected family members. Linkage studies fall within this category.
4. Research related testing that is usually conducted under a protocol approved by an Institutional Review Board.
5. Testing done by insurance companies for the purpose of excluding individuals from coverage.
6. Presymptomatic testing to predict a child's future risk of developing a genetic disease or having a predisposition for which no treatment or prevention exists.
7. Carrier testing at an age when the child cannot procreate.

This section will address genetic counseling issues pertinent to the adolescent with either a family history of a genetic condition or genetic condition in him or herself, as well as testing issues (noted above) that are applicable.

Genetic Counseling and Testing Issues for Family History of a Disorder

The two types of tests that apply to this situation are carrier testing and predictive testing. Carrier testing is performed to determine whether an individual carries either a chromosome rearrangement (e.g., balanced translocation) or single copy of an altered gene for a particular disorder inherited in autosomal recessive or X-linked recessive manner. Predictive testing is done to determine whether a healthy individual will develop a certain disorder that is usually inherited in an autosomal dominant manner and for which there is usually a positive family history. Predictive testing could also apply

to conditions that have complex inheritance, and for which testing for one or more genes involved in the disease process is available, for example, apolipoprotein E (APOE) testing and predisposition to heart disease.[17]

Several hypothetical situations will be used to convey the issues involved. These are not meant to provide all the answers, but rather to provoke thought and demonstrate how complex some of these issues may be.

CASE 1

A mother relates to you that her husband is affected with "some sort of genetic colon cancer." She wants her 13-year-old son tested. Although the child has no evidence of being affected, should DNA testing be done on him? You realize that there are several conditions that fall within the category of "genetic colon cancer." You seek more information and find that the father is 38 years old and has numerous polyps, as did several of his family members (Chap. 10). You know that in the case of familial adenomatous polyposis (FAP), which can have onset as early as 10 years, testing should be offered by age 10–12 years.[18] However, a second condition, attenuated familial adenomatous polyposis (AFAP) generally has onset in the 30s, and the recommendation is for DNA testing to not be done until the at-risk individual is 18 years of age.[19] Of course, at this point referral to a cancer genetics unit could be done; however, that is not a logistically possible option in this case, so the burden of arranging for testing falls on you. What should you do?

The ethical guidelines put forth by several authors would suggest that if testing is associated with a medical benefit to the child, such as in the case of FAP, testing be offered now. If however the father has AFAP, testing would not be indicated using current testing guidelines.[19-21] You seek more information on the father's condition and find that affected individuals in his family, including himself, did not have the appearance of polyps until age 25 years or later, and generally had around 20–30 polyps. Although this is likely AFAP, molecular testing can determine the father's mutational status and further clarify whether he had FAP or AFAP,[19] as well as identify if molecular testing is an available option for your patient, whenever testing is done.

CASE 2

A 17-year-old boy who has two brothers with Down syndrome due to a familial 14; 21 translocation asks you to do his karyotype to determine whether he carries the balanced translocation. He is sexually active and concerned that if an unplanned pregnancy in his girlfriend occurred prenatal testing might be an option she would consider. It can be argued that since he is asking the question, testing should be available to him.[15]

CASE 3

Your patients are siblings, a 13-year-old female and her 15-year-old brother. Their parents recently delivered a baby with autosomal recessive polycystic kidney disease. They would like to have prenatal diagnosis in a future pregnancy. However, DNA analysis only identified one mutation, maternal in origin, which is not surprising given the complexity of the gene.[22] Linkage studies need to be done to determine which of the paternal chromosomes carries the other mutant allele. To do this, your patients need to be tested to determine whether the paternal chromosome 6 with the mutant allele can be identified. It is known that testing will identify whether they are likely carriers or not. Should testing be done? Who should consent? Should the parents consent for the younger child and the older child provide his own consent? What are other ramifications of linkage testing, beyond that of potentially receiving

results on carrier status that need to be considered? See Fanos[23] for a detailed discussion of linkage analysis and the well sib.

CASE 4

Your patients are a 16-year-old boy and his 13-year-old sister whose two brothers have autism. The family has been approached by a research group that is studying genes predisposing to autism. Blood samples would need to be obtained on all family members, including the unaffected teens. The family is considering participating, but wants to discuss the situation with you. Pertinent issues include who can and must consent, and who should receive results of the study, should they become available.

CASE 5

(These situations are only rarely likely to occur, but are included for completeness and to provoke thought). Your 14-year-old patient's mother reports that her insurance company requests that her daughter be tested for BRCA1, a breast cancer-predisposing gene present in the family. They want this information before determining rates. A second insurance-related scenario could be a situation in which the insurance company has increased rates based on family history alone, and your patient's mother wants testing so that if it were negative, the rates could be reduced. Although you state that testing is inappropriate, the mother accuses you of being paternalistic and vows she will find a way to get testing done. As a side note, Wertz and Reilly[24] surveyed several DNA diagnostic laboratories and found that among 105 labs that were surveyed, the majority had tested children (some younger than 12 years of age) for late-onset disorders (e.g., familial polyposis coli, Huntington disease), and almost half had provided tests directly to the consumer.

CASE 6

Your 16-year-old male patient's mother recently determined that she has the gene for Huntington disease, having inherited it from her mother. She wants her child tested to determine whether he has the gene or not. She states that she would feel "better" if she knew whether she had transmitted the gene to him or not. You ask him whether he wants testing to be done, and he states that he does not really know much about Huntington disease—he has not had much contact with his grandmother since she was diagnosed.

CASE 7

One of your patients is a 12-year-old girl whose younger brother has Duchenne muscular dystrophy (DMD). She is not sexually active, nor dating anyone. The mother requests testing to determine whether she is a carrier for DMD, because she does not want to worry about it when her daughter does start dating.

In cases 6 and 7 most would agree that testing should not be offered or condoned, though in case 6 it could be argued that if after counseling the boy wanted testing, it should perhaps be offered.[25] In case 7 the nature of the test and the age of the patient would proscribe against doing the testing at this point in time.

The American Society of Human Genetics and the American College of Medical Genetics have published a detailed position paper on genetic testing in children and adolescents. The key points include discussion on impact of potential benefits and harm on decisions about testing, the family's involvement in decision making, and considerations for future research. The reader is referred to this work for more detail about these various points (and see also the American Academy of Pediatrics statement on genetic testing in children, as well as the work by Ross and Moon for a discussion of ethical issues in genetic testing in children).[21,25,26]

However, there are still situations that have not been adequately addressed. Consider these two situations. In the first situation, one of your patients is a 17-year-old boy who is known to be a carrier for a 7;13 balanced translocation by virtue of his mother having had amniocentesis during her pregnancy. You have asked his mother whether her son knows his chromosome status, to which she replies no. You then ask her when she plans to tell her son of his situation. Mother replies that she will tell him when he gets married and starts thinking about having children. You then ask how many teenagers in her community are sexually active. In 2002, 3% of girls aged 15–19 became pregnant[27] (Chap. 26). As pointed out by Burke,[28] if this boy's girlfriend becomes pregnant and delivers a baby with multiple major anomalies secondary to an unbalanced karyotype, might not she or her family have the right to sue either him or his family for their failure to act on knowledge or suspected knowledge of an increased risk for an adverse outcome?

The second case situation illustrates what will likely become a testing dilemma, particularly for conditions with complex inheritance. For example, recent studies have suggested that those with the ε4 allele of APOE may be at higher risk for having a poor outcome following head trauma.[29] An individual may choose to not participate in a high-contact sport (e.g., football, boxing) if he or she has one or two copies of this allele. However, the ε4 allele is also associated with a higher risk of developing Alzheimer disease (for which there are no preventative measures). Clearly APOE testing would not be indicated for predicting the risk of developing Alzheimer disease, but if determination of APOE status could identify those at significantly higher risk for poor outcome following head trauma, and those individuals would choose to avoid high-contact sports, might not testing be viewed as beneficial under these circumstances?

Based on what we learning about gene function, it is likely that similar situations where testing for a particular genetic variation could be both contraindicated and useful will arise. Policies addressing who can request testing and who should have access to the results will need to be developed.[29]

Genetic Counseling And Testing For An Individual Affected With A Genetic Disorder

For the adolescent affected by a genetic disorder or congenital anomaly, the risks delineated in Table 21-1 apply. In the situation where the adolescent has an autosomal recessive disorder, the risk to offspring is 1/2 times the carrier frequency. For example, if an adolescent female has cystic fibrosis (CF), the chance of her child also being affected is 1/50 (1/2 times the carrier frequency of 1/25). The chance that her child will be a carrier for CF is 100%.

However, in addition to counseling conveying reproductive risks, discussion should also include information about potentially adverse effects on offspring, where applicable.

In some cases, there is thought to be an increased risk for congenital anomalies in general in offspring born to mothers with certain conditions (e.g., maternal inflammatory bowel disease, diabetes, and obesity).[30–32] In many cases mechanism of malformation is unknown, and interventions may not be available. In other cases there is an increased risk to offspring of mothers with certain conditions, but for a specific set of problems for which appropriate interventions to reduce risk exist. The paradigm of this situation is maternal phenylketonuria (PKU).

In 1980, Lenke and Levy[33] reported that offspring born to untreated pregnant women with PKU had a frequency of mental retardation of 92%, microcephaly of 73%, low birth weight of 40%, and heart defects in 12%. Treatment during pregnancy was found to reduce these frequencies, and virtually eliminate them if the blood phenylalanine levels are between 120–360 µmol/L from conception onward.[34–36] However, it has become apparent that there appears to be a relationship between level of control and outcome,[37] and dietary control is not always achieved.[38] However, development of novel approaches to treatment (e.g., oral administration of phenylalanine ammonia lyase and enzyme replacement therapy[34]) may ameliorate these risks.

Although the counseling issues can be more difficult, the testing issues are generally less problematic. In many cases, a test has already been done to make the diagnosis or determine the cause of the physical symptoms. If the diagnosis was based on clinical manifestations, testing for prenatal diagnosis purposes is now often available.

MANAGEMENT ISSUES FOR THE ADOLESCENT WITH A GENETIC SYNDROME OR CONDITION

In this section management issues for the adolescent with a syndrome or other genetic condition will be briefly reviewed. The entities selected for inclusion in this section are those that are either discussed in more detail in *Management of Genetic Syndromes*[39] or listed in a recent article by Cadle et al.[40] These conditions are:

1. Achondroplasia
2. Beckwith-Wiedemann syndrome
3. CHARGE syndrome
4. Down syndrome
5. Fragile X syndrome
6. Klinefelter syndrome
7. Marfan syndrome
8. Neurofibromatosis, type 1
9. Noonan syndrome
10. Osteogenesis imperfecta
11. Prader-Willi syndrome
12. Sotos syndrome
13. Stickler syndrome
14. Turner syndrome
15. Velocardiofacial syndrome
16. Williams syndrome

Achondroplasia

Achondroplasia is caused by a mutation in the fibroblast growth factor receptor (FGFR) 3 gene, and is inherited as an autosomal dominant trait. In some cases, there is no family history and thus the occurrence of achondroplasia in a child born to a family with no prior history is the result of a new mutation. A recent review by Hunter et al.[41] described the medical complications in a group of individuals with achondroplasia. During adolescence, health issues that should be addressed include hearing loss, orthodontic problems, and complications associated with skeletal abnormalities. Hunter et al.[41] found that approximately 28% of individuals will have hearing loss by age 20, with approximately 5% developing hearing loss between the ages 12 and 19 years. Hearing loss is more often conductive, but the frequency of sensorineural hearing loss can also be increased. Orthodontic problems affected 22% of those by age 20, with problems generally related to malocclusion secondary to the disproportionate growth of the cranial base. Although it is recommended that children with achondroplasia be evaluated during mid-childhood, in most cases treatment does not occur until the teens or adulthood. Tibial bowing is perhaps one of the most common orthopedic problems, affecting 26% by age 20. Cervicomedullary compression affects 12.5% by age 20. Symptoms in these individuals include apnea and arm and/or neck neurologic signs. Finally, although lumbosacral spinal stenosis becomes an issue of concern generally during adulthood, in Hunter et al.'s[41] series, 20% of adolescents had neurologic leg signs and 29% had leg pain. Therefore evaluations should be considered during adolescence, and include a thorough motor and sensory evaluation of the legs. Symptoms can include numbness, clumsiness, leg weakness, or bladder and/or bowel incontinence.[42]

An individual with achondroplasia has, at each pregnancy, a 50% chance of producing a child with achondroplasia and a 50% chance of having a child unaffected with achondroplasia.

Beckwith-Wiedemann syndrome

This condition is characterized by congenital macrosomia, macroglossia, umbilical hernia or omphalocele, and minor craniofacial anomalies. There are no specific recommendations for managing the adolescent with Beckwith-Wiedemann syndrome (BWS). BWS is a condition characterized by congenital overgrowth, macroglossia, minor craniofacial anomalies, and abdominal wall defects.[43] By the time an individual with BWS has reached adolescence, there are few, if any, medical management issues, though preliminary findings have suggested that surveillance of renal function, particularly for hypercalciuria, should be done on perhaps a regular

basis.[44] Because BWS can have several causes, recurrence risks depend on the cause. 85% of BWS is associated with a negative family history and normal chromosomes. If within this group the cause of BWS is paternal uniparental disomy for all or part of chromosome 11 or hypomethylation of KCNQ1OT1, the risk to offspring is low. If, however, the cause is a CDKN1C mutation, risk could be as high as 50% if affected parent is female, and somewhat less if affected parent is male. If the chromosomes are normal and there is a positive family history, the cause is likely a CDKN1C mutation, and risks are as above. If there is a chromosome anomaly (e.g., duplication, inversion, translocation) involving 11p15, risks are dependent on the nature of the chromosome abnormality.[45]

Charge Syndrome

Most of the cardinal signs of the CHARGE syndrome (C = coloboma, H = heart defects, A = atresia choanae, R = retardation of growth and/or development, G = genital defects, E = ear anomalies and/or deafness) are congenital anomalies and recognized at or soon after birth. The main adolescent issue for individuals with CHARGE syndrome is delayed puberty, occasionally associated with abnormalities of the hypothalamic-pituitary-gonadal axis.[46] Hypoadrenalism has also been described.[47] The chance of an individual with CHARGE syndrome having a similarly affected child is as high as 50%. In addition, a recent review found that one or two component manifestations of CHARGE syndrome occur significantly more often among family members.[48]

Down Syndrome

Several articles have detailed the medical management of individuals with Down syndrome (DS), and will be summarized here.[49–51]

Audiology

Almost half of individuals with DS have hearing loss, and hearing tests should be performed every 1 or 2 years. Sensorineural hearing loss is most common, followed by conductive and mixed loss. Otitis media can also still be a problem in adolescence.

Ophthalmology

Annual exams are recommended, because more than half of DS patients have either a refractive disorder, strabismus, or nystagmus by adolescence. Adolescents with DS are also more likely to develop keratoconus and corneal opacities or cataracts. Blepharitis is another common concern.

Dental

Although dental caries is less common in DS, periodontal disease is extremely common, and thought to be related to poor chewing function and poor oral hygiene.

Cardiac

Perhaps the most common cardiac issue in adolescents is the development of mitral valve prolapse (Chap. 9). Appropriate evaluation is indicated, with institution of SBE prophylaxis if valvular insufficiency is found.

Pulmonary

Pulmonary problems are frequent in individuals with DS, and include aspiration, upper and lower respiratory tract infections, and obstructive sleep apnea. A study of 53 children and adolescents with DS found that all of the symptomatic individuals (21/53) had abnormal polysomnograms, and 60% of the asymptomatic group had abnormal polysomnograms.[52]

Gastrointestinal

Swallowing function is often impaired in adolescents with DS, and may lead to aspiration and eventual pulmonary infection. Individuals with DS are more prone to celiac disease, and appropriate screening should be done, even if symptoms are not present. Screening should be repeated every three years; if symptoms such as constipation, diarrhea, bloating, or weight loss occur, screening should be done more often.

Orthopedic

The most debilitating orthopedic condition in DS is atlantoaxial instability, which is symptomatic in 1%–2% of individuals with DS. It is clear that in those with symptoms (including loss of motor skills, loss of bowel and/or bowel control, neck pain, torticollis, or abnormal deep tendon reflexes) appropriate evaluation (e.g., radiographs, MRI) is indicated. However, it is controversial whether evaluation of asymptomatic individuals is indicated, in large part because most asymptomatic individuals with or without subluxation and with or without activity limitation usually do not go on to become symptomatic. Other orthopedic problems include dislocations, subluxations, and scoliosis and appropriate evaluations should be done.

Endocrinology

The two most common endocrinologic problems in adolescents with DS are diabetes mellitus and hypothyroidism. Annual screening for thyroid disease is indicated; if clinical indications of diabetes occur, further evaluation is recommended, though regular monitoring may not be indicated. Obesity is an extremely common occurrence in those with DS, and management is complicated by the lower resting metabolic rate and lower bone density. If caloric intake is restricted, vitamin supplements are recommended to provide the necessary micronutrients.

Skin

Over half of DS individuals will develop folliculitis during adolescence. Dermatitis (both atopic and seborrheic), skin or nail fungal infections, and dry skin are all more common in DS adolescents. Vitiligo and alopecia, though still relatively rare, do occur more frequently in those with DS.

Development and Behavior

Adolescents with DS have been found to have a mental age of 4–5 years. Expressive language is deficient, even when compared to mental age. It has been recommended that speech and language therapy be offered to adolescents with DS with focus on expressive language and articulation. Approximately 18% have a psychiatric or behavioral disorder, with conditions including disruptive behavior, aggression, attention deficit, and autism. Depression is fairly common in adolescents. A common finding (80%) in adolescents with DS is self-talk (talking to oneself), and may be misinterpreted as a sign of psychosis.

Males with DS generally do not reproduce; females with DS have an increased chance of having a child with DS.

Fragile X

Fragile X is caused by an expanded trinucleotide region within the fragile X gene on the X chromosome. The main issues in adolescents concern behavior and cardiac anomalies.

Over half of the males and females with fragile X have mitral valve prolapse, which is believed to develop during adolescence and early adulthood. Mild dilatation of the aorta has also been described, though this dilatation does not appear to be progressive.[53,54] Auscultation of the heart at clinical visits is appropriate, with further referral to a cardiologist if a murmur or click is heard (Chap. 9).

The second area of concern is behavior. Merenstein et al.[55] described high frequencies of hyperactivity, aggression, shyness, anxiety, violent outbursts, and tactile defensiveness among males with fragile X. A more detailed review of behavioral issues and recommended therapeutic interventions can be found in Hagerman and Cronister.[53]

Finally, males with fragile X show a decline in IQ scores and adaptive behavior scores. This does not mean that there is a loss or regression; rather, males with fragile X develop at a slower rate, and fall further behind their age-matched peers as they become older.[56] It may therefore be worthwhile to perform a neurocognitive assessment in an adolescent male with fragile X if one had not been done for some time.

Unlike other X-linked conditions, the risks to offspring are dependent on the number of repeats, particularly in the mother. If the mother's repeat size is <60, risk is less than 1% that the premutation will expand to a full mutation. However, if repeat size is above 90, the risk of expansion to a full mutation is approximately 99%.[57] Most males with the full mutation do not reproduce.[53] A male with a premutation will generally not have a child with a full mutation, since repeat number changes very little when transmitted through a male.

Klinefelter Syndrome

Klinefelter syndrome is caused by polysomy of the X chromosome in a male. The most common karyotype is 47 XXY, but other forms include 48 XXXY, 48 XXYY, and 49 XXXXY. The diagnosis should be suspected in an adolescent with hypogonadism; decreased facial, axillary, and pubic hair; and tall stature for his family (Chap. 15). Supportive manifestations include a history of speech and language deficits and/or learning disabilities.[58] Gynecomastia is described as a common feature, though reported frequencies range from 15%–88%,[39,58] and may be related to the technique used to assess for this feature. Hormone evaluation will reveal elevated FSH and LH levels with low testosterone levels. Timely diagnosis is important so that testosterone therapy can be instituted. Testosterone therapy has been shown to not only maintain secondary sexual characteristics, but also increase muscle mass, contribute to increased energy, maintain bone density, and improve psychological well being.[59,60] In males diagnosed either prenatally or prior to puberty, testosterone therapy should be considered around the age of 11 or 12.[59,60] Some autoimmune disorders, diabetes, venous disease, and osteoporosis are all more common in men with Klinefelter syndrome.[58]

Infertility is a virtually constant manifestation, so recurrence risks are generally not applicable.

Marfan Syndrome

Marfan syndrome is an autosomal dominant condition caused by mutation in the fibrillin-1 gene. Although the gene has been identified, diagnosis is still made on clinical grounds as opposed to DNA diagnosis. Manifestations include effects on the ocular (especially lens dislocation), skeletal (arachnodactyly, pectus excavatum, arm span greater than height, scoliosis, and so on), and cardiovascular systems (aortic root dilatation involving the sinuses of Valsalva, Chap. 9); and diagnostic criteria[61,62] to aid in clinical diagnosis have been published. Most cases are inherited from an affected parent, but 25%–30% is the result of new mutation. It is in these latter cases that diagnosis may be difficult, particularly since some of the manifestations important for diagnosis develop over time.[63,64] However, the goal of the primary care clinician should be to identify those individuals that merit referral for evaluation for the Marfan diagnosis, and to coordinate care for those that have been diagnosed with Marfan.[65,66] Recent articles have addressed reasons for referral, and note that these reasons include the finding by a physician of one or more typical physical findings (primarily skeletal, ocular, or cardiac), a positive family history of the condition, or recent publicity prompting an inquiry by the family or physician.[67] In addition, the appearance of striae unrelated to weight gain around the time of puberty is another fairly frequent manifestation in the adolescent with Marfan syndrome.[63]

In individuals already diagnosed with Marfan syndrome, the cardiovascular system merits the most attention (Chap. 9), but the skeletal and ocular systems also merit evaluation. It is recommended that echocardiograms be done routinely, attention be paid to the spine (to rule out scoliosis), joints, and chest (pectus excavatum is most likely to cause problems), and blood pressure be monitored.[63]

Marfan syndrome is an autosomal dominant condition, and affected individuals have a 50% chance at each pregnancy of having a child with Marfan syndrome. Women with Marfan syndrome are at significant risk of aortic dissection, even if the aorta was not significantly dilated prior to pregnancy[68] and may warrant monitoring by various subspecialists during the pregnancy.

Neurofibromatosis

Neurofibromatosis is an autosomal dominant condition caused by mutations in the *NF1* gene on chromosome 17. The condition is a fully penetrant condition, but with variable expressivity and age-dependent development of several of the diagnostic manifestations. Nonetheless, almost all affected individuals can be diagnosed using standard criteria by the age of 10 years.[39] The diagnosis is made in an individual who has two or more of the following criteria.[69]

1. Six or more café au lait macules that are 5 mm or more in diameter prepuberty or 15 mm or more in diameter after puberty.
2. Two or more neurofibromas of any type, or one or more plexiform neurofibromas
3. Axillary and/or inguinal freckling
4. Optic nerve glioma
5. Two or more Lisch nodules (iris hamartomas)
6. Osseous lesion such as sphenoid wing dysplasia or long bone bowing
7. Affected first degree relative, using the above criteria.

Guidelines for management of the adolescent with neurofibromatosis have been published,[69] and include evaluation for scoliosis, monitoring for development of plexiform neurofibromas (these should be suspected in cases of soft tissue asymmetry or unusual skin pigmentary or hair growth patterns), and monitoring for hypertension.

Since neurofibromatosis is inherited as an autosomal dominant condition, risk to offspring is 50%.

Noonan Syndrome

Noonan syndrome is an autosomal dominant condition characterized by the combination of characteristic facial appearance (e.g., hypertelorism, downslanting palpebral fissures, diamond-shaped eyebrows, and low set ears with thickened helix), short stature, congenital heart defect (Chap. 9), chest abnormality consisting of pectus carinatum superiorly and pectus excavatum inferiorly, and variable developmental delay. Noonan syndrome is heterogeneous. One causative gene (*PTPN11*) maps to the long arm of chromosome 12 and is responsible for 50% of the cases; the other gene or genes have not yet been identified. Manifestations pertinent to the adolescent pediatrician include growth monitoring and referral to endocrinology for possible institution of the growth hormone therapy;[70,71] and assessment for clotting dysfunction, if not already done.

This latter recommendation is based on the presence of a bleeding diathesis attributable to various coagulation factor abnormalities in 30%–50% of individuals with Noonan syndrome.[72,73]

Noonan syndrome is inherited as an autosomal dominant condition, thus risk to offspring is 50%.

Osteogenesis Imperfecta

There are as many as seven types of osteogenesis imperfecta (OI), with one of them, OI II, lethal in the newborn period.[74,75] The other types are compatible with life span into adulthood. Type I is considered a relatively mild form of OI, characterized by blue sclerae, easy bruising, mild short stature, increased frequency of hearing loss, and occasional dentinogenesis imperfecta. Type II is a perinatal lethal form with numerous in utero fractures, minimal calvarial mineralization, and early death or stillbirth being the rule. Type III is the progressively deforming type, with multiple congenital fractures, progressive deformity of bones, short stature, normal sclerae, hearing loss, and dentinogenesis imperfecta common. Type IV is considered to be more severe than type I, with mild to moderate bowing of bones, normal sclerae, short stature, and hearing loss as a relatively common finding. Type V is characterized by short stature, dislocated radial head, white sclera, and no dentinogenesis imperfecta. Type VI is associated with short stature, fish scale pattern of bone lamellation, white sclera, and no dentinogenesis imperfecta. Type VII also has short stature, white sclera and no dentinogenesis imperfecta as component manifestations, but also has short humeri and femora and coxa vara as features.[74,75] The causes of types I–IV are gene mutations in collagen chains *1A1* or *1A2*; the causes of types V–VII are unknown.

Orthopedic issues are the most significant concern for the adolescent. Although fracture frequency tends to decrease after puberty, the development of scoliosis and/or kyphosis is a major concern. Recently growth hormone and biphosphonates have been used as treatments to reduce the frequency of fractures.[74–76] Hearing loss is a common occurrence in late adolescence or early adulthood, and is often a combination of sensorineural and conductive loss.

Dental issues primarily related to dentinogenesis imperfecta can be troublesome, and the primary health care provider needs to insure the individual seeks regular dental care.

OI types I–V are inherited as an autosomal dominant condition, therefore risk to offspring is 50%, and is for the same type of OI (that is, a parent with OI type I will have a child with type I, but not type III). OI type VII is inherited as an autosomal recessive trait, and the mode of inheritance of type VI is unknown.[75]

Prader-Willi Syndrome

Prader-Willi syndrome (PWS) is a multisystem, mental retardation syndrome caused by insufficiency of paternally inherited chromosome 15 material. Although infants with PWS are often described as failing to thrive, the child and adolescent with PWS is characterized by obesity and hyperphagia. Most of the medical complications in PWS are the result of obesity, and include hypertension, diabetes, thrombophlebitis, and sleep apnea. Management of obesity is key, but it has been noted that it may be impractical to aim for an "ideal" body weight.[39] Other pertinent issues include hypogonadism with delayed or abnormal pubertal development, short stature, scoliosis, and osteoporosis.[77] Treatment with pituitary or gonadal hormones may be indicated;[77,78] indeed, some consider growth hormone therapy a standard of care element in the management of the child with Prader-Willi syndrome.[79] Other treatment options, too numerous to list here, are reviewed by Goldstone.[80] Dermatologic concerns, such as those secondary to chronic skin picking, are common. The pediatrician should examine the skin and mucosal membranes for evidence of picking and its complications.

Males with Prader-Willi generally do not reproduce; a female with Prader-Willi caused by deletion would theoretically have a 50% chance of having a child with Angelman syndrome.

Sotos Syndrome

Sotos syndrome, also known as cerebral gigantism, is characterized by overgrowth (pre- and postnatal), advanced bone age, developmental delay, and characteristic face, which is long with a high forehead, downslanting palpebral fissures (after midchildhood), and prominent jaw (after the age of two). The only significant medical issue is the possibility of the development of scoliosis.[39]

Inheritance of Sotos syndrome is autosomal dominant; risk to offspring is 50%.

Stickler Syndrome

Stickler syndrome is an autosomal dominant condition characterized by effects on the ocular, craniofacial, and skeletal system. This is a heterogeneous condition, caused by at least three different genes. Manifestations pertinent to the adolescent include ocular manifestations and skeletal changes. Significant myopia is a common feature of Stickler syndrome, and many individuals are at risk of retinal detachment. Many individuals with Stickler syndrome have a mild spondyloepiphyseal dysplasia. In addition, joint pain and stiffness is a fairly common complaint, and should be treated accordingly.[39]

Offspring born to an individual with Stickler syndrome have a 50% chance of being similarly affected.

Turner Syndrome

Turner syndrome is caused by the lack of two normal X chromosomes in a female. The most common karyotype is 45 X, but other variants, including deletions, also occur. Medical management issues include the cardiovascular, endocrine, auditory, and gastrointestinal systems. Aortic coarctation is a known manifestation of Turner syndrome, but recently there have been reports of aortic dissection occurring in some women with Turner syndrome. Almost all reportedly have predisposing factors, including repaired or unrepaired coarctation of the aorta, hypertension, or bicuspid aortic valve (Chap. 9). For the newly diagnosed adolescent, an echocardiogram is strongly recommended. Gonadal dysgenesis is a constant feature of Turner syndrome. 90% will need estrogen and progesterone to initiate puberty and maintain menses. However, it is important to note that approximately 5% of young women with Turner syndrome will be fertile and achieve pregnancy. In one study, the frequency of Down syndrome among the offspring of a woman with Turner syndrome was 3%.[81] Other endocrine manifestations include increased frequencies of hypothyroidism and diabetes. Hearing loss is also more common in Turner syndrome; in one study, 10% of children had sensorineural hearing loss whereas 90% of middle aged women were reported to be affected.[82] Individuals with Turner syndrome are also more prone to gastrointestinal tract vascular malformations and inflammatory bowel disease. There are no recommendations for routine screening, but symptoms such as rectal bleeding or chronic diarrhea should prompt further evaluations.

See above for genetic counseling issues.

Velo-Cardio-Facial Syndrome

Velo-cardio-facial syndrome (VCFS) is also known as Shprintzen syndrome, 22q deletion syndrome, DiGeorge syndrome, and with less frequency, CATCH-22. The cause is a microdeletion of chromosome 22. Many, if not most, of the manifestations are congenital, and thus are likely to have been diagnosed and treated prior to adolescence. However, hypocalcemia is common, and intermittent, not becoming evident until the second (or third) decade. Serum calcium monitoring on a yearly basis has been recommended. A second issue important to the adolescent is the relatively high risk of developing psychiatric disorders, either during adolescence or early adulthood. Individuals with VCFS should therefore be monitored for behavioral or psychiatric problems, with referral to a psychiatrist for diagnosis and management. For a detailed review of the condition, see Emanuel et al.[83]

The chance of an individual with VCFS having a similarly affected child is 50%.

Williams syndrome

Williams syndrome is caused by a microdeletion of chromosome 7. Cardinal manifestations include a characteristic facial appearance, cardiovascular disease, mild mental retardation in most, and idiopathic hypercalcemia. Adolescents with Williams syndrome are prone to several health issues that require assessment and management. Recommendations for evaluations include blood pressure measurement, cardiology evaluation, vision and hearing screening, GI evaluations to rule out diverticulitis/diverticulosis, cholelithiasis, and chronic constipation in the patient with chronic abdominal pain, and various laboratory evaluations. These evaluations should include yearly urinalysis and, if symptomatic, yearly calcium levels; calcium-creatinine ratio and serum creatinine levels every two years; and thyroid function, total calcium (if asymptomatic), and bladder and renal ultrasonography (done at puberty for baseline) every four years.[84] In addition, it has been recommended that if surgery is to be done, a pediatric anesthesia consultation be obtained, in that there have been reports of anesthesia-related deaths in individuals with Williams syndrome.[85]

The chance of an affected individual for having a child with Williams syndrome is 50%.

References

1. Harper PS: *Practical Genetic Counseling*. 5th ed., Woburn, MA: Butterworth Heimann, 1998.

2. Lin T, Lewis RA, Nussbaum RL: Molecular confirmation for carriers of Lowe syndrome. *Ophthalmology* 106:119, 1999.

3. Kerrison JB, Vagefi MR, Barmada MM, et al.: Congenital motor nystagmus linked to Xq26-q27. *Am J Hum Genet* 64:600, 1999.

4. Wynne-Davies R: Familial (idiopathic) scoliosis. *J Bone Joint Surg* 50B:24, 1968.

5. Wynne-Davies R: Family studies and aetiology of club foot. *J Med Genet* 2:227, 1965.

6. Strober M, Freeman R, Lampert C, et al.: Controlled family study of anorexia nervosa and bulimia nervosa: evidence of shared liability and transmission of partial syndromes. *Am J Psychiatr* 157:393, 2000.

7. King RA, Rotter JI, Motulsky AG, eds.: *The Genetic Basis of Common Diseases*. New York: Oxford University Press, 2002.

8. Monsén U, Broström O, Nordenvall B, et al.: Prevalence of inflammatory bowel disease among relatives of patients with ulcerative colitis. *Scand J Gastroenterol* 22:214, 1987.

9. Hall JG: Nontraditional inheritance. *Growth, Genet Horm Res* 6:1, 1990.

10. Harper PS, Harley HG, Reardon W, et al.: Anticipation in myotonic dystrophy: new light on an old problem. *Am J Med Genet* 51:10, 1992.

11. Langbehn DR, Brinkman RR, Falush D, et al.: A new model for prediction of the age of onset and penetrance for Huntington's disease based on CAG length. *Clin Genet* 65:267, 2004.

12. Brinkman RR, Mezei MM, Theilmann J, et al.: The likelihood of being affected with Huntington's disease by a particular age, for a specific CAG repeat size. *Am J Hum Genet* 60:1202, 1997.

13. Baker DL, Schuette JL, Uhlmann WR, eds.: *A Guide to Genetic Counseling*. New York: Wiley-Liss, 1998.

14. Rich EC, Burke W, Heaton CJ, et al.: Reconsidering the family history in primary care. *J Gen Intern Med* 19:273, 2004.

15. Wertz DC, Fanos JH, Reilly PR: Genetic testing for children and adolescents. *JAMA* 272:875, 1994.

16. Hoffman DE, Wulfsberg EA. Testing children for genetic predispositions: Is it in their best interest? *J Law Med Ethics* 23:331, 1995.

17. Eichner JE, Dunn ST, Perveen G, et al.: Apolipoprotein E polymorphism and cardiovascular disease: a HuGe review. *Am J Epidemiol* 155:487, 2002.

18. Laxova R: Testing for cancer susceptibility genes in children. *Adv Pediatr* 46:1, 1999.

19. Knudsen AL, Bisgaard ML, BÅlow S: Attenuated familial adenomatous polyposis (AFAP). A review of the literature. *Fam Cancer* 2:43, 2003.

20. Kodish ED: Testing children for cancer genes: the rule of earliest onset. *J Pediatr* 135:390, 1999.

21. Ross LF, Moon MR: Ethical issues in genetic testing of children. *Arch Pediatr Adolesc Med* 154:873, 2000.

22. Rossetti S, Torra R, Coto E, et al.: A complete mutation screen of PKHD1 in autosomal-recessive polycystic kidney disease (ARPKD) pedigrees. *Kidney Int* 64:391, 2003.

23. Fanos JH: The missing link in linkage analysis: the well sib revisited. *Genet Testing* 3:273, 1999.

24. Wertz DC, Reilly PR: Laboratory policies and practices for the genetic testing of children: a survey of the Helix network. *Am J Hum Genet* 61:1163, 1997.

25. Anonymous: ASHG/ACMG report. Points to consider: Ethical, legal, and psychosocial implications of genetic testing in children and adolescents. *Am J Hum Genet* 57:1233, 1995.

26. American Academy of pediatrics committee on bioethics: Ethical Issues with genetic testing in pediatrics. *Pediatrics* 107:1451, 2001.

27. Martin JA, Hamilton BE, Sutton PD: Births: Final data for 2002. *NVSS* 52(10):1, 2003.

28. Burke BM: Genetic testing for children and adolescents. *JAMA* 273:1089, 1995.

29. Caulfield TA: The law, adolescents, and the APOE ε4 Genotype: A view from Canada. *Genet Test* 3:107, 1999.

30. Michlin R, Oettinger M, Odeh M, et al.: Maternal obesity and pregnancy outcome. *Isr Med Assoc J* 2:10, 2000.

31. Nørgård B, Puho E, Pedersen L, et al.: Risk of congenital abnormalities in children born to women with ulcerative colitis: a population-based, case-control study. *Am J Gastroenterol* 98:2006, 2003.

32. Versiani BR, Gilbert-Barness E, Giuliani LR, et al.: Caudal dysplasia sequence: severe phenotype presenting in offspring of patients with gestational and pregestational diabetes. *Clin Dysmorphol* 13:1, 2004.

33. Lenke RR, Levy HL: Maternal phenylketonuria and hyperphenylalaninemia. An international survey of outcome of treated and untreated pregnancies. *N Engl J Med* 303:1202, 1980.

34. Clarke JTR: The maternal phenylketonuria project: A summary of progress and challenges for the future. *Pediatrics* 112:1584, 2003.

35. Rouse B, Azen C: Effect of high maternal blood phenylalanine on offspring congenital anomalies and developmental outcome at ages 4 and 6 years: the importance of strict dietary control preconception and throughout pregnancy. *J Pediatr* 144:235, 2004.

36. Widaman KF, Azen C: Relation of prenatal phenylalanine exposure to infant and childhood cognitive outcomes: results from the international maternal PKU collaborative study. *Pediatrics* 112:1537, 2003.

37. Antshel KM, Waisbren SE: Timing is everything: executive functions in children exposed to elevated levels of phenylalanine. *Neuropsychology* 17:458, 2003.

38. Brown AS, Fernhoff PM, Waisbren S, et al.: Barriers to successful dietary control among pregnant women with phenylketonuria. *Genet Med* 4:84, 2002.

39. Cassidy SB, Allanson JE, eds.: *Management of Genetic Syndromes.* New York: Wiley-Liss, 2001.

40. Cadle RG, Dawson T, Hall BD: The prevalence of genetic disorders, birth defects and syndromes in central and eastern Kentucky. *KMA Journal* 94:237, 1996.

41. Hunter AG, Bankier A, Rogers JG: Medical complications of achondroplasia: A multicentre review. *J Med Genet* 35:705, 1998.

42. Pyeritz RE, Sack GH, Udvarhelyi GB: Thoracolumbar laminectomy in achondroplasia: long term results in 22 patients. *Am J Med Genet* 28:433, 1987.

43. Bayly EM, Cole T, Temple IK, et al.: Clinical features and natural history of Beckwith-Wiedemann syndrome: presentation of 74 new cases. *Clin Genet* 46:168, 1994.

44. Goldman M, Shuman C, Weksberg R, et al.: Hypercalciuria in Beckwith-Wiedemann syndrome. *J Pediatr* 142:206, 2003.

45. Shuman C, Weksberg R: Beckwith-Wiedemann syndrome. In *GeneReviews at GeneTests: Medical Genetics Information Resource* (database online). Seattle, WA: University of Washington, 1997–2004. Available at *http://www.genetests.org* (updated April 10, 2003).

46. Khadilkar VV, Cameron FJ, Stanhope R: Growth failure and pituitary function in CHARGE and VATER associations. *Arch Dis Child* 80:167, 1999.

47. James PA, Aftimos S, Hofman P: CHARGE association and secondary hypoadrenalism. *Am J Med Genet* 117A:177, 2003.

48. Tellier AL, Cormier-Daire V, Abadie V, et al.: CHARGE syndrome: Report of 47 cases and review. *Am J Med Genet* 76:402, 1998.

49. Bosch JJ: Health maintenance throughout the life span for individuals with Down syndrome. *J Am Acad Nurse Pract* 15:5, 2003.

50. Roizen NJ: Medical Care and monitoring for the adolescent with Down syndrome. *Adolesc Med* 3:345, 2002.

51. Roizen NJ, Patterson D: Down syndrome. *Lancet* 361:1281, 2003.

52. Marcus CL, Keens TG, Bautista DB, et al.: Obstructive sleep apnea in children with Down syndrome. *Pediatrics* 88:132, 1991.

53. Hagerman RJ, Cronister A, eds.: *Fragile X syndrome. Diagnosis, treatment, and research.* 2d ed., Baltimore, MD: Johns Hopkins University Press, 1996.

54. Loehr JP, Synhorst DP, Wolfe RR, et al.: Aortic root dilatation and mitral valve prolapse in the fragile X syndrome. *Am J Med Genet* 23:189, 1986.

55. Merenstein SA, Sobesky WE, Taylor AK, et al.: Molecular-clinical correlations in males with an expanded FMR1 mutation. *Am J Med Genet* 64:388, 1996.

56. Fisch GS, Simensen RJ, Schroer RJ: Longitudinal changes in cognitive and adaptive behavior scores in children and adolescents with fragile X mutation or autism. *J Autism Dev Disord* 32:107, 2002.

57. Fu Y, Kuhl DPA, Pizzuti A, et al.: Variation of the CGG repeat at the fragile site results in genetic instability: resolution of the Sherman paradox. *Cell* 67:1047, 1991.

58. Visootsak J, Aylstock M, Graham JM Jr.: Klinefelter syndrome and its variants: An update and review for the primary pediatrician. *Clin Pediatr* 40:639, 2001.

59. Smyth CM, Bremner WJ: Klinefelter syndrome. *Arch Intern Med* 158:1309, 1998.

60. Manning MA, Hoyme HE: Diagnosis and management of the adolescent boy with Klinefelter syndrome. *Adolesc Med* 13:367, 2002.

61. Beighton P, dePaepe A, Danks D, et al.: International nosology for heritable disorders of connective tissue, Berlin, 1986. *Am J Med Genet* 29:581, 1988.

62. DePaepe A, Devereux RB, Dietz HC, et al.: Revised diagnostic criteria for the Marfan syndrome. *Am J Med Genet* 62:417, 1996.

63. Lipscomb KJ, Clayton-Smith J, Harris R: Evolving phenotype of Marfan syndrome. *Arch Dis Child* 76:41, 1997.

64. Knirsch W, Haas NA, Bauerle K, et al.: Difficulties in diagnosing Marfan syndrome in childhood and adolescence. *Klin Padiatr* 215:262, 2003.

65. Cushing V, Slocumb E: Identification of Marfan syndrome in primary care. *Adv Nurse Pract* 12:87, 2004.

66. Committee on genetics: Health supervision for children with Marfan syndrome. *Pediatrics* 98:978, 1996.

67. Hamod A, Moodie D, Clark B, et al.: Presenting signs and clinical diagnosis in individuals referred to rule out Marfan syndrome. *Ophthalmic Genet* 24:35, 2003.

68. Rahman J, Rahman FZ, Rahman W, et al.: Obstetric and gynecologic complications in women with Marfan syndrome. *J Reprod Med* 48:723, 2003.

69. Gutmann DH, Aylsworth A, Carey J, et al.: The diagnostic evaluation and multidisciplinary management of neurofibromatosis 1 and neurofibromatosis 2. *JAMA* 278:51, 1997.

70. Ogawa M, Moriya N, Ikeda H, et al.: Clinical evaluation of recombinant human growth hormone in Noonan syndrome. *Endocr J* 51:61, 2004.

71. MacFarlane CE, Brown DC, Johnston LB, et al.: Growth hormone therapy and growth in children with Noonan syndrome: results of a 3 years' follow-up. *J Clin Endocrinol Metab* 86:1953, 2001.

72. Bertola DR, Carneiro JDA, D'Amico EA, et al.: Hematological findings in Noonan syndrome. *Rev Hosp Clin Fac Med S Paulo* 58:5, 2003.

73. Sharland M, Patton M, Chittolie A et al.: Coagulation factor deficiencies and abnormal bleeding in Noonan syndrome. *Lancet* 339:19, 1992.

74. Antoniazzi F, Mottes M, Fraschini P, et al.: Osteogenesis imperfecta. Practical treatment guidelines. *Paediatr Drugs* 2:465, 2000.

75. Rauch F, Glorieux FH: Osteogenesis imperfecta. *Lancet* 363:1377, 2004.

76. Kanaka-Gantenbein C: Present status of the use of growth hormone in short children with bone diseases (diseases of the skeleton). *J Pediatr Endocrinol Metab* 14:17, 2001.

77. Nativio DG: The genetics, diagnosis, and management of Prader-Willi syndrome. *J Pediatr Health Care* 16:298, 2002.

78. Burman P, Ritzen EM, Lindgren C: Endocrine dysfunction in Prader-Willi syndrome: a review with special reference to GH. *Endocrin Rev* 22:787, 2001.

79. Lee PDK: Disease management of Prader-Willi syndrome. *Expert Opin Pharmacother* 3:1451, 2002.

80. Goldstone AP: Prader-Willi syndrome: advances in genetics, pathophysiology and treatment. *Trends Endocrin Metab* 15:12, 2004.

81. Tarani L, Lampariello S, Raguso G, et al.: Pregnancy in patients with Turner syndrome: Six new cases and review of the literature. *Gynecol Endocrinol* 12:83, 1998.

82. Hultcrantz M, Sylvén L, Borg E: Ear and hearing problems in 44 middle-aged women with Turner syndrome. *Hear Res* 76:127, 1994.

83. Emanuel BS, McDonald-McGinn D, Saitta SC, et al.: The 22q11.2 deletion syndrome. *Adv Pediatr* 48:39, 2001.

84. Committee on genetics: Health care supervision for children with Williams syndrome. *Pediatrics* 107:1192, 2001.

85. Bird LM, Billman GF, Lacro RV, et al.: Sudden death in Williams syndrome: report of ten cases. *J Pediatr* 129:926, 1996.

SEXUAL AND GYNECOLOGIC HEALTH

22

ADOLESCENT SEXUALITY

Ellen S. Rome

At the age of 14, he was a married man,
At the age of 15, the father of a son;
At the age of 16, his grave it was green,
And death put an end to his growing.

Joan Baez

Adolescent sexuality has changed much since the time about which Joan Baez sang. No longer are most teens married in early to middle adolescence, though teen parenthood at 15 years remains a possibility. The number of current high school students that have ever had sexual intercourse has dropped, with the majority going off to college not having had sexual intercourse. According to the 2003 Youth Risk Behavior Survey (YRBS), rates of adolescents who have ever had sexual intercourse are now 46.7%, down from 54% in 1991 (Grunbaum, 2004).

The risk of sexual intercourse in adolescence increases in minority youth and with age/grade, with two-thirds of the 15 million new sexually transmitted diseases in the United States each year occurring in the 25 years or younger age group (Braverman, 2001). Of those teens who are sexually active, one in four acquires a sexually transmitted disease annually. By 1998, gonorrhea rates had begun rising after a 13-year decline, with the highest increase in the Midwest (a 16.4% increase) (Chap. 24). By 2002, chlamydia rates showed a 37% increase since 1996, rising to 1483 cases per 100,000 (Irwin, 2004). Some of this rise may be due to better screening techniques, the advent of urine testing, the initiation in 2000 of universal reporting of chlamydia as a reportable sexually transmitted infection to public health departments, and the addition of screening for chlamydia as a Health Plan and Employer Data Information Set (HEDIS) measure as a quality of care indicator for health plans (Irwin, 2004).

In the United States, 7.4% of students have had sexual intercourse by age 13 (10.4% male, 4.2% female, with African American males as high as 31.8%, Hispanic males 11.6%, African American females 6.9%, Hispanic females 5.2%). Not all of this sexual activity is consensual, with 9.0% having reported that they were physically forced to have sexual intercourse against their will. This number is likely an underestimation, as adolescents will not always classify a sexual encounter as either rape or unwanted contact, when they feel that they did not clearly say no. In other words, despite some improvement in trends in adolescent sexual activity and in teen pregnancy rates, we have ways to go toward the goal of raising teens with a healthy sexuality.

In the national health objectives for 2010, responsible sexual behavior among adolescents remains one of the 10 leading health priorities. From 1991 to 2001, the prevalence of sexual experience decreased 16% among high school students. Simultaneously from 1991 to 2001, condom use increased and then has leveled off. There was also a simultaneous decrease in adolescent rates of gonorrhea, teen pregnancy, and birth rates over that decade, with these positive trends likely the result of the combined efforts of health care providers, parents, families, communities and schools, religious organizations, government agencies, and the media working together to reduce the risks. (Ventura et al., 2001). Teen pregnancy rates reached a peak in 1991, at which time the rate was 116.5/1000. By 1997, that rate had lowered to 94.3/1000, the lowest rate since 1976. In 2002, girls aged 15–19 years had the lowest teen birth rate ever reported in the United States, 42.9/1000, down from a peak of 61.8/1000 in 1991. The majority of these births occurred out of wedlock, rising steadily since the 1960s, and parallel to the fall in available jobs that could provide a young family with adequate income and with the rise in college opportunities for minority youth. Adolescent pregnancy and abortion are reviewed in Chap. 26.

The good news is that smaller proportions of teens are having sex at all, and those adolescents engaging in intercourse have a declining pregnancy rate (National Campaign to Prevent Teen Pregnancy, 2001). Rates of oral contraceptive use have remained relatively constant, with 17% of sexually active high school students reporting birth control use at their most recent sexual intercourse (MMWR, 2004). This rate has varied from 16% to 18% since 1993, with non-Hispanic Caucasian girls more likely to report oral contraceptive use. Another factor may be the choice to be abstinent after having had a prior sexual encounter, coincident with the campaign for "secondary virginity," or deciding to be abstinent after having had sexual intercourse previously.

BARRIERS TO ACHIEVING A HEALTHY SEXUALITY

Developmental Barriers

Developmental barriers exist that can lead teens to unhealthy sexual choices. The adolescent mindset, or the view that "it can't happen to me," predominates from early until late adolescence. Abstract thought, or the ability to foresee consequences, occurs in late adolescence, if at all (Chap. 2). Concrete thought processes predominate in early and mid adolescence. One true example comes to mind: the young girl comes into the physician's office, pregnant at age 15. Her clinician, who has followed her and had convinced her to use condoms every time she had sex with her boyfriend, asked what had happened. The young girl replied, "But I wasn't with my boyfriend!" Here lies the difficulty—helping teens extrapolate "the rules" to all situations, while simultaneously encouraging abstinence but tempering with practicality: "If you are going to have sex, you need to use a condom every time, and a second method for contraception" (unless counseling on same-sex activity, where contraception is less relevant yet disease prevention remains imperative). Simultaneously, the adolescent experiences the drive to discover his or her own sexual identity, which in turn can lead to experimentation.

It is the job of the clinician, the family, and the community to ensure that this experimentation proceeds in a way that leads to sexual health, high self-esteem, and ability to make healthy choices. Complicating the social milieu is the adolescent's shift in focus in middle adolescence to an emphasis on peers rather than parents; if teen pregnancy is highly visible and normative in a school or community, it becomes an "ok thing to do." In communities with high sanctions against early sexual activity, more pressure exists not to have sex, and more shame potentially ensues if a teen pregnancy occurs.

BIOLOGIC AND CULTURAL BARRIERS

Biologic barriers also exist, with the prominent exocervix of the adolescent serving as the perfect breeding ground for *Chlamydia*, human papillomavirus (HPV), and other diseases (Chap. 24). Other barriers to care include fear of a pelvic exam, which the American College of Obstetricians and Gynecologists has now mandated within 3 years of initiating sexual activity, as opposed to before or immediately after starting, as most teens perceive.

Fear of disclosure of sexual activity to parents may impede access to care, as can misperceptions of "risk" associated with use of various contraceptives by adolescents, their families, and by clinicians themselves. Religious beliefs may condemn premarital sex or homosexual exploration. Adolescents may not use a condom or any form of contraception as such usage implies that they intended to have sex, which may be in conflict with their religious, personal, or family values; rather, they can rationalize that it "just happened." Biologic and social factors also intermingle to add complexity to adolescent sexual health: biologically, girls reach menarche by $12^{1}/_{2}$ years, and boys can also ejaculate sperm by age 13. However, culturally, young people are not expected to marry or be in their "forever" relationship until they are in their mid twenties, or older. Thus, a decade of disconnect exists, when the media messages say "Go!" and the school, community, parents, and society say, "Wait!"

Which Teens Are More Likely to Have Sex?

The younger the adolescent initiates sexual activity, the less likely to use condoms, and the more likely the teen will have multiple partners. Despite this fact, serial monogamy remains the rule for most youth, though a "long-term relationship" may mean 3 weeks in duration. Younger teens, in particular, report curiosity as a reason to initiate sexual intercourse, because "everyone's doing it." Many youth are surprised to hear that the majority of adolescents going off to college have not had sexual intercourse (53.3%). Helping an adolescent feel that he or she is not the only one choosing to wait can be a useful strategy in delaying initiation or next sexual encounter.

Approximately one-third (34.3%) of American high school students had sexual intercourse in the 3 months prior to the 2003 YRBS (Grunbaum, 2003). Table 22-1 reflects risk factors that may be associated with adolescent sexual activity. Table 22-2 describes risk factors associated with early onset of sexual activity. Among the third of students that were sexually active on the 2003 YRBS, almost two-thirds (63%) reported that either they or their partners had

TABLE 22-1

FACTORS ASSOCIATED WITH TEENS WHO ARE MORE LIKELY TO HAVE SEXUAL INTERCOURSE

Low self-esteem
Low academic achievement
Learning problem
Other social/emotional/behavioral problems
Low income families
Ethnic minorities (socioeconomic status related)
Victims of sexual or physical abuse
In families with marital discord
In families with less parental supervision

used a condom during the last sexual intercourse. Condom use at last sexual intercourse was reported in 68.8% of males, and 57.4% of female students. One out of four students (25.4%) drank alcohol or used drugs before last intercourse. Cultural context and expectations can mediate sexual risk-taking behavior. Although a majority of youth in the

TABLE 22-2

RISK FACTORS FOR EARLY INITIATION OF SEXUAL ACTIVITY

Being African American
Being male
Living in a low income family
Nonsupportive parents with little supervision
Lack of connectedness to school
Less religiosity
External locus of control
Use of drugs and alcohol
Easily influenced by peers
Long-term dating relationships, especially
  at younger ages
Having peers who have sex, use drugs/alcohol
Victims of sexual or physical abuse

Source: American Academy of Pediatrics, Sexuality Education, Pediatrics 2001; 108:498–502; Donovan P. *The Politics of Blame: Family Planning, Abortion and the Poor.* New York: Alan Guttmacher Institute, 1995; Alan Guttmacher Institute. *Sex and America's Teenagers.* New York: Alan Guttmacher Institute, 1994.

Caribbean (65.9%) reported not having had sexual intercourse, fewer than 30% regularly used contraception (Halcon and Blum, 2003).

What About Just Dating?

Currently, 10th and 12th graders are less likely to date than teens reported a decade ago. More dating has been associated with higher self-esteem, being seen as "popular," but it can result in lower academic achievement and less academic motivation. Teens who date may have more conflict with parents over curfew issues or rules on sexuality, and they also may be more depressed than their nondating peers, especially when the relationship turns sour. Another modern phenomenon is the "Hook Up," which a generation ago may have been called, "The One Night Stand." The difference is that many youth, especially college age adolescents, may intentionally seek out a sexual relationship without the entanglements of commitment, reflecting a growing sense of emancipation on a sexual front. This view can also result in sexual experimentation or reflect a disconnect between emotional connection and sexual experience, with potential negative consequences, including sexually transmitted diseases, HIV, pregnancy with an unwanted partner, depression, and anxiety.

Trends in Dating Violence and Rape

About 1.5 million women in the United States are physically or sexually assaulted each year by a current or former intimate partner (Tjaden and Thoennes, 2000). Girls and women aged 16–24 years have the highest rates of nonfatal intimate partner violence (Rennison, 2001). In the most recent YRBS 2003, 8.9% of students nationwide had been hit, slapped, or physically hurt on purpose by their boyfriends or girlfriends during the 12 months prior to survey (Grunbaum, 2004). The prevalence was higher among African American (9.3%) than Caucasian (7.0%) students, and highest among African American female students (14.0%), as opposed to Hispanic female (9.2%) and white female (7.5%) students. African American male students were subjected to 13.7% episodes of

dating violence, in contrast to Hispanic males at 9% and Caucasian male students at 6.6%. Rape was reported by 9.0% of students, with more girls than boys having been raped (11.9% vs. 6.1%). These numbers may be an underestimation, as they only reflect answers of students currently attending school, and traumatic experiences may contribute to school dropout or runaway youth. An estimated 18%–32% of female adolescents have been the victims of dating violence, with 8%–27% of adolescent and young adult women estimated to have been raped (Halpern et al., 2001).

In a study by Taylor and Sorenson, 3679 Californian adults from 6 distinct ethnic groups were given an experimental vignette and asked about it via structured interview (Taylor and Sorenson, 2004). As expected, 97% of adults felt that most forms of teen dating violence are wrong, and 81% felt that teen dating violence should be illegal. Although a majority of adults supported interventions such as calling the police or issuing a restraining order, Asian Americans were least likely to support police intervention for teen dating violence, and those adults born outside of the United States were less likely to support police intervention. These findings highlight the disparities between judgment that teen dating violence should not occur and the common legal interventions used to avert this behavior, specifically restraining orders and police involvement. Prevention programming needs to take these findings into account, as well as building on innate strengths of various populations, such as traditional Asian values of order, harmony, and family closeness that may contribute to the minimization of domestic violence or other risk behaviors.

What Do We Know About Oral Sex?

A developmentally challenged adolescent discovers that she gets a lot of male attention if she performs oral sex on the guys who ask; she is caught in a stairwell of the local high school, with a number of adolescent boys lined up waiting their turn. Parents of 7th and 8th graders at a local girls' school ask how to protect their daughters from the dangers, physically and emotionally, of oral sex.

Their sons tell them that they "aren't ready, but the girls expect it." A 7th grader propositions an 8th grader on a bus, promising oral sex at the back of the bus; he refuses, but does not tell his peers that he has done so. They both have consequences at school, his for not promptly sharing the truth, due to embarrassment, and hers for her proposition. A 15-year-old girl suffers posttraumatic stress disorder after a boy on whom she had a crush comes over to her house and performs cunnilingus on her.

All of these examples have occurred. Simultaneously, some high school girls (and some boys) state that oral sex is "gross," but that they will have vaginal intercourse with a partner. Others prefer oral sex since they can remain virgins. Still others will acquiesce to anal sex, as it still "maintains their virginity," with anal sex in this group rarely occurring with use of a condom. In the 1990s, President Clinton publicly stated that he "did not have sex with that woman," despite much graphic media depicting the details of their acts of oral sex. Again, the implicit message is that oral sex is not sex. In 2003, local pop artist Liz Phair released an album containing a song entitled "HWC," which is not given radio time due to its explicit content extolling the medicinal values of oral sex. (Note: HWC refers to the "hot white" ejaculate produced by males during sexual release). We have moved from innuendo to graphic representtation, with little left to the imagination for today's teens.

Little data exist on the prevalence of oral sex among adolescents. One study of 212 10th graders in a suburban New England high school found that 37.9% of boys and 42.1% of girls reported having had oral sex; 72.7% of boys and 67.9% of girls reported never using a condom (Prinstein et al., 2003). In this same cohort, 22.2% of the boys and 35.2% of the girls reported having had sexual intercourse. Interestingly, adolescents who reported sexual activity had high levels of reputation-based popularity, but were not necessarily seen as "likeable." As numbers of partners increased, popularity decreased, as well. In a study of 580 ninth grade adolescents in San Francisco, 19.6% had engaged in oral sex, as opposed to 13.5% engaging in vaginal sex; 31.5% of these teens intended to have oral sex in the next six months, while 26.3% intended to have vaginal sex during this same time period (Halpern-Fisher et al, 2005). In other studies of 9th to 12th graders, prevalence of oral sex has ranged from 33% to 59%, with 7%–24% of adolescent virgins reporting that they had given or received oral sex (Gates and Sonenstein, 2000; Schuster et al., 1996). Some adolescents view oral sex as less risky than vaginal sex with respect to health outcomes as well as social and emotional consequences.

Biologic risks of oral sex include sexually transmitted diseases such as HPV, HIV, gonorrhea, herpes simplex virus, and syphilis. Dentists cringe at the sight of fulminant HPV in the mouths of their immunocompromised young adult patients. Adolescents should be advised to use a nonlubricated condom or dental dam when participating in oral sex. Attempts to make use of condoms more palatable have met with limited success; flavored condoms, and other forms of nonlubricated condoms suitable for oral sex have gained limited market share. This failure in the United States may be a reflection of the lack of media advertising for condoms in most public forums other than MTV.

ADOLESCENT SEXUALITY AND THE MEDIA

Today's American youth are bombarded with ambiguous messages about their own sexuality. Popular TV shows talk openly about sexuality and demonstrate behaviors such as extramarital sexual activity, casual sex, three-way sexual encounters, and other expressions of sexual thoughts and behaviors. Adolescents can be immunized against such exposure by discussions with adults helping them to clarify their own values and ascertain/ interpret what explicit and implicit messages are portrayed in a particular episode or show. Same-sex preference role models are also available through the media, with both negative and positive stereotypes. By the age of 18, the average American youth will have viewed 14,000 sexual references on television per year, with only 170 of these references dealing with birth control, abstinence, or self-control (Strasburger and Donnerstein, 2000).

The media traditionally claims merely to reflect society rather than shape it. Four decades of research on media violence contradicts this view, showing a direct causal effect between media violence and real-life violence (Strasburger and Donnerstein, 2000). Similar data likely will emerge longitudinally with respect to sexual behaviors and the media. Two-thirds of prime time television shows contain sexual content, with only 9% of incidents including any mention of the risks or consequences of sexual activity or the need for contraception (Kunkel et al., 1999). Each time there is mention of contraception, or the reference is framed in terms of a healthy sexuality, there is a strong likelihood that a public health expert or adolescent medicine specialist joined forces with the media industry to carefully craft that message; they do not occur "by accident." As youth advocates, we can continue to put positive pressure on the media to decrease or minimize risk behavior rather than glamorize it, such as changing the norm on-screen away from having a cigarette after sex. Ongoing content analyses are needed to measure the impact of television sex on the trends in sexual behavior.

Both boys and girls require sophisticated media literacy skills. Exposure to R-rated material that depict women as willingly being raped has been shown to increase men's beliefs in myths about women desiring rape or deserving sexual abuse (Malamuth and Check, 1981). In a study of 522 African American females aged 14–18, 29.7% had seen an X-rated movie, and exposure was associated with the following: (1) more negative attitudes toward condom use (OR 1.4), (2) multiple sexual partners (OR 2.0), (3) to have sex more frequently (OR 1.8), (4) to have not used contraception during the last act of intercourse (OR 1.5), (5) to have not used contraception in the 6 months prior to the study (OR 2.2), (6) to have a strong desire to conceive (OR 2.3), and (7) to test positive for chlamydia (OR 1.7) (Wingood et al., 2001). Teachers, clinicians, and public health interventions can enhance media literacy by deconstructing the stated and implied messages of various advertisements, commercials, television shows, or movies. These efforts can occur in the classroom, in the doctor's office or waiting room, through public

service advertisements and media campaigns, and through other public health avenues. Clinicians need to correlate health or behavioral concerns with media use, e.g., adverse sexual health consequences (Wingood et al., 2001).

The Role of the Clinician

Despite the fact that two-thirds of American youth report that they want information about sexually transmitted diseases and pregnancy from their physicians, physicians often miss opportunities to raise these topics for discussion during office visits (Kapphahn et al., 1999). Some primary care clinicians will ask about sexual activity, but rarely about sexually transmitted diseases, condom use, sexual orientation, number of partners, or sexual/physical abuse despite the fact that *BRIGHT FUTURES* (the AAP guidelines to preventive care) and GAPS (the guidelines for adolescent preventive services, from the AMA) both recommend obtaining a comprehensive sexual history from each teen annually. Only slightly greater than half of teens who had seen a doctor in the past year received the opportunity to talk alone with their doctor without a parent in the room.

Clinicians caring for children and adolescents should provide longitudinal sexuality education to their patients, as well as provide parents with the vocabulary with which to begin or continue these ongoing dialogues with their children. Clinicians can help put sexuality into a lifelong context, using proper words for anatomic parts, handling questions such as, "Why does Sally have two mommies?" and help parents find ways to discuss sensitive areas with grace if not ease. Clinicians should help parents to clarify their own values and beliefs without imposing the practitioner's beliefs. Pediatricians and other clinicians are particularly well suited to provide education and advocacy in schools, at parent programming, and in their communities. For those clinicians feeling that they lack the skills for such presentations, the American College of Obstetricians and Gynecologists has published the Adolescent Sexuality Kit: Guides for Professional Involvement (ACOG, 1992). Examples of ways to take a confidential sexual history can be seen in Table 22-3. Pediatricians and other clinicians

TABLE 22-3

QUESTIONS THE CLINICIAN SHOULD ASK ADOLESCENTS ABOUT THEIR SEXUAL HEALTH

After establishing confidentiality, ask:

Have you ever had sex? What did you use for protection? If condoms, did you use them sometimes, always, or most of the time? What about a second method of contraception used? (If not using a second method, motivational interviewing can be used here to introduce the concept of a second method and get them to action phase to initiate a second method.)

Are you attracted to guys, girls, or both? (Can add a qualifier, "I ask everyone this question, don't be embarrassed, I ask so that I can best counsel you on your own health.")

Has anyone ever done anything to you sexually that made you uncomfortable? Tell me about that. Have you ever had sex when you said, "No"?

Have you ever had a sexually transmitted disease? Have you ever been pregnant?

For girls, are your periods regular? Cramps, no cramps? Duration of flow? Any vaginal discharge?

For boys, have you had any discharge from your penis? Any pain? Any problems with erection or ejaculation? If so, are you having wet dreams ever? (Again, the clinician can qualify these questions, saying, "I ask because there are many factors that can affect your health, including your sexual health.")

The HEADS questions (Home, Education, Activities, Drugs/Depression, Sex/Suicide) should also be asked confidentially.

should also link with subspecialists providing care to children with chronic illness, allowing the subspecialist to attend to the disease process, and the primary care clinician to address issues of risk behaviors, sexuality, and other psychosocial risks that may be missed if the teen is seeing solely the subspecialist.

The Role of the Family

As quoted by Iris Litt in 2003, "Parents are 'in' again" (Litt, 2003). In the early 20th century, children were chattel, little more than property; by the last quarter of that century, children and adolescents had earned certain privileges, some of which were deemed none of the parents' business! In fact, in treating certain patients who were victims of domestic violence, a "parentectomy" was prescribed, with the "cure" including emancipation and helping provide the adolescents with a healthy set of survival skills. Now, the pendulum has turned, and in the 21st century, successful treatment includes the families and empowerment of teens to make healthy sexual choices, which when done well, involves a strong parental component. Discussion between parents and adolescents that occurred early (prior to the first sexual activity) has

been associated with greater condom use with first sex and greater condom use with subsequent sexual activity. Trust established between an adolescent girl and her parents appears to protect against participation in risky behaviors but seems to have little effect on adolescent boys (Borawski et al., 2003). In helping adolescents learn to make healthy decisions for themselves, individuation with increasing responsibility should be an expected developmental outcome; parents and other caring adults need to be mindful not to provide too much unsupervised time before trust is warranted.

Parent-child connectedness is associated with lower youth violence and alcohol use regardless of socioeconomic strata, and with less sexual activity in some neighborhoods or communities. Parent-child communication on sexual risk taking has been associated with more conservative sexual attitudes, later onset of coitarche, and greater use of condoms (Hutchinson et al., 2003; Whitaker and Miller, 2000).

Primary care clinicians can help parents by demystifying sex education and helping them find and use "teachable moments." Such moments can include a baby's first erection noted in the office or at home, or the birth of a sibling or pet. Developmentally appropriate language and interventions can be used to allow children to appreciate their own bodies, take responsibility for their own behaviors, and act on their own beliefs and values when they conflict with those of their peers. Parents (and clinicians) should be counseled to be nonjudgmental, as well as be aware of their own innate biases, strengths, and weaknesses.

Clinicians can encourage parents to use proper terms for anatomic parts in a matter of fact way, and to help parents initiate discussions about sexuality with children at relevant times. Clinicians can help discuss masturbation, wet dreams, and other sexual behaviors as part of normal sexuality, while teaching that private parts are private, reinforcing stranger danger, and ways to keep safe from abuse. Parents should be encouraged to discuss explicitly their values and goals for their children with respect to abstinence and sexuality, and not have the discussion as a one-time occurrence; the talk is of more value over several iterations, just as many aspects of learning taking repetition, in order to make it stick. Single parents should also be advised to use caution in their own dating and sexual practices, so that they do not reflect a "do as I say, not as I do" attitude. Clinicians need to remind parents of children with developmental disabilities or with chronic illness that their offspring are sexual beings as well, and that they still need counseling and frank discussion on sexual choices. Developmentally delayed youth

may also require special counseling or services to ensure that they are not abused or placed in coercive situations, to which they may acquiesce to fit in.

Definitions of Sexuality (Box 22-1). Gender identity and gender role can be simple or confusing to an adolescent. "I am a boy, attracted to girls," is relatively straightforward. But if you have a transgender boy whose gender identity is female, then he may feel trapped in the wrong body, and confused as to how to identify himself sexually. To complicate matters further, his sexual identity could be heterosexual, homosexual, or bisexual; thus, he can be attracted to males, females, or both. To give a concrete example from real life, he could be male, feeling as if he should be female, attracted to males, but as a woman would be attracted to males—sound confusing? Try explaining that to your peers, parents, or others at age 16!

Transsexual means believing one's self to be a different gender than his or her assigned biologic gender, in other words gender identity does not match biologic identity. So, using the last scenario, gender identity is female, biologic identity (assuming normal 46,XY chromosomes) is male, and sexual identity is female attracted to male, which in his current body appears to be a homosexual sexual identity, but is actually heterosexual in identity if he comes at it from a woman's gender identity. As

---

BOX 22-1
DEFINITIONS OF SEXUALITY

Sexuality encompasses the sexual knowledge, attitudes, beliefs, and behaviors of individuals, including the physiologic response plus the thoughts, feelings, and relationships.

Sexual health involves the ability to express affection, love, and intimacy in respectful ways that are consistent with one's values, with an ability to develop and maintain meaningful interpersonal relationships.

Sexual orientation describes one's erotic, romantic, and affectionate attraction to someone of the same sex, someone of the opposite sex, or both.

Sexual identity involves the inner sense of oneself as a sexual human being, including how one identifies oneself in terms of gender and sexual orientation.

Gender identity involves the personal sense of one's maleness or femaleness, which a child usually can determine by age 3. Gender identification describes the understanding of the values, duties, and responsibilities of being a man or a woman.

Gender role is the public expression of gender identity, the actions, and choices that signal to others whether one is male or female.

one couple who had gone through counseling prior to surgery for gender reassignment stated, "It's not who you go to bed with, it's who you go to bed as that matters." In a heterosexually biased world with homophobia prevalent in certain segments of society, children and adolescents with gender identity or sexual preference questions may not feel safe exploring their feelings. The resulting drive into hiding can lead to depression, or to some risky behaviors in sexual explorations in adolescence and young adulthood. Sexual risk-taking may be heterosexual despite homosexual orientation, or vice versa.

A transvestite has a gender identity that matches his or her biologic identity, but derives pleasure from dressing in the clothing of the opposite gender. In little girls, our society affectionately labels these girls "tomboys"; that same society will often frown on the young boy who prefers wearing dresses. The skilled clinician can help individuals with dysphoric gender identities (again, determined by age 3), and sexual identity (determined by age 14, but potentially not acted upon until much later), to become comfortable with themselves, and "come out" to loved ones and others when ready.

Sexual orientation does not always translate directly into sexual behavior. Many adults who identify themselves as heterosexual report a sexual experience with a same sex partner during adolescence, and heterosexual intercourse in adolescence or young adulthood has been reported by homosexual adults (Bell and Weinberg, 1978). Homosexual, bisexual, and transgender youth are at higher risk of school dropout, of being "pushed out" of homes ("throwaway youth" rather than "runaway youth"), self-medicating with substances such as marijuana, alcohol, or other illegal drugs at earlier ages than their heterosexual peers (Garofalo et al., 1998). Adolescents who identify themselves as gay are two to seven times as likely to attempt suicide and two to four times more likely to be threatened with a weapon at school (Russell et al., 2001; Remafedi et al., 1998; Garofalo, 1999).

Same-sex or bisexual risk-taking behavior may also occur as part of the sexual tourism industry, seen both in the United States and abroad. Same-sex relationships may be an economic choice,

rather than one of sexual orientation, as has been noted in the Caribbean (Halcon and Blum, 2003) as well as in Thailand and other countries.

The clinician caring for adolescents needs to ask question about sexual health, sexual orientation, and sexual behaviors in a nonjudgmental, caring, and confidential way. Examples of questions on sexual health can be seen in Table 22-3. When an adolescent reveals a same-sex or bisexual orientation, the clinician needs to assess and reassess over time that adolescent's sense of well being; a critical or homophobic environment may lead to a profound sense of isolation and fear of discovery, which may interfere with the expected adolescent developmental tasks of achieving a positive self-identity and ability to maintain healthy, intimate relationships (Frankowski, 2004).

Clinicians should have educational brochures and resource lists with phone numbers or Web sites available in the office to provide information on local GLBT (gay, lesbian, bisexual, and transgender) support groups for youth available where a teen or his/her parents can pick them up privately or publicly. If a clinician has personal barriers that prevent him or her from being able to deliver nonjudgmental care to GLBT youth, that clinician should refer the patient to a more neutral clinician. Negative body language or overt discomfort can be devastating to a youth who sees his or her physician as the professional whose judgment matters. Parents of GLBT youth may require support, as well; projection of their own vision of how their child's life should be can cause intense family conflict (the same could be said for the parent of a pregnant teen, or other teen choosing a path not consistent with the parent's vision/choice). Myths may need to be dispelled; the parents may not realize that their lesbian daughter or gay son can still be a wonderful parent and have a committed, positive relationship with shared life dreams and goals. Most states have chapters of Parents and Friends of Lesbians and Gays (PFLAG) to which parents can be referred (Frankowski, 2004).

Sexual Dysfunction in Adolescents

Adolescent sexual dysfunction remains an ignored topic that can derail a teen's quest for the achievement of a healthy adult sexuality. Negative sexual experiences in the early years, ranging from the most serious sexual abuse to the far less drastic experience of being ridiculed by a partner can interfere with an adolescent's ability to form intimate, trusting relationships. These negative experiences can also color an adolescent's lifetime attitudes and sexual behaviors. Commonly encountered types of sexual dysfunction are described below.

Chronic Anxiety or Depression

Underlying anxiety or depression most likely causes most cases of adolescent sexual dysfunction. Responses may range from withdrawal from contact with subsequent isolation or to acting out sexually, also often with lack of intimacy. Both anxiety and depression can prevent future development of warm, trusting, and lasting relationships.

Erectile Dysfunction

Erectile dysfunction in adolescents and young adults is most frequently psychologic in origin (Greydanus et al., 1996). This diagnosis is usually suggested by having compromised sexual performance in the face of normal nocturnal erections and emission. Several studies of college-age males have found a significant prevalence of erectile dysfunction. Responses ranged from erections during foreplay but difficulty maintaining erections during intercourse, to lack of achievement of an erection at all. Needless to say, this problem can be embarrassing and an assault to the male ego.

Physical factors can include prostatic enlargement, as can occur with gonorrheal or chlamydial infection. Prescription drugs such as antihypertensives, imipramine, cimetidine, propranolol and other beta blockers, phenothiazines, along with drugs of abuse such as alcohol, marijuana, amphetamines, opiates, and hallucinogens may produce the unwanted side effect of impotence. Other less common conditions include diabetic neuropathy with concomitant retrograde ejaculation, as well as fibrosis of the corpora cavernosa secondary to sickle cell disease-induced priapism.

Ejaculatory Dysfunction

Premature ejaculation can be a common problem in adolescence, with 20% of teen males reporting having experienced this problem at least once, especially in the early days of their sexual experience. This problem is often very responsive to specific mental health therapy because it usually stems from psychologic and educational factors. Less easy to fix is the retrograde ejaculation that can occur in adolescent diabetics.

Orgasmic Dysfunction

Early adolescent girls in particular commonly do not experience orgasm. In fact, orgasm may not be a goal of sexual activity for the young girl, who may be choosing to initiate sexual activity to please or keep a partner. Orgasmic dysfunction may be more frequent in young girls, but it also occurs in older girls and young adults who may consider it the norm. Causal factors include depression, guilt, anxiety, and other psychologic factors, along with lack of partner skill. Use of alcohol or drugs may also interfere with sexual response, as can local irritations and infection. Management includes education on normal male and female sexual responses and counseling to address perceived psychologic barriers. Removing alcohol and drugs from the sexual experience and treating for any detected infections can also help. Use of KY jelly or other vaginal lubricants can help decrease friction.

Dyspareunia

Another common phenomenon in adolescent girls and young women, dyspareunia may accompany orgasmic dysfunction. Girls with dyspareunia may also early on have difficulty with tampon insertion. The principal causes of dyspareunia include lack of vaginal lubrication due to insufficient foreplay and anxiety about engaging in sexual activity. Local chemical or mechanical irritation and sexually transmitted infections can also be causative. Dyspareunia can also be associated with endometriosis, positional problems, adnexal masses, pelvic infections, and anatomical factors such as a retroflexed uterus. Management depends on the cause and should be addressed with sensitivity. Education on the normal human sexual response, reassurance, and appropriate use of lubricant may solve much of the problem, but specific medical conditions need to be addressed.

Successful resolution of all problems of sexual dysfunction require a trusting relationship between patient and clinician, allowing the adolescent to communicate openly and honestly. Questions on sexual abuse as well as sexual dysfunction need to be asked in a sensitive way, with reassurance that these problems can occur commonly in teenagers and can be reversible. A complete physical examination should include pelvic or genital examination, along with inspection of the perianal area. Screening for sexually transmitted infections should occur. For those adolescents and young adults who show signs of depression, anxiety, or have been sexually abused, counseling should be recommended.

Sexuality Education: Room to Improve

Despite the fact that over 90% of teens reported having received HIV prevention education in school from YRBS in 1997 and beyond, many children continue to lack sufficient knowledge, motivation, and skills to prevent HIV infection. School-based interventions may lack opportunities for confidential questions, individual risk assessment, or targeted prevention. Although two-thirds of adolescents seeing a physician report wanting information about STDs and pregnancy from their physician, relatively few have ever discussed these issues with their physicians (Kapphahn et al., 1999). Over half of primary care providers neglect to routinely ask adolescents about sexual activity, with fewer still asking about STD, condom use, second method of protection used, sexual orientation, number of partners, or sexual abuse (Millstein et al., 1996), despite the fact that GAPS and BRIGHT FUTURES have routinely recommended obtaining comprehensive sexual histories from adolescents for the past decade (Green, 1994; Elster and Kuznets, 1994).

What Have We Learned?

Three types of programs have been shown to be effective at reducing teen pregnancy: programs that focus on sexual antecedents, those that focus on nonsexual antecedents, and those that focus on both (Kirby, 2001). Nonsexual antecedents include positive youth development programs, with a paradigm shift from youth as problems to be solved to youth as assets, with individual strengths to be cultivated. The view is that positive youth development protects or insulates youth from engaging in risk behaviors (Vesely et al., 2004). In an analysis of cross-sectional, in-home interview data from randomly selected inner city teenagers in two Midwestern cities, several developmental assets were associated with a lower likelihood of ever having had sexual intercourse, including increasing parental income, two-parent households, having at least one parent who has earned a bachelor's degree. Never having had sexual intercourse was associated with having positive nonparental adult role models, peer role models, good family communication, time spent engaging in religious activities, community involvement, future aspirations, and responsible choices (Vesely et al., 2004). Two assets, peer role models and family communication, were positively correlated with use of birth control.

Several sexuality education programs have been evaluated using experimental or quasiexperimental designs and have been shown to have impact on adolescents' sexual behavior (Frost and Forrest, 1995). Effective programs tend to teach practical skills such as communication and negotiation, using role playing and interactive discussion (AAP, Committee on School Health and Committee on Adolescence, 2001). Abstinence-only programs have not demonstrated successful outcomes with regard to delay of sexual debut or of safer sex practices (Frost and Forrest, 1995; Kirby et al., 2004). However, abstinence education, promoted as the best option but combined with education on HIV, STDs, and contraceptive options for adolescents who choose to have sex, has been shown to delay first sexual activity and increase the proportion of sexually active adolescents using birth control, with both efforts combining to decrease teen pregnancy and STD rates (AAP, 2001). When programs link reproductive health services with sexuality education including both abstinence and contraceptive counseling and comprehensive community-based interventions, decreases in teen pregnancy rates have been demonstrated (Zabin, 1988a,b).

In the area of teen pregnancy prevention, sex and family-life programs can be divided into three categories: teen-focused skills-building models, family-focused communication-building models, and community-focused information-building models (ACOG, 1997). Teen-focused programs help adolescents develop skills in postponing sexual involvement, resisting perceived peer pressure to become sexually active, and enhancing skills for responsible sexual decision making. These programs have not been shown to increase sexual activity. Family-focused programs arose with a goal of improving parent-child communication while promoting abstinence and encouraging a delay in sexual activity. Both family-focused and teen-focused programs have been implemented in schools since 1955; however, with no consensus on national standards for sexuality education in the United States, great variability exists in what gets covered. No state currently explicitly requires the provision of information about where to obtain birth control, or how to use a method correctly. Community-based programs can also vary in content, with some offering pregnancy and contraceptive information, some solely abstinence-based, and some offering a combination of abstinence and family-planning counseling. Abstinence-based messages work best with 5th and 6th graders, and groups who have not yet initiated sexual activity.

Effective programs share common features, including: (1) a clear focus on reducing one or more sexual behaviors that lead to teen pregnancy; (2) use of age-appropriate and culturally relevant behavioral goals, teaching methods, and materials that coincide with the sexual experience level of the participants; (3) use of a theoretical approach with demonstrated effectiveness at reducing other health-related risk behaviors; (4) allowance of sufficient time for presentation of information and interactive learning; (5) personalization of the material through use of interactive learning techniques; (6) provision of basic and scientifically accurate information about the risks of sexual activity without protection and about ways to avoid participating in unprotected sexual intercourse; (7) addressing of peer pressure; (8) modeling of skills for improved communication, negotiation, and refusal; and (9) use of teachers and peer-leaders who are committed to the program, seen as credible leaders, and have received adequate skills-training to facilitate the program effectively (ACOG, 1997). Further details of specific programs are beyond the scope of this chapter but can be found elsewhere (ACOG, 1997; Kirby, 2001).

Uganda has been one of the few countries to demonstrate a significant reduction in HIV seroprevalence over the past decade, effected by its explicit national policy teaching Abstinence, Be faithful, and Condoms (Blum, 2004). In contrast to the United States' experience, where abstinence education is targeted toward teen pregnancy reduction, Uganda's abstinence education focuses on HIV reduction. Moreover, during abstinence education class in an elite Christian school in Uganda, students felt safe to raise questions and were given appropriate answers on homosexuality, masturbation, abortion, and forced sex. In the United States, on the other hand, abstinence-only education would likely not cover as wide-ranging a set of adolescent concerns. In the United States, all educators agree that abstinence is the safest message; politicians and others differ in their views on the alternatives to abstinence appropriate for adolescents, and on complex issues of reproductive rights and confidentiality. Access to nonjudgmental care as well as to contraceptives themselves can be a barrier in many countries, including China, where the majority of traditional family planning service providers view sexual activity as an acceptable activity only for married couples and may be perceived as hostile by youth trying to obtain contraceptive advice (Lou et al., 2004).

Helping Guide Adolescents to Responsible Decision Making

In contrast to risk behaviors such as substance abuse where the goal is permanent abstinence, the adult recipe for a healthy sexuality usually includes intercourse or other form of sexual expression. Thus, our message for teens shifts more to, "We want you to enjoy this some day, just not yet!" To that end, even a delay in initiation of sexual activity can be considered a valid and worthwhile goal, with school programs such as Postponing Sexual Involvement designed to delay initiation of risk-taking behavior and improve condom use if sexual activity occurs. Even a 9-month delay in sexual initiation, especially with younger adolescents, has been associated with fewer partners and improved condom use.

In 15–17-year olds, virginity pledges have been shown to delay sexual intercourse by 18 months, a finding well received by the popular press despite the fact that these findings did not generalize to all groups, ages, or ethnicities (Dailard, 2001). These pledges worked best when not all adolescents endorsed the behaviors, giving participants a sense of belonging to their own special group. In one southern high school, once the virginity pledges became normative, they seemed to lose their appeal and hence some of their efficacy. Such pledges also carry another set of inherent risks: teens who break their pledges are one-third less likely than non-pledgers to use contraceptives when they do become sexually active, putting them at even greater risk for unintended pregnancy and sexually transmitted diseases. A similar finding is found in teens who embrace religious views condemning premarital intercourse, with planning of contraception not acceptable since it means that intention was involved in their sin or violation of a religious rule.

Lessons can be learned from other developed countries, whose rates of teen pregnancy are far lower than in the United States despite similar levels of sexual activity (Darroch et al., 2001). In the Netherlands and Sweden, contraceptive use is normative and acceptable; as a Dutch public health official said, "Having sex without a condom is like driving through a red light, and that is something that you don't do—you simply don't do it" (Rome et al., 2001). These countries tend to have higher societal acceptance of sexual activity among young people, but the context is expected to be between committed older adolescents in monogamous, loving relationships with delayed childbearing.

Different levels of intervention need to be implemented throughout communities. The primary care clinician must remember to ask the right questions in a confidential setting, then have knowledge and access to appropriate resources as needed. The family requires interventions that build parent-child communication about risk-taking behavior, capitalizing on teachable moments, specific to each child's developmental level, weaving in the moral context, and reinforcing both knowledge and the "safety net" around each child (DiClemente and Wingood, 2000). Family interventions and other school or community-based interventions must be culturally sensitive and theory based in order to promote lasting change. Interventions need to be sustained and coupled with efforts to avoid complacency leading to political or cultural expectations that a problem is solved, resulting in withdrawal of needed resources to continue to address the problem.

JoAnn Deak talks of the protective value of the three C's: Competence, Confidence, and Connectedness (Deak, 2003). In raising kids with a healthy sexuality, one could add several more C's: Caring Community, including school, home, physician's offices, the surrounding neighborhood(s), and the religious community. Add a sixth C, Core Knowledge and Skills, and we get at the educational component necessary to make healthy sexual choices. A seventh C might be Communication, particularly sexual-risk communication between parent and child. Parents need to articulate their values explicitly with their teens, not just assuming that the adolescent knows their values. Parents should also proactively seek out pediatricians who communicate well with teens and can help open the lines of communication between parent and child. Clinicians need to take the time to establish confidentiality (another C) and respond to teens' concerns. Cultural context comprises the next set of C's, with messages better received if constructed and delivered with these factors taken into account. Combine all of these C's, and we may succeed in helping teens find the motivation to pursue healthy choices, synthesizing what they know and expect into a healthy sexual identity.

Bibliography

American Academy of Pediatrics, Committee on Psychosocial aspects of child and family health and Committee on Adolescence. Sexuality education for children and adolescents. *Pediatrics* 2001;108: 498–502.

American College of Obstetricians and Gynecologists, Committee on Adolescent Health Care. *Adolescent Sexuality Kit: Guides for Professional Involvement*, 2d ed. Washington, DC: American College of Obstetricians and Gynecologists, 1992.

American College of Obstetricians and Gynecologists. *Strategies for Adolescent Pregnancy Prevention.* Washington, DC: American College of Obstetricians and Gynecologists, 1997.

Bell AP, Weinberg MS. *Homosexualities: A Study of Diversity among Gay Men and Women.* New York: Simon & Shuster, 1978.

Blum RW. Uganda AIDS prevention: A, B, C and Politics. *J Adolesc Health* 2004;34:428–432.

Borawski EA, Ievers-Landis CE, Lovegreen LD, Trapl ES. Parental monitoring, negotiated unsupervised time, and parental trust: The role of perceived parenting practices in adolescent health risk behaviors. *J Adolesc Health* 2003;33:60–70.

Braverman PK. Sexually transmitted diseases. *Adolesc Health Update* 2001;14(1):1–12.

Dailard C. Recent findings from the "Add Health" Survey: Teens and Sexual Activity. *The Guttmacher Report on Public Policy.* New York: The Alan Guttmacher Institute, 4(4):1–3, 2001.

Darroch JE, Frost JJ, Singh S. *Teenage Sexual and Reproductive Behavior in Developed Countries: Can more Progress be made?* Occasional report No. 3 New York: The Alan Guttmacher Institute, 2001.

Deak JoAnn. *How Girls Thrive: An Essential Guide for Educators (And Parents).* Hudson, Ohio: The Deak Group, 2003

Deak JoAnn. *Girls Will Be Girls: Raising Confident and Courageous Daughters.* Hudson, Ohio: The Deak Group, 2003

DiClemente R, Wingood G. Expanding the scope of HIV prevention for adolescents: Beyond individual-level interventions. *J Adolesc Health* 2000;26:377–378.

Dilorio C, Kelley M, Hockenberry-Eaton M. Communication about sexual issues: Mothers, fathers, and friends. *J Adolesc Health* 1999;24:181–189.

Elster AB, Kuznets NJ (eds.). *AMA Guidelines for Adolescent Preventive Services (GAPS): Recommendations and Rationale.* Baltimore, MD: Williams & Wilkins, 1994.

Frankowski BL. Committee on Adolescence, American Academy of Pediatrics. Sexual orientation and adolescents. *Pediatrics* 2004;113:1827–1832.

Frost JJ, Forrest JD. Understanding the impact of effective teenage pregnancy prevention programs. *Fam Plann Perspect* 1995;27:188–195.

Garofalo R, Wolf RC, Kessel S, Palfrey SJ, DuRant RH. The association between health risk behaviors and sexual orientation among a school-based sample of adolescents. *Pediatrics* 1998;101:895–902.

Garofalo R, Wolf RC, Wissow LS, Woods ER, Goodman E. Sexual orientation and risk of suicide attempts among a representative sample of youth. *Arch Pediatr Adolesc Med* 1999;153:487–493.

Gates GJ, Sonenstein FL. Heterosexual genital sexual activity among adolescent males: 1988 and 1995. *Fam Plann Perspect* 2000;32:295–297, 304.

Ginsburg KR, Jablow M. *But, I'm Almost 13!: An Action Plan for Raising a Responsible Adolescent.* New York: McGraw-Hill, 2001.

Gordon T. *Parent Effectiveness Training.* New York: Three Rivers Press, 2000.

Green M (ed.). *Bright Futures: Guidelines for Health Supervision of Infants, Children, and Adolescents.* Arlington, VA: National Center for Education in Maternal and Child Health, 1994.

Greydanus DE, Pratt HD, Baxter T. Sexual dysfunction and the primary care physician. *Adolesc Med* 1996; 7(1):9–26.

Grunbaum JA, Kann L, Kinchen S, Ross J, Hawkins J, Lowry R, et al. Youth risk behavior surveillance—United States, 2003. *MMWR* 2004;53 (SSO2):1–96.

Halcon L, Blum RW. Adolescent health in the Caribbean: A regional portrait. *Am J Publ Health* 2003;93: 1851–1857.

Halpern C, Oslak S, Yooung M, et al. Partner violence among adolescents in opposite sex romantic relationships: Findings from the national longitudinal study of adolescent health. *Am J Public Health* 2001;91: 1679–1685.

Halpern-Fisher BL, Cornell JL, Kropp RY, et al: Oral versus vaginal sex among adolescents: Perceptions, attitudes, and behavior. Pediatrics 2005;115: 845–851.

http://www.agi-usa.org/index.html

http://www.childtrendsdatabank.org/

http://www.isna.org (Intersex Society of North America)

http://www.siecus.org/index.html

http:www.sxetc.org/ (this is a useful website geared toward teen readers)

Hutchinson MK, Jemmott JB, Jemmott LS, Braverman P, Fong GT. The role of mother-daughter sexual risk communication in reducing sexual risk behaviors among urban adolescent females: A prospective study. *J Adolesc Health* 2003;33:98–107.

Irwin C. Adolescent sexuality and reproductive health: Where are we in 2004? *J Adolesc Health* 2004;34: 353–355.

Kapphahn CF, Wilson KM, Klein JD. Adolescent girls and boys' preferences for provider gender and confidentiality in their health care. *J Adolesc Health* 1999; 25:131–142.

Kirby D. Emerging Answers: Research Findings on Programs to Reduce Teen Pregnancy. *The National Campaign to Prevent Teen Pregnancy* 2001:1–186.

Kirby DB, Baumler C, Coyle KK, et al. The "safer choices" intervention: Its impact on sexual behaviors of different subgroups of high school students. *J Adolesc Health* 2004;35:442–252.

Kunkel D, Cope KM, Farinola WJM, et al. *Sex on TV: Content and context.* Santa Barbara, CA: Henry J. Kaiser Family Foundation, 1999.

Litt I. Parents are "In" Again. *J Adolesc Health* 2003; 33:59.

Lou CH, Wang B, Shen Y, Gao ES. Effects of a community-based sex education and reproductive health service program on contraceptive use of unmarried youths in Shanghai. *J Adolesc Health* 2004;34:433–440.

Malamuth N, Check J. The effects of mass media exposure on acceptance of violence against women: A field experiment. *J Res Pers* 1981;15:436–446.

Millstein SG, Igra V, Gans J. Deliver of STD/HIV preventive services to adolescent by primary care physicians. *J Adolesc Health* 1996;19:249–257.

National Campaign to Prevent Teen Pregnancy. *What's Behind the Good News: The Decline in Teen Pregnancy Rates during the 1990's,* 2001. Available at: *http:// www.teenpregnancy.org/inew.htm*

Parents and Families and Friends of Lesbians and Gays (PFLAG website) *http://www.pflag.org*

Prinstein MJ, Meade CS, Cohen GL. Adolescent oral sex, peer popularity, and perceptions of best friends' sexual behavior. *J Pediatr Psychol* 2003;28:243–249.

Remafedi G, French S, Story M, Resnick MD, Blum RW. The relationship between suicide risk and sexual orientation: Results of a population-based study. *Am J Publ Health* 1998;88:57–60.

Rennison CM. *Intimate Partner Violence and Age of Victim, 1993–1999.* Washington, DC: US Department of Justice, Office of Justice Programs, Bureau of Justice Statistics, 2001.

Rome ES, Camlin K, Cromer BA. Messages heard loud and clear: Four countries' perspectives on society's role in adolescent pregnancy. Abstract presented at *Annual Meeting of the Society for Adolescent Medicine,* March 2001, San Diego, CA.

Russell ST, Franz BT, Driscoll AK. Same-sex romantic attraction and experiences of violence in adolescence. *Am J Publ Health* 2001;91:903–906.

Schuster MA, Bell RM, Kanouse DE. The sexual practices of adolescent virgins: Genital sexual activities of high school students who have never had vaginal intercourse. *Am J Publ Health* 1996;86:1570–1576.

Strasburger VC, Donnerstein E. Children, adolescents, and the media in the 21st century. *Adolesc Med* 2000; 11(1):51–68.

Taylor CA, Sorenson SB. Injunctive social norms of adults regarding teen dating violence. *J Adolesc Health* 2004;34:468–479.

Tjaden P, Thoennes N. *Full Report of the Prevalence, Incidence, and Consequences of Violence against Women: Findings from the National Violence Against Women Survey.* Washington, DC: US Department of Justice, Office of Justice Programs, National Institute of Justice, 2000.

Ventura SJ, Mosher WD, Curtin SA, Abma JC. Trends in pregnancy rates for the United States, 1976–1997: An update. *Nat Vital Stat Rep* 2001;49:1–12.

Vesely SK, Wyatt VH, Oman RF, Aspy CB, Kegler MC, et al. The potential protective effects of youth assets from adolescent sexual risk behaviors. *J Adolesc Health* 2004;34:356–365.

Whitaker D, Miller K. Parent-adolescent discussions about sex and condoms: Impact on peer influences of sexual risk behavior. *J Adolesc Res* 2000;15: 251–273.

Wingood GM, DiClemente RJ, Harrington K, Davies S, Hook WE, Oh MK. Exposure to X-Rated movies and adolescents' sexual and contraceptive-related attitudes and behaviors. *Pediatrics* 2001;107:1116–1119.

Zabin LS, Hirsch MB, Smith EA, et al. The Baltimore pregnancy prevention program for urban teenagers II. What did it cost? *Fam Plann Perspect* 1988a;20:188–192.

Zabin LS, Hirsch MB, Streett R, et al. The Baltimore pregnancy prevention program for urban teenagers. I. How did it work? *Fam Plann Perspect* 1988b;20:182–187.

23

SEXUAL ABUSE AND THE ADOLESCENT PATIENT

Joyce A. Adams

INTRODUCTION

The prevalence of different kinds of abuse in children and adolescents (i.e., child sexual abuse, sexual molestation, sexual assault, and "date rape") is so high as to demand attention from all health care professionals who treat adolescents. While prevalence rates vary depending on how and from whom the data are collected, national data from the *Year 2001 Youth Risk Behavior Survey* revealed self-reported rates of forced sexual intercourse among high school girls at 10%, and 5% for high school boys.[1]

Sexual abuse at any age will have a profound impact upon the victim and the family, but adolescents are particularly vulnerable because they are still developing their own sense of identity. For a young woman or man who is the victim of sexual assault, the change is dramatic: before the rape, a young woman may think of herself as "Mary, who is quiet but friendly." After the rape, she is "Mary, who has been raped." This is called the integration of the rape experience into the individual's sense of self. It is not uncommon for a rape victim to never tell anyone about their sexual abuse, whether it happened as a young child, or during adolescence. However, many of the symptoms, conditions, or

behaviors that may bring an adolescent into the health care system can be thought of as possible "red flags," which should alert the health care provider to the possibility of past abuse. Table 23-1 lists some of the known associations with past or current sexual abuse.

DEFINITIONS AND PREVALENCE

Child Sexual Abuse

Child sexual abuse is usually defined as sexual abuse that occurred prior to age 12 or prior to the onset of puberty. Sexual abuse includes non-contact exposure, contact involving touching or fondling only, and contact between the abuser's hand, mouth, or genital organ and the child's mouth, breasts, genital, or anal area. Sexual contact between an adult and a child is always considered abusive, no matter the type of contact or the relationship of the abuser to the child.

While the definition of "child" may vary from one legal jurisdiction to another, most consider a child under the age of 12–14 years to be incapable of consenting to sexual activity. Sexual contact between minors of the same or similar age is also considered abusive if force or coercion is used or threatened.

TABLE 23-1

ASSOCIATIONS WITH HISTORY OF PAST SEXUAL ABUSE

Behaviors	Symptoms	Conditions/Diagnosis
Running away	Abdominal pain	Depression
Truancy	Headaches	Anxiety disorders
Delinquent behavior	Muscle pain	Eating disorders
School failure	Pelvic pain	Obesity
Substance abuse	Recurrent vaginal complaints	Posttraumatic stress disorder
Suicide attempts	Sexual dysfunction	Sexually transmitted diseases
Cutting	Numbness of body parts	Pregnancy as an adolescent
Binge-purge behavior	Sleep problems	
Overeating	Fatigue	
Early onset of	Irritability	
consensual sexual	Seizures	
activity		
Multiple sexual partners		
Nonuse of contraception		
Nonuse of condoms		

The National Violence Against Women Survey, published in 2000[2] found that 1 in 6 women and 1 in 33 men reported having experienced, attempted, or completed rape. More than half of the rapes occurred before age 18 years, and 22% occurred before age 12.

In the Adverse Childhood Experiences (ACE) study, when data were collected from 17,337 adult health plan members receiving an initial medical evaluation at Kaiser Permanente in Southern California, the rates of sexual abuse before age 12 were 25% among women and 16% among men.[3] Child sexual abuse was only one of the ACEs; others included physical abuse, emotional abuse, witnessing mother being abused, substance abuse in a parent, parent's divorce, parent incarcerated, and mental illness in a parent. The ACE score ranged from 0 to 8, and sexual abuse increased by two- to fourfold the likelihood of a person having another ACE. The severity, duration, and frequency of the sexual abuse were significantly related to the total ACE score.

In all studies that are based on surveys, whether they are administered through questionnaires or by telephone or personal interviews, sexual abuse may be defined differently; thus, it is difficult to compare reported rates from one study to another. There is also the problem of recall bias, since adults may be less likely than adolescents to recall specific events. On the other hand, adults may be more willing than adolescents to acknowledge past sexual abuse, if it occurred.

Adolescent Sexual Abuse

Adolescents are sometimes sexually assaulted by strangers, but more commonly, the assailant is someone they know. The National Survey of Adolescents, an in-depth telephone survey of 4023 young people between 12 and 17 years of age was conducted in 1995. In this survey, 13% of girls and 3% of boys reported having been sexually assaulted. In 74% of the cases, the assailant was someone they knew well, and of those, 21% were family members.[4] This study also revealed that 86% of the sexual assaults were not reported by the adolescent to anyone, prior to their being surveyed.

In many states in the United States, as well as other countries, any sexual contact between a minor under the age of 17 or 18 and someone over age 17 or 18 is prohibited by statute; hence the term "statutory rape." Whether or not the sexual contact, when reported to police, is then investigated, varies from one jurisdiction to another. There seems to be a growing trend in many communities in the United States to criminalize sexual activity between adolescents, even if it is consensual; this is a practice which may prevent some adolescents from seeking needed contraceptive and other reproductive health services. Clinicians should check with the Office of the District Attorney or local law enforcement agencies in their own communities, to become familiar with local reporting laws.

Groups at Risk

Women are 16 times more likely than men to experience sexual assault, and adolescents between the ages 12 and 24 are at the highest risk. It is known that alcohol and other substance abuse increases the chances of a young woman being sexually assaulted, as does being mildly mentally retarded. In addition, sexual or physical abuse as a younger child is associated with sexual assault as an adolescent and as an adult.

A study of 1000 women attending primary care clinics in England, using anonymous questionnaires, found that those women who were sexually abused or physically abused as children, were two to three times more likely to report having experienced sexual assault or domestic violence as an adult, compared to women without such histories.[5]

Adolescents may also be at higher risk of sexual assault because of their sense of being invulnerable. Just like youth may be convinced that automobile accidents will not happen to them because they are good drivers, some may feel that sexual assault is something that just will not happen to them because they are too smart or too careful. In addition, there is a stigma attached to sexual assault, and many girls feel that if they are the victim of rape, it is because they did something wrong, dressed too provocatively, stayed too late at the party, or ignored their parent's warnings about drinking alcohol. These factors may also contribute to adolescents' reluctance to report sexual assault.

For the adolescent male who was sexually abused by another male, there may be fear that the rape will cause the victim to become homosexual. Males may also be concerned that if the rape is reported, it will give the impression to others that he is homosexual. These fears probably prevent many young men from reporting their sexual assaults. Young men can also be assaulted by older females, and though sexual contacts may still qualify as statutory rape due to the differences in age, they are even less likely to be reported. Special issues related to male victims will be discussed later.

Factors Affecting Disclosure

Data from the National Survey of Adolescents (NSA), described previously, has been analyzed by a number of researchers. Both race and gender were significant factors affecting disclosure, with males and African American youth being significantly less likely to have told anyone about their abuse. Among girls, younger age at the time of the abuse (under age 6 years), knowing the perpetrator or the perpetrator being a family member, and never living with both parents, were all associated with nondisclosure.

Factors which were associated with immediate disclosure were older age at the time of the abuse, fear for one's life during the assault, injury during the assault, penetration during the assault, and being in a family with a drug abusing household member. While children under age 11 were more likely to disclose the abuse to an adult, adolescents aged 14–17 years were more likely to disclose to a peer.[6]

THE IMPORTANCE OF SCREENING

The Impact of Abuse on Behavior and Risk-taking

The NSA also asked many questions about behaviors and emotional difficulties. Rates of posttraumatic stress disorder (PTSD), substance abuse, and delinquent behavior between girls and boys with a history of child sexual abuse, were three to five times higher than among adolescents without such a history,[4] as shown in Table 23-2.

Physical abuse, as well as sexual abuse, is known to increase the likelihood of adverse behavioral outcomes in adolescents. Data from the *Commonwealth Fund Adolescent Health Study* revealed that girls who reported both types of abuse, compared with girls who did not report any abuse, were three to six times more likely to experience moderate to severe depressive symptoms, moderate to high levels of stress, regular smoking and alcohol consumption, use of other illicit drugs, and reports of fair to poor health status.[7] Other researchers have reported a significant association between physical and sexual abuse and binge-purge behaviors in both boys and girls, with the highest rates occurring in subjects who reported both types of abuse.[8] Sexual abuse is not a problem limited to the United States, of course, and studies from England, Australia, and New Zealand, among others, have shown similar high rates of abuse and correlations with adverse behavioral and psychological outcomes. One study of 1159 pairs of female twins and 832 pairs of male twins in Australia, all of whom were young adults at the time they volunteered for the study, showed the specific effects of child sexual abuse.[9] The self-reported rates of child sexual abuse were 16.7% among the women and 5.4% among the men; also, the abuse was reported more commonly if the subjects also reported parental alcohol-related problems.

Women who reported child sexual abuse had significantly higher risks for major depression, suicide attempt, conduct disorder, alcohol dependence, nicotine dependence, social anxiety, rape after the age of 18, and divorce. For men, the results were similar. In pairs where one twin reported sexual abuse and the other did not, the nonabused twin still had higher rates of adverse outcomes, compared to other nonabused subjects, revealing the strong influence of family factors. However, in the discordant pairs, the twin who reported abuse still had significantly higher rates of all eight adverse outcomes compared to their nonabused twins.

Other behaviors that may be particular warning signs of past abuse, among adolescents who seek medical care, include early onset of sexual activity, nonuse of condoms, poor use of contraception, avoidance of pelvic examinations, recurrent sexually transmitted infections (STIs), and pregnancy as a young teen. In a study of almost 4000 high school students, Raj et al. found that girls who reported past sexual abuse were twice as likely as girls who did not report sexual abuse to have had earlier first coitus, three or more sexual partners, and a pregnancy. Among boys, those reporting past sexual abuse were three times more likely to report having three or more sexual partners and to having caused a pregnancy.[10]

Sexual abuse as a child increases the risk that young women will experience sexual assault as an adolescent; likewise, sexual assault as a young adolescent increases the likelihood of sexual assault as a young adult. A survey of 1569 college women found that sexual assault before the age of 14 almost doubled the risk of later adolescent victimization.[11]

TABLE 23-2

ASSOCIATIONS BETWEEN SEXUAL ABUSE AND EMOTIONAL/BEHAVIORAL OUTCOMES[*]

	Sexual Abuse	No Sexual Abuse
Girls:		
PTSD (90)	30	7
Substance abuse (90)	27	5
Delinquent acts (90)	20	5
Boys:		
PTSD (90)	28	5
Substance abuse (90)	34	9
Delinquent acts (90)	47	17

[*]From National Survey of Adolescents.[4]

The rates of sexual victimization among college women who had experienced rape or attempted rape as a young adolescent were 4.6 times higher than the rates among non-victims.

When and How Should Adolescents be Screened?

The data from studies of college women indicate that a question about past experiences with sexual victimization should be a routine part of the pre-college physical examination, or at the first visit to college health services. The American Medical Association (AMA), in the *AMA Guidelines for Adolescent Preventive Services* or GAPS,[12] recommends that all adolescents, at their initial examination, and at yearly examinations, should be asked about past physical, sexual, and emotional abuse. If a questionnaire is used as a routine, and the adolescent is allowed to complete it in confidence, this questionnaire lets the patient know that the physician or other health care provider is open to discussing this topic. The questionnaires, in English and in Spanish, are available on the AMA's web site.[13]

Another method of screening is to include questions about sexual abuse and unwanted sexual intercourse in the sexual history (Chap. 2), taken as a part of the confidential HEADDSS interview (Home, Education, Activities, Drugs, Depression, Sex, Suicide), or to ask: "How old were you the first time you had any kind of sexual contact with someone, including anything that happened when you were a young child?" Some adolescents may answer "no" to a question like: "Have you ever been sexually abused?" but will give an age less than 11 or 12 years as the age at which their first sexual experience occurred.

Adolescents with symptoms of depression, anxiety, post traumatic stress disorder, and suicidal ideation should always be carefully interviewed about possible past or ongoing abuse, due to the known high prevalence of all types of abuse in these patients. When being informed about the confidentiality of the health care visit, most health care providers will include abuse, intent to self-harm, or intent to harm another, as the three exceptions to the confidentiality rule.

Will an adolescent admit that they have been, or are being abused, given that information? If they are ready to tell someone, adolescents will usually feel relief that the question was asked, and the fact that the abuse must be reported is not likely to deter them from making a disclosure. Asking the questions in person, in a confidential setting, may be better than paper questionnaires for some adolescents.

When to Report

If a patient reports ongoing abuse, an immediate report to either protective services or law enforcement, or both, must be initiated. In many jurisdictions, the child protective agency will only accept reports of abuse that is occurring in the home, or if it is felt that the family is not protective of a child who is being abused by a non-family member. If someone outside the home is abusing the adolescent, the report needs to be made to the law enforcement agency in the city, county, or area in which the abuse occurred or is occurring. Abuse which occurred some time in the past, but has stopped, should also be reported if it is determined that the alleged abuser still has access to minors who may be at risk of abuse.

Sexual contact between an adolescent and an older peer should be reported according to the local statutes. If an adolescent is found to be pregnant or to have contracted an infection that can only be spread by sexual contact, it is important to determine whether or not the sexual contact was forced or coerced. This can sometimes be very difficult, especially in a young adolescent who may not really understand that she/he actually had a choice to say "no" to the sexual contact. A young adolescent who is asked: "Was this something you wanted, or were you forced to have sex with this person?" may simply shrug her/his shoulders. If the young person is of the age that they are considered legally incapable of giving consent, the pregnancy or sexually transmitted disease must be reported, regardless of their response to questions about consent.

Case Examples

CASE 23-1

"This must be Herpes"

Marissa is an 11-year-old girl who tells her mother that she has a painful sore in her genital area. She allows her mother to take a look, and mother sees what looks like a blister on her labia. She brings her daughter to her primary care physician for an examination. Her doctor questions Marisa in private and asks about any type of sexual contact. Marisa vehemently denies that anyone has ever touched her or hurt her in her genital area. She says the sore has been there for about 4 days, that it hurts when she urinates, that she has no other sores anywhere else, and no history of "cold sores" in her mouth or on her lips. She has had no recent viral illnesses, and has had two menstrual periods, the first being 6 months prior, and the second 2 months prior to this visit.

Examination reveals a shy adolescent girl who is Tanner stage III for breast development and IV for pubic hair development. Genital inspection shows a 5-millimeter ulcer on the right labium majora which is painful when touched with a swab. A culture for viruses is obtained, as well as a screening test for syphilis. A urine pregnancy test is negative. Her doctor suspects herpes simplex, and makes a report to Child Protective Services of possible sexual abuse.

Marissa is interviewed in detail by the social worker, and again denies any sexual touching. She is referred to a Sexual Abuse Evaluation clinic, where additional cultures are taken. The results from the initial viral culture are available by this time, and the culture is negative for herpes. A routine bacterial culture is done, revealing *Escherichia coli*. She is treated with sitz baths and oral amoxicillin; the lesion resolves in 1 week.

Should the primary care physician have reported suspected sexual abuse before receiving the results of the herpes culture? In the absence of a history from the child, who is old enough to be interviewed and give a credible statement, another option would have been to wait for the results of the STD testing before making the report. However, in most states, only a suspicion of sexual abuse is required for a health professional to make a report.

CASE 23-2

"It was a Long Time Ago"

An 18-year-old girl, suffering from depression and anorexia nervosa, completing the GAPS (AMA) questionnaire at intake, checks "yes" on the question: "Have you ever been physically, sexually, or emotionally abused." Further questioning reveals that the abuse occurred at age 8, and involved fondling by a 10-year-old neighbor girl. The patient has never told her parents about this, and is adamant that she will not. She is in therapy, and agrees to tell her therapist about this abuse, understanding it is a possible contribution to her depression and eating disorder.

In this case, since the patient is not willing to give the name of the girl, and has no information as to her whereabouts, a report to law enforcement is not necessary. If the patient were under age 18 and was not already in therapy, it would have been important for her physician to encourage her to tell her parents, so they could help her access the necessary mental health counseling.

CASE 23-3

"I Need to Tell You Something"

Katherine is a 15-year-old girl who is being evaluated for possible sexual abuse after her 14-year-old sister committed suicide under suspicious circumstances. There had been multiple reports to protective services of physical abuse to both girls, though they always had other explanations for their bruises. Katherine admits to feelings of depression, and has been suicidal herself in the past. When questioned prior to her examination about whether anyone had ever touched or hurt her in her genital or anal area, she discloses that her mother had inserted a broom handle into her vagina once. She stated that this occurred about 3 months ago, and that she bled for 5 days afterward, even though she was not having a menstrual period. She denied any other type of sexual contact, either forced or consensual.

Her examination in the supine position revealed a redundant hymen with a large tag at the midline (Fig. 23-1). In the prone, knee-chest position, using a cotton swab, a complete, healed transection of the hymen was identified in the midline, corresponding to the 6 o'clock position if she were examined supine (Fig. 23-2). This is a finding that is clear evidence of blunt force penetration, consistent with the patient's disclosure. This abuse must be reported immediately, since social service intervention is needed to find a safe place for Katherine and her younger siblings, who are still in the home.

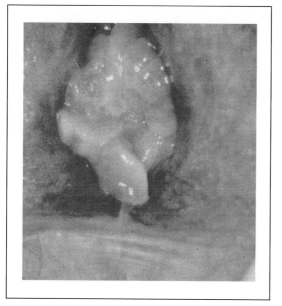

FIGURE 23-1

15-YEAR-OLD GIRL, EXAMINED IN THE SUPINE POSITION. LARGE HYMENAL TAG VISIBLE AT THE 6 O'CLOCK POSITION. COLPOSCOPIC PHOTO-GRAPH AT 10X MAGNIFICATION.

Source: This photograph, and figure 2-4, reprinted with permission of the North American Society for Pediatric and Adolescent Gynecology.[32]

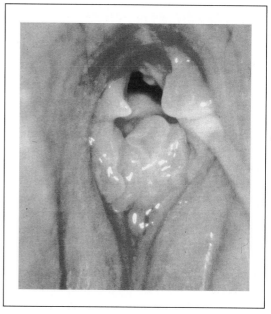

FIGURE 23-2

SAME PATIENT AS IN FIGURE 23-1, EXAMINED IN THE PRONE, KNEE-CHEST POSITION. A DEFECT IN THE HYMEN AT THE MIDLINE IS SEEN, REPRE-SENTING A HEALED TRANSECTION.

TIMING OF THE MEDICAL EVALUATION

The Acute Examination

If an adolescent reports that a sexual assault or unwanted sexual contact has occurred within the past 72 hours (the time frame in most states), an examination needs to be conducted in order to collect forensic evidence, such as semen, sperm, trace evidence, or DNA. Specially trained nurses or physicians in an emergency department, or at special rape crisis centers, usually perform these examinations. Local law enforcement agencies can be contacted to determine where or to whom the patient should be referred for the forensic examination. Both the American Academy of Pediatrics[14] and the American College of Emergency Physicians (ACEP)[15] have published guidelines and protocols for conducting the acute evidential examination of the victim of sexual assault.

The Non-acute Examination

For adolescent patients who reveal that a sexual assault has occurred outside the 72-hour time frame, but who are currently complaining of pain, bleeding, or signs of infection, an examination is necessary. For this type of examination, forensic specimens will usually not be taken, but the patient will need to be checked for sexually transmitted diseases, counseled about pregnancy prevention, and referred for mental health counseling.

Figures 23-3 and 23-4 are photos of a 16-year-old adolescent girl who described being sexually assaulted by an 18-year-old male 10 days prior to the examination. She reported the assault because she was "still bleeding," and was concerned she had sustained serious genital injury. She was having a menstrual period when examined, and had probably bled for 1 or 2 days from the assault, then 5 or 6 days from her period. However, because she gave a very detailed description of being assaulted, and because the examination showed clear evidence of penetrating genital trauma, the law enforcement agency was convinced to interview the alleged assailant. The 18-year-old male, under pressure, admitted to sexually assaulting the patient.

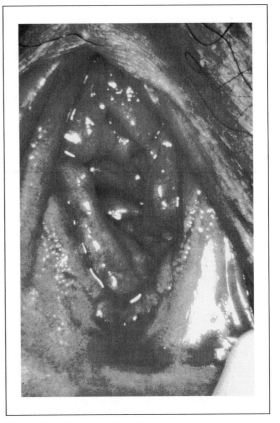

FIGURE 23-3

THIS 16-YEAR-OLD GIRL WAS EXAMINED 10 DAYS AFTER A SEXUAL ASSAULT, REPORTED BECAUSE OF CONTINUED BLEEDING. SHE IS ALSO ON HER MENSTRUAL PERIOD, AND THE HYMEN RIM IS NOT WELL DEFINED IN THIS PHOTOGRAPH.

Even in the absence of physical symptoms, an examination may be very helpful as a way to educate the young male or female patient that he or she is healthy, and should not experience any long-term negative effects, from a physical standpoint. When adolescent girls, who were being examined following a sexual assault, using video colposcopy, were allowed to view the examination on a video monitor, their anxiety scores after the exam were significantly lower than before the examination.[16] The reassurance of the examining physician or nurse that all the tissues appear to be healthy, or if injuries are found, are shown to be minor, is a very important benefit of the examination.

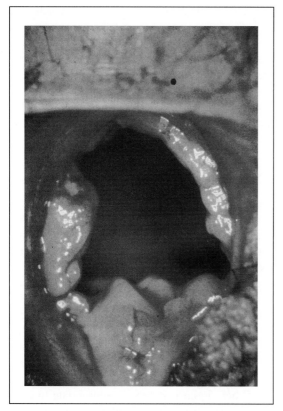

FIGURE 23-4

SAME PATIENT AS IN FIGURE 3, EXAMINED IN THE PRONE, KNEE-CHEST POSITION. A LOSS OF HYMENAL TISSUE IN THE POSTERIOR RIM, AND THE TORN EDGE OF THE HYMEN WITH YELLOW-WHITE GRANULATION TISSUE, ARE CLEARLY SEEN.

FREQUENCY OF PHYSICAL FINDINGS

Genital and Non-genital Trauma

Adolescents, who are examined within 72 hours of being sexually assaulted, may have signs of genital, anal, or non-genital trauma. One study of 819 women, aged 15 and older, who received a standardized acute forensic examination, showed that non-genital injuries were more common than either genital or anal injuries.[17] General body trauma was documented in 52% of the women, and was associated with being hit or kicked, with an attempted

strangulation, with oral or anal penetration, and with stranger assault. The same study found visible genital-anal trauma in 20% of women, and this type of trauma was more frequently documented in women under age 20 or over age 49, women who had never experienced intercourse prior to the assault, women reporting anal assault, and in women examined within 24 hours of the assault.

A similar study involving only adolescent women between the ages 12 and 17, examined acutely and using photo-colposcopy, found nongenital trauma in 58% of subjects and abrasions/lacerations of the fossa or posterior fourchette in 45%.[18] Anal injuries were significantly more common in women describing anal penetration compared to those who denied anal contact (14/31, 61% vs. 2/150, 1%; $P = 0.000$). There was also a significant correlation between the presence of non-genital trauma and the number and severity of genital or anal injuries.

Common Expectations of What the Examination Will Show

Many lay persons, as well as many medical professionals, assume that if an adolescent girl is sexually assaulted, and examined within a short period of time after that assault, there should be physical findings on her examination to support the allegation of rape. Specifically, there is an expectation that the examining physician will be able to know from the examination whether or not penile-vaginal intercourse occurred. This is possible only in a minority of cases, as for example, when pregnancy is confirmed, when sperm is found inside the vagina, when specific sexually transmitted diseases are documented, or when there are acute lacerations of the hymen.

The "myth of the hymen" holds that the hymen always tears the first time a young woman has penile-vaginal intercourse, and that the act will result in bleeding. Numerous studies have shown that this does not always happen, and two recent studies provide additional evidence. In a comparison of the appearance of the hymen in adolescent girls with and without a history of consensual vaginal intercourse, only 48% of subjects admitting intercourse had deep notches or complete clefts in the posterior hymen.[19] Even more convincing, a recent report on the appearance of the hymen in pregnant adolescents showed that only 2 out of 36 pregnant girls had healed transections (complete clefts) of the hymen[20] documented on photographs taken through a colposcope.

The hymen in adolescent women is a very elastic structure, and it can stretch to allow penile penetration, without tearing. This point needs to be explained to patients who are having a sexual assault examination and fear that they will not be believed if there is not "evidence" that penetration occurred as described. The elasticity of the hymen must also be explained over and over again by physicians and nurses who testify in court on sexual assault cases, where there is usually an absence of recent or healed trauma to the hymen.

Consensual versus Nonconsensual Intercourse

There have been very few studies comparing the frequency and type of physical findings in adolescent girls who describe being sexually assaulted and those who admit to having engaged in consensual sexual intercourse. One early study found no difference in the frequency of tears of the posterior fourchette, highlighted with Toluidine Blue dye, among adolescents examined at a sexual assault center, and a control group of adolescents who volunteered for an examination after having consensual sex.[21] In each group, 7 out of 25 subjects had this finding. More recently, Jones et al.[22] found no statistically significant difference in the percentage of adolescent girls with posterior fourchette tears between girls describing sexual assault, and those who were examined at the same center in the same manner, but stated that the intercourse was consensual. This latter group was made up of adolescents who were brought in by parents or police for evidential examinations, because they were below the age at which they could legally consent to intercourse.

These studies should cause physicians and nurses who perform evaluations on adolescents to be cautious in their conclusions, after examining an adolescent who states she was the victim of sexual assault. Posterior fourchette lacerations, erythema of the labia or hymen, edema of the hymen, and superficial abrasions of the perineum can all result from either consensual or nonconsensual sexual intercourse. Consent is an issue to be decided by the judge or jury, not by the examining physician or nurse. An example of a summary statement used by forensic nurse examiners on this issue is: "The presence or absence of physical findings does not speak to the issue of consent."

What to Tell the Patient or Family

Since it is usually not possible to determine from the examination whether or not a young woman has experienced penile-vaginal penetration, what should the clinician or nurse tell the patient who is referred for an evaluation to look for "evidence" of abuse? What if the family wants to know if their daughter is "still a virgin"? What if the family refuses to believe that a sexual assault took place if there are no injuries found?

There are several approaches that can be used. In cultures where virginity is so highly valued that the girl will be ostracized if she is known to have "lost" her virginity, it may be appropriate to reassure the patient and the family that your examination found no evidence of any injury to the genital tissues (which is usually the case, anyway). Some clinicians will tell a young patient that she is still a virgin until she has sex voluntarily with someone she loves. Parents can also be educated that sexual assaults do not always leave physical evidence or evidence of injury, and that the clarity and detail of the adolescent's description of the events is also evidence that he/she was assaulted.

Families often need advice on how to best help their child after the sexual assault is reported. Adolescents should not be questioned in detail by family members about the assault, but should be allowed to talk about the details when they are ready. The assault victim should also be reassured that no matter the circumstances leading up to the assault, they are not to blame for being assaulted. Families need to be careful that the comments they make do not imply blame, and that they protect the patient's privacy with friends or associates. It should also be pointed out to families that their child may have mood changes, may withdraw from friends and usual activities, or may begin acting out as part of the reaction to being abused. If behaviors change drastically, parents need to be sure the adolescent obtains necessary mental health referrals.

TREATMENT AND FOLLOW-UP

Adolescents who receive a forensic medical examination, with collection of samples using a "Rape Kit," are usually offered prophylaxis for several sexually transmitted diseases. Table 23-3 lists the infections and the recommended treatments, suggested by the Centers for Disease Control and Prevention.[23] If the patient is being examined weeks or months after the sexual assault, it is more appropriate to obtain cultures for gonorrhea and Chlamydia, and, for females, to perform a wet mount examination of any vaginal secretions to look for *Trichomonas vaginalis* organisms or for evidence of bacterial vaginosis (see Chap. 24). Serologic testing for syphilis and HIV can also be performed, if the patient so requests. Adolescent girls may request a pelvic examination and PAP test, but they may also be very reluctant to undergo these examinations because of anxieties related to the sexual assault experience. If that is the case, urine polymerase chain reaction tests can be done for gonorrhea and Chlamydia, and the patient can even self-collect a vaginal swab for microscopic analysis.

Counseling is always recommended for victims of sexual assault, but adolescents may not be ready to see a therapist in the weeks or months following the assault or disclosure. Denial, "forgetting," and distraction, are all methods adolescents may use to cope with these experiences, and being asked to talk about their feelings related to the assault is sometimes too frightening. It may be months to a year later that the emotional and behavioral consequences develop, and that is when therapy is most likely to be accepted.

ADOLESCENT MALES AS VICTIMS AND PERPETRATORS

The true prevalence of sexual assault and sexual molestation among males in non-clinical populations is unknown. It is theorized that males may be abused at similar rates, but report the abuse much less frequently than women. The ACE study, mentioned previously, collected data from adult members of a large health maintenance organization. Of the 4127 male respondents, 15% self-reported a history of child sexual abuse, 32% reported physical abuse, and 11% reported that their mothers were battered.[24] A study of 2500 British men attending general physicians' offices showed rates of self-reported child sexual abuse of 5.4%, with another 2.9% reporting non-consensual experiences as adults.[25]

The reported rates of sexual abuse and sexual assault among males who self-identify as gay or bisexual vary according to the setting in which the data were collected. Studies of adult males attending STD clinics reveal self-reported rates of childhood sexual abuse of 34%–36%.[26,27] When subjects were recruited through community outreach, rather than in medical settings, the rates were lower: 14% reported sexual abuse before age 14, and another 14% reported abuse after age 14.[28] In the later study, subjects reporting sexual abuse were about three times more likely to abuse alcohol and to have attempted suicide.

Adolescent males, including young adults, are the most common perpetrators of sexual assault. It is known that adolescents who commit rape have a high incidence of past victimization, with 25%–50% of offenders reporting past physical abuse, and 10%–80% reporting past sexual abuse.[29] Other risk factors include family dysfunction, substance abuse, exposure to erotica, and co-morbid disorders such as conduct disorder, adjustment disorders, and attention deficit-hyperactivity disorders. For a comprehensive review of the topic of adolescent offenders and the role of the Pediatrician, see Pratt et al.[29]

PREVENTION

Primary prevention of adolescent sexual assault would also have to involve prevention of child physical and sexual abuse, since both of these are risk factors leading to increased vulnerability of the victim, as well as risk factors for perpetration. In addition, adolescents can be taught how to avoid situations where sexual assaults may be more

TABLE 23-3

TESTING AND TREATMENT OPTIONS

	If Prophylaxis is Not Given (And/Or At Follow-up Examination)	If Prophylaxis is Given	12-Week Follow-up Visit
Type of test			
Neisseria gonorrhea	Culture from cervix, urethra (males), and/or rectum	None	Culture as indicated
Alternative method for N. gonorrhea	Nucleic acid amplification test approved by FDA, if culture not available. Two tests using different segments of DNA as probe	None	If patient has had unprotected intercourse in the interim
Chlamydia trachomatis	Culture from cervix or urethra (males)	None	Culture as indicated
Alternative method for C. trachomatis	Nucleic acid amplification test approved by FDA, if culture not available. Two tests using different segments of DNA as probes	None	If patient has had unprotected intercourse in the interim
Syphilis	Serology	Serology	Serology
HIV	Serology	Serology	Serology
Hepatitis B	Serology if not immunized	Hepatitis B immunization, if not immunized	None
Trichomonas	Wet mount examination and culture if available	None	Wet mount examination if indicated by symptoms
Bacterial vaginosis	Wet mount examination if indicated	None	Wet mount if indicated
Pregnancy	Testing	Emergency contraception (plan B has less nausea and vomiting)	As indicated
Treatments			
N. gonorrhea	None	Ceftriaxone 125 mg IM	As indicated
C. trachomatis	None	Azithromycin 1 g orally, or Doxycycline 100 mg orally twice a day for 7 days	As indicated
Trichomonas/bacterial vaginosis	None	Metronidazole, 500 mg orally twice a day for 7 days	As indicated

likely to occur. The San Diego Police Department developed a sexual assault risk reduction curriculum for high school and middle school students, which is available at *http://www.sannet.gov/police/about/curriculum.shtml*. This resource includes teacher aids, slides, parent brochures, and booklets for males and female students heading to college. The evaluation of the project is also available on the web site.

Another program, called "Safe Dates," includes a theatre production performed by students, a curriculum consisting of 10 sessions taught by health and physical education teachers, and a poster contest for the students. This program has been evaluated in rural North Carolina, and has been shown to significantly decrease the perpetration of physical, psychological, and sexual abuse among participants compared to control students.[30]

Clinicians also have a role in the primary and secondary prevention of adolescent sexual assault. When parents are being counseled about the physical, emotional, and cognitive changes of puberty, a discussion of sexuality is also needed. Sexual abuse/assault prevention should be an important part of that discussion. A recent study by Thomas et al.[31] demonstrated that over 90% of parents surveyed were comfortable discussing these topics with their child's pediatrician; however, only 45% of their physicians had discussed sexuality, and only 29% had discussed sexual abuse prevention.

Sexual abuse is an uncomfortable topic for many people, but it is such a common phenomenon with so many negative emotional, behavioral, and physical consequences that it needs to be asked about on a routine basis. If the question is asked in such a way as to communicate the health provider's willingness to hear the answer, however uncomfortable or potentially time-consuming, adolescent patients will have the opportunity to tell someone, and so begin the process of recovery.

BIBLIOGRAPHY

1. Centers for Disease Control. Youth Risk Behavior Surveillance—United States, 2003. *MMWR Surveillance Summaries*. May 21, 2004/53(SS02);1–96. Available at: *http://www.cdc.gov/mmwr/PDF/SS/SS5302.pdf.*

2. Tjaden P, Thoennes N. *Full Report of the Prevalence, Incidence, and Consequences of Violence Against Women: Findings from the National Violence Against Women Survey.* Report for grant 93-IJ-CX-0012, funded by the National Institute of Justice and the Centers for Disease Control and Prevention. Washington, DC: National Institute of Justice, 2000.

3. Dong M, Anda RF, Dube SR, et al. The relationship of exposure to childhood sexual abuse to other forms of abuse, neglect, and household dysfunction during childhood. *Child Abuse Negl* 2003;27:625–639.

4. Kilpatrick DG, Saunders BE, Smith DW. *Youth victimization: Prevalence and implications.* National Institute of Justice, Research in Brief, 2003. Available at: *http://www.ojp.usdoj.gov/nij.*

5. Coid J, Petruckevitch A, Feder G, et al. Relationship between childhood sexual and physical abuse and risk of revictimisation in women: A cross-sectional survey. *Lancet* 2001;358:450–454.

6. Kogan SM. Disclosing unwanted sexual experiences: results from a national sample of adolescent women. *Child Abuse Negl* 2004;28:147–165.

7. Diaz A, Simantov E, Rickert VI. Effect of abuse on health: results of a national survey. *Arch Pediatr Adolesc Med* 2002;156:811–817.

8. Ackard DM, Neumark-Sztainer D, Hannan PJ, et al. Binge and purge behavior among adolescents: Associations with sexual and physical abuse in a nationally representative sample: The Commonwealth Fund survey. *Child Abuse Negl* 2001;25:771–785.

9. Nelson EC, Heath AC, Madden PA, et al. Association between self-reported sexual abuse and adverse psychosocial outcomes: Results from a twin study. *Arch Gen Psychol* 2002;59:139–145.

10. Raj A, Silverman JG, Amaro H. The relationship between sexual abuse and sexual risk among high school students: Findings from the 1997 Youth Risk Behavior Survey. *Matern Child Health* 2000;4:125–134.

11. Humphrey JA, White JW. Women's vulnerability to sexual assault from adolescence to young adulthood. *J Adolesc Health* 2000;27:419–424.

12. American Medical Association. *Guidelines for Adolescent Preventive Services Manual*, 1997. Available at: *http://www.ama-assn.org/ama/upload/mm/39/gapsmono.pdf.*

13. American Medical Association. *Guidelines for Adolescent Preventive Services, Questionnaires.* Available at: *http://www.amaassn.org/ama/pub/category/2280.html.*

14. Committee on Adolescence, American Academy of Pediatrics. Care of the adolescent sexual assault victim. *Pediatrics* 2001;107:1476–1479.

15. American College of Emergency Physicians. *Evaluation and Management of the Sexually Assaulted or Sexually Abused Patient*, 1999. Available at: *http://www.acep.org/download.cfm? resource=472.*

16. Mears CJ, Heflin AH, Finkel MA, et al. Adolescents' responses to sexual abuse evaluation including the use of video colposcopy. *J Adolesc Health Care* 2003;33:18–24.

17. Sugar NF, Fine DN, Eckert LO. Physical injury after sexual assault: findings of a large case series. *Am J Obstet Gynecol* 2004;190:71–76.

18. Adams JA, Girardin B, Faugno D. Adolescent sexual assault: documentation of acute injuries using photocolposcopy. *J Pediatr Adolesc Gynecol* 2001;14:175–180.

19. Adams JA, Botash AS, Kellogg N. Differences in hymenal morphology between adolescent girls with and without a history of consensual sexual intercourse. *Arch Pediatr Adolesc Gynecol* 2004;158: 280–285.

20. Kellogg ND, Menard SW, Santos A. Genital anatomy in pregnant adolescent girls: "normal" doesn't mean "nothing happened." *Pediatrics* 2004;113:e67–e69. Available at: *http://www.pediatrics.org/cgi/content/full/113/1/e67.*

21. McCauley J, Gorman RL, Guzinski G. Toluidine blue in the detection of perineal lacerations in pediatric and adolescent sexual abuse victims. *Pediatrics* 1986;78:1039–1043.

22. Jones JS, Rossman L, Hartman M, et al. Anogenital injuries in adolescents after consensual sexual intercourse. *Acad Emerg Med* 2003;10:1378–1383.

23. Centers for Disease Control: Sexually Transmitted Diseases Treatment Guidelines. *MMWR* 2002;51: 69–71.

24. Anda RF, Felitti VJ, Chapman DP, et al. Abused boys, battered mothers, and male involvement in teen pregnancy. *Pediatrics* 2001;107:e19.

25. Coxell A, King M, Mezey G, et al. Lifetime prevalence, characteristics, and associated problems of non-consensual sex in men: A cross-sectional survey. *BMJ* 1999;318:846–850.

26. Bartholow BN, Doll LS, Joy D, et al. Emotional, behavioral, and HIV risks associated with sexual abuse among adult homosexual and bisexual men. *Child Abuse Negl* 1994;18:747–761.

27. Doll LS, Joy D, Bartholow BN, et al. Self-reported childhood and adolescent sexual abuse among adult homosexual bisexual men. *Child Abuse Negl* 1992; 16:855–864.

28. Ratner PA, Johnson JL, Shoveller JA, et al. Non-consensual sex experienced by men who have sex with men: Prevalence and association with mental health. *Patient Educ Couns* 2003;49:67–74.

29. Pratt HD, Patel DR, Greydanus DE, et al. Adolescent sexual offenders: Issues for pediatricians. *Int Pediatr* 2001;16:73–80.

30. Foshee VA, Bauman KE, Ennett ST, et al. Assessing the long-term effects of the Safe Dates program and a booster in preventing and reducing adolescent dating violence victimization and perpetration. *Am J Public Health* 2004; 94:619–624.

31. Thomas D, Flaherty E, Binns H. Parent expectations and comfort with discussion of normal childhood sexuality and sexual abuse prevention during office visits. *Ambul Pediatr* 2004; 4:232–236.

32. Muram D, Harrison L, Adams J (eds.). *Sexual Abuse: Medical Evaluation for the Primary Care Physician.* [teaching CD-ROM] North American Society for Pediatric and Adolescent Gynecology, 2002. Available at: *www.NASPAG.org.*

24

SEXUALLY TRANSMITTED DISEASES IN THE ADOLESCENT

Jennifer Johnson

INTRODUCTION

Sexually active adolescents and young adults have the highest incidence of virtually all sexually transmitted diseases (STDs). About one in four sexually experienced adolescents aged 13–19 acquires an STD each year. Young people aged 15–24 were estimated to account for half of the 18.9 million new cases of major STDs in the United States in 2000. The estimated financial burden of these cases was $6.5 billion, with human papillomavirus (HPV) and human immunodeficiency virus (HIV) accounting for 90% of the total.

For a female, contracting an STD at the outset of her reproductive career may have devastating consequences for fertility and for pregnancy outcomes. Of bacterial infections, chlamydia and gonorrhea are by far the most common. Particularly in women, asymptomatic infections are more common than clinical illness. For example, 50%–70% of men and 70%–80% of women infected with *Chlamydia trachomatis*, a major cause of pelvic inflammatory disease (PID), never experience any symptoms. "Silent" PID occurs nonetheless, often leading to tubal scarring and subsequently higher rates of infertility and ectopic pregnancy. Prevalent viral STDs, such as herpes simplex virus (HSV) and HPV, also may be asymptomatic, or manifestations and complications of infection may be serious and/or long-lasting. Prevention, early detection and, when possible, treatment of asymptomatic STDs, are crucial for both personal and public health.

EPIDEMIOLOGY

Risk Factors

Behavioral, biologic, cognitive, psychologic, and social factors all contribute to the high risk for STDs in adolescents. Risk factors are listed in Table 24-1. There has been recent interest in biologic risk factors, which include immunologic naiveté in both sexes. In females, additional biologic risk factors appear to play a role, including cervical ectopy that is common in adolescent and young adult women. Ectopy represents a transitional state during cervical maturation. Endocervical columnar epithelial cells, which are preferentially infected by *Neisseria gonorrhoeae* and *C. trachomatis*, extend

TABLE 24-1

FACTORS ASSOCIATED WITH ADOLESCENT RISK FOR STDS

Category	Risk factors
Biologic susceptibility	Immunologic naiveté
	Cervical ectopy
	Possible decreased cervical mucus immunity (particularly in follicular phase)
	Vaginal douching
Sexual behaviors	<15 years old
	Early age at first intercourse
	Multiple lifetime sexual partners (adolescent or sexual partner)
	New sexual partner
	≥2 sexual partners in previous 6 months
	Males having anogenital, orogenital, or oroanal sex with other males
	Failure to consistently use condoms
Past history	Prior STD; prior unintended pregnancy or paternity
	Sexual molestation, abuse
Characteristics of "high-risk" youth	Use of illicit drugs, especially crack cocaine
	Poor school performance, dropout
	Delinquent behavior, juvenile offender
	Runaway, homelessness
Environmental	High prevalence of STDs in local area
Health knowledge, access to care,	Concerns about confidentiality
help-seeking behaviors	Fear about having an STD
	Not aware of need to screen for asymptomatic infection
	Signs and/or significance of infection not recognized or exaggerated
	Fear of exposure of genitals, pain, embarrassment
	Lack of access to appropriate health care services

onto the ectocervix that is exposed to the vaginal environment, and hence, more susceptible to infection. Also, adolescent girls show a more rapid decrease in cervical mucosal IgG during the follicular phase of the menstrual cycle than do adult women; this may increase the risk of acquiring an STD. The vaginal flora and pH of mature women (vs. girls in early puberty) may be protective against STDs. Douching disturbs the microbiologic environment of the vagina and increases the risk for chlamydial infection and PID.

Sexual Behaviors and STD Transmission

The likelihood of STD transmission varies with organism and sexual behavior. Orogenital sex, common in both heterosexual and homosexual couples, can transmit gonorrhea, *C. trachomatis*, syphilis, chancroid, and HIV. Fellatio (oral contact with a partner's penis; receptive orogenital sex) carries a small risk of HPV and possibly hepatitis C infection by the oral partner. Insertive orogenital contact is an important risk factor for acquisition of HSV-1. Cunnilingus (oral stimulation of the female genitals) predisposes to vulvovaginal candidiasis. Oroanal and orogenital contact is implicated in the transmission of enteric infections, including *Campylobacter jejuni*, *Shigella* sp., *Entamoeba histolytica*, and *Giardia lamblia*. Oroanal transmission can occur with hepatitis A and B. HIV is transmitted primarily through vaginal and anal intercourse. Although the risk is substantially less, HIV transmission also occurs through receptive and insertive oral intercourse and cunnilingus.

Epidemiology of Common Bacterial STDs

The epidemiology of the 3 major bacterial sexually transmitted organisms in adolescents is reviewed here. For other organisms, this is discussed together with the relevant clinical conditions later in this chapter.

Chlamydia and Gonorrhea

Gonorrhea and chlamydia are epidemiologically linked and they are discussed together here. Prevalence of chlamydia generally exceeds 5% in sexually active 15–19-year olds; as with young adults, gonorrhea is now less prevalent. Reported chlamydia prevalence ranges from 2% to 40% for young adults 15–24-years old; gonorrhea prevalence ranges from 0.1% to 12%. A recent large, nationally representative survey of young adults aged 18–26 years found the overall prevalence of chlamydia to be 4.2% (3.7% in men and 4.7% in women) and of gonorrhea, 0.43%, 0.44%, and 0.42%, respectively. Reported rates vary considerably by patient population. CDC data and other sources indicate that in general, the incidence of gonorrhea and chlamydia is higher in females, African Americans, those in southern states, medium to large metropolitan areas, and demographic areas of low socioeconomic status.

Coinfection with both organisms is probably 5% in high-risk 15–19-year olds, but is less common in older adolescents and young adults. Being infected with gonorrhea is associated with a high rate of infection with chlamydia (up to 55% in high-risk adolescent females ≤19 years old). Conversely, in this patient population, 25%–40% of those infected with chlamydia also have had gonorrhea. Importantly for screening and dual ("presumptive") treatment, factors that predict coinfection have not been identified.

The risk of adverse reproductive health complications of chlamydia infection increases significantly with repeated infections, which may occur in 15%–30% of young women within 6 months. During a recent 5-year period, of all women in the state of Washington <20 years old at the time of initial infection, 6% were reinfected by 6 months,

11% by 1 year, and 17% by 2 years after the index infection. In adolescent females diagnosed at a school-based clinic, the median time to a repeat positive test result (among those with repeat visits) was 4.8 months for gonorrhea and 6.3 months for chlamydia.

Syphilis

Primary and secondary syphilis rates in the United States declined by almost 90% from 1990 to 1999. In 2001, syphilis rates in men increased for the first time. It was associated with outbreaks in several urban areas among males having sex with male (MSM), high reported rates of HIV coinfection, and high-risk sexual behavior. In recent years, <500 cases/year of primary and secondary syphilis have been diagnosed in youth <20 years of age, representing about 8% of the United States total. Reported rates for adults 20–39 years old are approximately double those for 15–19-year olds.

The prevalence of syphilis infection varies widely between communities, geographical areas, patient groups ("social networks"), and patient populations. For example, the prevalence of syphilis infection differs by ethnicity (the prevalence of syphilis infection is higher in Hispanic and African American populations than it is in the Caucasian population) and by region (the prevalence of infection is higher in the southern United States and in some metropolitan areas than in the United States as a whole). In addition to those living in high-prevalence areas, MSM, commercial sex workers, and persons who exchange sex for drugs have a higher incidence of syphilis infection. In its 2004 review, the U.S. Preventive Services Task Force (USPSTF) did not find that, in general, individuals diagnosed with other STDs had been shown to be at increased risk for syphilis.

PREVENTION

Primary Prevention

Immunization

Hepatitis B and hepatitis A are the only sexually transmitted diseases for which a vaccine is currently licensed (Chap. 3). Hepatitis B immunization is currently mandated for elementary and/or middle school students in all but five states.[1] Hepatitis A vaccine is recommended for MSM and illegal drug users (both injection and noninjection). Vaccines for HSV and cervical-cancer-associated HPV are in phase III clinical trials. There is hope that eventually a chlamydia vaccine will become available. A number of phase II trials are underway for both preventive and therapeutic HIV vaccines.[2] With any vaccine for STD prevention, cost-effectiveness and acceptance by health care providers, patients, and parents will be particularly important.

Education and Counseling

Most youth in the United States receive some basic education about STDs and HIV/AIDS in schools and/or other venues. Funding restrictions generally prohibit in-school discussion of condom use, and school programs rarely incorporate the decision making and behavioral skills development necessary for them to be effective. All current guidelines recommend that anticipatory guidance for adolescents include STD and pregnancy prevention counseling. Simply helping adolescents feel comfortable disclosing that they are sexually active is important. Providers should ask all adolescents, sexually active or not, about risk behaviors and involve them in a discussion about how to protect themselves from STDs, HIV, and unintended pregnancy. The correct use of condoms should be routinely demonstrated, as many adolescents incorrectly believe that they know how to use them. Even in the best of circumstances, prevention counseling may be of limited effectiveness in increasing adolescent condom use and preventing first or repeat episodes of STDs. (Diagnosis of an STD does appear to be a "sentinel" event for some adolescents, however, in that consistent condom use is more likely afterward.) Providers should give adolescents information about community-based prevention and screening programs (available from local health departments and Planned Parenthood offices).

[1]Immunization Action Coalition: Hepatitis B Prevention Mandates. Available at: *http://www.immunize.org/laws/ hepb.htm.* Accessed 8/2/04.

[2]Department of Health and Human Services: AIDSinfo. Available at: *http://aidsinfo.nih.gov/vaccines/.* Accessed 8/8/04.

Condoms

Consistent use of the male latex condom has been demonstrably effective in preventing transmission of HIV. Recently, a 3-year follow-up study of sexually active women with PID, reported that consistent condom use (about 60% of sexual encounters) at time of diagnosis and persistent use of condoms during the study (vs. no condom use) reduced the risk of recurrent PID, chronic pelvic pain, and infertility by about 50%.

In laboratory studies, the female condom is an effective mechanical barrier to viruses, including HIV. Clinical data are scant. In one recent randomized controlled trial, women attending an STD clinic were given small-group education, and also free supplies of either female or male condoms. They were followed for STDs via medical records. Among women returning for subsequent screening, incidence rates for the first new postintervention STD were similar in both groups. If used consistently and correctly, the female condom may substantially reduce the risk for STDs.

Secondary Prevention: Early Detection and Treatment

Regular, routine screening of all sexually active adolescents, together with partner notification, evaluation, and treatment, are underutilized but are imperative methods for STD/HIV prevention. These are discussed in the following sections.

Screening and Testing

Early detection and treatment of the large proportion of STDs that are asymptomatic decreases the number of symptomatic cases, decreases the rates of severe disease (such as PID), and prevents further STD transmission. Recommendations from major groups regarding screening and testing of adolescents are currently undergoing revision. Health care providers should review the most recent guidelines from national and professional associations.

There is ample evidence that providers and health care organizations have largely not implemented recommendations for screening adolescents for STDs; this is even observed since the year 2000, when annual chlamydia screening of sexually active women between 15 and 25 years of age was added to the National Committee for Quality Assurance Health Plan Employer Data and Information Set (HEDIS) quality measures.

Chlamydia: Screening young women for chlamydia reduces the incidence of PID and is associated with reductions in prevalence of infection in uncontrolled studies. All major guidelines recommend screening sexually active females <25 years of age for chlamydia. The USPSTF in 2001 did not recommend a specific frequency. The overall prevalence of chlamydia in sexually active adolescent females <20 years of age is ≥5%. In recent publications, a number of authors have recommended screening these women more often than the traditional annual screening. Given the frequently short time period until reinfection, retesting of women <25 years old should take place in 4–6 months.

Because no studies were found to determine whether screening asymptomatic men would reduce transmission or prevent acute infections or complications, the USPSTF did not recommend routine screening of asymptomatic males. The feasibility, acceptability, and usefulness of screening of asymptomatic men is under investigation.

The high rates of coinfection previously described indicate that all youth and young adults found to have gonococcal infection should be screened or presumptively treated for chlamydia, as is recommended by the CDC.

Gonorrhea: In 1996, the USPSTF recommended screening of females <25 years old, males and females with two or more sex partners in the prior year, and high-risk groups such as women who have sex in exchange for money. Local epidemiology and patient population determine actual risk for infection. The feasibility, acceptability, and usefulness of screening of asymptomatic men are under investigation.

Syphilis: Syphilis screening is generally recommended for adolescents at highest risk for syphilis: intravenous (IV) drug use, MSM, and sex in exchange for drugs, money, or shelter. According to the 2004 USPSTF recommendation, though persons diagnosed with other STDs may be more likely than others to engage in high-risk behavior, placing them at increased risk for syphilis, there is no evidence that supports the routine screening of individuals diagnosed with other STDs for syphilis infection. It was recommended that health care providers use clinical judgment to individualize screening for syphilis infection based on local prevalence and other risk factors.

Detecting Infection

Chlamydia and gonorrhea: Before current tests for chlamydia and gonorrhea became available, considerable research documented the cost-effectiveness of initial screening of adolescent males with the urine leukocyte esterase dipstick (LE). This is no longer common. However, for adolescent males in juvenile detention facilities, and presumably for other groups of adolescent males with a high prevalence of chlamydia, LE screening appears to decrease the costs associated with diagnosis, treatment, and sequelae of urogenital chlamydial infection.

The newest generation of tests for gonorrhea and chlamydia is based on nucleic acid amplification technology (NAAT), such as ligase chain reaction and PCR. When urine or self-obtained vaginal smears are used as specimens, these tests are more sensitive than culture, specific, and more acceptable to patients than those using traditional endocervical and urethral samples. These tests are widely used in clinical settings; the majority of tests performed in public health laboratories employ DNA probes. They have also been utilized to screen high-risk populations in non-clinical settings such as schools, recreation centers, and shopping malls. The efficacy of such alternative testing strategies in reducing infection rates has not yet been demonstrated. This new technology will potentially make STD testing and prevention counseling more accessible and less dependent on the initiative of individual clinicians.

Syphilis: Screening continues to be based on serology, using the more sensitive but less specific nontreponemal tests, the VDRL (Venereal Diseases Research Laboratory) slide, or the RPR

(Rapid Plasma Reagin) card. False-positive tests, usually <1:8, occur in 1%–2% of the population. Transient false-positives are observed in pregnancy and acute febrile illnesses, and after most immunizations. A false-positive test can last >6 months in chronic intravenous drug users and in persons with autoimmune diseases.

Pelvic examinations: The advent of nucleic acid testing of urine and self-collected vaginal swabs for *C. trachomatis* or *N. gonorrhoeae* has initiated discussion regarding the speculum and bimanual examination of nonpregnant adolescent females, previously a sine qua non for detecting these STDs. Screening for bacterial vaginosis (BV) is not recommended for young women who are not pregnant. Although examination of vaginal fluid for trichomoniasis has traditionally been performed in conjunction with a pelvic exam, the current role of this test in asymptomatic females is unclear, given that use of nucleic acid-based tests for chlamydia and gonorrhea is widespread. NAAT-based tests for trichomonads in vaginal swabs and urine are becoming available. (See further discussion of trichomoniasis later in this chapter).

Discussion about the need for a pelvic examination in conjunction with routine, office-based screening for STDs in adolescents is enlivened by the opinion of a number of experts that a pelvic should not be a prerequisite for initiation of hormonal contraception (see Chap. 27). Randomized controlled trials have yet to be published. Because patients with PID may be asymptomatic but have uterine/adnexal and/or cervical motion tenderness, females with positive tests should be examined when they present for treatment. PID is discussed later in this chapter.

GENERAL PRINCIPLES OF EVALUATION AND MANAGEMENT

Legal and Forensic Aspects

The great majority of states allow minors to give their own consent for STD evaluation and treatment (Chap. 3). Clinicians should be familiar with specific provisions in their state, most easily accessed from the web sites of the Alan Guttmacher Institute (*http://www.agi.org*) and the National Center for Youth Law (*http://www.ncyl.org*). Further discussion about legal aspects of minors' consent, reporting requirements regarding sexual abuse and statutory rape, and applicable provisions of the Health Insurance Privacy and Portability Act (HIPAA) is found in Chaps. 3 and 23. The forensic evaluation for STDs after sexual abuse or forced intercourse has specialized requirements (Chap. 23).

Case Reporting

All states require that certain STDs (at a minimum, chlamydia, gonorrhea, syphilis, and AIDS) be reported by health care providers when they suspect that a case has occurred or they have laboratory confirmation. Providers can use confidential morbidity report systems that allow them to provide basic demographic information to the local or state health department, which routes data without personal identifiers to the Centers for Disease Control and Prevention (CDC). Although most jurisdictions accept a gonorrhea or chlamydia case report from either a clinician or a laboratory, some require that each case be reported from both sources, and reject case reports from a single source. Clinicians should be familiar with local reporting requirements, which can be obtained from local health departments or state STD programs.

Timely reporting is integral to disease control efforts. Local health authorities use data to target at-risk populations for preventive efforts. Depending on circumstances, including the specific infection, information from the health care provider, local patterns of infection, and current resources, trained health representatives may directly contact patients to facilitate treatment, identification, and notification of sex partners who may be infected. Before public health representatives conduct a follow-up of a positive STD-test result, they should consult the patient's health care provider to verify the diagnosis and treatment. Unavailability of the provider to review lab reports, notify patients, and initiate treatment may result in a public health representative contacting an adolescent patient at home before the patient is aware of test results.

General Guidelines

1. The clinician should notify patients immediately of any positive test results while maintaining confidentiality. A visit for education, counseling, and treatment should be scheduled as soon as possible. This decreases the likelihood of transmission but is also recommended on clinical grounds. Because patients with PID may be asymptomatic, females with positive tests should be examined when they present for treatment. When patients are contacted about a positive test, they should be instructed to abstain from sexual contact until after they and their partner(s) have been treated. Additional information can be found later in this chapter.
2. Unless testing for gonorrhea has been performed, all adolescents diagnosed with chlamydia or gonorrhea should be either tested for the other infection or treated for both.
3. Based on patient risk factors and local epidemiology, the provider should consider recommending syphilis screening. HIV testing should be offered whenever an STD is diagnosed.
4. Patients should be educated about their diagnosis, patterns of disease transmission, treatment, and follow-up recommendations. Specific recommendations for some diagnoses are provided later in this chapter. These adolescents should also receive counseling to address the psychologic impact of their diagnosis; this is discussed in the following section.
5. The clinician should facilitate identification, examination, testing, and treatment of all sexual contacts. In general, this applies to contacts within 60 days of symptom development or diagnosis. If the patient had not had sexual contacts in the last 60 days, this applies to the most recent sexual partner. Organism- and disease-specific recommendations are discussed in later sections.
6. When selecting a treatment regimen, health care providers should consider availability, cost, patient acceptance, and antimicrobial susceptibility. Single dose treatment is preferable to multidose treatment to enhance compliance.
7. Medication should be dispensed and/or administered on site whenever possible.

8. If there is a high index of suspicion for infection based on history, examination, or other factors, presumptive treatment should be considered if diagnostic test results may be delayed, testing is not readily available, or follow-up by the patient is questionable.
9. Microbiologic/diagnostic "test of cure" is not generally recommended. Adolescents diagnosed with gonorrhea, chlamydia, and/or PID should be rescreened in 4–6 weeks to 4–6 months as determined by the health care provider.
10. General and disease-specific prevention education and counseling should be provided. Ideally this is done both before and after testing.

Counseling

Individual reactions to an STD diagnosis vary greatly, depending upon STD knowledge, personal factors, characteristics of the relationship with sexual partner(s), and the presence or absence of symptoms. Adolescents may believe that they can "tell" whether a partner has an STD and be surprised when a test is positive. The concept of having been asymptomatically infected by a prior asymptomatic partner, and subsequently infecting a partner who develops symptoms, is difficult for everyone involved to understand. Consequently, "blaming" not infrequently leads to a break-up. Adolescents may also focus on blaming themselves, rather than coping more positively with development of problem-solving skills. Adolescents seeking care for a suspected STD may be relieved that the diagnosis is a different one, but may nonetheless persist in the belief that a sexual partner has done something wrong. Thus, health care providers should assess knowledge level and individual circumstances, beliefs, and concerns when sharing STD test results with patients.

Patient-Delivered Partner Treatment

Sexual partner(s) of females with trichomoniasis are sometimes prescribed or provided with medication without direct contact by a health care provider. Such *patient-delivered partner treatment*, also known as *expedited partner treatment*, has been evaluated in two randomized controlled trials. Risk of reinfection at follow-up in patients with chlamydia (both studies) or gonorrhea (1 study) was lower or no higher than after traditional self-referral (women were asked to refer their sex partners for treatment). Additional data regarding efficacy and safety are needed, and concerns regarding legal issues must be addressed. As of January 2001, California legislation allows medical providers, if necessary, to prescribe or dispense antibiotic therapy for the sex partners of patients infected with genital chlamydia infection. Providers are, however, not protected from liability in the event of adverse outcomes.

KEY ORGANISMS, DISEASES, AND SYNDROMES

The following sections provide information about the most common sexually transmitted organisms, diseases, and syndromes. Information about other infections transmitted through intimate contact and related conditions is also presented.

Gonorrhea

Epidemiology

N. gonorrhoeae may be transmitted at birth as well as by sexual contact. The epidemiology was discussed earlier in this chapter.

Clinical Presentations

Males: *Common*—Asymptomatic in 10%–40% (especially rectal); urethritis (purulent penile discharge, dysuria). *Less common*: Epididymitis (unilateral scrotal pain, groin pain, fever, chills, and tender swelling above a nontender testis); prostatitis (primarily MSM; rectal pain, perineal discomfort, enlarged, and tender prostate).

Females: *Common*—Asymptomatic in 50%–80%. *Less common*—PID; urethritis; Bartholinitis.

Males and females: *Not common*—Pharyngitis (pharyngeal colonization commonly asymptomatic).

Rare—Disseminated gonococcal infection (see below).

Laboratory Diagnosis

Gram stain: Because it is inexpensive, yields immediate results, and is 90% sensitive and 95% specific in symptomatic males, Gram stain of a urethral smear is useful in clinical settings where microscopy is directly available. Gonorrhea is diagnosed if kidney bean shaped, gram-negative diplococci are seen within, or directly adjacent to, polymorphonuclear cells (PMNs). *Neisseria meningitidis* may be difficult to differentiate from *N. gonorrhoeae* on Gram stain. Culture or testing is not necessary given a positive Gram stain but should be performed if the Gram stain is negative or equivocal. Gram stain of cervical discharge is not adequately sensitive or specific.

Culture: Culture, the conventional method for detection of gonorrhea, is inexpensive but requires invasive sampling and stringent specimen transport conditions. The expiration date of the Thayer-Martin media should be checked prior to plating. False-negative cultures from the male urethra (with positive Gram stains) may occur. Sites for culture should be determined based on reported sexual practices and clinical findings or complaints. Colonization of any site may be symptomatic or asymptomatic.

Nucleic acid amplification techniques (NAAT): These are discussed elsewhere in this chapter.

Management

Antimicrobial treatment: Treatment is outlined in Table 24-2.

Additional recommendations: Recommendations for follow-up and management of sex partners are found in Table 24-3.

Complications

Perihepatitis and periappendicitis: Perihepatitis (Fitz-Hugh-Curtis syndrome) and periappendicitis

TABLE 24-2

TREATMENT FOR GONORRHEA

Uncomplicated gonococcal infections of the cervix, urethra, and rectum

Recommended regimens

1. Antigonococcal treatment with one of the following in a single dose:

   a. Ceftriaxone 125 mg intramuscularly or cefixime 400 mg orally (cefixime tablets not available in the United States at time of writing) *or*

   b. Ciprofloxacin 500 mg orally, or ofloxacin 400 mg orally, or levofloxacin 250 mg orally* *plus*

2. If chlamydial infection is not ruled out, azithromycin 1 g orally in a single dose or doxycycline 100 mg orally twice a day for 7 days

Alternatives

1. Antigonococcal treatment with one of the following:

   a. Spectinomycin 2 g in a single, IM dose or

   b. Single-dose cephalosporin regimen other than those above: ceftizoxime (500 mg, IM), or cefoxitin (2 g, administered IM with probenecid 1 g orally), or cefotaxime (500 mg, IM) or

   c. Single-dose quinolone regimen* other than above: gatifloxacin 400 mg orally, or norfloxacin 800 mg orally, or lomefloxacin 400 mg orally *plus*

2. If chlamydial infection is not ruled out, either azithromycin 1 g orally in a single dose or doxycycline 100 mg orally twice a day for 7 days

Uncomplicated gonococcal infections of the pharynx†

Recommended

1. Either ceftriaxone‡ 125 mg IM in a single dose or ciprofloxacin*,‡ 500 mg orally in a single dose plus

2. If chlamydial infection is not ruled out, either azithromycin 1 g orally in a single dose or doxycycline 100 mg orally twice daily for 7 days

*Precautions regarding use of quinolones are: (1) *administration of quinolones to adolescents*: Fluoroquinolones have not been recommended for persons aged <18 years because studies have indicated that they can damage articular cartilage in some young animals. However, no joint damage attributable to quinolone therapy has been observed in children treated with prolonged ciprofloxacin regimens. Thus, the CDC recommends that children who weigh >45 kg be treated with any regimen recommended for adults. (2) *quinolone resistance*: Rates of quinolone-resistant NG strains have recently increased in some populations and in some geographic areas. As of April 30, 2004, the CDC recommends that fluoroquinolones no longer be used to treat proven or suspected gonococcal infections (a) in MSM in the United States or (b) acquired in California, Hawaii, Asia, the Pacific, and other areas, such as England and Wales, with increased QRNG prevalence. If antimicrobial susceptibility testing or tests of cure are available, use in such patients could be considered.

†Gonococcal infections of the pharynx are more difficult to eradicate than infections at urogenital and anorectal sites. Few antimicrobial regimens can reliably cure >90% of infections. Although chlamydial coinfection of the pharynx is unusual, coinfection at genital sites sometimes occurs. Therefore, treatment for both gonorrhea and chlamydia is recommended.

‡Persons who cannot tolerate cephalosporins or quinolones should be treated with spectinomycin. Because spectinomycin is unreliable against pharyngeal infections, patients who have suspected or known pharyngeal infection should have a pharyngeal culture evaluated 3–5 days after treatment to verify eradication of infection.

Source: Sexually Transmitted Disease Treatment Guidelines, 2002.

MEDICATION ADMINISTRATION, ABSTINENCE, FOLLOW-UP, AND PARTNER REFERRAL/TREATMENT BY DISEASE

Diagnosis	Medication Administration / Resumption of Sexual Activity	Partner(s)	Follow-up
Gonorrhea	Patients should abstain from sexual intercourse until therapy is completed and until they and their sex partners no longer have symptoms.	Evaluate and treat partner for NG and CT if last sexual contact with patient was within ≤60 days before patient's onset of symptoms or diagnosis. If patient's last sexual intercourse was >60 days before onset of symptoms or diagnosis, patient's most recent sex partner should be treated.	Patients with uncomplicated anogenital gonorrhea treated with a CDC-recommended regimen need not return for a "test of cure." Patients who have symptoms that persist after treatment should be evaluated by culture for *N. gonorrhoeae*. Any gonococci isolated should be tested for antimicrobial susceptibility.
Chlamydia	Medications should be dispensed on site and the first dose directly observed. Patients should abstain from sexual intercourse for 7 days after single-dose therapy or until completion of a 7-day regimen and until 7 days after partner treatment.	Evaluate and treat partner if last sexual contact with patient was within ≤60 days before patient's onset of symptoms or diagnosis.*	Retest for chlamydia 3–4 months after treatment.
Trichomoniasis	Patients should avoid sex until they and their partners have completed therapy and patient and partner(s) are asymptomatic.	Sex partners should be treated. It has been common practice for providers to prescribe antibiotics for sexual partners without personal contact with them.	Follow-up is unnecessary for men and women who become asymptomatic after treatment or who are initially asymptomatic.
Nongonococcal urethritis	Patients and their sex partners should abstain from sexual intercourse until therapy is completed, as for Chlamydia (above).	Sex partners should be evaluated and treated if their last sexual contact with a symptomatic patient was within 30 days of symptom onset.	Patients should be instructed to return for evaluation if symptoms persist or recur after completion of therapy.

(Continued)

PID	Patients should abstain from coitus until they and their sex partner(s) are asymptomatic and have completed therapy, and for 7 days after partner treatment with single-dose Chlamydia.	Male sex partners should be examined and treated if they had sexual contact with the patient during the 60 days preceding the patient's onset of symptoms. Sex partners should be treated empirically with regimens effective against both NG and CT, regardless of the etiology of PID or pathogens isolated from the infected woman.	If primary therapy is outpatient, follow-up examination within 72 h of initiation. If not improved†: hospitalize, initiate parenteral therapy, evaluate further. Consider rescreening for CT and NG 4–6 weeks after therapy is completed if documented infection.
MPC	Patients and their sex partners should abstain from sexual intercourse until therapy is completed (i.e., 7 days after a single-dose regimen or after completion of a 7-day regimen).	Partners should be notified, examined, and treated for identified or suspected STD. In and of itself, MPC is not a reportable STD.	Follow-up should be conducted as recommended for the infections for which a woman is being treated. If symptoms persist, women should be instructed to return for reevaluation and to abstain from sexual intercourse, even if they have completed the prescribed therapy.
HSV	Please refer to Table 24-8.	If symptomatic: evaluate and treat same as patients with genital lesions. If asymptomatic: ask about history of genital lesions, teach about asymptomatic infection, clinical manifestations, and offer type-specific serologic testing for HSV infection. If infected, counsel as for patients with genital lesions.	

*California state law allows health care providers to treat sex partners of individuals infected with genital *Chlamydia trachomatis*, even if they have not been able to perform an examination of the patient's partner(s). Guidelines available at: *http://www.dhs.ca.gov/ps/dcdc/STD/docs/PDT_GUIDELINES_19.pdf*.

†As indicated by defervescence; reduction in direct or rebound abdominal tenderness; reduction in uterine, adnexal, and cervical motion tenderness.

(serositis not involving the intestinal mucosa) are commonly associated with PID and occur primarily in young women. Intraabdominal spread of gonorrhea or chlamydia can cause inflammation of serosal surfaces. In perihepatitis, the liver capsule and adjacent peritoneum are inflamed in association with PID. PID symptoms may be minimal and may not manifest until after the development of acute, severe right-upper-quadrant pain. Signs and symptoms mimic pleuritis or cholecystitis; perihepatitis is in fact more common than these entities in adolescent and young adult women.

Disseminated gonococcal infection (DGI):
Gonococcal bacteremia occurs in 1%–3% of untreated infections (Chap. 19). Some strains of *N. gonorrhoeae* that cause DGI may cause minimal genital inflammation. The most common sequelae are asymmetric migratory arthralgias followed by characteristic skin lesions that may be accompanied by tenosynovitis and septic arthritis of large joints. Gonococcal arthritis is the most common form of septic arthritis in adolescents (Chap. 11). Occasionally, perihepatitis and rarely, endocarditis or meningitis may occur. Gram stain and culture are most commonly positive on samples from the primary site of infection and large septic joints. Adolescents should initially be hospitalized for intramuscular (IM) or intravenous (IV) treatment. As usual, patients should be tested for concurrent *C. trachomatis* infection and their sex partners referred for evaluation and treatment. Details are provided in the 2002 CDC STD Treatment Guidelines.

Chlamydia

Epidemiology

C. trachomatis is sexually transmitted; neonatal transmission (conjunctivitis, pneumonitis) can also occur. Epidemiology is discussed earlier in this section.

Clinical Presentations

Males: *Common*—Asymptomatic in 25%–50% of males; urethritis with mild dysuria and absent or scant mucoid penile discharge. Urethritis not caused by gonorrhea is most commonly due to chlamydia, for which specific diagnosis was not previously possible; thus the term "nongonococcal" urethritis [NGU] or "postgonococcal" urethritis. Other common causes of NGU are *Ureaplasma urealyticum* (20%–40%) and *Trichomonas vaginalis*. *Less common*—Epididymitis, prostatitis, Reiter syndrome (see Chap. 19).

Females: *Common*—Asymptomatic in >50% of females; endocervical inflammation with postcoital bleeding and/or increased vaginal discharge. *Less common*—PID, periappendicitis, and perihepatitis.

Males and females: *Uncommon*—Proctitis and pharyngitis.

Laboratory Diagnosis

Tissue culture: With the exception of forensic applications, tissue culture has largely been replaced by nonculture techniques in clinical practice. It is expensive and insensitive.

Direct testing methodologies: Tools such as direct fluorescent antibody testing and enzyme immunoabsorbent assays have been largely replaced by the nucleic acid amplification technologies discussed elsewhere in this chapter.

Treatment

Antimicrobial therapy: The treatment currently recommended by the CDC is:

1. Azithromycin 1 g orally in a single dose, *or*
2. Doxycycline 100 mg orally twice a day for 7 days (equally effective).

Although not recommended by the CDC, testing and/or presumptive treatment for gonorrhea should be considered in adolescents and young adults. Results of ongoing studies will provide additional information regarding advisability.

Additional recommendations: Recommendations for follow-up and management of sex partners are found in Table 24-4. Patient-initiated partner therapy is discussed elsewhere.

TABLE 24-4

CLINICAL CRITERIA FOR THE DIAGNOSIS OF ACUTE PELVIC INFLAMMATORY DISEASE

Minimum criteria
Uterine/adnexal tenderness
Cervical motion tenderness
Additional criteria supportive of diagnosis
Oral temperature >101°F (>38.3°C)
Abnormal cervical or vaginal mucopurulent discharge
Presence of white blood cells on saline microscopy of vaginal secretions*
Elevated erythrocyte sedimentation rate
Elevated C-reactive protein
Laboratory documentation of cervical infection with *N. gonorrhoeae* or *C. trachomatis*

*Most women with PID have either mucopurulent cervical discharge or evidence of WBCs on a microscopic evaluation of a saline preparation of vaginal fluid. If cervical discharge appears normal and no white blood cells are found on the wet prep, the diagnosis of PID is unlikely, and alternative causes of pain should be investigated.

Source: Sexually Transmitted Diseases Treatment Guidelines, 2002.

Pelvic Inflammatory Disease (PID)

PID comprises a spectrum of inflammatory disorders of the upper female genital tract. It may include any combination of endometritis, salpingitis, tubo-ovarian abscess, and pelvic peritonitis. PID is a significant cause of infertility, ectopic pregnancy, and chronic pelvic pain. Increasingly, the role of isolated endometritis in asymptomatic PID and its importance with regards to PID sequelae are being investigated.

Etiology

Sexually transmitted organisms, especially *N. gonorrhoeae* and *C. trachomatis*, are implicated in many cases of PID; one or both are isolated from 25% to 75% of young women with PID. However, PID has also been associated with microorganisms that comprise the vaginal flora (e.g., anaerobes, *G. vaginalis, Haemophilus influenzae*, enteric gram-negative rods, and *Streptococcus agalactiae*). Although etiologic roles for viruses or protozoa have been postulated, current evidence does not

support this. While they are commonly present in the lower genital tract of women with PID, the role of genital mycoplasmas is unclear. Anaerobic bacteria, gram-negative facultative bacteria, and streptococci have been isolated from the upper reproductive tract of women who have PID, and data from in vitro studies have revealed that certain anaerobes (e.g., *Bacteroides fragilis*) can cause tubal and epithelial destruction. In addition, bacterial vaginosis (BV) is present in many women who have PID. Precisely what precipitates the development of PID in an individual with a lower reproductive tract STD is not yet well defined.

Epidemiology

It is estimated that 15%–20% of females with *N. gonorrhoeae* and 10% with *C. trachomatis* will develop PID. Risk factors for PID are the same as those for other STDs (Table 24-1). Most PID occurs in women <24 years old; the majority of cases are in girls <19 years of age.

Clinical Presentation, Findings, and Diagnosis

As initially recognized from retroactive analyses of women with infertility, many cases of PID are asymptomatic. Subclinical PID, as defined by the presence of histologic endometritis, may be present in as many as 25% of adolescent and adult women with chlamydia or gonorrhea. Additional episodes of PID go undiagnosed because the patient or the health care provider fails to recognize the implications of mild or nonspecific symptoms or signs (e.g., abnormal bleeding, dyspareunia, and vaginal discharge). Because of the difficulty of diagnosis and the potential for damage to reproductive health, even by apparently mild or atypical PID, health care providers should maintain a low threshold for the diagnosis of PID.

Even in symptomatic PID, diagnosis is imprecise. No single historical, physical, or laboratory finding is both sensitive and specific for the diagnosis of acute PID (i.e., can be used both to detect all cases of PID and to exclude all women without PID), as determined by laparoscopic evidence of salpingitis; laparoscopy does not detect endometritis and may not detect subtle inflammation of the fallopian tubes.

Negative endocervical tests for *N. gonorrhoeae* or *C. trachomatis* do not preclude upper reproductive tract infection with these organisms. Diagnostic criteria for PID recommended by the CDC are listed in Table 24-4.

Management

Antimicrobial treatment: To lessen the chances of long-term consequences and in the absence of some other established cause, empirical treatment should be instituted immediately when minimum criteria are present. Until further data are available, recommended regimens should provide anaerobic coverage. Currently recommended antimicrobial regimens are summarized in Table 24-5.

No currently available data compare the efficacy of parenteral with oral therapy or of inpatient with outpatient treatment settings in adolescents. In adults, a single multicenter study of more than 800 women with mild to moderate PID randomized to either inpatient or outpatient treatment did not find

TABLE 24-5

TREATMENT REGIMENS FOR PELVIC INFLAMMATORY DISEASE

Initial parenteral therapy followed by oral therapy*

Regimen A

1. Cefotetan 2 g intravenously every 12 h or cefoxitin 2 g intravenously every 6 h *plus*
2. Doxycycline 100 mg orally or intravenously every 12 h[†] until 24 h after clinical improvement, *followed by*
3. Oral therapy with doxycycline (100 mg twice a day) to complete 14 days of therapy[‡]

Regimen B

1. Clindamycin 900 mg intravenously every 8 h *plus*
2. Gentamicin loading dose intravenously or intramuscularly (2 mg/kg of body weight) followed by maintenance dose (1.5 mg/kg) every 8 h[§] until 24 h after clinical improvement, *followed by*
3. Doxycycline 100 mg orally twice a day or clindamycin 450 mg orally four times a day to complete a total of 14 days of therapy

Oral treatment only*

Regimen A

1. *Either* of the following orally for 14 days: ofloxacin 400 mg twice a day *or* levofloxacin 500 mg once daily, *with or without*
2. Metronidazole 500 mg orally twice a day for 14 days

Regimen B

1. One of the following intramuscularly in a single dose
   a. Ceftriaxone 250 mg *or*
   b. Cefoxitin 2 g, with probenecid, 1 g orally administered concurrently *or*
   c. Other parenteral third-generation cephalosporin (e.g., ceftizoxime or cefotaxime), *plus*
2. Doxycycline 100 mg orally twice a day for 14 days, *with or without*
3. Metronidazole 500 mg orally twice a day for 14 days[¶]

*Refer to text for discussion of parenteral vs. oral treatment and outpatient vs. inpatient treatment.

†Similar bioavailability; because of pain associated with infusion, doxycycline should be administered orally when possible, even for inpatients.

‡For tubo-ovarian abscess, may use clindamycin or metronidazole with doxycycline for more effective anaerobic coverage.

§Daily dosing acceptable.

¶Clinical trials have demonstrated that a single dose of cefoxitin is effective in obtaining short-term clinical response in women who have PID; however, the theoretical limitations in its coverage of anaerobes may require the addition of metronidazole to the treatment regimen. Metronidazole also will effectively treat BV, which is frequently associated with PID.

Source: Sexually Transmitted Diseases Treatment Guidelines, 2002.

any statistically significant differences between groups in the outcome of time to pregnancy or in the proportion of women with PID recurrence, chronic pelvic pain, or ectopic pregnancy. In the past, many specialists recommended that all adolescents with PID be hospitalized for initial parenteral therapy and to ensure bed rest and compliance. The decision of whether hospitalization is necessary should be based on the discretion of the provider. Recommended criteria for hospitalization include inability to exclude surgical emergencies (e.g., appendicitis), severe illness (i.e., nausea and vomiting, high fever), tubo-ovarian abscess, pregnancy, lack of clinical response to oral antimicrobial therapy, inability to follow or tolerate an outpatient oral regimen, and uncertainty about the patient's returning for follow-up examination within 72 hours.

Both parenteral and oral regimens have demonstrated effectiveness. Transition to oral therapy can usually be initiated within 24 hours of clinical improvement. Most clinicians recommend at least 24 hours of direct inpatient observation for patients who have tubo-ovarian abscesses, after which time home antimicrobial therapy is adequate.

Additional recommendations: Please refer to Table 24-3.

Complications and Sequelae

A palpable adnexal mass, indicating pyo- or hydrosalpinx or tubo-ovarian abscess, is found in 10%–15%. As previously discussed, perihepatitis (Fitz-Hugh-Curtis syndrome) occurs in 15%–30% of cases.

One measure of the sequelae of PID is the risk of postinfection tubal dysfunction (tubal-factor infertility and an ectopic pregnancy as the first one after PID). A single mild episode of PID in a woman <25 years old does not appear to significantly increase her relative risk. However, the relative risk increases to 2.4, 8.5, and 16.2 after moderate or severe single episodes of PID and 2 episodes, respectively. Chronic pain lasting >6 months occurs in about 12% of women after one episode of PID and 30% after two episodes. The risk of severe tubal damage is greater with *C. trachomatis* infection.

Diseases Characterized by Genital Ulcers

In the United States, genital ulcers are caused primarily by HSV. In the current decade, rates for all stages of syphilis have been below 12/100,000, compared with almost 300/100,000 for chlamydia. Rates for the "minor" STDs (chancroid, granuloma inguinale [donovanosis] and lymphogranuloma venereum) have all been below 0.1/100,000. For that reason, the minor STDs are not discussed here.

Patients with genital ulcers are more likely to contract HIV than others, presumably due to easier viral entry through an open lesion. Reciprocally, when patients who already are infected with HIV and immunosuppressed do contract a genital ulcer disease, they have a more protracted course and are more difficult to treat.

Genital Herpes Simplex Virus Infection

Epidemiology: Genital HSV, caused by serotypes 1 and 2, is a recurrent, lifelong infection (Chap. 19). It is transmitted by vaginal, oro- and anogenital contact; autoinoculation is possible. Transmission to neonates at delivery may occur. It is estimated that some 650,000 new infections occur annually in persons 15–24 years old. Most genital herpes infections are transmitted by persons unaware that they have the infection or who are asymptomatic when transmission occurs. Up to 30% of first-episode cases of genital herpes are caused by HSV-1.

Clinical presentations: Typically, multiple painful vesicular or ulcerative lesions, but these are absent in many infected persons. In fact, the clinical diagnosis of genital herpes is both insensitive and nonspecific. Lesions may be located on the external genitalia, internal genitalia (females), urethral meatus, perianal region, and oropharynx. Other symptoms include tender local lymphadenopathy, fever, or malaise, especially with primary infections. Rarely, first-episode genital herpes is manifested by severe disease that may require hospitalization. In fact, most persons with genital herpes have not been diagnosed, having remained asymptomatic or had only mild or unrecognized symptoms.

Recurrent symptomatic episodes occur within 12 months in 90% of persons with HSV-2 and 55%

of those with HSV-1 infection. Repeat episodes tend to be less severe than the initial one. Patients may shed virus and can be infectious even in the absence of lesions. Asymptomatic viral shedding is more frequent in genital HSV-2 infection than genital HSV-1 infection and is most frequent in the first 12 months of acquiring HSV-2.

Laboratory diagnosis: Because differences between HSV serotypes influence prognosis and counseling, any clinical diagnosis of genital herpes should be confirmed by laboratory testing. Both virologic tests and type-specific serologic tests for HSV should be available in clinical settings that provide care for patients with STDs or those at risk for STDs.

Virologic tests: Isolation of HSV in cell culture is the preferred virologic test in patients who present with genital ulcers or other mucocutaneous lesions. The sensitivity of culture declines rapidly as lesions begin to heal, usually within a few days of onset. False-negative HSV cultures are common, especially in patients with recurrent infection or with healing lesions. Some HSV antigen detection tests, unlike culture and the direct fluorescent antibody test, do not distinguish HSV-1 from HSV-2. Tzanck preparations from genital lesions and cervical Papanicolaou (Pap) smears are too insensitive and unspecific to be useful.

Type-specific serologic tests: Both type- and non-specific antibodies to HSV develop during the first several weeks following infection and persist indefinitely. Because almost all HSV-2 infections are sexually acquired, type-specific HSV-2 antibody indicates anogenital infection, but the presence of HSV-1 antibody does not distinguish anogenital from orolabial infection. Guidelines for utilization of HSV-2 serologies for diagnosis and screening are provided in Table 24-6.

Accurate type-specific assays for HSV antibodies must be based on the HSV-specific glycoprotein G2 for the diagnosis of infection with HSV-2 and glycoprotein G1 for diagnosis of infection with HSV-1. These serologic type-specific IgG-based assays should be specifically requested when serology is performed, as older, inaccurate assays are not based on this glycoprotein. An HSV-2

TABLE 24-6

RECOMMENDED USE OF HSV-2 SEROLOGIES FOR DIAGNOSIS AND SCREENING*

Diagnosis of genital lesions/symptoms
Type-specific serology tests should be available for diagnostic purposes in conjunction with virologic tests at any clinical setting where patients are evaluated for STDs.
Serology tests may be helpful in the following settings:
Culture-negative recurrent lesion
History suggestive of herpes/atypical herpes without lesions to culture
Suspected primary herpes or first presentation of genital symptoms, if culture or antigen detection testing is negative or not available and acquisition likely more than 6 weeks prior
Screening
Should be offered to select patients
Patients at-risk for STD/HIV (current STD, recent STD, high-risk behaviors)
Should generally be offered to:
HIV-positive patients
Patients in partnerships or considering partnerships with HSV-2-infected persons

*Herpes education and prevention/transmission counseling is necessary for all persons being tested or screened for HSV-2.
Source: California Sexually Transmitted Diseases Controllers Association, California Department of Health Services: Guidelines for the Use of Herpes Simplex Virus (HSV) Type 2 Serologies. Berkeley, CA: California STD/HIV Prevention Training Center, 2003.

assay that provides results for HSV-2 antibodies from capillary blood or serum during a clinic visit is available. The sensitivities of these tests for detection of HSV-2 antibody vary from 80% to 98%, and false-negative results may occur, especially at early stages of infection. The specificities of these assays are >96%. False-positive results can occur, especially in patients with low likelihood of HSV infection. Therefore, repeat testing or a confirmatory test (e.g., an immunoblot assay if the initial test was an ELISA) may be indicated in some settings.

Management

Systemic antiviral medication: Antiviral drugs partially control the symptoms and signs of herpes episodes when used to treat first and/or recurrent clinical episodes or when used as daily suppressive therapy. Three antiviral medications are of clinical benefit: acyclovir, valacyclovir, and famciclovir. However, they neither eradicate latent virus nor affect the risk, frequency, or severity of recurrences after the drug is discontinued. Topical therapy with antiviral drugs offers minimal clinical benefit and its use is not recommended. Recommended treatment regimens are listed in Table 24-7.

First clinical episode: Many patients with first-episode herpes present with mild clinical manifestations but later develop severe or prolonged symptoms. Therefore, most patients with initial genital herpes should receive antiviral therapy. If begun within 6 days of the onset of lesions, it shortens duration and may reduce severity of systemic symptoms and degree of viral shedding.

Recurrent episodes: Antiviral therapy for recurrent genital herpes can be administered either episodically, to ameliorate or shorten the duration of lesions, or continuously as suppressive therapy to reduce the frequency of recurrences. Many patients, including those with mild or infrequent recurrent outbreaks, benefit from antiviral therapy; therefore, options for treatment should be discussed with all patients.

Effective *episodic* treatment of recurrent herpes requires initiation of therapy within 1 day of lesion

TABLE 24-7
ANTIVIRAL THERAPY FOR GENITAL HERPES

First clinical episode of genital herpes*.†

One of the following taken orally for 7–10 days:

- Acyclovir 400 mg three times a day; or
- Acyclovir 200 mg five times a day; or
- Famciclovir 250 mg three times a day; or
- Valacyclovir 1 g twice a day.

Treatment may be extended if healing is incomplete after 10 days of therapy.

Recurrent episodes of HSV disease

Episodic therapy

For 5 days administration of one of the following oral regimens:

- Acyclovir 400 mg three times a day, or 200 mg five times a day, or 800 mg twice a day; or
- Famciclovir 125 mg twice a day; or
- Valacyclovir 1.0 g once a day or valacyclovir 500 mg twice a day.

Suppressive therapy

One of the following oral regimens:

- Acyclovir 400 mg twice a day; or
- Famciclovir 250 mg twice a day; or
- Valacyclovir 500 mg once a day or valacyclovir 1.0 gram once a day‡

*It is not known whether first episodes of herpes proctitis and/or oral infection require higher doses of acyclovir than those used for genital herpes. Valacyclovir and famciclovir probably are also effective in treating these manifestations.
†IV acyclovir should be administered to those who have severe disease or complications that necessitate hospitalization, such as disseminated infection, pneumonitis, hepatitis, or complications of the central nervous system (e.g., meningitis or encephalitis).
‡Valacyclovir 500 mg once a day might be less effective than other valacyclovir or acyclovir dosing regimens in patients who have >10 episodes per year.

onset, or during the prodrome (regional tingling and irritation) that precedes some outbreaks. The patient should be provided with a supply of drug or a prescription for the medication with instructions to self-initiate treatment immediately when symptoms begin.

Suppressive therapy reduces the frequency of genital herpes recurrences by 70%–80% among patients who have frequent recurrences (i.e., >6 recurrences per year), and many patients report no symptomatic outbreaks. Treatment probably is also effective in patients with less frequent recurrences, though definitive data are lacking. Safety and efficacy have been documented among patients receiving daily therapy with acyclovir for as long as 6 years, and with valacyclovir or famciclovir for 1 year. Quality of life often is improved in patients with frequent recurrences who receive suppressive compared with episodic treatment.

The frequency of recurrent outbreaks diminishes over time in many patients, and the patient's psychologic adjustment to the disease may change. The need for continued suppressive therapy should be reviewed with the patient on an annual basis. Suppressive antiviral therapy reduces but does not eliminate subclinical viral shedding. The extent to which suppressive therapy prevents HSV transmission is unknown.

Additional recommendations

Counseling: Counseling of infected persons and their sex partners is critical to management of genital herpes. The goals of counseling are: (1) to help patients cope with the infection and (2) to prevent sexual and perinatal transmission. Although initial counseling can be provided at the first visit, many patients benefit from learning about the chronic aspects of the infection after the acute illness subsides.

The psychologic impact of HSV infection often is substantial and not necessarily correlated with clinical severity. Common concerns about genital herpes include the severity of initial clinical manifestations, recurrent episodes, sexual relationships and transmission to sex partners, and ability to bear healthy children. The misconception that HSV causes cancer should be dispelled, because the role of HSV-2 in cervical cancer is at most that of a cofactor, not a primary etiologic agent.

Management of sex partners: See Table 24-3.

Syphilis

Epidemiology: The epidemiology of syphilis, which is caused by *Treponema pallidum*, is reviewed earlier. Syphilis can be transmitted by nonsexual contact with open lesions and infected tissues. Infected persons can transmit *T. pallidum*

to others as early as 3 weeks after contracting syphilis and can continue to do so, regardless of symptom status, until treatment is completed.

Clinical presentations

Primary syphilis: Syphilitic chancres are classically nontender, indurated, nonpurulent ulcers. However, that triad was present in only 31% of syphilis patients in a recent study. The presence of induration was 95% specific but only 47% sensitive. Chancres may not be noticed or may be located where they cannot be visualized, particularly in the vagina or anus. The chancre typically appears 3 weeks (range, 10–90 days) after infection, lasts 2–6 weeks if not treated, and then spontaneously resolves.

Secondary syphilis: Symptoms, appearing 6 weeks to 6 months after the primary chancre has cleared, last for 10–14 days and then also resolve without treatment. "The Great Imitator" can cause fever, malaise, diffuse adenopathy, sore throat, headache, rhinitis, arthralgias, hepatosplenomegaly, anogenital condylomata lata, alopecia, and a polymorphic rash.

Later stages: These include early and late latent as well as tertiary stages. If untreated, persons remain infectious through the early latent stage, which ends 1 year after the initial infection.

Laboratory diagnosis

Direct techniques: Direct fluorescent antibody testing (DFA-TP) of smears or direct examination of scrapings or washings from a lesion with dark field microscopy are seldom available and insensitive, though useful in some specific situations (e.g., prior to seroconversion).

Serologic testing: Serologic methods are usually used for both screening and diagnosis. Nontreponemal tests measure antilipoidal antibodies to lipid on the surface of the treponeme; treponemal tests identify antibodies to its cellular components. Nontreponemal tests are used for screening, while treponemal tests are used for confirmation of the diagnosis.

The nontreponemal tests (VDRL and RPR) become reactive approximately 14 days after the appearance of a chancre and are virtually always positive in secondary syphilis. Titers are followed to assess response to therapy; they should decline approximately fourfold 3 months after therapy and eightfold after 6 months. In primary syphilis, nontreponemal tests generally become negative within 1 year of treatment and are negative within 2 years of treatment of secondary syphilis. However, a substantial minority remain positive 3 years after treatment. False-positives are discussed elsewhere.

For treponemal tests, the fluorescent treponemal antibody absorption (FTA-ABS) and the microhemagglutination assay (MHA–TP) are commonly used. In the majority of cases, they remain positive for life.

Differential diagnosis: An extensive list of entities to consider is reviewed by Golden (2003).[3]

Primary syphilis: Among many others, genital herpes, chancroid, lymphogranuloma venereum, and granuloma inguinale should be considered.

Secondary syphilis: The long list includes infectious mononucleosis, infectious hepatitis, fungal infections, "id" eruptions, drug sensitivity reactions, pityriasis rosea, psoriasis, erythema multiforme, condylomata acuminata, and alopecia from any other cause.

Management

Antimicrobial treatment: These recommendations are adapted from 2002 CDC recommendations.

Primary, secondary, or early latent syphilis:[4] The recommended regimen is benzathine penicillin G, 2.4 million units in a single dose, intramuscularly; or, in the case of penicillin allergy: doxycycline, 100 mg by mouth twice daily for 14 days.[5,6]

A 2-g dose of azithromycin may be considered for penicillin-allergic patients, but only with close follow-up; the treatment efficacy of this regimen is not well documented, has been associated with treatment failure, and has not been studied in persons with HIV infection.

Late latent syphilis, tertiary syphilis, neurosyphilis: Management of these forms is discussed in the CDC 2002 STD Treatment Guidelines and in a recent review article.[7]

Additional recommendations: All patients who have syphilis should be tested for HIV infection. In geographic areas in which the prevalence of HIV is high, patients who have primary syphilis should be retested for HIV after 3 months if the first HIV test result was negative.

Serologic tests for syphilis should be repeated 3 and 6 months after treatment for primary and secondary syphilis and at 6 and 12 months for latent disease.

Management of sex partners: Persons exposed sexually to a patient who has syphilis in any stage should be evaluated clinically and serologically according to the following recommendations.

1. Persons who were exposed within the 90 days preceding the diagnosis of primary, secondary, or early latent syphilis in a sex partner might be infected even if seronegative; therefore, such persons should be treated presumptively.

2. Persons who were exposed >90 days before the diagnosis of primary, secondary, or early latent syphilis in a sex partner should be treated presumptively if serologic test results are not available immediately and the opportunity for follow-up is uncertain.

3. For purposes of partner notification and presumptive treatment of exposed sex partners

---

[3]Golden MR, Marra CM, Holmes KK: Update on syphilis: Resurgence of an old problem. *JAMA* 290:1510, 2003.
[4]Latent syphilis is defined as seroreactivity without other evidence of disease. Early latent syphilis is diagnosed in patients infected within the preceding year as defined by 1 of the following: (1) a documented seroconversion; (2) unequivocal symptoms of primary or secondary syphilis; or (3) a sex partner documented to have primary, secondary, or early latent syphilis.

[5]Pregnant women should not be treated with doxycycline.
[6]Patients with non-life-threatening allergies to penicillin should ideally be desensitized.
[7]Golden MR, Marra CM, Holmes KK: Update on syphilis: Resurgence of an old problem. *JAMA* 290:1510, 2003.

only, patients with syphilis of unknown duration who have high nontreponemal serologic test titers (i.e., >1:32) can be assumed to have early syphilis.

4. Long-term sex partners of patients who have latent syphilis should be evaluated clinically and serologically for syphilis and treated on the basis of the evaluation findings.

5. For identification of at-risk partners, the time periods before treatment are (a) 3 months plus duration of symptoms for primary syphilis, (b) 6 months plus duration of symptoms for secondary syphilis, and (c) 1 year for early latent syphilis.

6. Sexual partners should have a physical examination and serologic testing if exposure was within 90 days prior to identification of the index case if in the primary or secondary stage; 1 year if in the latent stage. Even if seronegative, contacts still may be in an incubating phase and should be treated empirically.

Diseases Characterized by Vaginal Discharge

Trichomoniasis

Epidemiology: *T. vaginalis* is primarily sexually transmitted, rarely by fomites. It occurs frequently in adolescents and is not uncommonly associated with gonorrhea or chlamydia in females.

Clinical presentations

Males: Usually asymptomatic. May cause nongonococcal urethritis (NGU), see prior discussion under Chlamydia.

Females: Asymptomatic in 25%–50% of cases. Typically presents with frothy, yellow-green, foul-smelling vaginal discharge. On examination, the cervix may be erythematous, rarely with microhemorrhages, which give the "strawberry cervix" its name. Occasionally causes urethritis.

Laboratory diagnosis: Motile trichomonads (see Fig. 24-1) and numerous white blood cells are found on normal saline wet mount of vaginal

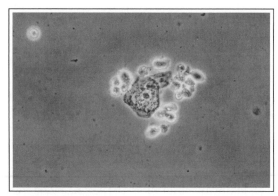

FIGURE 24-1

TRICHOMONADS.
This phase contrast wet mount micrograph of a vaginal discharge reveals the presence of *T. vaginalis* protozoa.
Source: Centers for Disease Control and Prevention, Public Health Image Library, image ID 5238.
http://phil.cdc.gov/phil/search.asp, accessed 7/16/04.

secretions or spun sediment of urine (male and female). Culture is rarely necessary in clinical practice. Trichomonads also are sometimes seen on Pap smears and routine urinalyses. A PCR test is available but not widely used.

Management

Antimicrobial treatment: Metronidazole (Flagyl) is the only drug readily available in the United States and approved by the FDA for treatment of trichomoniasis. Recommended regimen is 2 g orally as a single dose or, alternatively, 500 mg twice daily for 7 days. Metronidazole gel is not recommended. Although approved for treatment of bacterial vaginosis, it is ≤50% effective for treatment of trichomoniasis. If treatment failure occurs with either regimen, the patient should be re-treated with metronidazole 500 mg taken orally twice daily for 7 days. If treatment failure occurs again, the patient should be treated with a single, 2-g dose of metronidazole once a day for 3–5 days. Nausea and vomiting are common side effects of metronidazole, and it should be taken with food. Alcohol ingestion exacerbates these side effects and should be avoided until 24 hours after completion of treatment.

Management of sex partners: Sex partners should be treated. Some providers use patient-initiated partner therapy (prescription for partner given to patient or "double dose" prescription written for patient). Patients should be instructed to avoid sexual intercourse until they and their sex partners are cured (i.e., when therapy has been completed and patient and partner(s) are asymptomatic [in the absence of a microbiologic test of cure]).

Vulvovaginal Candidiasis (VVC)

Epidemiology: About 10%–20% of women of childbearing age have vaginal colonization with yeast, mostly *Candida albicans* strains, but sometimes *Torulopsis glabrata* or other *Candida* sp. Sexual behavior does not play a role in the pathogenesis of vulvovaginal candidiasis, though frequent orogenital sex increases colonization rates.

Lifetime incidence of VVC is about 75%; almost half of women have two or more episodes. Colonization and the rate of symptomatic vaginitis are hormonally dependent, so that rates are much lower in premenarchal girls and symptoms typically develop premenstrually. Antibiotic use predisposes to development of vaginitis in some colonized females.

Clinical presentations

Males: Occasionally candida causes urethritis or balanitis.

Females: Vulvar pruritus is the most frequent symptom and is commonly accompanied by increased vaginal discharge, dysuria, and dyspareunia. Clinical signs and symptoms of vulvovaginal candidiasis are relatively nonspecific, so that the diagnosis should not be made on history and clinical findings alone.

The white discharge may be thin and/or homogeneous, though it is classically described as thick and lumpy. In contrast to BV and trichomoniasis, the discharge is not malodorous and vaginal pH is normal (<4.5). Physical examination reveals the vulva and vagina to be erythematous; perineal excoriations or dermatitis may be present.

VVC is classified as uncomplicated or complicated based on the presence of one of several factors:

- Severity (mild-to-moderate vs. severe [extensive vulvar erythema, edema, excoriation, and fissure formation]), *or*
- Frequency (sporadic or infrequent vs. recurrent [≥4 episodes/year]), *or*
- Causative organisms (likely *C. albicans* vs. nonalbicans candidiasis), or
- Host factors (nonimmunocompromised vs. compromised host [pregnancy or uncontrolled diabetes, debilitation, or immunosuppression])

Approximately 10%–20% of women will have complicated VVC; its prevalence in adolescent females is unknown. Risk factors for recurrence include a history of bacterial vaginosis, use of panty liners or pantyhose, and consumption of cranberry juice or acidophil-containing products.

Laboratory diagnosis: VVC can be diagnosed in young women with typical signs and symptoms by demonstration of yeasts or pseudohyphae in either a wet preparation (saline, 10% potassium hydroxide) or Gram stain (Fig. 24-2). Yeast and mycelia are more easily visualized on a potassium hydroxide wet preparation, which has a sensitivity of about 75% in

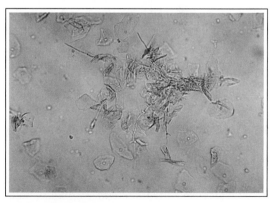

F I G U R E   2 4 - 2

CANDIDA ALBICANS.
This photomicrograph of a vaginal smear identifies *Candida albicans* while using a wet mount technique.
Source: Centers for Disease Control and Prevention, Public Health Image Library, image ID 2035.
http://phil.cdc.gov/phil/search.asp, accessed 7/15/04.

women with typical symptoms. If the potassium hydroxide preparation is negative, fungal culture may confirm the presence of yeast. Because yeast colonization may be asymptomatic, and because symptoms are relatively nonspecific, it is important to confirm the absence of clue cells, excess PMNs, and trichomonads. Candida vaginitis is associated with a normal vaginal pH (<4.5). In addition to trichomoniasis, any other STD can occur concomitantly with VVC.

Management: Treatment regimens are listed in Table 24-8. Topical therapy is preferred for uncomplicated VVC because of the low rate of side effects. A single dose or a 1- to 3-day course of an azole drug is more effective than nystatin and provides an 80%–90% rate of clinical and microbiological cure. Treatment with a single fluconazole 150 mg oral tablet is also effective. Women with vulvitis due to VVC may respond best to a combination of intravaginal and topical vulval therapy (available as a combination package).

A number of topical products are available over-the-counter (OTC) (see Table 24-8). Unnecessary or inappropriate use of OTC preparations is common and can lead to delay of treatment of other etiologies of vulvovaginitis that could result in adverse clinical outcomes. Self-medication with OTC preparations should be advised only for those who have been diagnosed previously with VVC and who have a recurrence of the same symptoms. If symptoms persist after using an OTC preparation or if symptoms recur within 2 months, the patient should seek medical care.

Bacterial Vaginosis (BV)

Etiology: BV is a clinical syndrome resulting from replacement of the normal H_2O_2-producing *Lactobacillus* sp. in the vagina with high concentrations of anaerobic bacteria (e.g., *Prevotella* and *Mobiluncus* sp.), *Gardnerella vaginalis*, and *Mycoplasma hominis*. The cause of the microbial alteration is not fully understood.

Epidemiology: BV is the most prevalent cause of vaginal discharge or malodor. BV is associated with having multiple sex partners, douching, and lack of

TABLE 24-8

TREATMENT OF VULVOVAGINAL CANDIDIASIS (VVC)*

Intravaginal agents	
Butoconazole	• 2% cream 5 g intravaginally for 3 days[†]
	• 2% cream 5 g (butoconazole sustained release), single vaginal application
Clotrimazole	• 1% cream 5 g intravaginally for 7–14 days[†]
	• 100 mg vaginal tablet for 7 days
	• 100 mg vaginal tablet, 2 tablets for 3 days
	• 500 mg vaginal tablet, 1 tablet in a single application
Miconazole	• 2% cream 5 g intravaginally for 7 days[†]
	• 100 mg vaginal suppository, 1 suppository for 7 days[†]
	• 200 mg vaginal suppository, 1 suppository for 3 days[†]
Nystatin[‡]	• 100,000-unit vaginal tablet, 1 tablet for 14 days
Tioconazole	• 6.5% ointment 5 g intravaginally in a single application[†]
Terconazole	• 0.4% cream 5 g intravaginally for 7 days
	• 0.8% cream 5 g intravaginally for 3 days or
	• 80 mg vaginal suppository, one suppository for 3 days
Oral agent	
Fluconazole	• 150 mg oral tablet, 1 tablet in a single dose

*Only one method of administration, one medication, one vehicle, and one dose should be used.
[†]Available without prescription.
[‡]Not as effective as other regimens.
Source: Sexually Transmitted Disease Treatment Guidelines, 2002.

vaginal lactobacilli; it is unclear whether BV results from acquisition of a sexually transmitted pathogen. Women who have never been sexually active are rarely affected. Treatment of the male sex partner has not been beneficial in preventing the recurrence of BV.

Clinical presentations: Up to 50% of women with BV may not report symptoms of BV. It is characterized by a thin white vaginal discharge. Dysuria and vulvar discomfort are not typical.

Laboratory diagnosis: The presence of *G. vaginalis* in a vaginal culture is not diagnostic; it is prevalent in adolescents who are not sexually active and in women who do not have BV. BV can be diagnosed by the use of clinical or Gram stain criteria. Clinical criteria require three of the following symptoms or signs:

1. Homogeneous, white, noninflammatory discharge that smoothly coats the vaginal walls
2. Clue cells on microscopic examination (see Fig. 24-3)
3. Vaginal fluid pH >4.5
4. Fishy odor of vaginal discharge before or after addition of 10% potassium hydroxide (i.e., the whiff test)

A Gram stain can be used to diagnose BV by determining the relative concentration of the bacterial morphotypes characteristic of the altered flora.

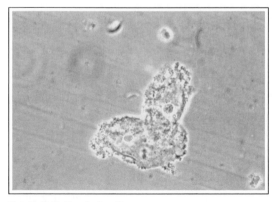

FIGURE 24-3

CLUE CELLS.
This photomicrograph reveals bacteria adhering to vaginal epithelial cells known as "clue cells." Clue cells are epithelial cells that have had bacteria adhere to their surface, obscuring their borders, and imparting a stippled appearance. The presence of many such clue cells is a sign that the patient has bacterial vaginosis.
Source: Centers for Disease Control and Prevention, Public Health Image Library, image ID 3720.
http://phil.cdc.gov/phil/search.asp, accessed 7/15/04.

Culture of *G. vaginalis* is not specific, and Pap tests are insensitive. A DNA probe based test for high concentrations of *G. vaginalis* may have clinical utility. Other commercially available tests that may be useful for the diagnosis of BV include a card test for the detection of elevated pH and trimethylamine and proline aminopeptidase.

Management: The established benefits of therapy for BV in nonpregnant women are to (a) relieve vaginal symptoms and signs of infection and (b) reduce the risk for infectious complications after hysterectomy. Other potential benefits include the reduction of other infectious complications (e.g., HIV and other STDs). All women who are symptomatic should be treated. The bacterial florae that characterize BV have been recovered from the endometria and salpinges of women who have PID.

Antimicrobial treatment: CDC-recommended regimens include metronidazole taken orally (500 mg twice a day for 7 days) or metronidazole gel 0.75%, one full applicator (5 g) intravaginally once a day for 5 days, and clindamycin cream 2%, one full applicator (5 g) intravaginally at bedtime for 7 days. The recommended metronidazole regimens are equally efficacious. The vaginal clindamycin cream appears less efficacious than the metronidazole regimens. Patients should be advised to avoid consuming alcohol during treatment with metronidazole and for 24 hours thereafter. Clindamycin cream and ovules are oil-based and might weaken latex condoms and diaphragms.

Alternative regimens with lower efficacy for BV are: metronidazole 2 g orally in a single dose (less effective than a 7-day course), or clindamycin 300 mg orally twice a day for 7 days, or clindamycin ovules 100 g intravaginally once at bedtime for 3 days. Although FDA has approved metronidazole 750-mg extended release tablets once daily for 7 days, no data have been published on the clinical equivalency of this regimen with other regimens.

Studies are currently underway to evaluate the efficacy of vaginal lactobacilli suppositories in addition to oral metronidazole for the treatment of BV.

No data support the use of nonvaginal lactobacilli or douching for the treatment of BV.

Follow-up: Follow-up visits are unnecessary if symptoms resolve. Because recurrence of BV is not unusual, women should be advised to return for additional therapy if symptoms recur. Another recommended treatment regimen may be used to treat recurrent disease. No long-term maintenance regimen with any therapeutic agent is recommended.

Management of sex partners: Response to therapy and likelihood of relapse or recurrence are not affected by treatment of sex partner(s). Therefore, routine treatment of sex partners is not recommended.

Human Papillomavirus Infection

Genital Warts

Epidemiology: HPV is transmitted sexually, by autoinoculation, and at delivery to neonates, which may result in laryngeal papillomatosis. More than 30 types of HPV can infect the genital tract. Persons who have visible genital warts can be infected simultaneously with multiple HPV types. Visible genital warts usually are caused by HPV types 6 or 11. HPV types 16, 18, 31, 33, and 35 are found occasionally in visible genital warts and have been associated with external genital (i.e., vulvar, penile, and anal) squamous intraepithelial neoplasia as well as internal genital (i.e., vaginal, anal, and cervical) intraepithelial dysplasia and squamous cell carcinoma. These HPV types have been strongly associated with cervical neoplasia. In addition to the genital area, HPV types 6 and 11 have been associated with conjunctival, nasal, oral, and laryngeal warts.

Clinical presentations: Most HPV infections are asymptomatic, unrecognized, or subclinical (Chap. 19). When present, genital warts are firm, gray to pink, and fimbriated. They may be single or multiple, varying in size from several millimeters to several centimeters. Most patients have <10 genital warts. Depending on the size and anatomic location, genital warts can be painful, friable, and pruritic, though they are commonly asymptomatic.

In addition to the external genitalia (i.e., the penis, vulva, scrotum, perineum, and perianal skin), genital warts can occur on the uterine cervix and in the vagina, urethra, anus, and mouth; these warts are sometimes symptomatic. Intraanal warts are seen predominantly in patients who have had receptive anal intercourse; these warts are distinct from perianal warts, which can occur in men and women who do not have a history of anal sex.

Laboratory diagnosis: Laboratory diagnosis is rarely needed.

Biopsy: Biopsy is needed only under certain circumstances (e.g., if the diagnosis is uncertain; the lesions do not respond to standard therapy; the disease worsens during therapy; the patient is immunocompromised; or warts are pigmented, indurated, fixed, and/or ulcerated).

Nucleic acid tests: No data support the use of type-specific HPV nucleic acid tests in the routine diagnosis or management of visible genital warts.

Differential diagnosis: This includes condyloma lata (secondary syphilis), molluscum contagiosum, micropapillomatosis labialis of labia minora, and pearly penile papules.

Treatment

Therapies: The primary goal of treating visible genital warts is the removal of symptomatic warts. If left untreated, visible genital warts may resolve spontaneously, remain unchanged, or increase in size or number. Currently available therapies for genital warts may reduce, but probably do not eradicate, infectivity. No evidence indicates that either the presence of genital warts or their treatment is associated with the development of cervical cancer.

Treatment of genital warts should be guided by patient preference, available resources, and the experience of the health care provider. No definitive evidence suggests that any of the available treatments is superior to the others, and no single treatment is ideal for all patients or all warts. Because of uncertainty regarding the effect of treatment on future transmission and the possibility for spontaneous resolution, some patients may reasonably choose to forego treatment and await spontaneous resolution.

Most patients have <10 genital warts, with a total wart area of 0.5–1.0 cm², which respond to most treatment modalities. Many patients require a course of therapy rather than a single treatment. In general, warts located on moist surfaces and/or in intertriginous areas respond better to topical treatment than do warts on drier surfaces.

External genital warts: Both patient-applied therapies and provider-administered therapies are available; recommended treatment regimens are summarized elsewhere (Chap. 19). The risk-benefit ratio of treatment should be evaluated throughout the course of therapy to avoid overtreatment. Complications rarely occur if treatments are employed properly.

Warts in other locations: For women who have exophytic cervical warts, high-grade squamous intraepithelial lesions (SIL) must be excluded before treatment is initiated. Management of exophytic cervical warts, vaginal, urethral meatus, anal, and rectal warts is discussed in the *Sexually Transmitted Diseases Treatment Guidelines, 2002.*

Additional recommendations

Education and counseling: Education and counseling are important aspects of managing patients with genital warts. Key messages for patients are summarized below.

1. Genital HPV infection is a viral infection that is common among sexually active adolescents and young adults.
2. Infection is almost always sexually transmitted, but the incubation period is variable and it is often difficult to determine the source of infection. Sex partners usually are infected by the time of the patient's diagnosis, though they may have no symptoms or signs of infection.
3. The natural history of genital warts is generally benign. The HPV types that usually cause external genital warts are not associated with cancer. Recurrence of genital warts within the first several months after treatment is common and usually indicates recurrence rather than reinfection.
4. The likelihood of transmission to future partners and the duration of infectivity after treatment are unknown. The use of latex condoms has been associated with a lower rate of cervical cancer, an HPV-associated disease.
5. Because genital HPV is common among persons who have been sexually active and because the duration of infectivity is unknown, the value of disclosing a past diagnosis of genital HPV infection to future partners is unclear. Candid discussions about other STDs should be encouraged and attempted whenever possible.

Follow-up: A follow-up evaluation 3 months after warts have cleared may be helpful in detecting recurrences, which occur most frequently during this time period; it also helps in providing an additional opportunity for patient education and counseling. Pap screening should be scheduled as recommended for women without genital warts.

Management of sex partners: Examination of sex partners is not necessary for the management of genital warts because no data indicate that reinfection plays a role in recurrences. Sex partners of patients who have genital warts may benefit from examination to assess the presence of genital warts and other STDs.

Human Immunodeficiency Virus/Acquired Immunodeficiency Syndrome (HIV/AIDS)

Epidemiology

Virtually all HIV infections in the United States are caused by HIV-1, while HIV-2 is prevalent in West Africa. HIV is transmitted sexually, in breast milk, and through needle sharing. Half of all new HIV infections in the United States occur among persons <25 years old; most are acquired through sexual contact. African Americans and Hispanic adolescents have been disproportionately affected by the HIV/AIDS epidemic. In the United States in 2001, 15% of the adolescent population was African American, yet 61% of reported AIDS cases in 13–19-year olds were in African Americans. Hispanics accounted for 15% of the population, yet 21% of reported AIDS cases in adolescents were in Hispanics. These patterns will probably continue because recent reports of HIV infection from states that report HIV infection also show that young racial/ethnic minority persons are disproportionately affected by HIV.

In earlier years, most cases of AIDS in adolescents and young adults were in men. However, as heterosexual contact has accounted for an increasing proportion of HIV infections, particularly in women, the proportion of cases reported in women has increased. The ratio of men to women with AIDS varies by age at diagnosis. Of 372 adolescents aged 13–19 years at AIDS diagnosis in 2001, 48% were women; of 1,461 persons 20–24 years of age, 41% were women. In contrast, the majority of reported AIDS cases that year in those ≥25 years were men (75%).

Data from HIV infection case surveillance present a more complete view of the HIV/AIDS epidemic in the United States than data from AIDS surveillance alone. In 2001, 37 areas (including Guam, the Virgin Islands, and some Pacific Islands) conducted name-based confidential HIV infection surveillance of adults and adolescents. Similar to the ratio seen with AIDS, the ratio of male to female adolescents and young adults with HIV diagnosed increases with age at diagnosis. In 2001, women accounted for 56% of the adolescents aged 13–19 years who were reported with HIV, compared with 40% of young adults aged 20–24 years and 30% of persons aged 25 and older. Heterosexual transmission and injection drug use are the primary risk categories for new HIV infections in young women, whereas MSM and injection drug use are most common among men. AIDS cases attributed to injection drug use are less common in adolescent than in young adult women.

Published data report exposure categories for all AIDS cases in adolescents and young adults who have been diagnosed since the beginning of the epidemic; similar analyses are not available for recently reported cases of HIV.

Clinical Presentations

Acute retroviral syndrome is characterized by fever, malaise, lymphadenopathy, and skin rash. This syndrome frequently occurs in the first few weeks after HIV infection, before antibody test results become positive. Suspicion of acute retroviral syndrome should prompt nucleic acid testing (HIV plasma RNA [i.e., viral load]) to detect the presence of HIV. As this test is not approved for diagnostic purposes, a positive test should be confirmed by another HIV test. Current guidelines suggest that persons with recently acquired HIV infection might benefit from antiretroviral drugs, and such patients may be candidates for clinical trials. Therefore, patients with acute HIV infection should be referred immediately to an HIV clinical care provider.

Laboratory Diagnosis

HIV antibody testing: HIV infection usually is diagnosed by tests for antibodies against HIV-1 and HIV-2 (HIV-1/2). Antibody testing begins with a sensitive screening test such as enzyme immunoassay (EIA). Reactive screening tests must be confirmed by supplemental test (e.g., the Western blot [WB]) or an immunofluorescence assay (IFA). If confirmed by a supplemental test, a positive antibody test result indicates that a person is infected with HIV and is capable of transmitting the virus to others. HIV antibody is detectable in at least 95% of patients within 3 months after infection. Rarely does seroconversion not occur until ≥12 months after infection. Although a negative antibody test result usually indicates that a person is not infected, antibody tests cannot exclude recent infection.

HIV-2 testing should be performed when clinical evidence of HIV exists but tests for antibodies to HIV-1 are not positive, or when HIV-1 Western blot results include a certain unusual indeterminate pattern. HIV-2 is endemic in West Africa, and persons have sex partners from this area or who are known to be infected with HIV-2 should be tested for HIV-2. This is also the case for individuals who received a blood transfusion or a nonsterile injection in a West African country.

Point-of-care rapid tests for HIV antibodies in oral fluid or a capillary blood sample are highly sensitive and specific. They have been approved as a waived test under Clinical Laboratory Improvement Amendments (CLIA) regulations. Reactive rapid HIV tests must be confirmed with either WB or immunofluorescent assay IFA, even if a subsequent EIA test is negative. If such confirmatory testing yields negative or indeterminate results, follow-up testing should be performed on a blood specimen collected 4 weeks after the initial reactive rapid HIV test result.

Plasma HIV RNA: Plasma HIV RNA testing can be used to diagnose HIV infection in patients with a syndrome consistent with acute HIV infection when HIV antibody tests are negative or indeterminate. A diagnosis made by HIV RNA testing should be confirmed by standard methods (e.g., Western blot serology performed 2–4 months after the initial indeterminate or negative test).

Treatment

HIV-infected adolescents should be referred to HIV/AIDS specialists immediately upon diagnosis, preferably to those with expertise in treating adolescents. Most state and local health departments provide clinical services for HIV-infected persons. Therapeutic advances and treatment protocols for HIV infection evolve too rapidly for textbooks to remain current. The most recently updated recommendations from the CDC and the National Institute of Health are available online (*http://www.cdc.gov/hiv/dhap.htm* and *http://aidsinfo.nih.gov/guidelines*, respectively) and from state and local health departments.

Antiretroviral therapy is recommended for asymptomatic patients with <200 CD4+ T cells/mL. As of April 2005, the Department of Health and Human Services expert panel recommends that treatment be offered to asymptomatic patients with CD4+ T cell counts of 201–350 cells/mL. Some HIV/AIDS experts also consider treatment for asymptomatic patients with CD4+ T cell counts of

>350 cells/mL and plasma HIV RNA >100,000 copies/mL. Preferred initial treatment regimens use combinations of antiretroviral agents in the same class. Combination treatment based on non-nucleoside reverse transcriptase inhibitors (NNRTI) includes efavirenz, lamivudine or emtricitabine, and zidovudine or tenofovir DF. Alternatively, a regimen based on protease inhibitors uses lopinavir and ritonavir in a co-formulation, lamivudine or emtricitabine, and zidovudine. For asymptomatic patients with CD4+ T cell counts of <200 cells/mL, randomized clinical trials indicate that such protocols improve survival and reduce disease progression. Antiviral therapy has rendered HIV/AIDS to a chronic condition rather than an invariably fatal infection/disease.

Testing Adolescents

All sexually active teenagers should be offered HIV testing and those at high and highest risk (see Table 24-1) should be encouraged to obtain it. All youths also should be counseled about how to reduce the risk of AIDS through safe sex practices or abstinence. The frequency of testing should be determined by a young person's own particular vulnerability factors, but testing should be offered as often as the risk of positivity remains, no matter how many times the young person has been screened before. Testing always should be confidential and performed only after (1) the adolescent has given his or her informed consent, (2) pretest counseling has been given, and (3) posttest counseling has been arranged. The following guidelines outline the contents of counseling at each point. All counseling sessions should be conducted with the adolescent in person and in confidence in a comfortable setting.

Pretest counseling

1. Discussion of the medical, psychologic, and social implications of HIV testing.
2. Evaluation of the adolescent's coping skills and external support system.
3. Explain confidentiality protections.

4. Review meaning of informed consent; assess adolescent's ability to give same; if deemed competent, obtain adolescent's written consent for testing.
5. Plan for immediate testing of high-risk individuals.

Posttest counseling for negative results

1. Careful explanation of negative results.
2. Further counseling on ways to reduce risk and importance of doing so. Advise adolescent that he or she is still vulnerable despite the negative test. (Negative results may reinforce teenagers' tendencies to perceive themselves as immune from risk.)
3. Include a plan by which a support person can assist the adolescent in modifying high-risk behaviors and following risk-reduction principles.

Posttest counseling for positive results: (May take several visits to accomplish all objectives)

1. Careful and sensitive explanation of meaning of positive results; optimistic discussion about new therapeutic modalities delaying the onset of AIDS and offering considerable promise for rendering AIDS a chronic rather than fatal disease.
2. Establish plans for involvement of parents or some other supportive adult.
3. Review conflicting issues regarding confidentiality rights and partner notification; assist youth in making decision about what to do (encourage partner notification).
4. Discuss follow-up issues, for example, where to go from here and what to do.
5. Discuss essential need for use of condoms if adolescent decides to continue sexual activity.
6. Develop a plan for ongoing social and emotional support, ongoing primary care, and HIV subspecialty care.
7. Arrange for immediate referral to skilled HIV services if not available on-site.
8. Plan to see adolescent in several days to review the previous issues again. There is a great deal to be accomplished, and young people who

may be in a state of shock are not able to grasp all the implications or make all the necessary plans without some time to adjust.

OTHER SEXUALLY TRANSMITTED ORGANISMS, RELATED CONDITIONS, AND OTHER GENITAL CONCERNS

A number of other conditions are either sexually transmitted or transmitted by some other means but commonly seen in the genital area. They are mentioned here to complete the spectrum of genital infections.

Enteric Organisms

Campylobacter jejuni, Shigella sp., *Entamoeba histolytica*, and *Giardia lamblia* all may be transmitted by oroanal or orogenital contact. They may cause proctitis and/or enterocolitis and present primarily men who have sex with men (MSM). Some individuals infected with enteric organisms remain asymptomatic. Diagnosis is confirmed by stool culture and examination for parasites or ova.

Epstein-Barr Virus

The Epstein-Barr virus, which causes infectious mononucleosis, can be transmitted to a sexual partner through intimate contact with oral or genital secretions (Chap. 20).

Hepatitis

Hepatitis A and B are both transmitted sexually (see Table 26-1). New hepatitis B infections continue to be a problem, despite recommendations for universal immunization in children. Hepatitis C may probably also be transmitted through sexual contact, though not all reports are in agreement (Chap. 10).

Hemolytic Streptococci

Group A streptococci may be transmitted by autoinoculation or sexual contact from a pharyngeal site (Chap. 7) and may cause vaginitis on rare occasions in prepubertal girls. When organisms are cultured from the vagina, treatment with penicillin, 250 mg orally for 10 days, is indicated whether patient is symptomatic or not. Group B and other types of streptococci usually constitute normal vaginal flora but may be involved in PID and postpartum infections. When group B streptococcus is present during pregnancy, treatment with penicillin and continuous monitoring of mother and newborn are indicated.

Pinworms

Pinworms may invade the vagina and cause itching, particularly at night. Diagnosis is by stool examination or an early morning and cellophane tape test. Treatment is with pyrvinium pamoate (Povan) or mebendazole.

Pediculosis pubis

Either the eggs ("nits") or active adult forms of *Pthirus pubis* are evident on examination of pubic hair with a hand lens (Chap. 19). They also may be found on perineal and axillary hair or eyelashes. Extensive excoriations also may be present due to intense pruritus. Treatment of sexual partners should not be overlooked.

Scabies

This presents as an intensely pruritic, papular rash caused by burrowing and egg laying of the mite *Sarcoptes scabiei*. Common sites of involvement include intertriginous areas, external genitalia, buttocks, belt line, breasts, and between digits. Involved areas commonly exhibit extensive excoriations and, sometimes, secondary infection due to scratching (see Chap. 19).

Tinea cruris

This common superficial fungal infection is most often seen in male athletes. The fungi from tinea cruris, or "athlete's foot," may be carried to the groin by autoinoculation or on underwear. Also colloquially

known as "jock itch," this condition manifests as a flat, contiguous, erythematous, pruritic rash involving the scrotum and adjacent thighs and groin (Chap. 19).

Molluscum contagiosum

Asymptomatic white- to pearly-colored, umbilicated papules measuring 2–3 mm in diameter may be seen. There may be only a single lesion but occurs much more commonly in crops variably scattered over the body. They may be located on pubic region and external genitals, as well as other sites (Chap. 19).

Physiologic Leukorrhea

Physiologic leukorrhea due to estrogen stimulation begins well before menarche and persists for years. It is not uncommonly a source of concern to adolescent girls. It also is apt to increase with the use of estrogen dominant oral contraceptives. The discharge varies from clear to white in color, mucoid to watery in consistency, and scant to moderate in amount, usually without causing any irritation or odor. Variations in character often parallel the menstrual cycle. Teenagers may also complain of yellowish staining of their underwear, which can be prevented by pretreating laundry with an enzyme-based bleach.

Contact Dermatitis

Dermatitis of the external genitals, urethra, vagina, or anus may result from exposure and/or sensitization to spermicides, sexual lubricants, latex condoms or diaphragms, or other agents such as scented or deodorant soaps, bubble bath and bath salts, "feminine hygiene" sprays or suppositories, douches, dyes in underclothing, patterned toilet tissue, or saliva. Treatment is by identifying and eliminating the source or recommending a less allergenic alternative. Topical compresses (Burow's solution), sitz baths, or mild topical steroids may be used for symptomatic relief (Chap. 19).

Foreign Bodies

A forgotten, retained tampon or other foreign body in the vagina may produce an extremely malodorous vaginal discharge. Treatment is by removing the foreign material, which generally requires its visualization.

Bibliography

Alter MJ: Epidemiology and prevention of hepatitis B. *Semin Liver Dis* 23:39, 2003.

Alter MJ: Prevention of spread of hepatitis C. *Hepatology* 36:S93, 2002.

Alter MJ: Protecting future generations through immunization against hepatitis B. *Ann Intern Med* 135: 835, 2001.

Anderson MR, Klink K, Cohrssen A: Evaluation of vaginal complaints. *JAMA* 291:1368, 2004.

Bauer HM, Chartier M, Kessell E, et al.: Chlamydia screening of youth and young adults in non-clinical settings throughout California. *Sex Transm Dis* 31: 409, 2004.

Berg AO: Screening for chlamydial infection. Recommendations and rationale. *Am J Prev Med* 20:90, 2001.

Bolu OO, Lindsey C, Kamb ML, et al.: Is HIV/sexually transmitted disease prevention counseling effective among vulnerable populations? A subset analysis of data collected for a randomized, controlled trial evaluating counseling efficacy (Project Respect). *Sex Transm Dis* 31:469, 2004.

Branson B: Point-of-care testing for rapid HIV antibodies. *J Lab Med* 27:288, 2003.

Braverman PK, Rosenfeld WD, (eds.): Sexually transmitted diseases. *Adolesc Med Clinics* 15:201–428, 2004.

Celentano D: It's all in the measurement: Consistent condom use is effective in preventing sexually transmitted infections. *Sex Transm Dis* 31:161, 2004.

Centers for Disease Control and Prevention, National Center for HIV, STD and TB Prevention, Divisions [sic] of HIV/AIDS Prevention: Rapid HIV testing. *http://www.cdc.gov/hiv/rapid_testing/*. Accessed 8/10/04.

Centers for Disease Control and Prevention: Heterosexual transmission of HIV–29 states, 1999–2002. *JAMA* 291:1317, 2004.

Centers for Disease Control and Prevention: HIV transmission among black college student and non-student men who have sex with men—North Carolina, 2003. *MMWR* 53:731, 2004.

Centers for Disease Control and Prevention: Incidence of acute hepatitis B—United States, 1990–2002. *MMWR* 52:1252, 2004.

Centers for Disease Control and Prevention: Primary and secondary syphilis—United States, 2002. *MMWR* 52: 1117, 2003.

Centers for Disease Control and Prevention: Revised guidelines for HIV counseling, testing, and referral and revised recommendations for HIV screening of pregnant women. *MMWR* 50:1, 2001.

Centers for Disease Control and Prevention: Sexually transmitted diseases treatment guidelines 2002. *MMWR* 51(RR-6):1, 2002.

Chesson HW, Blandford JM, Gift TL, et al.: The estimated direct medical cost of sexually transmitted diseases among American youth, 2000. *Perspect Sex Reprod Health* 36:11, 2004.

Cohen J, Powderly W (eds.): *Infectious Diseases.* 2d ed. Edinburgh, Scotland: Mosby, 2004.

Crosby RA, Diclemente RJ, Wingood GM, et al.: Associations between sexually transmitted disease diagnosis and subsequent sexual risk and sexually transmitted disease incidence among adolescents. *Sex Transm Dis* 31:205, 2004.

Crosby RA, Diclemente RJ, Wingood GM, et al.: Value of consistent condom use: A study of sexually transmitted disease prevention among African American adolescent females. *Am J Public Health* 93:901, 2003.

Department of Health and Human Services (DHHS), Panel on Clinical Practices for Treatment of HIV Infection: Guidelines for the use of antiretroviral agents in HIV-1-infected adults and adolescents. Electronic publication, *http://aidsinfo.nih.gov/guidelines/adult/ AA_040705.pdf*, April 7, 2005. Accessed 4/27/05.

Diclemente RJ, Wingood GM, Sionean CP, et al.: Association of adolescents' history of sexually transmitted disease (STD) and their current high-risk behavior and STD status: A case for intensifying clinic-based prevention efforts. *Sex Transm Dis* 29: 503, 2002.

Eng TR, Butler WT (eds.): *The hidden epidemic: Confronting sexually transmitted diseases.* Washington, DC: Institute of Medicine, 1997.

Fortenberry JD: Clinic-based service programs for increasing responsible sexual behavior. *J Sex Res* 39: 63, 2002.

French PP, Latka M, Gollub EL, et al.: Use-effectiveness of the female versus male condom in preventing sexually transmitted disease in women. *Sex Transm Dis* 30:433, 2003.

Futterman DC: HIV and AIDS in adolescents. *Adolesc Med Clin* 15:369, 2004.

Garnett GP, Dubin G, Slaoui M, et al.: The potential epidemiological impact of a genital herpes vaccine for women. *Sex Transm Infect* 80:24, 2004.

Gershon AA, Hotez PJ, Katz SL (eds.): *Krugman's Infectious Diseases of Children,* 11th ed. Philadelphia, PA: Mosby, 2004.

Golden MR, Marra CM, Holmes KK: Update on syphilis: Resurgence of an old problem. *JAMA* 290:1510, 2003.

Golden MR, Whittington WLH, Handsfield HH, et al.: Effect of expedited treatment of sex partners on recurrent or persistent gonorrhea or chlamydial infection. *N Engl J Med* 352:676, 2005.

Gross M: HIV topical microbicides: Steer the ship or run aground. *Am J Public Health* 94:1085, 2004.

Haggerty CL, Ness RB, Amortegui A, et al.: Endometritis does not predict reproductive morbidity after pelvic inflammatory disease. *Am J Obstet Gynecol* 188: 141, 2003.

Holmes KK, Sparling PF, Mardh PA, et al. (eds.): *Sexually Transmitted Diseases,* 3d ed. New York: McGraw-Hill, 1999.

Holzman C, Leventhal JM, Qiu H, et al.: Factors linked to bacterial vaginosis in nonpregnant women. *Am J Public Health* 91:1664, 2001.

Johnson RE, Newhall WJ, Papp JR, et al.: Screening tests to detect *Chlamydia trachomatis* and *Neisseria gonorrhoeae* infections–2002. *MMWR Recomm Rep* 51: 1, 2002.

Kahn JA, Bernstein DI: Human papillomavirus vaccines. *Pediatr Infect Dis J* 22:443, 2003.

Kahn JA, Hillard PA: Human papillomavirus and cervical cytology in adolescents. *Adolesc Med Clin* 15:301, 2004.

Ledger WJ, Monif GR: A growing concern: Inability to diagnose vulvovaginal infections correctly. *Obstet Gynecol* 103:782, 2004.

Leone P, Fleming DT, Gilsenan AW, et al.: Seroprevalence of herpes simplex virus-2 in suburban primary care offices in the United States. *Sex Transm Dis* 31:311, 2004.

Lum PJ, Ochoa KC, Hahn JA, et al.: Hepatitis B virus immunization among young injection drug users in San Francisco, Calif.: The UFO study. *Am J Public Health* 93:919, 2003.

Miller WC, Ford CA, Morris M, et al.: Prevalence of chlamydial and gonococcal infections among young adults in the United States. *JAMA* 291:2229, 2004.

Mitchell H: Vaginal discharge–causes, diagnosis, and treatment. *BMJ* 328:1306, 2004.

Morse SA, Ballard RC, Holmes KK (eds.): *Atlas of Sexually Transmitted Diseases and AIDS,* 3d ed. Edinburgh, Scotland: Mosby, 2003.

Moscicki AB, Ellenberg JH, Farhat S, et al.: Persistence of human papillomavirus infection in HIV-infected and -uninfected adolescent girls: Risk factors and differences, by phylogenetic type. *J Infect Dis* 190:37, 2004.

Moscicki AB: Human papillomavirus, Papanicolaou smears and the college female. *Pediatr Clin North Am* 52:163–177, 2005.

Ness RB, Randall H, Richter HE, et al.: Condom use and the risk of recurrent pelvic inflammatory disease, chronic pelvic pain, or infertility following an episode of pelvic inflammatory disease. *Am J Public Health* 94:1327, 2004.

Ness RB, Soper DE, Holley RL, et al.: Effectiveness of inpatient and outpatient treatment strategies for women with pelvic inflammatory disease: Results from the pelvic inflammatory disease evaluation and clinical health (PEACH) randomized trial. *Am J Obstet Gynecol* 186:929, 2002.

Nsuami M, Cammarata C, Brooks BN, et al.: Chlamydia and gonorrhea co-occurrence in a high school population. *Sex Transm Dis* 31:424, 2004.

Page-Shafer KA, Cahoon-Young B, Klausner JD, et al.: Hepatitis C virus infection in young, low-income women: The role of sexually transmitted infection as a potential cofactor for HCV infection. *Am J Public Health* 92:670, 2002.

Patel D, Gillespie B, Sobel J, et al.: Risk factors for recurrent vulvovaginal candidiasis in women receiving maintenance antifungal therapy: Results of a prospective cohort study. *Am J Obstet Gynecol* 190:644, 2004.

Peipert JF: Genital chlamydial infections. *N Engl J Med* 349:2424, 2003.

Quint EH, Bacon J: HPV in teenagers. *J Pediatr Adolesc Gynecol* 16:147, 2003.

Rimsza ME: Sexually transmitted infections: New guidelines for an old problem on the college campus. Pediatric Clin N Am 2005;52:217–228.

Rosen T: Update on genital lesions. *JAMA* 290:1001, 2003.

Rylander E, Berglund A-L, Krassny C, et al.: Vulvovaginal candida in a young sexually active population: Prevalence and association with oro-genital sex and frequent pain at intercourse. *Sex Transm Infect* 80: 54, 2004.

Schillinger JA, Kissinger P, Calvet H, et al.: Patient-delivered partner treatment with azithromycin to prevent repeated chlamydia trachomatis infection among women: A randomized, controlled trial. *Sex Transm Dis* 30:49, 2003.

Schwebke JR, Desmond RA, Oh MK: Predictors of bacterial vaginosis in adolescent women who douche. *Sex Transm Dis* 31:433, 2004.

Serlin M, Shafer M-A, Tebb K, et al.: What sexually transmitted disease screening method does the adolescent prefer? Adolescents' attitudes toward first-void urine, self-collected vaginal swab, and pelvic examination. *Arch Pediatr Adolesc Med* 156:588, 2002.

Shain RN, Piper JM, Holden AE, et al.: Prevention of gonorrhea and chlamydia through behavioral intervention: Results of a two-year controlled randomized trial in minority women. *Sex Transm Dis* 31:401, 2004.

Shlay JC, Mcclung MW, Patnaik JL, et al.: Comparison of sexually transmitted disease prevalence by reported level of condom use among patients attending an urban sexually transmitted disease clinic. *Sex Transm Dis* 31:154, 2004.

Shrier L: Sexually transmitted diseases in adolescents: Biologic, cognitive, psychologic, behavioral, and social issues. *Adolesc Med Clin* 15:215, 2004.

Spigarelli MG, Biro FM: Sexually transmitted disease testing: Evaluation of diagnostic tests and methods. *Adolesc Med Clin* 15:287, 2004.

Steinbrook R: The AIDS epidemic in 2004. *N Engl J Med* 2004;351:115–120.

Swygard H, Sena AC, Hobbs MM, et al.: Trichomoniasis: Clinical manifestations, diagnosis and management. *Sex Transm Infect* 80:91, 2004.

U.S. Preventive Services Task Force: *Screening for syphilis infection: Recommendation statement.* Rockville, MD: Agency for Healthcare Research and Quality (AHRQ), 2004.

Weinstock H, Berman S, Cates W Jr: Sexually transmitted diseases among American youth: Incidence and prevalence estimates, 2000. *Perspect Sex Reprod Health* 36:6, 2004.

25

CONTRACEPTION IN THE ADOLESCENT

Mary Ellen Rimsza

INTRODUCTION

Sexually active adolescents are at high risk of unintended pregnancy if they fail to use effective contraception. Despite the widespread availability of contraception, approximately 35% of teens do not use contraception at the time of first intercourse. The most effective contraceptive methods are hormonal contraceptives, though the use of barrier methods should also be encouraged to prevent sexually transmitted infections (STIs). This chapter discusses the commonly used contraceptive methods including oral contraceptive pills (OCPs), transdermal patches, vaginal contraceptive ring, emergency contraceptives, condoms, spermicides, vaginal barrier methods, and intrauterine devices (IUDs).

CONTRACEPTIVE EFFICACY

A sexually active adolescent has an 85% chance of becoming pregnant within 1 year if no method of contraception is used. Using a highly efficacious contraceptive method (e.g., OCPs) can reduce this pregnancy risk to 0.1%. Even contraceptive methods that are traditionally thought to be less effective such as male condoms can reduce the risk of

pregnancy to 2% per year if used consistently and correctly (Table 25-1). Pregnancy rates are influenced by frequency of intercourse, age, and user compliance with the method. For the adolescent, the most important influence is compliance (correct and consistent use of the method). Younger women can be expected to have higher contraceptive failure rates with typical use than older women. For example, among adolescents the typical failure rate for OCPs has been estimated to be as high as 15% in the first year of use whereas the typical failure rate among women of all ages is only 3%. Since fertility declines with age, older women also are less likely to become pregnant if they fail to use their contraceptive properly. For these reasons, it is especially important to provide the adolescent with counseling and appropriate information on the proper use of the method.

In general, methods that protect the adolescent from pregnancy for a long time (e.g., injectable hormonal contraceptives) tend to be associated with a lower pregnancy rate with typical use because there is less likelihood of user error. Contraceptive efficacy can also be improved by the simultaneous use of two contraceptive methods (e.g., combined OCPs and condoms) since the failure of one of the two methods (e.g., broken condom) will be mitigated

CONTRACEPTIVE EFFICACY DURING FIRST YEAR OF USE

Method	Pregnancy/100 Woman-Years
No contraception (chance)	85
Combined oral contraceptive pill	0.1–3
Contraceptive patch	0.4–1.3
Contraceptive ring	0.65–2
Progestin-only pill	0.5–3
Medroxyprogesterone	0.3
Diaphragm	6–20
Male condom	2–14
Female condom	5–21
Vaginal spermicides	6–26
Vaginal sponge	6–28
Cervical cap	9–40
Intrauterine device	0.1–2

by the second method. It is especially important that two methods of contraception be used when adolescents are taking teratogenic medications (e.g., isotretinoin) or are at risk for serious medical complications if they become pregnant. For adolescent women who are taking isotretinoin it is recommended that they use a hormonal method of contraception and an additional method. It is also recommended that they have a negative pregnancy test before starting the drug, begin taking the drug on the third day of a normal menses, and have the prescription refilled monthly only after a negative monthly pregnancy test.

Combined Oral Contraceptive Pills

OCPs are the method of contraception used by 44% of adolescents 15–19 years old. OCPs consist of a synthetic estrogen and progestin. They prevent pregnancy by inhibiting gonadotropin-releasing hormone and thus ovulation. Other secondary mechanisms of contraception include thickening of the cervical mucus, endometrial atrophy, and changes in tubal transport. If used correctly, less than 1% of women taking OCPs will become pregnant per year of use. However, the typical failure rate is approximately 3% in adults and 5%–15% in adolescents. The estrogen component of combined OCPs usually is ethinyl estradiol in dosages ranging from 20 to 50 µg/day. Mestranol is another synthetic estrogen that is rarely used today. The progestin component of OCPs is more variable; currently available progestins in the United States include ethynodiol diacetate, norethindrone acetate, norethindrone, norgestrel, levonorgestrel, desogestrel, norgestimate, and drospirenone. Norethindrone and those progestins that metabolize to norethindrone (i.e., norethindrone acetate, ethynodiol diacetate) are classified as estranes. Levonorgestrel, norgestrel, norgestimate, and desogestrel are classified as gonanes. Drospirenone is a new synthetic progestin chemically related to spironolactone. OCPs containing drospirenone (e.g., Yasmin) have an antimineralocorticoid effect, which can cause potassium retention. Because of this, OCPs containing drospirenone should not be prescribed for women taking spironolactone or who are at risk for hyperkalemia due to underlying disease (e.g., renal failure). Comparison studies of women taking OCPs containing either drospirenone or levonorgestrel showed no difference between the groups in weight gain and the effect on acne appears to be similar to that of other OCPs.

Most currently available OCPs consist of 21 days of hormonal pills followed by 7 days of placebo per 28-day cycle (Tables 25-2 and 25-3). Two OCPs (Mircette and Kariva) have 21 days of combined estrogen and progesterone (20 µg ethinyl estradiol and 0.15 µg desogestrel) followed by 5 days of a lower dose of estrogen (10 µg ethinyl estradiol) and only 2 days of placebo. This type of pill may be beneficial for women who are estrogen deficient and have estrogen deficiency symptoms (e.g., hot flashes, vaginal dryness) when taking placebos.

EXTENDED CYCLING OF OCPS

For some adolescents, extending the length of the menstrual cycle by prescribing hormonally active pills containing both estrogen and progestin for more than 21 days may be beneficial. Extended

MONOPHASIC ORAL CONTRACEPTIVE AVAILABLE IN THE UNITED STATES: 2004

Estrogen	Progestin	Product Name
50 μg mestranol	1 mg norethindrone	Necon 1/50 Norinyl 1 + 50 Ortho-Novum 1/50
50 μg ethinyl estradiol 50 μg ethinyl estradiol	1 mg norethindrone 1 mg ethynodiol diacetate	Ovcon-50 Demulen 1/50 Zovia 1/50E
50 μg ethinyl estradiol	0.5 mg norgestrel	Ovral-28 Ogestrel 0.5/50
35 μg ethinyl estradiol	1 mg norethindrone	Ortho-Novum 1/35 Necon 1/35 Nortrel 1/35 Norinyl 1 + 35
35 μg ethinyl estradiol	0.5 mg norethindrone	Brevicon Modicon Necon 0.5/35 Nortrel 0.5/35
35 μg ethinyl estradiol	0.4 mg norethindrone	Ovcon-35
35 μg ethinyl estradiol	0.25 mg norgestimate	Ortho-Cyclen Mononessa Sprintec
35 μg ethinyl estradiol	1 mg ethynodiol diacetate	Demulen 1/35 Zovia 1/35E
30 μg ethinyl estradiol	1.5 mg norethindrone acetate	Loestrin Fe 1.5/30 Microgestin Fe 1.5 Junel Fe 1.5/30
30 μg ethinyl estradiol	0.3 mg norgestrel	Lo/Ovral Low-Ogestrel Cryselle
30 μg ethinyl estradiol	0.15 mg desogestrel	Desogen Ortho-Cept Apri
30 μg ethinyl estradiol	0.15 mg levonorgestrel	Nordette Levlen Levora 0.15/30 Portia Seasonale
30 μg ethinyl estradiol	3 mg drospirenone	Yasmin 3/0.03
20 μg ethinyl estradiol	1 mg norethindrone acetate	Loestrin Fe 1/20 Loestrin 1/20 Microgestin Fe 1/20 Junel 1/20
20 μg ethinyl estradiol	0.1 mg levonorgestrel	Alesse Levlite Aviane Lessina

TABLE 25-3

MULTIPHASIC ORAL CONTRACEPTIVES AVAILABLE IN THE UNITED STATES: 2004

Product	Phase 1	Phase 2	Phase 3
Tri-Norinyl	0.5 mg norethindrone, 35 µg ethinyl estradiol	1 mg norethindrone, 35 µg ethinyl estradiol	0.5 mg norethindrone, 35 µg ethinyl estradiol
Ortho-Novum 7/7/7 Necon 7/7/7	0.5 mg norethindrone, 35 µg ethinyl estradiol	0.75 mg norethindrone, 35 µg ethinyl estradiol	1 mg norethindrone, 35 µg ethinyl estradiol
Tri-Levlen TriPhasil Enpresse	0.05 mg levonorgestrel, 30 µg ethinyl estradiol	0.075 mg levonorgestrel, 40 µg ethinyl estradiol	0.125 mg levonorgestrel, 30 µg ethinyl estradiol
Trivora	0.05 mg levonorgestrel, 30 µg ethinyl estradiol	0.075 mg levonorgestrel, 40 µg ethinyl estradiol	0.125 mg levonorgestrel, 30 µg ethinyl estradiol
Ortho Tri-Cyclen Tri-Sprintec Trinessa	0.18 mg norgestimate, 35 µg ethinyl estradiol	0.215 mg norgestimate, 35 µg ethinyl estradiol	0.25 mg norgestimate, 35 µg ethinyl estradiol
Estrostep Fe Estrostep 21	1 mg norethindrone acetate, 20 µg ethinyl estradiol	1 mg norethindrone acetate, 30 µg ethinyl estradiol	1 mg norethindrone acetate, 35 µg ethinyl estradiol
Cyclessa	0.1 mg desogestrel, 25 µg ethinyl estradiol	0.125 mg desogestrel, 25 µg ethinyl estradiol	0.15 mg desogestrel, 25 µg ethinyl estradiol
Ortho Tricyclen Lo	0.18 mg norgestimate, 25 µg ethinyl estradiol	0.25 mg norgestimate, 25 µg ethinyl estradiol	0.25 mg norgestimate, 25 µg ethinyl estradiol

cycling involves prescribing hormonally active pills continuously for two to four 21-day cycles (6–12 weeks of hormonally active OCPs) followed by a 7-day hormone-free interval. Gynecologic indications for extended cycling in adolescents include dysmenorrhea, endometriosis, premenstrual syndrome, and dysfunctional uterine bleeding (DUB). Adolescents who have chronic medical conditions that are exacerbated by menses such as bleeding disorders (e.g., factor IX deficiency, von Willebrand's disease), catamenial epilepsy, and rheumatoid arthritis also may benefit from extended cycling. Even for the healthy adolescent, extended cycling may be desirable to accommodate their lifestyle (e.g., athletes, dancers). Extended cycling can be accomplished by prescribing 21-day OCPs continuously. One approach is to initially prescribe 42 days of continuous pills. If breakthrough bleeding (BTB) does not occur, the duration of the cycle can be extended by an additional 21 days each consecutive cycle up to a maximum of 12 weeks.

An OCP that is monophasic and contains 20–35 µg of ethinyl estradiol and a progestin with a long half-life (e.g., norgestimate, levonorgestrel) should be used for extended cycling. Alternatively, a new OCP specifically designed for extended cycling (Seasonale) can be prescribed. This OCP contains 84 days of hormonally active pills and 7 days of placebo pills.

Benefits of OCP Use

In addition to preventing pregnancy, there are many noncontraceptive benefits of OCP use (Table 25-4). Discussing these noncontraceptive benefits with the adolescent may help improve compliance, especially if the teen feels they are at low risk for pregnancy. Most teens are "serially monogamous" and may decide to stop using OCPs when they end a sexual relationship. If they are aware of the noncontraceptive benefits of OCPs, they may be more likely to continue them and thus be protected when

TABLE 25-4

BENEFITS OF ORAL CONTRACEPTIVE PILLS

Gynecologic Benefits	Nongynecologic Benefits
Less dysmenorrhea	Less acne
Less menorrhagia	Less iron deficiency anemia
Less premenstrual syndrome	Less rheumatoid arthritis
Less ectopic pregnancy	Less duodenal ulcer
Less dysfunctional uterine bleeding	Increased bone density
Less ovarian cancer	
Less uterine cancer	
Less pelvic inflammatory disease	
Less fibrocystic breast disease	
Less ovarian cysts	

they begin a new sexual relationship. For the adolescent, some of the most important noncontraceptive benefits to discuss with them are lighter and more predictable menses, decreased dysmenorrhea, and improvement in acne.

DUB is common in adolescent girls and usually is caused by anovulatory cycles. OCPs can be used to regulate the menstrual cycle and decrease menses-associated blood loss by decreasing endometrial proliferation. OCPs decrease bleeding days and amount of blood loss. Women who are taking OCPs have 45% lower incidence of iron deficiency anemia compared with women who are not taking OCPs and 48% reduction in menorrhagia. Approximately 60%–90% of adolescents experience dysmenorrhea. OCPs decrease menstrual pain by decreasing the production of prostaglandin F_2 alpha by the endometrium. OCPs are effective in reducing dysmenorrhea in 90% of patients who have primary dysmenorrhea but it may take 3 months of use before maximum benefit is obtained.

Acne vulgaris is the result of obstruction of sebaceous follicles by excessive amounts of sebum. Because sebaceous glands are androgen-dependent, estrogen and antiandrogens suppress sebum production. Estrogen also raises the levels of sex hormone binding globulin, which decreases the levels of biologically active free testosterone. In theory, OCPs containing higher doses of ethinyl estradiol and nonandrogenic progestins (e.g., norgestimate, desogestrel, drospirenone) are more likely to be effective than other OCPs. Randomized double-blind controlled studies have demonstrated improvement in acne in patients who were prescribed a multiphasic norgestimate/ethinyl estradiol OCP (OrthoTriCyclen) for 6 months. OCPs may be as effective as benzoyl peroxide, retinoic acid, and antibiotics (topical or systemic) in controlling acne.

Multiple studies have shown that OCPs reduce the risk of ovarian cancer. While the exact biologic effect leading to reduced risk of ovarian cancer is not known, it is likely related to the suppression of ovulation and lowering of gonadotropin secretion. Women who used OCPs for as little as 3–6 months experienced a 40% reduction in risk of ovarian cancer and those who used OCPs long-term (>10 years) experienced an 80% reduction. This risk reduction persists after stopping OCPs.

The risk of endometrial cancer also is reduced with OCP use. Protection against endometrial cancer increases with duration of use from 56% at 4 years to 72% at 12 or more years of use. This reduction in risk may be due to the suppression of endometrial mitotic activity by OCPs.

OCPs improve bone mineral density (BMD) in young women who are hypoestrogenic due to anorexia nervosa, exercise-induced amenorrhea, gonadal dysgenesis, or premature ovarian failure. The average woman acquires 98% of her bone mass by age 20. After peak bone mass is attained, natural aging reduces bone mass by approximately 1% per year until menopause. Even use of OCPs is associated with 25% reduction in hip fractures for women over age 50 years.

Another benefit of OCPs is the prevention of pelvic inflammatory disease (PID). The progestins in OCPs thicken cervical mucus, which resists penetration by bacteria. The use of OCPs for at least 12 consecutive months is associated with a 60% reduction in hospitalization for PID.

PRESCRIBING PRINCIPLES

Most adolescents can safely take any OCP containing 35 μg or less of ethinyl estradiol. There have been several studies suggesting that desogestrel-containing OCPs increase the risk of venous thromboembolism (VTE). Since this is one of the few serious complications of OCP use, some experts recommend that desogestrel be avoided. A 20 μg OCP may be desirable if there is a history of vascular headaches or past history of nausea while on OCPs. Newly released gonanes (e.g., norgestimate) and drospirenone have less androgenic effects than many other progestins, and are preferred if the patient has acne, hirsutism, or hyperlipidemia. If the patient is interested in extended cycling, it is best to use a monophasic pill in order to minimize spotting. The most important factors to consider in choosing an OCP for the healthy adolescent are cost, patient preference, and past experience using OCPs.

Pelvic Examination

Although many physicians require patients to have a pelvic examination prior to prescribing OCPs, these examinations are not necessary and may reduce the adolescent's access to effective contraceptive methods. Numerous professional organizations, including WHO, American College of Obstetricians and Gynecologists (ACOG), and the U.S. Agency for International Development have stated that a pelvic examination is not necessary for safe use of OCPs (Stewart et al., 2001). Although a sexually active adolescent should be screened for cervical cancer and STIs, these tests are not necessary prior to prescribing OCPs. If a pelvic examination is mandated prior to prescribing OCPs, many teens that fear this examination will delay seeking effective contraceptive services. If a teen is not sexually active, OCPs can be prescribed indefinitely without mandating a pelvic examination. The sexually active teen should be counseled regarding the benefits of screening for cervical cancer and STIs and also encouraged to have a pelvic examination. Many adolescent centers now allow the sexually active teen to defer the pelvic examination for up to 1 year if they wish. Using this approach, over 80% of teens return for follow-up and do obtain a pelvic examination within this time period.

Laboratory Testing

No laboratory tests are needed routinely prior to starting OCPs. The increased risk of VTE in OCP users who have prothrombotic mutations has led to questions about the value of screening for these mutations before OCPs are prescribed. However, even screening for the most common mutation, factor V Leiden, which occurs in 5% of the Caucasian population, is not cost-effective. Indeed, >500,000 women would need to be screened to avoid a single death.

A pregnancy test is not necessary if the OCPs are started during or on the Sunday after menses begin. In order to avoid inadvertently prescribing OCPs to a teen that is already pregnant, many physicians prefer to start OCPs on the Sunday after the beginning of the next menses or on the first day of the next menses rather than at the time of the medical visit. However, recent studies have suggested that compliance may be improved by starting OCPs on the day of the visit. If this "quick start" approach is used, it is advisable to perform a urine pregnancy test at the time of the visit (Lara-Torre, 2004). By using the quick start approach, the adolescent may be more likely to remember how to take the pills but unless the pills are started within 6 days of menses, a backup contraceptive (e.g., condoms) should be used for the first 3 weeks since ovulation may still occur. For the adolescent who has very irregular cycles or prolonged amenorrhea, it is usually best to start OCPs on the day of the visit.

Side Effects of OCPs

Compliance with OCP use can be improved by reviewing the common side effects and their management with the adolescent when OCPs are prescribed because side effects are the most commonly reported reason why adolescents discontinue OCPs. Although some side effects (e.g., venous thrombosis) can be explained by the medication's pharmacologic action, others (e.g., mood changes) cannot. Many of the symptoms commonly attributed to OCPs have not been shown to occur with greater frequency in pill users compared with a placebo control group. In a recent review of placebo-controlled studies on OCP side effects, there was no difference in reported rates of headache, weight gain, breast pain, depression, or emotional lability between OCP users and the placebo group. There was a significant difference in incidence of nausea and vomiting in the OCP users in only one study in which the OCP prescribed contained 100 mg of ethinyl estradiol.

For adolescents, the potential side effect of OCPs that most concerns them is weight gain. This concern may deter them from starting OCPs or lead to premature discontinuation of OCPs. In a placebo controlled study of triphasic ethinyl estradiol/norgestimate there was no significant weight gain noted in either OCP users or the placebo group. Risser compared the weight change at 1 year between adolescents taking OCPs or medroxyprogesterone and found that 70% of the teens had either lost weight or gained less than 5% of baseline weight. Unfortunately, fear of gaining weight is one of the most common reasons given by women for not using OCPs for contraception.

At a minimum, the practitioner should discuss management of BTB, nausea, and amenorrhea when prescribing OCPs. In one study, 33% of women who discontinued OCP use did so because of BTB (Rosenberg et al., 1995). This is more likely to occur with lower dose OCPs and if pills are skipped. Because this bleeding is not harmful and tends to resolve within 4 months of OCP use, it is rarely necessary to discontinue OCPs because of this side effect. If the bleeding is heavy or very bothersome, switching to another OCP with higher endometrial activity may help. Nausea occurs most often during the first cycle and is more common in underweight women. This symptom also tends to resolve with increasing duration of use. Taking the OCP with a meal or at bedtime sometimes helps reduce the nausea. If nausea is persistent and thought to be due to OCPs, changing to an OCP with 20 mg of estrogen may decrease the symptom.

SKIPPED PILLS

The average adolescent will forget to take her OCP three times a month. In general, if she is less than 24 hours late in taking a pill, she should take the missed pill as soon as she is aware of it and continue with their regular pill-taking routine. If she is more than 24 hours late, she should be advised to take both the missed pill and the pill for the current day. If two or more pills have been skipped on consecutive days, an additional method of contraception should be used for the rest of the cycle to prevent pregnancy.

Medical Conditions that are Contraindications to OCP Use

Most adolescents who have chronic medical conditions also can safely take OCPs. However, OCPs are contraindicated in women who have hypercoagulability disorders, history of thromboembolic disease (e.g., venous thrombosis, pulmonary embolism), liver disease, breast cancer, coronary artery disease, congestive heart failure, cerebrovascular disease, or severe hypertension (>160/110 mmHg) (Table 25-5). Systemic lupus erythematosus (SLE) associated with vascular disease, nephritis, or antiphospholipid antibody is also a contraindication. In addition to these absolute contraindications for OCP use, there are other medical conditions for which OCPs usually are contraindicated unless there are no other

TABLE 25-5

ORAL CONTRACEPTIVE PILL CONTRAINDICATIONS

Venous thromboembolic disease
Thrombophilia
Migraine with focal neurologic deficits
Severe hypertension (160/110 mmHg)
Coronary artery disease
Hemorrhagic or ischemic stroke
Breast cancer
Diabetes mellitus with vascular or neurologic complications
Active or chronic liver disease
Systemic lupus erythematosus with vascular complications
Pregnancy
Adrenal disease (Drospirenone-containing OCPs only)
Kidney disease (Drospirenone-containing OCPs only)

contraceptives methods available and/or acceptable such as gall bladder disease.

Diabetes Mellitus

It is especially important for adolescents who have type I diabetes to use effective contraception. Although the adolescent who has nephropathy, retinopathy, neuropathy, or other vascular disease should not be placed on OCPs, the diabetic adolescent who does not have these complications can safely use OCPs. In a study of young women who had diabetes, hemoglobin A1C levels were similar in OCP users and nonusers and OCP use did not accelerate the development of diabetic vascular disease.

Migraine Headaches

Adolescents who have migraine headaches associated with focal neurologic deficits (e.g., hemiplegic migraine) should not use OCPs because they may be at increased risk for stroke. Some physicians also recommend that women who have migraine headaches without focal neurologic deficits use another method of contraception because OCPs elevate the risk for ischemic but not hemorrhagic stroke (Daniel and Mishell, 2000).

Venous Thromboembolism

A history of deep vein thrombosis or pulmonary embolism is a contraindication to the use of OCPs because OCPs increase the risk of VTE by a factor of 3–6 (Vandenbroucke et al., 2001). The absolute risk for the healthy young woman taking OCPs, however, is low (3–4/10,000) and the mortality risk of VTE among 15–24-year-old OCP users is 0.3 per 100,000 women per year (Dickey, 2000). The increased risk of VTE due to OCP use is approximately half the risk of VTE associated with pregnancy (Daniel and Mishell, 2000). Because the symptoms of VTE and pulmonary embolism often are vague, it is wise to discuss them with the OCP user so that they are aware of them and can seek medical attention promptly if symptoms of VTE occur. The risk of VTE is increased in OCP users who have factor V Leiden mutation, obesity, immobility, and family history of VTE. Factor V Leiden mutation occurs in 5%–7% of the healthy Caucasian population and 20%–40% of patients who have VTE. Women who have factor V Leiden mutation have 28.5/10,000 woman-years incidence of VTE while using OCPs compared with a 5.7/10,000 woman-years incidence if they are not taking OCPs.

Cardiovascular Disease

In women without other risk factors, OCP use does not increase the risk of myocardial infarction or ischemic or hemorrhagic stroke. Because the risk of myocardial infarction is low in women <35 years and the excess risk for MI due to OCPs among smokers is small, OCPs can be prescribed to young women even if they smoke cigarettes (Daniel and Mishell, 2000). Adolescents who have mild hypertension can also safely take OCPs, but their blood pressure should be monitored regularly.

Pregnancy and Lactation

There is no evidence that OCPs are teratogenic, but OCPs should not be prescribed during pregnancy and they should be stopped whenever pregnancy is diagnosed. There is also no evidence for increased chromosomal abnormalities or congenital malformations in children of women who used OCPs within 1–3 months prior to becoming pregnant. After stopping OCPs, there is an average 2-month delay in return of fertility, but some women will become pregnant without delay. OCPs should not be prescribed until 21 days after delivery because of the increased risk for VTE in the postpartum period. Because the estrogen in OCPs decreases volume of milk production and the caloric and mineral content of the breast milk, it is not the first choice for contraception for breastfeeding mothers. However, OCPs can be used once milk flow is well established, beginning at 6 weeks postpartum.

Female Athlete

Intense athletic activity can impact the menstrual cycle. Young women who train extensively in sports that promote leanness (e.g., gymnastics, long distance running) are especially at risk for amenorrhea. The prevalence of amenorrhea is 4–20 times higher in athletes compared to other women. This athletic amenorrhea is the result of hypothalamic dysfunction and associated with low estrogen levels, which may reduce bone mass (Eliakim and Beyth, 2003). Because OCPs help preserve BMD in the hypoestrogenic athlete and restore menses, they may be an excellent method of contraception for the female athlete.

Systemic Lupus Erythematosus

Effective contraception is important for teens that have SLE because of the high risks associated with pregnancy complicated by SLE. However, OCPs should be avoided in women who have SLE complicated by vascular disease, nephritis, or antiphospholipid antibodies (ACOG, 2000). VTE have been reported in women who have SLE and antiphospholipid antibodies. It is preferable to use other methods of contraception that do not contain estrogen (e.g., progesterone-only mini pill) in teens who have SLE.

Sickle cell disease

Effective contraception is also important for women who have sickle cell disease (SCD) because there is an increased risk for maternal complications. The vasoocclusive episodes associated with SCD differ from intravascular thromboembolism and there are no well-controlled studies assessing whether VTE risk is higher in OCP users who have SCD than in other OCP users. The ACOG clinical management guidelines state that pregnancy carries a greater risk than OCP use for women who have SCD and thus OCPs can be used in these women. However, depot-medroxyprogesterone acetate (DMPA) is a better contraceptive option for women who have SCD because DMPA reduces the incidence of painful crises and does not increase the risk for VTE (ACOG, 2000).

Drug Interactions

Concomitant use of OCPs and other drugs may affect contraceptive efficacy. Unfortunately, most of the available information on drug interactions is anecdotal and there have been few prospective, well-designed, pharmacokinetic, or population-based studies on the interactions of OCPs and other medications. Possible drug interactions have been reported for antibiotics, anticonvulsants, acetaminophen, aspirin, and St. John's Wort (Greydanus et al., 2001; ACOG, 2000). Anticonvulsants that induce hepatic enzymes (e.g., barbiturates, phenytoin, carbamazepine, felbamate, topiramate, vigabatrin) can decrease serum concentrations of estrogen and/or progestin. Other anticonvulsants such as valproic acid, gabapentin, or tiagabine do not affect serum levels. Although many physicians believe that antibiotics decrease OCP efficacy, clinical reports of contraceptive failure associated with antibiotic use are not supported by pharmacokinetic data. Indeed, pharmacokinetic studies have shown that plasma levels of OCP steroids are unchanged with the concomitant use of ampicillin, ciprofloxacin, clarithromycin, doxycycline, metronidazole, and tetracycline. Three retrospective studies of OCP users who were taking antibiotics (tetracycline, minocycline, penicillins, and cephalosporins) for dermatologic conditions failed to show an increased pregnancy rate compared to a control group. However, there is pharmacokinetic data to support decreased efficacy of OCPs in women who are taking rifampin and griseofulvin.

TRANSDERMAL HORMONAL CONTRACEPTION

A transdermal contraceptive patch is 20 cm^2 and contains ethinyl estradiol and norelgestromin. The patch can be placed on any area of the body except the breast or genital area. It is applied once each week for 3 consecutive weeks followed by 1 week without use of the patch to allow for withdrawal bleeding.

The contraceptive patch provides efficacy, cycle control, and safety comparable to OCPs of similar dosage (Creasy et al., 2001). Perhaps because the patches only need to be changed weekly, perfect compliance with the method has been reported to be as high as 90% (Smallwood et al., 2001). Although the pregnancy rate was only 0.7%, there may be an increased risk for pregnancy in women who weigh >90 kg because four of the five pregnancies in a study of 1664 women occurred in women who weighed >90 kg. Thus, the contraceptive patch may not be as effective a method for women who weigh >90 kg. The incidence of BTB may be higher in the first two cycles in women who use the contraceptive patch compared to those who use OCPs, but in subsequent cycles there is no difference in incidence of BTB. When compared to women using OCPs, the contraceptive patch users have a higher incidence of breast tenderness in the first two cycles of use and dysmenorrhea. Local skin irritation may occur with the transdermal patch but in only 1% of patients is it severe enough to cause discontinuation of the method. The contraceptive patch's adhesion to the skin is excellent with only 1.8%–2.9% of patches requiring replacement due to complete or partial detachment. The starter kit for patients contains an extra patch, which can be used if a patch falls off. Heat, humidity, and exercise do not seem to affect adhesion.

Contraceptive Ring

A contraceptive vaginal ring containing ethinyl estradiol and etonorgestrel (NuvaRing) was approved for use in the United States in 2001 (Johansson, 2004). Etonorgestrel is the biologically active metabolite of desogestrel. The ring has a diameter of approximately 2 in. and is made of flexible plastic. It is inserted into the vagina and left in place for first 3 weeks of the menstrual cycle and removed during the fourth week so that menses will occur. A new ring is inserted after the fourth week. The efficacy, cycle control, and side effects of the contraceptive ring are similar to OCPs. Absorption of the contraceptive steroids through the vaginal epithelium is efficient and rapid. The ring provides steady blood levels of hormones, releasing approximately 15 mg of ethinyl estradiol per day. There is a higher incidence of vaginal discomfort, vaginitis, and leukorrhea among women using the ring compared to OCPs. Since the ring can be left in place for 3 weeks, compliance may be better than with OCPs. The contraindications are the same as for OCPs.

Progestin-only Pills

Progesterone-only pills (POPs) prevent conception by thickening cervical mucus and inducing endometrial atrophy but do not reliably inhibit ovulation. Because POPs do not inhibit ovulation, skipping even one pill or a delay of even a few hours in taking a pill can result in contraceptive failure. If an adolescent who is taking POPs is more than 3 hours late in her pill taking, recommend a back-up method for the next 2 days. Because they do not contain estrogen, POPs do not increase the risk of VTE. Lactating women also can use them because lactation is not suppressed once milk production has been established (Trussell, 1998).

Injectable Hormonal Contraceptive

DMPA, a 3-month progestin-only medication containing 150 mg of medroxyprogesterone acetate (MPA) per 1 cc injection (Depo-Provera), is a highly effective contraceptives that prevent pregnancy by suppressing levels of follicle stimulating hormone and luteinizing hormone, thus inhibiting ovulation (Westhoff, 2003). The ideal time to start DMPA is within 5 days of the onset of menses so that ovulation can be prevented during the first month of use. DMPA can be started immediately postpartum or after induced or spontaneous termination of pregnancy in the first or second trimester. Because DMPA does not affect lactation, breastfeeding mothers can also be started on DMPA immediately after delivery. Repeat injections of DMPA are given every 12 weeks, but because ovulation does not occur for at least 14 weeks after a 150-mg injection of DMPA, there is a 2-week grace period.

There are many noncontraceptive health benefits associated with the use of DMPA (Table 25-6). These benefits include decreased risk of iron deficiency anemia, PID, ectopic pregnancy, and endometrial cancer. DMPA use is associated with an 80% risk reduction for endometrial cancer. The majority of DMPA users will experience amenorrhea, which can be of benefit to women who have menses-related disorders such as dysmenorrhea, menorrhagia, premenstrual syndrome, and migraine (Westhoff, 2003). Amenorrhea may also be desirable for the mentally retarded adolescent who has difficulty managing menstrual hygiene. Adolescents who have SCD may have decreased painful crises during treatment with DMPA. Adolescents who have epilepsy are also good candidates for DMPA because DMPA efficacy is not affected by concomitant anticonvulsant medication use and data indicate that DMPA has intrinsic anticonvulsant activity (Kaunitz, 2002). DMPA is not associated with increased risk of stroke of any type, acute myocardial infarction, or VTE, and does not adversely affect blood pressure in adolescents or adults. Changes in menstrual pattern are common among DMPA users. Approximately 70% of DMPA users will be amenorrheic after 12 months of use. However, in the initial 3 months of use, 46% of women report irregular bleeding or spotting. These menstrual changes are the most common reason cited for discontinuing this method of contraception (Harel et al., 1996).

TABLE 25-6

BENEFITS OF INJECTABLE
MEDROXYPROGESTERONE ACETATE

Gynecologic Benefits	Nongynecologic Benefits
Less dysmenorrhea	Less anemia
Less pelvic inflammatory disease	Less painful sickle cell crises
Less premenstrual syndrome	Less seizures
Less ectopic pregnancy	
Less endometrial cancer	

Weight gain also is often cited by adolescents as the reason they discontinue DMPA. However, the data regarding weight gain with DMPA use suggests no consistent effect on weight. Some women will indeed gain weight but others will maintain or lose body weight on DMPA. Postpartum adolescents, women who have high BMI, Native American and African American women are more likely to gain weight while using DMPA.

Since DMPA is a long-acting contraceptive, there is a delay in the return of fertility after stopping DMPA. This may be of benefit for the young adolescent who does not wish to become pregnant but delays returning for follow-up injections. For patients who discontinue DMPA because they wish to become pregnant, the median time to conceive is 10 months after the last injection of DMPA (Westhoff, 2003).

DMPA suppresses estradiol production, which raises concern that it may decrease bone mineralization in adolescence and lead to osteopenia and fractures in later life. Prospective studies have shown that adolescents using DMPA have a slight decrease in BMD at an age when teens normally are increasing their BMD. There was a 1.5% decrease in BMD after 1 year and 3.1% decrease in BMD over 2 years in contrast to a 2.9% increase at 1 year and a 9.5% increase at 2 years in controls (Cromer et al., 1996). However, this loss of BMD is reversible with cessation of use. Changes in BMD do not appear to be affected by whether the woman is amenorrheic or not (Tang et al., 1999). Until more research clarifies this issue, DMPA users should be advised to optimize their BMD by taking an adequate amount of calcium, engaging in weight-bearing and muscle-strengthening exercise, and avoiding alcohol and cigarettes. DMPA probably should not be used by teens that are at increased risk for osteoporosis (e.g., chronic renal disease, anorexia nervosa).

The majority of published reports indicate that DMPA does not cause depressive symptoms (Westhoff, 2000). A 12-month prospective study of adolescents using DMPA showed that there was no emergence of depressive symptoms or significant change in affect (Gupta et al., 2001). Another study showed that even in women who had depressive symptoms at the time they started using DMPA, there was no increase in these symptoms during DMPA use (Westhoff et al., 1998).

Combined injectable contraceptives containing both estrogen and progestin have been used successfully in other countries for many years and a monthly injectable hormonal contraceptive containing 5 mg estradiol cypionate and 25 mg MPA (Lunelle) had been approved by the FDA for use in the United States. In October 2002 the manufacturer, Pharmacia, suspended distribution of Lunelle due to quality control issues (Johansson, 2004). The side effects and contraindications are similar to OCPs. Because these combined injectable contraceptives contain estrogen, BMD is not affected and menses are regular. However, these combined injectable contraceptives require a monthly injection, which makes them less popular with adolescents than DMPA, which requires only four injections per year.

HORMONAL EMERGENCY CONTRACEPTIVE PILLS

Emergency contraceptive pills (ECPs) can be used to prevent pregnancy after unprotected intercourse or when regular contraceptive methods fail. Use of emergency contraception (EC) after unprotected intercourse can reduce the risk of pregnancy to 1%–2% (Westhoff, 2003). A single act of unprotected intercourse occurring 1–2 days before ovulation is associated with an 8%–50% chance of pregnancy. Since sperm can survive in the female genital tract for 5–6 days, fertilization may occur days after sexual activity.

Combined ECPs are ordinary OCPs that are taken in higher dosages. Although a single mechanism of action of ECPs has not been established, they most likely work by inhibiting or delaying ovulation. ECPs do not interrupt an implanted pregnancy and there is no evidence that ECPs increase the risk of ectopic pregnancy.

The OCPs most commonly prescribed for EC are those containing ethinyl estradiol and levonorgestrel. The amount of ethinyl estradiol prescribed is

100–120 μg per dose and the amount of levonorgestrel prescribed ranges from 0.50 to 0.60 mg per dose. The first dose is taken as soon as possible after unprotected intercourse and a second dose is taken 12 hours later (Trussel, 2004). The FDA has approved two hormonal contraceptive methods specifically for EC. The Preven emergency contraceptive kit consists of four pills each containing 0.25 mg of levonorgestrel and 50 μg of ethinyl estradiol, a urine pregnancy test, and an information booklet. The first two pills are taken as soon as possible after unprotected intercourse and the second two pills are taken 12 hours later. The other EC is a progestin-only method (Plan B). It consists of two tablets, each containing 0.75 mg of levonorgestrel.

Several factors complicate the calculation of efficacy of ECPs including when intercourse occurred in the menstrual cycle and how soon after intercourse the ECP was taken. The sooner ECPs are taken after intercourse, the more effective they will be. When taken within 12 hours of intercourse, the pregnancy rate is <1% compared to over 3% when given between 61–72 hours. Because there is also evidence that ECPs continue to be effective up to 120 hours after unprotected intercourse, they should be offered to women who have experienced any episode of unprotected intercourse in the previous 5 days (Ellerston et al., 2003). Since the length of menstrual cycle and day of ovulation is so variable in adolescents, ECPs should be offered regardless of the cycle day on which unprotected intercourse occurred. The progestin-only method (Plan B) appears to be up to three times more effective in preventing pregnancy than the combination-pill methods. Plan B also can be administered as a single dose of two 0.75-mg pills whereas administering combined OCPs or Preven in a single dose cannot be recommended due to lack of data on its efficacy.

Hormonal EC is very safe. There are no absolute contraindications for its use, even in women who have contraindications to the long-term use of daily OCPs. However, some physicians may prefer to prescribe a progestin-only ECP such as Plan B for these women. No laboratory tests or physical examination are needed prior to prescribing ECPs. Although not indicated for a woman who is already pregnant, there is no evidence that taking ECPs or Plan B is harmful to the woman or her fetus. However, if existing pregnancy is suspected, a pregnancy test prior to administration could be helpful in facilitating management of the pregnancy. There also is no good evidence of an increased risk of ectopic pregnancy in women who use ECP.

The most common side effects of ECPs are nausea and vomiting, which are less likely to occur if a progestin-only method is used since it does not contain estrogen. Although there might be some benefit in prescribing an antiemetic to be taken prior to taking the ECP, this usually is not necessary with progestin-only methods. About 10% of patients will have mild menstrual bleeding during the cycle in which they use ECPs. Especially if taken early in the cycle, ECPs also may result in earlier than expected menses (Webb et al., 2004). Routine follow-up is not necessary but if menses do not occur within one week after their usual time, the patient should be advised to return for follow-up.

Because adolescent sexual activity is often sporadic and unplanned, increased knowledge and availability of ECPs may help reduce the number of unwanted adolescent pregnancies. The approaches advocated to help make ECPs more available include increased education of physicians and patients about ECPs, advance provision of ECPs, and over the counter distribution without a prescription. Some states now allow pharmacists to dispense ECPs without a prescription and the American College of Obstetrics and Gynecology as well as many major medical organizations have petitioned the FDA to allow progestin-only ECPs to be sold without prescription. Direct access to ECPs has been shown to increase their use (Bajos et al., 2002). Advanced supply of ECPs to postpartum women also has been shown to significantly increase their use. These women were no more likely to change to a less effective method of contraception because of the advance supply of ECPs or have increased episodes of unprotected intercourse. A similar study among adolescents showed that advance provision of EC was not associated with more unprotected intercourse or less condom or hormonal contraception use compared to the control group participants. At follow-up, the group that had received advance

provision of EC reported significantly higher condom use than the control participants and had begun the EC on average 10 hours sooner than adolescents who were not given EC in advance. They also reported fewer pregnancies and no increase in the number of STIs compared to the control participants (Gold, 2004a,b,c).

NONHORMONAL CONTRACEPTIVES

Vaginal Spermicides

Vaginal spermicides are available as a gel, foam, cream, film, or suppository. They contain a chemical that kills sperm. In the United States the chemical agent is nonoxyl-9 (N-9), a surfactant that destroys the sperm cell membrane. In other countries, other surfactant products, including octoxynol and benzalkonium chloride, are available. These agents must be placed into the vagina no more than one hour before intercourse. Pregnancy rates when vaginal spermicides are used alone range from 5% to 50% (Trussel, 1998). Thus, it is usually recommended that these spermicides be used with other barrier methods (e.g. diaphragm) in order to improve efficacy. Although N-9 has in vitro activity against STIs and human immunodeficiency virus infection, a recent evidence-based review found no evidence that N-9 is of benefit in preventing HIV infection or other STIs (Wilkinson, 2002). Indeed, frequent use of spermicides containing N-9 has been associated with genital lesions, which may be associated with increased risk of HIV transmission (Wilkinson, 2002; Prevention CDC, 2002).

Vaginal barrier contraceptives include the diaphragm, cervical cap, vaginal cap, cervical sponge and female condom. All of the vaginal barriers have similar efficacy for nulliparous women but parity significantly affects the efficacy of the sponge and cap. The per cent of nulliparous women who experience unintended pregnancy within the first year of typical use is 20% for the sponge, female condom, diaphragm, and cap. For parous women, however, 40% experience unintended pregnancy within the first year of typical use of the sponge or cap. There are few serious medical problems associated with the use of vaginal barriers. Use of vaginal barriers with spermicide does increase the risk for urinary tract infection, bacterial vaginosis, and vaginal candidiasis, and there is an increased risk of toxic-shock syndrome if barrier methods are left in the vagina for a prolonged time. Latex allergy may occur in adolescents who use a latex cap or diaphragm and some women are allergic or sensitive to N-9. Minor problems with vaginal barriers include vaginal irritation, odor, and discharge, especially if the barrier is left in the vagina for a prolonged time. Some adolescents may have difficulty inserting or removing a vaginal barrier.

The female condom is a loose-fitting polyurethane bag that is approximately 8 cm in diameter and 17 cm long. It contains two flexible polyurethane rings. One of the rings fits inside the vagina and the other remains outside the vagina. It is sold without prescription and is intended for one-time use. It can be inserted up to 8 hours before intercourse. It cannot be used with the male condom because when used together the two condoms may adhere to each other, causing displacement of one or both of the condoms. It is an effective mechanical barrier to viruses, including HIV, and should provide protection from other STIs that is at least as good as male condoms (Prevention CDC, 2001).

The diaphragm is a dome-shaped latex rubber cup that has a flexible rim. It should be used with spermicidal cream or jelly. It is inserted before intercourse and is effective for up to 6 hours. After intercourse, the diaphragm should be left in place for 6 hours and then removed, washed and stored in a cool place. The diameter of diaphragms range from 50 mm to 95 mm. A pelvic examination is required to determine the proper size diaphragm. Although manufacturer labeling for diaphragms recommend refitting after a gain or loss of weight of 10 lb or more, weight change does not commonly require a change in diaphragm.

The contraceptive sponge is a disposable polyurethane device that contains N-9 spermicide. It is approximately 2×5 cm in size and available without prescription. The sponge should be moistened and placed in the vagina before intercourse. It is effective for up to 24 hours and does not require the vaginal insertion of additional spermicide with prolonged use. A recent Cochrane review concluded that the sponge is significantly less effective than the diaphragm and its discontinuation rate at 12 months was higher as well (Kuyoh et al., 2003).

The Prentif cervical cap is a latex rubber cup that fits snugly over the cervix. It should be used with a spermicide and provides continuous contraceptive protection for 48 hours. Cervical caps sizes range from 22 mm to 31 mm and a pelvic examination is required for fitting. Approximately 10% of women cannot be fitted either due to the limited sizes available or the physical characteristics of their cervix.

The FemCap is an anatomically designed silicone rubber vaginal barrier that looks like a sailor's cap. It was approved for use in the United States in 2003 and its efficacy is comparable to the diaphragm. It should be used with spermicide on the inside and outside surfaces and can be reused for up to 2 years. It must remain in place for at least 6 hours after intercourse, but no longer than 48 hours. The FemCap comes in 3 sizes but does not require a pelvic examination for fitting. The smallest size (22 mm) is intended for women who have never been pregnant, women who have miscarried or had caesarean section should use the 26 mm cap and the largest (30 mm) cap should be used by women who have had a vaginal delivery of a full-term baby.

Male Condoms

The male condom consists of a thin sheath, which is placed over the glans and shaft of the penis. It prevents pregnancy by preventing the deposition of semen into the vagina during intercourse. Condoms are available in a wide variety of shapes, sizes, colors, and thickness. Some are lubricated and/or contain spermicides. When used consistently and correctly, condoms are an effective method of contraception. Calculated on a "per use" basis, the pregnancy rate for couples that use male condoms per episode of intercourse is very low (0.04%). However, because couples that use condoms as their sole method of contraception do not always use them consistently and correctly, the typical pregnancy rate with condom use is 14% within the first year of use. Although condom users fear that the condom will break or fall off during sexual activity, studies have shown that this is a rare occurrence. Breakage rates range from 0% to 6.7% and complete slippage ranges from 0.6% to 5.4% (Trussell, 1998). Indeed, the most common error associated with condom use among university students is failure to have a condom available when needed followed by applying the condom after sex had begun (Crosby et al., 2003).

Most condoms are made of latex, but about 5% are made from the intestinal cecum of lambs (natural or lambskin condoms). When used consistently and correctly, latex condoms are effective in preventing the sexual transmission of HIV infection and can reduce the risk of other STIs. They are more effective in preventing the transmission of STIs transmitted by fluids from mucosal surfaces (e.g., gonorrhea, chlamydia, trichomonas, HIV) than STIs transmitted by skin-to-skin contact (e.g., herpes simplex virus, human papilloma virus, syphilis). A Cochrane Review of data regarding HIV serodiscordant heterosexual couples demonstrated that HIV seroconversion was reduced by 80% with condom use (Weller, 2002). Nonlatex condoms are slightly more likely to break during use but their contraceptive efficacy is similar to latex condoms (Gallo et al., 2003). Condoms lubricated with spermicides are no more effective than other lubricated condoms in protecting against transmission of STIs. Condoms lubricated with N-9 spermicide cost more, have a shorter shelf life and are associated with urinary tract infections in young women (Prevention CDC, 2002).

Intrauterine Device

IUDs are a highly effective, long-acting method of contraception when used effectively. IUDs primarily prevent pregnancy by preventing fertilization. Progesterone-releasing IUDs also thicken cervical mucus, alter endometrial lining, and impair tubal motility. The first year failure rate with IUDs varies with the type of IUD used, but is very low (0.1%–1.5%). The American Academy of Pediatrics recommends that they be reserved for adolescent females who cannot use other methods of contraception and are not at risk for STIs (Committee, 1999). Appropriate candidates for IUD use are adolescents who are in a mutually monogamous sexual relationship for the duration of use and desire a long-acting method of contraception. IUDs do not interfere with breastfeeding. Adolescents who have active, recent (past 3 months), or recurrent pelvic infection should not use any IUD because of the increased risk of upper genital tract infection and subsequent infertility. An adolescent who has a distorted uterine cavity (e.g., bicornuate uterus) also should not use an IUD because these anatomic abnormalities can cause difficulties with insertion and increase the risk of uterine perforation.

IUDs currently available in the United States include a levonorgestrel IUD (Mirena) that is approved for 5 years continuous use, copper IUD (ParaGard) that is approved for 10 years continuous use, and progesterone IUD (Progestasert) that must be replaced annually.

Bibliography

American College of Obstetrics and Gynecology. The Use of Hormonal Contraception in Women with Coexisting Medical Conditions. *ACOG Pract Bull* 2000;95(18):1–18.

Bajos N, Goulard H, Job-Spira N, et al. Emergency contraception: from accessibility to counseling. *Contraception* 2002;67:39–40.

Committee on Adolescence. Contraception and adolescents. *Pediatrics* 1999;194:1161–1166.

Creasy G, Abrams L, Fisher A. Transdermal Contraception. *Semin Reprod Med* 2001;19(4):373–380.

Cromer BA, Blair JM, Mahan JD, et al. A prospective comparison of bone density in adolescent girls receiving depot medroxyprogesterone acetate (DMPA), levonorgestrel (Norplant), or oral contraceptives. *J Pediatr* 1996;129:671–676.

Cromer BA, Stager MB, Bonny A, et al. Depo medroxyprogesterone acetate, oral contraceptives and bone mineral density in a cohort of adolescent girls. *J Adolesc Health* 2004;35:434–441.

Crosby R, Sanders S, Yarber WL, et al. Condom-use Errors and Problems. A neglected aspect of studies assessing condom effectiveness. *Am J Prev Med* 2003; 24(4):67–370.

Daniel R, Mishell J. Oral contraceptives and cardiovascular events: Summary and application of data. *Int J Fertil* 2000;45(Suppl 2):121–133.

Dickey RP. *Managing Contraceptive Pill Patients,* 10th ed. Dallas, TX: EMIS Medical Publishers, 2000.

Eliakim A, Beyth Y. Exercise training, menstrual irregularities and bone development in children and adolescents. *J Pediatr Adolesc Gynecol* 2003;16(4):201–206.

Ellerston C, Evans M, Ferden S, et al. Extending the time limit for starting the Yuzpe regimen of emergency contraception. *Obstet Gynecol* 2003;101:1168–1171.

Gallo MF, Grimes DA, Schulz KF. Nonlatex vs. latex male condoms for contraception: a systematic review of randomized controlled trials. *Contraception* 2003;68:319–326.

Gold MA, Bachrach LK. Contraceptive use in teens: A treat to bone health? *J Adolesc Health* 2004a;35:427–429.

Gold MA, Sucato GS, Conrad LAE, et al. Provision of emergency contraception to adolescents. Position paper of the Society for Adolescent Medicine. *J Adolesc Health* 2004b;35:66–70.

Gold MA, Wolford JE, Smith JA, et al. The effects of advance provision of emergency contraception on adolescent women's sexual and contraceptive behaviors. *J Pediatr Adolesc Gynecol* 2004c;17(2):87–96.

Greydanus DE, Patel DR, Rimsza ME. Contraception in the adolescent: An update. *Pediatrics* 2001;107(3):562–573.

Greydanus DE, Rimsza ME, Matytsina L. Contraception for college students. *Pediatr Clin North Am* 2005;52:135–161.

Gupta N, O'Brien R, Jacobsen LJ, et al. Mood changes in adolescents using depot-medroxyprogesterone acetate for contraception: A prospective study. *J Pediatr Adolesc Gynecol* 2001;14:71–76.

Harel Z, Biro FM, Killar LM, et al. Adolescent's reasons for and experience after discontinuation of the long-acting contraceptives DMPA and Norplant. *J Adolesc Health* 1996;19:118–123.

Johansson EB. Future developments in contraception. *Am J Obstet Gynecol* 2004;190(Suppl 4):S69–S71.

Kaunitz AM: Current concepts regarding the use of DMPA. *J Repro Med* 2002;47 (9 Suppl):785–789.

Kuyoh MA, Toroitich-Ruto C, Grimes DA, et al. Sponge versus diaphragm for contraception: A Cochrane review. *Contraception* 2003;67:15–18.

Lara-Torre E. "Quick Start," an innovative approach to the combination oral contraceptive pill in adolescents. Is it time to make the Switch? *J Pediatr Adolesc Gynecol* 2004;17(1):65–67.

Prevention CDC. Sexually transmitted diseases treatment guidelines 2002. *MMWR Morb Mortal Wkly Rep* 2002;51:1–77.

Rimsza ME. Counseling the Adolescent about Contraception. *Pediatr Rev* 2003;24(5):162–170.

Rosenberg MJ, Waugh MS, Meehan TE. Use and misuse of oral contraceptives: Risk indicators for poor pill taking and discontinuation. *Contraception* 1995;51:283–288.

Smallwood GH, Meador ML, Lenihan JP, et al. Efficacy and safety of transdermal contraceptive system. *Obstet Gynecol* 2001;98:799–805.

Stewart FH, Harper CC, Ellertson CE, et al. Clinical breast and pelvic examination requirements for hormonal contraception. current practice vs. evidence. *JAMA* 2001;285(17):2232–2239.

Tang OS, Tang G, Yip P, et al. Long-term depot-medroxyprogesterone acetate and bone mineral density. *Contraception* 1999;59:25–29.

Trussell J. Contraceptive efficacy. In: Hatcher RA, Trussell J, Stewart FH WC Jr, Stewart GK, Guest F, et al. (eds.), *Contraceptive Technology,* 17th ed. New York: Ardent Media, 1998, pp. 779–845.

Trussell J, Ellertson C, Stewart F, et al. The role of emergency contraception. *Am J Obstet Gynecol* 2004;190(4S):S30–S38.

Vandenbroucke JP, Rosing J, Bloemenkamp KWM, et al. Oral Contraceptives and the Risk of Venous Thrombosis. *N Engl J Med* 2001;344(20):1527–1534.

Webb A, Shochet T, Bigrigg A, et al. Effect of hormonal emergency contraception on bleeding patterns. *Contraception* 2004;69:133–135.

Weller S. Condom effectiveness in reducing heterosexual HIV transmission (Cochrane Review). *Cochrane Database Syst Rev* 2002.

Wilkinson D, Tholandi M, Ramjee G, Rutherford GW. Nonoxynol-9 spermicide for prevention of vaginally acquired HIV and other sexually transmitted infections: systematic review and meta-analysis of randomized controlled trials including more than 5000 women. *Lancet Infect Dis* 2002; 10.

Westhoff C, Truman C, Kalmuss D, et al. Depressive symptoms and DMPA. *Contraception* 1998;57:237–240.

Westhoff C. Depot-medroxyprogesterone acetate injection (Depo-Provera): a highly effective contraceptive option with proven long-term safety. *Contraception* 2003;68:75–87.

Westhoff C. Emergency contraception. *N Engl J Med* 2003;349(19):1830–1835.

C H A P T E R

26

ADOLESCENT PREGNANCY AND ABORTION

Renée R. Jenkins and Tina R. Raine

EPIDEMIOLOGY

Trends in Pregnancy, Births, and Abortions

Birth rates among adolescents 15–19 years old in the United States have declined since the early 1990s, predominantly fueled by the fall in the pregnancy rate. Pregnancy rates are calculated as the sum of births, miscarriages, stillbirths, and abortions. Birth rates have dropped most dramatically in the 15–17 years old and among African American adolescents (Fig. 26-1).[1] The rates in these teenagers dropped 40% since 1991, to a rate of 23.2/1000. Repeated pregnancies accounted for the lower rates in the early 1990s, but in the later 1990s, first pregnancies accounted for the drop.[2] Abortion rates have also declined gradually, with about 33% of teens choosing to terminate a pregnancy by a legal abortion. They represented about 18.8% of all abortions in 2000, down from 21% in 1991. Young Caucasian women above 20 years report abortions at slightly higher rates than African Americans and other ethnic groups at 19%, compared to 17.5% and 18%, respectively.[3]

An analysis by the Alan Guttmacher Institute attributes the decline in pregnancies to increased abstinence among teenagers, and the increased use of contraceptives in general, and most specifically, the use of long-acting hormonal methods among sexually active adolescents (Chap. 25). The improvement in the U.S. rates of teen pregnancy still pales when compared to low rates in other industrialized countries. For example, the U.S. rate is twice those in Canada and Great Britain, and almost four times those in France and Sweden.[4]

FACTORS ASSOCIATED WITH TEEN PREGNANCY AND CHILDBEARING

Adolescents who become pregnant are impacted upon by multiple factors ranging from policy and environmental influences to family and individual factors (Chap. 22). Some of the factors protect against unintended early pregnancy, while other increase the risk. In industrialized countries with lower adolescent birth rates, cultural norms for adolescent sexuality, and policies supporting access to protection against sexually transmitted infections and pregnancy, adolescents use hormonal contraceptives and condoms at higher rates.

In the United States, states with fewer restrictions on contraceptive access and more coordinated programs addressing teen pregnancy, demonstrate a protective effect in ameliorating the risks

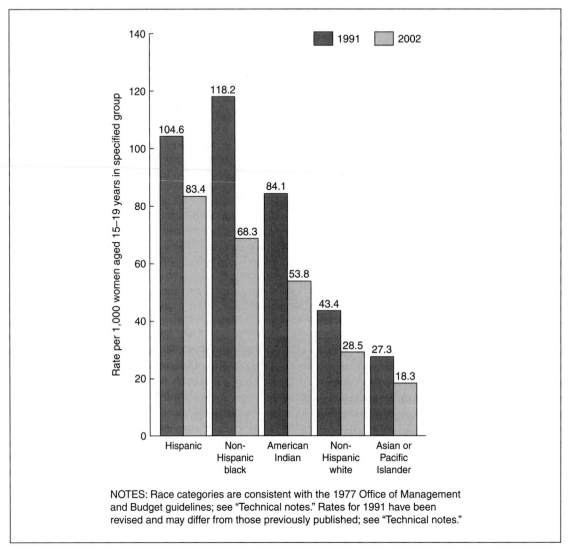

FIGURE 26-1
BIRTH RATES FOR TEENAGERS BY RACE AND/OR HISPANIC ORIGIN FOR 1991 AND 2002.
Source: Martin JA, Hamilton BE, Sutton PD, et al. Births: final data for 2002. Natl Vital Stat Rep 2003;52(10).

associated with teen births. Schools with programs designed to increase school attachment and reduce school dropout, demonstrate effects in delaying the onset of sexual initiation and reducing teen pregnancy, even when the program's intent is not directed toward sexual behavior outcomes. In spite of these protective factors, poverty, disorganized schools, poor school performance, and families with prior histories of teen childbearing, still have a negative differential impact in placing young people on the path to adolescent childbearing.[5] Hispanic and African American youths are more likely to face such factors, and have higher rates of adolescent childbearing than their Caucasian peers.

PREVENTION STRATEGIES

Prevention strategies are based on clinical approaches and community/school-based approaches. Given the broad multifaceted factors associated with teen pregnancy, these strategies should be implemented simultaneously. In the clinical setting, the identification of the sexually active adolescent through a confidential interview is the initial step in a clinical intervention aimed at providing factual, balanced, and realistic information to the adolescent and guiding her/him through the decision-making process in selecting an appropriate contraceptive (Chaps. 2, 3, 22, and 25). The clinical setting also provides the opportunity to reinforce the behavior of adolescents remaining abstinent and encourage them to continue to do so.

Program interventions that have demonstrated efficacy were reviewed in a monograph, "Emerging Answers", distributed by the National Campaign to Prevent Teen Pregnancy. Their review identified three types of programs: (1) those that address the sexual antecedents of sexual risk taking, (2) those that address nonsexual antecedents (i.e., service learning programs), and (3) those addressing both groups of antecedents.[5] The selected points in their findings are listed in Table 26-1. Youth development programs addressing social and psychologic skills in children through their youth, coupled with a multilevel intervention with the key adults, have demonstrated an impact on reducing adolescent pregnancy rates.

CLINICAL PRESENTATIONS AND DIAGNOSIS

Common Presentations

Every clinician who cares for an adolescent female, irrespective of the nature of the practice or specialty, should raise the question: "Is she sexually active?" When there are any aberrations in menses or report of unprotected intercourse, the provider should also consider the diagnosis of pregnancy. The diagnosis of pregnancy is ordinarily very easy to establish, provided there is an index of suspicion and the appropriate test is performed. In some circumstances, particularly when adolescents are in denial or fear for loss of confidentiality, they may present with vague complaints such as abdominal pain or weight gain.

TABLE 26-1

RESEARCH FINDINGS ON PROGRAMS TO REDUCE TEEN PREGNANCY[5]

Both the studies of antecedents and the evaluations of programs indicate that there are no single, simple approaches that will dramatically reduce adolescent pregnancy across the country.

Abstinence and use of contraception are compatible goals and topics.

Relatively little is known about the impact of programs that stress abstinence as the only acceptable behavior for unmarried teens.

Studies of some sex and HIV education programs have produced credible evidence that they reduce sexual-risk-taking either by delaying the onset of sex, reducing the frequency of sex, and reducing the number of sexual partners, or by increasing the use of condoms or other forms of contraception.

Family planning clinics probably prevent a large number of teen pregnancies, although there is remarkably little evidence to support this common sense view.

Several studies have consistently indicated that when clinics provide improved educational materials, discuss the adolescent patient's sexual and condom or contraceptive behavior, and incorporate other components into the clinic visit, clinics can increase condom or contraceptive use, although not always for a prolonged period of time.

School-based and school-linked clinics and school's condom-availability programs do not increase sexual activity, but it is not clear whether they increase condom and contraceptive use.

Generally, however, the adolescent is aware of the likelihood or at least the possibility of pregnancy before presenting to the clinical setting. Data from the 1995 National Survey of Family Growth indicate that 16% of sexually active girls of 15–19 years had visited a family planning clinic or physician for a pregnancy test in the previous 12 months.[6] In fact, for many teens, the precipitating reason for making the first visit to a family planning clinic is pregnancy testing. Data by Zabin et al. demonstrated that 37% of teenage clinic patients reported the need for a pregnancy test as the precipitating reason for a first clinic visit.[7] Adolescents may be more likely to use family planning clinics for pregnancy tests because of the cost of over-the-counter tests and to avoid care with a private provider through their parents' insurance. In a convenient sample of about 3000 adolescents from 52 clinics presenting for a pregnancy test, 36% of tests were positive.[8] Clinicians need to realize that the majority of adolescents will have negative pregnancy test results, and this serves as an opportunity to educate as well as initiate more effective hormonal contraceptive methods (Chap. 25).

The diagnosis of pregnancy can be established by detection of human chorionic gonadotropin (hCG) in the urine or blood. hCG is a glycoprotein hormone, produced by the syncytiotrophoblast in the developing placenta. The production of hCG in the trophoblast begins very early with implantation and can be detected by 8 or 9 days after ovulation. Most commercially available urine pregnancy tests, both for home and clinical use, utilize antibodies to the hCG molecule and have high accuracy rates. These tests detect hCG in a urine specimen containing 25 mIU/mL hCG or more, and generally will be positive on the day of a missed period. Evaluation of blood hCG levels should be done in women with abnormal bleeding or clinical situations when it is necessary to exclude the possibility of abnormal intrauterine or ectopic pregnancy. The blood hCG level is less than 3 mIU/mL in the absence of pregnancy.

Physical Examination

During the first few weeks of pregnancy, the increase in size of the uterus is minimal; at about 6–8 weeks after the first day of the last menstrual period, the uterus becomes slightly enlarged and globular. By 12 weeks of gestation, the uterus can be palpated as a soft pelvic structure measuring about 8 cm. It is not until 12 weeks that the uterus can be palpated above the pubic symphysis as an abdominal organ.[9] Thereafter, gestational weeks can be estimated by measuring the height of the uterine fundus above the symphysis in centimeters.

Determining Gestational Age

In addition to calculation of gestation age by weeks since the first day of the last menstrual period, gestational age can be estimated using a number of methods. A normal intrauterine pregnancy may be demonstrated by vaginal ultrasonography at about 4–5 weeks after the first day of the last menstrual period. A gestation sac should be visible at this time when the blood hCG level is about 1500–2000 mIU/mL. Ultrasound dating performed within the first half of pregnancy is accurate within 10 days.[10] Pregnancy dating can also be estimated by auscultation of the fetal heart. The heartbeat can be detected by auscultation with fetal echo Doppler generally by the 10th week of gestation and by the 17th week with a stethoscope.[9]

PREGNANCY COUNSELING

Once the diagnosis of a pregnancy is confirmed, the adolescent needs to be counseled about her decision to continue or legally terminate the pregnancy. The decision of whether to continue the pregnancy and place the baby for adoption is not immediate. The gestational staging of the pregnancy is a key determinant of the options available to the adolescent. The options are often limited when the pregnancy has progressed beyond 16 weeks or reached the acceptable limits for abortion service providers accessible in the community. The context of counseling should be supportive and nonjudgmental with the purpose of giving the adolescent complete information in order to make an informed decision (Chap. 2). The adolescent should have the option of voluntarily involving a responsible adult or partner and should be encouraged to do so. Confidentiality, however, should be protected for adolescents during the decision-making counseling process (Chaps. 2 and 3).

Important background information that helps to guide the process include (1) whether the pregnancy was intended or unintended, (2) the presence of a chronic medical condition (i.e., diabetes, sickle cell disease, cardiac disease, and others), developmental disability, or psychiatric diagnosis, (3) the age and status of the partner, (4) the presence of lifestyle risks (i.e., smoking, illicit drugs, and others), (5) family context and anticipated support, and (6) the evaluation for sexually transmissible infections as a result of unprotected intercourse (Chap. 24).[11]

The adolescent's response to the pregnancy, whether definitive or ambivalent, is often related to whether the pregnancy was intended or unintended. Counseling should not proceed with the assumption that adolescent pregnancy is always unintended. The age and status of the partner is most critical in counseling. Early adolescents may be victims of sexual abuse or statutory rape (Chap. 23). Statutory rape laws and reporting requirements vary by state and should be known to the health professional providing the counseling. Conversely, older adolescents may be in stable, supportive, or cohabitation relationships. Anticipation of a negative or positive family response can vary by whether the pregnancy was intended or unintended. Unintended pregnancies are most often associated with negative responses from parents and partners. Parent or sibling patterns of early childbearing may be associated with more acceptance and support from family members.[12]

Follow-up after the initial counseling session is the key to confirm that the adolescent has implemented the decision made at the time of counseling. Up to 20% of adolescents may delay the first prenatal visit for up to 4 months. Legal access and financial barriers may delay the adolescent's abortion choice. Over one-third of adolescents remain ambivalent after the initial counseling and feel that they need more time to make a decision.[13] The younger, less mature adolescent needs to identify an adult support person by the end of the initial session

with whom one can maintain contact, ensuring that the adolescent is not "lost to follow-up" because of any of these barriers; such barriers include the fear to communicate her pregnancy status resulting in a delay in medical care.

MEDICAL MANAGEMENT OF THE PREGNANT ADOLESCENT

The objective of prenatal care is to improve the health and well-being of the mother and unborn fetus by dealing with medical, psychologic, social, and environmental variables that affect health.[9] As the majority of adolescent pregnancies are unintended and unplanned, few adolescents are afforded the benefits of preconception counseling. The pregnant adolescent should be seen at routine intervals ranging from 1 to 4 weeks, based on the needs of the teen and gestational age, with shorter intervals later in the pregnancy. In addition to routine, indicated tests, and procedures recommended by the American College of Obstetricians and Gynecologists (Table 26-2), adolescents should receive developmentally appropriate and comprehensive services targeted toward the psychosocial needs of adolescents (Chaps. 2 and 3).[14] Ideally this care should be provided by a multidisciplinary team of providers including physicians and/or midwives, nutritionists, and social workers. In addition to potential medical complications, antenatal care should address critical psychosocial issues including support systems, preparation for parenting, school retention, postpartum nursing, and contraception (Chap. 25).

Complications

In the developing world, where a third of women give birth before the age of 20, complications from pregnancy and childbirth are the leading causes of death in young women aged 15–19.[15] In contrast, while adolescent childbearing in the United States is associated with poorer pregnancy outcomes, this is largely related to the social, economic, and behavioral factors that predispose some young women to pregnancy.[16] The risk of having a medical

TABLE 26-2

RECOMMENDED TESTS DURING PRENATAL CARE[14]

Gestational Age (weeks)	Assessment
Initial (6–8 weeks)	Hematocrit or hemoglobin levels
	Hemoglobin electrophoresis (risk based*)
	Urinalysis and urine culture
	Blood group, Rh type, and antibody screen
	Rubella antibody titer
	Syphilis screen
	Cervical cytology (if sexually active >3 years)
	Hepatitis B screen
	Chlamydia and gonorrhea testing
	Human immunodeficiency virus antibody testing
16–18 weeks	Maternal serum marker screening
16–20 weeks	Ultrasound (risk based*)
26–28 weeks	Diabetes screening (risk based*)
28 weeks	Repeat antibody test for unsensitized Rh-negative patients
	Prophylactic administration of Rho (D) immune globulin
32–36 weeks	Repeat testing for sexually transmitted diseases
36–37 weeks	Genital culture for group B *Streptococcus*

*Testing indicated by physical examination, personal or family history indicating increased risk.

condition during pregnancy does differ by maternal age. For example, teenage mothers are nearly twice as likely to have anemia during pregnancy compared with women aged 40 and above (36 compared with 19.8 per 1000). Older mothers, conversely, are more prone to chronic conditions; these disorders include diabetes (71.7 for mothers 40 years and over compared with 9.2 for mothers under 20); chronic hypertension (25 compared with 2.9); and cardiac disease (9.5 compared with 2.7). Some risk factors, such as pregnancy-associated hypertension, however, follow a U-shaped pattern with the highest levels at the extremes of the maternal age distribution.[17]

Adolescent childbearing is also associated with unfavorable pregnancy outcomes, including low birth weight (LBW) infants, preterm delivery, small for gestational age, and maternal and prenatal deaths.[18] As a mother's age increases, the frequency of LBW infants decreases progressively in all racial groups. A logistic regression analysis of 54,447 linked birth certificates in California from 1980 to 1987 found that younger teenage mothers were 3.4 times more likely to deliver preterm compared with women in their twenties.[19] Where adverse effects of teenage pregnancy exist, they are more prominent in the younger teenagers compared to older teenagers, who differ very little from adults.[20,21] Several investigators have compared adolescent (≤19 years) to adult mothers in an attempt to clarify the risk factors associated with adverse pregnancy outcomes in adolescents.[22,23] Teenage pregnancy is strongly associated with a large number of social, economic, educational, and behavioral factors. The complex interaction of these effects on teenage pregnancy is still poorly understood. Furthermore, these socioeconomic and behavioral factors associated with becoming pregnant as a teenager, are independently associated with adverse obstetric and neonatal outcomes.[24]

PREGNANCY TERMINATION

While unintended pregnancy is a universal problem in the United States, cutting across all ages and classes of women of reproductive age, it occurs disproportionately in adolescents. Approximately 78% of pregnancies to adolescents are unintended and about half of these pregnancies end in abortion.[25] Whether these pregnancies end in abortion or unintended births, they pose a significant personal, social, and economic burden.

Surgical Abortion

Since the 1973 Supreme Court decision that made abortion legal, abortion has become one of the most common surgical procedures performed in the United States.[25,26] Since legalization, mortality, and morbidity from abortions has declined dramatically, making complications from abortion less common than those from childbirth. More than half (58%) of reported legal induced abortions were performed during the first 8 weeks of pregnancy; 88% were performed during the first 12 weeks of pregnancy. Adolescents are slightly more likely to present at later gestations for pregnancy termination. In 1998 and 1999, the most recent data are available, where a total of 14 maternal deaths related to legal induced abortion were reported, for a rate of approximately 0.6 deaths per 100,000 abortions.[27,28]

After appropriate counseling and informed consent is obtained, first trimester procedures can be completed in 1 day with oral analgesics or conscious sedation. Dilation of cervix is achieved using laminaria or mechanical dilation with Pratt-type dilators. The uterus is then evacuated using either electrical or manual vacuum aspiration. Potential complications include infection, injury to the uterus (perforation), and hemorrhage. Major complications requiring further surgical intervention occur less than 1% of the time and are directly correlated with advancing gestational age.[26] Second trimester procedures are generally performed over the course of 1–2 days, allowing for slow cervical dilation either with laminaria or chemical ripening agents such as misoprostol.

Medical Abortion

Medical abortion is an abortion that is induced by taking medications that will end a pregnancy. A medical abortion is done without entering the uterus. Usually mifepristone, previously known by its abbreviated company code name "RU 486," a progesterone antagonist, is used together with another medication, misoprostol. Since progesterone is essential to early human pregnancy, mifepristone has abortifacient properties. Methotrexate, an antimetabolite, used in cancer therapies, is toxic to rapidly dividing cells including the trophoblast, and can be used instead of mifepristone. Prostaglandins are fatty acid derivatives with uterotonic and cervical ripening properties. Misoprostol, the synthetic

prostaglandin of choice in the United States, is taken a few days after mifepristone or methotrexate, and causes uterine contractions and expulsion of the uterine contents.

Medical abortions can be performed up to 9 weeks (63 days) from the first day of the last menstrual period.[29] A medical provider must confirm the pregnancy and determine the exact gestational age using ultrasonography. Medical abortion can take anywhere within 3 days to 3 weeks and requires several visits to a clinic or doctor's office. With mifepristone, 95%–97% of women will abort within 2 weeks. About 1 in 20 women who have a medical abortion will not spontaneously expel the uterine contents and will need to have a surgical procedure (dilation and curettage) to complete the abortion.[29]

The advantages of medical abortion for the adolescent are:

It can be performed as soon as a pregnancy is identified by ultrasound (4–5 weeks).
It avoids surgical and anesthetic risk.
It is psychologically preferable to women for reasons that include greater autonomy and privacy; also it is perceived as being more natural.

However, because of the small risk of incomplete abortion with vaginal hemorrhage, a woman having a medical abortion must have access to acute emergency care. For this reason, adolescents with transportation or confidentiality concerns may not be suitable candidates for medical abortion. Adverse effects include side effects from the medications, i.e., vomiting, diarrhea, fever/chills, potential teratogenicity after an incomplete procedure, infection, and heavy bleeding.

ADOPTION

Estimating the proportion of adolescents who relinquish the care of their children through adoption is difficult. National formal adoption statistics ceased being collected in 1992, leaving the National Survey of Family Growth (NSFG) as the only source of a nationally representative sample collecting information on adoption. Prior to 1982, the NSFG only collected data on ever married women, thus limiting the ability to gather data on adolescent women. Data on older women, 18–44 years old, between 1989 and 1995, show very little evidence that relinquishing an infant for adoption is common, with less than 1% of African American and 1.7% of Caucasian never married women placing their babies for adoption.[30] Informal adoption by real or fictive kin remains a common yet untracked option for African American adolescents, further obscuring any opportunity to reliably estimate infants born to adolescents who are cared for by others.

Older studies on the impact of adolescents relinquishing their infants fail to show any consistently adverse outcomes of this choice. There are some evidence of transient psychologic trauma; but most of the small, nonrepresentative studies show that adolescents who give up their infants are more likely to complete their education, become employed, and delay a second pregnancy, when compared to adolescents who chose to parent. [31,32] Today, alternatives such as kinship adoption and open adoption, in which the adolescent plays a more active role in determining the adoptive family, have yet to be studied with sufficient rigor to determine the impact on the adolescent or the infant. Adolescents who may be interested in adoption should be referred to trained counselors at crisis pregnancy centers, family planning clinics, or adoption agencies for several counseling sessions prior to making a decision.

ADOLESCENT PARENTING

Confidentiality and Legal Rights of Minors

Confidentiality of care is at the crux of the provision of reproductive care to adolescents and it is determined by the individual rendering the care (Chap. 3 and 25).[33] On the other hand, a minor's right to consent for health care is determined by state statutes for reproductive services, such as pregnancy diagnosis, prenatal care, and abortion services. States also govern statutes that allow a minor to consent for their child's care or to place the child for adoption. Statutes governing the right to an abortion are the most restrictive and variable, while those allowing a minor to consent to the pregnancy diagnosis and prenatal care are the most liberal and consistent across states. Only 2 states and the District of Columbia allow a minor to consent for an abortion, while 31 states mandate parental involvement, 16 of those requiring consent, and 15 requiring that the parent(s) be notified prior to the abortion. Several of the parental involvement states allow a judicial bypass, where a judge can give authorization for an abortion without informing the parent(s). None of the states require parental consent for prenatal care, and only five require parental consent to place a child for adoption.[34]

Psychosocial Outcomes for Adolescent Mothers

The adverse psychosocial outcomes for young adolescents who bear children can have long-term effects on family formation. Younger teens are more likely to remain single parents, and if they do not return to school, the lack of education results in poor employment opportunities and consequent poverty. Repeated pregnancies occur in 35% of the adolescents within 2 years of the first pregnancy, with almost 20% of those adolescents bearing a second child as a result of the pregnancy. Early repeated pregnancies occur more frequently if the adolescent mother fails to return to school within 6 months, if she marries or lives with the male partner, and if her mother provides major child care assistance.[35]

In addition to the medical complications of pregnancy, adolescent pregnancy is closely linked to a host of other critical poor outcomes for the mother and the child; these factors include out-of-wedlock births, high school dropout, welfare dependency, poor school performance for the child, and higher rates of child abuse and neglect.[24]

Adolescent Males and Pregnancy Issues

Young men below 20 years account for approximately 35% of the males who are fathers to babies of adolescent mothers. Since the highest birth rate occurs in 18–19 years old adolescents, the traditional

2–3 years age difference between partners would place most fathers older than 20 years of age. In younger mothers, aged 15–17 years, about 27% of the male partners are 5 or more years older than their partners. Nonetheless, these young adult males still carry economic and educational disadvantages, which impact on the adolescent mother and her infant's psychosocial status.[36]

Most of the risk factors for young fathers are extensions of the vulnerabilities preceding the pregnancy and not an impact of the pregnancy alone. In a survey, young men who acknowledged causing a pregnancy, also acknowledged multiple sexual partners, a history of a sexually transmitted disease, and the use of an illegal substance. Compared to their peers, young men who become fathers are more likely to be 1–2 years behind in school, be high school dropouts, and have higher rates of involvement in illegal activities. The lack of economic resources in these young men translates into continuing family poverty as an outcome in adolescent pregnancies.[36]

Infants of Adolescent Mothers

Young adolescent mothers generally lack the maturity and skills to provide optimal infant care. It is not unexpected that without strong social support, cognitive and social developmental deficits occur in children of adolescents that may persist into the child's adolescence. These young mothers often have unrealistic developmental expectations for their infants, compared to older mothers with similar backgrounds, and demonstrate fewer positive bonding behaviors. However, when social support is strong, young mothers adapt less punitive parenting methods. In addition, when biologic fathers are involved with their infants, long-term benefits accrue to them later in the form of better educational and employment outcomes, and less risk of becoming a teen parent themselves.

Reducing the Risks of Early Adolescent Parenting

The risks of early parenting can be reduced through programs focused on the adolescent family. The most consistently successful approaches are directed toward getting the adolescent mother to successfully complete her education. Returning to school is one of the strongest determinants of long-term success for the adolescent and her child. Comprehensive multidisciplinary programs emphasizing life skills, medical care, and psychosocial support are associated with higher employment, higher income, and less likelihood of becoming welfare dependent for those involved in the program compared to adolescent mothers not exposed to these programs.[35]

The goal of the public health approach to adolescent pregnancy is to continue reducing the rates of pregnancy and its adverse effects through sex education, prevention programs, and access to reproductive health services.[37,38] When a birth occurs, a support program to reduce negative family outcomes, and to delay a second pregnancy is the next level of intervention. The fundamental objective following a birth is to improve the life course for the adolescent mother, father, and the infant.

Bibliography

1. Martin JA, Hamilton BE, Sutton PD, et al. Births: final data for 2002. Natl Vital Stat Rep 2003; 52(10):1–113.
2. Papillo AR, Frenzett K, Manlove J, et al.: Child Trends. Facts at a glance. 2003:1–6.
3. Elan-Evans LD, Strauss Lt, Herndon J, et al. Abortion Surveillance U.S. 2000. MMWR 2003; 52(SS12):1–32.
4. Alan Guttmacher Institute. Teen pregnancy: trends and lessons learned. Issues in Brief 2002;(1):1–4.
5. Kirby D. *Emerging answers: Research Findings on Programs to Reduce Teen Pregnancy*. Washington, DC: National Campaign to Prevent Teen Pregnancy, 2001.
6. Abma JC, Chandra A, Mosher WD, Peterson LS, Piccinino LJ. Fertility, family planning, and women's health: New data from the 1995 National Survey of Family Growth. Vital Health Stat 1997;23:1–114.
7. Zabin LS, Clark SD. Why they delay: A study of teenage family planning clinic clients. Fam Plann Perspect 1981;13:205–217.
8. Zabin LS, Emerson MR, Ringers PA, Sedivy V. Adolescents with negative pregnancy test results, an accessible at-risk group. JAMA 1996;275:113–117.
9. Cunningham FG. *Williams Obstetrics*, 21st ed. New York: McGraw-Hill, 2001.

10. P, Hiilesmaa V. Predicting delivery date by ultrasound and last menstrual period in early gestation. Obstet Gynecol 2001;97:189–194.

11. American Academy of Pediatrics: Committee on Adolescence. Counseling the adolescent about pregnancy options. Pediatrics 1998;101(5): 938–940.

12. Alan Guttmacher Institute. Teenagers' Pregnancy Intentions and Decisions: A Study of Young Women in California Choosing to Give Birth, 1999.

13. Polaneczky M, O'Connor K. Pregnancy in the adolescent patient. Pediatr Clin No Amer 1999;46(4): 649–670.

14. American College of Obstetrics and Gynecology: Guidelines for Perinatal Care, 5th ed. Committee on Obstetrics, 2002.

15. Mayor S. Pregnancy and childbirth are leading causes of death in teenage girls in developing countries. Br Med J 2004;328:1152.

16. Cunnington AJ. What's so bad about teenage pregnancy? J Fam Plann Reprod Health Care 2001;27: 36–41.

17. Martin JA, Hamilton BE, Ventura SJ, Menacker F, Park MM, Sutton PD. Births: Final data for 2001. Natl Vital Stat Rep 2002;18:1–102.

18. Fraser AM, Brockert JE, Ward RH. Association of young maternal age with adverse reproductive outcomes. N Engl J Med 1995;332:1113–1117.

19. Maynard RA (ed.). *Kids Having Kids: A Robin Hood Foundation Special Report on the Costs of Adolescent Childbearing*. New York: The Robin Hood Foundation, 1996.

20. DuPlessis HM, Bell R, Richards T. Adolescent pregnancy: Understanding the impact of age and race on outcomes. J Adolesc Health 1997;20: 187–197.

21. Scholl TO, Hediger ML, Belsky DH. Prenatal care and maternal health during adolescent pregnancy: A review and meta-analysis. J Adolesc Health 1994;15: 444–456.

22. Scholl TO, Miller LK, Salmon RW, Cofsky MC, Shearer J. Prenatal care adequacy and the outcome of adolescent pregnancy: Effects on weight gain, preterm delivery, and birth weight. Obstet Gynecol 1987;69:312–316.

23. Blankson ML, Cliver SP, Goldenberg RL, Hickey CA, Jin J, Dubard MB. Health behavior and outcomes in sequential pregnancies of black and white adolescents. JAMA 1993;269:1401–1403.

24. The National Campaign to Prevent Teen Pregnancy. *Not Just another Single Issue: Teen Pregnancy Prevention's Link to Other Critical Social Issues*. Washington, DC, 2001.

25. Henshaw S. Unintended pregnancy in the United States. Fam Plann Perspect 1998;30:24–29.

26. Darney PD. *Protocols for Office Gynecologic Surgery*. Cambridge, MA: Blackwell Science, 1996.

27. Trussell J, Leveque JA, Koenig JD, et al. The economic value of contraception: A comparison of 15 methods. Am J Public health 1995;85:494–503.

28. Centers for Disease Control and Prevention. Surveillance Summaries. MMWR 2003;52(SS-12).

29. Spitz IM, Bardin CW, Benton L, Robbins A. Early pregnancy termination with mifepristone and misoprostol in the United States. N Engl J Med 1998;338: 1241–1247.

30. Chandra A, Abma J, Maza, Bachrach C. Adoption, adoption seeking, and relinquishment for adoption in the Unites States. Adv Data 1999;11(306):1–16.

31. Donnelly BW, Voydanoff P. Parenting versus placing for adoption: Consequences for adolescent mothers. Fam Relat 1996;45(4):427–434.

32. McLaughlin SD, Manninen DL, Winges LD. Do adolescents who relinquish their children fare better or worse than those who raise them? Fam Plann Perspect 1988;20(1):25–32.

33. Ford C, English A, Sigman G. Confidential health care for adolescents: Position paper of the Society for Adolescent Medicine. J Adolesc Health 2004;35: 160–167.

34. Boonstra H, Nash E. Minors and the right to consent to health care. The Guttmacher Report on Public Policy, 2000;3(4). Available at: *www.guttmacher.org/ pubs/journals/gr030404.html*.

35. American Academy of Pediatrics, Committee on Adolescents and Committee on Early Childhood Adoption, and Dependent Care, 2001, Vol. 1072, pp. 429–434, 2002.

36. Elfenbein DS, Felice ME. Adolescent pregnancy. Pediatr Clin North Am. 2003;781–800.

37. Santelli JS, Abma J, Ventura S, et al. Can changes in sexual behaviors among high school students explain the decline in teen pregnancy rates in the 1990s? J Adolesc Health 2004;35:80–90.

38. Sonenstein FL. What teenagers are doing right: Changes in sexual behavior over the past decade. J Adolesc Health 2004;35:77–78.

27

BREAST DISORDERS

Paritosh Kaul and Roberta K. Beach

INTRODUCTION

Breast concerns are very common among adolescents, whether or not they mention them initially during the office visit. Breast budding heralds the onset of puberty and the anxieties that accompany adolescent development. In our culture, breasts are highly symbolic of femininity and sexuality. Adolescent boys may therefore be frightened by the temporary gynecomastia the majority of them experience. Adolescent girls typically worry about appearance and are concerned about breast size and shape. Breast cancer will affect one in seven adult women, and mothers may be anxious about genetic risk factors for their daughters.

Due to the frequency of breast masses, pain, and numerous common minor abnormalities, most of the adolescents in a primary care provider's practice will have breast concerns at some point. Sensitive treatment of breast problems is an excellent chance to establish trust and rapport with adolescent patients and to offer reassurance and support that will extend into many other areas of health promotion. While the majority of adolescent breast concerns will prove benign, some are pathologic and require a diagnostic evaluation. This chapter will review the essentials of the breast examination and discuss breast issues and disorders seen in primary care clinical settings.

ANATOMY AND ENDOCRINOLOGY

Anatomy of the Breast

Breasts are modified, milk-producing apocrine glands, which lie over the anterior chest wall and pectoralis major muscle from the second to the sixth intercostal space (Fig. 27-1). Each breast consists of 15–20 wedge-shaped lobes and excretory ducts, each of which open into the nipple. These lobes in turn consist of 10–100 alveoli, which are the structural units of the breast. The lobes are surrounded by dense fatty connective tissue, which gives the breast its smooth contour. Fibrous bands called Cooper's ligaments extend from the skin to the underlying pectoralis muscle and provide some support to the breast. Laterally from the upper outer quadrant the breast extends into the axilla in a long portion called the axillary tail of Spence (see Fig. 27-2). During pubertal growth and pregnancy this tissue may enlarge and mimic an axillary tumor that then resolves once the physiologic hormonal surge abates. Toward the center of the breast is the darkened areola that contains sebaceous glands called Montgomery tubercles. The nipples extend above the areola containing the minute openings of the lactiferous ducts. The breast develops in the sixth week of intrauterine life as an ectodermal thickening bilaterally along what is known as the "nipple line" or

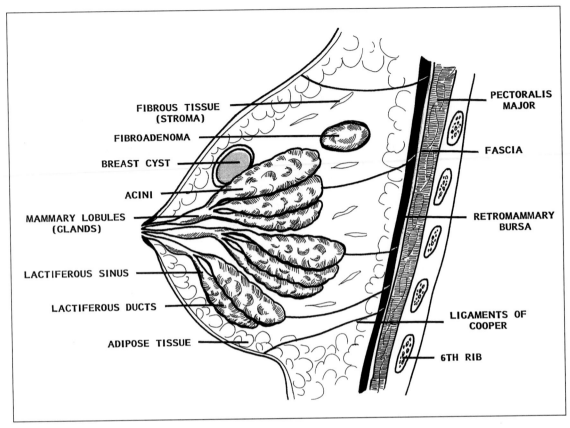

FIGURE 27-1

INTERNAL ANATOMY OF THE BREAST (SAGITTAL VIEW).

Source: Reprinted from Beach RK: Breast disorders. In: McAnarney ER, et al. (eds.), *Textbook of Adolescent Medicine.* Philadelphia, PA: W.B. Saunders, 1992.

"milk line" from the axilla to the groin, though at birth only the two breasts at the mammary ridge develop. The male breast is similar to the female in structure and development until puberty, when further growth stops in the absence of hormone stimulation.

Endocrinology of the Breast

The physiologic development of the breast occurs during two stages, puberty and pregnancy, under the influence of various hormones (see Fig. 27-3). During puberty, estrogen secretion results in increase in adipose tissue and stromal growth in the breast. Progesterone influences the growth of the alveolar components of the lobule resulting in lobular growth, alveolar budding, and alveolar secretory development. Other important hormones for optimum breast development include prolactin, growth hormone, insulin, cortisol, and thyroxine. Prolactin plays a pivotal role in normal production of breast milk. It is secreted by the lactotroph cells of the anterior pituitary. These cells are under dual control of the hypothalamus through the hypothalamic-pituitary portal circulation. Prolactin is stimulated by hypothalamic hormone thyrotropin-releasing hormone. The predominant signal from the hypothalamus is inhibitory and is mediated by the neurotransmitter dopamine. Stress, sucking, sexual stimulation, and dehydration also stimulate prolactin secretion. Medications that block the dopamine pathway or cause depletion of catecholamines result in stimulation of low levels of prolactin and can lead to galactorrhea.

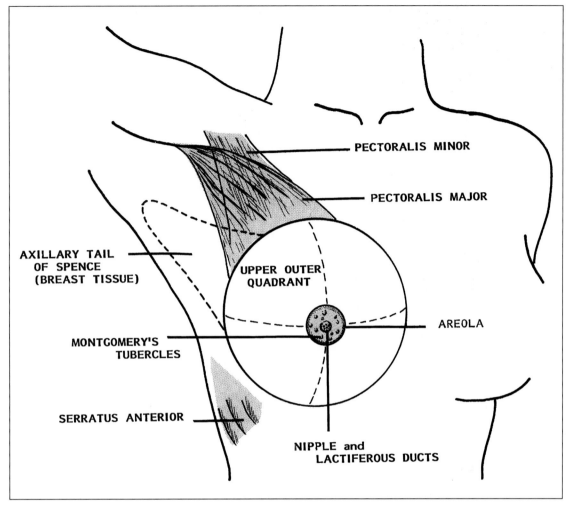

FIGURE 27-2

EXTERNAL ANATOMY OF THE BREAST WITH MAJOR MUSCLES AND AXILLARY TAIL OF SPENCE.

Source: Reprinted from Beach RK: Breast disorders. In: McAnarney ER, et al. (eds.), *Textbook of Adolescent Medicine.* Philadelphia, PA: W.B. Saunders, 1992.

BREAST EXAMINATION

Thelarche is the term used to describe the onset of breast development and is usually the first sign of puberty in girls (Chap. 1). The average age at thelarche has decreased slightly in the last decade in the United States to 9.6 with a range of 7–13 years for 99% of the population (Kaplowitz and Oberfield, 1999). Examination of the breasts should begin at the time of thelarche, which can also serve as anticipatory guidance for sexual development for both the teen and her parents. Thelarche is a good reminder for the clinician to check for scoliosis since the teen will begin her growth spurt within a year.

Before examining the patient, the clinician should obtain a thorough history including breast symptoms, family history of breast disease, menstrual history, substance abuse history, medications the adolescent is currently taking, and specific past

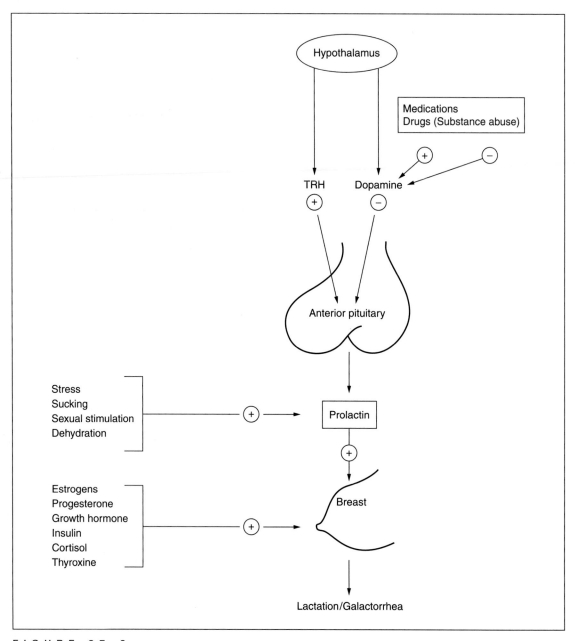

FIGURE 27-3

ENDOCRINOLOGY OF LACTATION AND GALACTORRHEA.

local risk factors like chest surgery and radiation. It is very important to be sensitive to the anxious young patient and appreciate concerns a teen girl might have regarding the examination of the breast. These issues are magnified when the clinician is a male and a chaperone (who might be the teen's mother) should be present during the physical examination in those circumstances. Giving the patient a gown, drape, privacy to change, and a brief explanation of the examination process and its importance are simple but effective methods to reassure the teenager (Chap. 2).

Technique of Breast Examination

Routine examination of an asymptomatic adolescent can be performed with the patient in the supine position. After inspection, the teen places her arm under her head while the examiner palpates the breast on that side. Palpation is performed with the fat pads of the clinician's middle three fingers using firm but gentle pressure. Several methods have been described to palpate from the sternum to the axilla (see Fig. 27-4). They include palpating in concentric circles from outer or inner margins, dividing the breast into spokes of a wheel and palpating along each spoke, or palpating as either horizontal or vertical strips (often the preferred method). The axilla is palpated in each case. The examiner then presses the nipple to detect masses or discharge.

Sexual maturity rating (SMR), developed by British anthropologist JM Tanner in 1962, is used to classify the stage of breast development and is noted on the chart. (The SMR stages are discussed in Chap. 2 on Growth and Development and the section on precocious puberty in Chap. 15 on Endocrinology.) The size of the areola is race dependent and does not form part of the SMR. The breast should be inspected for symmetry, size, shape, and skin findings. Palpation detects breast masses, inflammatory lesions, and lymph node enlargement. Any abnormalities should be documented verbally and visually (words and diagrams) in the patient medical record. Minor anomalies and normal variations should be discussed with the teen even if she has not openly expressed concern about these issues.

Teaching Breast Self-Examination

Teaching routine breast self-examination (BSE) in teens is debatable for various reasons. The incidence of breast cancer in adolescents is rare. BSE takes time to teach, requires specific techniques to be effective, and needs to be reviewed yearly to ensure that the skills are not lost. The heightened anxiety and attention may result in increased use of health care visits and surgical biopsies. The same

amount of time could be spent in counseling the teen about high-risk behaviors that cause more morbidity and mortality during adolescence. On the other hand, BSE opens the door to discussion of women's health issues, serves to increase comfort with the teenager's body, and the clinical examination of the breast. The decision to teach BSE is left to the caregiver and the specific circumstances of the individual teen and her family.

CONGENITAL AND DEVELOPMENTAL ANOMALIES OF THE BREAST

Polythelia and Polymastia (Accessory Breast Tissue)

Polythelia is the presence of supernumerary nipples and polymastia the presence of other accessory breast tissue. The typical finding is a small pigmented macule that may arise anywhere from the axilla to the thigh along the embryonic milk line and this occurs in 1%–2% of adolescents. These anomalies usually do not present clinical issues except transient enlargement during pregnancy and lactation. Occasionally, these conditions are associated with congenital syndromes and renal and cardiovascular abnormalities. Surgical removal is indicated for cosmetic reasons.

Amastia and Athelia (Absence of Breast Tissue)

The lack of either a breast (amastia) or a nipple (athelia) is a rare but disturbing congenital abnormality in an adolescent. Amastia is associated with other abnormalities of the chest wall, such as Poland syndrome, which includes aplasia of the pectoralis muscles, ipsilateral rib deformity, webbed fingers, and radial nerve palsy. Rarely is amastia due to past chest wall surgery or trauma in infancy or childhood that resulted in inadvertent removal of the breast bud.

Breast Asymmetry

Unequal rates of breast growth are normal and breast asymmetry is often seen during early puberty. The teen can be reassured that there is

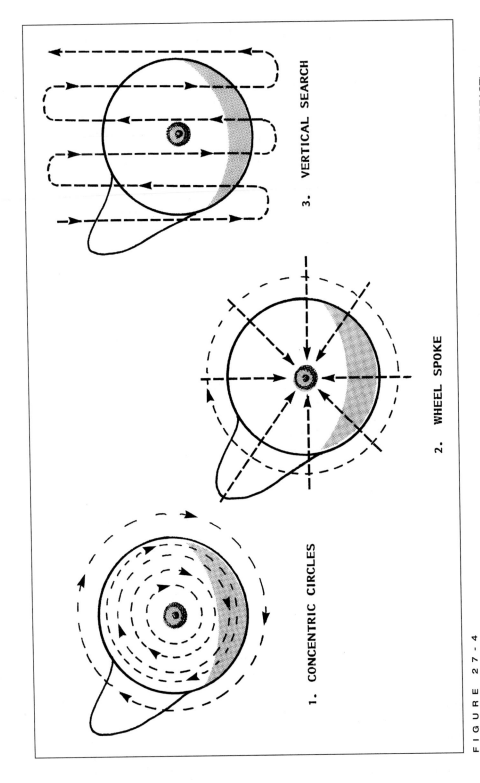

FIGURE 27-4
THREE METHODS OF PALPATION DURING BREAST EXAMINATION, INCLUDING THE AXILLARY TAIL (SHOWN ON RIGHT BREAST).
Source: Reprinted from Beach RK: Breast disorders. In: McAnarney ER, et al. (eds.), *Textbook of Adolescent Medicine*. Philadelphia, PA: W.B. Saunders, 1992.

good likelihood of catch-up growth and symmetry. However, almost 25% persist to be noticeably asymmetrical into adulthood. A careful examination should rule out asymmetry due to hypomastia, hypermastia, or a giant fibroadenoma. Corrective surgery is an option in cases of significant asymmetry. Surgical reduction or augmentation should be performed after completion of breast development (SMR 5) since earlier correction may result in inadvertent removal of normal breast tissue.

Tuberous Breast Deformity

Tuberous breast deformity occurs when the base of the breast is underdeveloped and the nipple-areola complex is overdeveloped giving the breast the appearance of a tuberous root. The glandular elements are present in the distended nipple-areola complex. Adolescents who have taken exogenous hormones for treatment of gonadal dysgenesis, premature ovarian failure, or abnormalities of gonadotropin-releasing hormone secretion may present with this type of deformity, but it may occur in patients in the absence of hormonal treatment. The condition can usually be managed conservatively with reassurance and counseling services. Cosmetic surgery is reserved for severe cases.

Areola Hair

Noticeable hairs growing around the areola are not uncommon and while disturbing to the teen, areola hair is a benign condition. It may be hereditary in some women. Repeated plucking can result in ingrown hairs and infection. The teen should be advised to clip the hair if she desires removal.

Hypomastia and Atrophy

There are no normal standards for breast size. Normal size is a function of societal norms. Final breast size is determined primarily by heredity. Small breast size is usually familial but can be indicative of other disease processes. Atrophy is caused by loss of both fat and glandular elements of the breast and is associated with weight loss, dieting, and eating disorders. Lack of development

could also be due to factors such as destruction of tissue by radiation therapy, inadvertent biopsy of a breast bud, gonadal dysgenesis, and endocrine disorders such as congenital or late-onset adrenal hyperplasia. Scleroderma may cause unilateral or localized breast atrophy. Small breast size is a cosmetic concern for many women due to perceived societal standards of feminine attractiveness. The commercial creams, supplements, and exercise programs that adolescent girls see advertised have no proven effectiveness in increasing bust size. Augmentation mammoplasty with silicone gel implants should be delayed till breast maturation (SMR 5) is reached and after legal age of consent. Complications, poor cosmetic outcomes, and issues regarding breastfeeding should be discussed in detail with the patient prior to such procedures.

Macromastia

Increased breast size or macromastia is usually familial and is also related to obesity. It is associated with symptoms of fungal intertrigo, back pain, shoulder grooving, and postural problems. Adolescents report significant psychological distress due to macromastia. Surgical correction is achieved by reduction mammoplasty. Follow-up studies evaluating symptoms and activity levels after reduction surgery have found improved outcomes.

Virginal or Juvenile Hypertrophy

Virginal or juvenile hypertrophy is a significant diffuse enlargement of the breast, usually symmetrical, occurring around the time of menarche. The etiology of this condition is not clearly understood but it is thought to be an abnormal response of the breast to estrogen. The hormonal levels in these patients are normal. The condition can also occur during pregnancy, with exogenous hormones, androgens, corticosteroids, and insulin. There is sudden explosive enlargement of the breast. The adolescent may present with the symptoms seen with macromastia only much more severe. The accompanying psychological problems and anxiety can often be extreme.

Since the breast tissue does not regress conservative management is not an option. Treatment standards have not been determined and the patient is best referred for specialty care. Surgical options include reduction mammoplasty or subcutaneous mastectomy with prosthesis implantation. Hormonal treatments include medroxyprogesterone, dyhydrogesterone, or danazol, but all carry risks of significant side effects. The combination of surgical reduction mammoplasty followed by hormone suppression to prevent recurrences is another modality. Adolescent girls with this condition may suffer severe psychological trauma and should be offered continuing supportive psychotherapy.

GYNECOMASTIA

P.J., a 14-year-old middle-school student, comes to the school-based clinic for a sports physical. During the interview process he mentions that he has a painful swelling on his left breast that he discovered when he was in the shower. What could be the reasons for this swelling? What are some of the pertinent questions to ask this teen? What are the specific areas the clinician should observe during the physical examination? What studies should be ordered?

Gynecomastia, an increase in palpable subareolar breast tissue in males, affects up to 70% of adolescent boys and usually is physiological in etiology. It is often a source of distress to the teenager who might be shy in expressing his concern when he presents to the clinician. Breast disorders are usually associated with females, and hence it is important not to neglect this area when evaluating adolescent males. This condition occurs in the pubertal male during SMR 2 to 4 and peaks around 14 years of age. Gynecomastia that occurs prior to puberty or after complete pubertal development needs a meticulous evaluation for underlying endocrine etiology.

Pathophysiology

The male breast is similar to the prepubertal female breast both in its anatomy and its response to hormones. Estrogen stimulates breast tissue development while androgens antagonize these effects. The relative imbalance of estrogen and androgen activity at the level of the breast tissue leads to gynecomastia. Thus in the male teen, gynecomastia could occur due to a temporary increase in levels of estrogens, decrease in androgen production, or alterations with end-organ estrogen and androgen receptors.

Clinical Features

Our patient in the case vignette is often the classic presentation of gynecomastia in the adolescent. The teen has a unilateral tender breast lump found on breast self-examination. Typically the lump is painful at onset. The swelling may be unilateral or bilateral, and can present sequentially starting on one side first. The lump is rubbery or firm, mobile, subareolar in position and usually about 2–3 cm in diameter. In rare circumstances, the size may enlarge beyond the areola to resemble a small (SMR 3) breast and in very rare circumstances the patient may present with galactorrhea.

Differential Diagnosis

While most cases of gynecomastia are physiological, the differential diagnosis is given in Table 27-1. The significant pathological causes of gynecomastia, particularly if galactorrhea is present, are drugs and hormone producing tumors.

Diagnostic Evaluation

The clinician should document a thorough history including substance abuse or use of medications and any history suggestive of liver, testicular, renal, or thyroid disease. The breast examination is performed and should rule out pseudogynecomastia from fatty adipose tissue seen in overweight boys (no mobile mass will be palpable). A physical examination with particular attention to the above systems (thyroid, liver, and testes) is prudent. The primary care provider should also consider the possibility of endocrine disorders such as Klinefelter syndrome, primary testicular failure, and partial androgen sensitivity (Chaps. 15 and 21). No laboratory

DIFFERENTIAL DIAGNOSIS OF GYNECOMASTIA

1. **Physiologic gynecomastia**
2. **Pseudogynecomastia**
3. **Increased estrogen production**
   a. Increased estrogen secretion from tumors
      i. Testicular Leydig cell tumors
      ii. Adrenal tumors
   b. Increased activity of estrogen aromatase or estrogen bioavailability
      i. Systemic diseases (hyperthyroidism, liver disease, starvation)
      ii. Increased body fat (obesity)
      iii. Drugs (spironolactone, ketoconazole)
   c. Exogenous intake of estrogens
      i. Estrogen containing cosmetics
      ii. Estrogen containing foods
      iii. Oral contraceptive pills and other hormonal agents
4. **Decreased androgen production**
   a. Congenital decreased production of testosterone
      i. Primary hypogonadism (Klinefelter syndrome)
      ii. Secondary hypogonadism
   b. Acquired testicular failure
      i. Viral orchitis (mumps)
      ii. Trauma
      iii. Castration
      iv. Granulomatous disease
   c. Androgen resistance syndromes
   d. Renal disease and dialysis
   e. Drugs (ketoconazole, spironolactone, metronidazole, and cimetidine)
   f. hCG secreting tumors leading to reduction in testosterone biosynthesis (liver, kidney, lung cancer)
   g. Increased in SHBG which results in ↓ in free testosterone (liver disease)
5. **Alteration in estrogen and androgen receptors**
   a. Androgen receptor pathology (androgen insensitivity syndromes)
   b. Drugs interfering with androgen receptors (spironolactone, flutamide, and cimetidine)
   c. Drugs interfering with estrogen receptors (digoxin, phytoestrogens in some preparations of marijuana)
6. **Drugs with unknown mechanism of action**
   a. Substance abuse
      i. Marijuana
      ii. Heroin
   b. Psychiatric medications
      i. Antipsychotics
      ii. Tricyclic antidepressants
   c. GI medications
      i. Omeprazole
      ii. Metoclopramide
   d. Others
      i. Human growth hormone
      ii. Antiretroviral drugs
      iii. Gabapentin
      iv. Calcium channel blockers
7. **Breast masses (rare)**
   a. Cancer
   b. Dermoid cyst
   c. Lipoma
   d. Neurofibroma

Adapted with permission from Rosen DS: Adolescent gynecomastia. Pediatr Rev 24(9):317, 2003.

studies are required in healthy teens with no history of substance abuse, medications, or likely systemic illness and who have a negative physical examination. The teen needs to be reassured in a developmentally appropriate manner that he is normal and not becoming a woman.

Those teens with positive findings would need to be investigated depending on the system involved. Those with a hepatic or renal disease need a complete metabolic panel and referral to the appropriate subspecialist. Males with a suspected testicular mass would usually be evaluated with a serum human chorionic gonadotropin (hCG) and ultrasound of the testes. Other endocrine causes are evaluated by measurement of LH, serum testosterone, estradiol, dehydroepiandrosterone sulfate, and appropriate imaging studies. If abnormal, it is best to refer these patients to an endocrinologist for further evaluation and management.

Treatment

In most cases of pubertal gynecomastia, reassurance from the health care provider and an explanation of the condition and prognosis are all that is required. The caregiver should validate the feelings of discomfort and embarrassment that the adolescent might have. Within 6 months to a year, pubertal gynecomastia will usually resolve. Medications including danazol, tamoxifen, clomiphene, dihydrotestosterone, and testolactone have been tried, with either no success or only mild improvement, but data among teens is minimal. The U.S. Food and Drug Administration has not approved any of these drugs for treatment of gynecomastia in adolescents. Those rare patients who have an SMR 4 size breast or greater may need surgical treatment for cosmetic and psychological benefits. Gynecomastia that persists beyond 2 years is unlikely to resolve (permanent stromal fibrous tissue has likely developed) and surgical removal is an option.

The patient in our school-based clinic denied any history of substance abuse or taking any medications. He did not have any history suggestive of hepatic, renal, or testicular disease.

The only positive finding on physical examination was a small left subareolar mass about 2 cm in diameter. P.J. was reassured that this was normal and no studies were ordered. This opportunity was used to discuss issues regarding sexuality, substance abuse, and testicular self-examination.

BREAST PAIN

A.G., a 16-year-old adolescent, comes to the clinic complaining of pain in her breast. She has no significant medical history and is not sexually active. On inquiry, the pain seems to be worse before her periods and 2 days into her menses the pain resolves. Sometimes she can feel some nodularity when she does a breast self-exam. What is the cause of the breast pain? Is this normal or are the nodules she feels a disease process? How would you treat A.G.? What are the other causes of breast pain?

Breast pain (mastodynia or mastalgia) is a common complaint among female adolescents. The etiology is extensive and includes psychological causes (usually cyclic), drug use (often noncyclic), inflammation, and breast masses. The pain may actually be from the underlying chest wall muscles. The challenge for the primary care clinician is to sort out the issue with a careful history and physical examination. Mastodynia affects 30%–40% of women in their reproductive years and for 8% of them may affect their daily activity.

Clinical Evaluation

Patients should be asked about the pattern of their pain (cyclic or noncyclic), their menstrual history, possibility of being pregnant, if they are postpartum or breastfeeding, and any use of hormones, medications, or drugs (assure confidentiality). Since musculoskeletal pain can present as breast pain, ask about local trauma to the chest wall during exercise or sex and consider possible sources of infection including those secondary due to nipple piercing. Perform a careful breast examination to identify any masses or inflammatory lesions. Palpate the chest and pectoral muscles for tenderness. During the examination it is essential that galactorrhea be ruled out since sometimes the only symptom the patient may have is breast pain. Pregnancy must always be ruled out in a teenage girl with breast pain. The history and examination will indicate if the presumptive diagnosis is physiological, musculoskeletal, or inflammatory pain.

Fibrocystic Changes of the Breast

The physiological response to cyclical hormonal changes is called fibrocystic changes of the breast. This condition was previously called fibrocystic disease of the breast but since it is not a disease process, the term fibrocystic changes is more appropriate. It has been identified in 54% of autopsies of clinically normal breasts. The exact pathophysiology of this process is not clear but an imbalance between estrogen and progesterone has been suggested. On histopathology, there are proliferative breast changes with obstruction and persistent secretory material in the alveoli and terminal ducts leading to enlargement and cyst formation. The role of methylxanthines (caffeine) previously implicated has not been confirmed by case-controlled and randomized trials.

The adolescent patient often presents with self-discovered breast pain or discomfort. Symptoms begin about 1 week prior to menstruation and subside after menstruation. Teens rarely present with the chronic lumpy breasts or recurrent multiple cysts seen in women in their middle decades. On examination, the breasts have the characteristic nodularity often without the presence of a discrete mass. These physical findings are seen most often during the luteal phase and resolve during the proliferative phase of the menstrual cycle. Some patients may have multiple cysts or a painful "thickening" without well-defined borders, and diffuse nodular lesions.

Treatment of this condition depends on severity. Mild cyclical breast pain prior to menses is normal and for most teenagers reassurance, advice to wear a well-fitted brassiere (which helps to prevent inflammation and stretching of the supportive ligaments), and mild analgesics (acetaminophen or ibuprofen) are adequate to control the pain. In more severe cases oral contraceptive pills (OCPs) are of benefit in 70%–90% of patients. The OCPs lessen the incidence of breast cysts and at the same time provide contraception for the adolescent. Among adolescents there is little experience with danazol or other drugs used in adult women.

Drug-Related Breast Pain

Most of the drugs associated with galactorrhea and gynecomastia can also cause breast pain (see the drugs listed in Tables 27-1 and 27-2). If the teenager gives a history of using illicit substances, she should be offered treatment services and counseling support (Chap. 34). If she is taking necessary prescribed medication, understanding its relationship to breast pain may provide the reassurance she needs.

Musculoskeletal and Chest Wall Pain

Postviral Tietze syndrome can cause inflammation of the costochondral junctions (Chap. 8). Weight training and many sports can cause muscle strain to the pectoral and intercostal muscles. Trauma from sports or even vigorous horseplay or sexual activity can cause muscle bruising, hematomas, and mild dislocations of the intercostal sternal joints. Once the cause has been localized, treatment may include rest, heat, and mild analgesics.

Brea-1st Inflammation and Infection

Mondor Disease

Superficial thrombophlebitis or Mondor disease is uncommon but has been reported in adolescents. It may be caused by local trauma or friction from repeated upper extremity exercises. The patient presents with breast pain and a palpable tender venous cord along the lateral aspect of the breast. This condition is benign and self-limited, resolving within a few weeks with treatment by heat and analgesics.

T A B L E   2 7 - 2

CAUSES OF GALACTORRHEA

Physiologic states	3. Antihypertensives
1. Pregnancy	a. Atenolol
2. Lactation	b. Methyldopa
3. Sleep	c. Reserpine
4. Stress	d. Verapamil
5. Mechanical stimulation	4. Phenothiazines
Central nervous system disease	a. Chlorpromazine
1. Tumors of the pituitary	b. Procholpzine
a. Prolactinomas	5. Antipsychotics
b. Gonadotropin or non-secreting adenomas	a. Risperidone
c. Other pituitary adenomas causing stalk compression	6. Hormones
2. Hypothalamic/pituitary stalk tumor or mass	a. Medroxyprogesterone acetate (Depo Provera)
a. Craniopharyngioma	b. Oral contraceptive pills
b. Rathke cleft cyst	c. Antiandrogens (danazol)
c. Epidermoid or colloid cyst	d. Dihydroergotamine
d. Chordoma	7. Substance abuse
e. Meningioma	a. Marijuana
f. Granulomatous disease especially sarcoidosis	b. Amphetamine
g. Metastatic carcinoma	c. Opiates
h. Cranial irradiation	8. Others
Drugs	a. H_2 receptor blockers (cimetidine famotidine, ranitidine)
1. Selective serotonin reuptake inhibitors	b. Valproic acid
a. Citalopram (Celexa)	c. Isoniazid
b. Fluoxetine (Prozac)	d. Cisapride
c. Paroxetine (Paxil)	e. Sumatriptan
d. Sertraline (Zoloft)	**Systemic disease**[*]
2. Antidepressants and anxiolytics	1. Renal failure
a. Tricyclic antidepressants	2. Liver failure
b. Alprazolam	3. Hypothyroidism
c. Buspirone	**Idiopathic**
d. MAOI	**Miscellaneous**
	1. Chest wall trauma (surgery and herpes)
	2. Spinal cord injury and lesions

[*]1 and 2 alter prolactin metabolism.

Breast Infection

Inflammation of the breast tissue presents with breast pain as an initial symptom. Clinically the patient could have cellulitis, mastitis, or a true breast abscess. Breast infection is usually associated with lactation but is also found as a cutaneous spread from superficial skin lesions, folliculitis, or trauma. Trauma occurs during sports, nipple piercing, sexual activity, or plucking of periareolar hair. The infection usually develops beneath the areola and at the margin between the areola and the adjacent skin.

Staphylococcus aureus is found in 80% of adolescent breast infections. Other organisms that cause mastitis include *Streptococcus pyogens, Micrococcus, Escherichia coli*, and *Pseudomonas aeruginosa*. The history and physical findings of pain, erythema, induration, or a fluctuant mass (late-stage finding) confirm the diagnosis of breast infection. Purulent drainage should be cultured for organisms and antibiotic sensitivities. The differential diagnosis includes trauma to the breast causing hematoma or fat necrosis, superficial thrombophlebitis of the skin (Mondor disease), and duct ectasia with nipple discharge.

If the breast infection is superficial it can be managed conservatively. The infection is treated with warm compresses and a full course of appropriate antibiotics to cover the most common organisms. A first generation cephalosporin (e.g., cephalexin or cephradine) or dicloxicillin for 4–6 weeks is given, with serial follow-up examinations to ensure the infection has completely resolved. If significant cellulitis is present, intravenous antibiotics should be considered in the initial stages of the infection. If a fluctuant abscess is present, the patient should be referred for surgical incision and drainage. This procedure should not be attempted in the office since the abscess often runs deep and drainage is difficult. If the patient is breastfeeding, she can be encouraged to continue to do so, unless there is a purulent nipple discharge. Breastfeeding prevents abscess formation and preserves milk supply.

The cause of the breast pain in our patient A.G. is fibrocystic changes of the breast. The changes she feels are normal and the nodules she feels are not a disease process. The treatment of this condition depends on the severity of the pain. A.G. has a mild case and she is advised to use simple analgesics and a properly fitted bra. If A.G. were sexually active and also needed contraception then oral contraceptive pills would be the first choice. This appointment is used as an opportunity to reinforce A.G.'s healthy sexual choices and encourage regular office visits for any future concerns.

BREAST MASSES

S.K., a 16-year-old Caucasian teen, presents to your office with her mother complaining of a lump in her right breast. There is no history of pain, trauma, nipple discharge, or constitutional symptoms. There is no family history of breast cancer or significant past medical or surgical history. Her last menstrual period was almost 3 weeks ago. In her interview alone, she discloses that she has recently become sexually active, has tried smoking cigarettes, but denies any other substance use. She also mentions that she would like to start on birth control pills but her friend told her that birth control pills could increase her chances of breast cancer. On examination, there is a 2 cm mass in the upper outer quadrant of the breast. The mass is firm, mobile, and discrete with no signs of inflammation or presence of any axillary lymph nodes.

What is the most common diagnosis? What investigations would you order today? How would you manage this patient? What are the other breast masses that could occur in this teenager? What are the chances that this could be a malignant mass? Are her concerns regarding birth control pills and breast cancer valid?

Breast masses in adolescent girls are cause for concern and anxiety with the inevitable fears of cancer. It is reassuring that in the adolescent population breast cancer is extremely rare. Most breast masses in teenagers are either fibroadenomas or breast cysts. Malignancies of adjoining structures in the chest wall, ribs, and dermal tissue can be mistaken for breast cancer, especially in thin girls.

Clinical Evaluation

The approach to an adolescent with a breast mass includes a history and a physical examination that reassures the patient (and parent) of sincere concern. The history should include when the mass was noticed, any subsequent changes in size, relationship to the menstrual cycle, and symptoms such as pain. Ask about a past history of radiation to the chest, trauma to the breast, and any family history (e.g., mother, maternal aunt, maternal grandmother) of breast cancer. Pregnancy should be ruled out. Obtain a thorough medication and substance abuse history. The examination of the breast, described previously, includes inspection and palpation of both breasts and axillae. Diagram the size and location of the lesion in the patient record. The history and physical findings will usually suggest a presumptive diagnosis of cyst versus solid tumor and suggest if any further studies are indicated (see Fig. 27-5). In most cases, observation is appropriate, and the adolescent should return for follow-up 1 week after her next menses. The mass is then remeasured and a more conclusive diagnosis and treatment plan determined.

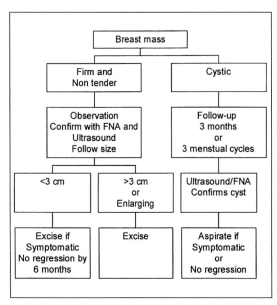

FIGURE 27-5

EVALUATION OF BREAST MASS IN ADOLESCENTS.
Source: Adapted from Kaul P, Coupey SM: Breast disorders. In: Coupey SM (ed.), *Primary Care of Adolescent Girls*. Philadelphia, PA: Hanley & Belfus, 2002.

Imaging Studies

Ultrasonography is the radiological investigation of choice among adolescent girls with breast masses. This procedure differentiates between a solid and cystic tumor. In addition, the breast cyst can be aspirated directly under ultrasound guidance.

Computerized tomography (CT) is used to assess the origin of the mass. In thin girls it can be difficult to differentiate if the mass is arising from the chest wall or the surrounding tissue. Tumors arising from the chest wall and surrounding structures tend to be fixed masses unlike breast masses.

Mammography is not recommended for diagnosis of breast tumors among adolescent girls. The adolescent breast differs from the adult in having larger amounts of fibroglandular tissue than fatty tissue, and the density makes detection of breast masses in adolescents difficult by mammography.

Breast Cysts

Breast cysts are the most common cause of painful breast lumps in adolescence and account for about 60% of breast masses seen in office practice. The cysts form from the terminal ducts and acini. The pathophysiology of these cysts is not well understood. They often present as a single, tender, soft, spongy, mobile mass. The cysts are painful and the maximum intensity of pain occurs prior to the menses and subsides after. The chronic lumpy breasts seen in women in their fourth decade are unusual among teens (see the previous discussion of Fibrocystic Changes of the Breast).

The diagnosis is confirmed when the painful lump regresses after the menses. Half will completely resolve within two to three menstrual cycles. A persistent or enlarging cyst needs a definitive diagnosis. The diagnosis is confirmed by ultrasound and the cyst can also be aspirated under ultrasound guidance. Breast cysts should be differentiated from breast abscess and fibrocystic changes of the breast.

Simple cysts can be managed conservatively with observation and analgesics like acetaminophen and ibuprofen. Larger or persistent cysts may need aspiration. Oral contraceptives decrease the incidence of recurrent breast cysts and may be useful in teens, especially those who also desire birth control. Treatment with medications like danazol, bromocriptine, and tamoxifen have been disappointing because of their adverse effects, high costs, and relapse rates.

Fibroadenomas

Among adolescents, fibroadenomas are the most common breast masses reported in diagnostic studies, accounting for 70%–90% of all biopsied lesions. Histologic features are variable and may include stromal proliferation, aggregates of elongated and distorted ducts, fibrosis, and epithelial hyperplasia. The etiology is not clear but may be related to abnormal sensitivity of breast stromal tissue to estrogens. Typically there are no associated symptoms of pain or nipple discharge. On examination, the mass is usually single, unilateral, and found in the upper outer quadrant. Multiple lesions in one or both breasts may be found in 10%–25% of adolescents. Classically the mass is a slow growing, nontender, firm, rubbery, well-demarcated, mobile lesion less than 5 cm in diameter with an average size of 2–3 cm (range 1–10 cm). The presumptive diagnosis is made on history and clinical findings. Ultrasonography shows classical features of a well-circumscribed, homogenous, hypoechoic mass. The diagnosis is confirmed by fine needle aspiration (FNA) cytology or biopsy.

FNA is a simple, safe office procedure, which does not require local anesthesia. The breast mass is immobilized between the thumb and the forefinger and a 20-gauge needle inserted while pulling on the syringe to create negative pressure. The material that is aspirated is sent for cytopathology to look for malignant cells.

Fibroadenomas less than 3 cm can be managed conservatively with close follow-up if the FNA is negative. However, if the mass is greater than 3 cm, symptomatic, suspicious for malignancy, or enlarging, the patient should be referred to a surgeon for an excision biopsy, which would be diagnostic. The biopsy can usually be performed under local anesthesia and mild sedation. Excision biopsy removes

both the mass and the anxiety in the patient and her family. Most fibroadenomas do not increase in size and 70% will eventually either regress or resolve. Fibroadenomas do not become malignant and are not associated with an increased risk of breast cancer.

Giant or Juvenile Fibroadenomas

This benign variant of fibroadenoma is usually seen at a younger age than common fibroadenomas and has a higher prevalence among African American adolescents. Giant fibroadenomas have potential to grow to greater than 5 cm in size and their growth is rapid and asymmetrical, leading to distortion of the breast parenchyma and/or pressure necrosis of the skin. Treatment is excision, which results in normalization of breast architecture. Mastectomy is not indicated and most patients do not require reconstructive surgery.

Cystosarcoma Phyllodes

Cystosarcoma phyllodes is an uncommon but well-documented cause of a large breast mass in adolescents. Histologic features are similar to the fibroadenomas, except the stroma is more cellular. This tumor is usually benign but malignant variations are reported, and malignant forms are more likely in adolescents than in older women. Malignant classification is determined by features of stromal cellularity, nuclear atypia, mitotic activity, necrosis, and tumor margins.

On clinical examination these masses are large (average size 6 cm) and can be massive (up to 20 cm). Palpation reveals a firm, mobile, well-defined mass with a smooth or slightly irregular surface. Due to rapid tumor growth, the breast skin tends to be shiny with venous engorgement. Other findings may include skin retraction, nipple discharge, and nipple retraction. If lymphadenopathy is present, the diagnosis is usually a lymphoma rather than a primary breast malignancy.

Treatment of cystosarcoma phyllodes is complete wide-margin excision with continued patient follow-up. There is no need for mastectomy or radical surgical procedures if the tumor is found to be benign. In the rare cases of malignancy or metastatic spread, surgery, adjuvant chemotherapy, and radiation have been recommended.

Malignant Breast Disease

Health care professionals taking care of adolescents are fortunate that malignancy of the breast is extremely rare in this age group (Hindle and Sarkis, 2002; Kalyani and Sekhon, 2001). Breast cancer is found in less than 1% of all breast tumors among teens. It is reassuring that almost 98% of reported breast cancer is found in women older than 25 years. Only one third of the breast cancers diagnosed in teens are primary breast tumors, mainly adenocarcinomas and malignant cystosarcoma phyllodes. The other two thirds are either tumors of nonbreast tissue or metastatic disease. Other malignancies presenting as breast masses in adolescents include secondary sarcomas (fibrosarcoma and liposarcoma) and secondary metastases from lymphomas, Hodgkin's disease, leukemia, and multiple myeloma.

When breast cancer does occur, more than 90% of malignant lesions in adolescents present as palpable breast masses. The typical lesion is hard, nontender, indurated, subareolar, and fixed to the underlying tissues. It is usually unilateral and single. The mass is often asymptomatic, painless, and with no axillary lymphadenopathy. Advanced cases and metastatic disease may present with axillary lymph nodes, constitutional symptoms, hepatosplenomegaly, and masses elsewhere in the body.

Since breast cancer is rare among teens, our knowledge about this disease is limited. Up to 30% of patients have a family history of breast cancer that includes first-degree relatives (mothers, sisters, and aunts). The risk is increased three to four times if that cancer occurred before menopause. Those patients who have been identified with mutations of the breast cancer gene BRCA-1 or BRCA-2 account for 80% of hereditary breast cancers and for about 5% of all breast cancers. Routine screening for BRCA-1 or -2 is not yet recommended. Other risk factors for adolescent breast cancer include a history of childhood Hodgkin's disease and radiation treatment to the chest during childhood (Robinson and Bhatia, 2003). The association and/or causality of hormonal contraception (specifically oral contraceptives) with breast cancer have been a controversial issue. However, large studies by both the World Health Organization and the Centers for Disease Control and Prevention have found no evidence of increased risk of breast cancer with use of oral contraceptives and it is likely that modern low-dose formulations will prove even safer in future long-term studies.

Treatment of adolescent breast cancer depends on the stage of the disease and the histologic classification of the tumor, and may include surgery, radiation therapy, and chemotherapy. Given limited data and newer treatment regimens, prognosis for the adolescent is uncertain as to whether her outcome will be better, worse or similar to that of older patients. While these tumors appear to be more aggressive on histology, it is not clear if this leads to poorer clinical prognosis or a worse long-term survival.

In our patient S.K., the most likely diagnosis is fibroadenoma. No studies need to be done today and the mass can be observed. She should be asked to follow-up after her menstrual period. Other masses that can occur are giant fibroadenomas and cystosarcoma phyllodes. The chances that this tumor is malignant are extremely rare in view of the history and clinical findings. Her concern regarding increased incidence of breast cancer after taking birth control pills is not valid and time should be spent in reassuring her about this fact. Contraceptive counseling should include birth control options and condom use. This opportunity should also be used to discuss tobacco cessation with S.K.

NIPPLE DISCHARGE AND GALACTORRHEA

Nipple discharge can be a distressing complaint for the adolescent girl. Although the fluid will usually be galactorrhea (milk production), it may be from physiologic causes or be a symptom of breast pathology. The presumptive cause of nipple discharge is based primarily on the color of the fluid (see Fig. 27-6).

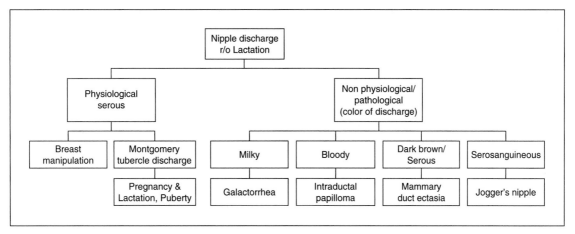

FIGURE 27-6

CAUSES OF NIPPLE DISCHARGE, SHOWING PRESUMPTIVE DIAGNOSIS BASED ON COLOR AND CHARACTERISTICS OF FLUID.

Physiological Causes of Nipple Discharge

Physiological Nipple Discharge

Physiological nipple discharge is typically unilateral and serous in nature. It often occurs from excessive manipulation of the breast either by the patient or her sexual partner. It can also occur due to local irritation of the breast from tight clothing or a poorly fitting brassiere. The stimulation of the breast results in neurologic reflexes via the anterior and the posterior pituitary. The reflex via the anterior pituitary inhibits dopamine resulting in release of prolactin, whereas the reflex via the posterior pituitary results in stimulation from release of oxytocin.

Montgomery Tubercle Discharge

Montgomery tubercles on the areola occasionally produce a benign whitish discharge for a few weeks during puberty or during pregnancy and lactation. This resolves spontaneously and requires no treatment.

Nonphysiological or Pathological Causes of Nipple Discharge

Mammary Duct Ectasia

Mammary duct ectasia produces a dark brown or grayish green nipple discharge. This is a clinical syndrome of nipple discharge, nipple inversion, breast mass, and/or nonpuerperal periareolar mastitis. On physical examination, there may be fibrosis of the underlying breast and skin dimpling. These patients may have elevated prolactin levels and undiagnosed prolactinomas. The treatment of choice is surgical excision of the duct and any associated mass.

Intraductal Papilloma

Intraductal papilloma often presents with a bloody nipple discharge. Abnormal proliferation of the mammary epithelium occurs, which then projects into the duct lumen causing a blockage of the duct. When local trauma occurs, it causes avulsion of the vascular stalk, producing the bloody discharge. These patients should be referred for surgical excision of the duct, and about 50% will have an associated ductal mass. The lesion is an infrequent finding in adolescents, mainly seen in women ages 20 through 40.

Jogger's Nipple

"Jogger's nipple" is associated with a serosanguineous discharge. This injury is caused by prolonged contact with an irritating material like a brassiere or other rough-surfaced clothing during running or other exercises. During exercise, moisture from perspiration evaporates and wind chill lowers the temperature of the nipple resulting in nipple soreness and sensitivity. In early stages, the nipple becomes thickened and scaly. With repeated trauma, nipple discharge can develop. Abrasions can be treated conservatively by wound care and if infection occurs by use of local antibiotics. "Bicyclist nipple" is similar to the jogger's nipple. Nipple trauma in athletes can be prevented by the use of wind-breaking material over the chest, properly fitted sport brassieres, lubricants such as petroleum jelly over the nipple, and avoidance of cold weather if possible.

Galactorrhea

Galactorrhea is milk-like discharge from the nipple, though the discharge is not always milky but can occasionally be thin and watery. The clinical objective when an adolescent presents with galactorrhea is to methodically determine the cause, which will most likely be due to pregnancy, drugs, or neuroendocrine disorders. Lactation is by far the most common cause of nipple discharge and is a normal, benign process. Galactorrhea that is not from pregnancy-related lactation must be evaluated.

Clinical Evaluation

An accurate history is essential to assess sexual activity, nipple stimulation, and any possibility of pregnancy or recent spontaneous or therapeutic abortion. Assure confidentiality to obtain a thorough drug history, including psychotropic medications, hormonal contraceptives, street drugs, substance abuse, and the other drugs listed on Table 27-2. The menstrual history may reveal amenorrhea, luteal phase defects, or dysfunctional uterine bleeding. Ask about neuroendocrine symptoms such as goiter, visual field defects, and headaches. The physical examination should include a thyroid assessment and neuroendocrine exam specifically checking for visual field defects and signs of hirsutism. On breast examination, attempt to express any nipple discharge by firmly stroking from axilla to nipple, and pressing firmly on the areola. If fluid is obtained, note the

color. A microscopic exam for fat globules will confirm galactorrhea.

Diagnostic Evaluation

The first step is to get an hCG pregnancy test (see Fig. 27-7). It is essential to rule out current or recently terminated pregnancy in all patients who present with galactorrhea. Postpartum milk production (in the absence of breast feeding) may continue for several months after termination of pregnancy, and up to a year in adolescents on hormonal contraceptives. The hCG pregnancy test may remain positive for 2–4 weeks after termination and may help confirm a recent pregnancy. Adolescents with a positive pregnancy test may be offered appropriate options counseling. For patients who have a negative pregnancy test, the clinician should proceed with further laboratory studies consisting of a prolactin level and thyroid-stimulating hormone (TSH).

If the TSH and prolactin level are normal, drugs that cause galactorrhea need to be carefully considered (see the list in Table 27-2). In adolescents,

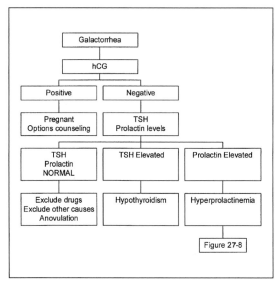

F I G U R E   2 7 - 7

EVALUATION OF GALACTORRHEA IN ADOLESCENTS. PREGNANCY AND LACTATION SHOULD ALWAYS BE CONSIDERED FIRST.

hormonal contraceptives, antidepressants, and heavy use of marijuana are the most likely drug-related causes. The galactorrhea usually resolves within several months after the medications are changed or discontinued. If the TSH level is elevated, a diagnosis of hypothyroidism is confirmed (Chap. 15). If the prolactin level is elevated, the diagnosis is hyperprolactinemia, which needs further evaluation.

Hyperprolactinemia

As reviewed in the previous section on the physiology of lactation, prolactin is under chronic inhibition by dopamine from the hypothalamus. As shown in Table 27-2, an extensive list of factors can affect prolactin levels. Prolactin levels are highest during sleep and are normally <20 ng/mL (or <20 μg/L). These levels are increased during pregnancy, stress, exercise, and sexual intercourse. The prolactin level should be measured before examination of the breast and when the patient is relaxed. However, physiological or psychological stress does not increase the levels beyond 40 μg/L. Since the secretion of prolactin is pulsatile in nature, levels between 25 and 40 μg/L should be repeated before a diagnosis of hyperprolactinemia is made. A level of >200 μg/L is almost always associated with a prolactin-secreting tumor.

Management of Hyperprolactinemia

Figure 27-8 explains the management of patients with hyperprolactinemia (Schlechte, 2003; Serri et al., 2003). Imaging studies to detect tumors are an essential part of the investigation when the other causes of hyperprolactinemia have been ruled out. Gadolinium-enhanced MRI is the imaging study of choice. While CT scan with intravenous contrast is also valuable, the MRI is more effective in revealing small adenomas and tumor extension. The MRI may detect no lesions or reveal a pituitary adenoma (Pickett, 2003). Adenomas are classified by their size as microadenomas (<10 mm) or macroadenomas (>10 mm). Macroadenomas are associated with prolactin levels of >250 μg/L.

Adolescents with a normal MRI who are symptomatic and those with microadenomas can be managed medically with serial prolactin levels and imaging studies. Those patients who undergo medical therapy should have the prolactin levels measured every 4–6months and MRI done every 2 years.

Macroadenomas may be intrasellar or suprasellar. Intrasellar microadenomas can be treated medically with dopamine agonists since they do not enlarge during pregnancy. Suprasellar tumors usually need to be treated surgically, followed by medical treatment with dopamine agonists.

Bromocriptine is a dopamine receptor agonist that results in normal prolactin levels in 80%–90% of patients, with a decrease in size of the tumor and return to normal menses. It is also safe during pregnancy. The medication has frequent side effects including nausea, vomiting, orthostatic hypotension, and depression. Bromocriptine has a short half-life and needs to be taken twice a day. Cabergoline is a long acting dopamine agonist that has been available in the United States for several years. Its advantage over bromocriptine is twice-weekly dosage and decreased side effects. However, it is more expensive. Pergolide is another dopamine agonist used extensively in Europe but not yet approved by the FDA to treat prolactinomas. It is less expensive than bromocriptine and is taken once a day. Surgical management is indicated in those patients who do not respond adequately to medications or are truly intolerant of drugs. Surgery is usually performed via the transsphenoidal route and for microadenomas has a success rate of almost 75%.

Uncommon Causes of Galactorrhea

Rarely an adolescent presents with galactorrhea who has no history of pregnancy or drug use and all initial studies are negative. Management then depends on menstrual history. If menses are normal, observation with repeat prolactin levels every 6–12 months should be considered to rule out a slow-growing pituitary adenoma. If the patient has amenorrhea, consider other neuroendocrine disorders such as polycystic ovarian syndrome, anorexia nervosa, or hormone producing adrenal or ovarian tumors.

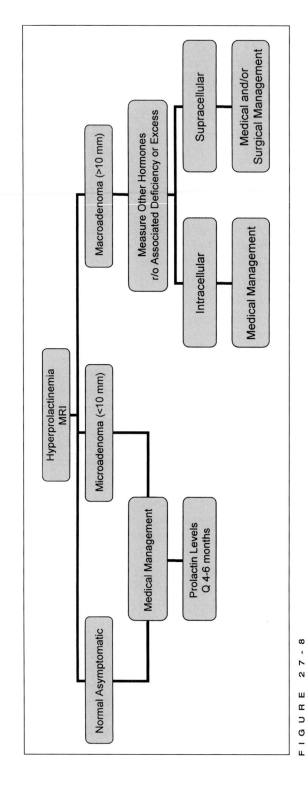

FIGURE 27-8

EVALUATION OF HYPERPROLACTINEMIA IN ADOLESCENTS, WITH PITUITARY ADENOMAS BEING THE SUSPECTED ETIOLOGY.

Source: Derived from Schlechte JA: Clinical practice. Prolactinoma. *N Engl J Med* 20; 349(21):2035,2003.

Bibliography

Arca MJ, Caniano DA: Breast disorders in the adolescent patient. *Adolesc Med* 15:473–485, 2004.

Beach RK: Breast lump in adolescent girls. In: Berman S(ed.), *Pediatric Decision-Making*. 4th ed. Philadelphia, PA: Mosby, 2003, p. 6.

Beach RK: Galactorrhea (nipple discharge) in adolescent girls. In: Berman S(ed.), *Pediatric Decision-Making*, 4th ed. Philadelphia, PA: Mosby, 2003, p. 32.

Beach RK: Breast pain in adolescent girls. In: Berman S(ed.), *Pediatric Decision-Making,* 4th ed. Philadelphia, PA: Mosby, 2003, p. 8.

Beach RK: Breast disorders. In: McAnarney ER, Kreipe RE, Orr DP, Comerci GD (eds.), *Textbook of Adolescent Medicine*. Philadelphia, PA: W.B. Saunders, 1992, p. 720.

Bland KI, Copeland III EM(eds.): *The Breast: Comprehensive Management of Benign and Malignant Disorders*. Philadelphia, PA: W.B. Saunders, 2004, p. 1694.

Cox EM, Seigel DM: Mondor disease: An unusual consideration in a young woman with a breast mass. *J Adolesc Health* 21(3):183, 1997.

Collaborative Group on Hormonal Factors in Breast Cancer: Breast cancer and hormonal contraceptives: Collaborative reanalysis of individual data on 53,297 women with breast cancer and 100,239 women without breast cancer from 54 epidemiological studies. *Lancet* 347:1713, 1996.

Foxcroft LM, Evans EB, Hirst C, et al: Presentation and diagnosis of adolescent breast disease. *Breast* 10(5): 399, 2001

Govrin-Yehudain J, Kogan L, Cohen HI, et al: Familial juvenile hypertrophy of the breast. *J Adolesc Health* 35(2):151, 2004.

Greydanus DE: Breast and gynecological disorders. In: Hofmann AD, Greydanus DE (eds.), *Adolescent Medicine*, 3d ed. Norwalk, CT: Appleton & Lange, 1997, p. 520.

Greydanus DE, Patel DR, Baxter TL: The breast and sports: Issues for the clinician. *Adolesc Med* 9(3): 533, 1998.

Hackshaw AK, Paul EA: Breast self-examination and death from breast cancer: A meta-analysis. *Br J Cancer* 88(7):1047, 2003.

Haddy TB, Mosher RB, Dinnodorf PA, et al: Second neoplasms in survivors of childhood and adolescent cancer are often treatable. *J Adolesc Health* 34(4):324, 2004.

Hindle WH, Sarkis N: Breast cancer and masses in women 22 years of age and younger. *Clin Obstet Gynecol* 45(3):758, 2002.

Kalyani K, Sekhon MS: Bilateral breast cancer-under age 20 years. *J Adolesc Health* 28:353, 2001.

Kaul P, Coupey SM: Breast disorders. In: Coupey SM(ed.), *Primary Care in Adolescent Girls*. Philadelphia, PA: Hanley & Belfus, 2000, p. 203.

Kaplowitz PB, Oberfield SE, Drug and Therapeutics and Executive Committees of the Lawson Wilkins Pediatric Endocrine Society: Reexamination of the age limit for defining when puberty is precocious in girls in the United States: Implications for evaluation and treatment. *Pediatrics* 104:936, 1999.

Marchant DJ: Benign breast disease. *Obstet Gynecol Clin North Am* 29(1):1, 2002.

McRath MH, Schooler WG: Elective plastic surgical procedures in adolescence. *Adolesc Med* 15:487–502, 2004.

Neinstein LS: Breast disorders. In: Neinstein LS (ed), *Adolescent Health Care: A Practical Guide*, 4th ed. Philadelphia, PA: Lippincott Williams & Wilkins, 2002, p. 1063.

Neinstein LS, Joffe A: Gynecomastia. In: Neinstein LS (ed), *Adolescent Health Care: A Practical Guide*, 4th ed. Philadelphia, PA: Lippincott Williams & Wilkins, 2002, p. 264.

Niebyl JR: Mastitis: Treating breast infections. In: Queenan JT, Hobbins JC(eds.), *Protocols for High Risk Pregnancy*, 3d ed. Boston, MA: Blackwell, 1996, p. 432.

Pickett CA: Diagnosis and management of pituitary tumors: Recent advances. *Prim Care* 30(4):765, 2003.

Rainer C, Gardetto A, Fruhwirth M, et al.: Breast deformity in adolescence as a result of pneumothroax drainage during neonatal intensive care. *Pediatrics* 111:80–86, 2003.

Robinson LL, Bhatia S: Late-effects among survivors of leukemia and lymphoma during childhood and adolescence. *Br J Haematol* 122(3):345, 2003.

Rosen DS: Question from the clinician: Adolescent gynecomastia. *Pediatr Rev* 24(9):317, 2003.

Sariego J, Zrada S, Byrd M, et al.: Breast cancer in young patients. *Am J Surg* 170(3):243, 1995.

Saslow D, Hannan J, Osuch J, et al: Clinical breast examination: Practical recommendations for optimizing performance and reporting. *CA Cancer J Clin* 54(6):327, 2004.

Schlechte JA: Prolactinoma clinical practice. *N Engl J Med* 349:2035, 2003.

Serri O, Chik CL, Ur E, Ezzat S: Diagnosis and management of hyperprolactinemia. *CMAJ* 169(6):575, 2003.

Spack NP, Neinstein LS: Galactorrhea. In: Neinstein LS (ed.), *Adolescent Health Care: A Practical Guide*, 4th ed. Philadelphia, PA: Lippincott Williams & Wilkins, 2002, p. 1043.

Winchester DP: Breast cancer in young women. *Surg Clin North Am* 76:279, 1996.

28

MENSTRUAL DISORDERS IN ADOLESCENTS

Tatiana Pavlova Greenfield and Margaret J. Blythe

INTRODUCTION

This chapter presents a *clinically-based* overview and an *easy-to-use* approach to the identification and management of menstrual disorders in adolescents. Its primary focus and objective is to provide the pediatrician, primary care practitioner, and other adolescent health care providers with the knowledge to assess and initiate the evaluation and treatment of such disorders in this age group. Often young women and their families may need reassurance about the normal variation in menstrual patterns and cycles. While normal menstrual bleeding and menstrual cycles should not produce a negative physical or emotional impact on the adolescent patient, some abnormalities of the menstrual pattern and/or cycles, may lead to serious complications or indicate the worsening of a preexisting or undiagnosed disease and/or condition.

This chapter reviews: (1) normal menstrual patterns, (2) premenstrual disorders and dysmenorrhea, (3) variations of the menstrual cycle and menstrual bleedings, (4) polycystic ovary syndrome, and (5) ovarian tumors. A review of these disorders, together with case studies and approaches provide a step-by-step guide for the management and recommended treatment of menstrual disorders in adolescents.

NORMAL MENSTRUAL PATTERNS

Menstruation or menses is physiologic uterine bleeding, which should be a fairly regular and repetitive event for each individual with variations in cycles occurring between individuals. The first period or menarche should take place usually 2 years after the onset of puberty (range 1–3 years). Menarche is preceded by breast development (thelarche), growth spurt, and pubic hair development (adrenarche). Usually thelarche occurs first, but adrenarche may first occur with the growth spurt usually early in puberty (Chap. 1). Menarche is one of the major latest developmental events of female puberty. In the United States, menarche normally occurs between ages 9 and 16 with the mean age 12.4 years. The age of menarche depends on many factors such as nutrition, socioeconomic status, weight, heredity, and race to name a few. During the last century in the United States and other industrialized countries, the age at menarche has gradually decreased with some groups affected more than others.[1,2]

The menstrual interval is defined as the time between the first days of two consecutive menstrual bleedings. The normal interval is 28+/7 days, but may not normalize for 2–3 years after periods begin. The menstrual period usually lasts no more than 7 days with the average flow 2–4 days. Estimated blood loss usually does not exceed more than 80 mL or about 5 tablespoons for each cycle. Variation from a normal pattern of the menstrual cycle and menstrual bleeding or excessive pain or dysphoria may be abnormal and should be investigated and treated appropriately.

PREMENSTRUAL CONDITIONS IN ADOLESCENTS

Definitions

Premenstrual syndrome (PMS) (ICD-9: 626.4) is a cluster of symptoms occurring cyclically and repetitively in the premenstrual interval, resolving during menstrual flow, and being followed by a symptom-free postmenstrual interval.[3]

Premenstrual dysphoric disorder (PMDD) is a disorder with distinct symptoms regularly occurring during the week before flow or the luteal phase of the menstrual cycle and occurring fairly consistently over one year before each period. Symptoms include markedly depressed mood, marked anxiety, marked affective lability, and decreased interest and ability to perform activities. The symptoms are cyclical and begin to disappear after the onset of menses and are gone the week after the period.[4]

Epidemiology

Approximately 75%–95% of women experience some premenstrual symptoms. Thirteen percent of women of reproductive age report impaired efficiency at work and 17% will seek treatment because of premenstrual symptoms.[4,5] Premenstrual symptoms can occur in adolescents as early as during the first postmenarchal year. Premenstrual dysphoric disorder should be considered present when the symptoms are severe enough to result in decreased productivity, missed school days, avoidance of school activities, and impaired efficiency at school/work. The symptoms may worsen with age. Only about 3%–5% of women of reproductive age experience premenstrual symptoms that can meet the criteria for the PMDD.[4-6]

Etiology

The etiology of premenstrual conditions remains unknown. Estrogen-progesterone imbalances as well as beta-endorphins and neurotransmitters like gamma-aminobutyric acid (GABA) and serotonin are considered as the main players in the mechanisms of premenstrual conditions.

Diagnosis and Differential Diagnosis

Diagnostic and Statisticla Manual of Mental Disorders-Fourth Edition DSM-IV criteria for PMDD require that five or more of the symptoms be present and cyclical: feeling sad, hopeless, or loss of self-worth; feeling tense, anxious, or "on edge"; marked lability of mood interspersed with frequent tearfulness; persistent irritability, anger, and increased interpersonal conflicts; decreased interest in activities, and withdrawal from social relationships. Other reported symptoms or findings are suicidal thoughts, increased muscle tension, joint and muscle pain, or feeling bloated or having swelling.[4-6] More than 60 different scales/questionnaires, measuring almost 200 signs and symptoms are reported in the literature.[6] There are no approved diagnostic tests or procedures. The evidence of the cyclic pattern of symptoms for at least 2 consecutive months can suggest the diagnosis. PMDD should be distinguished from symptoms of premenstrual syndrome or depression or other mental health disorders.[4]

Treatment

Several groups of medications have been tried for the treatment of premenstrual dysphoric disorder. Published controlled clinical trials suggest that selective serotonin reuptake inhibitors (SSRIs) (e.g., fluoxetine), anxiolytics (e.g., alprazolam), danazol, diuretics (e.g., spironolactone) gonadotropin-releasing hormone (GnRH) agonists (e.g., Lupron), and anti-inflammatory drugs (e.g., ibuprofen) have all demonstrated some clinical efficacy.[5,7,8] Other medications such as beta-blockers, lithium, bromocriptine, dietary supplements (calcium, magnesium), chlorthalidone, Evening Primrose Oil, oral contraceptives, low dose estrogens and progestins, and pyridoxine (vitamin B6) have had limited to no clinical effect in the treatment of premenstrual symptoms.[5,8] Psychotherapy may be recommended for unresponsive cases with positive effects confirmed by well controlled, randomized clinical trials.[5,8,9] Other available treatment options have included:

1. Life-style changes: stress reduction, smoking cessation, behavioral modification, and aerobic exercise.
2. Dietary modifications: increased consumption of fish, whole grains, fruits, vegetables, nuts, and ground flax seed.
3. Nutritional supplements: calcium, vitamins B6 and E, magnesium, essential fatty acids, zinc, tryptophan, and vitamin A.
4. Herbal medicines: Chasteberry (vitex agnus-castus) and ginkgo biloba have been shown to be effective in controlled clinical trials. Other herbs like black cohosh, kava, St. John's Wort, and primrose oil have been demonstrated to be effective in small clinical studies.[8]
5. Use of acupuncture, homeopathy, light therapy, reflexology, and relaxation therapy has been reported in the literature.[5,8,10]

DYSMENORRHEA

Definitions

Primary dysmenorrhea (ICD-9: 625.3) is painful menstrual bleeding with no underlying pelvic pathology; this is the most common type for adolescents and young women under the age of 20. Secondary dysmenorrhea is painful menstrual bleeding secondary to some underlying pelvic pathology. Dysmenorrhea is associated with painful cramping sensations in the lower abdomen often accompanied by other symptoms, which may include any or all of the symptoms of headaches, nausea, vomiting, diarrhea, sweating, and myalgias and occurs just before or during the menses.[11]

Epidemiology

It is estimated that between 75% and 90% of women of all ages experience dysmenorrhea during their menstrual cycles. Severe dysmenorrhea, reported in 10% of these women, results in increased missed school and work days. Primary dysmenorrhea indicates the beginning of ovulatory menstrual cycles in adolescents. Family history of dysmenorrhea may help support the diagnosis.[11–13]

Etiology

The most popular theory of the cause of primary dysmenorrhea includes increased production of prostaglandins, in particular F-2-alpha, which leads to increased uterine contractility and intrauterine pressure. Secondary dysmenorrhea is a result of a pelvic condition and/or pathologic process. Secondary dysmenorrhea may be misdiagnosed as a primary. Emphasis has been on early diagnosis of endometriosis in the adolescent population over the last decade with other diagnoses that must be considered listed in Table 28-1.

Evaluation and Management

The management of dysmenorrhea in teens is determined by its cause. Adolescents with primary dysmenorrhea have been successfully treated with combined hormonal pills or patches. Nonsteroidal anti-inflammatory drugs (NSAIDs), specifically the prostaglandin synthetase inhibitors, can be used alone or in the combination with combined hormonal products (Fig. 28-1, Table 28-2). Other suggested changes may include exercise, relaxation techniques, vitamins, and intake of foods low in sodium. The treatment of secondary amenorrhea in adolescents should be directed to identification and treatment of underlying pelvic pathology or condition.[12–14]

Specific Conditions in Adolescents with Secondary Dysmenorrhea

Endometriosis (ICD-9: 617.9)

Endometriosis is defined as the presence of functional endometrial glands and stroma outside the normal anatomic location in the uterus. Endometriosis may cause significant functional impairment at a time in life when attention to academics and work experience are critical. The clinical presentation of endometriosis in adolescents may include

TABLE 28-1

DIFFERENTIAL DIAGNOSIS OF DYSMENORRHEA

System	Common Possible Etiology
Reproductive organs	Endometriosis
	Genital tract malformations and/or obstruction
	Mittelschmerz
	Ovarian cyst
	Pelvic inflammatory disease (acute or chronic)
	Pelvic serositis
	Postoperative adhesions
Gastrointestinal	Constipation
	Irritable bowel
	Food intolerance
	Infections
	Inflammatory bowel disease
Urinary system	Infection
	Congenital/acquired obstruction
Musculoskeletal	Disc disease/ malalignment
	Inflammation
	Neoplasms
Psychosomatic	Stress fractures—pubis, vertebral body

Source: Adapted with permission from Joffe A, Blythe MJ. Handbook of adolescent medicine. *Adolesc Med* 2003;14(2):303, Table 4.

acyclic pain, gastrointestinal symptoms, and irregular uterine bleeding. Different than adults, the pelvic examination may be difficult to perform and thus contribute only limited information. But even when the pelvic exam is performed satisfactorily, it is most often normal in teens with endometriosis.[14,15] Having endometriomas and advanced forms of the disease are rare in teens.[15,16] Direct visualization during laparoscopy or laparotomy is considered the gold standard to diagnose endometriosis. Laparoscopy is considered after treatment with NSAIDs and

combined hormonal methods are tried and failed. In studies of teens with chronic pelvic pain, endometriosis was documented in percentages of 25%–38.3% teens undergoing laparoscopy.[17] In another study, the diagnosis of endometriosis was confirmed in 69.6%–73% in adolescents with pelvic pain who were screened for nongynecologic disorders and were unresponsive to a combination of NSAIDs and oral contraceptives OCPs.[16] Two cases of endometriosis have been reported as early as at 1 month after menarche.[18]

Treatment approach is outlined in Fig. 28-1. The goals of treatment are symptom control, prevention of further progression, and preservation of fertility using a nonsurgical approach in adolescents with endometriosis whenever possible.[14–16,19] There are no data about the regression of endometriosis in adolescents treated with combined hormone methods and NSAIDs. Depot medroxyprogesterone acetate (DMPA) every 4–12 weeks has been shown to be effective in the treatment of endometriosis symptoms in adult patients who have not responded to OCPs and NSAIDs and more effective than were OCPs combined with Danazol.[14,15] Surgery has been shown to be effective for varying percentages of patients (38%–100%) with symptomatic endometriosis.[14–16,19] As opposed to adults, no radical surgery should be used in adolescents. The recurrence of endometriosis after surgical intervention is not uncommon.[14–16] The high rate of coexistence of endometriosis and obstructive Mullerian anomalies has been reported.[15]

Other Conditions

Pelvic adhesions, secondary to sexually transmitted infections (gonorrhea, chlamydia, other infections) or an intrauterine device (IUD), is a possible cause of chronic pelvic pain in sexually active adolescents, as well as past surgeries or conditions resulting in intra abdominal adhesions.

Cervical stenosis should be suspected if severe cramping and scant menstrual flow are present. Diagnosis is confirmed by the inability to pass a thin probe of a few millimeters' diameter through the internal os.[11] Pelvic congestion syndrome is a rare condition in which the chronic pelvic pain is due to vascular

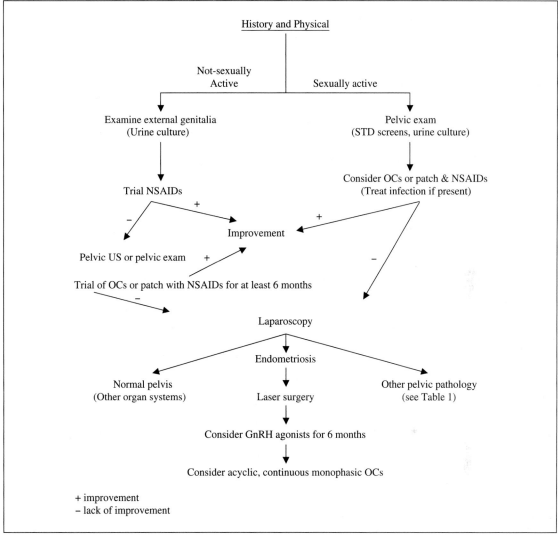

FIGURE 28-1

EVALUATION AND TREATMENT FOR DYSMENORRHEA AND ENDOMETRIOSIS.
Source: Adapted with permission from Blythe MJ. Common menstrual problems of adolescence. In: Braverman PK, Strasburger VC (eds.), *Office-Based Adolescent Health Care. Adolesc Med* 1997;8(1):107, Fig. 2.

malformations. Mittelschmerz is a recurrent midcycle pain or discomfort (ovulatory pain) of unknown cause. Dull, crampy, and sometimes very severe pain may last from a few minutes to hours and may persist for 2–3 days during the midcycle. Diagnosis can be made using the menstrual calendar. Adolescents should receive an appropriate explanation and reassurance. NSAIDs with and without a combined hormone method are found to be helpful. Nongynecologic causes like constipation and irritable bowel syndrome should be ruled out in adolescents with chronic pelvic pain and/or dysmenorrhea (Table 28-1).

TABLE 28-2

TREATMENT OF PRIMARY DYSMENORRHEA IN TEENS

Drug	Usual Dose
Aspirin	650 mg qid (max: 4000 mg/24 h)
Acetaminophen	650–1000 mg qid (max: 4000 mg/24 h)
Ibuprofen	200–800 mg qid (max: 3200 mg/24 h)
Ketoprofen (Orudis)	75 mg tid (max: 300 mg/24 h)
Naproxen (Naprosyn)	500 mg initially, then 250–375 mg tid (max: 1500 mg /24 h
Naproxen sodium (Alleve)	440 mg initially, then 440 mg tid (max: 1320 mg/24 h)
Combined hormone methods	
Oral contraceptives Patch	

Note: Aspirin and NSAIDs not recommended in aspirin sensitive patients with asthma, or ulcers or inflammatory bowel disease.
Source: Adapted with permission from Joffe A, Blythe MJ. Handbook of adolescent medicine. *Adolesc Med* 2003;14(2):303, Table 5.

VARIATIONS IN MENSTRUAL CYCLES

Amenorrhea, Oligomenorrhea, Hypomenorrhea, Irregular Menses

Irregular menstrual bleeding (ICD-9: 626.4) is one of the most common concerns for young adolescents, their families, and pediatricians. "When should the first period occur? Why has the period not started yet?" are common questions that may occur with the first signs of puberty. Menstrual irregularities considered abnormal in older women of reproductive age may be just a normal variation for the first 2 years after menarche. In the majority of these cases, the cause of menstrual irregularities in adolescents is anovulation due to the immaturity of biofeedback regulation of the menstrual cycle at the level of the hypothalamus-pituitary-ovaries. On the other hand, early menstrual irregularities or absence of menarche in adolescents

may be a result of a previously undiagnosed eating disorder or a chronic disease, such as inflammatory bowel disease, or the first sign of an endocrine disorder, such as polycystic ovarian syndrome (PCOS). All of these disorders have the potential to affect both general and reproductive health (Table 28-3).

Primary amenorrhea (ICD-9: 626.0) may be the first sign of a very serious, sometimes silent, underlying condition or disease (Table 28-4). Early and correct diagnosis during puberty may tremendously affect not only future reproductive and sexual function, but also general physical and psychosocial health. As examples, the diagnosis of uterine agenesis or Turner syndrome, or androgen insensitivity or hypogonadotropic hypogonadism as Kallmann syndrome, are devastating and may come as a shock for both the adolescent and her family because of limited or no potential for fertility or even normal sexual function. Secondary amenorrhea (ICD-9: 626.0) or oligomenorrhea (ICD-9: 626.1) may present just as primary amenorrhea except for when the cause is a congenital or chromosomal abnormality. Beyond a

TABLE 28-3

DEFINITIONS OF MENSTRUAL CYCLE IRREGULARITIES (ICD-9 CODES)

Amenorrhea (626.0)
Primary amenorrhea: Absence of menarche with no history of prior spontaneous uterine bleeding by age 16 or lack of initiation of menses after presence of puberty for more than 3 years or lack of initiation of menses with no signs of puberty by age 14.
Secondary amenorrhea: Cessation of menstrual cycles for more than three menstrual cycles after having experienced menses for more than 2 years.

Oligomenorrhea (626.1)
Infrequent, irregular menses consistently occurring at >42-day intervals for the last 6 months or more after having experienced menses for more than 2 years.

Hypomenorrhea (626.1)
Decreased amount of menstrual blood loss at each cycle but menses occurring at regular intervals.

Irregular menses (626.4)
Menstrual bleeding occurring at varying intervals at >21 days and <42 days, usually not requiring evaluation or intervention.

TABLE 28-4

CAUSES OF PRIMARY AND SECONDARY AMENORRHEA

Physiologic
Early puberty
Pregnancy
Lactation and postpartum period
Anatomic
Congenital abnormalities:
  Müllerian abnormalities:
  Uterine agenesis, imperforate hymen, transverse
    intravaginal septum, vaginal agenesis
Other:
  Endometriosis, bilateral ovariectomy, uterine
    adhesions
Genetic and chromosomal abnormalities
Gonadal dysgenesis:
  Turner syndrome (classic 45,XO) and mosaicism
    (e.g., 45,X/47,XXX)
  Swyer syndrome (mixed 46,XY)
  Androgen insensitivity syndrome (XY)
Hypothalamic-pituitary
Eating issues: weight loss, female athlete triad,
  excessive exercise
Depression
Misuse and abuse of illegal and prescribed drugs
PCOS
Medications: contraceptives, steroids, drugs inducing
  elevated prolactin (e.g., antipsychotics)
	Hypogonadotropic hypogonadism: idiopathic,
	  Kallmann syndrome, isolated GnRH-deficiency
	Tumors: craniopharyngioma, adenoma, carcinoma
	Chronic diseases: cystic fibrosis, chronic renal disease,
	  rheumatologic disorders, inflammatory bowel disease,
	  chronic liver disease
	Structural Damage: hemochromatosis, tuberculous,
	  granuloma, meningoencephalitis, aneurysm
	Radiation and/or chemotherapy
	Ovarian
	PCOS
	Severe pelvic inflammatory disease
	Ovarian cysts and tumors
	Gonadal dysgenesis or absence of ovarian tissue
	Premature ovarian failure
	Total or partial resection
	Pelvic radiation and/or chemotherapy
	Uterine
	Uterine agenesis and other Mullerian abnormalities
	Endometritis
	Pelvic radiation
	Other diseases and conditions
	Hypothyroidism
	Hyperandrogenism as adrenal disorders
	Diabetes mellitus
	Chronic liver disease

good history and physical and urine pregnancy test, menses defined as hypomenorrhea (ICD-9: 626.1) and/or irregular menses (ICD-9: 626.4) usually requires no further workup but observation using a menstrual calendar for documentation (Table 28-3). The primary care physician's role is important in providing appropriate reassurance and explanations about puberty and menses to the young adolescent and her family. An understanding about menstrual irregularities will help to determine when to initiate appropriate evaluation and treatment and/or to refer to a specialist.

Etiology

In some cases the cause of amenorrhea may not be well defined. The major categories of either primary or secondary amenorrhea are defined by either the cause or the level of functional or structural damage (Table 28-4). Hypogonadotropic or hypergonadotropic refers to low or high levels of FSH and LH and suggests the etiology of the amenorrhea. Hypogonadism refers to the function of the ovary and indicates low levels of estradiol.

Evaluation

A detailed history, a careful assessment of general and pubertal development, and the correlation between the clinical findings and the individual patient's chronologic age are the most important initial steps to be undertaken by the primary care provider. An expensive and sometimes unnecessary workup in adolescent females with amenorrhea may be avoided.

Step 1. Rule out the physiologic causes of amenorrhea in young adolescents: The adolescent may be too early in her pubertal sequence to have menarche (prepubertal or early pubertal). Both the presence and sequence of the major pubertal events should be documented and correlated with chronological age: breast development, the growth spurt and pubic hair development, then menses. For some teens, pubic hair occurs first before breast development, growth spurt, and menses. In the evaluation of any young patient with primary amenorrhea, the initial evaluation should include history with detailed birth, past medical, family, social histories along with the physical examination assessing pubertal development, and the staging of secondary sexual characteristics. The diagnosis of physiologic amenorrhea of puberty if present avoids unnecessary tests or interventions.

Step 2. Adolescent may be pregnant: The absence of menarche and denial of sexual activity by a young pubertal adolescent should not discourage a pediatrician from checking a urine pregnancy test in the office. It is necessary to exclude pregnancy as a possible cause of secondary and, in rare cases, of primary amenorrhea in adolescents. A urine pregnancy test first becomes positive after the first 7–10 days of pregnancy or implantation or after 1–2 weeks of a missed period.

Step 3. There may be no menstrual outflow tract: An initial or reexamination of the external genitalia should be performed by the pediatrician, at least once during puberty before the onset of menses. If present, an imperforate hymen may indicate other congenital anomalies of the vagina, cervix, and uterus referred to as Müllerian abnormalities. The presence of a hymen and even its patency as determined by probe with a small Q-tip cannot exclude other vaginal anomalies such as transverse septum, agenesis of the upper vagina, or uterine abnormalities as agenesis of uterus. An MRI of the pelvis best evaluates the anatomy of the reproductive system to exclude the possibility of congenital anomalies.

Step 4. Adolescent is too stressed or too thin or too overweight: Family, school, social, and nutritional history, as well as exercise patterns and recent weights are necessary to obtain in any young patient with amenorrhea or irregular menses. The presenting BMI (body mass index)[*] may be the best clue. BMIs <15% and >85% place teens at risk for period problems. Primary or secondary amenorrhea may be the presenting symptom of an eating disorder, depression, drug use, physical/sexual abuse, and/or other psychosocial issues affecting the teen.

Step 5. Adolescent is compulsive exerciser or competitive athlete or a professional dancer or skater: Areas of nutrition, exercise, and recent weights should be emphasized. The patient may have symptoms of an eating disorder along with the syndrome of the Female Athlete Triad (disordered eating, amenorrhea, and decreased bone mineral density [BMD]).[20] In sports demanding low body weight, a combination of factors including intensity of exercise, insufficient calories, mental stress, and genetic factors result in "energy drain" and hypothalamic dysfunction.[20]

Step 6. Adolescent may have a chromosomal disorder: Turner syndrome and testicular feminization are the most common genetic causes of primary amenorrhea in adolescents and may not be diagnosed until the time of the expected menarche during puberty.

Step 7. Adolescent has signs and symptoms of endocrine disorder: Especially if the findings of hirsutism, acne, acanthosis nigricans, breast discharge, thyroid nodule or enlargement, and/or clitoromegaly are present. Thyroid disorders, prolactinoma, or hyperandrogenism are associated with amenorrhea, oligomenorrhea, and irregular menses in adolescents.

Step 8. Adolescent has a previous diagnosis or undiagnosed chronic condition or disease that requires treatment and intervention: A variety of chronic diseases and conditions present during adolescence and childhood. As an example, chemotherapy and/or pelvic radiation may have a major impact on normal puberty and menstrual function (Table 28-4). A diagnostic workup for adolescents with secondary amenorrhea and oligomenorrhea and a normal history and examination is summarized in Fig. 28-2.

---

[*]BMI = weight in pounds/height in inches/ height in inches × 703

CASE STUDY 28-1

Primary Amenorrhea in a 16-Year-Old Female with Congenital Hypogonadotropic Hypogonadism or Kallmann Syndrome

History: This 16-year-old female presents with the history of no menses. She had a normal birth history and development. She just finished her sophomore year of high school on the honor roll. Family history includes an intact family with the biologic mother (63 inches.) and father (69 inches) and two older female sibs with menarche at age 13. Her mother's menarche was at age 11. Her past medical history is unremarkable except for irritable bowel. Alone she denies use of substances such as tobacco alcohol or marijuana. She has never been sexually active. Of note on the review of systems is anosmia or the inability to smell, as has the mother's half-brother who has two children.

Physical: Her height 63 inches. at the 25th percentile, her weight 103 pounds at the 10th percentile, and a BMI of 18 (25%) were normal. Her blood pressure was 101/67 mmHg and her pulse was 74/min. She was Tanner B1 for breasts and Tanner P4 for her pubic hair. The remainder of her examination was unremarkable including her external genitalia, which demonstrated vaginal patency.

Laboratory/treatment: Her thyroid tests, complete blood count (CBC) tests, and prolactin were unremarkable while her follicle-stimulating hormone (FSH) of 3.5 mU/mL, leutinizing hormone (LH) of 0.3 mU/mL, and estradiol of <25 pg/mL were prepubertal levels. Her bone age was delayed at age 13 years. Her pelvic ultrasound and MRI of brain and reproductive organs were unremarkable except for prepubertal appearance of the ovaries and uterus. Her chromosomes were normal. A probe for the *anosmin* gene on the X chromosome was sent and a GnRH stimulation test was scheduled by the endocrinologist. Treatment with hormones was initiated.

CASE STUDY 28-2

Secondary Amenorrhea in a 16-Year-Old Female with Acquired Hypogonadotropic Hypogonadism

History: This 16–year-old female presents with secondary amenorrhea for 14 months with a history of menarche at age 13 with periods described as always irregular, but occurring every 2 months. Over the last year her weight had decreased about 7–10 lbs with "more careful attention to eliminating foods with fat." She does not eat any dairy products and will usually eat meat such as chicken and turkey when her mom serves it. Pertinent family history includes an older female sib in college with a past history of anorexia nervosa. Exercise includes aerobic activity every day without missing a day as "I just don't feel good unless I exercise." Past medical history includes a stress fracture of her lumbar spine when she was playing competitive volleyball year-round the previous year. The remainder of her review of systems was unremarkable.

Physical: Her physical was unremarkable with her weight 134 pounds (50%–75%), her height 69.5 inches. (>95%), and her BMI of 19.5 at the 50%. Her Tanner staging was B5 P5. Her external genitalia appeared normal. Her CBC, electrolytes, glucose, Ca^{2+}, liver functions, and kidney functions were normal as was her thyroid functions. Her FSH was 5 mU/mL, LH 0.5 mU/mL, and her estradiol <25 pg/mL, all prepubertal levels. Her free testosterone and prolactin were normal. She did not respond to the progestin challenge. Her BMD study did not reveal any abnormalities.

Treatment: A nutrition referral was made with a food diary requested. Discussion ensued regarding her food and exercise obsession and a suggestion for counseling was made. Hormone replacement was not recommended at this time. Periods will often disappear in young women with eating issues before the BMI <15%.

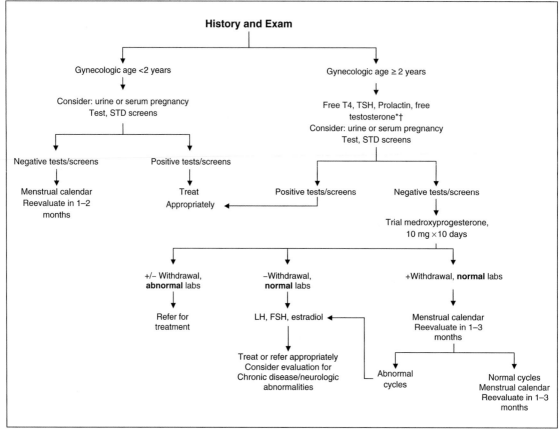

FIGURE 28-2
EVALUATION OF SECONDARY AMENORRHEA AND OLIGOMENORRHEA IN THE ADOLESCENT PATIENT.
Source: Adapted with permission from Joffe A, Blythe MJ. Handbook of adolescent medicine. *Adolesc Med* 2003;14(2):296, Fig. 2.

Dysfunctional Uterine Bleeding, Menorrhagia, Metrorrhagia

Prolonged, heavy and frequent menses is a very common reason for presentation to the primary care provider for teens, particularly during the first 2 years after menarche. The most likely cause of excessive uterine bleeding in adolescents is anovulatory dysfunctional uterine bleeding (DUB) with the variations of bleeding patterns and ICD-9 codes in Table 28-5.

Classification of DUB

DUB is divided into two major categories: anovulatory and ovulatory. Anovulatory DUB is the most common type of DUB in adolescents (90%) and usually presents during the first 2 years after

menarche. Based on the degree of anemia and the associated clinical findings, anovulatory DUB is subdivided as: mild, moderate, and severe. If occurring within the first 2 years after the onset of periods, DUB is associated with anovulation due to the lack of maturity of regulation of the menstrual cycle at the hypothalamic-pituitary-ovarian level.

Evaluation

Excessive, prolonged, and irregular menses may be accompanied by anxiety, fears, and frustrations in the patient and her family. In some cases, excessive blood loss may lead to severe anemia and hemodynamic instability, and require immediate intervention including hospitalization. Primary care provider may initiate the evaluation and management of prolonged,

TABLE 28-5

DEFINITIONS OF DYSFUNCTIONAL UTERINE BLEEDING AND RELATED DISORDERS (ICD-9 CODES)

Dysfunctional uterine bleeding (626.8)
Prolonged, excessive (>8 days), irregular (<21 days), painless uterine bleeding in the absence of any other uterine pathology.

Menorrhagia (626.2)
Excessive amount and increased duration uterine bleeding occurring at regular intervals (>21 days, <42 days).

Metrorrhagia (626.6)
Intermenstrual irregular bleeding between regular periods (>21 days, <42 days)

Polymenorrhea (626.2)
Frequent regular or irregular bleeding at <21 day intervals.

heavy, irregular menstrual bleeding in adolescents. A detailed history and physical examination is the first step to appropriate treatment. Consider the following suggestions, using a routine approach to the evaluation and management of a teen with excessive and irregular menses (Fig. 28-3).

Step 1. Determine if this adolescent patient is hemodynamically stable: The general rule in the evaluation of any adolescent with excessive irregular menses is to determine the degree of anemia and hemodynamic instability. The clinical classification defines three types of DUB based on severity of anemia and clinical findings of hemodynamic instability including obtaining hemoglobin (Hgb) and hematocrit (Hmt):

Mild: characterized by the normal hemoglobin (Hgb) (>12 g/dL) and Hmt (38%), in clinically stable patient.
Moderate: characterized by decrease in the Hgb (10–12 g/dL) and Hmt ((28–35%) in clinically stable patient.
Severe: characterized by significant decreases in the Hgb (<10g/dL) and Hmt (<28%), tachycardia, orthostatic changes, hypotension, and delayed capillary refill.

Occasionally mild to moderate DUB may be associated with signs and symptoms of hemodynamic instability and require immediate intervention including hospitalization. Always check orthostatics in a patient with history of prolonged, excessive bleeding.

Step 2. Determine pregnancy status: Abnormal uterine bleeding in an adolescent may be the result of pregnancy and its complications. Young age and denial of sexual activity should not interfere with obtaining a pregnancy test. Previous sexual contact(s) may have been unwanted, unreported, and unrecognized. Recent potential delivery, miscarriage, or termination of a pregnancy may have occurred. The results of a pregnancy test should be documented on all patients with irregular menses.

Step 3. Determine if any there has been any use of hormonal products either with or without parental knowledge: Inquire about the current or recent use of estrogen and/or progesterone containing products, including pills, shots, patches, rings, or creams. Irregular uterine bleeding may be due to noncompliance or a side effect of a method.

Estrogen withdrawal bleeding is the result of a sudden decrease in estrogen levels.
Example: anovulation or noncompliance with oral contraceptive pills.
Progesterone breakthrough bleeding is the result progesterone-induced atrophy of the endometrium.
Example: irregular bleeding in patients on progestin-only containing products (e.g., injectable progestin)

Step 4. Determine if there has been any use of prescribed or over-the counter or street drugs: Drug-drug interactions between combined hormones and other medications like anticonvulsants, antipsychotics, antifungals, and the antibiotic rifampin. Inquiry should be made with the family about medications (prescribed and over-the-counter), and with the teen alone about drug use and abuse (illegal and banned) such as with nutritional supplements or herbal products.

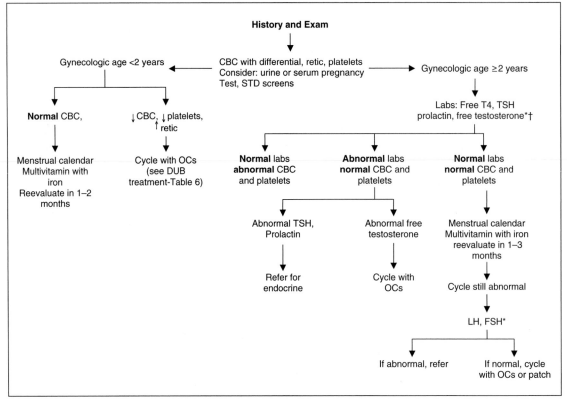

FIGURE 28-3

EVALUATION OF DYSFUNCTIONAL UTERINE BLEEDING IN ADOLESCENT PATIENTS.
Source: Adapted with permission from Joffe A, Blythe MJ. Handbook of adolescent medicine. *State Art Rev* 2003;14(2):294, Fig. 1.

Step 5. Determine if any local pathology or structural abnormalities in the reproductive system

Example:

Urethral trauma: accident, rape, first intercourse
Vaginal or cervical bleedings: pregnancy, sexually transmitted infectious, foreign body, cervical or uterine polyps.
Nongenital bleeding: fissures, hemorrhoids, polyps, and so forth.

Step 6. Determine if menarche is premature:

Menarche is the last event in the sequence of female pubertal development. In girls menarche usually occurs between 10.5 and 14.5 years of age, usually during Tanner Stage 3 or 4 of both breast and pubic hair development. Breast development, growth spurt, and pubic hair development always precede

menarche during normal puberty. Staging of secondary sexual characteristics, correlation with chronological and bone age, and the hormonal profile (e.g., FSH, LH, estradiol) are the part of diagnostic workup. If menarche appears before other signs of puberty, conditions associated with precocious puberty like ovarian tumors or McCune-Albright syndrome should be ruled out.

McCune-Albright syndrome is a condition when premature menarche occurs prior to breast and pubic hair development due to estrogen secreting ovarian cysts (GnRH [gonadotropin]-independent). Abnormal stimulation of the growth and function of gonads due to a gene mutation is considered the most likely cause. The other clinical findings are café au lait type skin pigmentation, usually unilateral on the upper spine and buttocks associated with bone changes (Chap. 15).

Step 7. Determine if pelvic or abdominal mass: If pelvic or abdominal mass is found, the pelvic ultrasound (or possibly MRI) should be obtained to rule out as an ectopic or uterine pregnancy, ovarian cyst or tumor, or congenital anomalies of reproductive tract. The pelvic ultrasound is the first step to rule out ovarian lesions.

Step 8. Determine if other endocrine disorders present: Hypothyroidism and hyperthyroidism may cause a DUB. History of weight loss and palpitations (hyperthyroidism) or weight gain and fatigue (hypothyroidism) should alert the provider about possible thyroid dysfunction. The physical examination of thyroid may detect tenderness, enlargement, or a node. Thyroid function tests should be included in the evaluation of adolescents with irregular bleeding. If galactorrhea is present consider a prolactinoma, hypothyroidism, or use of medication as antipsychotics or use of illicit drugs that may result in increased prolactin production.

Step 9. Determine if signs of hirsutism or virilization present: Often disorders like PCOS, congenital adrenal hyperplasia (late-onset 21-OHase deficiency), Cushing syndrome, androgen-producing tumors, use of steroids, or exogenous hormone-containing products are other hormonal causes of a DUB in adolescents (Chap. 15).

Step 10. Determine if coagulation problems present: Von Willebrand's disease is the most common inherited bleeding disorder (Chap. 17). In girls, this disorder may be diagnosed later in life, shortly after menarche. Other conditions (e.g., renal and liver failure, leukemia, idiopathic thrombocytopenic petechiae (ITP), inherited bleeding disorders) as well as medications and therapies (e.g., chemotherapy, warfarin, aspirin) are associated with bleeding disorders, and may result in abnormal blood coagulation and prolonged and excessive uterine bleeding. A variety of tests are currently available to determine bleeding disorders.

Step 11. Determine chronic disease or condition that may affect adolescent's menstrual cycle: Epilepsy, systemic lupus erythematosus (SLE), liver disease, cystic fibrosis, and inflammatory bowel disorder are chronic diseases associated with increase frequency of menstrual irregularities from prolonged bleedings to amenorrhea. Past or current use of chemotherapy or radiation may have a negative impact on all levels of menstrual cycle regulation.

Step 12. Determine the presence of stress or weight changes: Due to anovulation, irregular menses may be the result of stress, excessive exercise, and eating disorders (Chap. 30).[20]

Step 13. Determine if the gynecologic or postmenarcheal age of adolescents is less than 2 years: Within the first 2 years after menarche, mild irregular bleeding may occur without any identifiable cause, signs, or other symptoms except for anemia. It is thought to be due to the immaturity of the biofeedback regulation mechanisms for the menstrual cycle. This diagnosis does not require an intensive laboratory workup or any intervention.

Recommended evaluation and treatment options for adolescents with prolonged, heavy, irregular menses are summarized in Table 28-6 and Figure 28-3.

CASE STUDY 28-3

Severe Uterine Bleeding in a 17-Year-Old Female with SLE-Induced Anemia

History: A 17-year-old, previously healthy, Caucasian female with no pertinent family history, social history, drug history, past medical history, weight or nutritional or exercise history. She reported the recent onset of symptoms of epistaxis, a rash on her cheeks following sun exposure, fatigue, and joint swelling. She was referred by her pediatrician to a community hospital because of heavy vaginal bleeding lasting for more than 2 weeks. Her CBC revealed hemoglobin of 3.6 mg% and a platelet count of 2000. An antinuclear antibody (ANA) titer was 1:640. She was transferred to the Children's Hospital at the university with possible diagnosis of hemolytic anemia secondary to SLE.

Physical Examination: She was very pale with no acute distress. Vital signs included a pulse of 110/min, RR 16/min, BP 134/60 mmHg, with her O_2 saturation documented at 100%. Her weight was 104 pounds (10%–25%) and her height was 65 inches (50%). Her BMI of 17.8 places her at the 10%–25%. The remainder of her examination was unremarkable except for a pierced tongue, tachycardia with a 3/6 systolic murmur at the left sternal border with good pulses, and a few petechiae on her legs. Her pelvic examination revealed the normal anatomy and evidence of severe uterine bleeding.

Laboratory values on admission: Her CBC showed a Hgb 3.5 gm/dL, hematocrit (Hct) 10.9%, platelet count 4000 k/cubic mm, and WBCs 4000 k/cubic mm with the differential of polys 80%, lymphs 18%, and monos 2%. Her iron of 3 µg/dL (50–160) was low with normal total iron binding capacity (TIBC) of 376 µg/dL, thus the iron saturation was low at 1%. Her ferritin was low at 5 ng/dL (10–106). Her clotting functions were normal with partial thromboplastin time (PTT) 23, prothrombin time (PT) 13.9, and International Normalized Ratio (INR) 1.15. Her electrolytes, kidney, and liver functions were unremarkable except for her complements, which showed a decreased C4 but normal C3. Her ESR was slightly elevated at 22 with her crithidia-nDNA Ab test positive for Lupus. Her antiphospholipids tests were positive. Her serum pregnancy test was negative. The pelvic ultrasound was unremarkable except for some fluid in the cul-de-sac. Her rheumatoid factor was negative. Her peripheral smear was consistent with microcytic, hypochromic anemia, and thrombocytopenia. Her bone marrow aspirate revealed hypocellular marrow. Her screens for sexually transmitted infections were negative.

Treatment: She was admitted to the hematology oncology ward. Several services were consulted including rheumatology, adolescent medicine for her vaginal bleeding, ophthalmology for possible uveitis and iritis, and the adolescent psychiatry for depression. IV conjugated estrogen (25 mg) was administered every 4 hours and a monophasic oral contraceptive in multiple doses was initiated. She was given 4 units of packed red blood cells. Her vaginal bleeding stopped after 36 hours of treatment with the IV estrogen, while the oral contraceptives were continued, while iron and Prednisone treatments were initiated. After 6 days she was discharged home in stable condition. Her CBC revealed Hgb of 7.3 g/d/, Hct of 23.9%, WBC of 8500 k/cubic mm, platelet count of 176,000 k/cubic mm, and reticulocyte count of 5.6%. Her return appointments included rheumatology clinic, adolescent medicine, and psychiatry. She was switched to the injectable progestin to control her periods as an outpatient.

POLYCYSTIC OVARIAN SYNDROME (ICD-D: 256.4)

One of the most common causes of amenorrhea in adolescents is PCOS. Menstrual irregularities, secondary amenorrhea, hirsutism, and specific morphologic changes in ovaries were described in 1935 by Stein and Levental as a PCOS.

Definition

There is a general consensus that PCOS is a syndrome because no single diagnostic criteria is sufficient for clinical diagnosis.[8,11,21–25] PCOS also remains a diagnosis of exclusion.[22,23,25] PCOS seems to be a part of general metabolic and endocrine disorder with the key features of insulin resistance, resulting in hyperinsulinemia that affects ovarian function resulting in the production of excess androgens and abnormal gonadotropin secretion.[25]

In 1990, the NIH Conference defined the clinical criteria for diagnosis of PCOS as chronic anovulation and androgen excess having no other identifiable cause. In a recent consensus workshop conducted in 2003, the suggestion was that PCOS be diagnosed when two of three criteria are present: oligomenorrhea/and or anovulation, clinical or biochemical signs of hyperandrogenism, and ultrasound

TABLE 28-6

TREATMENT OF DUB OR METROMENORRHAGIA IN ADOLESCENT PATIENTS

Mild anemia

Hct >33% or Hgb >11 g/dL

Acute treatment

Menstrual calendar

Iron supplementation

Consider: oral contraceptives (OCs) or patch if patient is sexually active and desires contraception
(standard once-daily dose)

Long-term treatment

Monitor: Iron status (Hgb/Hct)

Follow-up: 1–2 months

Moderate anemia

Hct 27%–33% or Hgb 9–11 g/dL

Acute treatment

Begin: OCs (30 μg EE monophasic) + antiemetics

Regimen:

Two pills/day × 13–19 days (1 bid)

Withdrawal bleeding × 7 days

Long-term treatment

OCs cycle for 3 months

Begin OCs one pill a day the Sunday after withdrawal bleeding begins

Length of use dependent on resolution of anemia. Iron supplementation

Monitor: Iron status

Follow up: 2–3 weeks and every 3 months

Severe anemia

Hct <27% or Hgb <9 g/dL(or dropping)

Acute treatment

Begin: OCs (30 μg EE monophasic) + antiemetics

4 pills/day × 4 days   (1 qid)

3 pills/day × 4 days   (1 tid)

2 pills/day × 13–19 days   (1 bid)

Withdrawal bleeding × 7 days

Long-term treatment

Cycle with OCs, one pill a day starting the Sunday after withdrawal bleeding begins

Length of OC use dependent on resolution of anemia. Iron supplementation

Monitor: Iron status

Follow-up: 2–3 weeks and every 3 months

Source: Adapted with permission from Blythe MJ. Common menstrual problems of adolescence. In: Braverman PK, Strasburger VC (eds.), *Office-based Adolescent Health Care. Adolesc Med* 1997;8(1)94, Table 7.

findings of polycystic ovaries. Clinically, it has been recognized that some women with polycystic ovaries and evidence of ovarian dysfunction do not have *clinical evidence* of androgen excess, or women with hyperandrogenism and polycystic ovaries may have normal ovulatory function.[22,23]

Epidemiology

As the most common endocrine disorder in women, PCOS, probably affects between 4% and 10% of women of reproductive age.[21-23] There is no significant difference in prevalence between Caucasian and African American women.[24]

Etiology and pathophysiology

After more than seven decades of research, the etiology and pathophysiology of PCOS still remain unclear.

Diagnosis

PCOS is a clinical diagnosis with variety of signs and symptoms of anovulation, hyperandrogenicity, and metabolic abnormalities.[8,21,23,25]

Chronic anovulation, the key feature of the PCOS, is the primary cause of menstrual irregularities.[11,23] Long-term chronic unopposed estrogenization of the endometrium increases risk for endometrial cancer in women with PCOS, if untreated. Menstrual irregularities usually start during puberty. Amenorrhea is the most common type (50%) of menstrual disorder in women with PCOS. Heavy and irregular uterine bleeding is reported in 30%. An elevated LH and normal to low FSH results in an increased LH/FSH ratio, with elevated free testosterone and androstenedione levels. On the other hand, 20%–40% of women with PCOS do not have elevated LH levels, but all have elevated levels of one or more androgens documented biologically.

Hyperandrogenism has been considered a necessary diagnostic criteria for PCOS. Other causes should be carefully evaluated. Android obesity, elevated blood pressure, and skin changes as acne and acanthosis nigricans may be present. The standardized Ferriman and Gallwey scoring system can be used for the assessment of hirsutism.[26] Androgen excess presents in overweight children with early pubic hair, body odor, and acne, and may be an early clinical sign of PCOS prior to puberty.[21,23]

Metabolic abnormalities include hyperinsulinemia, hyperglycemia, impaired glucose tolerance test, and abnormal lipid profile (elevated total cholesterol, low-density lipoprotein [LDL], very low-density lipoprotein [VLDL], triglycerides, and low high-density lipoprotein [HDL]) and are the most commonly associated metabolic abnormalities reported in women with PCOS. The lipid abnormalities occurring early in women with PCOS are a potential risk for atherosclerosis later in life.[11,21,23,25,27] Insulin resistance is considered the principal metabolic abnormality in patients with PCOS. Many studies suggest that insulin resistance may be the primary process leading to anovulation in women with PCOS. Most women with PCOS have normal fasting glucose concentrations, yet are at risk for impaired glucose tolerance and type II diabetes (Chap. 15). This suggests that fasting glucose levels are poor predictors of the future onset of noninsulin dependent diabetes mellitus in patients with PCOS.[25,27] But a fasting glucose to insulin ratio (glucose/insulin) of <4.5 in adults has suggested PCOS.

Acanthosis nigricans is associated with insulin resistance and hyperandrogenism.[11,21,26,28] Acanthosis nigricans is a velvety brownish black or gray discoloration of the skin at the neck, groin, and axillae (Chaps. 15 and 19). This clinical sign, in some cases indicates PCOS, but is not an absolute marker for hyperandrogenism. Acanthosis nigricans may be found in normal women.

Ovarian changes documented by ultrasound may be normal or indicate bilaterally enlarged ovaries with numerous follicles in varying early stages of development including atretic follicles. Histologically, on cut section, the ovary exhibits 8–10 discrete subcapsular follicles 4–8 mm in diameter and peripherally arrayed to resemble a necklace in PCOS.[25]

Evaluation

Any adolescents with reported irregular menstrual cycle with and without clinical features of hyperandrogenism and obesity should be evaluated for possible PCOS. The key points in the evaluation and the clinical laboratory criteria for PCOS in adolescents are summarized in Table 28-7. The "typical" findings of polycystic ovaries on ultrasound may be present in only in 54%–66% of women with PCOS and present in 23% of normal women.[8,11,22,23,25]

Management of PCOS

For many years the treatment objectives for those patients with PCOS were directed at the problems of infertility, hirsutism, and irregular menses. Currently, the commonly used therapeutic interventions can be divided into two major groups:

1. Symptomatic therapy(e.g., hyperandrogenism, irregular menses)
2. Prevention and management of health risks (e.g., cardiovascular, metabolic abnormalities, diabetes)

The clinical studies have demonstrated that metformin and combined hormone use as pills or patch can regulate both menstrual and the metabolic abnormalities.[28,29] Metformin serves to improve insulin sensitivity, decrease insulin levels, and thus lessen the symptoms associated with hyperinsulinemia including ovarian hyperandrogenism, acne, hyperlipidemia, and acanthosis nigricans. Antiandrogens such as spironolactone and cimetidine[21,23,28–30] can be used for the treatment of acne and hirsutism but must be used in combination with contraceptives (Table 28-7). Patient education, lifestyle modifications, stress-control therapy, exercise, nutritional supplements, herbs, and acupuncture have been used in the management of women with PCOS. Surgery is no longer considered as a first line of therapy in patients with PCOS.[8, 21,25]

Long-term complications of PCOS documented in clinical and basic research conducted in the last two decades indicates that women with PCOS are at the increased risk for infertility, endometrial cancer, type II diabetes, lipid abnormalities, hypertension,

---

TABLE 28-7

POLYCYSTIC OVARIAN SYNDROME IN ADOLESCENTS

Evaluation of adolescents with possible PCOS

A detailed history and physical examination

A pregnancy test

Staging of secondary sexual characteristics

A gynecologic examination (at least external genitalia)

Laboratory assessment

   FSH, LH, total and free testosterone, prolactin, and TSH

   Liver functions as SGOT (AST), SGPT (ALT), and bilirubin (direct and indirect)

   Fasting glucose and insulin level (ratio glucose/ insulin <4.5 suggestive of hyperinsulinemia)*

   Fasting lipid profile

   If patient hirsute, need fasting DHEA-S, 17-OH progesterone, and cortisol to rule out adrenal gland disorders or adrenal or ovarian tumors

A progestin challenge test if no menses in the last 2 months or more

Clinical and biologic criteria suggesting PCOS in adolescents

An increased ratio of serum LH/FSH

An increased serum free testosterone (97% specific and 70% sensitive)

A positive response to a progestin challenge test (uterine bleeding)

Treatment

Counsel the patient in weight reduction if appropriate.

Treat the menstrual disorder with combination hormonal methods as the oral contraceptives or the patch.

Use antiandrogens for accompanying symptoms of acne and/or hirsutism.

Consider use of metformin 1500–2000 mg daily in divided doses for treatment of hyperinsulinemia.

*Legro RS. *J Clin Endocrinol Metab* 1998; 83: 2694-8.

---

and cardiovascular disease.[22,23,27] In summary, early diagnosis of PCOS in adolescents allows not only the early assessment and treatment of teens but education about the long-term reproductive, hormonal, and metabolic consequences associated with this disorder.

CASE STUDY 28-4

Amenorrhea in a 15-Year-Old Female with PCOS

History: A 15-year 10-month-old female appeared in clinic with the general complaints of not feeling well. Menarche was at age 8 with irregular menses with her last period 11 months before her presentation. Her mother's gynecologic history was unremarkable. Family history included the patient as the only child. Her biologic father has a history of weight problems and high blood pressure and type II Diabetes mellitus. Her social history was unremarkable including no history of sexual activity. She excelled in her academic work. She also had symptoms of depression but denied use or misuse of any substances.

Physical examination: Her vital signs were weight 152 pounds (75th–90th percentile) and her height of 61.25 inches (10th–25th percentile) placed her BMI of 28 at the 90%–95%. The remainder of the examination was unremarkable including no evidence of acne, thyroid enlargement, acanthosis nigricans, hirsutism, striae, and clitoromegaly. She was Tanner Stages B5 and P5. Her blood pressure and heart rate were normal.

Laboratory: Her LH was elevated at 24 mU/mL and her FSH was normal at 6.7 mU/mL. Her fasting glucose was 98 mg% and insulin was 43.5 MCIU/mL with an decreased glucose to insulin ratio (98/43.4=2.25). Her thyroid functions were normal including her free thyroxine and thyroid-stimulating hormone (TSH) as was her CBC. Her free testosterone was elevated at 3.5 pg/mL (normal 0.6–2.6). She had normal liver functions including a total bilirubin, serum glutamic oxaloacetic transaminase (SGOT), alkaline phosphatase, serum glutamic pyruvate transaminase (SGPT), and γ-glutamyl transpeptidase (GGT). Her fasting cholesterol was 216 mg% with LDL 123 mg%, triglycerides 135 mg%, and HDL 66 mg%. She had a normal transabdominal ultrasound that showed normal ovarian size and normal follicular activity. She was seen by the dietician and counseled on appropriate nutrition. Her urine pregnancy test was negative.

Treatment: Her trial of oral progestins resulted in a menstrual period and she was started on oral contraceptives and metformin and fluoxetine. Over the next 12 months with dietary counseling and mental health assessment, she was able to decrease her weight by 40 lb while remaining on all of her medications.

OVARIAN TUMORS IN ADOLESCENTS

Menstrual irregularities, premature menarche, with and without abdominal pain and/or pelvic mass, may be the result of benign and/or malignant ovarian disorders in adolescents. Although ovarian tumors are more common in women of reproductive or postmenopausal age, several types of benign or malignant ovarian tumors may occur during adolescence (Table 28-8).

TABLE 28-8

MALIGNANT OVARIAN TUMORS AND THEIR MARKERS IN ADOLESCENTS

CELL Origins/ Tumor Type	Tumor Markers
Germ cell malignancies	
Dysgerminoma	Alpha-fetoprotein (AFP)
Choriocarcinoma	Serum hCG
Mixed germ cell tumor	LDH
Sex cord-stromal tumors	
Juvenile granulose cell	Elevated estrogen
Sertoli cell tumor	Elevated estrogen, and/or progesterone or testosterone
Sertoli-Leydig cell tumor	Elevated testosterone

Benign Ovarian Cysts/Tumors

1. *Follicular ovarian cysts* are the most common type of ovarian cysts found with the onset of puberty and through adolescence. Irregular menses, abdominal pain, and/or pelvic mass should alert the pediatrician as to the possibility of an ovarian lesion. Follicular ovarian cysts are observed in 12.2% in healthy adolescents, and most cysts will regress within a 3-month period with no surgical or hormonal treatment.[8,25,31] Malignant transformation is rare but may occur in 4.4% of teens.[31]

2. *Dermoid cyst* or *mature cystic teratoma* is very common in children, adolescents, and young women. Due to the specific histologic origin of dermoid cysts (presence of ecto-, meso-, and endodermal tissues), hair, teeth, bone, and skin fragments can be found within the tumor. The clinical presentation is usually asymptomatic except for the presence of a unilateral (60%) mass or bilateral (10.8%) mass. If a large size tumor is present, the symptoms of acute abdominal pain, nausea, and vomiting may indicate ovarian torsion of the affected side. Also, ovarian tumors have ruptured. Rare cases of virilization reported the presentation of dermoid cysts.[8,25,31] Another complication, hemolytic anemia, has been reported but resolved after surgery.[8,25] Malignant cells can be present in 19% of dermoid cysts.[8,25] A node within a tumor, Rokitansky's protuberance, is a common site of malignancy. Management is directed (1) ruling out malignancy and (2) performing surgery.

3. *Ovarian fibroma* is a benign ovarian tumor with cellular origins from the sex cord stroma. The tumor is rare representing only 1%–3% of all ovarian tumors, usually presenting as a unilateral and asymptomatic pelvic mass.[8,31] For no known reason, the left ovary is the more commonly affected. This tumor may be associated with a very rare condition called the classic Meig syndrome (e.g., ascites, ovarian tumor, hydrothorax), or the pseudo-Meig syndrome (ascites only). Malignancy is more likely present with these findings. Serum CA-125, a tumor marker, can be elevated and thus a marker of malignancy.[8,25,32]

Management is (1) to rule out malignancy and (2) surgery. Reoccurrence of ovarian fibroma is common.

4. *Serous cystadenoma* is a benign ovarian tumor of epithelial origin, usually unilateral and asymptomatic. Serous cystadenoma may occur in children but the most common age group is women of the reproductive age. Reaching large sizes, the presenting symptoms may be abdominal and pelvic discomfort along with increasing abdominal girth. Serous cystadenoma can be diagnosed by ultrasound, however MRI is recommended because of its significantly higher sensitivity and capacity for differential diagnosis of malignancy.[8,25,32] Management is (1) to rule out malignancy and (2) surgery.

5. *Endometrioma* is an extremely rare ovarian tumor of endometrial origin, usually presenting unilaterally in women of menopausal age. Cases in adolescents have been reported. Management is a surgery.

Malignant Ovarian Neoplasm in Adolescents

Malignant ovarian tumors are rare in children and adolescents, representing less than 1% of all cancers of childhood. A family history positive for ovarian cancer and the onset of early puberty are among the risk factors for ovarian cancer.[25,32]

Malignant Ovarian Germ Cell Tumors

Malignant germ cell tumors are rare (only 5% of all ovarian tumors), and may occur in children and adolescents. Gonadal location versus extragonadal presentation is considered to be more common in adolescents and to be associated with a more favorable prognosis. Two categories of metastases may occur and are divided into pulmonary and nonpulmonary. Surgery based on the staging and chemotherapy is the therapeutic options. Survival rate for gonadal presentation is almost 100% for stage I and approximately 95% for stages II, III, and IV. The survival rate for extragonadal location is slightly lower; approximately 95% in the early stages and 75% for stages III and IV.[825] Monitoring of tumor markers are indicated before, during, and after chemotherapy.

1. *Dysgerminoma* is the most common type of germ cell malignant ovarian tumor, associated with gonadal dysgenesis (e.g., Turner syndrome, mosaicism). Endometrial bleeding, acute abdominal pain, and palpable pelvic or abdominal, mass are the most common clinical findings. Fever and rare cases of isosexual precocious puberty have been reported. Malignant germ cell tumors may reach a gigantic size and are known for rapid growth and possible complications of torsion, rupture, necrosis, hemorrhage, and hematoperitoneum. Elevated lactate dehydrogenase (LDH) is a tumor marker found in this disorder. Liver, lungs, and lymph nodes are the most common sites for metastases.

2. *Choriocarcinoma* may occur at any age. Isosexual precocious puberty is the most common (50%) clinical presentation in children. Elevated serum human chorionic gonadotropin (hCG) is a tumor marker found in this disorder. Normal pregnancy and ectopic pregnancy should be ruled out with cases of pregnancy and tumor coexistence documented.

3. *Ovarian mixed germ cell tumors* are the most common of all germ cell tumors in children and adolescents with a mean presenting age of 16 years.[33] Abdominal pain is the presenting symptom reported in 90% of the cases. Elevated tumor marker is LDH.

Ovarian sex cord-stromal tumors in adolescents are rare, hormone producing tumors (5%–8% of all ovarian tumors). Estrogen producing tumors may cause premature menarche, isosexual precocious puberty, abnormal uterine bleeding, endometrial hyperplasia, and endometrial cancer. Acne, hirsutism, and clitoromegaly are the result of hyperandrogenism induced by sex cord-stromal tumors that may be associated with Maffucci syndrome (enchondromatosis with vascular anomalies as hemangiomas), Ollier disease (enchondromatosis without vascular anomalies), and Peutz-Jeghers syndrome (e.g., gastrointestinal hamartomas, melanin spots

on buccal mucosa and lips).[34] Conservative surgery and combination chemotherapy are the therapeutic options in young patients.[25,32–34]

1. *Juvenile granulosa cell tumor* is a unilateral (98%), estrogen-producing ovarian tumor in predominantly young patients with a mean age of 13 years.[8,35] A genetic predisposition, such as having trisomy or extra abnormal chromosome 12, has been reported.[36] Abnormal uterine bleeding, amenorrhea, abdominal pain and discomfort, a pelvic mass, and acute abdomen may be the presenting symptoms and findings in adolescent girls. Elevated estradiol levels are the most common clinical laboratory findings and can be used for the purpose of monitoring. The size of this tumor may vary from 11/2 to 14 in. The survival rate is higher with the early stage (IA) but dramatically decreases with advanced stages.[8,25,31] The late reoccurrence of juvenile granulosa cell tumors is possible, and lifelong monitoring is recommended. In young patients, conservative surgery with the preservation of the uterus and other ovary is the most common approach complemented by chemotherapy.

2. *Sertoli cell tumors* are rare (less than 1% of all ovarian tumors) hormone secreting tumors (e.g., androgen, estrogen, progesterone) with the clinical presentation of symptoms and findings of hyperestrogenism, hyperandrogenism, or a combination. In some cases ovarian Sertoli tumor may be hormone inactive. Abnormal uterine bleeding, amenorrhea, galactorrhea, virilization, isosexual precocious puberty, pelvic and abdominal pain, abdominal or ovarian mass, increased abdominal girth, or swelling are the clinical findings. Elevated estradiol, progesterone, or testosterone can be used for the monitoring.

3. *Sertoli-Leydig cell tumors* are very rare (0.5% of all ovarian tumors), primarily unilateral, androgen-producing (40%), ovarian malignant neoplasms, most likely to occur in women of 30 years or younger (75%), as early as age 2.[8,25,32,33,37] Abdominal pain, pelvic and/or abdominal mass, and signs of hyperandrogenism

are the most common findings. In most cases, this tumor is diagnosed at a very early stage (stage I in 97.5%). Elevated testosterone level is the tumor marker. Tumor calcification can be found. A list of ovarian tumors and their markers are listed in Table 28-8.

CASE STUDY 28-5

Abdominal Mass Presenting in a 13-Year-Old with Multiple, Comple Benign Ovarian Cysts

History: This 14-year-old female presented with a history of right lower quadrant pain preceding her menses over the last 6 months. She had menarche at age 12 with regular menses. She had been evaluated in an emergency room three different times in the last 6 months. She was hospitalized for observation only the month before presentation. Alone she admitted to sexual activity with three different partners in the last year. Her last sexual contact was in the last 2 days. There was no remarkable family history of gynecologic diseases or cancers. Her mother and father had been divorced since she was an infant. She attended middle school but had been expelled for using marijuana on school property. She admitted to polydrug use, both street drugs and prescription. She had spent a month in juvenile detention before her last hospitalization.

Physical: Her weight was 106 pounds (25th–50th percentile), her height was 59.5 inches (10th percentile), and with her BMI of 21 was at the 50th–75th percentile). Her vital signs, including temperature, blood pressure, and heart rate, were unremarkable. Her examination was only positive for a large mass extending from her umbilicus into her lower abdomen. Her pelvic was remarkable for a large mass about the size of a 24-week pregnancy. She had no clinical evidence of infection.

Laboratory: Her CBC showed mild anemia with Hgb 11.1 g/dL, Hmt 32%, platelet count 173,000 k/cumm, and WBC 6300 k/cumm with

a normal distribution. Her urine pregnancy test was negative as was her DNA-amplification tests for chlamydia and gonorrhea. On vaginal ultrasound she had evidence of multiple cysts in both ovaries. Her tumor marker tests were unremarkable before surgery.

Treatment: She was given emergency contraception and placed on the birth control patch as an outpatient before surgery. At surgery, multiple large cysts were confirmed. The ovaries were conserved with excision only of the cysts. Her pathology reports were consistent with large multi follicular cysts of the ovaries.

Bibliography

1. Chumlea WC, Schubert CM, Roche AF, Kulin HE, Lee PA, Himes JH, Sun SS. Age at menarche and racial comparisons in US girls. *Pediatrics* 2003;111: 110–113.
2. Herman-Giddens ME, Slora EJ, Wasserman RC, et al. Secondary sexual characteristics and menses in young girls seen in office practice: A study from the Pediatric Research in Office Setting Network. *Pediatrics* 1997;99:505–512.
3. Gomel V, Munro MG, Rowe TC. *Gynecology: A Practical Approach*. Baltimore, MD Williams & Wilkins, 1990.
4. American Psychiatric Association. *DSM-IV: Diagnostic and Statistical Manual of Mental Disorders*, 4th ed. Washington, DC: American Psychiatric Association, 1994.
5. Endicott J, Amsterdam J, Eriksson E, et al. Is premenstrual dysphoric disorder a distinct clinical entity? *J Womens Health Gend Based Med* 1999;8: 663–679.
6. Budeiri DJ, Li WP, Dornan JC. Clinical trials of treatments of premenstrual syndrome: Entry criteria and scales for measuring treatment outcomes. *Br J Obstet Gynaecol* 1994;101:689–695.
7. Cohen LS, Miner C, Brown E, et al. Premenstrual daily fluoxetine for premenstrual dysphoric disorder: A placebo-controlled clinical trial using computerized diaries. *Obstet Gynecol* 2002;100:435–444.
8. Ostrzenski A. *Gynecology: Integrating Conventional, Complementary, and Natural Alternative Therapy*. Philadelphia, PA: Lippincott Williams & Wilkins, 2002.

9. Blake F, Salkovskis P, Gath D, et al. Cognitive therapy for premenstrual syndrome: A controlled trial. *J Psychosom Res* 1998;45:307–318.

10. Stevinson C, Ernst E. Complementary/alternative therapies for premenstrual syndrome: A systematic review of randomized controlled trials. *Am J Obstet Gynecol* 2001;185:227–235.

11. Speroff L, Glass RH, Kase NG. *Clinical Gynecologic Endocrinology and Infertility*, 5th ed. Baltimore, MD: Williams & Wilkins, 1994.

12. Harel Z. A contemporary approach to dysmenorrhea in adolescents. *Paediatr Drugs* 2002;4(12): 797–805.

13. Klein JR, Litt IF. Epidemiology of adolescent dysmenorrhea. *Pediatrics* 1981;68:661–664.

14. Laufer MR, Sanfilippo J, Rose G. Adolescent endometriosis: Diagnosis and treatment approaches. *J Pediatr Adolesc Gynecol* 2003;16:S3.

15. Black AY, Jamieson MA. Adolescent endometriosis. *Curr Opin Obstet Gynecol* 2002;467–474.

16. Laufer MR, Goitein BA, Bush M, et al. Prevalence of endometriosis in adolescent women with chronic pelvic pain not responding to conventional therapy. *J Pediatr Adolesc Gynecol* 1997;10:199–202.

17. Kontoravdis A, Hassan E, Hassiakos D, et al. Laparoscopic evaluation and management of chronic pelvic pain during adolescence. *Clin Exp Obstet Gynecol* 1999;26:76–77.

18. Yamamoto K, Mitsuhashi Y, Takaike T, et al. Tubal endometriosis diagnosed within one month after menarche: A case report. *Tohoko J Exp Med* 1997; 181:385–387.

19. Sutton J, Ewen SP, Whitelaw N, Haines P. Prospective, randomized, double blind, controlled trial of laser laparoscopy in the treatment of pelvic pain associated with minimal, mild and moderate endometriosis. *Fertil Steril* 1994;64:696–700.

20. Papanek PE. The female athlete triad: An emerging role for physical therapy. *J Orthop Sports Phys Ther* 2003;33:594–614.

21. Salmi DJ, Zisser HC, Jovanovic L. Screening for and treatment of polycystic ovary syndrome in teenagers. *Exp Biol Med* 2004;229:369–377.

22. The Rotterdam ESHRE/ASRM-Sponsored PCOS consensus workshop. Revised 2003 consensus on diagnostic criteria and long-term health risks related to polycystic ovary syndrome (PCOS). *Hum Reprod* 2004;19:41–47.

23. Azziz R. PCOS: A diagnostic challenge. *Reprod Biomed Online* 2004;8:644–648.

24. Knochenhauer ES, Key TJ, Kahsar-Miller M, Waggoner W, Boots LR, Azziz R. Prevalence of the polycystic ovary syndrome in unselected black and white women of the southeastern United States: A prospective study. *J Clin Endocrinol Metab* 1998; 83:3078–3082.

25. Altchek A. *Diagnosis and Management of Ovarian Disorders*, 2d ed. London: Academic Press, 2003.

26. Ferriman D, Gallwey JD. Clinical assessment of hair growth in women. *J Clin Endocrinol* 1961; 21:1440–1447.

27. Legro RS, Castracane VD, Kauffman RP. Detecting insulin resistance in polycystic ovary syndrome: Purposes and pitfalls. *Obstet Gynecol Surv* 2004; 59:141–154.

28. Harborne L, Fleming R, Lyall H, Sattar N, Norman J. Metformin or antiandrogen in the treatment of hirsutism in polycystic ovary syndrome. *J Clin Endocrinol Metab* 2003;88:4116–4123.

29. Elter K, Imir G, Durmusoglu F. Clinical, endocrine, and metabolic effects of metformin added to ethinyl estradiol-cyproterone acetate in non-obese women with polycystic ovarian syndrome: A randomized controlled study. *Hum Reprod* 2002;17:1729–1737.

30. Farquhar C, Lee O, Toomath R, Jepson R. Spironolactone versus placebo or in combination with steroids for hirsutism and/or acne. *Cochrane Database Syst Rev* 2003 ;(4):CD000194.

31. Strickland JL. Ovarian cysts in neonates, children and adolescents. *Curr Opin Obstet Gynecol* 2002; 14:459–465.

32. Raney Jr RB, et al. Malignant ovarian tumors in children and Adolescents. *Cancer* 1987;59:14–20.

33. Gershenson DM. Management of early ovarian cancer: Germ cell and sex cord-stromal tumors. *Gynecol Oncol* 1994;55:S62–S72.

34. Outwater EK, Wagner BJ, Mannion C, McLarney JK, Kim B. Sex cord-stromal and steroid cell tumors of the ovary. *Radiographics* 1998;18:1523–1546.

35. Young RH, Dickersin GR, Scully RE. Juvenile granulosa cell tumor of the ovary. A clinicopathological analysis of 125 cases. *Am J Surg Pathol* 1984;8: 575–596.

36. Fletcher JA, Gibas Z, Donovan K, Perez-Atayde A, Genest D, Morton CC, Lage JM. Ovarian granulosa-stromal cell tumors are characterized by trisomy 12. *Am J Pathol* 1991;138:515–520.

37. Stepanian M, Cohn DE. Gynecologic malignancies in adolescents. *Adolesc Med Clin* 2004;15: 549–568.

PART

IV

EATING DISORDERS

29

ADOLESCENT NUTRITION

Maija Petersons, Mozhdeh B. Bruss, and Jon B. Bruss

Adolescence is a time of rapid physical growth as well as emotional and psychologic development affecting every aspect of a person's future adult life. Stature, weight, muscle mass in boys, and fat distribution in girls, in part due to hormonal changes, all undergo dramatic change as a child transitions into adulthood during the adolescent years. In addition, this transition involves the maturation to formal operational thought, internalization of a personal set of values and standards, and the development of self-identity in relation to society and the surrounding world. All of these processes and changes are dependent on the chemical composition of the body and by necessity place a high demand on nutrition. Aside from the immediate nutritional needs, patterns of nutritional consumption set during the adolescent years will have significant health consequences for individuals in their adult life, including lifelong food habits. This chapter will present (1) an overview of adolescent physical growth and development, (2) nutritional conditions relevant to adolescents, (3) adolescent diet, and important factors to be considered in promoting healthy eating among adolescents, (4) screening and assessment of nutrition status and risk factors, (5) dietary reference intakes (DRI) for adolescents, (6) a discussion of key macro- and micronutrients necessary for good adolescent health, growth, and development, and (7) nutrition considerations for adolescent athletes.

ADOLESCENT PHYSICAL GROWTH AND DEVELOPMENT

During puberty, there is a 15% increase in height and a 45% increase in skeletal mass.[1] At the peak of the growth spurt in height, boys increase in height by about 10.3 cm/year and girls by about 9.0 cm/year.[1] The growth spurt in both boys and girls is followed by a rapid increase in bone mass. In the 2 years of peak skeletal growth, adolescents accumulate over 25% of their adult bone mass and length.[2] In boys, the peak in weight velocity occurs simultaneously with the peak in height velocity, while in girls, the peak in weight velocity occurs 6–9 months before the rapid change in height.[1] The increase in skeletal mass is primarily the result of mineralization of bone due to the deposition of calcium and other minerals. Weight gain during this time accounts for approximately 50% of the adult weight, assuming ideal body weight in both the adolescent and adult years.[1]

Body composition changes from the childhood pattern to that of adulthood due the appearance of sex-related hormones. The testosterone promotes growth and stimulates increases in lean body mass. As a result, boys develop a heavier skeleton, grow taller, and lay down more muscle tissue than girls.[1] Estrogen and progesterone in contrast promote more deposition of fat than of muscle tissue. By the end of adolescence, girls' body fat percentage has increased from about 19% to about 23% of total body weight. For boys the percent body fat remains at about 15%.[1] At the age of 11, boys and girls deposit an average of 48 mg/kg/day and 35 mg/kg/ day of protein, respectively. On average, girls stop depositing protein by 17 years of age, while boys continue protein deposition into their 18th year.[3] Social and emotional development during adolescence centers on preparation for adulthood. According to Erickson, early adolescence is a time for learning to relate with peers according to rules; mastering basic skills in reading, writing, and arithmetic; and learning self-discipline required for successful completion of schoolwork.[4] The development of identity and skills in intimacy are the next developmental tasks to be mastered. Adolescents explore roles and identities that may lead them into alternative diets such as vegetarianism. Peers and role models outside of the family increase in importance. According to Piaget, concrete operations skills have developed by age 11 and there is evidence of organized, logical thought.[5] Between the ages 11 and 15, thought becomes more abstract, incorporating the principles of formal logic.[5]

Adequate nutrition is needed not only for physical growth, but for providing energy and nutrients for learning and interacting with others that is essential for development. In particular, iron deficiency has been shown to decrease learning in adolescents. These dramatic physical and developmental changes, particularly increases in height, weight, and bone mass, place a high demand for appropriate nutrients. Inadequate nutrition can lead to a number of nutritional conditions in adolescents. In addition, nutritional habits, and in particular, nutritional excesses leading to overweight and obesity can have serious health consequences for individuals in their adult years (Chap. 31). Despite the complexity of this age group, there are some practical approaches to counseling on nutrition and dietary requirements.

NUTRITIONAL CONDITIONS RELEVANT TO ADOLESCENTS

Inadequate nutrition can lead to a number of nutritional conditions in adolescents, including iron deficiency anemia, decreased bone mass accrual, folate deficiency in girls of child bearing capacity, displacement of vitamins and minerals due to large amounts of nonnutrient foods such as soft drinks, and nutrient depletion from fad diets and inadequate vegetarian diets as well as conditions such as anorexia and bulimia (Chap. 30). Table 29-1 presents a list of these conditions and recommended interventions.

Iron deficiency anemia may decrease growth and increase fatigue (Chap. 17). Even in the absence of anemia, iron deficiency has been shown to reduce work capacity. Among adolescents, the prevalence of iron deficiency is 16% for girls aged 16–19.[6] The iron deficiency state is characterized by depletion of iron stores, including a reduction in functional iron. Erythropoiesis may not be affected, and measurable anemia may not be manifest until late in the condition. The prevalence of anemia due to iron deficiency is 2% in 12–19-year-old girls.[6]

Mineral deposition in bone reaches its peak during the adolescent years, achieving maximal bone density just before adulthood. Diet, heavy alcohol abuse, and the use of oral contraceptive pills may have significant impact on the rate of bone deposition. Sexually active females taking oral contraceptives should be counseled about their diets to help minimize this impact. An adolescent diet low in calcium, leading to decreased bone density, may lead acutely to an increased rate of fractures,[7] and chronically to an increased rate of osteoporosis, as discussed later in this chapter. Diet plays a critical role in an adolescent female's ability to receive adequate amounts of calcium. Wyshak[8] reported that high calcium intakes protected against fractures in both boys and girls. The consumption of carbonated soft drinks has been associated with a greater incidence of fractures.[8] Fractures taking weeks to heal impact an adolescent's participation in active sports and even affect their performance in school and extracurricular activities. This is an example of how nutrition can have a broad impact on the life of an adolescent.

Periconceptual folate supplementation has been shown to reduce the risk of neural tube defects in infants including spina bifida and anencephaly.[9] Because adolescent females who become pregnant did so unintentionally, prenatal planning is often too late for prevention of the defects. A healthy diet, rich

TABLE 29-1

CRITICAL NUTRITION BEHAVIORS

Critical Nutrition Behaviors	Nutrition Concerns	Recommended Interventions
Chronic dieting practices	Iron deficiency anemia; reduced bone mass	Referral to a psychologist to focus on body image
Excessive consumption of colas	Displacement of vitamin and mineral from diet; increased risk of overweight/obesity	Referral to dietitian
Sedentary lifestyle	Increased risk of overweight/obesity and chronic diseases	Negotiate strategies in reducing television and computer use
Alternative dieting practices	Imbalanced food intake	Promote use of food guide pyramid with follow-up referral to dietitian
Excessive supplement use	Imbalanced nutrients intake	Educate client with information about toxicity levels of certain vitamins and minerals
Excessive consumption of low nutrient dense food	Nutrient depletion; increased risk of overweight/obesity and diabetes	Referral to a dietitian; negotiate use of food guide pyramid and strategies to modify diet
Omitting food and food groups	Nutrient depletion; increased risk of overweight/obesity and diabetes	Referral to a dietitian; negotiate use of food guide pyramid and strategies to modify diet
Inappropriate portion sizes	Increased risk of overweight/obesity and diabetes	Referral to a dietitian; negotiate use of food guide pyramid and strategies to modify diet
Skipping meals	Nutrient depletion; increased risk of overweight/obesity and diabetes	Negotiate behavior change in eating healthy choices of convenient foods and high nutrient density foods

in fruits and vegetables, and dietary supplementation are important for adolescent girls, especially if they are sexually active.

Adolescents are experimenting with fad and vegetarian diets, which for the uninformed may lead to nutrient depletion. Unless these diets are carefully planned they may be deficient in iron, folate, calcium, energy, vitamin B12, and other nutrients. Vegetarian diets vary in the number of foods included in the diet. A lacto-vegetarian consumes milk products while the lacto-ovo vegetarians also include eggs in the diet. The vegan diet is the most restrictive and the one most likely to result in nutrient deficits since it excludes all animal products. Vitamin B12, vitamin D, calcium,

and iron are the nutrients of concern. Vegetarian diets require significant knowledge about foods and nutrients in order to achieve a balanced source of certain vitamins, minerals, and amino acids. Adolescents may not have the knowledge or the discipline to manage such diets appropriately. However, with guidance in planning meals, the vegetarian diet can provide adequate nutrition for the adolescent.

In addition correlations between dieting and substance abuse in adolescents have been observed.[10] Conditions of anorexia and bulimia are psychologic disorders that may present even more serious health risks due to nutrient depletion than fad and vegetarian diets (Chap. 30).

ADOLESCENT NUTRITION AND ADULT CHRONIC DISEASE

Adolescence is a time of great importance for the prevention of chronic diseases in adulthood.[11] Nutrition patterns established during this period can influence a person's health later in adulthood. In particular, chronic conditions such as overweight and obesity, eating disorders, osteoporosis, diabetes type II, and cardiovascular diseases are all affected by eating and nutritional patterns established during the adolescent years. Table 29-2 presents the nutrition concerns and recommended interventions associated with each of these conditions.

Adolescent obesity is a risk factor for adult obesity, which increases the risk of chronic diseases such as diabetes[12,13] (Chaps. 15 and 31). As shown in Fig. 29-1 there is an increase in the prevalence of adolescent obesity defined as body mass index (BMI) at or above 95th percentile for age and sex using data from National Center for Health Statistics (NCHS),[14] National Health and Nutrition Examination Survey (NHANES), Hispanic Health and Nutrition Examination Survey (HHANES, 1982–1984), and National Health Examination Survey (1963–1965 and 1966–1970). Physical inactivity measured by television viewing and computer use, is a risk factor for overweight and obesity.[15] In 1999, 42.8% of adolescents reported to have watched 3 or more hours of television per day on an average school day. In addition, less than 10% of adolescents reported not participating in any vigorous or moderate physical activity during the past 7 days.[16] Overweight and obesity in adults have been associated with increased rates of diabetes, cardiovascular disease, stroke, hypertension, and some cancers. Management of overweight and obesity during the adolescent years can have significant impact on health patterns later in life (Chap. 31).

In 2002, the total prevalence of diabetes in the United States for all ages was 18.2 million or 6.3% of the population[17] (Chap. 15). As mentioned above, there is an increased risk for the development of diabetes in overweight and obese individuals. In addition to increasing rates of overweight and obesity among adolescents, which may lead to diabetes in adulthood, there are trends indicating increasing rates of type II diabetes among adolescents. While the rate of diabetes is still low among adolescents (0.25%), they often go undiagnosed. Although, there are no national monitoring systems in place to track type II diabetes among adolescents, an increase in the number of diagnosed cases of adolescents with diabetes has been observed in clinic-based and regional data reports especially among ethnic minority populations such as African Americans, Native Americans, and Hispanics.[17]

Slightly less than 30% of the population according to NHANES reported to have hypertension (Chaps. 9 and 16). This figure is about 4% higher than a decade earlier.[18] A small percentage of children (about 1%) are diagnosed with hypertension.[19]

TABLE 29-2

ACUTE AND CHRONIC CONDITIONS

Nutritional Disorders	Nutrition Concerns	Recommended Interventions
Underweight	Depletion of vitamin and minerals and caloric reserves; iron deficiency anemia	Referral to a dietitian
Overweight and obesity	Increased risk of adult obesity and chronic diseases	Referral to a team involving psychologist, dietitian, and primary care physician
Eating disorders	Increased risk of osteoporosis; vitamin depletion; iron deficiency anemia; reduced bone mass	Referral to a team involving psychologist, dietitian, and primary care physician
Diabetes, type II	Increased risk overweight/obesity; poor diet planning; physical inactivity	Referral to diabetes educator

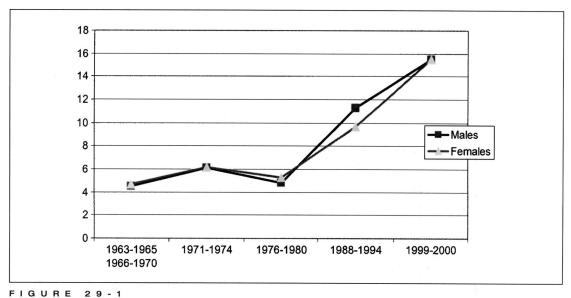

FIGURE 29-1

PERCENT OVERWEIGHT FOR 12–19 YEARS OLD FOR ALL RACE GROUPS.
Source: Adapted from reference 14.

Overweight and obesity increases the risk of adult obesity and chronic diseases such as hypertension.[12,13] An increase in the rates of hypertension in adults has been reported by Center for Disease Control (CDC). In 1995, age-adjusted rates of hypertension was reported as 46.2 per 100 adults with diabetes as compared to 52.9 per 100 adults in 2001, which may be linked to increasing rates of overweight and obesity.[16]

Some cancers, particularly colon cancer have been linked to diet. Some of these dietary behaviors may first become manifest during adolescence. For instance, there is an increased risk of colon cancer with moderate alcohol consumption,[20,21] a dietary pattern that often starts in adolescence, particularly binge drinking (Chap. 34). Studies suggest that consuming folate rich foods found in dark green leafy vegetables and orange juice can reduce the risk of developing cancers such as colon cancer.[22] This is particularly concerning given recent trends in the adolescent diet. According to the Youth Risk Behavior Surveillance System (YRBSS), only 23.9% of students in 1999 and 21.4% in 2001 reported to have consumed five or more servings of fruits and vegetables per day during the past 7 days.[16]

As mentioned in a previous section, the consumption of calcium is important in preventing acute fractures in adolescents, but it is also important in preventing osteoporosis later in adult life. Consumption of calcium rich foods and engaging in weight bearing exercise are protective factors in the prevention of osteoporosis. In addition to tobacco use, excessive alcohol consumption characterized by chronic heavy drinking during adolescence has been shown to increase the risk of osteoporosis especially in women.[23] According to the YRBSS, only 18% of students in 1999 and 16% in 2001 reported drinking three or more glasses of milk per day during the past 7 days.[16] In addition, nearly a third of adolescents report consuming five or more drinks of alcohol within 2 hours (binge), on one or more occasions in the past 30 days.[16]

THE ADOLESCENT DIET

The current adolescent diet is of concern because of the short- and long-term impact of dietary habits and current impact on health in later life. NHANES[25] and the Continuing Survey of Food Intakes of Individuals

(CSFII)[26] show that some nutrients are consumed in excess while the intake of others is below recommendations (Table 29-3). Among the nutrients consumed in excess are sodium, total fat, and saturated fat. In addition, total energy consumption for 9–13-year-old males was higher than the recommended amount. Calcium was inadequate in the diets of both males and females, while folate and iron were low in the diets of females.

When the Food Guide Pyramid based on CSFII data is used to assess the food intake of adolescents, results are consistent with NHANES. Males reported more than the recommended number of daily servings of meats and/or meat alternatives, while females reported fewer daily servings of vegetables and dairy products. Discretionary fats contributed to 25% of the total kcal, while added sugar contributed to 20% of the total kcal for both males and females (see Table 29-4).

Results suggest that majority of the adolescents do not consume the specified numbers of pyramid servings for fruits. Females consumed less of the specified number of pyramid servings for any food than males. In fact, less than one-third of the 12–19-year-old females reported consuming the specified numbers of pyramid servings of fruits, dairy, and meat and/or meat alternates (see Fig. 29-2). Consumption of low nutrient-density foods is a negative predictor of intake of the nutrient rich foods recommended by the pyramid guide.[27] Using data from the NHANES survey, Kant determined that more than 30% of the daily energy intake was from low nutrient-density foods. The highest intake was among 13–18-year-old girls. Furthermore, with increasing low-density food intake, the reported consumption of total energy increased, but consumption of protein, fiber, vitamin A, vitamin B6, folate, calcium, iron, zinc, and magnesium decreased proportionately.

As mentioned previously, an adolescent diet low in calcium may lead acutely to an increased rate of fractures, and chronically to an increased rate of osteoporosis. Diet plays a critical role in an adolescent female's ability to receive adequate amounts of calcium. The low consumption of calcium related to bone density has raised concern whether low bone mass may be contributing to some fractures in children.[7] A lower intake of calcium was reported by 11–15-year-old girls with fractures compared with girls of the same age without fractures.[28] Wyshak reported that high calcium intakes protected against fractures in both boys and girls. Furthermore, a greater incidence of fractures has been reported for adolescents consuming carbonated beverages.[8] In a cross-sectional retrospective study of 460 females in

TABLE 29-3

TEN KEY NUTRIENTS FOR 12–19 YEARS OLD INDIVIDUALS: UNITED STATES

	Recommended DRI[24]				Mean Intake ± SEM 1999–2000 (25) (N = 2208)			
	Males (years)		Females (years)		Males		Females	
Nutrients	9–13	14–18	9–13	14–18	MEAN	SEM*	MEAN	SEM
Calcium (mg)	1300	1300	1300	1300	1081	31.9	793	26.5
Folate (µg)	300	400	300	400	421	15.0	323	10.3
Iron (mg)	8	11	8	15	18.3	0.65	13.4	0.44
Zinc (mg)	8	11	8	9	14.3	0.50	9.6	0.29
Energy (kcal)	2279	3152	2071	2368	2686	56.4	1993	45.7
Cholesterol (mg)	<300 mg/day				296	12.4	203	9.1
Sodium (mg)	No more than 2400 mg/day				4124	125.8	3041	90.1

*SEM = Standard error of the mean.

TABLE 29-4

FOOD PYRAMID FOR 12–19 YEARS OLD INDIVIDUALS

	Mean Daily Servings Intake		Recommended	Sample One-Day Diet		
				Lower	Moderate	Higher
Food Groups	Male	Female	Servings	1600 kcal	2200 kcal	2800 kcal
Grains	9.2	6.3	6–11	6	9	11
Vegetables	3.7	2.7	3–5	3	4	5
Fruits	1.4	1.3	2–4	2	3	4
Dairy	2.4	1.5	2–4	2–3	2–3	2–3
Meat or meat alternative	5.9	3.7	2–3	5	6	8
Discretionary fat and added sugars (kcal)	2716	1841				
% of total kcal from	25.5	25.0				
Discretionary fat	20.0	20.0				
Added sugar						

Source: Adapted from reference 26.

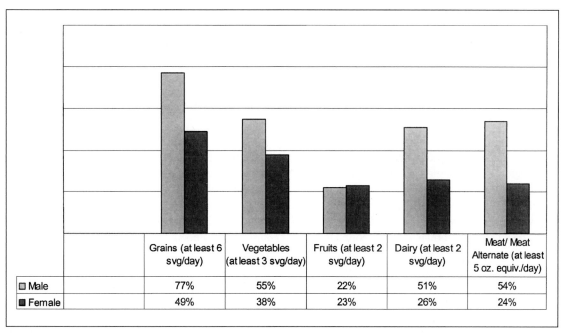

	Grains (at least 6 svg/day)	Vegetables (at least 3 svg/day)	Fruits (at least 2 svg/day)	Dairy (at least 2 svg/day)	Meat/ Meat Alternate (at least 5 oz. equiv./day)
☐ Male	77%	55%	22%	51%	54%
■ Female	49%	38%	23%	26%	24%

FIGURE 29-2

PERCENTAGE OF 12–19 YEARS OLD INDIVIDUALS CONSUMING SPECIFIED NUMBERS OF PYRAMID SERVINGS.
Source: Adapted from reference 26.

grades 9 and 10, 79% reported consuming some type of carbonated beverage drink. In this sample, active girls who consumed both cola and noncola carbonated beverages were at higher risk (OR = 7) for bone fracture than those who did not drink carbonated beverages.[8] Further evidence that the increased soft drink consumption is of concern was provided by Whiting et al. and McGartland et al. who reported that in girls, bone accrual was negatively correlated with soft drink consumption, which may be due to the replacement of calcium rich drinks such as milk.[2,29] Whiting et al. consider that the replacement of calcium-rich milk by low nutrient density beverages is a plausible mechanism for some of the effects of soft drinks on bone accrual. Although, boys' intake of calcium also decreased with soft drink consumption, their total calcium intake still averaged above 1000 mg/day.[29] The girls' intake averaged less than 900 mg/day and may be below the threshold for maximal bone accrual.[2]

There is a growing concern for the increasing rates of adolescent overweight and obesity, a risk factor for adult obesity and chronic diseases such as diabetes.[30] Limited vigorous physical activity combined with a physically inactive lifestyle and prevalent dieting behavior often associated with increasing concern for a certain body image is an important consideration for adolescents of all ages, gender, and ethnicity. Food intake is influenced by concerns about weight and body image. For example, in a nationally representative sample of more than 6000 adolescents, 45% of girls and 20% of the boys reported affirmatively to the question of ever being on a diet. Additionally, 68.8% of girls and 54.3% of boys rated "not being overweight" as very important. Although dieting behavior was more common among those who were either overweight or at risk for overweight, those who were also normal weight reported to have dieted. Dieting was also observed in both older and younger adolescents. Among all ethnic groups dieting was reported. However, the prevalence of dieting was highest among Caucasian non-Hispanic females followed by other ethnic group males. African American, non-Hispanic girls had the lowest prevalence of dieting as compared to the other groups. For females, BMI and ethnicity was found to be a predictor of dieting, whereas for males only BMI was found to be a predictor of dieting. Socioeconomic status and grade level were not found to be a predictor of dieting in either of the two gender groups.[10]

The pressure to conform to a certain body image puts adolescents at risk for dieting practices that may result in nutrient depletion. From 1999 to 2001, findings from the YRBSS suggest a slight increase (12.6%–13.5%) in students who reported having gone without eating for 24 hours or more to lose weight or to keep from gaining weight during the past 30 days.[16] Some adolescents also experiment with fad diets and vegetarian diets, which for the uninformed may lead to nutrient depletion. Vegetarian diets require significant knowledge about foods and nutrients in order to achieve a balanced source of certain vitamins, minerals, and amino acids. Adolescents do not also have the knowledge or the discipline to manage such diets appropriately. Less than 1% of the adolescents in the Minnesota Adolescent Health Survey reported to be vegetarian. More than 80% of the vegetarian respondents were female. Results showed that vegetarians were twice as likely to consume fruit and vegetables and 30% less likely to consume sweets as compared to nonvegetarians. However, vegetarian adolescents were at greater risk for chronic dieting and disordered eating as compared to the nonvegetarians.[31]

PROMOTING HEALTHY EATING AMONG ADOLESCENTS

The current status of the adolescent dietary intake and practices suggest the need for health care professionals to develop effective counseling strategies that can empower the adolescent to make appropriate dietary changes. From a developmental perspective, adolescents are making an important transition from childhood to being young adults (Chaps. 1 and 2). During this time the adolescent implicitly and explicitly demonstrates the need for independence and freedom. Figure 29-3 presents an ecologic perspective on the four main factors that influence the diet of the adolescent. These include (1) geophysical factors, (2) sociocultural factors, (3) familial factors, and (4) physiologic and psychosocial factors. These factors are not independent of each other; rather there is ongoing interaction between the factors in influencing the adolescent diet.

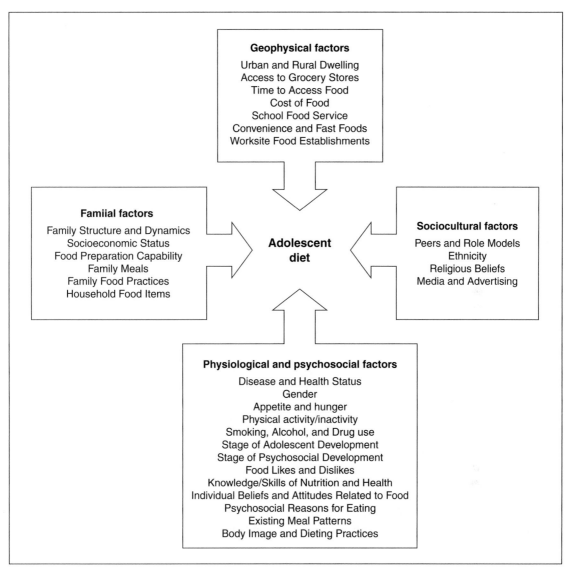

FIGURE 29-3

ECOLOGIC PERSPECTIVE ON THE ADOLESCENT DIET.

Geophysical Factors

Urban or rural dwelling of an adolescent, cost of food, and the time it takes to access the food are examples of geophysical factors. Although some aspects of these factors may be out of the adolescent's control, it can influence food choices and overall dietary intake. Other examples of geophysical factors include access to convenience foods, fast foods, and vending machine foods, which are often frequented by adolescents of all ages and a critical part of their diet. In fact, many of these foods can now be found in public schools. High calorie, high-fat, low nutrient branded foods are now sold directly in schools. Additionally, because adolescents are beginning to seek employment, access to work site food establishments can also influence their diets. Health care providers can influence school communities with regard to geophysical factors by advocating on behalf of the adolescents to ensure a more health promoting environment.

Sociocultural Factors

During adolescence, peers play an important role in influencing each other. With regard to food behavior, adolescents may spend more time eating with their peers than with their families. Peer influences on foods such as soft drinks, fast foods, snack foods, and alcohol have been observed. Media and advertising are a powerful sociocultural influence on adolescent body image and dietary habits. Many food and beer companies actually target adolescents as first entrants into their markets, knowing that they will have customers for life. For this they use role models to promote products and reinforce perceptions of weight normalcy images among adolescents. For some adolescents, ethnic and religious beliefs, attitudes and practices, may influence dietary behavior. Adolescents' interaction with media intensifies during this time either through the use of television and/or computer. The peer group may further reinforce the influence of advertising on the adolescent's food-related attitudes and behavior. Recognizing the complex interrelated influence of these sociocultural factors on the dietary habits of adolescents is the first step in identifying the challenges that face adolescents during this critical time. Helping adolescents develop media literacy skills along with strategies that can aid them in effectively using positive peer support to promote health and well-being is a necessary element of successful counseling with regards to sociocultural factors.

Familial Factors

Because, adolescence is a time where individuals are searching for their identity, this process often involves seeking independence from the family and a desire to establish an independent way of life. Previously the choices of food were made for the children by the parents. During adolescence the need for independence may result in food-related behaviors that are typically out of the parent's control.

Parents can make healthy breakfast and lunch food items available for the adolescent-on-the-run. Additionally, recognizing that adolescents are social beings and desire family get-togethers that are positive and fun emphasizes the role of parents in creating family meals that are warm and welcoming. Because of the many stresses that adolescents may be experiencing during this time, they need a family mealtime that is pleasant, supportive, and friendly. Stressful topics discussed at mealtime may result in short mealtimes and/or avoiding family mealtime all together. The role of the parent during this time is to make nutritious foods available and accessible to the adolescent and to plan at least one family meal a day. Families can identify and develop a weekly family dinner, lunch, or brunch with routines around food preparation and meal service. Every effort should be made to make this a memorable event for the adolescent. Even though, both the adolescent and the family may be busy, taking the time to have a family meal can enhance familial relationships and provide for at least one-third of the recommended dietary allowance (RDA) requirements for the day. Recognizing the need to support the adolescent's desire for independence, parents can engage the older adolescent who drives in purchasing the family foods and the younger adolescent in planning the family meals. Making food lists and requesting that the adolescent purchase the foods is also an important training for the transition away from the family home.

Physiologic and Psychosocial Factors

There are a number of physiologic and psychosocial factors that interact with the diet of the adolescents (Chaps. 1 and 2). Disease and health status, gender, appetite and hunger, frequency and level of physical activity and inactivity, smoking, alcohol, and substance use, and the stage of adolescent development are examples of physiologic factors. Psychosocial factors include food likes and dislikes, knowledge and skill of nutrition and health, individual beliefs and attitudes related to food, psychosocial reasons for eating, existing meal patterns, body image and dieting practices, and stage of psychosocial development.

Adolescence is a time when individuals may be learning time and resource management. This includes (1) the time it takes to access food, (2) existing meal patterns, and (3) cost of food. Other considerations with regard to the adolescence are the desire for the adolescent to look attractive while eating popular foods that is pleasing to their taste. Helping adolescents gain the knowledge and skills of health and nutrition in a socially supportive environment can be beneficial to making healthier choices. This can be done by offering curriculums through the schools that offer skill building activities in media literacy, reading nutrition labels, food preparation, selecting from a list of foods at fast food restaurants, convenient stores, and vending machines.

SCREENING AND ASSESSMENT OF NUTRITION STATUS

There are two sources for guidelines for nutritional screening and assessment of adolescents: *Bright Futures: Guidelines for Health Supervision of Infants, Children, and Adolescents*[32] and *Guidelines for Adolescent Preventive Services*[33] (Chap. 2). These guidelines recommend that all adolescents receive annual health supervision or preventive services. Implementation of such services complement, but do not replace, the health education provided by family, school, and the community.[33] Annual visits allow early detection of nutrition-related health issues and offer opportunities for nutrition guidance that can have a significant impact on life-long health. Such supervision should include comprehensive screening for nutrition risk factors[34] so that those adolescents who have poor nutrition status and those at risk for developing nutrition-related problems in the near term or later in life can be identified. Adolescents who are found to be at risk should be given an in-depth assessment to determine what specific behaviors need to be addressed through education and counseling with referral to a registered dietitian and other health professionals as appropriate. When possible parents need to be engaged and informed with regard to findings from the assessment

so they can support the overall nutrition needs of the adolescent if this does not violate confidentiality (Chap. 3).

SCREENING FOR NUTRITION RISK FACTORS

The main components of screening include the adolescent's (1) history of growth and development (Chap. 1), (2) current acute or chronic conditions that may alter requirements for nutrients or impair nutrient metabolism, (3) dietary patterns, and (4) socioeconomic status.

History of Growth and Development

A history of heights and weights plotted on CDC growth charts will show growth progress and can reveal deviations that may be attributable to nutrition inadequacy or excess (Chaps. 1 and 15). Alternatively, BMI-for-age tables (CDC) can also be used to screen for under- and overweight. A BMI-for-age at or above the 95th percentile is indicative of overweight, but being between the 85th and 95th percentile indicates risk of overweight. Underweight is indicated by a BMI-for-age at or below the 5th percentile. A sexual maturity rating will indicate stage of physical growth and changes in nutrient needs. A key question to ask adolescents is about their level of satisfaction with weight and body image and dieting practices.

Current Acute or Chronic Conditions

A personal history of acute or chronic conditions can affect not only growth and development, but also requirements for energy and nutrients, and lifelong health. In addition chronic diseases can alter nutrient digestion, transport, or metabolism so that nutrition status becomes impaired. In addition, the family history of heart disease, diabetes overweight and obesity, cancer, eating disorders, depression, and substance abuse form a context for the adolescent's own history. Table 29-2 shows examples of acute and chronic conditions, nutrition-related concerns, and recommended interventions.

Dietary Patterns

Critical components of dietary patterns include the number and timing of meals and snacks, the number of meals eaten with the family, the number of meals consumed away from home, and avoidance of any foods or food groups. A food frequency questionnaire can identify the number of times dairy products, fruits, vegetables, and whole grains are consumed. Frequency of sweetened beverages and other low nutrient density foods can also be determined with this tool. Table 29-5 presents examples of low and high density nutrient foods. Frequency and dose of prescribed and over-the-counter supplements needs to be included. Information on weight control strategies and practices need to be included in view of the commonly expressed concern about weight and body image. A history of weight changes due to dieting practices should also be noted. Table 29-1 presents examples of critical nutrition behaviors, nutrition concerns, and recommended interventions.

Economic Status

Food sufficiency, adequate housing, and availability of food storage and cooking facilities have an obvious role in determining food and nutrient intake. Availability of transportation and nearness to food stores also should be noted. As presented earlier, the economic status of the family and the adolescent has an impact on food choices made in the household and away from the home environment. Additionally studies suggest that individuals from families with low socioeconomic status are at higher risk of overweight and obesity.[35] Conversely, economic status may also impact priorities in purchasing among adolescents, with food and nutrition being sacrificed before other nonfood priorities.

DIETARY REFERENCE INTAKES

In 1995, fundamental changes were made in the criteria used to develop dietary recommendations and ways in which they are reported. The Food and Nutrition Board of the Institute of Medicine, National Academy of Sciences initiated the use of DRI as a generic term that encompasses a range of reference values, based on the best available scientific data and are more closely related to optimum health indicators than the previous criterion of preventing nutrient deficiencies.[36] The term RDA is reserved for those nutrients for which the intake level that will meet the requirements of 97%–98% of the healthy U.S. population can be determined. Adequate intake (AI) is a recommended average daily intake level based on estimates of nutrient intake by a group of people when there is not sufficient data to determine an RDA. The DRI for the first time also includes tolerable upper intake level (UL). This is the highest average daily nutrient intake level that is likely to pose no risk of adverse health effects to almost all individuals in the general population. As intake increases above the UL, the potential risk of adverse effects may increase.

DRI are still based on age and sex groups each with a median height and weight. Children and adolescents are divided into the age groups of 9–13 and 14–18 years. Nineteen year olds are classified with those up to 30 years of age. No allowance or adjustment is made for maturational stage, which makes interpretation and use of the DRI more complex. When determining an adolescent's nutrition needs, height, weight, BMI, growth stage, and physical activity level should be taken into account as well as

TABLE 29-5

EXAMPLES OF LOW AND HIGH NUTRIENT DENSITY FOODS

Low Nutrient Density Foods	High Nutrient Density Foods
Soft drinks, sugared beverages, salty snack foods, snacks foods with added sugar, fatty snack foods, refined cereals, breads, and so forth	Skim milk, cheese, yogurt, plain popcorn, plain pretzels, fruits, green and yellow vegetables, roots and tubers, legumes, walnuts and almonds, whole grain cereals and breads, fish, lean poultry, and so forth

presence of any chronic conditions that may affect absorption, excretion, or altered metabolism of nutrients. Lifestyle and hereditary risk factors should also be considered.

DRI FOR ADOLESCENTS

Daily dietary intake of the adolescents needs to supply sufficient energy, fat, protein, carbohydrate, vitamins, minerals, water, and fiber to meet the demands for growth, development, and daily activities. Particular attention needs to be devoted to iron, folic acid, sodium, dietary fat, sugar, and energy intake to prevent such common conditions as iron deficiency, anemia, dental caries, heart disease, and obesity with the associated risk of diabetes mellitus

Energy

Recommended energy intakes for adolescents represent the average dietary energy intake that is predicted to maintain energy balance in a healthy individual of a defined age, gender, weight, height, and level of physical activity[37] and includes the energy needs for growth. The recommendations were made assuming the individual is physically active and either 11 years old (younger adolescent group) or 16 years old (older adolescent group). The values listed are estimated energy requirements (EER).

RDA values were not calculated for energy since intakes above an individual's EER would result in undesirable and potentially hazardous weight gain [37]. The values for 9–13-year-old and 14–18-year-old males are 2270 kcal/day and 3152 kcal/day, respectively, while for females in the same age categories, the values are 2071 and 2368, respectively (Table 29-6). The levels would need to be adjusted downward for adolescents who are physically inactive.

Carbohydrate

Dietary carbohydrate is composed of starch and sugars and is readily digested and absorbed. Starches include amylose and amylopectin while sugars include mono- and disaccharides. Furthermore, sugars can be classified as naturally occurring or added sugars. Examples of naturally occurring sugars are the lactose in milk and the sugars in fruits, fruit juices, and some vegetables. Added sugars are refined sugars used in food processing and preparation and include brown sugar, white sugar, honey, molasses, and syrups. High-fructose corn syrup has become the most widely used food and beverage additive. Its use has increased from less than a pound per capita in 1972 to more than 62 lb per capita in 2001.[38]

The RDA for carbohydrates is set at 130 g/day for adults and children.[37] This level is based on the average minimum amount of glucose utilized by the brain, which is the major carbohydrate-dependent

TABLE 29-6

MACRONUTRIENTS

	9–13 Years Old		14–18 Years Old	
Protein (RDA)	0.95 g/kg		0.85 g/kg	
Carbohydrate (RDA)	130 g/day		130 g/day	
Total fat	ND		ND	
	Male	*Female*	*Male*	*Female*
n-3 (AI) g/day	1.2	1.0	1.6	1.1
n-6 (AI) g/day	12	10	16	11
Dietary fiber/g/day	31	26	38	36
Total energy kcal/day	2279	2071	3152	2368

organ in the body. The Food and Nutrition Board has concluded that no more than 25% of the daily kcal should be provided by sugar. This is in sharp contrast to the recommendation of the WHO/FAO report *Nutrition, Diet, and Chronic Disease*. In an effort to stem the epidemic of obesity, this joint expert report recommends less than 10% of kcal come from added sugar.[39]

Protein

Protein needs are dependent upon the adolescent's specific stage of growth and development. The recommendations are the sum of the needs for maintenance based on body weight and the estimated amount needed for protein deposition.[37] For younger adolescents the RDA is set at 0.95 g/kg body weight/day. For older adolescents it is 0.85 g/kg/day. This is equal to about 34 g of protein a day (equivalent to 5 oz of meat). The amount for those 13–18 years is 46 g/day (6.5 oz meat) for girls and 52 g/day (7.5 oz meat) for boys.

Fat

Total Dietary Fat

There is no RDA or adequate intake (AI) for total fat consumption for those above the age of 2 due to lack of data for a defined level of intake at which risk of inadequacy or prevention of chronic disease occur.[37] Instead, acceptable macronutrient distribution ranges (AMDR) has been set at 20%–35% of kcal for fat.[37] The American Academy of Pediatrics, Committee on Nutrition recommends that for adolescents, no more than 30% and no less than 20% of kcal be supplied by fat.[40] The Committee further recommends that saturated fat should provide less than 10% of total kcal. Dietary changes to meet these recommendations are safe and acceptable and have the potential to reduce atherosclerotic heart disease, if carried into adult life.[40]

GAPS[33] recommends lipid profile screening for adolescents who have a positive family history of early cardiovascular disease or hyperlipidemia and that they be followed up with the protocol developed by the Expert Panel on Blood Cholesterol levels in Children and Adolescents.

Polyunsaturated Fatty Acids

Besides being a major source of kcal, dietary fat is needed for absorption of fat-soluble vitamins and as a source of polyunsaturated fatty acids that cannot be made by the body. Humans can synthesize neither the omega-6 nor the omega-3 fatty acids. The omega-6 fatty acids (such as linoleic acid) are found in corn and other vegetable oils and have been shown to decrease blood cholesterol levels when they replace saturated fats in the diet. In the body, omega-6 fatty acids are found in cell membranes and serve as precursors for eicosanoids, such as prostaglandins and thromboxanes. Omega-3 fatty acids (α-linolenic acid) are found most abundantly in fatty fish. They are components of membranes and neural structures and precursors to another family of eicosanoids. A dietary lack of either one results in characteristic symptoms of rough scaly skin, dermatitis, failure to grow, and an elevated triene/tetraene ratio.

Research studies have shown that populations that consume a diet high in fatty fish have higher intakes of α-linolenic acid and other omega-3 fatty acids and have a reduced risk of cardiovascular disease. Individuals who consume diets naturally high in linoleic acid-containing oils have higher levels of high-density lipoprotein (HDL) cholesterol, which is protective of heart disease. For these reasons, AI for omega-6 and omega-3 fatty acids has been established (Table 29-6). Linolenic acid recommendations can be met by consuming 1–2 tablespoon of canola oil/day in cooking or as a salad dressing, an ounce of walnuts, or butternuts.[41] Alternatively, consuming 2–4 ounces of fatty fish such as salmon will provide sufficient amounts of the long-chain omega-3 fatty acids derived from linoleic acid. Linoleic acid is found in vegetable oils such as corn oil, sunflower oil, and safflower oil and 2 tablespoons are sufficient to meet the AI. Margarines made from these oils can be sources if hydrogenated fat is not the major ingredient.

Trans-Fatty Acids

Trans-fatty acids are not essential to the diet and no DRI has been established for them. In fact, intake of trans-fatty acids is associated with increased levels of low-density lipoprotein (LDL) cholesterol, which is a known risk factor for heart disease. No UL was set for trans-fatty acid since any intake incrementally increases LDL levels.[37] Because these fatty acids are widely distributed in the food supply, a 0% intake cannot be recommended either without major changes in food habits and food supply. Trans-fatty acid intake should be kept as low as possible by limiting the intake of baked goods and other commercially prepared items, such as cookies, crackers, and snack cakes. Liquid, nonhydrogenated margarines and fats are preferable to hydrogenated products. The median trans-fatty intake is higher in 12–19-year-old males than in any other age group.[42]

Cholesterol

Cholesterol is not an essential nutrient and no DRI has been set. Similar to trans-fatty acids, no UL was set either because any incremental intake increases LDL concentration and CHD risk.[36] Cholesterol is found in animal products only. A reduced intake of saturated fats will also result in a decrease in cholesterol intake. Of the commonly eaten foods, egg yolks contain the most cholesterol (212 mg/egg)[43] and should be limited to maintain the recommended intake of less than 300 mg of cholesterol/day (Chap. 9).

Dietary Fiber

Dietary fiber is the nondigestible carbohydrate and lignin found intact in plants while functional fiber is isolated nondigestible carbohydrate that may have beneficial physiologic effects in humans. Total fiber is the sum of these two categories. Intake of viscous fiber can have a variety of effects based on delay of gastric emptying time. This effect may produce a feeling of fullness, slow down the absorption of digestible carbohydrate, and reduce the absorption of dietary fats, cholesterol, and enterohepatic circulation of bile salts. All of these are potentially beneficial effects in that they could reduce food intake, reduce postprandial blood glucose levels, and reduce the absorption and plasma levels of cholesterol.[37] Intake of nonviscous fiber that is not fermented in the colon, can increase fecal bulk and enhance elimination.

AI levels have been established for total fiber.[37] For the 9–13-year-old, the AI is 31 g/day and 26 g/day for boys and girls, respectively. For those 14–18 years of age, the AI for boys and girls is 38 g/day and 26 g/day, respectively. Sources of dietary fiber include whole grain products, fruits (especially with the peel), vegetables, and legumes.

IMPORTANT MICRONUTRIENTS FOR ADOLESCENTS

Iron

In adolescents, the need for iron is based on the demands of growth as well as on basal iron losses. Hemoglobin mass increases along with the blood volume during growth and the absolute numbers of red blood cells increase.[37] The growth of muscle and other lean tissue during the growth spurt creates the need for more iron, which is needed for myoglobin and for the several hundred iron-dependent enzymes.[9] About 1.0 mg/day of iron is lost through shedding of skin and other epithelial cells. With menarche, girls lose additional iron in the menses. The amount lost is estimated to be 0.45 g/day, but menstrual losses are highly variable among women. Some may have losses three times the median.[44] In addition, iron losses due to bleeding may significantly increase if the adolescent is using intrauterine devices. Oral contraceptive use, however, will significantly decrease menstrual iron loss.

The RDA for 9–13-year-old is 8 mg/day, but increases to 11 mg/day and 15 mg/day for 14–18-year- old males and females, respectively.[37] These recommendations do not include iron allowance for storage. If an adolescent enters puberty with reduced iron stores, the accelerated growth rate will stress the existing stores and they will be at increased risk of iron deficiency and iron-deficiency anemia.

Prevention of iron deficiency can be achieved by dietary means. Including or increasing the amount of lean meat, fish, and poultry in the diet will increase the intake of the more absorbable heme iron. Plant foods such as legumes, dried fruits, and whole grain or enriched grain products are also good sources of iron, though it is in the form of nonheme iron, which is poorly absorbed. Including an excellent source of vitamin C, such as citrus or fortified fruit juices in the same meal with iron-containing plant foods will significantly improve nonheme iron absorption.[45]

Treatment of iron deficiency anemia is effectively treated with one to two tablets of 60 mg of elemental iron, preferably ferrous sulfate[32] (Chap. 17). Absorption can be increased by consuming the supplement between meals and avoiding taking iron with substances that impair iron absorption, such as dairy products, calcium supplements, coffee, tea, and whole grains.[32]

Folate

Folic acid functions as a coenzyme in metabolism of amino acids and for the conversion of dUMP to dTMP. Because of the latter reaction, folate is essential for replication and translation of DNA, thereby for cell division and protein synthesis. Among the folate-requiring enzymes is methionine synthetase, which methylates homocysteine to regenerate methionine. The cobalamin coenzyme is also required for this reaction. From 2%–16% of the white population are homozygous for the 5, 10-methylenetetrahydrofolate reductase (MTHFR) C667T allele, which results in a significantly elevated plasma homocysteine level. These individuals have a higher requirement for folate than do others.[45]

Folate metabolism can be significantly affected by medications. Very large therapeutic doses of nonsteroidal anti-inflammatory drugs can have antifolate activity. Chronic use of the anticonvulsants diphenylhydantoin and phenobarbital has been reported to be antifolate in activity.[47,48] Methotrexate may be used for nonneoplastic conditions such as rheumatoid arthritis. It is recommended that folate supplements are needed with chronic use of methotrexate. Additionally, alcohol use may also impair folate absorption putting the individual at higher risk of folate deficiency.

Folate supplementation in the amount of 400 µg/day was recommended for women in the childbearing years by the Public Health Service in 1992 in and effort to reduce the incidence of neural tube defects, such as spina bifida. To be effective, the supplement must be used prior to conception since the folate is needed for processes that occur during the embryonic period, a time when most women are not even aware of the pregnancy. Folate fortification of cereal products has been mandatory since 1996. Besides fortified breads and cereals, excellent sources of folate are orange juice, papayas, and green leafy vegetables such as spinach, broccoli, and legumes.

The RDA for 9–13-year-old and 14–18-year-old is, respectively, 300 and 400 µg/day of dietary folate equivalents (DFE).[46] The DFE unit of measure was introduced to account for the greater bioavailability of synthetic folate, which is used in supplements and food fortification. One DFE is equivalent to 1 µg of food folate or 0.5 µg of supplemental folate taken on an empty stomach or 0.6 µg taken with food. Folic acid fortification of grain products became mandatory in 1998 at a level of 140 µg/100 g grain product.

Calcium and Vitamin D

Ninety-nine percent of the calcium in the body is found in bones and teeth. The accrual process begins in utero and continues through childhood and adolescence into young adulthood. Calcium supports the growth of bones in length and width, a process that is completed during late adolescence. Calcium, along with weight bearing exercise, is needed for development of peak bone mineral density (BMD). Providing there is sufficient calcium intake, BMD continues to increase into the fourth decade.[49]

For bone mineralization and development of peak BMD, calcium levels must be maintained within a narrow range. Vitamin D and parathyroid hormone (PTH) are required in addition to sufficient dietary calcium. PTH activates vitamin D, which stimulates calcium absorption. If sufficient calcium is not consumed, vitamin D and PTH will stimulate removal of calcium from bone. For adolescents, the AI for calcium is set at 1300 mg/day for both males and females from 9 to 18 years of age.[36] The AI was used since there is not sufficient information about calcium requirements to determine the RDA.

Exposure to sunlight provides some of the vitamin D through photoconversion, but the amount produced is highly variable and depends on climate, season, latitude, skin pigmentation, age, the amount of skin area exposed to sunlight, and the use of sunscreen. The RDA was set assuming that photo-conversion contributes to vitamin D.

Sodium, Chloride, Potassium, and Water

Sodium is the main extracellular cation and along with other electrolytes is required to maintain extracellular volume and serum osmolality. For adolescents, the AI of sodium is set at 1.5 g/day to ensure that the overall diet provides AI of other nutrients.[50] This level is meant to cover sweat losses in unacclimatized individuals who are exposed to high temperatures or who become physically active. The Food and Nutrition Board/National Academy of Sciences (FNB/NAS) states that this AI does not apply to highly active people, such as endurance athletes who lose large amounts of sweat every day. The UL of sodium is set at 2.2 g and 2.3 g in younger and older adolescents, respectively. The reason for this setting an UL is the well-known adverse effects of higher levels of sodium intake on blood pressure. The AI for chloride is set at the molar equivalent to sodium, 65 mmol/day or 2.3 g/day.[50] This is equivalent to 3.8 g/day of sodium chloride. Potassium is the major intracellular cation. It is required for normal cellular function including neuromuscular activity. The AI for adolescents is 4.5 g/day and 4.7 g/day for younger and older adolescents, respectively.[50] Consumption of potassium sources from foods is recommended because the foods providing this mineral also provide organic acids as the anion. When potassium is added to food it is usually paired with chloride. The AI for potassium should be sufficient for healthy people and should maintain lower blood pressure, reduce the risk of kidney stones, and possibly reduce bone loss. No UL has been established since a potassium intake from foods above the AI level poses no potential for risk in a healthy population with normal kidney function.

Water is needed in both intracellular and extracellular compartments as a solvent, transport medium, and coolant. Dietary water, or total water intake, includes the water found in nearly all foods as well as in beverages. The AI for water is set based on the median total water intake from U.S. survey data. For adolescents the AI is 2.4 L/day in 9–13-year-old boys

and 2.1 L/day for girls of the same age.[50] The AI for 14–18-year-old boys and girls is 3.3 L/day and 2.3 L/day, respectively.[50] Body water deficits occur because of decreased intake of water or increased water loss due to physical activity and/or heat exposure. There is no UL for water intake.

THE ADOLESCENT ATHLETE AND NUTRITION

Physical activity such as that involved in recreational and competitive sports requires optimal nutrition to enhance performance and to support growth. The key concern is meeting energy, protein, carbohydrate, and fluid needs. If these needs are not met, the athlete may lose body weight and lean body mass, which will reduce strength and endurance. Besides the effect on performance, failure to meet nutrition needs may impact growth, menstrual function, and development of bone mass. In addition, inadequate nutrition can cause fatigue, which can result in injury or illness.[51]

There is no evidence that the energy distribution among carbohydrate, fat, and protein needs to be different for athletes. Sufficient energy to maintain weight and support growth consumed in the pattern suggested by *Dietary Guidelines for Americans* will generally provide enough carbohydrate for maintenance and restoration of glycogen stores.[51] Protein needs of athletes are higher than those of nonathletes, approximately 1.2–1.4 g/kg body weight for endurance activities and 1.6 g/kg for resistance and strength training. Nevertheless, a diet providing 12%–15% of kcal as protein will be sufficient as long as energy needs are met. Efficacy and safety of supplements of individual amino acids as performance enhancers has not been established.[51]

Risk of vitamin and/or mineral deficiencies is greatest for those restricting energy intake and using severe weight loss techniques to make weight. Deficits of the micronutrients can not only impair performance, but also compromise nutrition status. With strenuous daily physical activity (as in organized athletics), especially in hot weather, protocols are essential to ensure maintenance of hydration. The athlete's sweat rate, sport dynamics, environmental factors, acclimatization state, exercise duration, and exercise intensity need to be considered in developing a rehydration strategy.[52] Fluid replacement beverages should be easily accessible and flavored to the preference of the athletes. Fluid replacement should be approximately equal to sweat and urine losses and sufficient to avoid losses of more than 2% of body weight. Following exercise, rehydration should include carbohydrate and electrolytes and should be completed within 2 hours. Sodium chloride may be added to fluid replacement beverages when access to meals is limited (or meals are not eaten), duration of physical activity is more than 4 hours, or during the first days of hot weather. The addition of 0.3–0.7 g of salt per 1 L can replace sweat losses and minimize cramping.[52]

Bibliography

1. Spear BA: Adolescent growth and development. *J Am Dietetic Assoc* 102:23s, 2002.
2. Whiting SJ, Vatanparast H, Baxter-Jones A, et al.: Factors that affect bone mineral accrual in the adolescent growth spurt. *J Nutr* 134:696s, 2004.
3. Panel on Micronutrients, Standing Committee on the Scientific Evaluation of Dietary Reference Intakes: *Dietary Reference Intakes for Vitamin A, Vitamin K, Arsenic, Boron, Chromium, Copper, Iodine, Iron, Manganese, Molybdenum, Nickel, Silicon, Vanadium, and Zinc.* Washington, DC: National Academy Press, 2002.
4. Erikson E: *Childhood and Society*, 2d ed. New York: Norton & Co., 1963.
5. Cook JL, Cook G: *Child Development: Principles and Perspectives*. Boston, MA: Pearson Allyn & Bacon, 2005.
6. Centers for Disease Control: Iron deficiency–United States, 1999–2000. *MMWR* 51:897, 2002.
7. Committee on Nutrition, American Academy of Pediatrics: Calcium requirements of infants, children, and adolescents. *Pediatrics* 104:1152, 1999.
8. Wyshak G: Teenaged girls, carbonated beverage consumption, and bone fractures. *Arch Pediatr Adolesc Med* 154:610, 2000.
9. Stipanuk MH: *Biochemical and Physiological aspects of Human Nutrition*. Philadelphia, PA: W.B. Saunders, 2000.
10. Neumark-Sztainer D, Hannen PJ: Weight-related behavior among adolescent girls and boys. *Arch Pediatr Adolesc Med* 154:569, 2000.
11. Lytle LA: Nutritional issues for adolescents. *J Am Dietetic Assoc* 102:8s, 2002.
12. Serdula MK, Ivery D, Coates RJ, et al.: Do obese children become obese adults? A review of the literature. *Prev Med* 22:167, 1993.
13. National Institute of Health: Clinical guidelines on the identification, evaluation, and treatment of overweight and obesity in adults–the evidence report. *Obes Res* 6:51s, 1998.
14. Centers for Disease Control and Prevention, National Center for Health Statistics: *National Health and Nutrition Examination Survey, Hispanic Health and Nutrition Examination Survey (1982–84), and National Health Examination Survey (1963–65 and 1966–70).* Revised 1/14/2003. Available at: *http://www.cdc.gov/nchs/data/hus/tables/2002/02hus 071.pdf.*
15. Andersen RE, Crespo CJ, Bartlett SJ, et al.: Relationship of physical activity and television watching with body weight and level of fatness among children. *J Am Med Assoc* 279:1561, 1998.
16. Youth Risk Behavior Surveillance System: Adolescent and school health. National Center for Chronic Disease Prevention and Health Promotion, Center for Disease Control. Available at: *http://apps.nccd.cdc. gov/YRBSS/ChangeByQuestionV.asp?Cat=5*, Accessed on May 1, 2004.
17. Diabetes Surveillance System, Diabetes Public Health Resource, National Center for Chronic Disease Prevention and Health Promotion, Center for Disease Control: Data and Trends. Available at: *http://www. cdc.gov/diabetes/statistics/prev/national/tablebyage. htm.* Accessed on May 1, 2004.
18. Hajjar I, Kotchen TA: Trends in prevalence, awareness, treatment, and control of hypertension in the United States 1988–2000. *JAMA* 290:199, 2003.
19. Penn State Children's Hospital: Health and Disease Information. Available at: *http://www.hmc.psu.edu/ childrens/healthinfo/h/hypertension.htm.* Accessed on May 1, 2004.
20. Lieberman DA Prindiville S, Weiss DG, et al.: Risk factors for advanced colonic neoplasia and hyperplastic polyps in asymptomatic individuals. *JAMA* 290:2959, 2003.
21. Cho E, Smith-Warner SA, Ritz J, et al.: Alcohol intake and colorectal cancer: A pooled analysis of 8 cohort studies. *Ann Intern Med* 140:603, 2004.

22. Harvard School of Public Health: Fruits and Vegetables. Available at: *http://www.hsph.harvard.edu/ nutritionsource/fruits.html*. Accessed on May 1, 2004.

23. Bohannon AD, Hanlon JT, Landerman R, et al.: Association of race and other potential risk factors with nonvertebral fractures in community-dwelling elderly women. *Am J Epidemiol* 149:1002, 1999.

24. Dietary Reference Intakes Series, Food and nutrition Board, National Academy of Sciences. National Academies Press. 1997, 1998, 2000, 2001. Washington, DC.

25. Wright JD, Wang C, Stephens-Kennedy J, et al.: *Dietary Intake of Ten Key Nutrients for Public Health, United States: 1999–2000. Advance Data from Vital and Health Statistics #334*. Hyattsville, MD: National Center for Health Statistics, 2003.

26. USDA: Continuing Survey of Food Intakes by Individuals, 1994–1996. Available at: *http://www. barc. usda.gov/bhnrc/foodsurvey/Products.html*. Accessed on May 1, 2004.

27. Kant AK: Reported consumption of low-nutrient-density foods by American children and adolescents. Nutritional and health correlates, NHANES III, 1988–1994. *Arch Pediatric Adolesc Med* 157:789, 2003.

28. Goulding A, Rockell JEP, Black RE, et al.: Children who avoid drinking cow's milk are at increased risk for prepubertal bone fractures. *J Am Dietetic Assoc* 104:250, 2004.

29. McGartland C, Robson PJ, Murray L, Cran G, et al.: Carbonated soft drink consumption and bone mineral density in adolescence: The Northern Ireland Young Hearts Project. *J Bone Miner Res* 18:1563, 2004.

30. Manson JE, Skerrett PJ, Greenland P, et al.: The escalating pandemics of obesity and sedentary lifestyle. *Arch Intern Med* 164:249, 2004.

31. Neumark-Sztainer D, Story M, Resnick MD, et al.: Lessons learned about adolescent nutrition from the Minnesota Adolescent Health Survey. *J Am Dietetic Assoc* 98:1449, 1998.

32. Bright Futures: *Guidelines for Health supervision of infants, children, and adolescents,* 2d ed. Arlington, VA: National Center for Education for Maternal and Child Health, 2003.

33. American Medical Association: *Guidelines for Adolescent Preventive Services*. Chicago, IL: American Medical Association, Department of Adolescent Health, 1992.

34. Stang J: Assessment of nutritional status and motivation to make behavior changes among adolescents. *J Am Dietetic Assoc* 102:13s, 2002.

35. Townsend MS, Peerson J, Love B, et al.: Food insecurity is positively related to overweight in women. *J Nutr* 131:1738, 2001.

36. Standing Committee on the Scientific Evaluation of Dietary Reference Intakes: *Dietary reference intakes for calcium, phosphorus, magnesium, vitamin D, and fluoride*. Washington, DC: National Academy Press, 1997.

37. Panel on Macronutrients, Standing Committee on the Scientific Evaluation of Dietary Reference Intakes: *Dietary Reference Intakes for Energy, Carbohydrate, Fiber, Fat, Fatty Acids, Cholesterol, Protein, and Amino Acids (Macronutrients)*. Washington, DC: National Academy Press, 2002.

38. Economic Research Service: Food Consumption (per capita) Data System. Available at: *http://ers.usda.gov/ data/foodconsumption/DataSystem.asp?ERSTab*=3. Accessed on May 1, 2004.

39. Report of the Joint WHO/FAO Expert Consultation: *Diet, Nutrition and the Prevention of Chronic Diseases*. Geneva, World Health Organization, 2003.

40. Committee on Nutrition, American Academy of Pediatrics: Cholesterol in childhood. *Pediatrics* 101: 141, 1998.

41. Nettleton JA: Omega-3 fatty acids: Comparison of plant and seafood sources in human nutrition. *J Am Dietetic Assoc* 91:331, 1991.

42. Allison DB, Egan SK, Barraj LM, et al.: Estimated intake of trans and other fatty acids in the U.S. Population. *J Am Dietetic Assoc* 99:166–174, 1999.

43. Food Data Laboratory, United States Department of Agriculture: Available at: *http://www.nal.usda.gov/ fnic/foodcomp/search/*. Accessed on April 29, 2004.

44. Hallberg L, Hogdahl A, Nilsson L, et al.: Menstrual blood loss—a population study. *Acta Obstet Gynecol Scand* 45:320, 1966.

45. Skikine B, Baynes RD: Iron absorption. In: Brock JH, Halliday JW, Pippard MJ, Powell LW eds., *Iron Metabolism in Health and Disease*. London: W.B. Saunders, 1994.

46. Panel on Folate, Other B Vitamins, and Choline, Standing Committee on the Scientific Evaluation of Dietary Reference Intakes: *Dietary Reference Intakes for Thiamin, Riboflavin, Niacin, Vitamin B6, Folate, Vitamin B12, Pantothenic Acid, Biotin, and Choline*. Washington, DC: National Academy Press, 1998.

47. Priest DG, Bunni MA: Folate and folate antagonists in cancer chemotherapy. In: Bailey LB (ed.), *Folate in Health and Disease*. New York: Marcel Dekker, 1995.

48. Morgan SL, Baggot JE: Folate antagonists in non-neoplastic disease: Proposed mechanism of efficacy and toxicity. In: Bailey LN (ed.), *Folate in Health and Disease*. New York: Marcel Dekker, 1995.

49. Recker RR, Davies KM, Hinders SM, et al.: Bone gain in young adult women. *JAMA* 268:2403, 1992.

50. Panel on Dietary Reference Intakes for Electrolytes and Water, Standing Committee on the Scientific Evaluation of Dietary Reference Intakes: *Dietary Reference Intakes for Water, Potassium, Sodium, Chloride, and Sulfate*. Washington, DC: National Academy Press, 2004.

51. American Dietetic Association, Dietitians of Canada, and the American College of Sports Medicine: Nutrition and Athletic performance. *J Am Dietetic Assoc* 100:1543, 2000.

52. Casa DJ, Armstrong LE, Hillman SK, et al.: National Athletic Trainers' Association position statement: Fluid replacement for athletes. *J Athl Train* 35:21, 2000.

30

EATING DISORDERS:

Anorexia Nervosa and Bulimia Nervosa in the Adolescent

Neville H. Golden

Eating disorders are prevalent in the adolescent age group and may be associated with potentially life-threatening complications. Current fashion trends have resulted in alarming number of adolescents who are concerned about their weight and who are dieting. Despite the large number of adolescents dieting, only a relatively small number of them actually develop a clinically significant eating disorder. Concerned parents will turn to the pediatrician to differentiate between relatively harmless dieting and a more serious eating disorder.

Eating disorders are complex biopsychosocial disorders that have significant medical and psychologic morbidity. Once thought to be diseases predominantly affecting Caucasian middle class young women, we now know that no socioeconomic or ethnic group is immune from the development of an eating disorder. Furthermore, increasing number of boys and younger children with eating disorders are being identified. Both anorexia nervosa and bulimia nervosa classically have their onset during the adolescent years, though their symptoms may continue well into adulthood. It is widely believed that early intervention is associated with improved outcome. The primary care clinician is in a unique position to recognize the problem early and initiate intervention.

The aim of this chapter is to describe the major eating disorders seen in children and adolescents, identify the warning signs and medical complications, and describe the role the primary care clinicians can play in management.

EPIDEMIOLOGY AND ETIOLOGY OF EATING DISORDERS

Most eating disorders begin in adolescence and over 90% of patients with eating disorders are diagnosed before the age of 25 years. For anorexia nervosa, the peak age of onset is in mid adolescence (13–15 years) and for bulimia nervosa it is in late adolescence or early adulthood (17–25 years). Prepubertal anorexia nervosa does occur but is uncommon, while bulimia nervosa developing before puberty is rare. Eating disorders primarily affect young women; only 5%–10% of cases are male.

Over the past two decades there have been interesting trends in the epidemiology of eating disorders with rising rates in adolescents, minority groups, and in those of lower socioeconomic status. While the incidence of anorexia nervosa among adult women has remained relatively stable, in 15–19-year-old girls it has increased dramatically from 1935 to 1989.[1] In the United States, the prevalence of anorexia nervosa in adolescent females is estimated to be 0.5%, making it the third most common chronic disease of adolescence following obesity and asthma.[2] Similar prevalence rates have been documented in the United Kingdom and Europe.[3] Lifetime prevalence rates of bulimia nervosa range from 1% to 4%.[4] Epidemiologic studies from developing countries have demonstrated that prevalence rates in Japan, China, South Africa, and Iran now parallel those seen in the United States, United Kingdom, and Europe.[5–8] The general consensus is that prevalence rates most likely reflect socioeconomic development rather than ethnicity.

Eating disorders arise from a complex interplay between hereditary, biologic, and sociocultural factors. There is an increasing body of literature demonstrating a genetic predisposition to the development of an eating disorder. Studies have consistently demonstrated increased concordance rates for anorexia nervosa in monozygotic as compared to dizygotic twins; there is also increased prevalence of eating disorders in female relatives of probands with both anorexia nervosa and bulimia-nervosa.[9–10] No single gene or set of genes has, as yet, been identified but recent research has suggested that certain areas of the human genome may harbor susceptibility genes for AN on chromosome 1 and for BN on chromosome 10p.[11,12]

Neurotransmitter abnormalities in serotonin, dopamine, and noradrenalin pathways have been identified in patients with eating disorders. Many patients respond to medications that affect central neurotransmitter levels. Most of the abnormalities resolve with refeeding, suggesting that they are secondary to malnutrition. Some have been found to persist after long-term weight gain, implying that they may have predated the development of the eating disorder and may even have predisposed to its onset. The role of disturbances in serotonin transmission in anorexia nervosa has received particular interest in recent years. Serotonin is known to play a role in modulation of appetite. Recently, Kaye et al. have proposed that increased serotonergic activity (present in low weight patients with anorexia nervosa

and persisting after weight restoration) contributes to the core features of perfectionism, obsessionality, anxiety, and body image distortion. The authors suggest that dieting reduces plasma levels of tryptophan, an essential amino acid that is the precursor of serotonin. Dietary deficiency of tryptophan may be one mechanism whereby the patient reduces brain serotonergic activity to decrease anxiety and modulate mood.[13]

Adolescents with certain personality traits such as perfectionism, obsessionality, extreme compliance, harm avoidance, poor self-esteem, and feelings of ineffectiveness are more susceptible to develop anorexia nervosa. Many of these traits persist after recovery. These young women are often very bright, high achieving, and not uncommonly, are good athletes. However, despite their achievements they feel inadequate and often describe a feeling of loss of control. In contrast to anorexia nervosa, patients with bulimia nervosa are more likely to have problems with impulse control and to engage in risk-taking behaviors such as alcohol and substance abuse, promiscuity, and shoplifting.

Earlier theories described family dysfunction in affected families evidenced by rigidity, over protectiveness, enmeshment, and lack of conflict resolution.[14] Boundaries within the family are often blurred. For example, the patient may act as a "parentified child" or a parent may act more like a friend rather than a parent. While many families may exhibit these characteristics, more recent research does not support the existence of any "typical" anorexia nervosa family. Also, the relationship between childhood sexual abuse and subsequent development of an eating disorder is complex with some, but not all studies finding an increased risk for developing an eating disorder in those who have been sexually abused.[15] Purging behaviors, in particular, should arouse suspicion of this possibility.

Weight concerns and societal emphasis on thinness are pervasive in westernized societies and adolescents tend to be more vulnerable to fashion trends than adults. More than half of middle and high school girls have dieted at one time or another.[2] Dieting is common to all of the eating disorders and there is good evidence from clinical and epidemiologic studies that dieting and a slim body ideal is a risk factor for development of an eating disorder. The slim body ideal for women is thought to be the key contributor to gender differences seen in both anorexia nervosa and bulimia nervosa. Prolonged starvation itself can result in predictable physiologic responses. In their classic experiments after the second World War, Keys et al. demonstrated that semi-starvation in previously healthy male volunteers resulted in many of the psychologic as well as physiologic disturbances seen in patients with anorexia nervosa. Subjects became preoccupied with food, dreamt about food, and collected recipes. They became progressively more depressed and irritable and lost their sexual drive.[16]

Adolescence itself is a risk factor for development of an eating disorder. It is a period during which there are marked changes in body weight and shape and there is an intense need to conform to peer pressure (Chap. 1). The perfectionist young girl who had previously excelled academically and athletically now has to deal with a changing body, changing emotions, and changing expectations regarding issues like emerging sexuality, establishing independence from her family, and choosing a career (Chap. 1). Feeling overwhelmed and out of control, she focuses on what she eats, when she eats, and how she eats, and in doing so, feels more in control. She has difficulty in mastering the normal developmental tasks of adolescence and resolution of these tasks may be delayed for many years.

In summary, current research suggests that in a biologically predisposed individual, a feeling of loss of control during adolescence may cause her to diet to regain control. Family and friends may meet initial weight loss with approval. Continued dieting leads to a cycle of further preoccupation with shape and weight and the features of malnutrition that perpetuate the illness. It is important to recognize, however, that the etiology of an eating disorder in an individual patient depends on many factors and may vary for different individuals.

DIAGNOSTIC CRITERIA

The most widely used definitions of eating disorders are those provided by the American Psychiatric Association's Diagnostic and Statistical Manual of Mental Disorders, Fourth Edition (DSM-IV), Table 30-1.[17] Anorexia nervosa is a condition characterized by dietary restriction, marked weight loss, preoccupation with weight and shape, and a profound distortion in body image. Amenorrhea (defined as lack of menses for three or more cycles) is one of the cardinal features for the diagnosis. The key features of bulimia nervosa are cycles of bingeing followed by unhealthy compensatory mechanisms, such as self-induced vomiting, excessive exercise, starvation, and the use of laxatives, diuretics, or diet pills. In contrast to those with anorexia nervosa, most patients with bulimia nervosa are of normal weight. There is a spectrum of eating disorders and 10%–30% of patients cross over from one disorder to another at some time in their illness. The most frequent change among diagnostic categories is from anorexia nervosa to bulimia nervosa, though the reverse can occur.

There are problems with these diagnostic criteria, particularly with respect to children and adolescents. Firstly, there is wide variability in the rate of weight gain during puberty, the amount of weight that is gained, and the timing of increase in both height and weight. A growing child who fails to meet expected weight gain during a period of growth would fulfill the first criterion even in the absence of weight loss. With regard to the second and third criteria, many younger adolescents are unable to express abstract concepts such as fear of weight gain, distortion of body image, preoccupation with food and weight, and feelings of self-worth. In addition, an eating disorder may delay the onset of menarche; even in healthy adolescents, menses are characteristically irregular during the first 2 years after menarche, limiting the applicability of the fourth criterion. Finally, adolescents may develop pubertal delay, growth retardation, or impaired bone mineral acquisition at subclinical levels of eating disorders.

The majority of adolescents who present to the primary care clinician or to referral centers do not meet formal criteria for either anorexia nervosa or bulimia nervosa, yet their symptoms may be severe enough to warrant intervention. These patients are classified as eating disorder not otherwise specified (EDNOS). Included in this poorly-defined group are

TABLE 30-1

DSM-IV DIAGNOSTIC CRITERIA FOR ANOREXIA NERVOSA AND BULIMIA NERVOSA

Anorexia nervosa

A. Refusal to maintain body weight over a minimally normal weight for age and height (e.g., weight loss leading to maintenance of body weight less than 85% of the expected), or failure to make expected weight gain during period of growth, leading to body weight less than 85% of the expected.

B. Intense fear of gaining weight or becoming fat, even though underweight.

C. Disturbance in the way in which one's body weight or shape is experienced, undue influence of body shape and weight on self-evaluation, or denial of the seriousness of current low body weight.

D. In postmenarcheal females, amenorrhea, i.e., the absence of at least three consecutive menstrual cycles. (A woman is considered to have amenorrhea if her periods occur only following hormone, e.g., estrogen, administration.)

Restricting type: During the current episode of anorexia nervosa, the person does not regularly engage in binge eating or purging behavior (i.e., self-induced vomiting or the misuse of laxatives, diuretics, or enemas).

Binge eating/purging type: During the current episode of anorexia nervosa, the person has regularly engaged in binge eating or purging behavior (i.e., self-induced vomiting or the misuse of laxatives, diuretics, or enemas).

Bulimia nervosa

A. Recurrent episodes of binge eating. An episode of binge eating is characterized by both of the following:

  1. Eating, in a discrete period of time (e.g., within any 2-h period), an amount of food that is definitely larger than most people would eat during a similar period of time and under similar circumstances

  2. A sense of lack of control over eating during the episode (e.g., a feeling that one cannot stop eating or control what or how much one is eating).

B. Recurrent inappropriate compensatory behavior in order to prevent weight gain, such as self-induced vomiting; misuse of laxatives, diuretics, or other medications; fasting; or excessive exercise.

C. Both binge eating and inappropriate compensatory behaviors occur, on average, at least twice a week for 3 months.

D. Self-evaluation is unduly influenced by body shape and weight.

E. The disturbance does not occur exclusively during episodes of anorexia nervosa.

Purging type: The person regularly engages in self-induced vomiting or the misuse of laxatives or diuretics.

Nonpurging type: The person uses other inappropriate compensatory behaviors, such as fasting or excessive exercise, but does not regularly engage in self-induced vomiting or the misuse of laxatives or diuretics.

Source: American Psychiatric Association. Diagnostic and Statistical Manual for Mental Disorders, 4th ed. Washington, DC: APA Press, 1994.

those who purge daily to maintain a "normal weight" but do not binge, those who have lost weight but have not yet lost enough weight to meet the 85% cutoff, and those who have lost their periods but have not yet been amenorrheic for 3 months. A particularly interesting group of patients, frequently considered as part of the EDNOS category, is of the female athletes. The "female athlete triad" refers to three interrelated conditions sometimes seen in female athletes—disordered eating, amenorrhea, and osteoporosis.[18] In these young women, caloric intake is insufficient for energy needs, resulting in hypothalamic amenorrhea, osteoporosis, and increased fracture risk. Although some of these women may meet criteria for an eating disorder, most do not. Most of them do not have body image distortion and body weight is often in the normal range. These athletes are using unhealthy methods to control body weight with the belief that a lower body weight will improve athletic performance.

Given that the DSM IV criteria are not always applicable to children and adolescents, researchers at the Hospital for Sick Children at Great Ormond Street in the United Kingdom have developed a different set of diagnostic criteria, particularly applicable for children or younger adolescents.[19,20] In this diagnostic system, anorexia nervosa and bulimia nervosa still exist but, in addition, there are new diagnoses that further categorize the EDNOS group. Food avoidance emotional disorder (FAED) refers to a condition seen in children 8–13 years old where a child refuses to eat. There is no fear of becoming fat and no distortion in body image. This condition may be accompanied by growth retardation and weight loss. Selective eating disorder (SED) refers to those younger patients who limit their foods to one or two foods for a prolonged period of time. They are unwilling to try new foods, which can be a major source of frustration for their parents. Similar to those with *FAED*, they do not have the cognitive distortions regarding weight or shape. Their weight and height are usually appropriate for age. *Functional dysphagia* refers to a group of children and younger adolescents who will avoid certain foods because of a fear of swallowing, choking, or vomiting. Often there is a history of an episode of choking on a specific food, which is then avoided. These latter three groups can be associated with weight loss, family distress, and the medical consequences of malnutrition, but they are not associated with the fear of weight gain or the cognitive distortions seen in anorexia nervosa and bulimia nervosa.

PRESENTING FEATURES

The warning signs of anorexia nervosa and bulimia nervosa are listed in Table 30-2. Most adolescents are reluctantly brought to the primary care clinician because the parents have noticed weight loss or have suspected that their child may be vomiting. Sometimes it is the school guidance counselor who makes the referral. Denial of the illness is universal and the patient herself will do her best to hide the weight loss by wearing multiple layers of clothing. Occasionally a teenager may be brought in for evaluation of short stature or delayed puberty (Chap. 15).

TABLE 30-2

WARNING SIGNS OF ANOREXIA NERVOSA AND BULIMIA NERVOSA

Warning signs of anorexia nervosa

Excessive weight loss or resistance to gain weight when advised to do so

Preoccupation with food and weight

Highly active, exercises compulsively

Strange rituals at mealtimes, unusual eating habits

Social isolation, depression, and irritability

Feels cold all the time, wears multiple layers of clothing

Constipation

Hair thinning or hair loss

Unexplained amenorrhea

Delayed puberty or growth retardation

Warning signs of bulimia nervosa

Marked fluctuations in weight

Suspicion of vomiting (smell of vomit, spends a long time in the bathroom with the faucet running)

Finding diet pills, laxatives, or diuretics in the teenager's room

Food disappearing from the refrigerator or cupboards

Finding hidden food or candy wrappers

Mood swings

Parotid hypertrophy

Calluses over the knuckles (Russell's sign)

Erosion of dental enamel

When an adolescent seeks help voluntarily, it is usually because of amenorrhea, hair loss, or a frightening event such as an episode of hematemesis. Sometimes medical attention is sought because the adolescent is "fed up" with the eating disorder.

A good history and physical examination can provide an accurate diagnosis; laboratory tests are usually normal, but do help exclude other conditions. The adolescent should be interviewed with her family as well as alone (Chap. 2). It is important to explore the patient's feelings about her current weight, her desired weight, and whether or not she is concerned about the weight loss. Even the most complex of adolescents will openly admit that they feel too fat and that they would like to lose further weight. If there is denial of feeling too fat, the clinician can then ask, "Is there any part of your body that you consider too fat?" The patient usually will admit that she perceives her abdomen, thighs, or buttocks to be too large.

Information should be obtained about the amount, duration, rate, and methods of weight loss, the patient's highest and lowest weights, the amount of exercise performed, and the duration of amenorrhea. The weight at which menses were lost should be noted because this can help predict the weight necessary for menses to resume. An average 24-hour dietary recall should be obtained. In review of systems, the adolescent should be asked about cold intolerance, bowel habits, and episodes of hematemesis or fainting. Some assessment should be made regarding coexistent depression and social isolation.

Physical Examination

Patients with anorexia nervosa are hypothermic and wear multiple layers of clothing in order to keep warm and to hide the weight loss. It is essential to obtain an accurate height and weight. Height should be measured using a wall-mounted stadiometer; weight should be measured postvoiding with the patient undressed and wearing only underwear and a hospital gown. Height and weight should be plotted on the standard growth charts for children and adolescents and should be compared to previous heights and weights. Body mass index (BMI) can be calculated by dividing the patient's weight in kilograms by the square of the height in meters (BMI = weight in kg/height in m^2) and can be plotted on the Centers for Disease Control charts (Chap. 29).[21]

In anorexia nervosa, the most notable findings on physical examination are the features of malnutrition. There is loss of subcutaneous tissue, muscle wasting, and prominence of bony protuberances. The extremities may be cold and blue (acrocyanosis), while the skin may be dry and scaly with a yellow discoloration secondary to carotenemia. There may be evidence of easy bruising. The hair may be dry and listless and the nails brittle; lanugo may be present over the back, abdomen, and extensor surfaces of the extremities. There may be evidence of dehydration, or less frequently, dependent edema; core body temperature may be very low.

Bradycardia may be profound with resting heart rates of 30–50 beats/minute; there may be hypotension with or without postural changes. The most common postural change found is an increase in the heart rate over 20 beats/minute when changing from a supine to a standing position. The breasts may be atrophic, while the abdomen is scaphoid and the posterior abdominal wall easily felt through the weak abdominal musculature. Stool may be palpable in the left lower quadrant. There may be generalized muscle weakness and evidence of peripheral neuropathy. In severely malnourished patients there may be confusion and psychomotor retardation with slowing of speech and difficulties in concentration.

Patients with bulimia nervosa are usually of normal weight. The three clinical signs to look for on physical examination are parotid hypertrophy, erosion of dental enamel, and calluses over the knuckle of the index finger (Russell's sign). Parotid hypertrophy occurs in 10%–30% of patients with bulimia nervosa; it is usually bilateral.[22] The exact etiology is not clear but it is thought to be secondary to hypertrophy as a result of the frequent binges. Erosion of dental enamel is most apparent on the lingual aspects of the anterior teeth and is caused by dissolution of the dental enamel by acidic gastric contents. Calluses over the knuckles are formed by abrasions from the incisors when the fingers are used to induce vomiting.

Laboratory Investigation

Recommended laboratory tests on initial presentation are listed in Table 30-3. Despite marked cachexia, the laboratory tests are usually normal. The complete blood count may show mild anemia, leukopenia, or thrombocytopenia, reflecting suppression of the bone marrow. The erythrocyte sedimentation rate is characteristically very low secondary to decreased hepatic production of fibrinogen. The presence of an elevated sedimentation rate should raise the suspicion of another diagnosis.

Electrolyte disturbances may occur with fluid restriction, vomiting, laxative, or diuretic use. Hypokalemia is seen in those who are vomiting or using laxatives. Hyponatremia can occur in the presence of water loading practiced by some

TABLE 30-3

RECOMMENDED LABORATORY AND ANCILLARY
TESTS FOR THE EVALUATION OF ADOLESCENTS
WITH EATING DISORDERS

Complete blood count
Erythrocyte sedimentation rate
Urinalysis
Chemistry profile including liver function tests
Serum amylase—if vomiting
Thyroid function tests
LH, FSH, estradiol, and prolactin—if amenorrheic
Electrocardiogram
If amenorrheic for >6 months, bone densitometry

patients either to suppress feelings of hunger or to achieve a desired weight in the doctor's office. Both hypernatremia and hyperkalemia can occur in the presence of dehydration. Hypochloremic alkalosis develops with recurrent vomiting. Serum phosphorus levels are usually normal on presentation but may drop precipitously on refeeding or after a binge. Serum transaminases are elevated in 4%–38% of patients with anorexia nervosa, probably because of fatty necrosis of the liver secondary to malnutrition.[23–25] In those who are bingeing and purging, serum amylase may be elevated. In contrast to other forms of malnutrition, total protein and serum albumin levels are usually normal. Cholesterol levels may be high but most frequently are normal.[26,27] Serum carotene levels are elevated in 13%–62% of cases, probably due to a combination of increased dietary intake of carrots and other pigmented vegetables, as well as derangement of hepatic conversion of beta-carotene to vitamin A.[25,28]

The urinalysis may show ketones, mild proteinuria, and alkaline urine. Specific gravity may be high in the presence of dehydration but low if the adolescent has been water loading prior to the office visit. Thyroid function tests may show a low triiodothyronine (T3) and occasionally a low thyroxine (T4) level (Chap. 15). Abnormalities in thyroid function tests, which reflect adaptive changes to malnutrition, respond to nutritional rehabilitation and should not be treated with thyroid hormone

replacement. Luteinizing hormone (LH), follicle-stimulating hormone (FSH), and estradiol levels are all low, secondary to suppression of the hypothalamic-pituitary-ovarian axis. A normal prolactin level helps rule out a prolactinoma.

The electrocardiogram usually shows sinus bradycardia and low voltage complexes; however, there may be a prolonged QTc interval, nonspecific ST segment depression or T wave changes, first and second degree heart block, and various atrial as well as ventricular arrhythmias.[24,29] A prolonged QTc interval is of particular concern because it has been identified preceding ventricular arrhythmias and sudden death in patients with anorexia nervosa.[30] In normal weight bulimics, arrhythmias may occur secondary to electrolyte and acid-based imbalance due to vomiting, laxative, or diuretic abuse. Bulimics who use ipecac to induce vomiting may develop a cardiomyopathy due to the toxic effect of emetine, the active alkaloid component in syrup of ipecac. The initial cardiac manifestations of ipecac cardiomyopathy are tachycardia, a prolonged QTc interval, inverted T waves, and depressed ST segments.[31] In those patients who have been amenorrheic for more than 6 months, bone densitometry of the lumbar spine and hip should be performed to measure bone mineral density and evaluate for the presence of reduced bone mass.

MEDICAL COMPLICATIONS

The medical complications of anorexia nervosa and bulimia nervosa are listed in Table 30-4. Most of the complications result from physiologic adaptations to the effects of malnutrition on different organ systems. Complications also occur as a result of aberrant weight-control behaviors. Many, but not all of the complications, are reversible with nutritional rehabilitation and improvement of the eating disorder symptoms; however, in the adolescent whose growth and development are not yet complete, the medical consequences of eating disorders can be long-lasting and potentially irreversible. Complications of particular concern in a teenager include growth retardation if the disorder commenced prior to closure of the epiphyses, pubertal

T A B L E   3 0 - 4

MEDICAL COMPLICATIONS OF EATING DISORDERS

	Anorexia Nervosa	*Bulimia Nervosa*
Weight	Low	Usually in normal range
Fluid and electrolytes	Increased blood urea nitrogen (BUN)	Hypokalemia
	Hyponatremia	Hypochloremia
		Metabolic alkalosis
Cardiovascular	Bradycardia	Ipecac cardiomyopathy
	Orthostatic hypotension	
	ECG abnormalities	
	Pericardial effusion	
	Congestive heart failure	
Gastrointestinal	Constipation	Parotid hypertrophy
	Delayed gastric emptying	Esophagitis
	Intestinal immotility	Erosion of dental enamel
	Fatty infiltration of the liver	Bloody diarrhea
	Acute pancreatitis	Mallory-Weiss tears
	Superior mesenteric artery syndrome	Esophageal or gastric rupture
	Gallstones	Barrett esophagus
Skin	Acrocyanosis	Calluses on back of hand
	Lanugo	Edema
	Hypercarotenemia	
	Edema	
Endocrine	Amenorrhea	
	Pubertal delay	
	Growth retardation	
	Low T3 syndrome	
	Hypercortisolism	
Skeletal	Osteopenia	
	Fractures	
Hematologic	Anemia	
	Thrombocytopenia	
	Leukopenia	
	Low ESR	
Neurologic	Seizures	
	Cortical atrophy	Syncope

delay or arrest, impaired acquisition of peak bone mass predisposing to osteoporosis and increased fracture risk, and the structural brain changes noted on cerebral tomography and magnetic resonance imaging.

In adolescents who develop anorexia nervosa prior to completion of growth, growth retardation and short stature can be prominent findings (Chap. 15). Danziger et al. plotted growth curves of 15 subjects who developed anorexia nervosa during the prepubertal and pubertal period. They found that, in every case where the disease had been present for at least 6 months and a growth curve could be reconstructed, growth arrest was observed.[32] Patients are shorter than expected[33] and growth stunting can even be the presenting feature.[34,35] Growth retardation as a major feature of anorexia nervosa is more likely to occur in adolescent boys because boys grow, on average, for 2 years more than girls (Chap. 1). Adolescents with anorexia nervosa have diminished growth hormone action resulting in decreased secretion of insulin-like growth factor-1 (IGF-1), the hormone that mediates cell proliferation and protein synthesis. Levels of growth hormone are normal or increased with low levels of growth hormone binding protein, suggesting an adaptive state of growth hormone resistance. These findings revert to normal after nutritional rehabilitation.[36] Peak height velocity is lower than expected, occurs later than expected, and menarche occurs significantly later than in healthy peers. Catch-up growth can occur with nutritional rehabilitation but, even with intervention, these adolescents may not reach their genetic height potential.[37]

Pubertal delay is a frequent finding in those developing anorexia nervosa prior to completion of puberty. Palla and Litt found pubertal delay in 17% of adolescents with anorexia nervosa.[24] Russell found failure of breast development in 14 out of 20 subjects who developed anorexia nervosa before menarche. Thirteen among the 20 had their first menstrual period after the age of 18 years.[38] Amenorrhea, either primary or secondary, is associated with a disturbance in the regulation of gonadotropin-releasing hormone secretion by the hypothalamus (Chap. 28). Serum levels of LH, FSH, and estradiol are low. In most instances, amenorrhea is associated with weight loss, but in approximately 20% cases, loss of menses may precede significant weight loss.[39] Weight gain is usually accompanied by restoration of normal hypothalamic-pituitary-ovarian function and resumption of spontaneous menses; however, in many cases, amenorrhea may be prolonged.

The most serious complication of prolonged amenorrhea and a low estrogen state is osteopenia or reduced bone mass (Chap. 29). In anorexia nervosa, osteopenia may occur after a relatively short duration of illness[40] and can be severe.[41] Recent studies have demonstrated that more than 90% of adolescents and young adults with anorexia nervosa have reduced bone mass at one or more skeletal sites.[42,43] There is both a decrease in the markers of bone formation and an increase in the markers of bone resorption.[44] Adolescence is a critical time for bone mass acquisition. The development of osteoporosis in later life depends not only on the rate of bone loss in adulthood, but also on the amount of bone present at skeletal maturity, often referred to as "peak bone mass." Approximately 60% of peak bone mass is accrued during adolescence and there is very little net gain in bone mass after 2 years following menarche.[45–48] A woman who develops anorexia nervosa during adolescence will not reach her peak bone mass. Even though she may recover fully from the eating disorder, her increased fracture risk can persist because she started off with a lower peak bone mass. A recent study conducted on 19 women who had fully recovered from anorexia nervosa for an average of 21 years, found that bone mineral density of the hip remained lower than controls and two of the subjects had experienced pathologic fractures.[49]

A number of computed tomography (CT) and magnetic resonance imaging (MRI) studies have demonstrated structural brain changes in malnourished patients with anorexia nervosa.[50–53] The cerebral ventricles and cortical sulci are enlarged and there are volume deficits of both grey and white matter, suggesting loss of brain substance or cerebral atrophy. In addition, using radioisotope scans, evidence of reduced regional blood flow to the brain in anorexia nervosa was demonstrated in 13 out of 15 children and adolescents aged 9–14 years.[54] Neuropsychologic testing has demonstrated impairment of attention, concentration, and memory with deficits in visuospatial ability; however, it is not clear whether the cognitive deficits are directly related to the structural brain changes.[55] The potential impact of these findings on the developing brain is not clear. While the ventricular enlargement and white matter changes revert to normal after weight restoration,[52,56] the grey matter volume deficits and regional blood flow disturbances may persist, suggesting that these changes may even have predated the illness.[52,54,56] Similarly, some but not all, of the cognitive deficits improve with weight restoration.[55]

TREATMENT

Both the American Academy of Pediatrics[57] and the Society for Adolescent Medicine[58] encourage early intervention for adolescents with eating disorders. In its position paper, the Society for Adolescent Medicine specifically states that the threshold for intervention in adolescents with eating disorders should be lower than that for adults.[58] The primary care clinician caring for children and adolescents is in a unique position to detect the onset of an eating disorder and to prevent its progression. The vast majority of patients can be managed as outpatients and the clinician can assume an important role in the management.

Early or Mild Anorexia Nervosa or Bulimia Nervosa

For the patient with recent onset of the disorder who is dieting and has lost some weight but not an excessive amount, the pediatrician can educate the patient about the dangers of eating disorders and establish a weight loss limit. Basic nutritional advice can be given regarding caloric requirements, taking into account age and activity level. To prevent daily weighing and preoccupation with weight, the patient should be advised to give away the scale and should instead, be monitored by the pediatrician every 2–4 weeks, as clinically needed. At each visit, weight should be measured in the same manner (postvoiding, wearing only a hospital gown) and on the same scale. Urine specific gravity should be measured for water loading or dehydration. If the patient responds to the intervention and cognitive distortions are not severe, the pediatrician can comfortably manage the adolescent without referring him or her to a mental health professional.

Established or Moderate Anorexia Nervosa or Bulimia Nervosa

If, on the other hand, the patient has a clinically significant eating disorder, a team approach is advised. Patients in this category would include those with significant weight loss, those who are using unhealthy methods to control weight (i.e., restricting caloric intake to less than 1000 kcal/day, exercising excessively, bingeing, purging, using laxatives or diuretics) even without significant weight loss, and those who have marked cognitive distortions.

In such youth, no single professional can be proficient in all aspects of the patient's care. The team usually comprises of the primary care clinician, a nutritionist, and a mental health professional. Frequent communication with clear delineation of roles is the key to success. It should be the clinician's responsibility to determine the treatment goal weight, the rate of weight gain, and to evaluate for medical complications. Patients may need to be monitored every 1–2 weeks; at each visit the patient should be weighed, examined, and the urine specific gravity checked. A rate gain of approximately 1–2 lb per week is encouraged. For those who have been severely restricting their caloric intake, prescribed caloric intake should be low initially (1200–1400 kcal/day) but should be slowly increased by 200–300 kcal/day at each visit. Ultimately intakes of 2400–3600 kcal/day may be necessary for adequate weight gain. Extracurricular activities such as ballet, gymnastics, and team sports may need to be curtailed. When medically appropriate, a return to sports can be used as a motivating factor for weight gain.

Treatment goal weight should be individualized and should take into account age, height, Tanner stage, premorbid weight, and previous growth charts. In postmenarcheal girls, resumption of menses can be used as an indicator of return to biologic health and a weight 90% of average body weight can be used as a reasonable treatment goal weight, since 86% of patients who achieve this weight resume menses within 6 months.[39] In growing children and adolescents, the treatment goal weight should be reevaluated every 6 months, based on changing height and weight.

The nutritionist can convert the caloric prescription into an actual meal plan incorporating some of the patient's food preferences. The nutritionist can educate the patient about the nutritional requirements for growth and development during adolescence and the relatively high-energy intake required during nutritional rehabilitation. Nutritional myths should be dispelled and "forbidden foods" can be slowly introduced into the diet.

Most patients will require individual psychotherapy to address the issues that led to the development of the eating disorder, to build self-esteem, and to develop better coping strategies. The therapist should be familiar with working with adolescents and should have expertise in treating eating disorders. For younger patients who still live at home, family-based therapy has been shown to be very effective.[59–62] Cognitive behavioral therapy has been used successfully in adults with anorexia nervosa, but has not been evaluated in adolescents. Despite limited scientific research on the use of psychotropic medications in anorexia nervosa, in some cases they may be useful to treat comorbid depression or obsessive-compulsive disorder. There is some evidence to suggest that fluoxetine may prevent relapse in older adolescents who have been weight restored.[63]

In bulimia nervosa, cognitive behavioral therapy, which focuses on changing the specific eating attitudes and behaviors, is the most effective form of psychotherapy.[64,65] Antidepressants, particularly the selective serotonin reuptake inhibitors (SSRIs; Chap. 36) are very effective in reducing the frequency of bingeing and purging episodes.[66,67] These same medications (SSRIs) can also treat comorbid depression and anxiety (Chaps. 36 and 37).

Severe Anorexia Nervosa or Bulimia Nervosa

Patients with more severe symptoms may require more intensive treatment in inpatient, partial hospitalization (day hospital), or intensive outpatient programs (IOPs). The choice of program will depend on the severity of the symptoms and the type of programs available in the area.

Indications for inpatient hospitalization are shown in Table 30-5. Such programs may be located

TABLE 30-5

INDICATIONS FOR HOSPITALIZATION IN AN ADOLESCENT WITH AN EATING DISORDER

One or more of the following justify hospitalization:

1. Severe malnutrition (Weight ≤75% average body weight for age, sex, and height)
2. Dehydration
3. Electrolyte disturbances (hypokalemia, hyponatremia, and hypophosphatemia)
4. Cardiac dysrhythmia
5. Physiologic instability

   Severe bradycardia (heart rate <50 beats/min daytime; <45 beats/min at night)

   Hypotension (<80/50 mmHg)

   Hypothermia (body temperature <96°F)

   Orthostatic changes in pulse (>20 beats/min) or blood pressure (>10 mmHg)

6. Arrested growth and development
7. Failure of outpatient treatment
8. Acute food refusal
9. Uncontrollable bingeing and purging
10. Acute medical complications of malnutrition (e.g., syncope, seizures, cardiac failure, pancreatitis, and so forth.)
11. Acute psychiatric emergencies (e.g., suicidal ideation, acute psychosis)
12. Comorbid diagnosis that interferes with the treatment of the eating disorder (e.g., severe depression, obsessive compulsive disorder, and severe family dysfunction)

Source: Golden NH, Katzman DK, Kreipe RE, Stevens SL, Sawyer SM, Rees J, et al. Eating disorders in adolescents: position paper of the Society for Adolescent Medicine. J Adolesc Health 2003; 33(6):496–503.

on general pediatric, adolescent medicine, or psychiatric units or they may be free standing eating disorder programs. Wherever the location, it is important that the staff has expertise in working with adolescents and is knowledgeable about adolescent physical and emotional development (Chap. 1). The backbone of most inpatient programs is a behavior modification contract aimed at weight restoration and reversal of the abnormal eating-related behaviors. Such programs have been shown to be both safe and effective.[68] Weight gain is an important early goal in the treatment process and is associated with improvement in mood and enhanced cognitive functioning. Nasogastric feeding is required infrequently and should only be used when the patient is unable to tolerate oral intake or is unable to consume enough food required for weight gain. On inpatient units a rate of weight gain of 2–4 lb per week is appropriate. On most units, meals are supervised in a nurturing environment and patients receive a combination of individual, family, and group psychotherapies.

In severely malnourished patients, care should be taken to advance caloric intake slowly in order to prevent the refeeding syndrome. This condition consists of serious cardiac, neurologic, and hematologic complications, which develop during nutritional rehabilitation.[69] During starvation, total body stores of phosphorus are low, but serum phosphorus levels are maintained. With refeeding, phosphorus is driven into the cells and is rapidly used for the production of high-energy phosphorus-containing compounds necessary for protein synthesis and cell regeneration. Serum phosphorus levels, which were previously normal, may drop to dangerously low levels. This can occur after oral, enteral, or parenteral refeeding. The major danger of hypophosphatemia is that it is thought to predispose to ventricular arrhythmias and sudden death. In anorexia nervosa, the refeeding syndrome can be prevented by slow refeeding with careful monitoring of heart rate and serum electrolytes (especially phosphorus) during the first 7–10 days of nutritional rehabilitation.[70,71] Phosphorus can be supplemented as needed if levels drop[71] or it can be administered prophylactically during the first 5 days of refeeding, as some authors have recommended.[72]

Day hospital programs offer a level of intensity intermediate between that of the inpatient program and outpatient programs. Typically, patients spend 5–8 hours a day, 4–6 days a week in the program. Some, but not all, of the meals are supervised and patients receive similar therapy to that provided in the inpatient program. Partial hospitalization programs provide the ideal transition from inpatient programs but can also be used to avoid inpatient hospitalization in someone who is on a progressively downhill course. IOPs meet in a group setting for 3–4 hours, 3–4 times per week and offer more intensive treatment and support for those being treated as outpatients.

Treatment of Osteopenia

The treatment of osteopenia in anorexia nervosa remains unresolved. Body weight, in particular, lean body mass, is the major determinant of bone mass.[40–42,73–76] In anorexia nervosa, weight gain is associated with an increase in bone mineral density, although bone mineral density will not necessarily return to normal levels.[42,49,77,78] Calcium supplementation has been shown to increase bone mass in healthy children and adolescents,[79–81] but has not been studied in subjects with eating disorders. Similarly, both weight-bearing and resistance exercises are known to increase bone mass in normal children, adolescents, and young women[82,83] but have not been evaluated in patients with anorexia nervosa. In runners, the protective effect of exercise is lost if the patient becomes amenorrheic. Current recommendations for the treatment of reduced bone mass in anorexia nervosa include weight restoration with resumption of spontaneous menses, calcium (1200–1500 mg/day) and vitamin D (400 IU/day) supplementation, and carefully monitored weight-bearing exercise (Chap. 29).[58] Excessive exercise that results in weight loss, is accompanied by amenorrhea, or prevents adequate weight gain, should be avoided.

Hormone replacement therapy, while commonly prescribed for the treatment of osteopenia,[84] has not been shown to improve bone mass in anorexia nervosa.[42,85] In fact, the monthly induced menstrual bleeding will obscure resumption of menses, the objective criterion used by many to determine the patient's individualized treatment goal weight. On hormone replacement therapy, the patient will be having monthly hormone-induced menstrual bleeding even at a low body weight. This fact may feed into the patient's denial about her appropriate treatment goal weight. Ongoing studies are evaluating the use of dehydroepiandrosterone,[86] IGF-1,[87] and the bisphosphonates for the treatment of osteopenia in anorexia nervosa.

SUMMARY

Anorexia and bulimia nervosa are prevalent in adolescents and are associated with significant medical as well as psychologic morbidity. Most adolescents with clinically significant symptoms do not meet rigid diagnostic criteria for either anorexia nervosa or bulimia nervosa, but their symptoms still warrant treatment. Early intervention is associated with improved outcome and prevents chronicity. The primary care clinician is in a unique position to identify the eating disorder problem early and can play an important role in the management of the patient and her family.

Bibliography

1. Lucas AR, Crowson CS, O'Fallon WM, Melton LJ, III. The ups and downs of anorexia nervosa. Int J Eat Disord 1999; 26(4):397–405.

2. Fisher M, Golden NH, Katzman DK, Kreipe RE, Rees J, Schebendach J, et al. Eating disorders in adolescents: a background paper. J Adolesc Health 1995; 16:420–437.

3. Hoek HW, van Hoeken D. Review of the prevalence and incidence of eating disorders. Int J Eat Disord 2003; 34(4):383–396.

4. Fairburn CG, Beglin SJ. Studies of the epidemiology of bulimia nervosa. Am J Psychiatry 1990; 147(4): 401–408.

5. le Grange D, Telch CF, Tibbs J. Eating attitudes and behaviors in 1,435 South African Caucasian and non-Caucasian college students. Am J Psychiatry 1998; 155(2):250–254.

6. Lee S, Lee AM. Disordered eating in three communities of China: a comparative study of female high school students in Hong Kong, Shenzhen, and rural Hunan. Int J Eat Disord 2000; 27(3):317–327.

7. McClelland L, Crisp A. Anorexia nervosa and social class. Int J Eat Disord 2001; 29(2):150–156.

8. Nakamura K, Yamamoto M, Yamazaki O, Kawashima Y, Muto K, Someya T, et al. Prevalence of anorexia nervosa and bulimia nervosa in a geographically defined area in Japan. Int J Eat Disord 2000; 28(2): 173–180.

9. Walters EE, Kendler KS. Anorexia nervosa and anorexic-like syndromes in a population-based female twin sample. Am J Psychiatry 1995;152(1): 64–71.

10. Strober M, Freeman R, Lampert C, Diamond J, Kaye W. Controlled family study of anorexia nervosa and bulimia nervosa: evidence of shared liability and transmission of partial syndromes. Am J Psychiatry 2000;157(3):393–401.

11. Bulik CM, Devlin B, Bacanu SA, Thornton L, Klump KL, Fichter MM, et al. Significant linkage on chromosome 10p in families with bulimia nervosa. Am J Hum Genet 2003;72(1):200–207.

12. Grice DE, Halmi KA, Fichter MM, Strober M, Woodside DB, Treasure JT, et al. Evidence for a susceptibility gene for anorexia nervosa on chromosome 1. Am J Hum Genet 2002;70(3):787–792.

13. Kaye WH, Barbarich NC, Putnam K, Gendall KA, Fernstrom J, Fernstrom M et al. Anxiolytic effects of acute tryptophan depletion in anorexia nervosa. Int J Eat Disord 2003;33(3):257–267.

14. Minuchin S, Baker L, Rosman BL, Liebman R, Milman L, Todd TC. A conceptual model of psychosomatic illness in children: family organization and family therapy. Arch Gen Psychiatry 1975;32(8): 1031–1038.

15. Herzog DB, Staley JE, Carmody S, Robbins WM, van der Kolk BA. Childhood sexual abuse in anorexia nervosa and bulimia nervosa: a pilot study. J Am Acad Child Adolesc Psychiatry 1993;32(5):962–966.

16. Keys A, Brozek J, Henschel A, et al. *The Biology of Human Starvation*. Minneapolis, MN: University of Minnesota Press, 1950.

17. American Psychiatric Association. Diagnostic and Statistical Manual for Mental Disorders, 4th ed. Washington, DC: APA Press, 1994.

18. Golden NH. A review of the female athlete triad (amenorrhea, osteoporosis and disordered eating). Int J Adolesc Med Health 2002;14:9–17.

19. Lask B, Bryant-Waugh R. Childhood Onset Anorexia Nervosa and Related Eating Disorders. Melksham, Wiltshire, UK: Redwood Press Limited, 1993.

20. Nicholls D, Chater R, Lask B. Children into DSM don't go: a comparison of classification systems for eating disorders in childhood and early adolescence. Int J Eat Disord 2000;28(3):317–324.

21. Kuczmarski RJ, Ogden CL, Grummer-Strawn LM, Flegal KM, Guo SS, Wei R, et al. CDC growth charts: United States. Advance Data from vital and health statistics No.314 2000;1–27.

22. Ogren FP, Huerter JV, Pearson PH, Antonson CW, Moore GF. Transient salivary gland hypertrophy in bulimics. Laryngoscope 1987;97(8 Pt 1):951–953.

23. Mickley D, Greenfeld D, Quinlan DM, Roloff P, Zwas F. Abnormal liver enzymes in outpatients with eating disorders. Int J Eat Disord 1996;20(3): 325–329.

24. Palla B, Litt IF. Medical complications of eating disorders in adolescents. Pediatrics 1988;81(5): 613–623.

25. Sherman P, Leslie K, Goldberg E, Rybczynski J, St Louis P. Hypercarotenemia and transaminitis in female adolescents with eating disorders: a prospective controlled study. J Adolesc Health 1994;15(3): 205–209.

26. Arden MR, Weiselberg EC, Nussbaum MP, Shenker IR, Jacobson MS. Effect of weight restoration on the dyslipoproteinemia of anorexia nervosa. J Adolesc Health Care 1990;11(3):199–202.

27. Mehler PS, Lezotte D, Eckel R. Lipid levels in anorexia nervosa. Int J Eat Disord 1998;24(2): 217–221.

28. Boland B, Beguin C, Zech F, Desager JP, Lambert M. Serum beta-carotene in anorexia nervosa patients: a case-control study. Int J Eat Disord 2001;30(3): 299–305.

29. Galetta F, Franzoni F, Cupisti A, Belliti D, Prattichizzo F, Rolla M. QT interval dispersion in young women with anorexia nervosa. J Pediatr 2002; 140(4):456–460.

30. Isner JM, Roberts WC, Heymsfield SB, Yager J. Anorexia nervosa and sudden death. Ann Intern Med 1985;102(1):49–52.

31. Schiff RJ, Wurzel CL, Brunson SC, Kasloff I, Nussbaum MP, Frank SD. Death due to chronic syrup of ipecac use in a patient with bulimia. Pediatrics 1986;78(3):412–416.

32. Danziger Y, Mukamel M, Zeharia A, Dinari G, Mimouni M. Stunting of growth in anorexia nervosa during the prepubertal and pubertal period. Isr J Med Sci 1994;30(8):581–584.

33. Nussbaum M, Baird D, Sonnenblick M, Cowan K, Shenker IR. Short stature in anorexia nervosa patients. J Adolesc Health Care 1985;6(6):453–455.

34. Root AW, Powers PS. Anorexia nervosa presenting as growth retardation in adolescents. J Adolesc Health Care 1983;4(1):25–30.

35. Modan-Moses D, Yaroslavsky A, Novikov I, Segev S, Toledano A, Miterany E, et al. Stunting of growth as a major feature of anorexia nervosa in male adolescents. Pediatrics 2003;111(2):270–276.

36. Golden NH, Kreitzer P, Jacobson MS, Chasalow FI, Schebendach J, Freedman SM, et al. Disturbances in growth hormone secretion and action in adolescents with anorexia nervosa. J Pediatr 1994;125(4): 655–660.

37. Lantzouni E, Frank GR, Golden NH, Shenker RI. Reversibility of growth stunting in early onset anorexia nervosa: a prospective study. J Adolesc Health 2002; 31(2):162–165.

38. Russell GF. Premenarchal anorexia nervosa and its sequelae. J Psychiat Res 1985;19:363–369.

39. Golden NH, Jacobson MS, Schebendach J, Solanto MV, Hertz SM, Shenker IR. Resumption of menses in anorexia nervosa. Arch Pediatr Adolesc Med 1997; 151(1):16–21.

40. Bachrach LK, Guido D, Katzman D, Litt IF, Marcus R. Decreased bone density in adolescent girls with anorexia nervosa. Pediatrics 1990;86(3):440–447.

41. Grinspoon S, Miller K, Coyle C, Krempin J, Armstrong C, Pitts S, et al. Severity of osteopenia in estrogen-deficient women with anorexia nervosa and hypothalamic amenorrhea. J Clin Endocrinol Metab 1999;84(6):2049–2055.

42. Golden NH, Lanzkowsky L, Schebendach J, Palestro CJ, Jacobson MS, Shenker IR. The effect of estrogen-progestin treatment on bone mineral density in anorexia nervosa. J Pediatr Adolesc Gynecol 2002; 15(3):135–143.

43. Grinspoon S, Thomas E, Pitts S, Gross E, Mickley D, Miller K, et al. Prevalence and predictive factors for regional osteopenia in women with anorexia nervosa. Ann Intern Med 2000;133(10):790–794.

44. Grinspoon S, Baum H, Lee K, Anderson E, Herzog D, Klibanski A. Effects of short-term recombinant human insulin-like growth factor I administration on bone turnover in osteopenic women with anorexia nervosa. J Clin Endocrinol Metab 1996;81(11): 3864–3870.

45. Golden NH, Shenker IR. *Amenorrhrea in Anorexia Nervosa: Etiology and Implications. Adolescent Nutrition and Eating Disorders.* Philadelphia, PA: Hanley & Belfus, 1992, pp. 503–518.

46. Katzman DK, Bachrach LK, Carter DR, Marcus R. Clinical and anthropometric correlates of bone mineral acquisition in healthy adolescent girls. J Clin Endocrinol Metab 1991;73(6):1332–1339.

47. Bonjour JP, Theintz G, Buchs B, Slosman D, Rizzoli R. Critical years and stages of puberty for spinal and femoral bone mass accumulation during adolescence. J Clin Endocrinol Metab 1991;73(3):555–563.

48. Theintz G, Buchs B, Rizzoli R, Slosman D, Clavien H, Sizonenko PC, et al. Longitudinal monitoring of bone mass accumulation in healthy adolescents: evidence for a marked reduction after 16 years of age at the levels of lumbar spine and femoral neck in female subjects. J Clin Endocrinol Metab 1992;75(4):1060–1065.

49. Hartman D, Crisp A, Rooney B, Rackow C, Atkinson R, Patel S. Bone density of women who

have recovered from anorexia nervosa. Int J Eat Disord 2000;28(1):107–112.

50. Enzmann DR, Lane B. Cranial computed tomography findings in anorexia nervosa. J Comput Assist Tomogr 1977;1(4):410–414.

51. Nussbaum M, Shenker IR, Marc J, Klein M. Cerebral atrophy in anorexia nervosa. J Pediatr 1980;96(5): 867–869.

52. Golden NH, Ashtari M, Kohn MR, Patel M, Jacobson MS, Fletcher A, et al. Reversibility of cerebral ventricular enlargement in anorexia nervosa, demonstrated by quantitative magnetic resonance imaging. J Pediatr 1996;128(2):296–301.

53. Katzman DK, Lambe EK, Mikulis DJ, Ridgley JN, Goldbloom DS, Zipursky RB. Cerebral gray matter and white matter volume deficits in adolescent girls with anorexia nervosa. J Pediatr 1996;129(6): 794–803.

54. Gordon I, Lask B, Bryant-Waugh R, Christie D, Timimi S. Childhood-onset anorexia nervosa: towards identifying a biological substrate. Int J Eat Disord 1997;22(2):159–165.

55. Kingston K, Szmukler G, Andrewes D, Tress B, Desmond P. Neuropsychological and structural brain changes in anorexia nervosa before and after refeeding. Psychol Med 1996;26(1):15–28.

56. Katzman DK, Zipursky RB, Lambe EK, Mikulis DJ. A longitudinal magnetic resonance imaging study of brain changes in adolescents with anorexia nervosa. Arch Pediatr Adolesc Med 1997;151(8):793–797.

57. American Academy of Pediatrics Policy Statement. Identifying and treating eating disorders. Pediatrics 2003;111(1):204–211.

58. Golden NH, Katzman DK, Kreipe RE, Stevens SL, Sawyer SM, Rees J, et al. Eating disorders in adolescents: position paper of the Society for Adolescent Medicine. J Adolesc Health 2003;33(6):496–503.

59. Eisler I, Dare C, Hodes M, Russell G, Dodge E, le Grange D. Family therapy for adolescent anorexia nervosa: the results of a controlled comparison of two family interventions. J Child Psychol Psychiatry 2000;41(6):727–736.

60. Geist R, Heinmaa M, Stephens D, Davis R, Katzman DK. Comparison of family therapy and family group psychoeducation in adolescents with anorexia nervosa. Can J Psychiatry 2000;45(2): 173–178.

61. Robin AL, Siegel PT, Moye AW, Gilroy M, Dennis AB, Sikand A. A controlled comparison of family versus individual therapy for adolescents with anorexia nervosa. J Am Acad Child Adolesc Psychiatry 1999; 38(12):1482–1489.

62. Russell GF, Szmukler GI, Dare C, Eisler I. An evaluation of family therapy in anorexia nervosa and bulimia nervosa. Arch Gen Psychiatry 1987;44(12): 1047–1056.

63. Kaye WH, Nagata T, Weltzin TE, Hsu LK, Sokol MS, McConaha C, et al. Double-blind placebo-controlled administration of fluoxetine in restricting- and restricting-purging-type anorexia nervosa. Biol Psychiatry 2001;49(7):644–652.

64. Agras WS, Walsh T, Fairburn CG, Wilson GT, Kraemer HC. A multicenter comparison of cognitive-behavioral therapy and interpersonal psychotherapy for bulimia nervosa. Arch Gen Psychiatry 2000;57(5):459–466.

65. Fairburn C. A cognitive behavioral approach to the treatment of bulimia. Psychol Med 1981;11(4): 707–711.

66. Fluoxetine Bulimia Nervosa Collaborative Study Group. Fluoxetine in the treatment of bulimia nervosa. A multicenter, placebo-controlled, double-blind trial. Arch Gen Psychiatry 1992;49(2): 139–147.

67. Walsh BT, Wilson GT, Loeb KL, Devlin MJ, Pike KM, Roose SP, et al. Medication and psychotherapy in the treatment of bulimia nervosa. Am J Psychiatry 1997;154(4):523–531.

68. Solanto MV, Jacobson MS, Heller L, Golden NH, Hertz S. Rate of weight gain of inpatients with anorexia nervosa under two behavioral contracts. Pediatrics 1994;93(6 Pt 1):989–991.

69. Solomon SM, Kirby DF. The refeeding syndrome: a review. JPEN J Parenter Enteral Nutr 1990;14(1): 90–97.

70. Kohn MR, Golden NH, Shenker IR. Cardiac arrest and delirium: presentations of the refeeding syndrome in severely malnourished adolescents with anorexia nervosa. J Adolesc Health 1998;22(3):239–243.

71. Ornstein RM, Golden NH, Jacobson MS, Shenker IR. Hypophosphatemia during nutritional rehabilitation in anorexia nervosa: implications for refeeding and monitoring. J Adolesc Health 2003;32(1):83–88.

72. Rome ES, Ammerman S. Medical complications of eating disorders: an update. J Adolesc Health 2003; 33(6):418–426.

73. Glastre C, Braillon P, David L, Cochat P, Meunier PJ, Delmas PD. Measurement of bone mineral content of the lumbar spine by dual energy x-ray absorptiometry in normal children: correlations with growth parameters. J Clin Endocrinol Metab 1990;70(5): 1330–1333.

74. Gordon CM, Goodman E, Emans SJ, Grace E, Becker KA, Rosen CJ, et al. Physiologic regulators of

bone turnover in young women with anorexia nervosa. J Pediatr 2002;141(1):64–70.

75. Henderson NK, Price RI, Cole JH, Gutteridge DH, Bhagat CI. Bone density in young women is associated with body weight and muscle strength but not dietary intakes. J Bone Miner Res 1995;10(3): 384–393.

76. Soyka LA, Misra M, Frenchman A, Miller KK, Grinspoon S, Schoenfeld DA, et al. Abnormal bone mineral accrual in adolescent girls with anorexia nervosa. J Clin Endocrinol Metab 2002;87(9):4177–4185.

77. Bachrach LK, Katzman DK, Litt IF, Guido D, Marcus R. Recovery from osteopenia in adolescent girls with anorexia nervosa. J Clin Endocrinol Metab 1991;72(3):602–606.

78. Rigotti NA, Neer RM, Skates SJ, Herzog DB, Nussbaum SR. The clinical course of osteoporosis in anorexia nervosa: a longitudinal study of cortical bone mass. JAMA 1991;265(9):1133–1138.

79. Cadogan J, Eastell R, Jones N, Barker ME. Milk intake and bone mineral acquisition in adolescent girls: randomised, controlled intervention trial. Br Med J 1997;315(7118):1255–1260.

80. Johnston CC, Jr, Miller JZ, Slemenda CW, Reister TK, Hui S, Christian JC, et al. Calcium supplementation and increases in bone mineral density in children. N Engl J Med 1992;327(2):82–87.

81. Lloyd T, Andon MB, Rollings N, Martel JK, Landis JR, Demers LM, et al. Calcium supplementation and bone mineral density in adolescent girls. JAMA 1993;270(7):841–844.

82. McKay HA, Petit MA, Schutz RW, Prior JC, Barr SI, Khan KM. Augmented trochanteric bone mineral density after modified physical education classes: a randomized school-based exercise intervention study in prepubescent and early pubescent children. J Pediatr 2000;136(2):156–162.

83. Snow-Harter C, Bouxsein ML, Lewis BT, Carter DR, Marcus R. Effects of resistance and endurance exercise on bone mineral status of young women: a randomized exercise intervention trial. J Bone Miner Res 1992;7(7):761–769.

84. Robinson E, Bachrach LK, Katzman DK. Use of hormone replacement therapy to reduce the risk of osteopenia in adolescent girls with anorexia nervosa. J Adolesc Health 2000;26(5):343–348.

85. Klibanski A, Biller BM, Schoenfeld DA, Herzog DB, Saxe VC. The effects of estrogen administration on trabecular bone loss in young women with anorexia nervosa. J Clin Endocrinol Metab 1995;80(3): 898–904.

86. Gordon CM, Grace E, Emans SJ, Feldman HA, Goodman E, Becker KA, et al. Effects of oral dehydroepiandrosterone on bone density in young women with anorexia nervosa: a randomized trial. J Clin Endocrinol Metab 2002;87(11):4935–4941.

87. Grinspoon S, Thomas L, Miller K, Herzog D, Klibanski A. Effects of recombinant human IGF-I and oral contraceptive administration on bone density in anorexia nervosa. J Clin Endocrinol Metab 2002; 87(6):2883–2891.

31

OBESITY IN THE ADOLESCENT

John D. Rowlett

...Obesity is one of the commonest ailments to which the flesh is heir, and is of importance to the individual in proportion to its degree and its association with other diseases

... (JH Means, *Cecil's Textbook of Medicine*, 1927).

EPIDEMIOLOGY

Obesity and overweight have become two of the most important and preventable health conditions affecting youths and adults. There are no universal definitions for overweight and obesity. Numerous measures of body fat have been proposed and tested; for the practicing clinician, the body mass index (BMI) is the most accepted and useful measure.

The "obesity epidemic" affects all age, race, gender, and socioeconomic groups. The prevalence of overweight and obesity has more than doubled in the United States in the past two decades; 16.1% of youths between the ages of 12 and 19 years are at or above the 95th percentile for BMI (based on standard growth charts with reference data from the 1970s). In subpopulations of minority and poor children, the numbers are still higher. An additional

30.9% of this group is considered "at-risk" for overweight (BMI between the 85th and 95th percentile). Even more dramatic increases in adult obesity are emerging; for example, an astounding 65.7% of U.S. adults are either overweight (BMI >85th percentile) or obese (BMI >95th percentile). Within the subgroup of adults most likely to have teenage children, one parent in three is obese (BMI >95th percentile).

ETIOLOGY

...The fundamental cause of obesity is a positive energy balance. That is, the caloric value of food absorbed is greater than the total expenditure of energy. A comparatively slight disproportion between fuel intake and combustion may, over a period of years, result in a marked grade of obesity ... The extraordinary thing is not that so many persons become obese, but rather that more do not ... The normal appetite ordinarily adjusts intake so accurately that it just meets, but does not exceed, the requirements of energy expenditure. When this adjustment loses its delicacy and eating falls under the rule of habit, obesity may develop

... (Means, 1927).

Means' eloquent description of the causes of obesity contains three critical elements. Obesity is the result of (1) too many calories consumed and/or (2) too few calories expended, and (3) obesity develops over time. In most persons, the process of becoming overweight is an insidious development. While it is possible for obesity to stem from dramatic changes in energy intake or expenditure, most persons, including children and adolescents, become overweight as a result of relatively minor imbalances in energy intake/expenditure. The first law of thermodynamics states that in an isolated system (such as in a teenager) total energy is conserved. Energy can be converted from one form to another (i.e., heat, motion, and growth); however, it cannot be created or destroyed, forming the fundamental basis for weight homeostasis. If a teenager consumes more calories than expended, the remaining calories are stored for later use. Conversely, if ongoing energy expenditure exceeds caloric intake, energy stores including short-term stores (glycogen) and long-term stores (i.e., adipose tissue, muscle) are utilized.

The "set point" theory states that much like glucose or temperature, there is a weight or "set point" that the body attempts to maintain. There may be a genetic predetermination to this set point, or it may simply be determined when a person maintains a particular weight for an extended period of time. Voluntary changes in energy intake or expenditure are counteracted by changes in satiety and metabolism to maintain the set point. Leptin, a hormone produced by fat cells in proportion to total fat mass, binds to hypothalamic nuclei that control energy expenditure and appetite. Changes in leptin levels initiate counter-regulatory hormones (i.e., insulin, thyroxine, and ghrelin) that return body weight to the set point. Elevated leptin levels, as seen in many obese patients, may lead to central receptor resistance (analogous to type II diabetes) and establish higher set points for weight and leptin levels. This makes weight loss particularly difficult unless the set point can be lowered.

While only about one-third of adult obesity is attributable to events in childhood, it is associated with significantly more long-term health risks than obesity that develops in adulthood. Three periods during childhood are particularly important to the development of obesity. The first period, prenatal, reflects endogenous intrauterine factors, including nutrients. High birth weight appears to be associated with increased risk of obesity, especially for infants of diabetic mothers. The exact mechanism(s) responsible for the effect of birth weight on obesity is unclear, but likely to involve a relationship between intrauterine nutrition and the hypothalamic set-point.

The second period, "adiposity-rebound," occurs around age 5–6 years. After a physiologic/developmental nadir, BMI begins to increase. Children who enter this rebound phase earlier are more likely to be obese as adults; higher BMI at the time of the rebound is also associated with higher adult BMI. The final period of risk for the development of obesity during childhood is adolescence; 50%–75% of overweight and obesity in adolescence will continue into adulthood. Particularly in boys, adolescence is associated with increased visceral fat deposition. Centripetal ("apple-shaped") obesity is associated with visceral fat deposition, which is associated with more physiologic complications than peripheral ("pear-shaped") obesity.

While there are many factors that contribute and modify this process, weight homeostasis remains a function of energy expenditure and energy (caloric) intake. Relatively minor changes in physical activity and diet, if sustained, have significant impact on weight homeostasis. A daily imbalance of only +50 kcal/day (equivalent to 4 oz of a sugared soft drink) or elimination of modest physical activity translates to about an annual 5-lb weight gain (1 lb = 3500 kcal). The current surge in obesity reflects adverse changes in both halves of the homeostasis equation—caloric intake is up and energy expenditure is down.

Changes in Caloric Intake

Dietary practices across the world have changed dramatically over the past century. Sustained excess caloric intake is, for the most part, a recent phenomenon. Though not yet entirely eliminated, hunger has greatly diminished as advances in production, processing, transportation, distribution, and refrigeration have increased worldwide food supply; this food, however is frequently high in extremely processed and less nutritious foods. While earlier diets revolved around a handful of staple items, modern supermarkets routinely carry more than 30,000 products (more than 12,000 new products introduced annually). Whole grains have been largely replaced by less nutritious, more lipogenic, and highly refined grains. As calorically dense foods have become abundant, portable, affordable, and widely available, total caloric intake has increased (particularly carbohydrates and less-healthy [trans] fats). Increased divorce rates, increased number of mothers entering the workforce, hectic schedules, urban sprawl, microwaves, and countless other things have greatly and often negatively changed food practices.

The emergence of the "fast food" industry closely parallels the modern obesity epidemic, and while it is not the sole cause, fast food consumption has contributed greatly to the changes in diets worldwide. More than 40% of the typical American family food budget is now spent on food away from home. This trend has adversely affected the nutritional quality of food; those substances consumed away from home by children and adolescents are typically higher in fat, particularly saturated fats, and lower in calcium and fiber. It has been estimated that if these nutriments consumed away from home had the same average nutritional content as food at home, the average American would consume almost 200 calories less per day, and would significantly decrease the intake of saturated fat while increasing dietary

calcium, fiber, and iron. Portion sizes of sugared beverages, entrees, and deserts have gone from modest to "super size." A typical adolescent meal of a hamburger, fries, and soft drink in the 1950s had about 500 calories; today's counterpart contains more than 1100 calories, and the majority of this increase is simple carbohydrates devoid of nutritional benefit (Table 31-1).

Among Caucasian or Hispanic youth in the United States, consumption of fast food more than twice per week is associated with an 86% increased risk of becoming obese compared to those who ate fast food less than once per week. Children who consumed fast food consumed more calories (187 kcal), more fat, more sugared beverages, less milk, and fewer fruits and vegetables. The fast food industry is under increasing pressure to become accountable for food practices. Most fast foods are high in energy density, trans and saturated fats, have high glycemic loads, and low fiber content. They are affordable, plentiful in abundant quantities, and taste good. Increased teen car ownership and the widespread availability, including 24-hour restaurants, have added to the long tradition of adolescents gathering at fast food restaurants. Recent changes in both menu selections and portion size are encouraging but much needs to be done to decrease the marketing of unhealthy foods to children and adolescents.

Consumption of sugar-added beverages is an increasingly recognized contributor to obesity. A single 12-oz sweetened, carbonated beverage

TABLE 31-1

FAST FOOD CHANGES*

	1954		2004	
Item	Ounces (oz)	Calories	Ounces (oz)	Calories
Burger King hamburger	2.8	202	4.3	310
McDonald's fries	2.4	210	7	610
Coca-cola	6.5	79	16	194
Total	491 calories		1114 calories	

*Assuming that everything else in an adolescent's diet and physical activity were the same and that fast food was only consumed once a week, this single change would result in a net increase of 623 calories per week, an extra 9 lb (3500 kcal/lb) per year.

contains 10 teaspoons of sugar and 150 kcal. In the past few decades, per capita consumption of sugar-sweetened beverages has increased several-fold, while average serving size has increased from 6.5 oz in the 1950s to 20 oz today; some convenience stores offer 44-oz servings with free or discounted refills. Over consumption is particularly easy when consumed in a liquid form and leads to a displacement of more nutritious caloric intake.

Milk consumption is gradually replaced by soft drinks between the 3rd and 8th grade with subsequent decrease in daily calcium intake. Phosphate in carbonated beverages (including "sugar-free") further depletes calcium stores. This is a particular problem for adolescent females as 40% of peak bone mass is accumulated during adolescence; a 5%–10% decrease in peak bone mass may translate to a 50% increased risk of hip fractures as an adult. Soft drinks also increase the risk of dental caries and enamel erosion. Revenue from vending machines has become a significant source of income for both public and private schools and provides ready access to a variety of food products, both healthy and unhealthy. A 2004 position paper by the American Academy of Pediatrics summarizes the problems associated with soft drinks (and vending machines) in schools. In short, sugared beverages should not be sold to children or adolescents during classroom hours; vending machines should offer lower-priced healthy alternatives to highly processed nutritionally depleted snacks.

Caloric Expenditure

The past century has seen the development of countless labor saving devices that have slowly and progressively decreased the amount of physical activity required for essential activities such as gathering and preparing food, transportation, heating and cooling homes, and most household duties. If it can be automated, it has been, or someone is working on it (probably with a remote control). Average caloric expenditure has decreased dramatically. As a mode of transportation, society walks less. Neighborhoods designed without sidewalks or safe access across major thoroughfares, increased distance to schools, heavy school backpacks, and

general safety concerns have contributed to the decline in the number of children (and adults) who walk to school, parks, or activities. Physical education (PE) classes, despite the Centers for Disease Control and Prevention's recommendation for PE of "every child, every day, every year" are poorly funded and too rarely mandated by local or state school authorities.

Although the percentage of high school students in the United States who are enrolled in PE has remained about 50%, prevalence of students reporting physical activity >20 minutes daily in PE dropped from 34% in 1991 to 21% in 1997. Recess has disappeared for many school children as curriculum demands have increased, funding (including for supervisors of playgrounds) has decreased, and safety concerns have been raised. Though the literature is mixed, many educators believe that lack of opportunities for physical activity during the school day contributes to poorer academic performance, particularly for students with disordered attention. As parents have become sedentary, there is less modeling of healthy activity behavior for children and adolescents. In addition to protecting against obesity, physical activity is an important determinant of childhood bone mineral density. As few as 10 additional minutes of vigorous physical activity per day is associated with statistically significant increases in bone density in prepubertal children.

Television viewing has been clearly demonstrated by various researchers to be a significant risk factor for obesity. Multiple factors associated with television viewing habits place children and adolescents (and adults) at increased risk for overweight and obesity. First, it is a sedentary activity; teens have been shown to burn more calories while sleeping than while watching television. By the time they graduate from high school, American adolescents have spent more time watching television and playing video games (15,000 hours) than in school (12,000 hours) or any other activity besides sleeping.

Despite recommendations to limit television to no more than 2 hours per day (and none during the school week), more than 33% of children watch more than 5 hours of television daily. Nearly one-third of children aged 2–7 years and two-thirds of those aged 8–18 years have a television set in their bedrooms; this is particularly a problem for students in lower income homes. Consumption of high caloric/low nutrient snacks while watching television is common; some children consume most of their meals in front of the TV. Shows watched by children and adolescents, in addition to often inappropriate content, contain heavy advertisements for fast food chains, candies, sugared beverages, and other less healthy food products. Controlled studies have demonstrated that reduced television viewing is associated with reduced weight gain and reduced prevalence of obesity. In addition to increasing the risk for obesity, high levels of television viewing by children and adolescents may be associated with violent behavior, attention disorders, and earlier initiation of high risk behaviors including cigarette smoking, alcohol consumption, and sexual activity.

GENETICS AND THE FAMILY

There is a strong genetic role in the determination of body weight; twin studies suggest that up to 67% of the variance (in a twin pair) in adiposity is genetic. Genes encoded for protein production are involved with basal metabolic rates, appetite, satiety, endocrine function, fat storage, and propensity toward diseases including type 2 diabetes. Genetics may determine whether an individual develops hyperplastic obesity (increase in the number of fat cells), hypertrophic obesity (increase in the size of individual fat cells), or a combination of both. Practical application of the increased understanding of genetics of weight homeostasis, satiety, and related items is minimal at this time. The epidemic of worldwide obesity has not been created by a change in genes, but genetic susceptibility to some complications may be manifested when persons are exposed to prolonged unhealthy diets (particularly simple carbohydrates). The marked increase in type 2 diabetes among native Americans and Hispanics is multifactorial in origin, but there is probably a genetic predisposition within these populations.

Parental obesity is highly predictive of obesity in their offspring. If both parents are obese, about 70% of their children will be obese. The prevalence of obesity is less than 50% if only one parent is obese, and less than 10% if neither is obese. Earlier studies suggest that about 20% of obesity at the age of 4 years will persist into adulthood; this number rises to about 80% persistence into adulthood for obese adolescents. The effect of the overall increase in prevalence of obesity on these numbers is unknown; it is likely to increase (particularly for younger children) the persistence of obesity into adulthood.

Economics

Americans spend an excess of 50 billion dollars per year on weight loss products (including foods) and services. Recent estimates suggest that obesity and related morbidity may be responsible for nearly 7% (117 billion dollars) of all healthcare costs in the United States; only smoking contributes more to mortality than obesity. Hospital charges for conditions attributable to pediatric obesity (i.e., sleep apnea, type II diabetes, gallbladder disease) have tripled over the past two decades and now exceed 125 million/year. Future charges related to obesity, will be astronomical; some estimate that as many as one in three children (one in two Latinos) will eventually develop diabetes.

MEDICAL CONDITIONS ASSOCIATED WITH OBESITY

...To the community, it (obesity) is of importance in that it may per se decrease human efficiency and shorten human life

... (Means, 1927).

Obesity is associated with numerous medical problems in childhood and adolescence (Table 31-2). Overweight and obesity are important and modifiable risk factors for many causes of adult morbidity and mortality. About 60% of overweight children and adolescents have at least one additional risk factor for cardiovascular disease (i.e., hypertension, hyperinsulinemia, and hyperlipidemia), more than 25% have two or more. Age-adjusted BMI and

TABLE 31-2

MEDICAL COMPLICATIONS ASSOCIATED WITH ADOLESCENT OVERWEIGHT/OBESITY

Short-term
Insulin resistance
Type II diabetes
Hyperlipidemia
Sleep apnea
Obesity-related hypoventilation
Fatty liver/nonalcoholic steato-hepatitis (NASH)
Cholelithiasis
Polycystic ovary disease
Advanced physical maturation (for age)
Eating disorders
Depression
Increased left ventricular mass
Pseudotumor cerebri
Blount's disease (tibia vara)
Slipped capital femoral epiphysis
Sedentary lifestyle

Long-term
Metabolic syndrome
Increased risk of cancers
   Breast, colon, prostate, and uterine
Cholecystitis
Depression
Eating disorders
Gastroesophageal reflux disease
Osteoarthritis
Cardiac disease
   Hypertension
   Coronary artery disease
   Cardiomyopathy
   Premature death

waist circumference values are predictive of the presence or absence of ≥3 age-adjusted risk factors (i.e., low high-density lipoprotein cholesterol, high low-density lipoprotein cholesterol, elevated triglycerides, elevated glucose, hyperinsulinemia, and hypertension). Elevated high-density lipoprotein-cholesterol (HDL-C) and C-reactive protein are the strongest predictors of peripheral arterial disease. Research suggests that increased adult carotid intimate-media thickness is associated with the persistence of childhood obesity into adulthood; this is not true for children who became obese as adults or for overweight children who were not obese adults.

Obesity is associated with earlier menarche; women who undergo early menarche are more likely to be obese adults (this may simply be a continuation of childhood obesity), polycystic ovary syndrome (Chap. 28), and type II diabetes. Obesity-related pulmonary problems include sleep apnea, obesity hypoventilation syndrome, and reactive airway disease. Overweight is associated with an increased risk of new onset asthma, particularly in boys and nonallergic children. Overweight/obese children with asthma have more exacerbations, medication use, and emergency room visits than nonobese children with asthma. Increasing BMI is associated with increased incidence of iron deficiency anemia. For children with low birth weights, increased weight gain after 2 years of age may also impart increased risk for diabetes and the metabolic syndrome.

THE METABOLIC SYNDROME

The metabolic syndrome (formerly "Syndrome X") has been shown in adults to impart significant risk for premature coronary artery disease and type II diabetes. Criteria for the metabolic syndrome are listed in Table 31-3. Initial estimates of prevalence included 4% of all adolescents, 6.8% of overweight adolescents, and nearly 30% of obese adolescents.

TABLE 31-3

CRITERIA FOR METABOLIC SYNDROME

Metabolic syndrome is defined as having at least three of the following:
- Systolic or diastolic blood pressure above the 95th percentile
- Serum HDL level below the 5th percentile
- Serum triglyceride level above the 95th percentile
- Impaired glucose tolerance
- BMI above the 97th percentile

Recent (2004) data suggest that the prevalence of the metabolic syndrome increases linearly with increasing BMI and approaches 50% in severely obese adolescents. Each of the five components of metabolic syndrome has been shown to increase with increasing obesity, independent of race, age, and pubertal status. C-reactive protein and interleukin 6 levels (biomarkers for inflammation and predictive of coronary artery disease in obese adults) increase with increasing obesity, while adiponectin levels (markers of insulin sensitivity and potentially important in the prevention of atheromatous plaques) decrease. Metabolic syndrome is associated with the development of nonalcoholic fatty liver disease.

Insulin resistance results in consumed calories being shunted more directly to adipose tissue. The resulting lack of energy contributes to a further sedentary lifestyle and accelerated weight gain. Insulin resistance leads to hyperinsulinemia, which contributes to both hypertension (increased sodium reabsorption in the renal tubule leading to increased intravascular volume; vascular overactivity due to sympathetic activation) and dyslipidemia. Acanthosis nigricans (velvety hyperpigmented skin on the neck and/or axillae) may be present in some individuals with insulin resistance, though it is neither a sensitive nor a specific physical finding.

Persons with metabolic syndrome need aggressive therapy to address all aspects of the disorder. In addition to lifestyle modification including a low fat diet and increased exercise, treatment may include antihypertensive agents, lipid-lowering drugs (statins), and metformin. Metformin decreases hepatic glucose production, increases the calories available for work versus storage, and may decrease insulin resistance and hyperinsulinemia. Metformin has been shown to prevent or delay diabetes in selected individuals.

Psychologic Complications

There are many psychologic/social consequences of obesity and overweight in children and adolescents. Media images and the actions of parents (particularly the father) may compound the cultural bias toward thinness that begins in early childhood. Obesity can be viewed as a social liability. Overweight children and adolescents are less popular than normal weight peers; also, they are more likely to be socially isolated and peripheral to social networks found in normal weight adolescents. Others may view obese persons as unattractive, lazy, unmotivated, and unable to demonstrate self-control. The recent increase in obesity has not changed the bias against heavier children/adolescents. Overweight and obese children and adolescents are more likely to be victims and perpetrators of bullying behaviors. Data are mixed regarding prevalence of depression and anxiety among obese and overweight youths. As adults, females who were overweight as adolescents are less likely to become married, are less educated, and have higher rates of poverty.

Decision to Treat

Adolescents at risk for overweight (BMI 85th – 95th percentile) should be evaluated annually. If significant risk factors for obesity and related complications are present, additional testing is indicated. Overweight teens (BMI >95th percentile) should be evaluated and referred for treatment. Adolescents may be reluctant to undergo treatment for many reasons including labeling by peers, fear of weight cycling, side effects of treatment plans, or economic reasons. Factors, which may encourage participation in treatment programs, include the presence of comorbidities (physical, medical, and social), greater magnitude or duration of overweight, older patients, and those with more supportive families or those whose family members have suffered complications of obesity.

Interventions should begin early and be gradual. Both the patient and the family must be ready to change detrimental behaviors. Education of patient and family regarding the complications of obesity is helpful; clinicians should emphasize permanent changes to promote healthy lifestyles over short-term fixes. Visits should be frequent, positive, and utilize other professionals (i.e., psychologists, trainers, nutritionists, educators, and/or social workers).

OFFICE EVALUATION OF THE OVERWEIGHT OR OBESE ADOLESCENT

Overweight or obese adolescents should have a thorough physical examination by a practitioner experienced in the care of adolescents. This should be done in a friendly, non-threatening manner with attention given to the unique psychologic needs of adolescents. Information regarding infant and childhood feeding practices may be of interest in the prevention of childhood obesity and overweight on the national level; however, minimal time should be focused on this element with adolescents.

Review of growth curves when available is useful in determining both the duration of overweight/obesity and any significant changes in weight patterns. Accurate weights may be obtained in a simple gown; some morbidly obese adolescents may require scales not typically found in pediatric offices; and teens may find this embarrassing. Accurate blood pressure readings require proper cuff placement. Additional measurements may include waist-hip ratio and waist circumference; neck circumference should be measured on morbidly obese teens as well as those suspected of having sleep apnea. All data should be plotted on current growth charts, which include BMI age-specific norms. These are available at *www.cdc.gov/growthcharts/* (accessed April, 2005).

Suggested laboratory evaluations for the obese or overweight adolescent are summarized in Table 31-4. Additional testing may be indicated by specific findings of the history or physical examination. Minimum testing should include a fasting glucose, complete blood count, insulin level, and complete lipid profile.

Management

> . . .The treatment of simple or exogenous obesity lies in the correction of the disproportion between intake and expenditure of energy . . . to that end, we may restrict food consumption and increase bodily activity.
>
> . . . (Means, 1927).

TABLE 31-4

SUGGESTED LABORATORY TESTING FOR THE OBESE/OVERWEIGHT ADOLESCENT

All patients
Fasting lipid profile
If abnormal, repeat after 6–12 weeks of intervention
Fasting glucose
Insulin level
Complete blood cell count
Serum electrolytes including liver function tests
If clinically indicated by history or physical examination
Thyroid stimulating hormone
Rarely indicated if child is of average or taller height
Pregnancy test
Urinalysis
A.M. cortisol level
Chromosome studies (only if genetic syndrome suspected—Chap. 21)

Successful weight management programs combine elements of behavioral change, nutritional change, and increased physical activity. Additional therapies, including pharmacologic agents and surgery, may have a role for some adolescents. The primary goal is the initiation of changes in food and activity behaviors. Secondary goals include weight stabilization (lack of further weight gain) and when appropriate, weight loss. For younger adolescents, simply stopping the weight gain and allowing them to "grow into the weight" may be all that is necessary. In most cases, weight loss goals should be no more than 1 or 2 lb per month. Long-term goals, such as a BMI >85th percentile, may not be initially appropriate. Improvement in comorbidities is generally evident with weight loss of 7%–10% of starting weight. Relapses are common and should be expected.

Behavioral Therapy

Changing behaviors related to food are essential to successful weight loss programs. Long-term weight loss maintenance is linked to behavioral changes more than specific dietary changes. Focus areas should include developing awareness of current eating and activity behaviors (including parents) and identifying as well as modifying problem behaviors by small, gradual changes. Essential to this is accurate reporting of food intake; overweight individuals tend to greatly under-report consumption. Behavioral goals should be simple and explicit (e.g., instead of "walk more," state "walk for 30 minutes 3 times a week"). Only one item should be changed at a time. Adolescents should be counseled on handling special situations such as meals away from home, restaurants, and holidays. Contracts may be useful.

Nutrition Therapy

Essential to all successful diets is an understanding of the types and quantities of foods to be consumed. Most adolescents overeat predictably—excessive portion size and excessive carbohydrates. Simple changes, such as switching from sugared to sugar-free beverages or not ordering "super-size" fries, may result in marked improvement. For most youths, gradual, relatively minor changes are helpful (Table 31-5). Limiting fast foods, including those prepared at home, is a good start.

> Dining with one's friends and beloved family is certainly one of life's primal and most innocent delights, one that is both soul-satisfying and eternal. In spite of food fads, fitness programs, and health concerns, we must never lose sight of a beautifully conceived meal.
>
> (Julia Child, 1989)

The adolescent and family members should be involved in meal planning, shopping, and when possible, meal preparation. Numerous diet plans are available for adolescents to consider. Most plans work to some degree, but the effect on lipid profiles, weight loss, and long-term success vary greatly. Many effective diets are simply difficult to maintain for adolescents or adults and are, therefore, of limited benefit. The long-standing recommendation of a diet high in carbohydrates and low in fats may not be as

TABLE 31-5

QUICK FACTS FOR TEENS AND DIETS

1. Avoid drastic changes and fads
2. Do not focus on diet and weight loss
3. Eat when you are hungry, not out of habit
4. Do not eat in front of the television, computer, while playing video games, and so forth.
5. Whenever possible, eat meals as a family
6. Limit sugared beverages
   a. Avoid sugared soft drinks
   b. Limit juice and related products
7. Limit prepared products including those
   a. High in unhealthy fats
   b. High in caloric density
8. Limit portion sizes
9. Limit fast food, never "super-size"
10. Eat breakfast
11. Limit snacks
12. "Bank" calories for special events by planning ahead

effective as previously thought. Excessive carbohydrates, particularly those with a high glycemic index (e.g., potatoes, rice, white flour) may contribute to the metabolic syndrome, increased insulin levels, and to some degree, hunger. More than 10% of youths skip breakfast; girls who skip breakfast consume significantly less calcium. Skipping breakfast is more likely to result in weight gain than weight loss. Breakfast foods with low-glycemic indices are preferred as they are more protective against mid-morning hunger than simple carbohydrates.

The "stoplight" diet promotes weight stabilization and loss in children and adolescents. It is simple, allows a variety of foods based on lipogenic/glycemic potential, and is maintainable. Persons may consume unlimited quantities of "green-light" foods (i.e., fresh fruits, nonstarchy vegetables, salads, low-fat dressing, fat-free dairy products, broiled/baked skinless chicken, and fish), may have cautious quantities of "yellow-light" foods (i.e., starchy vegetables such as peas, corn, potatoes, and rice, breads, pasta), and should seek to limit or completely avoid "red-light" foods (i.e., cakes, candies, concentrated sugars, most fast foods, juice, and pizza).

Diets promoting lower carbohydrate intake, particularly of those with high glycemic indices, are increasingly popular. Many varieties of these (e.g., Atkins, South Beach, The Carbohydrate Addict's Diet) are available; significant differences exist between specific low-carbohydrate diets, particularly regarding the consumption of types (saturated/unsaturated) and quantities of fat. Initial studies have shown these diets to be safe and effective in teens; long-term data, including compliance and potential increased cancer risks, are not available.

Very low calorie diets (VLCD) or protein modified fasts (PMF) should be considered for the treatment of morbidly obese adolescents with major complications of obesity (i.e., sleep apnea, pseudotumor cerebri, Blount's disease, and slipped capital femoral epiphysis). Youths must demonstrate weight maintenance (lack of further weight gain) prior to initiation of the PMF; those who cannot maintain weight are more likely to relapse. Extensive baseline and ongoing laboratory evaluation as well as patient and family counseling are necessary. Such diets should only be done under the supervision of highly experienced adolescent weight loss specialists.

Perhaps the best diet is no particular diet, just better nutritional habits. The presence of a parent at the evening meal is associated with increased intake of fruits, vegetables, and dairy foods along with decreased incidence of skipping breakfast. Parental control over eating behavior is not associated with obesity, and in fact may be protective against overweight. Preoccupation with diets, particularly for adolescent girls, may actually promote weight gain. Frequent dieting, including semistarvation diets, may lead to "yo-yo" (up and down) weights, guilt, binge eating, and frequent relapses.

Physical Activity

Increasing physical activity is central to effective weight loss/maintenance programs. In addition to increasing caloric expenditure, physical activity helps build lean muscle, strengthens bones, and reduces body fat. Physical activity may decrease anxiety and stress and increase self-esteem. Exercise improves blood pressure and cholesterol levels, reduces the risk of chronic diseases, and may be protective against some forms of cancer (i.e., breast, colon). Thirty minutes of sustained physical activity daily improves insulin resistance, raises metabolic rates, and may decrease or eliminate the need for oral diabetes agents and/or insulin. Programs should be entered into gradually, with slow increases in both duration and intensity of exercise. They do not have to be fancy, walking around the neighborhood is as effective as walking around a track. Participation in active sports (e.g., soccer) provides exercise and peer interaction.

"Verb, it's what you do!" is a multimedia campaign from the CDC aimed at promoting physical activity by encouraging people to spend less time in sedentary activities, such as watching television, playing video games, or using the computer. This program stresses simply doing something active. Simple solutions include taking the stairs when possible, walking to school or activities, parking cars further from destinations, and family walks. Inexpensive pedometers measure steps taken; the CDC suggests that everyone gets at least 10,000 steps per day. School-based interventions in PE classes have been effective in decreasing sedentary behavior (but not weight) in adolescent females. Persons who increase leisure time physical activity (LTPA) during adolescence have a lower risk of adult obesity. If possible, adolescents should get a minimum of 30–45 minutes of sustained physical activity at least five times per week. The intensity of physical activity is more important in lowering low density lipoprotein-cholesterol (LDL-C) in young women than the total calories expended on physical activity.

Pharmacologic Treatment

Pharmacologic agents in conjunction with lifestyle changes have been shown to be effective in weight reduction in adult populations. Though numerous medications have been used to facilitate weight loss, only two have current Food and Drug Administration (FDA) approval for long-term use in adults; only orlistat (Xenical) is currently approved in persons under the age of 18 years.

Sibutramine (Meridia) is a centrally acting agent that decreases appetite through inhibition of the synaptic reuptake of serotonin, norepinephrine, and dopamine. Randomized, double-blind, placebo-controlled studies in adults have shown a dose-dependent weight loss from 5% to 10% of initial body weight. With continued use, 80% of this weight loss was maintained for 2 years. Though not FDA approved for use in persons under the age of 18 years, published clinical trials have demonstrated the effectiveness of sibutramine in addition to behavioral therapy in promoting weight loss and controlling hunger in overweight and obese adolescents. The typical starting dose of sibutramine is 10 mg once a day. Side effects include dry mouth, insomnia, anxiety, headache, asthenia, depression, nausea, and constipation. Further, sibutramine use is associated with a small increase in pulse rate and blood pressure and may be contraindicated in selected subjects with heart disease. Sibutramine cannot be given with selective serotonin reuptake inhibitors or monoamine oxidase inhibitors.

In 2003, the FDA approved the use of orlistat for weight loss in adolescents 12–16 years of age. Orlistat is an inhibitor of pancreatic lipase and blocks absorption of dietary fat by about 30%. In addition to weight loss, the majority of which is maintained at 2 years, adults taking orlistat have demonstrated improvement in insulin sensitivity, glucose control, blood pressure, and lipid levels. Clinical trials in adolescents demonstrate that orlistat is effective in promoting weight loss in obese adolescents. Separate studies have demonstrated no adverse effects on selected macro and micronutrients. Due to its mechanism of action, orlistat is of little use in persons with minimal fat intake. Typical dosage of orlistat is 120 mg with meals. Principal side effects include steatorrhea, oily discharge, and an increased frequency and urgency of bowel movements; these tend to improve over time and with reduction of dietary fat as a part of the overall weight loss strategy. Because of the unpredictable nature of fat-soluble vitamin (A, D, E, and K) deficiency, a daily multivitamin is recommended. Orlistat is contraindicated in pregnant or lactating women and in persons with malabsorption syndromes.

Numerous medications are being studied that may have a role in promoting or maintaining weight loss. Some (e.g., metformin, bupropion,

and topiramate) are FDA approved for other indications and are being actively studied for potential efficacy in obesity treatment in children and adolescents. Metformin, an oral biguanide approved for use in type II diabetes since 1995, decreases hepatic gluconeogenesis and appears to improve cell membrane transport of glucose in skeletal muscle and adipose tissue (Chap. 15). In addition to improving hyperglycemia and lowering insulin levels, metformin may decrease weight gain or promote weight loss in adults with type II diabetes. Metformin induces modest weight loss in nondiabetic adult subjects. Limited studies in children and adolescents have been encouraging; randomized controlled trials of metformin in obese adolescents with hyperinsulinemia (metabolic syndrome) are ongoing. Typical starting doses are 500 mg twice a day; side effects, which tend to decrease over time, include nausea, diarrhea, bloating, and flatulence. Metformin use in adults has been associated with rare but life-threatening lactic acidosis and should therefore not be used in persons with renal insufficiency, congestive heart disease, liver disease, or hypoxia. Metformin should be withheld from any critically ill patient.

Leptin, a neuropeptide produced predominantly by adipose tissue, mediates the neuroendocrine response to food deprivation through a complex series of positive and negative feedback at multiple sites, including the arcuate nucleus of the hypothalamus. Leptin deficient mice and humans are hyperphagic and have an apparent inability to achieve satiety leading to severe obesity. Replacement of leptin in genetically leptin deficient mice and humans results in marked reduction in food intake and promotes weight loss. Most obese humans, however, have normal or supranormal leptin levels, which correlate closely with total body adiposity. Despite elevated leptin levels, obese individuals remain hyperphagic; the role of leptin resistance in such persons is unclear. Limited data on recombinant leptin supplementation in leptin sufficient humans have shown minimal efficacy; the long-term role of leptin treatment in obese persons without mutations in the leptin gene is unclear.

Among the additional agents being studied for potential use in obesity treatment in humans include bupropion (approved for treatment of depression), topiramate (approved antiepileptic medication), ciliary neurotrophic factor, neuropeptide Y, cholecystokinin, synthetic β-3 agonists, glucagon-like peptide-1, and the somatostatin receptor agonist octreotide.

Numerous over-the-counter medications have claimed to promote weight loss. The clinical evidence for such claims is largely absent from the peer-reviewed literature; as such no recommendations can be supported for the use of herbal products, including chromium picolinate, *Garcinia cambogia*, and chitosan. The FDA banned over-the-counter ephedrine containing compounds in 2004 after numerous reported complications including death. One herbal compound, *Ma huang*, is rich in ephedra alkaloids and is especially dangerous. Clinicians should counsel patients against using any weight loss agent that has not been proved efficacious in peer-reviewed, controlled clinical trials.

Bariatric Surgery

Surgical intervention to treat obesity, available for several decades, has now become a more common procedure. When performed on properly screened persons by experienced surgeons as a part of a multidisciplinary team approach, the procedures are both effective and generally safe. Because of widespread successful surgical treatment of obese adults, there is increasing interest in surgical treatment for morbidly obese adolescents who have failed traditional therapy.

Bariatric surgery has been shown to improve both serious (i.e., type II diabetes mellitus, sleep apnea) and less serious (i.e., hypertension, dyslipidemia, gastroesophageal reflux, and arthropathies) obesity-related conditions. Bariatric surgery is not indicated for persons with a medically correctable cause of obesity (i.e., hypothyroidism), substance abuse, current lactation, pregnancy (or planned pregnancy in the next 2 years), and psychosocial situations that would limit the patient and/or parent's ability to understand or comply with the long-term dietary and medical regimens that are necessary.

Three principal operations are currently offered by bariatric surgeons, vertical-banded gastroplasty (VBGP), adjustable gastric banding (AGB), and roux-en-y gastric bypass (RYGBP). Current practice favors the RYGBP or the AGB in adolescents. All have been shown to be successful in promoting varying degrees of weight loss and decreasing comorbid conditions. Each involves some elements of gastric reduction/restriction and is associated with different short- and long-term complications.

RYGBP is the most common bariatric procedure performed on adults; this procedure is increasingly performed laparoscopically. The stomach is divided to create a small (30 mL) pouch into which a segment of jejunum from below the ligament of Treitz is inserted. The proximal portion of jejunum, which drains the duodenum and remaining stomach, is then reanastomosed 50–75 cm distal to the gastrojejunostomy. In adults, weight loss is rapid and nearly 80% of cases of type II diabetes resolve. Data from adult populations suggest that long-term weight reduction and improvement in overall quality of life is greater in those patients who underwent RYGBP than those who had restrictive procedures. RYGBP has been shown to induce greater and longer weight loss, particularly in those patients previously "addicted" to carbohydrates. Early postoperative complications include wound dehiscence, staple line leaks, thrombophlebitis, pulmonary embolus, small bowel obstruction, and subhepatic abscess. Late complications of RYGBP include ulcers, incisional hernia, volvulus, small bowel obstruction, cholelithiasis, nutritional deficiencies (especially iron, calcium, and vitamin B_{12}), and stomal stenosis. Limited published trials of RYGBP in adolescents show similar efficacy and complications to adult studies.

AGB is the most recently available surgical procedure for weight loss. An adjustable silicone band is placed laparoscopically around the proximal stomach just below the gastroesophageal junction. A peripheral reservoir allows the injection of saline, which adjusts the band. The AGB is attractive as it is minimally invasive, adjustable, and has less adverse nutritional consequences compared to the RYGBP. As it does not significantly alter the esophagogastric anatomy, it is theoretically reversible. Adult data suggest that AGB is not as effective as RYGBP in inducing weight loss. Potential complications related to the device include failure due to product age, leakage, malposition, malfunction or slippage, foreign body related infection, and erosion of the band into the stomach or esophagus. The AGB device has not been approved by the FDA for use in persons under the age of 18 years.

The VBGP involves the creation of a small upper gastric pouch, which directly communicates with the rest of the stomach through a small outlet that is created. This is typically done laparoscopically and may be complicated by severe gastroesophageal reflux. It has become the least commonly performed operation in adolescents.

It is recommended that weight-loss surgery for adolescents should be performed only by experienced bariatric surgeons practicing at major medical centers, in conjunction with experts in adolescent medicine (including adolescent obesity), psychology, and nutrition. Additional expertise in adolescent gastroenterology, pulmonology, cardiology, endocrinology, and other specialties may be necessary. Until such time when there are long-term data demonstrating prolonged safety and efficacy of these procedures in adolescents, the procedure should only be done in highly selected patients. Adolescents to be considered for bariatric surgery must have failed to show adequate weight loss progress after a minimum of 6 months in a supervised program under the ongoing care of their primary physician. They and their parent(s)/guardian(s) must have the psychologic and decision-making capacity, necessary to understand the short- and long-term risks and commitments (including nutritional and dietary requirements, need for lifelong medical surveillance) of the proposed procedure. Adolescents must be at or near physiologic maturity (>95% of projected adult stature, bone age radiograph of wrist/hand may be helpful); females should not be lactating or considering pregnancy within 2 years. Adolescents with a BMI ≥40 and major obesity-related conditions (e.g., type II diabetes, sleep apnea, cor pulmonale, pseudotumor cerebri) or adolescents with BMI ≥50 who satisfy the other criterion may be considered for bariatric surgery.

Adolescents who undergo bariatric procedures must be followed for short-term as well as long-term medical and psychosocial conditions and complications of both the surgery and the underlying condition (obesity). Ongoing counseling with a bariatric nutritionist is essential for optimum success. The primary physician should monitor additional lifestyle modifications and other adolescent health issues. If careful surveillance demonstrates the ongoing safety and efficacy of bariatric surgery in adolescents, consideration of surgery in less obese teen patients without comorbid considerations may become appropriate.

Follow-up

Regular physician visits help reinforce goals and successes, however minor, and also help formulate future goals. The clinician should be a positive force of change; encouragement and empathy are preferred to criticism, even when mistakes have been made. It is important to keep the rest of the adolescent's life (and that of the family) in focus; weight management should be integrated into the family lifestyle and not necessarily a continued item of discussion. Weight loss attempts may be associated with unhealthy caloric restriction, resulting in loss of lean body mass, and may adversely affect growth. Preoccupation with weight may lead to problem of low self-esteem or rarely, overt anorexia or bulimia nervosa. Clinicians should caution against repeated weight loss and weight gain ("yo-yo" diets), as this may actually increase weight gain. Behavioral therapy may be necessary to help in conflicts between adolescents and family or peers.

Prevention

... Prophylaxis is better than treatment. It is easier to prevent obesity than to treat it ... to that end we may restrict food consumption and increase bodily activity

... (Means, 1927).

A single action or group of actions will not accomplish the prevention of overweight and obesity. Rather, it will only be possible to slow the progression, halt, and ultimately reverse the obesity epidemic by coordinated and sustained efforts in multiple aspects of modern life, beginning even before birth. Breastfeeding for a minimum of 6 months should be encouraged not only because it may protect against obesity in later life, but also because it is simply the best nourishment for the infant, and confers many protective and essential nutrients. Television viewing should be limited in lieu of physical activity with family and friends. Interventions in elementary school have been shown to improve eating and physical activity behaviors (CATCH: Child and Adolescent Trial for Cardiovascular Health); similar programs should be integrated early into school curriculums.

Suggested Readings

Abu-Abeid S, Gavert N, Klausner JM, et al. Bariatric surgery in adolescence. *J Pediatr Surg* 2003;38:137–182.

American Academy of Pediatrics, Committee on School Health. Soft drinks in schools. *Pediatrics* 2004;113:152–154.

American Academy of Pediatrics, Committee on Nutrition. Prevention of pediatric overweight and obesity. *Pediatrics* 2003;112:424–430.

Amisola RV, Jacobson MS. Physical activity, exercise, and sedentary activity: Relationship to the causes and treatment of obesity. *Adolesc Med* 2003;14:23–35

Austin SB, Field AE, Wiecha J, et al: The impact of a school-based obesity prevention trial on disordered weight control behaviors in early adolescent girls. *Arch Pediatr Adolesc Med* 2005;159:225–230.

Barlow SE. Bariatric surgery in adolescents: For treatment failures or health care system failures? *Pediatrics* 2004;114:252–253.

Berkowitz RI, Wadden TA, Tershakovec AM, et al. Behavior therapy and sibutramine for the treatment of adolescent obesity: A randomized controlled trial. *JAMA* 2003;289:1805–1812.

Bhargava SK, Sachdev HS, Fall CH, et al. Relation of serial changes in childhood body-mass index to impaired glucose tolerance in young adulthood. *N Engl J Med* 2004;350:865–875.

Bowman SA, Gortmaker SL, Ebeling CB, et al. Effects of fast food consumption on energy intake and diet quality among children in a national household survey. *Pediatrics* 2004;113:112–118.

Centers for Disease Control. Trends in intake of energy and macronutrients—United States, 1971–2000. *MMWR* 2004;53:80–82.

Cook S, Weitzman M, Auinger P, et al. Prevalence of a metabolic syndrome phenotype in adolescents: Findings from the third National Health and Nutrition Examination Survey, 1988–1994. *Arch Pediatr Adolesc Med* 2003;157:821–827.

Copperman N, Jacobson MS. Medical nutrition therapy of overweight adolescents. *Adolesc Med* 2003;14:11–21.

Freedman DS, Dietz WH, Tang R, et al. The relation of obesity throughout life to carotid intima-media thickness in adulthood: The Bogalusa heart study. *Int J Obes Relat Metab Disord* 2004;28:159–166.

Greydanus DE, Bhave S. Obesity in adolescence. *Ind Pediatr* 2004;41(6):545–550.

Inge TH, Krbs NF, Garcia VF, et al. Bariatric surgery for severely overweight adolescents: Concerns and recommendations. *Pediatrics* 2004;114:217–223.

Institute of Medicine. Preventing Childhood Obesity: Health in the Balance. Institute of Medicine, National Academies of Science, Washington, DC: National Academies Press, January, 2005.

Jamner MS, Spruijt-Metz D, Bassin S, et al. A controlled evaluation of a school-based intervention to promote physical activity among sedentary adolescent females: Project FAB. *J Adolesc Health* 2004;34:279–289.

Jolliffe D. Extent of overweight among US children and adolescents from 1971 to 2000. *Int J Obes Relat Metab Disord* 2004;28:4–9.

Katzmarzyk PT, Srinivasan SR, Chen W, et al. Body mass index, waist circumference, and clustering of cardiovascular disease risk factors in a biracial sample of children and adolescents. *Pediatrics* 2004;114:e198–e205.

Koon M, Booth M. The worldwide epidemic of obesity in adolescents. *Adolesc Med* 2003;14:1–9.

McDuffie JR, Calis KA, Uwaifo GI, et al. Efficacy of orlistat as an adjunct to behavioral treatment in overweight African American and Caucasian adolescents with obesity-related co-morbid conditions. *J Pediatr Endocrinol Metab* 2004;17:307–319.

Nead KG, Halterman JS, Kaczorowski, et al. Overweight children and adolescents: A risk group for iron deficiency anemia. *Pediatrics* 2004;114:104–108.

Neumark-Sztainer D. Childhood and adolescent obesity: An ecologic perspective. *Pediatr Basics* 2003;101:11–22.

Neumark-Sztainer D: Addressing obesity and other weight-related problems in youth. *Arch Pediatr Adolesc Med* 2005;159:290–291.

Rodgers B. Bariatric surgery for adolescents: A view from the American Pediatric Surgical Association. *Pediatrics* 2004;114:255–256.

Schwimmer JB. Managing overweight in older children and adolescents. *Pediatr Ann* 2004;33:39–44.

Swallen KC, Reither EN, Hass SA et al: Overweight, obesity, and health-related quality of life among adolescents: The National Longitudinal Study of Adolescent Health. *Pediatrics* 2005;115:340–347.

Urrutia-Rojas X, Menchaca J, Wadley W, et al. Cardiovascular risk factors in Mexican-American children at risk for type 2 diabetes mellitus. *J Adolesc Health* 2004;34:290–299.

Weiss R, Dziura J, Buget TS, et al. Obesity and the metabolic syndrome in children and adolescents. *N Engl J Med* 2004;350:2362–2374.

V

SPORTS MEDICINE

C H A P T E R

32

SPORTS PREPARTICIPATION EVALUATION

Dilip R. Patel, Donald E. Greydanus, and Eugene F. Luckstead, Sr.

The "sports physical" should be viewed as a process that qualifies the athlete for participation in a suitable sport. A preparticipation evaluation (PPE) is generally recommended at least once a year, about 6 weeks prior to the season to allow time for correction or rehabilitation of any identified problems. The primary objective of PPE is to detect conditions that may limit participation and/or predispose to an injury. Such an evaluation is not a substitute for a comprehensive health assessment, although it may provide a setting to initiate or motivate the student athlete for such an assessment. Office-based evaluation offers the advantages of physician-athlete familiarity, continuity of care, and privacy to explore sensitive adolescent health issues and counseling. On the other hand, station-based evaluation is useful to screen a large number of athletes in a reasonable time, is relatively cost-effective, and knowledgeable as well as interested nonphysician staff (i.e., athletic trainer, nurse) can effectively participate in the process. The recommendations for PPE and eligibility for participation in sports continue to evolve as our understanding of specific problems is enhanced by new research.

HISTORY

Medical history remains the cornerstone of the PPE and should help identify more than 70% of issues of concern. Such history should be obtained both from the athlete and the parents. Several areas of history are of specific relevance in the context of PPE and key elements of PPE history are listed in Table 32-1. *Cardiovascular history* may help identify young athletes with previously unrecognized cardiac problems (Chap. 9). More than 95% of sudden deaths in the young athletes are due to cardiac causes. Although the incidence of sudden cardiac death is estimated to be 1 to 2 per 200,000 athletes per year, such episodes receive much public attention. The most common cause of sudden cardiac death in the young athlete is hypertrophic cardiomyopathy. Other causes are aberrant coronary arteries, acute myocarditis, cardiac arrhythmias, aortic valve stenosis, long QT syndrome, and Marfan syndrome (Chaps. 9 and 21). A sudden precordial blow from a baseball or a hockey puck leading to fatal ventricular arrhythmias has been reported (*commotio cordis*). In the history, one should inquire about exercise-related presyncope and syncope, chest pain, palpitations,

TABLE 32-1

KEY ELEMENTS OF PPE HISTORY

Known medical conditions (e.g., asthma, epilepsy, diabetes)

Recent febrile illness

Major surgery (especially chest, abdomen, or spine)

Medications

Nutritional supplements

Known allergies

Exercise-induced presyncope or syncope

Chest pain, palpitations, undue fatigue, heart murmur, hypertension

Personal or family history of high cholesterol or lipid disorders

Family history of sudden cardiac death before age 50

Family history of Marfan syndrome or cardiomyopathy

Details of any head injury

Neck injury or burners

Exercised-related difficulty breathing, wheezing, cough

Hearing or vision problems

Eye surgery

Musculoskeletal injuries

Any weight control practices to either gain or lose weight

Immunizations

Menstrual history

undue fatigue, seizure-like episodes, and recent febrile illness. A personal history of high blood pressure or heart murmur, and a family history of premature cardiac death (before age 50) should be elicited. Any past history of surgery for congenital heart disease and follow up should also be ascertained.

The neurologic history should include a detailed history of previous head and neck injuries (including the severity of the injury), history of loss of consciousness, and recovery time. Inquire about persistent neurologic symptoms, such as headache, confusion, memory impairment, and new onset of academic difficulties. Ask the athlete about burners, transient quadriplegia, and persistent numbness, paraesthesia, or weakness of extremities following cervical injuries.

Musculoskeletal history should include questions about previous injuries, their treatment, and if fully rehabilitated (Chap. 11). Inadequately treated past injuries may predispose the athlete to recurrent injuries. A history of chronic musculoskeletal pain should be investigated further to rule out causes other than injuries, such as an infection or a neoplasm.

A history of *heat-related illness* in the past may help identify those athletes prone to heat illness. One should ask about muscle cramps or heat syncope. These athletes may be prone to recurrent heat illness. One should inquire about any *known medical disorder* the athlete may have (e.g., asthma, epilepsy, diabetes) and ascertain if it is adequately controlled and stable. A careful history of all the *medications* that the athlete might be taking is important so that side effects can be recognized, and the team physician can ensure that the athlete is continuing the medically recommended medications for any known medical condition. A history of over-the-counter medications that the athlete may be taking should be included. For example, antihistamines may predispose the athlete to heat illness and aspirin to increased bleeding. In the female athlete, menstrual history should be obtained. Exercise-related menstrual irregularities are known to be associated with long-term complications. Athletes with a history of previous eye injuries, surgery, retinal detachment, corneal grafting, and other eye disorders should have a thorough ophthalmologic evaluation.

PHYSICAL EXAMINATION

Height and weight measurements will help identify any significant deviation from the normal growth pattern, and may point to the need for further evaluation (Chaps. 1 and 15). A finding of significant weight loss or gain should lead inquiry into possible unhealthy weight control measures. Examination of *eyes and visual acuity* will help determine risk from sports participation (Chap. 7). Note any baseline anisocoria. Athletes with best-corrected visual acuity of less than 20/40 in one eye and a normal visual acuity in the other eye are considered functionally one-eyed. These athletes and their parents should be counseled as to the risk of participation in contact/collision and racquet sports. *Cardiovascular examination* should include correct measurement of blood pressure, feel femoral pulses (for coarctation of aorta), note systolic ejection murmur that intensifies with standing or Valsalva maneuver and decrease with squatting (for hypertrophic cardiomyopathy), and aortic (decrescendo diastolic) or mitral insufficiency (holosystolic) murmurs (Chap. 9). Note any abnormal pulse, presence of a murmur, and perform screening examination for Marfan syndrome (height, span, hypermobility, eyes, and musculoskeletal) when indicated (Chaps. 9 and 21).

Palpate the *abdomen* for hepatosplenomegaly. Persistent splenomegaly from recent acute illness, such as infectious mononucleosis predisposes the athlete to splenic rupture in contact/collision sports (Chap. 20). Examine for enlarged kidney. The athlete who has one normal kidney, or a diseased kidney should be counseled about significant risk from participation in contact/collision sports. *Skin* should be carefully examined for any contagious lesions, such as herpes, scabies, and impetigo (Chaps. 19 and 24). If any abnormality is detected from a screening orthopedic examination, a detailed focused examination of the area should be done. Examine *genitalia* for absent or undescended testis, or testicular mass (Chap. 16). Note any inguinal lymphadenopathy and hernia. Assess sexual maturity rating.

DETERMINING ELIGIBILITY FOR SPORT PARTICIPATION

Based on the information obtained from the history and examination, a determination of eligibility for participation in sports is made. The determination to allow an individual athlete with a specific medical condition to participate is influenced by a number of factors, including current health status of the athlete, level of competition, sport played, position played, psychologic maturity of the athlete, understanding of risks by the athlete and parents, and ability to modify aspects of sports; and the clinician's clinical judgment is essential in this

regard. Risks of injury vary depending on whether the sport is contact sports or noncontact sports, as well as the static and dynamic demands of the specific sport.

SPECIFIC CONDITIONS AND SPORTS PARTICIPATION

Concussions

Concussions are the most common head injury in sports. The highest number of concussions is seen in American football. Other sports in which concussions are common include soccer, rugby, ice hockey, snowboarding, martial arts, and lacrosse. The Second International Conference on Concussion: Concussion in Sport Group defined concussion as:

> Concussion is defined as a complex pathophysiological process affecting the brain, induced by traumatic biomechanical forces. Several common features that incorporate clinical, pathological, and biomechanical injury constructs that may be used in defining the nature of a concussive head injury include:
> a. Concussion may be caused by a direct blow to the head, face, neck, or elsewhere on the body with an "impulsive" force transmitted to the head.
> b. Concussion typically results in the rapid onset of short lived impairment of neurological function that resolves spontaneously.
> c. Concussion may result in neuropathologic changes, but the acute clinical symptoms largely reflect a functional disturbance rather than structural injury.
> d. Concussion results in a graded set of clinical syndromes that may or may not involve loss of consciousness. Resolution of the clinical and cognitive symptoms typically follows a sequential course.
> e. Concussion is typically associated with grossly normal structural neuroimaging studies.

The athlete who has sustained or is suspected of having a concussion should not be left alone, but should be carefully observed on the sidelines, because symptoms and signs may evolve gradually over several minutes following the head injury. In addition to *acute* symptoms and signs of concussion (Table 32-2), *delayed* symptoms and signs may develop over several weeks following head injury; this delayed presentation can include dizziness, headache, vision disturbances, light headedness,

TABLE 32-2

SYMPTOMS AND SIGNS OF ACUTE CEREBRAL CONCUSSION (CONCUSSION IN SPORT GROUP)

Cognitive features
Unaware of period, opposition, score of the game
Confusion
Amnesia
Loss of consciousness
Unaware of time, date, place

Typical symptoms
Headache
Dizziness
Nausea
Unsteadiness/loss of balance
Feeling "dinged" or stunned or "dazed"
"Having my bell rung"
Seeing stars or flashing lights
Ringing in the ears
Double vision

Physical signs
Loss of consciousness/impaired conscious state
Poor coordination or balance
Concussive convulsion/impact seizure
Gait unsteadiness/loss of balance
Slow to answer questions or follow directions
Easily distracted, poor concentration
Displaying unusual or inappropriate emotions, such as laughing or crying
Nausea/vomiting
Vacant stare/glassy eyed
Slurred speech
Personality changes
Inappropriate playing behavior, for example running in the wrong direction
Appreciably decreased playing ability

Source: Aubry M, Cantu R, Dvorak J, et al. Summary and agreement statement of the First International Conference on Concussion in Sport, Vienna, 2001. *Phys Sportsmed* 2002;30(2):57–63.

concentration and attention problems, academic difficulties, sleep disturbances, and mood disturbances. Neuropsychologic testing provides an effective sensitive and objective way of assessing and monitoring recovery in concussion. Neuroimaging studies are indicated in athletes with severe clinical symptoms, focal neurologic signs, and persistent symptoms and signs typically over 2 weeks.

Numerous concussion grading systems and management guidelines have been published; however, none of these have been validated by research. Management of concussion requires individual assessment and clinical judgment. The Concussion in Sport Group and the Canadian Academy of Sports Medicine recommend a stepwise approach to rehabilitation and return to play for athletes who have sustained concussion. The athlete should be removed from further participation and clinically evaluated. No activity is allowed until the athlete is asymptomatic both at rest as well as on exertion; this may take variable periods of time, depending on the initial severity of the concussion and progression of recovery. Initially light aerobic activity, such as walking or stationary cycling, is recommended, followed by sport-specific training. If the athlete at any stage has recurrence of symptoms, he or she must return to the previously asymptomatic level and rest for 24 hours. Following sports-specific training, the athlete progresses from noncontact activities to full contact activities. Effect of multiple concussions is cumulative and results in neurocognitive deficits. Anticipatory guidance and education of the athlete, parents, and coach are essential to prevent long-term adverse consequences of concussion.

Epilepsy

Adolescents with well-controlled epilepsy can participate in all sports (Chap. 13). Certain high-risk situations in which a seizure episode may result in significant harm to the athlete or others need individual assessment. High-risk activities include water sports (i.e., swimming, scuba diving), sports involving heights (i.e., parachuting, hang gliding, mountain climbing), archery, riflery, and parallel bars in gymnastics. Weight training and strength training have not been shown to precipitate seizures.

Cardiovascular Conditions

The 36th Bethesda Conference Guidelines provide details of specific guidelines for athletes with various cardiovascular conditions (Chap. 9). For the purpose of determining the level of participation allowed, sports are classified based on the static and dynamic demands and strenuousness of specific sport. For example, athletes with mitral valve prolapse may be allowed unrestricted sport participation in the absence of syncope, a family history of death from mitral valve prolapse, repetitive supraventricular tachycardia or complex ventricular arrhythmias, moderate-to-marked mitral regurgitation, or prior embolic event. On the other hand, athletes with mitral valve prolapse and any of the above criteria may be limited to class IA type of activities. For detailed guidelines for individual cardiovascular conditions, the reader is referred to the 26th Bethesda Guidelines.

Hematologic Disorders

Athletes with hemophilia are at risk for bleeding from injuries in contact or collision sports, and most experts recommend against participation in such sports. Athletes with well-controlled von Willebrand disease may participate in all sports without restrictions. Athletes with sickle cell trait should be educated in maintaining proper hydration and allowed unrestricted sport participation. Athletes with sickle cell disease may participate in most sports, but must be cautioned against severe physical exertion in very hot or cold environments, and at high altitudes. High intensity activity may lead to lactic acidosis and hypoxemia predisposing to sickling. General well-being of the athlete with sickle cell disease and presence of complications are important considerations in individual assessment of these athletes. Anemia can adversely affect sports performance because of decreased aerobic capacity. Athletes with anemia should be evaluated on an individual basis to determine the level and intensity of physical exertion allowed (Chap. 17).

Diabetes Mellitus

Most adolescents with diabetes mellitus have type 1 diabetes (Chap. 15). With aggressive control, education of the athlete, parents, and sport officials athletes with diabetes can participate in all sports with no restrictions.

Infectious Diseases

Acute viral upper respiratory infections (URIs) are the most common cause of morbidity in athletes. An athlete with URI not associated with constitutional symptoms may be allowed to continue participation in sports. Athletes with constitutional symptoms (such as fever, malaise, headaches, others) should be cautioned against continued physical exertion, because of small but significant risk of viral myocarditis and cardiac arrhythmias. Athletes with acute infectious mononucleosis may have splenomegaly and should avoid contact sports until clinical resolution of illness and splenomegaly (Chap. 20). This typically takes about 1 month.

Most experts agree that athletes with HIV infection who are feeling well, and are asymptomatic should be allowed full sports participation (Chap. 24). Risks to other athletes should be discussed with the athlete; the other players should be informed that there might be an athlete with HIV, while respecting the patient-doctor confidentiality. Patients with active hepatitis B may not be allowed to participate in contact sports until infectivity is lost (Chaps. 10 and 24). In the athletic setting, all universal precautions should be implemented to prevent transmission of infection via blood. All athletes should have their vaccinations up-to-date, especially tetanus, measles-mumps-rubella (MMR), and hepatitis B. Patients with acute streptococcal pharyngitis can participate in contact sports after 24 hours of antibiotic treatment.

Athletes with skin diseases, such as herpes, molluscum contagiosum, impetigo, scabies, and chicken pox must avoid contact sports until lesions are healed and the athlete is considered noncontagious (Chap. 19). Athletes with fungal infections of the skin should be on treatment and all lesions should be adequately covered before allowing contact sports. Athletes with active infectious pulmonary tuberculosis may not be allowed contact sports; however, the infectivity is lost within few weeks of starting treatment (Chap. 8). The athlete's general well-being is an important consideration.

Abdomen and Genito-Urinary Conditions

Uncomplicated inguinal hernia is not a contraindication to sports. A large hernia may be vulnerable to contact trauma. Incarceration during sports is extremely rare. The athlete may be allowed full participation pending definitive elective repair. Athletes with one testis can participate in all sports with use of protective cups. Athletes with one functioning kidney must be informed of significant risks of injury in contact sports. An athlete with significant renal disease should be evaluated on an individual basis in consultation with a nephrologist.

Exercise-related hematuria is benign and typically resolves within 24–48 hours of rest. Similarly exercise-associated proteinuria is a benign, self-limiting condition with resolution within 24–48 hours. Persistent hematuria or proteinuria should be investigated further (Chap. 16).

HYPERTENSION

The American Academy of Pediatrics has published guidelines of sport participation by athletes with hypertension. Athletes with significant hypertension (95th to 98th percentile for age and gender) and no evidence of target organ damage or other cardiovascular disease should be allowed full sports participation. Athletes with severe hypertension (99th percentile for age and gender) should be restricted from competitive sports and activities with high static loads until blood pressure is adequately controlled and there is no evidence of target organ damage (Chaps. 9 and 16).

Eyes

Athlete with one eye, or history of eye surgery, retinal problems must be evaluated individually in consultation with an ophthalmologist. Some experts recommend that all contact and racquet sports be avoided (Chap. 7).

Musculoskeletal Conditions

Athletes with mild-to-moderate degrees of scoliosis who have no pain can participate in all sports. Pain associated with scoliosis needs further assessment. Athletes with spondylolysis who are pain free can continue all sports; however, they should be instructed in core conditioning and caution against hyperextension activities. Athletes with low-grade spondylolisthesis with no pain can also continue all sports; high-grade spondylolisthesis should be referred for orthopedic consultation (Chap. 11).

Pulmonary Disease

Athletes with well-controlled asthma can participate in all sports with no restrictions. Athletes with cystic fibrosis should be evaluated for pulmonary function and capacity to determine the level of physical activity allowed (Chap. 8).

Bibliography

American Academy of Pediatrics, American Academy of Family Physicians, American Medical Society for Sports Medicine, American Orthopedic Society for Sports Medicine, American Osteopathic Association for Sports Medicine: Preparticipation Physical Evaluation Monograph. New York, NY: McGraw-Hill, 2005.

American Academy of Pediatrics: Committee on Sports Medicine and Fitness Position Statement. Athletic participation by children and adolescents who have systemic hypertension. *Pediatrics* 1997;99(4):637–638.

Aubry M, Cantu R, Dvorak J, et al. Summary and agreement statement of the first International Conference on Concussion in Sport. *Br J Sport Med* 2002;36: 6–10.

Beckerman J, Wang P, Hlatky M. Cardiovascular screening of athletes. *Clin J Sport Med* 2004;14:127–133.

36th Bethesda Conference. Recommendations for determining eligibility for competition in athletes with cardiovascular abnormalities. *J Am Coll Cardiol* 2005; 45:1–64.

Draznin MB, Patel DR. Diabetes mellitus and sports. *Adolesc Med* 1998;9:457.

Garrick JG. Preparticipation orthopedic screening evaluation. *Clin J Sport Med* 2004;14(3):123–126.

Greydanus DE, Patel DR, Luckstead EF, Pratt HD. Value of sports pre-participation examination in health care for adolescents. *Med Sci Monit* 2004;10(9):1–11.

Homnick DN, Marks JH. Exercise and sports in the adolescent with chronic pulmonary disease. *Adolesc Med* 1998;9:467.

Landry GL. Central nervous system trauma: Management of concussions in athletes. *Pediatr Clin North Am* 2002;49(2):723–744.

Luckstead EF. Cardiac risk factors and participation guidelines for youth sports. *Pediatr Clin North Am* 2002;49(2):681–708.

Maron BJ. Sudden death in young athletes. *N Engl J Med* 2003;349:1064–1075.

McCrory P, Johnston K, Meeunisse W, et al. Summary and agreement statement of the 2nd International Conference on Concussion in Sport, Prague, 2004. *Br J Sport Med* 2005;39:196–204.

Orenstein DM. Pulmonary problems and management concerns in youth sports. *Pediatr Clin North Am* 2002; 49(2):709–722.

Patel DR, Gordon RC. Contagious diseases in athletes. *Contemp Pediatr* 1999;16(9):139.

Patel DR, Torres AD, Greydanus DE. Kidneys and sports. *Adolesc Med Clin* 2005;16(1):111–119

Patel DR, Greydanus DE, Luckstead Sr EF: The college athlete. *Pediatr Clin North Am* 2005;52(1): 25–60.

Wingfield K, Matheson GO, Meeuwisse WH. Preparticipation evaluation. *Clin J Sport Med* 2004; 14(3):109–122.

Wojtys EM, Hovda D, Landry G, et al. Concussions in sports. *Am J Sport Med* 1999;27:676.

33

SPORTS INJURIES

Dilip R. Patel, Eugene F. Luckstead, Sr.,
and Donald E. Greydanus

INTRODUCTION

About 30 million children and adolescents in the United States participate in organized sports and many more in recreational activities. Sport participation carries with it an inherent risk of injury and about 80% of such injuries involve the musculoskeletal system. Epidemiologic data on sports injuries in children and adolescents are limited. Definition of an injury varies in different studies making it difficult to evaluate data across studies. One of the more accurate measures of injury is the injury rate per athlete exposure, defined as one athlete participating in one practice or game where there is the possibility of sustaining an athletic injury.

In interscholastic high school sports, the yearly incidence has been reported to be between 30 and 40%. The injury rates for males and females are similar for most high school sports, with the exceptions of soccer, football, and wrestling. Soft tissue injuries, namely sprains, strains, and contusions, are the most common injuries; also, overuse injuries are more common than acute injuries accounting for 35–50% of all sports-related injuries. Acute injuries more commonly occur in practice than in games.

Certain aspects related to growth and development are unique to adolescents in terms of sports participation. Normal physical growth and maturation (Chap. 1) in height, weight, muscle size, and strength during adolescence influence sports performance. Due to adolescent growth the athletes get bigger, have increased body mass, and increased momentum, which increases the risk of injury severity. Neuromuscular development continues through adolescence—improved motor skills, power, agility, coordination, and speed—all affect sports performance. During adolescence, body composition, in terms of fat mass (FM) and fat free mass (FFM), and body fat distribution undergo differential change in boys and girls during adolescent years, which also influence sports performance. Many athletes try to manipulate body composition and body weight by engaging in unhealthy weight control and dietary behaviors, predisposing them to increased risks for dehydration, excessive weight loss, menstrual irregularities, and deficiency in bone mineral density.

Musculotendinous flexibility changes during adolescence. Females are typically more flexible compared to males. Optimal load is necessary for normal bone growth and modeling. Because most of the bone mineral density is acquired during the adolescent years, inadequate dietary intake and caloric restriction may result in failure to accrue normal bone mineral density. Growth cartilage is present at the epiphyseal plate, articular surface, and apophysis. The growth cartilage is relatively weaker compared to adjacent ligaments and bone; hence, there is more susceptibility to injury.

GROWTH PLATE INJURIES

Acute Injuries of the Growth Plate

An estimated 15–20% of injuries to long bones involve the growth plate and a significant number of these injuries are sports injuries. Growth plate injuries are more common in soccer, alpine skiing, gymnastics, weight lifting, and baseball. Growth plate injuries are twice as common in the upper extremities than in the lower extremities. The peak incidence of growth plate injuries is during early adolescence. Some authors cite increased sports participation, and weakening of the growth plate as possible factors for an increased number of such injuries during the period of rapid growth. Acute injuries are commonly classified according to the Salter-Harris Classification based on radiographic appearance.

Possibility of an injury to the growth plate should be strongly considered when there is a moderate or severe injury to the adjacent ligaments. A localized swelling and tenderness over the site of the growth plate is elicited on palpation. In severe injuries one may note a deformity. Plain films in two views with comparison films of the uninjured extremity should be obtained.

The specific treatment depends on the type of the injury and any associated injury to the adjacent structures. Usually uncomplicated type I and II injuries can be treated with closed reduction and immobilization. It is important to restore the normal anatomic configuration in type III and IV injuries. The athlete should be referred to an orthopedic surgeon when an acute growth plate injury is suspected. A careful long-term follow up is essential to detect and treat delayed complications.

A partial or complete growth arrest is a known complication of injuries to the growth plate. Fortunately the majority of injuries heal without clinically significant growth disturbance. Growth arrest and deformity may result following type III or IV injuries, if anatomic configuration cannot be restored. Growth arrest commonly occurs after type V injuries.

A complete growth arrest in lower extremity may result in a clinically significant leg-length inequality requiring subsequent corrective surgery.

Stress Injuries of the Growth Plate

Chronic repetitive microtrauma from intense training and sports participation can result in an overuse type of injury of the growth plate. Commonly described stress injuries of the growth plate are injury to the distal radius in gymnasts, the proximal humerus in pitchers, and injuries to the distal femur and proximal tibia in runners. The athlete presents with localized pain of gradual onset, which may worsen with continued activity. Localized tenderness can be elicited over the area. Other important causes of chronic bone and joint pain, such as infection, tumor, or arthritis should be included in the differential diagnosis. A radiographic examination is indicated, which typically shows widening of the physis.

Prompt recognition of the injury followed by cessation of the offending activity, up to 3 months in many cases, usually results in a rapid resolution of symptoms; the majority of such injuries heal without complications. On resolution of the pain, the athlete can return to a gradually increasing level of activity and avoid excessively intensive training to prevent recurrence. Recurrence of pain should be evaluated promptly.

OVERUSE INJURIES: GENERAL CONCEPTS

Musculoskeletal overuse injuries are the most common injuries in the adolescent athlete. Overuse injury is a result of excessive stress to normal tissue leading to a localized chronic inflammatory reaction. Tendons and tendon-apophyseal junctions are common sites for such injuries in the young. Overuse injuries of bone manifest as stress fractures. Overuse injuries are commonly seen in the athlete who is engaged in regular training and exercise, and who has recently increased the intensity of training. Also, a poorly conditioned recreational athlete, and an athlete early in the sports season, are prone to such injuries. A number of factors have been postulated to contribute to overuse syndromes (Table 33-1); however, the most consistent factor contributing to an overuse injury is a rapid increase in overall intensity and volume of training.

Clinically, it is useful to consider the process of overuse as a spectrum of injuries on a continuum of clinical severity. In grade 1 injuries, the pain or soreness is diffuse and occurs hours after the activity, with mild diffuse tenderness. When pain follows immediately after the activity, it is considered a grade 2 injury. Pain is usually present for about 2–3 weeks and tenderness may localize to the affected area. This is the most common presentation of an overuse syndrome. In grade 3 injury, pain is felt during the activity, is well localized, severe, and persistent. In grade 4 injury, the pain is present at rest or before the activity, interfering with function; tenderness is severe and well localized.

TABLE 33-1
OVERUSE INJURIES: CONTRIBUTING FACTORS

Anatomical factors
Pes cavus, tarsal coalition, metatarsus adductus, hyperpronation
Genu valgus, varum, recurvatum
Femoral anteversion, leg-length inequality

Equipment-related factors
Inappropriate size balls, rackets grips, or string tension
Inappropriate size gymnastic dowel rings
Improper use of strength-training machines
Shoes with poor shock absorption

Environmental factors
Hard surface running
Jumping on hard surface

Training errors
Rapid increase in intensity, duration, frequency
Musculoskeletal imbalance in strength and flexibility
Inadequate sport-specific skills (throwing, serving, and so on)

Growth-related factors
Presence of growth cartilage
Myo-osseous disproportional growth

In grade 3 and 4 injuries, a stress fracture should be strongly considered.

Treatment of an overuse injury begins with a decrease in or cessation of the offending activity and control of pain. Local application of ice in the form of ice massage directly over the area of pain and tenderness, two to three times for 10–15 minutes maximum a day, is recommended. Short term use of anti-inflammatory medication may be considered. The application of ultrasound and other physical therapy modalities are effective in controlling pain and inflammation in some patients. The athlete should decrease the intensity, amount, duration, or frequency of the training to a level that does not produce the pain. This may mean a period of complete cessation of the particular activity. The athlete should be allowed to continue aerobic training and strength training of the uninjured extremity. Alternative activities, such as cycling and swimming, should be encouraged. The physician should work closely with a sports physical therapist or athletic trainer, and institute an individualized progressive rehabilitation program for the athlete, which will allow the athlete to return to gradually increasing level of activity. Preventive measures include education of the athlete regarding the proper training regimen, and identifying and correcting various contributing factors to the best possible extent, especially faulty techniques.

SPECIFIC INJURIES: BURNERS

Pinched nerve syndrome (burner or stinger) is a common brachial plexus injury in sports seen in almost half of all high school football players. It results from the stretching of brachial plexus when the head is forced to the opposite side in a collision, as for example during tackling in football or when the shoulder is forcefully depressed. The incidence is highest in defensive players—linebackers and defensive backs. There is an acute, burning pain radiating down the arm commonly associated with numbness. Depending on the specific nerve root involved, there may be weakness and decreased tendon reflexes in the upper extremity. Symptoms may be aggravated by passive movement of the head to the opposite side. Symptoms usually resolve within a few minutes of rest, but in some athletes, it may take a few weeks. In some athletes full recovery may take months and further medical evaluation is indicated for such athletes. Sometimes muscle weakness may develop gradually and careful long-term follow up is essential in such cases. The athlete should follow a program of neck and upper extremity range of motion and strengthening. A gradual return to sports participation is allowed when the athlete is pain free, has full range of motion, full strength, and no neurologic signs. The athlete who fails to recover fully should be referred for further evaluation. A thorough evaluation for cervical spine or cord injuries or lesions is warranted in any athlete presenting with bilateral symptoms or signs.

SHOULDER INJURIES: ACUTE TRAUMA

Acute shoulder injuries usually result from direct impact to the shoulder in a collision or from a fall on the shoulder. Shoulder injuries are the second most common injuries (after knee) seen in football; injuries also occur in bicycling, skiing, and wrestling. Acromioclavicular (AC) sprain and shoulder dislocation are common acute injuries. AC sprain typically results from a fall on the shoulder or a fall on the outstretched hand. The athlete presents with localized pain and tenderness over the AC joint, which is aggravated by adduction of the arm across the chest. These injuries are classified depending on the structures damaged. Treatment depends on the type of injury.

Type 1 injury is stable, with minimal damage to the joint capsule and the ligaments. Treatment is symptomatic with rest, nonsteroidal anti-inflammatory drugs (NSAIDs), local ice and return to sports as symptoms resolve. In type 2 injuries, there is partial tearing of the joint capsule as well as the coronoid and trapezoid ligaments. There is localized tenderness and plain x-ray with stress may show increased coracoclavicular interval of less than 50%. Treatment is similar to type 1; additionally, sling support may be considered and return to sports may be more gradual. In type 3

injuries, there is complete tearing of the AC and coracoclavicular ligaments and possible AC dislocation. The coracoclavicular interval is increased more than 50%. Treatment is controversial. Most authorities advocate a conservative, nonoperative approach with immobilization in a sling. Resolution may take up to 6 weeks. Type 4, 5, and 6 injuries are more severe and complex and orthopedic referral is recommended.

Anterior dislocation of the shoulder is the most common type of traumatic dislocation of the shoulder. A fall on an outstretched hand or any excessive force leading to sudden abduction, and external rotation is the typical mechanism of injury. The athlete presents with a history of immediate severe pain in the shoulder. On examination, one may notice obvious asymmetry of shoulder contours, prominent acromion, and an arm held in abduction and slight flexion supported by the other hand. Range of shoulder motion is limited and tenderness is noted over the shoulder. Neurovascular assessment is imperative. Axillary nerve injury is the most common complication and sensation over the lateral aspect of the upper arm should be tested. Plain x-ray films in AP, lateral, and transscapular views are indicated.

There are numerous methods described to reduce the dislocation. Use of any particular method depends on the individual physician's experience and preference. In the traction-countertraction method, the athlete is supine and traction is applied to the injured arm in abduction and slight flexion. The countertraction is applied with a sheet wrapped around the chest. In the Stimson method, the athlete lies prone with the arm hanging with weight suspended from the wrist. After reduction, the arm is immobilized in a sling for 2–4 weeks to allow for tissue healing. In the Hennepin technique with the patient supine, the arm is slowly externally rotated to 90° followed by elevation until reduction is achieved. A further period of gradually progressive rehabilitation is necessary and full pain-free range of motion and strength should be achieved prior to returning to sports. Adequate rehabilitation may take 6–12 weeks and return to full sports participation may take 3–6 months. An athlete with significant associated trauma or recurrent dislocations should be referred to an orthopedic surgeon.

OVERUSE INJURIES

Shoulder Impingement Syndrome

Shoulder impingement syndrome is uncommon in adolescents. Since there can be different mechanisms underlying the impingement, the term does not indicate a specific diagnosis. Because of the predominant involvement of the rotator cuff muscles in the pathophysiology, it is often referred to as rotator cuff impingement syndrome. Primary impingement can be external (anterior), in which the supraspinatus tendon impinges against the undersurface of the coracoacromial arch; this is primarily due to eccentric overload of the tendon and glenohumeral instability. Internal impingement refers to injury to the glenoid labrum and is typically associated with a history of acute trauma. The term secondary impingement indicates underlying pathology causing impingement, such as glenohumeral instability, rotator cuff tendonitis or tear, AC joint trauma, or other local trauma.

Mechanism

The rotator cuff consists of four muscles namely supraspinatus, infraspinatus, teres minor, and subscapularis. The main function of these muscles is to stabilize the head of the humerus in the glenoid. The rotator cuff muscles, along with the long head of the biceps, prevent the head of the humerus from moving upward when the arm is abducted. The long head of biceps and supraspinatus run underneath the arch formed by coracoacromial ligament. Glenohumeral instability and tendon overload lead to primary impingement in the young. Impingement of the supraspinatus tendon under the coracoacromial arch occurs when the arm is abducted, elevated, or externally rotated. Repetitive overuse mainly in overhead activities, as seen in pitchers, swimmers, or tennis players, can lead to chronic inflammation of the rotator cuff tendons leading to edema and swelling, compromising the available space. It is also seen in weight lifters and gymnasts where the mechanism seems to be sustained isometric muscle contractions. A vicious cycle of impingement, edema and swelling, and further impingement thus sets in. Other factors believed to contribute to the development of impingement are decreased vascularity of the rotator cuff tendons, shoulder joint laxity and instability, and muscle strength imbalance.

Clinical Features

Shoulder pain secondary to impingement is of gradual onset and gets progressively worse with continued activity. Pain is usually localized in the superolateral aspect of the shoulder, and is exaggerated by overhead movements of the arm. Athletes may experience shoulder or arm pain and stiffness, deterioration of performance, and decreased as well as painful range of shoulder motion, especially with overhead activities. Palpation may reveal tenderness under the acromion process. There may be tenderness over the long head of biceps tendon as it traverses the bicipital groove anteriorly, if it is also inflamed. Usually, a full range of motion is maintained with some pain specifically on abduction between 70 and 120°. The supraspinatus is tested for pain on resisted movement and weakness. Resistance is applied with arm abducted to 90°, forward flexed at 30°, and internally rotated. Pain is also elicited with abduction, internal rotation, flexion of the arm, and forward flexion of the internally rotated arm.

Glenohumeral stability should be assessed by moving the humeral head in anterior, posterior, and inferior directions in relation to the glenoid. In anterior subluxation, apprehension can be elicited when the shoulder is abducted and externally rotated. In the relocation test, shoulder pain is present when the arm is abducted and externally rotated; the pain improves when the humeral head is moved in a posterior direction. Diagnosis is based on the clinical findings; in a diagnostic test, pain is temporarily relieved by injection of xylocaine into the subacromial bursa with restoration of full range of arm movements without pain. Plain radiographs are normal in the majority of these young athletes. In the growing athlete, stress injury of the proximal humeral growth plate should be considered in differential diagnoses; in this situation, tenderness may be present over the proximal humerus and impingement signs are absent. Tear of the rotator cuff in a young athlete is a rare acute event, and should be referred for orthopedic evaluation; it presents with acute that is severe and localized pain along with tenderness, loss of motion, and weakness. Causes of chronic or recurrent shoulder pain in young athletes are listed in Table 33-2.

Treatment

Treatment of impingement syndrome in the young athlete is conservative. To alleviate the initial pain, complete rest from the offending activities may be necessary, along with local ice massage and analgesic anti-inflammatory medications. This will permit the athlete to begin a rehabilitation program; a progressive rehabilitation program specifically focuses first on restoration of full range of motion. Once pain-free range of motion is achieved, the athlete works on strength, balance, and endurance of the rotator cuff muscles. A careful review of the overall training program and techniques is an essential component of any prevention plan. Athletes should

TABLE 33-2

CAUSES OF CHRONIC/RECURRENT SHOULDER PAIN IN ADOLESCENT ATHLETES

Arthritis of glenohumeral joint
Arthritis of AC joint
AC joint sprain
Atraumatic osteolysis of distal clavicle
Brachial plexus injuries
Cervical rib
Cervical root impingement (referred pain)
Cervical disc herniation (referred pain)
Cervical cord syringomyelia, tumors (referred pain)
Glenohumeral joint instability
Long head of biceps tendonitis
Proximal humeral physeal stress injury
Rotator cuff impingement
Rotator cuff tendonitis
Rotator cuff tear
Scapular dyskinesis
Subacromial bursitis
Thoracic outlet syndrome

follow a preseason conditioning program in addition to learning and maintaining correct sport-specific techniques.

Proximal Humeral Physeal Stress Injury

The proximal humeral physis accounts for the 80% of upper extremity longitudinal growth; early recognition and treatment of any injuries to this growth plate are important to prevent complications. Chronic or stress injuries of the proximal humeral physis are seen in sports in which overhead activities are predominant, such as in volleyball, swimming, racquet, and throwing sports. The peak incidence is between 11 and 16 years of age. The athlete typically presents with gradual onset, activity-related, shoulder pain over a period of several weeks to months. There is a history of loss of throwing strength and significant pain associated with overhead activities. Tenderness can be localized on the lateral proximal humerus in 70% of patients. Plain films in internal and external rotation will show widening of the physis compared with the uninjured side. Treatment necessitates discontinuation of offending activity, up to 3 months in many cases, and gradual return to sports with limitations on throwing volume.

Atraumatic Osteolysis of the Distal Clavicle

Atraumatic osteolysis of the distal clavicle (AODC) is believed to be an overuse injury affecting the distal end of the clavicle. It is typically seen in young body builders or competitive weight lifters who have been engaged in weight lifting and weight training for a period of months to years. Excessive repetitive stress at the distal clavicular area produces a chronic inflammatory response. With continued activity, cumulative stress leads to loss of subchondral bone, development of microcysts, and eventually, osteolysis localized to distal clavicle. In addition to AODC in weight lifters, cases have been described in baseball pitchers, tennis players, swimmers, and football players. Although common in males, cases have been described in female volleyball and basketball players.

TABLE 33-4

INTRINSIC CAUSES OF CHRONIC WRIST PAIN IN ADOLESCENT ATHLETES

Relatively more common
Distal radial physis stress injury
Triangular fibrocartilage complex injury
De Quervain tenosynovitis
Dorsal soft tissue impingement syndrome

Relatively less common
Carpal instabilities
Distal radioulnar instability
Extensor tendonitis
Flexor tendonitis
Carpal tunnel syndrome (median nerve entrapment neuropathy)
Ulnar nerve entrapment neuropathy
Intersection syndrome
Kienbock's disease
Ganglion cysts
Wrist capsulitis
Stress fracture of scaphoid

Source: Patel DR, Greydanus DE. Overuse injuries of elbow and wrist in adolescent athletes. *Asian J Paediatr Pract* 2000;3(4):57.

complex (TFCC) disc is an intraarticular structure, susceptible to perforation or tear from repetitive loading, supination, and pronation movements, especially with ulnar deviation.

Injury to TFCC can be acute or chronic and is commonly seen in racquet sports, hockey, and gymnastics. The athlete presents with recurrent or chronic wrist pain, located on the ulnar side of the joint, aggravated by supination and pronation. Movements at the wrist may be associated with a clicking sensation. Full range of wrist motion is generally maintained and swelling is uncommon. Localized tenderness can be elicited over the ulnar side of the wrist joint line. Plain x-rays are usually normal; in some cases, there may be a positive ulnar variance. Magnetic resonance imaging (MRI) is the most useful imaging study for detecting a tear or perforation of the TFCC. The offending activity should be stopped and wrist immobilized initially for 4–6-week duration (sometimes longer).

TFCC injuries are difficult to heal and an orthopedic or hand surgery consultation may be required for arthroscopy as well as further management.

BACK INJURIES AND LOWER BACK PAIN

Injuries to the back can involve any of the soft tissue structures or the spine, most affecting the lumbosacral spine or lower back. Unlike in an acute injury, the cause and effect relationship between the chronic injury and symptoms or spine abnormalities is not always clearly established in many young athletes. It appears that the severity of the lower back pain and abnormal findings of the spine are relatively increased during the adolescent growth spurt. Some studies suggest that early age at onset and longer duration of sports participation may contribute to increased symptomatology. It is estimated that 80% of the injuries occur during practice, and acute injuries account for 60% of these.

Such injuries may result from a variety of mechanisms. Direct blows to the back can cause muscle contusions. Hyperextension of lumbar spine, as seen in football and gymnastics, is implicated in the development of spondylolysis (Chap. 11). In gymnasts, a higher level of competition is correlated with a higher incidence of back problems. Studies suggest that floor exercises, the balance beam, uneven parallel bars, flips, and vaulting dismounts contribute to back injuries in gymnasts. In throwing sports, musculotendinous avulsions may occur from forceful sudden muscle contractions. In the adolescent athlete, the immature vertebral end plates may be injured from improper weight lifting. Lifting with spine in flexion, and moving from flexion to extension causes significant stress to the spine. Improper lifting techniques may cause injuries in ballet and figure skating. Twisting motions in tennis can cause musculotendinous strains and avulsions. Chronic poor posture may result in chronic ligamentous strain.

Acute and chronic musculotendinous and spine injuries are a significant cause of back pain; however, in the young adolescent athlete with back pain, many other significant medical conditions not necessarily related to sports participation, should be considered (Chap. 11) in the differential diagnosis. A thorough history and physical examination will yield the most useful information needed to make the diagnosis.

Treatment of the athlete with low back injury and pain depends on the specific condition. The athlete with *acute back strain/sprain*, who is otherwise in good health, should expect full recovery. Absolute bed rest is no longer recommended. The athlete should be allowed to carry on daily activities as tolerated. Analgesics and muscle relaxants may help relieve pain during the acute phase. As the pain and general mobility improve, a back rehabilitation exercise program is started in consultation with a sports physical therapist. The goals of rehabilitation for acute back strains and sprains are to regain normal pain-free range of motion, improve strength of the back and abdominal muscles, and correct abnormal posture.

KNEE INJURIES

Acute Trauma

Knee injuries are common injuries seen in football, soccer, and basketball. *Evaluation* begins with an accurate history: ask the athlete how the injury occurred, whether the athlete was running, changing direction, or stopped suddenly at the time, and what was the position of the leg and the knee at the time. Injury to the meniscus or the anterior cruciate ligament (ACL) is associated with a sudden change in direction. Landing off balance may result in an anterior cruciate sprain, while direct force laterally or medially may injure the collateral ligaments. Isolated posterior cruciate ligament sprain may result following a direct impact against the tibia when the knee is flexed. Ask the athlete if there was a pop or a snap, usually associated with an anterior cruciate tear. Inquire about the rapidity with which the swelling occurred. Rapid onset hemarthrosis occurs in an ACL tear, patellar dislocation, or a fracture. With cartilage injury the swelling is minimal and gradual, although a peripheral meniscal tear can cause significant hemarthrosis. A history of locking suggests a meniscal injury or an intraarticular

loose body. A history of knee or leg giving away indicates joint instability. Pain is felt by the athlete immediately at the time of a ligamentous injury, dislocation, or a fracture.

On examination assess the extent of effusion, look for deformity, and assess active range of motion. Palpate carefully to localize tenderness and perform the apprehension patella test. Perform the Lachman test with the athlete supine and knee flexed at 15°; feel for increased forward motion of tibia over the femur and for the end-point of the movement.

MCL sprains result from a valgus or external rotation stress to the knee when the foot is planted. Athletes typically give a history of having sustained a sudden forceful hit on the lateral aspect of the knee from another athlete. The athlete has knee pain and is able to walk with some discomfort. There is usually no effusion while flexion and extension motions are normal. With the athlete supine, a valgus stress at 30° of knee flexion increases the medial knee pain and increased laxity may be noted. There is localized tenderness over the ligament. Uncomplicated MCL sprains heal well with a period of relative rest. A hinged brace prevents valgus or varus stress and allows early range of motion and strengthening exercises.

ACL sprain typically is a noncontact injury, which results from a twisting or hyperextension force to the knee, as seen in football and basketball. Athletes feel immediate pain and there is a rapid onset of hemarthrosis. The Lachman test is positive, the MRI is diagnostic, and the athlete should be referred to an orthopedic surgeon. Treatment in the skeletally immature athlete presents a unique dilemma, and most surgeons prefer to wait until skeletal maturity before performing reconstructive surgery. The athlete is fitted with a special brace, started on a rehabilitation program, and restricted from contact/collision and aggressive sport participation. Some surgeons with special expertise elect to perform surgical reconstruction using special techniques that avoids the growth plates. Sport-specific conditioning programs have been successful in preventing ACL sprains, especially in female athletes, and should be strongly recommended. Athletes should work with athletic trainers with expertise in such regimens.

A medial meniscus tear may be an isolated injury or may be associated with other ligamentous injuries. This athlete has knee pain, minimal swelling, locking, medial joint line tenderness, and may have a positive McMurray test. In McMurray test with the athlete supine, the hip and knee are flexed, followed by extension of the knee with concomitant external rotation; this elicits pain over the medial joint line or one may be able to feel the torn posterior horn of meniscus. Injury results from a deceleration force with a twisting motion leading to compression and tearing of the meniscus. MRI is helpful in this diagnosis and young athletes with medial meniscus tears should be referred to an orthopedic surgeon.

Acute patellar dislocation may result from direct impact to the patella, but more commonly from a forceful quadriceps contraction during a cutting motion. The patella is dislocated laterally, and associated with immediate severe pain, rapid onset of swelling, and apparent deformity; there is restriction of knee motion and significant tenderness over the knee. Treatment is immediate reduction and a short period of immobilization. Closed reduction can be achieved with the athlete relaxed and supine with leg flexed at the hip and knee; the knee is then gently extended with pressure over patella from a lateral to medial direction. Plain x-ray films should be obtained to assess the reduction and to detect any associated fracture. The knee is immobilized in a knee immobilizer for few days followed by a rehabilitation program before returning to sports.

Overuse Injuries of Knee: Idiopathic Anterior Knee Pain

There are a number of specific causes of anterior knee pain (Table 33-5) in a young athlete. In a subset of athletes, however, it is difficult to conclusively establish a specific etiology and the term idiopathic anterior knee syndrome is used to describe this condition.

Mechanism

Intense physical activity overloading the patellofemoral mechanism appears to be the most consistent factor leading to the development of anterior

TABLE 33-5

CAUSES OF CHRONIC OR RECURRENT KNEE PAIN IN ADOLESCENT ATHLETES

Anterior	Idiopathic anterior knee pain
	Patellar or quadriceps tendinitis
	Hoffa's fat pad syndrome
	Prepatellar or infrapatellar bursitis
	Osgood-Schlatter disease
	Multipartite patella
	Patellar stress fracture
	Osteochondritis dissecans
	Chondromalacia patellae
	Sinding-Larsen-Johansson syndrome
Posterior	Baker's cyst (associated with meniscal tear)
	Fabella syndrome
	Gastrocnemius tendinitis
	Hamstring tendinitis or chronic strain
Medial	Medial meniscal tear
	Pathologic medial plica
	Pes anserine bursitis/tendinitis
	Semimembranosus bursitis/tendinitis
Lateral	Iliotibial band friction syndrome
	Popliteus tendonitis
	Discoid lateral meniscus injury
Referred	Slipped capital femoral epiphysis
	Legg-Calve-Perthes disease
	Femoral neck stress fracture
	Spinal tumors
Other	Osteosarcoma, Ewing's tumor
	Osteoid osteoma, synovial tumors
	Connective tissue disease
	Sickle cell arthropathy
	Leukemia
	Osteomyelitis
	Reflex sympathetic dystrophy

knee pain. The patellofemoral unit provides the mechanism for knee extension and deceleration. The stability of the patella in the femoral groove is provided by the surrounding soft tissue attachments and the bony supporting structures. Malalignment and abnormal tracking of the patella has been postulated to contribute to anterior knee pain.

Vastus medialis obliquus plays an important role in stabilizing the patella in the femoral groove and its proper tracking. Many other factors have been postulated to contribute to the development of anterior knee pain in adolescents (Table 33-6). A chondromalacia patella is a pathologic diagnosis indicating softening and erosion of the cartilage of the patellofemoral joint; in some athletes, it is a cause of severe anterior knee pain.

Clinical Features

Anterior knee pain syndrome is typically seen in a young active athlete who presents either acute or gradual onset of pain that is unilateral or bilateral; the pain is usually seen following a recent increase in physical activity. The pain is increased after prolonged sitting (theater sign), going up and coming downstairs, and prolonged squatting. Usually the pain has been present for few weeks and the athlete might have tried pain medications intermittently. A worsening of pain, which adversely affects performance leads the athlete to seek medical attention. The athlete may give a history of the knee catching, pseudolocking, or giving way; a history of knee swelling is uncommon.

On examination, look for abnormal gait, increased lumbar lordosis, and any asymmetry of hips or lower extremities; also observe for atrophy and weakness of the quadriceps muscles by comparing it to the normal side. A decrease in flexibility of the hamstrings and quadriceps is a common finding. Isometric quadriceps contraction with the leg extended may reveal a subtle lateral patellar deviation. This can be assessed by placing a row of three dots in a straight line while the knee is relaxed (one several inches above the knee in the midline, one several inches below, and one at mid patellar point); then look for lateral displacement of the patellar dot on isometric quadriceps contraction. Knee effusion or soft tissue swelling is an uncommon finding. A full range of motion is maintained. In some athletes tenderness may be elicited by palpating and exerting pressure on the articular margins of the patella while displacing it medially or laterally. A crepitus may be felt in some athletes.

Plain x-ray films may help rule out other conditions causing anterior knee pain, such as osteochondritis dissecans of the patella or knee, or stress fracture of the patella. Radiographs are not indicated routinely. Abnormal tilt of the patella may indicate maltracking, best shown with a tangential view at 45–90° of flexion of the knee.

Treatment

Conservative treatment consists of relative rest, local ice, and judicious use of anti-inflammatory medications to help control the pain. Complete rest and cessation of all activities is generally not necessary and the athlete should be allowed to continue all activities as tolerated. Prolonged sitting, squatting, and climbing up or going downstairs, and full arc knee extension exercises should be avoided. Alternative activities, such as cycling with a proper fit, swimming, and walking are encouraged as tolerated. The effectiveness of different kinds of taping techniques and knee braces varies considerably; their use should be individualized. Rehabilitation exercises focus on increasing the flexibility, strength, and endurance of the quadriceps and hamstrings. Knee immobilization is not recommended, except when pain is severe affecting daily activities.

TABLE 33-6

ANTERIOR KNEE PAIN: POSSIBLE CONTRIBUTING FACTORS

Chondromalacia patellae
Chronic overuse
Patella alta
Abnormal Q angle
Abnormal patellar tracking
Quadriceps weakness
Decreased hamstring or quadriceps flexibility
Knee ligamentous laxity or generalized ligamentous laxity
Exaggerated lumbar lordosis
Genu varum or valgus
Hyperpronated feet
Decreased flexibility of Achilles tendon

Prognosis in young athletes is excellent for resolution of pain and ability to participate fully in sports.

Osgood-Schlatter Disease

Osgood-Schlatter disease results from chronic stress at the site of insertion of the patellar tendon over the tibial tuberosity. Rapid growth occurring during early adolescence, combined with increased physical activity, predisposes to the development of this condition. The immature patellar tendon-tibial tubercle junction is highly susceptible to repetitive tensile stress resulting from high level of activity. This leads to minor avulsions at the site and subsequent inflammatory reaction.

Osgood-Schlatter disease is commonly seen during Tanner stage 2 or 3 in adolescent boys. The incidence is higher in athletes compared to nonathletes, and symptoms are bilateral in 20–30% of patients. The athlete presents with anterior knee pain, aggravated by jumping, squatting, and kneeling, and relieved by a period of rest. There may be decreased range of knee motion because of pain, and accentuation of pain with extreme flexion and with resisted knee extension. There is localized tenderness, and sometimes swelling over the tibial tubercle. Plain radiographs are recommended to rule out other causes of localized pain, such as osteomyelitis or tumor. Plain films may show prominent and irregular tibial tubercle, fragmentation of tibial tubercle and sometimes, an ossicle in the patellar tendon.

Complications are rare, and include complete avulsion of patellar tendon (very rare), ossicle formation in the tendon, and genu recurvatum resulting from premature fusion of the anterior aspect of the proximal tibial physis. An enlarged tibial tubercle may have cosmetic significance, especially in female athletes. The pain improves on decreased activity and rest; local ice massage and short term use of nonsteroidal anti-inflammatory agents help relieve inflammation, edema, and pain. It is not uncommon for recurrent pain to last up to 2 years. This is a benign self-limited condition and over treatment should be avoided. The adolescent should be allowed all the tolerated activities. Typically, an acute episode lasts for about 4–6 weeks. Therapeutic exercises should focus on flexibility of hamstrings and quadriceps. Local injections of corticosteroids are contraindicated. Local padding or a neoprene knee sleeve can be protective to some extent. Knee immobilization is not necessary and generally not recommended.

LEG PAIN

Shin Splints

Shin splints or shin splint syndrome is a nonspecific term that generally refers to chronic anterior leg pain resulting from a variety of underlying causes; it is commonly seen in runners. Medial stress syndrome is the commonest cause of shin splints and is described here.

The underlying pathology is believed to be tibial periostitis or stress reaction secondary to chronic excessive stress at the bone-muscle junction. Repeated forceful dorsiflexion of the foot, repeated impact loading during foot strike, and excessive foot pronation can lead to micro tears at the soft tissue attachments to the periosteum of tibia. This results in a musculotendinous inflammatory reaction. Poor shock absorption from shoes, hard running surface, rapid increase in the intensity of training, muscular weakness and imbalances in strength of leg muscles, poor conditioning, and overweight are contributing factors.

Athletes present with anterior leg pain following a recent increase in activity. Pain and tenderness are localized along the middle third of the posteromedial border of the tibia. There may be weakness of the tibialis posterior and flexor hallucis longus muscles. A tibial stress fracture and chronic compartment syndrome should be considered in the differential diagnosis. There is exertional pain in compartment syndrome localized to the affected compartment, which is increased on passive stretching of the muscles of the compartment. Tenderness is elicited over the compartment affected. A definitive diagnosis is made by measurement of compartment pressure. If compartment syndrome is suspected, the athlete should be appropriately referred for further evaluation and treatment. Plains radiographs should be obtained if a stress fracture is suspected.

A period of relative rest from offending activities is essential and the most effective treatment for shin splints. Modification of current level and type of activity is needed. Generally, all nonweight bearing activities should be allowed. Local application of ice is recommended. Shoes with good shock absorbing capacity should be worn while excessive pronation should be corrected by using orthosis; a softer training surface should be preferred. The athlete should follow a regular program of stretching and strengthening of leg muscles, Achilles stretching, and strengthening of the anterior and posterior tibialis muscles. Prevention measures include a regimen of gradually increasing the level of activity, on-going stretching and strengthening exercises, and maintaining good shoe shock absorption.

ANKLE SPRAINS

Ankle sprain is the most common acute injury of the ankle and the most common acute sport-related injury, accounting for about 15% of all sports-related injuries. Previous ankle injury, inadequate rehabilitation, muscle weakness or ligamentous laxity, and poor Achilles tendon flexibility are noted as some of the contributing factors. Inversion injuries account for 85% of sprains resulting in injuries to the lateral ligaments. Such an injury usually occurs when the plantar flexed foot is suddenly inverted, causing sprain of the anterior talofibular ligament, calcaneofibular ligament, and posterior talofibular ligament in that order, with progressively severe injury. Eversion injuries are less common and require a significantly more force to injure the strong deltoid ligament. The foot goes into sudden forceful eversion and dorsiflexion. Ankle injuries tend to occur during sudden change in direction, landing from a jump, or sudden deceleration.

Clinical Features

The athlete presents with ankle pain and swelling following the injury. If ice was applied immediately, the swelling may be minimal. The athlete may or may not be able to bear weight, depending on the severity of the sprain and stability of the ankle joint.

There may be history of a pop or snap at the time of the injury. The athlete may not be able to continue to play in severe sprains. Examine for extent of swelling, localized ligament, and bony tenderness, and assess range of ankle motion. Assessment of ligament laxity and joint instability may be difficult with initial pain and swelling. Anterior drawer and inversion tests should be performed.

The anterior drawer test is performed with one hand holding the leg steady just above the ankle and the other hand around the heel attempts to move the foot forward. Feel for increased forward motion of the foot and the end-point of the movement while comparing to the uninjured side. The anterior drawer specifically tests for the integrity of the anterior talofibular ligament. A soft end point and excessive anterior motion of the foot compared to the uninjured ankle, indicates sprain of the anterior talofibular ligament. Compare bilateral inversion and talar tilt and assess side to side motion. Inversion stress at 90° or neutral position assesses the calcaneofibular ligament. The examiner also assesses the neurovascular status. Radiographic examination is indicated in severe injuries, inability to bear weight, when there is rapid onset of swelling, deformity, eversion injury, localized bony tenderness, penetrating injury, and joint instability. AP, lateral, and mortise views should be obtained. Occult fractures may be difficult to detect on plain radiographs and a CT scan may be needed.

In assessing the ankle sprain, carefully look for associated injuries. In the young athlete with open physes, there may be injury to the distal fibular physis. There may be fracture of the proximal fibula or the shaft of the fibula. On plain x-ray films, look for any talar dome fracture or avulsion at the base of the fifth metatarsal. Palpate the peroneal and Achilles tendons; peroneal tendon subluxation or dislocation may be associated with ankle sprains. Side to side movements at ankle and squeezing of malleoli may elicit pain in tibiofibular syndesmotic sprain.

Treatment

Ankle sprains are commonly graded as mild, moderate, or severe depending on the extent of the damage.

Most ankle sprains are mildly to moderately severe and not associated with other injuries or instability. Treatment of uncomplicated ankle sprains consists of immediate application of ice, and, compression dressing. Crushed ice is placed in a plastic bag and applied directly around the ankle. Ice should be kept in place for about 10–15 minutes at a time, 20–40 minutes apart; such cryotherapy should be used as long as there is ankle swelling. Depending on pain tolerance and severity of the injury, protected weight bearing may be allowed. While at rest the leg should be elevated. Early active range of motion exercises is encouraged. Different types of ankle braces have been used with varying success. Air stirrups prevent inversion and eversion movements and may help during the recovery phase. Depending on the initial injury, recovery may take anywhere from 2 to 6 weeks.

Once the pain is improved, additional specific exercises should be started. The athlete may do foot circles, which involves tracing small circles in the air with toes or print alphabet with foot using the big toe as a pointer. The athlete may practice picking up marbles with toes or curl towel. Further exercises involve stretching of Achilles tendon and calf muscles, toe raises, and heel raises. The next stage involves progressive strength-training exercises. Proprioception is enhanced by using balance board exercises. The final stage is to regain the coordination and agility and this involves a program of alternate jogging-walking, running in figure of eight, or zig-zag cutting. Working closely with a trainer or therapist is very helpful to develop an individualized rehabilitation plan and returning the athlete to sports. Follow up is important to detect residual weakness and development of chronic instability. Delayed recovery or chronic pain following ankle injury may result from soft tissue impingement, chronic synovitis, significant scarring, incomplete rehabilitation, unrecognized occult fracture, or tibiofibular diastasis.

Acknowledgments

The authors thank Ms. Cori Edgecomb for assistance in preparing this manuscript.

Bibliography

Anderson K, Strickland SM, Warren R. Hip and groin injuries in athletes. *Am J Sport Med* 2001;29: 521–533.

Baker RJ, Patel DR. Back injuries in athletes. *Primary Care Clinics in Office Practice* 2005;32:201–229.

Bono CM. Low-back pain in athletes. *J Bone Joint Surg* 2004;86A(2):382–396.

Clark KD, Tanner S. Evaluation of the Ottawa ankle rules in children. *Pediatr Emerg Care* 2003;19(2):73–78.

DeLee JC, Drez D Jr, Miller MD. *DeLee & Drez's Orthopaedic Sports Medicine: Principles and Practice*, 2d ed. Philadelphia, PA: W.B. Saunders, 2004.

Dormans JP. Evaluation of children with suspected cervical spine injury. *JBJS* 2002;84A:124–132.

Fulkerson JP. Diagnosis and treatment of patients with patellofemoral pain. *Am J Sport Med* 2000;30: 447–456.

Gomez J. Upper extremity injuries in youth sports. *Pediatr Clin North Am* 2002;49(3):593–626.

Greydanus DE, Patel DR. Back pain in adolescent athletes. *Asian J Pediatr Pract* 2000;3:83–94.

Greydanus DE, Patel DR. Knee injuries in the adolescent athlete. *Asian J Paediatr Pract* 2000;3:49–56.

Greydanus DE, Patel DR. Diagnosis and management of ankle sprains. *Asian J Paediatr Pract* 2000;3: 43–48.

Jackson AM. Anterior knee pain. *JBJS* 2001;83B: 937–948.

Kibler WB, McMullen J. Scapular dyskinesis and its relation to shoulder pain. *J Am Acad Orthop Surg* 2003;11:142–151.

Luckstead EF, Greydanus DE. *Medical Care of the Adolescent Athlete*. Los Angeles: PMIC, 1993, p. 325.

Luckstead EF, Patel DR. Catastrophic pediatric sports injuries. *Pediatr Clin North Am* 2002;49(3):581–592.

Luckstead EF (ed.). Pediatric sports medicine, parts I and II. *Pediatr Clin North Am* 2002;49(3):497–679, 49(4):681–876.

Patel DR, Greydanus DE. Overuse injuries of elbow and wrist in adolescent athletes. *Asian J Paediatr Pract* 2000;3:54–58.

Patel DR, Nelson TL. Sports injuries in adolescents. *Med Clin North Am* 2000;84:983–1007.

Reid DC. *Sports Injury Assessment and Rehabilitation*. New York, NY: Churchill-Livingstone, 1992.

Torg JS, Guille JT, Jaffe S. Injuries to the cervical spine in American football players. *JBJS* 2002;84A:112–122.

34

SUBSTANCE ABUSE IN THE ADOLESCENT

Donald E. Greydanus and Dilip R. Patel

INTRODUCTION

The use and abuse of illicit substances (Table 34-1) by adolescents and adults are among the most important biopsychosocial issues of our times. Increasing prevalence of the use of tobacco and alcohol by younger adolescents is a disturbing trend (Tables 34-2 to 34-4). It is not a new problem and not confined to any specific group of adolescents alone, or to any culture. Clinicians should join other groups seeking to heighten the awareness of authorities, including government, of the dangers of drug abuse to our society. Legitimate queries in this direction include why such drugs as tobacco are allowed to grow and why the widespread availability of drugs, such as cocaine or heroin, continues to occur. It is also important to look at whether we are becoming a drug-dependent culture, using medications of all kinds to solve all of our problems. These are not simple questions, nor are there easy solutions. However, our children and their future demand that we all explore such difficult challenges.

Table 34-5 lists some of the causes of drug use and abuse by adolescents. In early and middle adolescence (Chap. 1), teens may use chemicals as a rite of passage from their former childhood and ongoing process of becoming adults. Drug use can serve as proof of maturation and is consistent with anthropologic studies revealing classic rites of passage in human cultures, with various ways to celebrate these changes, sometimes with chemicals. Illicit drug use can be part of attempts to demonstrate rebellion against authorities, or to simply acquiesce to peer pressure that calls for drug experimentation. This call can be irresistible to many youth.

Drugs can provide many teens with the "courage" to engage in various peer-approved high-risk behaviors, such as sexual promiscuity. Illicit drug use may help an adolescent escape the chaos and dysfunctionality observed in the family, other peers, or society at large. This may be seen in abuse that may be occurring in the family or at school, marital problems in parents, academic difficulties, inability to find adequate employment, and others. The media (i.e., movies, cable, internet, others) has considerable effects in encouraging all members of society that drug use is acceptable, desired, and without adverse consequences. Table 34-6 provides some factors that are *protective* of drug use.

Though clinicians are under increasing pressure to see more patients in less time, it is critical that the teens' trusted clinician spend time to seek out whether the teen patient is experimenting with drugs. Various questionnaire forms are available, but

TABLE 34-1
DRUGS OF ABUSE

Inhalants
Tobacco
Alcohol
Marijuana
Amphetamine
Methamphetamine
MDMA (Ecstasy) (methylenedioxymethamphetamine)
Date rape drugs
MDMA (Ecstasy)
Flunitrazepam (Rohypnol)
GHB
Ketamine (Ketalar)
Hallucinogens
LSD
PCP
Tryptamines
Cocaine
Opiates (Heroin, others)
Barbiturates
Anabolic steroids

it is stressed that actively enquiring about the patient's potential high-risk behavior and if the patient needs help for any identified problem are the main points. The youth typically has limited education about the dangers of drug use and the clinician can provide teens with much critically important information about drugs. For example, adolescents may feel that they are simply experimenting with a drug in an "innocent" manner, but do not realize that most adult tobacco addicts began their addiction while they were teens; also they may not consider that some drugs can cause irreversible neuropsychiatric changes (as noted with *Ecstasy*), or that acute psychosis may be induced by some drugs (as noted with phencyclidine [PCP] or marijuana).

Table 34-7 reviews various risk factors for drug abuse to consider when evaluating youth, while Table 34-8 lists helpful, nonspecific indicators of drug abuse. Table 34-9 lists common comorbid disorders of substance abuse; these can be kept in mind as the assessment proceeds. The classic progression from experimentation to chronic drug abuse is reviewed in the McDonald Stages of Drug Abuse in

Table 34-10. Referral to experts in substance abuse treatment is suggested if the clinician does not have such expertise or the time to manage these potentially complex and difficult patients. However, the resolution of the issue is to identify if a problem of substance abuse exists, and if the youth is willing to accept help. Major specific illicit drugs that are abused by adolescents are reviewed here.

INHALANT DRUGS

Inhalant drugs (Table 34-11) are chemicals that depress the central nervous system (CNS). They are typically sniffed or inhaled by young, often male adolescents and the purpose is to have the users develop a sense of euphoria and joy, albeit short-lived. The term, inhalant drugs, refers to chemicals such as paints, sprays, or aerosol cans that are inhaled; glue sniffing is seen, with ingredients such as toluene found in airplane glue and some rubber cements. These drugs may be seen by the young teens as an inexpensive and ever-available substitute for other drugs, such as marijuana or alcohol (Table 34-2). Youth in rural America and Native American teens may concentrate on gasoline, while middle to late adolescents may use some chemicals for reported aphrodisiac effects of amyl nitrite, butyl nitrite, and other volatile substances.

These chemicals are put in a plastic bag or similar device and inhaled to develop psychoactive or intoxicating effects lasting from a few minutes to many hours. A mild stimulatory effect is described by abusers; unfortunately there is an inhibition reduction followed by unconsciousness. Specific complications are listed in Table 34-12. The usual young inhalant abuser stops this behavior, sometimes moving on to other illicit drugs. However, some remain with this drug class and become chronic inhalant abusers; these adolescents and adults usually present with many behavioral problems that may hinder management attempts.

TOBACCO

Despite the well-known dangers of tobacco addiction and the fact that smokers quickly become addicts until death, the acceptance of tobacco in

TABLE 34-2

PREVALENCE OF ILLICIT DRUG USE: 2003 MONITORING THE FUTURE SURVEY OF DRUG USE

Drug	Grade	Lifetime%	Annual%	30 Day%
Any illicit drug	8	22.8	16.1	9.7
	10	41.4	32.0	19.5
	12	51.1	39.3	24.1
Marijuana/hashish	8	17.5	12.8	7.5
	10	36.4	28.2	17.0
	12	46.1	34.9	21.2
Inhalants	8	15.8	8.7	4.1
	10	12.7	5.4	2.2
	12	11.2	3.9	1.5
Hallucinogens(all)	8	4.0	2.6	1.2
	10	6.9	4.1	1.5
	12	10.6	5.9	1.8
MDMA	8	3.2	2.1	0.7
	10	5.4	3.0	1.1
	12	8.3	4.5	1.3
Cocaine	8	3.6	2.2	0.9
	10	5.1	3.3	1.3
	12	7.7	4.8	2.1
Amphetamines	8	8.4	5.5	2.7
	10	13.1	9.0	4.3
	12	14.4	9.9	5.0
Alcohol	8	45.6	37.2	19.7
	10	66.0	59.3	35.4
	12	76.6	70.1	47.5
Cigarettes	8	28.4	No	10.2
	10	43.0	data	16.7
	12	53.7		24.4
Smokeless tobacco	8	11.3	No	4.1
	10	14.6	data	5.3
	12	17.0		6.7
Anabolic steroids	8	2.5	1.4	0.7
	10	3.0	1.7	0.8
	12	3.5	2.1	1.3

Source: Johnston LD, O'Malley PM, Bachman JG, Schulenberg JE (2004): *Monitoring the Future National Results on Adolescent Drug Use: Overview of Key Findings.* Bethesda, MD: National Institute on Drug Abuse, NIH Publication No. 04-5506, 2003.

TABLE 34-3

PERCENTAGE OF HIGH SCHOOL STUDENTS WHO INITIATED DRUG-RELATED BEHAVIORS BEFORE AGE 13 YEARS: YOUTH RISK BEHAVIOR SURVEY, 2003

	Smoked a Whole Cigarette	Drank Alcohol	Tried Marijuana
Female	16.4	23.3	6.9
Male	20.0	32.0	12.6

Source: Centers for Disease Control and Prevention. Youth Risk Behavior Surveillance: United States, 2003. *MMWR Morb Mortal Wkly Rep* 2004;53(SS2).

TABLE 34-4

PERCENTAGE OF STUDENTS REPORTING EPISODIC HEAVY ALCOHOL DRINKING: YOUTH RISK BEHAVIOR SURVEY, 2003*

Grade	Female	Male
9	20.9	18.8
10	27.2	27.7
11	29.4	34.1
12	34.5	39.5

*Episodic heavy drinking = drank 5 or more drinks of alcohols in a row on 1 or more of the 30 days preceding the survey.
Source: Centers for Disease Control and Prevention. Youth Risk Behavior Surveillance: United States, 2003. *MMWR Morb Mortal Wkly Rep* 2004;53(SS2).

TABLE 34-5

CAUSES OF SUBSTANCE ABUSE DISORDER

Rite of passage of puberty, from childhood to adulthood
Result of adolescent changes, especially in middle adolescence
Result of general societal chaos
Reflection of mirroring behavior of various adults
Encouragement of the media for euphoric drugs without sequelae
Availability and affordability of a wide range of illicit drugs
Result of dysfunctionality in the youth outside the range of normal

TABLE 34-6

FACTORS PROTECTIVE OF SUBSTANCE ABUSE IN ADOLESCENTS

Nurturing home environment
Good communication within family
Supportive parents, intact family, appropriate adult supervision
Positive self-esteem
Assertiveness
Social competence
Academic success
Good schools
Good general health
High intelligence
Positive adult role models
Peer group with positive personal attributes
Religious involvement
A personal sense of morality

Source: Patel DR, Greydanus DE: Substance abuse: A pediatric concern. *Ind J Pediatr* 1999;66:557–567.

the United States and the world is staggering. Governments around the world allow their citizens to grow, produce, and use tobacco products in various forms, whether as cigarettes, cigars, bidis, kreteks, or other forms. Cigars have enjoyed an increased popularity over the past decade, partly due to the promotion by famous sports stars in basketball and other sports that eagerly light up to signify a hard-won victory on the competitive trail. Baseball stars have likewise encouraged young, hopeful future stars to use smokeless tobacco, despite its dangers for mouth cancer and other adverse effects. Kreteks are clove cigarettes that contain a mixture of tobacco and cloves from Indonesia, while bidis (beddies) are hand-rolled, brown, tobacco flavored products popular in some countries, such as India.

The promotion by the tobacco companies and the media have contributed to the large number of adolescents who develop a lifetime addiction to tobacco, ensuring that the millions of adults who die each year from tobacco consumption are replaced by addicted youth who will smoke until the same fate consumes them years later; indeed, about 3000 adolescents start smoking cigarettes every day in the United States. High school seniors have a 58% life prevalence rate

TABLE 34-7

RISK FACTORS FOR SUBSTANCE ABUSE IN ADOLESCENTS

Genetics

Alcoholism among 1st or 2nd degree relatives

Male gender

Self/individual/personal

Abuse	Antisocial behavior	Parental rejection
Early onset of drug use	Aggressive temperament	Lack of self-control
Early sexual activity	Depression	Low self-esteem
Attention deficit disorders	Poor self-image	Euphoric/mood altering
Body modification (as cutting)	Learning disorders	Effects of drugs

Family

Dysfunctional family dynamics

Permissiveness

Authoritarianism

Parental conflict, divorce, separation

Poor supervision, lack of supervision

Poor parental role modeling

Community/environmental/societal

Easy availability of drugs and alcohol	Cultural and religious sanction
Acceptance of drug use behavior	Employment
Poor general quality of life in the neighborhood	
Media influence	Low religiosity
Criminal activities in neighborhood	Increased use of drugs and alcohol in certain ethnic groups

Peer group influence

Drug using peers	Curiosity
Rebellion	Desire to belong
Rites of passage of puberty	Independence
Risk-taking behavior	Early tobacco use

School/academic

Poor school performance

Poor school environment

Truancy

Source: Patel DR, Greydanus DE: Substance abuse: A pediatric concern. *Ind J Pediatr* 1999;66:557–567.

for cigarette smoking that represents a 22% daily consumption and a 37% use over the past survey in 2000. The lifetime prevalence has declined from 70.4% in 1999 to 58.4% in 2003 (Tables 34-2 and 34-3). Cigarettes remain the illicit drug most commonly consumed on a daily basis by teenagers in America and around many parts of the world. Nearly 10% of youth experiment with smokeless tobacco,

and the rate of cigar use during the previous 30 survey days in 2003 was 18.7% in high school students— 25.4% for males and 9.9% for females. The myth is common in adolescent groups that cigars are safer than cigarettes; data suggest that this is not the case.

Tobacco consumption is highly addictive due to nicotine. Tobacco consumption is often a drug consumed by young adolescents, and may signify future

TABLE 34-8

NONSPECIFIC INDICATORS OF SUBSTANCE ABUSE

Physical Indicators	Academic Indicators	Behavioral and Psychologic Indicators
Unexplained weight loss	Deterioration of short-term memory	Risk-taking behavior
Hypertension	Poor judgment	Mood swings
Red eyes	Falling grades	Depression, withdrawal
Nasal irritation	Frequent absence	Panic reaction
Frequent "colds" or "allergies"	Truancy	Acute psychosis
Hoarseness	Conflicts with teachers	Paranoia
Chronic cough	Suspension	Lying
Hemoptysis	Expulsion	Stealing
Chest pain		Promiscuity
Wheezing		Conflict with authorities and family members
Frequent unexplained injuries		Runaway behavior
Needle tracks		Altered sleep pattern
Blank stares into space		Altered appetite
Scratch marks		Poor hygiene
Tattoos		Loss of interest in extracurricular activities
Excessive acne		Drug using peers
Testicular atrophy		Preferences for dress, music, movies, identifying with drug using culture
Malaise		Drug paraphernalia

Source: Patel DR, Greydanus DE: Substance abuse: A pediatric concern. *Ind J Pediatr* 1999;66:557–567.

high-risk behaviors, such as sexual behavior, failure to use a condom, drinking and driving, and increased risk for other illicit drug consumption. A major risk factor for drunk driving is cigarette use before 14 years of age. Nicotine is absorbed over many areas, including the lungs, skin, gastrointestinal tract, and buccal mucosa. Smoking a cigarette allows

TABLE 34-9

COMORBID DISORDERS OF SUBSTANCE ABUSE DISORDER

Attention-deficit/hyperactivity disorder
Anxiety disorders
Conduct disorders
Mood disorders
Oppositional defiant disorder
Posttraumatic stress disorder
Psychosis

1–3 mg of nicotine to be absorbed by the smoker out of the 10 mg found in an average cigarette. Nicotine is quickly absorbed by the CNS nicotinic acetylcholine receptors. Other tobacco chemicals are dangerous as well, including tar, carbon monoxide, radioactive polonium, benzopyrene, carbon monoxide, others. Complications of chronic tobacco smoking are well-known and a partial list is provided in Table 34-13.

Nicotine Therapies

Tables 34-14 and 34-15 provide a list of medical products used to help tobacco addicts give up their drug, if motivated. Stopping the use of tobacco, once addicted, is difficult and the nicotine replacement products may double the chance of getting off this habit, perhaps from 15% to 30%. The use of bupropion in adults raises this to perhaps 40%, though studies in adolescents are limited. The clinician

TABLE 34-10

MCDONALD STAGES OF SUBSTANCE ABUSE

Stage	1. Learning Mood Swing	2. Seeking the Mood Swing	3. Preoccupation with the Mood Swing	4. Using Drugs to Feel Normal
Mood alteration	Euphoria Normal	Euphoria Normal Some pain	Euphoria Normal Definite pain	Euphoria Normal Marked pain
Feelings	Feels good; few consequences	Excitement Early guilt	Euphoric highs; doubts, including severe shame and guilt; depression, suicidal thoughts	Chronic guilt; shame, remorse, depression
Drugs	Tobacco Marijuana Alcohol	Tobacco, marijuana, alcohol plus inhalants, hashish, depressants, methamphetamine prescription drugs	All stages 2 and 3 plus psilocybin, PCP, LSD, cocaine	Whatever is available
Sources	Peers	Buying	Selling	Any possible way
Behavior	Little detectable change; moderate After-the-fact lying	Dropping extracurricular activities and hobbies; mixed friends (straight and drug users); dress changing; erratic school performance and truancy; unpredictable mood and attitude swings; manipulative behavior	"Cool" appearance; straight friends dropped; family fights (verbal or physical); stealing (police incidents); pathologic lying; school failure; truancy, expulsion, jobs lost	Physical deterioration (weight loss, chronic cough); severe mental deterioration (memory loss and flashbacks); paranoia volcanic anger; school dropout; frequent overdosing
Frequency	Progress to weekend use	Weekend use progressing to four to five times per week; some solo use	Daily Frequent solo use	All day, every day

Source: Patel DR, Greydanus DE: Substance abuse: A pediatric concern. *Ind J Pediatr* 1999;66:557–567.

should counsel the teen on a regular basis, when seen in the office, that tobacco consumption is dangerous and stopping is the best option. The adolescent female who is pregnant or the youth with asthma or repeated bronchitis may present special circumstances the clinician can use to enforce the need to stop tobacco as soon as possible. Though not recommended, youth may continue with tobacco consumption and the nicotine therapy (NT) product without clear negative consequences.

The patch is usually prescribed for 2 months in which the high dose patch is used the first month, and the lower strength the second month; it is changed once a day, usually in the morning. The patch is not placed over a hairy part of the body, and like other patch technologies, may induce local dermatitis that is usually controlled with topical hydrocortisone; apply the patch only while the youth is awake if insomnia or intense dreaming occurs. If the gum is chosen, tobacco addicts smoking over 25 cigarettes a day should start

TABLE 34-11

TYPES OF INHALANT DRUGS

A. Solvents
  1. Industrial or household solvents or
     solvent-containing products
    a. Paint thinners or solvents
    b. Degreasers (dry-cleaning fluids)
    c. Gasoline
    d. Glues
  2. Art or office supply solvents
    a. Correction fluids
    b. Felt-tip-maker fluid
    c. Electronic contact cleaners

B. Gases
  1. Gases used in household or commercial
     products
    a. Butane lighters
    b. Propane tanks
    c. Whipping cream aerosols or dispensers
     (whippets)
    d. Refrigerant gases
  2. Household aerosol propellant and associated
     solvents
    a. Found in spray paints
    b. Found in hair or deodorant sprays
    c. Found in fabric protector sprays
  3. Medical anesthetic gases
    a. Ether
    b. Chloroform
    c. Halothane
    d. Nitrous oxide

C. Nitrites (aliphatic nitrites)
    a. Cyclohexyl nitrite (available to general
     public)
    b. Amyl nitrite (available only with prescription)
    c. Butyl nitrite (illegal substance)

Source: Greydanus DE, Patel DR: Substance abuse in adolescents: A complex conundrum for the clinician. *Pediatr Clin North Am* 2003;59(5):1179–1223.

TABLE 34-12

EFFECTS OF INHALANTS

A. Hearing loss
  1. Toluene (paint sprays, glues, dewaxers)
  2. Trichloroethylene (cleaning fluids, correction
    fluids)
B. Peripheral neuropathies or limb spasms
  1. Hexane (glues, gasoline)
  2. Nitrous oxide (whipping cream, gas cylinders)
C. CNS or brain damage: toluene
D. Bone marrow damage: benzene (gasoline)
E. Liver and kidney damage
  1. Toluene-containing substances
  2. Chlorinated hydrocarbons
    a. Correction fluids
    b. Dry-cleaning fluids
F. Blood oxygen depletion
  1. Organic nitrites (*poppers, amyl, bold*, and *rush*)
  2. Methylene chloride
    a. Varnish removers
    b. Paint thinners
G. Death
H. Kaposi's sarcoma

Source: Greydanus DE, Patel DR: Substance abuse in adolescents: A complex conundrum for the clinician. *Pediatr Clin North Am* 2003;59(5):1179–1223.

gum and self-consciousness about chewing the gum in public prevent many youth from using this NT technology. Self-limiting adverse effects of this gum include hiccups, jaw ache, mouth soreness, and dyspepsia.

TABLE 34-13

ADVERSE EFFECTS OF TOBACCO USE

Severe addiction
Lung cancer
Emphysema
Laryngeal carcinoma
Other cancers (as oral cancer from chewing tobacco)
Heart disease
Keratosis of the mucosal
In utero effects: lower birth weight, ADHD
Increased cough and dyspnea
Worsening of preexistent asthma

with the 4 mg gum, eventually lowering to the 2 mg dose as improvement occurs. Avoid acidic liquids for 15 minutes before and during gum chewing, since absorption of the gum's nicotine may result. Table 34-16 provides an outline of instruction given to the patient using the gum. The bitter taste of the

TABLE 34-14

PHARMACOLOGIC PRODUCTS AVAILABLE IN THE UNITED STATES

Nicotine Medications	
Nicotine gum	Nicorette OTC
Nicorette	DS OTC
Nicotine patch	Nicoderm CQ (SmithKline Beecham) OTC
	Nicotrol Patch (McNeil) OTC
	Habitrol (Novartis)
	Prostep (Lederle)
Nicotine inhaler	Nicotrol Inhaler (McNeil)
Nasal spray	Nicotrol Nasal Spray (McNeil)
Nonnicotine medications	
Bupropion	Zyban SR (Glaxo Welcome) sustained-release tablets

Source: Patel DR, Greydanus DE: Office interventions for adolescent smokers. *Adolesc Med* 2000;11(3):1–11.

The purpose of the nicotine inhaler is to allow the smoker to copy the hand-to mouth habit of smoking; low nicotine levels are delivered via the buccal mucosa, but enough nicotine is provided with 80 inhalations over 20 minutes; 4 mg out of the cartridge's 10 mg of nicotine are usually delivered. The smoker uses the inhaler for about 3 months, and then tapers off over the next 3 months or so. Side effects include dyspepsia and irritation of the mouth, nose, or throat; coughing may also develop and like the other adverse effects, usually improves with time. The other NT method is the nasal spray that is used

TABLE 34-15

NICOTINE PATCH REGIMENS

Brand	*Duration*	*Dosage*
Nicoderm	4 weeks	21 mg/24 h
Habitrol	then 2 weeks	14 mg/24 h
	then 2 weeks	7 mg/24 h
Prostep	4 weeks	22 mg/24 h
	then 4 weeks	11 mg/24 h
Nicotrol	8 weeks	15 mg/24 h

Source: Patel DR, Greydanus DE: Office interventions for adolescent smokers. *Adolesc Med* 2000;11(3):1–11.

TABLE 34-16

RECOMMENDATIONS FOR USE OF NICOTINE GUM

Chew a piece each hour for 6 weeks.
Then, chew a piece every 2 h for 3 weeks.
Finally, chew a piece every 4 h for 3 weeks.
Maximum limit is 30 pieces per day for the 2 mg gum and 20 pieces per day for the 4 mg gum.
Chewing instructions:
  Chew slowly until a peppery taste appears (often after 15 chews)
  Then put the gum between the cheek and buccal mucosa until the peppery taste has disappeared (often 1 min)
  Start chewing again and repeat the above cycle
  Get rid of the gum when the peppery taste is gone (often 30 min).

from 8 to 40 doses per day or not over 5 inhalations per hour. Each dose provides 1 mg of nicotine and it is used for at least 3 months. Reported negative effects include bronchospasm (thus, is not used in those with asthma), cough, sneezing, watery eyes, nasal irritation, and rhinitis.

Bupropion

Bupropion may be used to reduce the tobacco addict's nicotine cravings while improving or preventing the problems of depression and weight gain noted in those stopping tobacco use without such pharmacologic help. The smoker is prescribed Zyban at 150 mg once a day for 3 days, and then twice daily (not over 300 mg a day). The medication is a sustained-release product that is given at least 8 hours apart and the patient may keep smoking for a temporary period while on this medication, if necessary. The clinician should always work with his patient to establish a quit date in the near future. Bupropion is contraindicated in epilepsy and situations that may increase seizure risks, including CNS tumor, eating disorder, medications that lower seizure threshold; it is also contraindicated in individuals taking monoamine oxidase (MAO) inhibitors. Adverse reactions include dry mouth, headaches, insomnia, tremors, and skin changes. Adult studies have shown some benefit for adult smokers placed on clonidine or nortriptyline in helping these individuals quit nicotine products. Others have been used, but not shown to be of help with adult or adolescent smokers: doxepin, oral dextrose, buspirone, naltrexone, and mecamylamine.

ALCOHOL

Alcohol is another commonly abused drug in adolescents, with high school seniors admitting to a lifetime prevalence of over 80%, over 50% use over the 30 days prior to a survey, and 4% daily drinking (Tables 34-2 to 34-4). The average age of alcohol initiation is 12 years and usually occurs in young adolescents who are also smoking cigarettes. Males tend to have higher rates of drinking than females and Caucasian teens more than African-American or Hispanic teens. This pattern also increases in college students. Binge drinking is officially defined as having 5 or more drinks in a row in males and 4 or more in females; such behavior may result in blacking out episodes. Further questioning of adolescents reveals that 13% have driven a motor vehicle after drinking alcohol and 31% have been in a vehicle with a driver under the influence of alcohol. In studies of those killed via suicide or a motor vehicle accident, approximately 50% were under the influence of alcohol. Since consumption of alcohol is a common pattern with many adolescents, clinicians should ask about this during examinations; established questionnaires, as the CRAFFT Screening Test for Adolescent Substance Abuse are helpful (Knight, 2002).

Alcohol is a chemical providing CNS depression that is favored by many for the transient euphoria that occurs to the drinker; continued use may lead to addiction, with the development of dependence (physiologic and psychologic) and tolerance. Beer usually contains 3%–6% alcohol, wine contains 12%, and "hard" liquors 50%. Impaired judgment for driving may occur at a blood alcohol concentration (BAC) of 0.10 g/dL or lower; legal intoxication is typically set at 0.05–0.10 g/dL. Consumption of large amounts of alcohol leads to acute alcohol intoxication with resultant respiratory depression, unconsciousness, and even death. Adolescents may continue with a drinking pattern that extends beyond the experimental phase and leads to more advanced stages of drug abuse. Alcohol abuse disorder is diagnosed mainly

based on a comprehensive history. Excessive drinking patterns are typically found in youth who come from both families where excessive drinking patterns occur and where abstinence is the rule.

Chronic excessive drinking patterns may lead to a variety of abnormal laboratory tests, including anemia, macrocytosis, and elevations in a variety of blood tests, such as uric acid, alkaline phosphatase, bilirubin, glutamic-oxaloacetic, or pyruvic transaminases and gamma glutamyl transpeptidase. Excessive drinkers may develop gastritis, pancreatitis, worsening health patterns of other chronic disorders (as diabetes mellitus or epilepsy), and death from intoxication. The alcohol withdrawal syndrome is characterized by seizures, tremors, hallucinations, and delirium tremens. The fetal alcohol syndrome is a well-known result of drinking while pregnant.

The adolescent who presents with acute alcohol intoxication is treated promptly with gastric emptying, rehydration with intravenous fluids, glucose, respiratory support, and, if necessary, dialysis. Clinicians should consider the possibility of additional drugs or of a complicating head injury, if the respiratory depression is more than what alcohol ingestion history suggests. A variety of medications have been used to help manage alcohol withdrawal syndrome; these include clorazepate, diazepam, various antipsychotics, lorazepam, and chlordiazepoxide. Approved medications in adults with alcohol dependence include naltrexone, tiapride, acamprosate, calcium carbimide, and disulfiram. Many other drugs have been used that are not approved for alcohol dependence in adults; these include selective serotonin reuptake inhibitors, tricyclic antidepressants, buspirone, carbamazepine, and nalmefene. Youth with excessive drinking patterns should be referred to experts in this disorder. There are a number of beneficial community programs, such as Mothers Against Drunk Drivers (MADD), Alcoholics Anonymous (AA), and Alateen.

MARIJUANA

Though marijuana does not have the status of being a legal drug for adults, like tobacco and alcohol, its classic euphoric and hallucinogenic effects have made it a very popular drug, one that many advocate should become legalized. Its many street names hints at its acceptance by the drug culture: *pot, weed, grass, hash, Ganja, doobs, BC Bud*, and many more. Pot accounts for three-quarters of the illicit drug use in the United States; in 2003, a lifetime use was reported by 46.1% of high school seniors, including 34.9% over the past survey year, and 21.2% over the past month of this survey (Tables 34-2 and 34-3).

The chemical at the heart of the drug abuser's fondness for marijuana is delta-9-tetrahydrocannabinol (THC). The pot product in the 1960s and 1970s contained 2–3% THC in contrast to the current versions ranging from 3% to 9%. Marijuana is smoked and the typical cigarette has about 20 mg of THC, though variations are noted. Marijuana remains for up to 1 month after even a single joint. A popular way to smoke this drug is with a blunt, which is a hollowed out cigarette filled with marijuana. The drug may be combined with other drugs to enhance its pleasure in the user; for example, marijuana may be combined with PCP while additives of the past included methaqualone and glutethimide. The marijuana cigarette (joint) or hand-rolled version is dipped into PCP that has been dissolved in an organic solvent (as formaldehyde); this mixture is then dried and smoked for enhanced euphoria. This concoction is called *wet, Sherms*, or *water*. Drugs like alcohol and diazepam augment marijuana's sedative effects, while other drugs, like amphetamines or cocaine, potentiate the stimulatory effects of marijuana. Marijuana can also be eaten in food prepared with this drug; such foods include brownies, spaghetti, or cookies made with THC. Dronabinol is a capsule of THC being researched to treat emesis induced by chemotherapy and to manage glaucoma by lowering the intraocular pressure.

Advocates for the legalization of marijuana are excited about the euphoria that THC causes within a few minutes of its use and may then enjoy for hours. Despite claims by THC enthusiasts of its safety, the record of this still illicit drug counters this claim. Chronic marijuana users develop a psychologic addiction and a withdrawal syndrome comparable to that seen with heroin addiction. Psychologic dependency and tolerance are seen in heavy pot smokers; after stopping pot, a flu-like reaction can be seen beginning in 24–60 hours, and lasting up to

14 days. Another complication of stopping this drug for these users is the development of persistent insomnia; this problem has been noted after stopping chronic benzodiazepine use as well. Trazodone has been helpful in some of these postpot insomnia cases.

Research has described cognitive impairment in chronic marijuana users that includes confusion, memory dysfunction, and altered time perceptions. Such problems can significantly interfere with successful adaptation to the demands of school, work, driving, and other issues. A variety of psychologic reactions have been reported in chronic pot users, including loss of interest in work or school, disinterest in social obligations, and extreme lethargy; some have called this the amotivational syndrome of marijuana use. Other psychologic sequelae of pot use include the development of anxiety, depression, overt hallucinations, violent behavior, and fear. In patients with known or unknown mental illness, the use of pot can lead to overt depression, mood shift, or an atypical psychosis.

Medial complications of marijuana use are also many and include amenorrhea, interference with DNA functioning, immunologic dysfunction, sperm reduction, chronic cough, bronchitis, and bronchospasm. The combination of pot and driving lead to many accidents, injuries, and deaths on the highways each year. The effects of second hand smoke and effects on the fetus are under investigation.

AMPHETAMINES

Amphetamine is classified as a CNS stimulant abused in hopes of becoming euphoric, reducing fatigue, shedding unwanted weight, extending sports energy/performance, and gaining a better attention span. The Monitor the Future study of 2003 noted that high school seniors had a 14.4% lifetime use that included 9.9% over the previous survey year and 5.0% over the past survey month (Table 34-2). Amphetamine can be abused orally, subcutaneously, or intravenously; street names include *meth, speed, chalk*, and others. Tolerance can occur with amphetamine abusers, and an overdose can induce hyperthermia, hypertension, seizures, cardiac arrhythmias, and death. An abstinence or withdrawal syndrome

TABLE 34-17

AMPHETAMINE ADVERSE REACTIONS

Tolerance
Withdrawal syndrome
Tachycardia
Hypertension
Anorexia
Exhaustion
Insomnia
Weight loss
Anxiety
Hyperactivity
Hyperhidrosis
Mydriasis
Personality changes
Psychotic experiences

can occur, resulting in symptoms such as severe apathy, hypersomnia, and depression. Complications of amphetamine use are multiple, including those listed in Table 34-17. Intravenous use of this and other drugs can lead to various infections, including endocarditis, HIV/AIDS, hepatitis, and others. Adolescents prescribed Adderall and Ritalin for attention-deficit/hyperactivity disorder (ADHD) should be monitored that this medication is not being abused or diverted to others for self-management of ADHD or for abuse. Short-acting methylphenidate (MPH) tablets can be crushed and the contents snorted; large doses can induce stroke, psychosis, and seizures. The long-acting preparations reduce the dispersion and abuse problems.

Methamphetamine

This drug is an *N*-methyl homolog of amphetamine and has a marked stimulant effect on the CNS. Its acceptance among drug users is suggested by the many street names for this chemical, such as *meth, ice, crystal, crank, fire, glass*, and others. Easily made in secret laboratories by amateur chemists, it becomes an odorless, white powder with a bitter taste and ready solvability in liquids. It can be produced as crystals that look like ice and is sold on the

streets or through illicit drug networks. In 1999, methamphetamine was tried by 2.5% of 8th graders, 4.0% of 10th graders, and 4.3% of 12th graders; there has been a gradual decrease in its use by adolescents, perhaps because of concerns over side effects.

Methamphetamine is consumed as a pill or its powder snorted, inducing a euphoria (*high*) that is addictive; when inhaled while smoking it or injecting it intravenously, a very intense and rapid "flash" or "rush" develops for a few minutes. Increasing dosage and frequency are needed to maintain this addictive feeling of pleasure. Dopamine is released in the CNS and thus, mood and body movements may be effected; a Parkinsonian-like movement disorder may develop. Under the influence of this drug, the person feels more awake, has less need for sleep, and increases the physical activity level; also, there may be anorexia (can be severe) with weight loss. Speech becomes more excited and vital signs are increased (i.e., increased temperature, pulse, and blood pressure). Since CNS cells with dopamine and serotonin are destroyed, low levels of dopamine can lead to cognitive dysfunction and depression. Some of the adverse effects of methamphetamine are listed in Table 34-18, and, if intravenous abuse occurs, includes endocarditis, HIV/AIDS, hepatitis B, other sexually transmitted diseases.

Management of meth addiction is difficult, and as with other substance abuse disorders, is dependent on the motivation of the addict to give up illicit medications. Research is seeking medication to block the euphoric effects of methamphetamine, including the development of an antibody to render the meth molecules benign.

TABLE 34-18

MAJOR ADVERSE EFFECTS OF METHAMPHETAMINE

Irritability, anxiety, confusion, memory loss, insomnia
Tremors, seizures
Hypertension, cardiac damage, cardiovascular
  collapse, death
Insomnia
Worsening aggressive and violent behavior
Paranoia and psychotic behavior

MDMA (Ecstasy)

3,4-Methylenedioxymethamphetamine (MDMA) is a phenethylamine that is part of a group of over 100 hallucinogenic chemicals; it resembles both a hallucinogen (mescaline) and a stimulant ([meth]amphetamine). A close conger of this drug is called Eve or 3,4-methylenedioxy-ethamphetamine (MDEA). Historically, MDMA was developed in 1912 in Germany as an appetite suppressant and was used 50 years later by psychotherapists to enhance their sessions; in 1985 the FDA made MDMA a schedule I drug. In 2003, high school seniors had an 8.3% lifetime experience with MDMA that included 4.5% over the past year and 1.3% over the past month of survey (Table 34-2).

MDMA is a "designer drug" that is a white, crystalline powder in its pure form, and red or brown if made with various impurities. It has many street names, such as *ecstasy, XTC, Adam, dex, bean, M, E, roll, diamonds, clarity, lover's speed, X*, and others. It leads to a high sense of energizing euphoria and sexuality that has become popular at all night dances called *raves* or *trances*; effects can last for several hours, sometime prolonged up to several days. It may be abused in a stacked pattern, with increasingly high doses being used. A number of side effects are described, as listed in Table 34-19.

The sensation of thirst is reduced and dehydration can result along with hyperthermia, hyponatremia, and cerebral edema. Unsuspecting youth taking high doses at raves may develop muscle breakdown, malignant hyperthermia, and failure of kidneys and the cardiovascular system. Abusers of this drug with undiagnosed vascular malformations may develop intracerebral hemorrhage. It is a popular date-rape drug. Its mescaline-like effects involved serotoninergic neuron destruction, with damage to thought and memory abilities. An anxious state of mind can develop with depersonalization, cognitive dysfunction, and behavioral problems. Anxiety, panic attacks, and paranoia may develop for weeks after stopping this drug. The risk for congenital anomalies increases if taken during pregnancy.

Drug abusers like to combine their drug of choice to enhance their pleasures and MDMA is no exception. For example, MDMA may be added to alcohol, marijuana, lysergic acid diethylamide (LSD), dextromethorphan, and others. Preparations with menthol, ephedrine, or camphor may be placed in the nose or on the chest while taking MDMA. Chemicals may be abused that are ecstasy-like in appearance, including ketamine, alpha-methyl fentanyl and ephedrine tablets (*Chinese ephedra, Ma Huang, herbal ecstasy*). The ephedrine found in herbal ecstasy has been banned by the FDA. Large amounts of these MDMA-like chemicals can lead to elevated blood pressure, cardiac arrhythmias, heart attacks, strokes, and death.

HALLUCINOGENIC DRUGS

Mood and state of mind are altered by hallucinogenic drugs and dissociative drugs (Tables 34-2 and 34-20). Drugs classified as hallucinogens classically induce visual, auditory, or tactile hallucinations; they include LSD, mescaline (peyote), psilocybin, and psilocin (mushrooms or *shrooms*). Drugs classified as dissociative drugs do not induce hallucinations per se, but lead to feelings of detachment called a dissociate reaction; they include PCP and ketamine (Greydanus, 2005). Trypamines (Table 34-14) refer to a number of naturally occurring chemicals classified as schedule I hallucinogens typically obtained from mushrooms found in South America, Mexico, and the United States; they can also be synthetically made.

TABLE 34-19

SIDE EFFECTS OF MDMA

Tachycardia and hypertension

Fatigue, sweating, and sleep disorders

Hyperthermia, dehydration and possible heat stroke

Confusion and paranoia

Muscle spasms

Depression, anxiety (including panic attacks)

Irreversible CNS damage with memory loss with
  chronic abuse

Intracerebral hemorrhage

Muscle breakdown

Organ dysfunction: CNS, liver, renal

LSD

PCP

Tryptamines
- Psilocybin (O-phosphoryl-4-hydroxy-N, N-ethyltryptamine)
- Psilocin (4-hydroxy-N,N-dimethyltryptamine)
- Dimethyltryptamine (DMT)
- Diethyltryptamine (DET)
- Alpha-ethyltryptamine (AET)
- N,N-diisopropyl-5-methoxytryptamine (Foxy-Methoxy)
- Alpha-methyltryptamine (AMT)
- 5-Methoxy-alpha-methyltryptamine (5-MeO-AMT) (alpha-O, alpha, O-DMS)
- Bufotenine (bufagin, 5-hydroxy-N, N-dimethyltryptamine)

Bufotenine is found in certain mushrooms, seeds, and the skin glands of the red and green Cane Toad (*Bufo marinus*).

Phencyclidine

PCP is an arylcyclohexalamine causing inhibition of neuronal catecholamines with resultant adrenergic potentiation. It can be made by amateur chemists in illegal laboratories as liquid, tablet, or powder; the powder can be added to joints (marijuana cigarettes) to enhance the THC euphoria. Street names for PCP include *pill, peace, peace pill, angel dust, hog, sheets, sternly*, and others. The drug sets up a powerful distortion of reality with sensory perception alterations (synesthesias involving sound and sight) and emotional changes involving euphoria and powerful fears; time and place are also altered. Tolerance to the drug develops and the mixture of changes can result in the perception of having a "good" trip or a "bad" trip. Cases of psychosis "flashbacks" are well-known; flashbacks may be precipitated by antihistamines or marijuana. An overdose can lead to profound respiratory depression, coma, and death.

The usual management of negative reaction to PCP ingestion is to keep the youth having the "bad" trip in a padded room that is dark and under close observation; diazepam (10–20 mg orally or 10 mg intramuscularly every 4 hours) or haloperidol is helpful for severe agitation. Patients die from PCP because of the development of hypothermia, seizures, trauma, blood pressure changes (hypotension or hypertension), respiratory depression, and/or psychotic delirium. D_3 agonists may be used for psychosis and research is seeking to find medication to inactivate PCP using an antibody mechanism.

Lysergic Acid Diethylamide

LSD is a well-known hallucinogenic drug that can induce its classic euphoria and hallucinogenic state in 20 μg placed on a sugar cube, postage stamp, paper blotter, or other small object. It is found naturally in morning glory seeds or on the rye fungus (*Ergot*); it is made in clandestine laboratories as an odorless, tasteless, colorless drug that is easily hidden and given at raves to unsuspecting victims. Street names include *acid, sugar, dots, cubes, L, big D, blotters*, and others. It increases serotonin and potentiates sympathetic activity, with resultant fever, mydriasis, tachycardia, and hypertension. Tolerance is well-known as is the classic "bad" trip and unpleasant flashback. Management of a youth having a negative experience is reassurance and observation until recovery occurs. If severe agitation or prolonged seizures occurs, haloperidol has been used.

DATE RAPE DRUGS

Various chemicals have been developed and identified as lowering inhibitions and/or consciousness so that sexual perpetrators can more easily sexually assault their victims. The so-called "date rape drugs" have potent sedative and hypnotic effects, especially combined with other drugs, like alcohol. Table 34-21 lists the date rape drugs, also known as club drugs or party drugs that are popular at raves and other gatherings where predators roam. These chemicals are available on the street, on the internet, and some are openly sold in so-called "health" or "nutrition" stores under such labels as "party drugs," "sleep aids," or "muscle builders." Adolescents must be warned

TABLE 34-21
CLUB (DATE RAPE) DRUGS

Rohypnol (Flunitrazepam)
LSD
Methamphetamine
Methylenedioxy-methamphetamine (Ecstasy, MDMA)
GHB
Gamma-butyryl lactone
Butanediol
Ketamine

about these drugs, about how they are quietly slipped into beverages, and subsequent sexual assault occurs with little if any later memory of the attack.

Flunitrazepam (Rohypnol)

This is a CNS depressant that has powerful anxiolytic, sedative, and anticonvulsant effects; drugs in this same class are Ambien, Xanax, Versed, Klonopin, and others. Flunitrazepam is made in Switzerland and available in Europe by prescription for treatment of insomnia and is also used as a presurgery anesthetic. It has a number of street names, including *Rope, Roche, Mexican valium, roofies*, and *forget-me pills.* Its use as date rape drug comes from its availability as a easily hidden chemical (colorless, odorless, and tasteless) that is easily slipped into the beverage of an unsuspecting victim; the drug decreases sexual inhibition and blackouts or short-term memory loss for events, such as a sexual assault. It induces anterograde amnesia, making it difficult for the assaulted victim to identify the attacker. Other adverse effects include drowsiness, confusion, dizziness, hypotension, visual disturbances, urinary retention, and others.

Flunitrazepam is also an addictive drug used as an adjunctive or alternative drug to LSD or marijuana; its popularity has increased 50% over the past several years. Increasingly higher doses are needed to achieve the desired euphoria; its effects are enhanced by alcohol.

Gamma-hydroxybutyrate (GHB)

There are many street names for this central nervous depressant, including *liquid ecstasy, liquid X,*

liquid E, liquid XTC, Oxy-Sleep, Scoop, fantasy, easy lay, soap, salty water, cherry meth, goop, and many others. GHB leads to reduced inhibition and heightened euphoria; as a colorless and odorless chemical, its ability to induce sedation and amnesia makes it another popular date-rape drug. It does have a soapy or salty taste, leading to its street names as *soap, salty water*, and others. The sedative effect develops within 20 minutes, peaks on 1–2 hours, lasts for 4 hours, and is quickly cleared from the body.

Individuals who take drugs in efforts to enhance their sports abilities or appearance use GHB; body builders and athletes believe it increases endogenous human growth hormone (HGH) while asleep, leading to increased muscle size and strength. It is also used in single doses to enhance or mimic the euphoric effects of alcohol; over time, higher doses are needed for this effect. GHB is a CNS depressant and respiratory depression along with seizures may occur, especially when adding other drugs, such as heroin, LSD, psilocybin, or alcohol. GHB was classified as a schedule I substance in 2000, though it is under study as possible management for cataplexy.

Gamma-butyrolactone (GBL)

As GHB becomes more difficult to get, precursors of GHB, such as GBL and 1-4-butanediol (BD)—an industrial solvent), are becoming popular in efforts to enhance sexuality and development of euphoria. A number of street names are noted for GBL, including *Blue Nitro, Blue Nitro Vitality, GH Revitalizer, Gamma G, Remforce*, and others. GHB and BD may be sold in health food stores and marketed as aphrodisiacs, dietary products, muscle-building chemicals, and others. BD has been banned by the FDA as a potentially life-threatening drug. Both are dangerous drugs and should be avoided.

Ketamine

Ketamine has been approved since 1970 for use as an injectable veterinary anesthetic. It is abused to produce dream-like, hallucinatory dissociate states. Its street names include *K, Special K, Cat Valium*, others. Abusers obtain it as a white powder to snort it and add it to marijuana or tobacco; intramuscular abuse is also noted. In low doses, it can lead to memory dysfunction, lowering of attention span, and learning impairment. In high doses, it can induce hypertension, delirium, amnesia, motor impairment, respiratory depression, and death.

COCAINE

Cocaine is an alkaloid derived from *Erythroxylon coca*, a South American plant. It is a CNS stimulant taken intranasally or intravenously; it can also be chewed (as coca leaves), swallowed, smoked, and inhaled. It was well-known as a crystalline, water-soluble powder produced from alkaloidal paste of coca leaves. Popular cocaine versions are "free base" and "crack" that are smoked. Free-based cocaine is vaporized in a bong (water pipe) or other object (as a soda can with a hole in it), while crack is named for pea-sized, cocaine bicarbonate pellets produced with ammonia or sodium bicarbonate (baking soda); the crackling sound is heard when it is heated to remove its hydrochloride component. Crack may be crushed, tobacco added, then smoked; mannitol, quinine, or marijuana can also be added.

In 2003, high school seniors reported a lifetime use of cocaine of 7.7% (vs. 9.5% in 1999); this included either crack, powder, or free-base cocaine. In 2003, 4.0% of seniors had tried cocaine over the previous 30 days of the survey versus 4.8% in 1999 (Table 34-2). The popularity of crack cocaine especially is due to its relative inexpensive price and its addictive ability. Over 50% of the street cocaine is crack cocaine.

Cocaine interferes with the reuptake of neuronal catecholamine and the reabsorption of dopamine. A powerful euphoria develops quickly if smoked or used intravenously (mainlined). Irritability and fatigue develop after the euphoria disappears. Severe psychologic and physiologic addictions develop in addition to tolerance. Table 34-22 lists some of the cocaine adverse reactions. Various chemicals are added to intensify the euphoria. Mixing alcohol with cocaine produces *cocaethylene* in the liver, leading to a more potent and longer-lasting euphoria as well as some blunting of cocaine side effects; however, the risk of sudden death is also increased. The risk of sudden death is also increased with *speedballing* or mixing cocaine with heroin.

TABLE 34-22

ADVERSE EFFECTS OF COCAINE

Aggressive paranoia
Angina pectoris
Anxiety
Confusion
Fontal lobe infarction
Hyperpyrexia
Hypertension
Intravenous needle complications (including endocarditis, hepatitis B, HIV/AIDS)
Irritability and restlessness
Peripheral blood vessel constriction
Pregnancy complications
Increased premature delivery
Abruption (bleeding between placenta and uterine wall)
Adverse neurodevelopmental sequelae in infant
Vascular spasm-induced limb reduction anomalies and strokes
Pupillary dilation
Myocardial infarction
Nasal septum infection and perforation
Tachycardia
Seizures
Ventricular arrhythmia and sudden death
Aggressive paranoia

Management of Cocaine Addiction

Short-acting beta-blockers and short-acting vasodilators (as esmolol) are used for cocaine-induced tachycardia and hypertension. Long-acting vasodilators are avoided, since they may induce severe hypotension in cocaine intoxication, a process that is usually a short, self-limited condition. Some cocaine addicts have ADHD and in using MPH find that MPH may reduce their use of cocaine.

Cocaine addiction is a CNS disorder that involves noradrenergic and dopaminergic pathways in the midbrain reward center; multiple reward centers are involved and medication for this difficult-to-treat CNS disorder must be effective in various areas of the brain. Table 34-23 identifies proposed psychopharmacologic mechanisms for treatment of

TABLE 34-23

POTENTIAL MECHANISM TO MANAGE COCAINE ADDICTION

Cocaine molecules are bound and prevented from movement into the CNS via the blood-brain barrier
Cocaine molecules are converted into harmless (inactive) particles
A vaccine using an antibody-type response eliminates the cocaine molecule
Cocaine molecules are changed into inactive fragments by "Catalytic" antibodies

cocaine addiction. If there is additional drug addiction, management of the other addictions may help with the cocaine disorder, as for example the use of naltrexone or disulfiram for coexistent alcoholism.

OPIOIDS

Table 34-24 provides a list of opiate narcotics, a group of illicit and legal drugs that have potent addiction potential. Some prescribed opiates are obtained by addicts from unsuspecting clinicians, stolen from home supplies of medicine, or bought on the streets. Oxycodone is abused by some in place of heroin, either by snorting the crushed pill or intravenous use after boiling the oxycodone powder. Street names for oxycodone include *oxycotton, OXY, OC*, and *killers*. Another narcotic with major addiction potential is fentanyl, a drug with 10 times the addiction potential of heroin.

TABLE 34-24

NARCOTIC OPIATES

Codeine
Heroin
Morphine
Methadone
Meperidine
Propoxyphene
Oxycodone
Fentanyl
Pentazocine

Heroin (named on the street as *smack, junk, China white, Mexican brown*) is identified by chemists as diacetyl morphine hydrochloride; it is used in a snuff form, subcutaneously (skin-popping), and intravenously. As the price of heroin dropped along with a 40% increase in drug purity, there was a doubling of high school seniors using heroin from 1990 to 1996. The mean age of heroin abuse was 27 years of age in 1988 and 19 years of age in 1995. The 2003 Monitor the Future survey noted that 1.5% of high school seniors had a lifetime use of heroin, including 0.8% over the past year and 0.4% over the past month of the survey. Heroin abuse increases as high seniors leave school and is also increased in school dropouts.

A heroin abuser often starts off snorting heroin, becomes addicted, and progresses to smoking or intravenous use leading to physical addiction, psychologic dependence, and a narcotic withdrawal syndrome. Youth who smoke or snort heroin may mistakenly assume this will not lead to intravenous use; the younger the user starts, the greater the risk for relapse with attempts at cessation. *Speedballing* refers to combining of heroin with cocaine to intensify the heroin euphoria while blunting its sedative effects.

Table 34-25 provides a list of medical complications of heroin abuse, including death from an overdose that causes respiratory depression and

TABLE 34-25

MEDICAL COMPLICATIONS OF HEROIN ABUSE

Amenorrhea
Endocarditis (from *Staphylococcus aureus*)
False positive VDRL
Fat necrosis
HIV/AIDS
Hepatitis (B and C)
Lipodystrophy
Osteomyelitis
Peptic ulcer disease
Pulmonary edema and pneumonia
Respiratory arrest
Skin infections
Tetanus

pulmonary edema. Clinicians can look for the use of tattoos to hide heroin-induced puncture wounds or needle-track marks. Newborns of mothers on heroin may develop a withdrawal syndrome; heroin withdrawal in utero may lead to meconium aspiration, bile pneumonitis, and severe respiratory distress.

Opioid dependence is a CNS disorder involving multiple brain receptors that become altered by addiction, leading to drug dependence and tolerance. Management of this complex neurobiologic disorder should not include incarceration, but efforts at multiple levels to help motivated addicts recover. Acute detoxification treatment is important followed by residential and outpatient management that includes community programs such as Narcotics Anonymous.

Table 34-26 lists medications that can be of help in managing heroin addiction. Naltrexone (*ReVia*, *Depade*) is an opiate antagonist used to manage opiate addiction that includes those with coexistent alcohol dependence. Methadone has been used since the 1960s to block narcotic effects and avoid providing the addict with opiate euphoria; it also is used to remove withdrawal symptomatology and reduce the need or desire for other drugs.

Methadone is given once a day to addicts that are officially 18 years of age or older in doses ranging from 40 to 400 mg. Longer-acting methadone alternatives include levomethadyl acetate and buprenorphine. The combination of buprenorphine/naloxone given sublingually provides help to addicts at least equal to that of methadone; naloxone is used to prevent diversion of buprenorphine to intravenous administration.

T A B L E   3 4 - 2 6

MEDICATIONS AVAILABLE FOR OPIOID ADDICTION

Naltrexone
Methadone hydrochloride
Levo-alpha-acetyl methadyl or levomethadyl acetate
  (LAAM)
Buprenorphine
Antidepressant drugs (as selective serotonin reuptake
  inhibitors)
Antistress medications (as buspirone)

BARBITURATES

Barbiturates, involving less than 3% of high school students, are sedative-hypnotic medications that are CNS depressants that enhance the neuroinhibitory actions of gamma-aminobutyric acid (GABA). They are classified as ultra-short-acting (thiopental), short-acting (pentobarbital [*yellow jackets*]), secobarbitals (*reds*), and long-acting (phenobarbital). Short-acting barbiturates have greater potential for abuse and can lead to death in overdoses or when combined with alcohol or opioids. Abuse can lead to physical addiction, abstinence, and discontinuation syndrome similar to that observed with alcoholism. Symptoms of acute use and overdose are similar to acute use and overdose noted with alcohol; this includes euphoria, lethargy, miosis, ataxia, and slurred speech. An overdose can lead to hypotension, bullous dermatologic lesions, respiratory depression, coma, and death. Barbiturates should be prescribed to youth only with extreme caution by clinicians.

SUMMARY

Substance abuse is a national and global threat to adolescents and young adults. Clinicians should screen all youth for drug use and abuse while also providing education to their patients about the severe complications of abuse. Management of substance abuse disorders is a complex task and involves education of all those involved, selective use of psychopharmacology, use of psychosocial and behavioral therapies, and use of community programs. Successful curtailment of drug abuse in youth involves intense commitment on the part of clinicians, parents, society, and governments toward education programs, prevention programs, and removal of drug availability (Greydanus, 2005). Research seeks to find medications to blunt or remove the euphoric and addictive potential of drugs of abuse.

Bibliography

American Academy of Pediatrics Policy Statement: Tobacco, alcohol, and other drugs: the role of the Pediatrician in prevention and management of substance abuse. *Pediatrics* 1998;101:125.

Baker F, Ainsworth DR, Burd L, Wilson H: Fetal, infant, and child mortality in a context of alcohol use. *Am J Med Genet* 2004;15:51–58.

Beyers JM, Toumbourou JW, Catalano RF, et al.: A cross-national comparison of risk and protective factors for adolescent substance use: The United States and Australia. *J Adolesc Health* 2004;35:3–16.

Cigarette use among high school students-United States, 1991–2003. *MMWR* 2004; 53:499–502.

Comerci GB, Schwebel R: Substance abuse. *Adolesc Med* 2000;11(1):79–101.

Donovan JES: Adolescent alcohol initiation: A review of psychosocial factors. *J Adolesc Health* 2004;35:529.

Doyon S: The many faces of ecstasy. *Curr Opin Pediatr* 2001;13:170–176.

Fiore MC, Bailey WC, Cohen SJ, et al.: Treating tobacco use and dependence. Clinical Practice Guideline. U.S. Department of Health and Human Services, 2000.

Galanter M, Kleber HD (eds.): The American Psychiatric Press Textbook of Substance Abuse Treatment. Washington, DC: American Psychiatric Association, p. 695, 2004.

Greydanus DE and Patel DR: Sports doping in the adolescent athlete. *Asian J Paediatr Pract* 2000;4(1): 9–14.

Greydanus DE, Patel DR: Sports doping in the adolescent: The hope, the hype and the hyperbole. *Pediatr Clin North Am* 2002;49(4):829–855.

Greydanus DE: Substance abuse in adolescents: Basic chemistry lessons gone awry. *Int Pediatr* 2002;17(1): 3–4.

Greydanus DE, Patel DR: Substance abuse in adolescents: A complex conundrum for the clinician. *Pediatr Clin North Am* 2003;59(5):1179–1223.

Greydanus DE, Patel DR: The adolescent and substance abuse: Current concepts. *Curr Probl Pediatr Adolesc Health* 2005;35(3):78–98.

Grunbaum JA, Kann L, Kinchen S, et al.: YRBS-U.S. 2003 in surveillance summaries. *MMWR Morb Mortal Wkly Rep* 2004;53:1–96.

Heischober BS, Hofmann AF: Substance abuse. In: Hofmann AF, Greydanus DE (eds.), *Adolescent Medicine*, 3d ed. Norwalk, CT: Appleton & Lange, Chap 32, pp. 703–739, 1997.

Hyman SE: A 28-year-old man addicted to cocaine. *JAMA* 2001;286:2586–2594.

Irwin CE: Tobacco use during adolescence and young adulthood: The battle is not over. *J Adolesc Health* 2005; 35:169–171.

Jenkins RR: Substance abuse. In: Behrman RE, Kliegman RM, Jenson HB (eds.), *Nelson Textbook of Pediatrics*, 17th ed. Philadelphia, PA: W.B. Saunders, Vol. 653–662, Chap. 105, 2004.

Johnston L, M'Malley PM, Bachman JG, et al.: National Survey Results on Drug Use from the Monitoring the Future Study, National Institute on Drug Abuse, US Department of Health and Human Services, NIH Publication 04-5506, 2004.

Knight J, Sherrit L, Shrier L: Validity of the CRAFFT substance abuse screening test among adolescent clinic patients. *Arch Pediatr Adolesc Med* 2002; 156:607.

Knight JR: A 35-year-old physician with opioid dependence. *JAMA* 2004;292:1351–1357.

Kulig JW: Tobacco, alcohol and other drugs: The role of the pediatrician in prevention, identification, and management of substance abuse. *Pediatrics* 2005; 115:816–821.

Landry DW: Immunotherapy for cocaine addiction. *Sci Am* 1997;276(2):42–45.

National Clearinghouse on Alcohol and Drug Information: *www.health.org.*

National Institute on Alcohol Abuse and Alcoholism: *www.niaaa.nih.gov,http://www.MonitoringTheFutur. org.*

National Institute on Drug Abuse: *www.nida.gov/NIDA Home.html.*

O'Connor PG: Treating opioid dependence—New data and new opportunities. *N Engl J Med* 2000;343(18): 193–195.

Patel DR, Greydanus DE: Office interventions for adolescents smokers. *Adolesc Med* 2000;11(3):1–11.

Patel DR, Greydanus DE: Substance abuse: A pediatric concern. *Ind J Pediatr* 1999.

Patel DR: Smoking and children. *Ind J Pediatr* 1999;66: 817–824.

Patel DR, Dalal K, Pimentel R: Nutritional supplement advertisements. *Int Pediatr* 2005;20:134–141.

Rimsza ME: Substance abuse on the college campus. *Pediatr Clin North Am* 2005;52:307–319.

Schydlower M (ed.): *Substance Abuse: A Guide for Health Professionals.* Elk Grove Village, IL: American Academy of Pediatrics, 2000.

Stevens LM, Lynm C, Glass RM: Cocaine addiction. *JAMA* 2002;287:146.

Vastag B: Brain sabotages sobriety, right on cue. *JAMA* 2004;291:1053–1055.

Wheeler KC, Fletcher KE, Wellman RJ, et al.: Screening adolescents for nicotine dependence: The hooked on nicotine checklist. *J Adolesc Health* 2004;35:225–230.

35

DISRUPTIVE BEHAVIOR DISORDERS IN ADOLESCENTS

Swati Y. Bhave and Amit Sen

INTRODUCTION

Disruptive disorders include a wide range of heterogeneous behavior disorders that include conduct disorders (CD), oppositional defiant disorder (ODD), and attention deficit hyperactivity disorder (ADHD, Chap. 38); less prevalent disruptive disorders are impulse control disorders (ICD), such as pyromania, kleptomania, and trichotillomania.

At the core of these disorders is an insensitivity toward the needs of others, and an apparent incapacity to learn from experiences; this results in behaviors that violate the basic rights of other people, major age-appropriate norms and rules set by society.[1,2] As a consequence, the emphasis in definition and diagnosis is laid on the impact of such behaviors on others, rather than the young person's subjective distress. Such behavior may arise in adolescence or continue from childhood, and needs to be assessed in the context of the youngster's life history and current circumstances. It must also be differentiated from ordinary mischief or pranks, and a degree of unreasonable behavior and poor impulse control that is not unusual during adolescence.[1]

Transient manifestations and occasional minor forms of public disorder must be distinguished from the persistent and pervasive symptoms of CD, which often disrupts normal development, and integration of the individual to the larger community. The manifest behaviors of CD almost invariably transgress social rules and norms; they may also break the law. In this respect, it may be helpful to clarify the difference among often-used terms, such as CD, the juvenile delinquent, and antisocial behavior. CD is a medical/psychiatric term defining a disorder characterized by persistent, aggressive, or defiant behavior that represents serious violations of age-appropriate social expectations. Juvenile delinquency is a legal term referring to juveniles committing offences against the law. The term antisocial is from a social perspective, referring to behavior that is hostile to principles and rules of society.

HISTORICAL VIEW

Traditionally, there have been two approaches to conduct/behavior problems in young people. The first one is a retrospective view derived from adults who show antisocial tendencies, often referred to as psychopathic. There is an understanding that such moral and social deficiencies are a result of a substantial defect in character formation during younger years. The second approach derives from the considerable experience of experts working with delinquent youth. A common assumption has been that such youngsters react with antisocial behavior on the face of the harsh and deprived environment of their families and community. This assumption has supported the belief that the younger individual may be more responsive to help and intervention.

However, there has always existed another lobby with the counter viewpoint that such deviance in behavior is primarily constitutional. William Healy, an obstetrician and founder of the first juvenile court clinics in Chicago and Boston, described in 1926 delinquents as having a "psychic constitutional deficiency." He stressed the importance of finding both physical and mental defects in such patients, emphasizing his belief in the hereditary nature of such behavior problems. The English psychologist, Cyril Burt, published a monumental treatise in 1925, recognizing the multiple biologic and social insults contributing to delinquency.[1]

Psychoanalytic ideas gained prominence in the 1940's and 50's. The concept of a poorly developed super ego attracted a great deal of speculation and some interesting therapeutic approaches. Cleckley's monograph, "The Mask of Sanity" published in 1941, provided detailed clinical description and a comprehensive assessment of both the constitutional and the psychodynamic theories of the psychopath. He arrived at his own list of cardinal features and believed that both hereditary and environmental factors were influential in its causation.[1] Bowlby, a psychoanalyst by training, was particularly interested in the affectionless character, and his intense interest in the developmental antecedents of this group, whose early histories are marked by "prolonged separations from their mothers and foster mothers." It became the inspiration for this subsequent work on attachment published in 1949.[1]

While the previous workers had focused on clinical description and causation, the work of Robins in 1966, provided a grasp of its natural history.

By tracing the adult outcomes of children who were initially seen in a child guidance clinic, a convincing link was established between childhood conduct problems and antisocial personality disorder (ASPD). This study has been replicated in several different samples and they highlight the seriousness and chronicity of antisocial disorders.[1]

CLASSIFICATION AND NOMENCLATURE

It was in the 1940s and 50s that badly behaved youngsters entered the lexicon of psychiatrists. Diagnostic categories like CD, and later ODD, highlighted the fact that not all antisocial children are delinquent. Although the first version of the Diagnostic and Statistical Manual of Mental Disorders (DSM) by the American Psychiatric Association (DSM)[3] included a category for adults termed as sociopathic personality: antisocial reaction, there was no mention of similar conditions in young people.

In DSM-II,[4] three categories of CD were recognized: (1) unsocialized, aggressive reaction of childhood; (2) group delinquent reactions; and (3) runaway reactions.

The behavior disorders described in DSM-III[5] included CD, ODD, and attention deficit disorder (ADD). CD was recognized to have four subtypes: *under socialized aggressive, under socialized nonaggressive, socialized aggressive, and socialized nonaggressive.*

The term, disruptive behavior disorders (DBD), was first used in DSM-III–R.[6] The same diagnostic categories, as DSM-III, were included with some changes in nomenclature and subcategories. ADD was renamed ADHD and the subcategories of CD was changed from the original four to three new types: *group solitary, aggressive, and undifferentiated.* There was some discomfort about the inclusion of ADHD in this group, as it was recognized that all young people with ADHD are not "disruptive." Consequently, DSM-IV[7] separated ADHD from the DBD group.

DSM-IV also redefined the subcategories of CD, using the age of onset on the defining criteria. The three types of CD in DSM-III-R gave way to two new types: *CD-childhood onset type and CD-adolescent onset type.* DSM-IV also introduced a new category in the DBD group called DBD-NOS *(non otherwise specified)*, which was defined as a disorder that qualified for a diagnosis of a DBD but did not fulfill criteria of either ADD or CD.

The DSM-IV-TR,[8] has maintained the DBD group of three disorders, but has introduced a new subcategory of CD, *not otherwise specified* (CD-NOS). It is to be used when the age of onset of CD cannot be determined adequately.

As the DSM has been refining the classification and diagnostic criteria of mental disorders over the years in the United States, a parallel evidence-based system has been developing in the form of the International Classification of Diseases (ICD). ICD-9[9] included *socialized and unsocialized CD*, but not ODD. Thereafter, there has been a concerted effort to bring the two classificatory systems closer. In keeping with this spirit, the ICD-10 and DSM-IV have the same list of symptoms and diagnostic criteria for CD and ODD. The fact that both systems view ODD as a milder and developmentally related form of CD forms the basis of this overlap.[10]

However, ICD-10 does not talk of a DBD group, but includes them under a broader group of CDs. Also, the disorders listed under CD are similar, but not the same as the DBD group disorders or their subcategories. It includes *socialized CD, unsocialized CD, CD confined to the family context, ODD,* and *unspecified CD.* The ICD-10 also recognizes a *hyperkinetic CD* (when criteria for both CD and ADHD are met); there is also a separate group of *mixed disorders of conduct and emotions*, which upholds the understanding that many adolescents who exhibit features of CD may also be emotionally disturbed or depressed.

EPIDEMIOLOGY

Disruptive/CD are the most frequently diagnosed behavior or psychiatric disorders of children and adolescence.[7] In research, prevalence rates have shown wide variations due to definitional and methodological differences in studies.[11] Large community-based studies in the United States and United Kingdom reflect a prevalence ranging between 4% and 8%.[1]

Past studies and recent reviews point toward a consistent pattern of increased prevalence of CD in boys.[12] The male: female ratio is stronger during childhood than in adolescence. By contrast, gender differences in ODD are less consistent. The prevalence of CD rises steadily with age in boys, while in girls, a sharp rise in prevalence is seen during the adolescent years. Overall, there is a 1.5- to 3-fold increase in CD during adolescence as compared to childhood.

The findings with ODD are less consistent, and, in fact, some studies show a decline in the prevalence of ODD during adolescence.[11] Among children who met diagnostic criteria of CD, status violations and other nonaggressive conduct problems increased with age, while aggressive symptoms became less common. Youngsters with disruptive disorders are more susceptible to developing other psychiatric disorders as compared to the normal population. The most common co morbidities are ADHD (Chap. 38), depression (Chap. 36), and anxiety disorders (Chap. 37).[11] It has been found that there is a significant rise in the prevalence of disruptive disorders in urban as compared to rural areas. A similar association is noticed with poverty, lower socioeconomic status, broken families, and harsh and abusive parenting.

CLINICAL MANIFESTATIONS

The central characteristic in the group of disruptive disorders is an egocentricity that severely limits the youngster's capacity to understand or sympathize with other peoples' needs. There is a tendency to blame others for their own misconducts, and an apathy toward their pain/discomfort; these adolescents exhibit a lack of regret for the acts.

As described in DSM-IV, CD involves a repetitive and persistent pattern of behavior in which the basic rights of others or major age-appropriate social norms or rules are violated; ODD is described in those with a persistent pattern of negativistic, defiant, disobedient, and hostile behavior toward authority figures.[7,8] Many experts believe that ODD is a developmental precursor of CD, and is therefore, more common in younger children, while the onset of CD peaks during late childhood and early adolescence.

A recent longitudinal study confirmed that ODD was a strong risk factor for CD in boys.[13] In girls, however, ODD provided no increased risk for later CD, but was associated with an increased risk for continued ODD, depression, and anxiety. ODD often begins during middle childhood and is developed by early adolescence. Some oppositional behavior is considered the norm during adolescence, but those adolescents with ODD have problems controlling their temper, curse frequently, and argue a lot. They are described as angry, spiteful, resentful, touchy, and easily annoyed by others. Other children may describe them as being bullies or being mean.

The majority of adolescents with CD exhibit symptoms of ODD. In addition, they may be deliberately cruel toward others and/or animals. Stealing at their house and outside is often accompanied by lying. Besides disruptiveness in the classroom, truancy becomes more common during adolescence. Although aggressive outbursts become less common with age, they may become more sinister and take the form of rape or systematic gang activity[11]; fire setting, vandalism, drug abuse, and sexual promiscuity also become more frequent at this age.

The DSM-IV subtype of childhood onset CD (i.e., onset before 10 years of age) is more commonly associated with ADHD, low IQ, positive family history, and frequent aggression. It appears to have similarities with the unsocialized subtype of ICD-10, as opposed to the socialized variety, which overlaps with the adolescent onset subtype of DSM-IV. Those of the latter variety may show loyalty to peer group, have shorter crime paths, and have more girls in the group. Gender-specific features become more prominent during adolescence; boys are usually more aggressive, while girls tend to get involved in covert crimes and prostitution.

It is important to remember the sociocultural context in which disruptive disorders are perceived. Different cultures show different levels of tolerance to deviant behavior. Consequently, what comes to the notice of the clinician may be skewed. For instance, it is understandable that CD features will be highly prevalent, even adaptive in the slum and street children of deprived urban areas; such children are often dealt with by the criminal justice system, particularly in developing countries where medical and mental health services for such children are woefully lacking.

ETIOLOGY AND RISK FACTORS

Disruptive disorders are a heterogeneous group and research into its etiology has thrown up a wide range of theories. The development of CD appears to be associated predominantly with disadvantaged backgrounds. There is evidence to suggest that psychosocial factors, particularly nonshared environmental influences are etiologically strong[14]; this refers to experiences that have unique effects on members of a family, e.g. life events, peer interactions, and differential parental treatment. However, some of the core vulnerabilities that predispose an individual to develop this disorder may be mediated through genetic and biologic processes.[15]

The major risks are genetic, biologic, environmental, and others. Under genetic risks, it is noted that males are more likely to suffer from disruptive disorders than females. There is familial aggregation and higher concordance rates in monozygotic twins as compared to dizygotic twins. Genetically influenced characteristics, such as low resting heart rate, hyperactivity, and difficult temperament show high association with CD. Under biologic factors, it is noted that low autonomic arousal has been repeatedly related to antisocial and criminal activity in both children and adults; low salivary cortisol is a correlate of severe and persistent aggression in male children and adolescents.[16] There is evidence that antisocial behavior in young people is associated with neuropsychological impairment, particularly involving executive functions. Other cognitive problems include language delay, lowered intelligence, and learning difficulties. Birth complications and minor physical anomalies (e.g., low set ears, adherent ear lobes, and furrowed tongue) are also associated with disruptive disorders.

In terms of biologic factors, studies note that abusive and rejecting parenting in families stricken with poverty and unemployment are likely to create a high risk of disruptive behavior in the family's vulnerable children.[15,17]

Other factors include insecure attachment, broken families, parental discord, parental psychopathology (especially maternal depression and paternal ASPD), parental alcohol or substance misuse, and delinquent peer affiliation. Table 35-1 lists factors noted to be protective of the development of disruptive disorders. The progressive accumulation of risk factors across development, along with a relative absence of protective factors, increases the likelihood that a disruptive disorder will develop. In adolescence, the role of family and parenting declines, and the influence of peers and the larger community (including school) becomes paramount.

Conduct and Differential Diagnosis

One of the most virulent co-morbid conditions of disruptive disorders is ADHD (Chap. 38). ICD-10 recognizes hyperkinetic CD as a separate entity; this diagnosis is made when the overall criteria of hyperkinetic disorders (ADHD) and the overall criteria for CD are met. In such cases, response to treatment is often much poorer and the outcome worse.[1]

Other frequent co morbidities are depression and anxiety.[11] This combination of emotional and conduct problems could be a reflection of the higher prevalence of depression and anxiety in disruptive disorders; or it could be emotional disorders masquerading as behavior problem during adolescence. It is established that emotional disorders, particularly depression (Chap. 36), can often present as behavior problems during adolescence and a potentially treatable condition may be misdiagnosed. Similarly, although less frequently, other conditions that can present as disruptive disorders include bipolar affective disorder, schizophrenic, and dissociative disorders. Topical features of these disorders are often hidden in the background of the more dramatic behavior problems and need to be carefully sorted out during assessment.

Several cross-sectional and longitudinal studies have found an association between DBD and alcohol/substance use disorders (SUD). In clinical populations the co morbidity of SUDs is substantial; up to 95% in some clinical samples.[17] The association between alcohol and DBD is prominent in males. However, it often becomes difficult to establish as to which disorder precedes which; the co morbid disorders of CD and mood disorders jointly characterize many adolescents with alcohol dependence. There is a range of neurodevelopmental conditions that are associated with DBD. Some of the common ones are specific learning difficulties, [18] mild mental retardation, and seizure disorders.[19]

COURSE AND OUTCOME

There is ample evidence to suggest that an early, severe behavioral problem is a strong risk factor for the development of subsequent DBD.[19] Several studies have reported that preschool behavioral problems and aggressive behavioral problems during middle childhood are predictive of disruptive disorders and serious delinquency in adolescence. Consequently, DSM-IV distinguishes two types of CD: an aggressive type starting in childhood and a nonaggressive type starting in adolescence. It is believed that the early onset variety has worse prognosis, particularly those who show severe aggressive and cruel behavior. In this context, the relationship between ODD and CD assumes a greater importance; the prevalence of ODD is higher during early childhood and the

TABLE 35-1

PROTECTIVE FACTORS FROM DISRUPTIVE DISORDERS

- High IQ
- An easy temperament
- At least one positive relationship with an adult
- Good work habits at school
- Areas of competence
- Prosocial peer group
- A school atmosphere that fosters success

rates fall significantly with age particularly in boys.[11] The rates of ODD in girls, however, do not decrease with age as significantly as noted with boys. There is now some evidence that there is a strong relationship between ODD and CD in boys, supporting the notion that ODD is a developmental precursor to CD. In girls the pattern of this association was markedly different.[13]

The prevalence of CD increases markedly during adolescence (8.6%–12.2%) in boys and (7.5%–9.5%) in girls.[20] About 40% of this population goes on to develop ASPD after age 18, the majority being the ones with an early onset. It also must be noted that all young people with CD who turn 18, do not automatically qualify for a diagnosis of APSD, which has a different and more stringent criteria (DSM-IV). The ones that do not fulfill such criteria continue with a label of CD until further development.

Childhood antisocial aggressive behavior predates and predicts later alcohol and other substance abuse problems. In clinical populations of adolescents, the co morbidity of SUD (Chap. 34) and CD is high, the correlation being more marked in males (up to 90%). The coexistence of CD and major depression is found to be more predictive of alcohol dependence in adolescents. It was traditionally believed that antisocial behavior is rare in adolescent girls, is sexual in nature if present, and runs a more benign course in adulthood.[20] However, reviews of recent studies have found nearly equal prevalence of CD in girls, an outcome not too dissimilar in boys; 35% developed ASPD as adults and 40–70% developed substance abuse problems.

It is known that young people with DBD are more prone to developing other psychiatric disorders including mood disorders, somatoform disorders, and psychoses. They also suffer higher mortality rates (58 times more than the normal population) and are at high risk of meeting with violent death during early adulthood.[1] They also exhibit a much higher crime rate during adulthood and widespread social malfunctions, such as having high divorce rates, and limited education, work history, as well as unsatisfactory social relationship.[19] As noted earlier (see subsection on co-morbidity), associated ADHD worsens the prognosis while

associated emotional disorder (depression and anxiety) are thought to improve outcome. The protective factors (listed in Table 35-1) are also likely to improve the prognosis.

ASSESSMENT/EVALUATION

Adolescents with DBD, due to the very nature of these disorder(s), are unlikely to seek help or volunteer much information. The referral often comes from affected parties, such as school, family, or the juvenile justice courts. The focus of the assessment may be guided by the needs of the referrer. However, any clinical assessment should be comprehensive and multidisciplinary in nature. The complexity of these DBDs and the various ways they can affect the individual's life and development necessitates a thorough assessment.[21]

It is important to obtain a detailed history of presenting complaints along with a comprehensive developmental and family history; this includes charting the chronology and evolution of reported difficulties. The clinician may have to use various sources of information, such as family, school, peers, and juvenile justice systems, to get the complete picture. A variety of rating scales and diagnostic tools are now available to supplement the clinical assessment; these include the Conner's Ratings Scale,[22] Child Behavior Checklist,[23] Diagnostic Interviews for Children and Adolescents (DICA),[24] and others.

A multidisciplinary team is an important part of the evaluation and management process. The patient's primary care clinician or neurologist should conduct a through physical and neurological examination; the assessment may include procedures such as an electroencephalogram (EEG) and MRI. A psychiatrist is helpful to help rule out any co morbid or masked psychiatric conditions. Psychologists are needed for testing of intelligence, assessment for any learning difficulty, and performing a neuropsychologic assessment. A special education teacher needs to be involved if there are any academic difficulties. A social worker needs to assess for family pathology and issues of abuse and neglect. An occupational therapist can help assess fine motor or sensory difficulties and disabilities. Other specialists can be added, depending on the conditions of each adolescent patient.

It is best if the team meets frequently to bring together their findings and plan appropriate interventions jointly and in a parallel manner. It is easy for a clinician to tick the checklist provided in the diagnostic criteria (DSM-IV) and make a diagnosis of DBD. However, such an approach is likely to be superficial and overlook the complex pathogenesis, treatable co morbid conditions, and the unique special needs of the young person; the comprehensiveness of a multidisciplinary team assessment, therefore, becomes an important part of the overall management strategy.

MANAGEMENT

A comprehensive multidisciplinary assessment remains the cornerstone of effective management plans. By their very nature, youth with DBDs produce much anxiety and stress on resources for both the family and the larger community. Therefore, it becomes imperative to differentiate between transient disturbances and long-term risks. Transient behavioral problems may be part of growing up or reflect co morbid conditions, such as mood disorders, adjustment disorders or drug abuse, and others; the management should be consistent with the severity and complexity of the identified disorder(s).

Individuals with embedded, long-term difficulties require carefully thought out interventions that are unique and in keeping with these adolescents' special needs. Implementation of treatment plans frequently includes various groups of people involved with the young person and need to occur in various physical settings (i.e., home, school, therapist's office, and others).[21] The management is often implemented by the same multidisciplinary team responsible for the initial assessment. Needless to say, the earlier the interventions start, the better is the outcome.

Many preventive programs have, therefore, become popular and are thought to be more effective both in terms of outcome and costs. Parenting programs and adolescent groups have been used effectively in the deprived and vulnerable population.[21] Many different treatment modalities have been tried to treat DBDs. It is not surprising that no single treatment has been effective in this heterogeneous group of complex etiology.

Although the success of most of these diverse modalities remains untested,[19] this chapter describes the range of interventions that may be available. These are often used in combination by a group of professionals, depending on available resources and the unique needs of these young persons. Any comprehensive management plan takes time to come together and show its effects. These plans, therefore, need to be long term with sustained efforts. The needs of the young person may change with time and this necessitates modification of active management plans. The therapists' beliefs and convictions in their approach and persistence in effort are often what make the difference in the final outcome.

Individual Therapy

Cognitive behavioral therapy (CBT) techniques are popular due to their problem focused approach and scientific basis of effectiveness. Cognitive problem solving skills training[25] helps adolescents to identify problems, recognize causation, appreciate consequences, consider alternative ways of handling difficult situations, and improve reality testing by cognitive means. CBT techniques are also used to enhance the patient's ability to handle anger and for social skills training. In addition, behavior modification techniques and relaxation as well as calming techniques, are often used.

Family Therapy

The role of the family in maintaining problematic behavior or conversely, in bringing about a positive change, cannot be over emphasized. Supportive family therapy, group therapy for families, group therapies for the adolescents, parenting training, therapy for the parents with mental disorders, and treatment of co morbid substance abuse disorders are all effective when used appropriately. In the event of absence or inadequacy of a family, an adoptive family is preferred over residential homes. There is evidence that youths with severe CD and with a chronic history of juvenile delinquency do better with group foster care than group residential care. [26]

Collaboration with Schools and College

Special education services are often involved in implementing individual education plans (IPE), which are based on the unique academic profile/abilities of the individual adolescent. Vocational training and rehabilitation may become part of the management plans of the older adolescents. Research also suggests that school-based behavioral interventions can be effective especially for very severely disturbed children.[27]

Multisystem Therapy

Good evidence exists for the efficacy of *multisystem therapy* (MST) in severely disturbed children and adolescents with CD.[28] MST is based on the theory that a multiplicity of systems influences a young person's adaptation, including adaptation to the family, peers, school, and community. Such treatment is varied, depending on the needs of the adolescent and family. A MST therapist works to reduce problem behavior by inducing change in the multiple systems in which the child or adolescent is embedded.[29]

At the family level, MST is designed to increase family structure and cohesion, while providing parents with the skills and resources necessary to monitor and discipline their children effectively. Besides learning to open lines of communication with their children and developing skills to diffuse conflictive family interactions, caregivers are encouraged to spend more time with their youth engaging in complementary and mutually desired activities. At the peer level, MST focuses on increasing the youth's association with prosocial peers (e.g., through organized games or religious youth groups), while helping parents disengage youth from deviant peers (e.g., gang members, school dropouts, or drug abusers).[30] It is, therefore, not surprising to learn that MST has been shown to be effective in several outcome studies,

given that it recognizes the individual and environmental vulnerabilities of severely delinquent adolescents, and attempts to address all of them.[20]

Pharmacologic Treatment

As with other forms of treatment, there is no single treatment or type of medication that has been shown to be specifically useful; medication is often not thought of as the first line of management. However, when used judiciously, it may form an important part of the overall management plan and often may help the implementation or effectiveness of other treatment modalities. Besides treating the co morbid conditions, such as depression or ADHD, medications are usually targeted at specific symptom clusters (e.g., aggressive behavior, impulsivity, mood swings, suicidal behaviors, and others). A wide variety of medicines have been tried, including stimulants, antidepressants, mood stabilizers, clonidine, and even beta blockers.[20] Out of these various medications, there is some evidence that risperidone[30] and lithium[31] may be effective in controlling severe aggressive tendencies, at least to some extent. This does not imply that the other medicines are never useful in some clinical settings. The only way to determine effectiveness of a medicine in a particular case is by choosing the symptom cluster carefully and trying out a drug that is likely to positively affect these symptoms.

Juvenile Justice System

From a clinical viewpoint, it seems that the juvenile justice system is often used as the last resort. It may become necessary to involve the law when these adolescents repeatedly place themselves and others at serious risk of harm. The assessment and management of such risk is often the domain of a forensic psychiatrist, psychologist, or social worker. The use of incarceration varies widely, according to the law of the land and facilities available within the juvenile justice system. It may be worthwhile consulting social services or a forensic expert, whenever there are concerns or worries about the potential for such a youth offending or harming others.

SUMMARY

Disruptive behavioral disorders are a wide range of heterogeneous group of disorders with complex biopsychosocial etiologies. Simply assigning a diagnosis to a badly behaved youngster is never going to do justice to the person's unique psychosocial and developmental needs. Neither can there be a prescribed management formula that matches the diagnosis. Effective management plans are therefore, invariably multilayered, tailored to the individual's unique needs, and often need to be modified, as needs change over time. Needless to say, putting together such an effort could deplete all available resources. In this scenario, what appears most urgent is early detection and prevention of disruptive behavioral disorders. Preventive work automatically places one in a position confronting sociocultural realities that influence the way badly behaved young people are perceived and dealt with in a community. Building awareness as well as advocacy, and using the broadening knowledge base and research data to influence the sociopolitical system may be the need of the hour to help our troubled young people. Further directions in management include cross-cultural research, extensive preventive programs, targeting vulnerable groups across sociocultural boundaries, and tapping into the dormant resources preserved in the traditions of different communities.

Bibliography

1. Earls F: Oppositional defiant and conduct disorders, in: Rutter M, Taylor E, Hersov L (eds.), Child and Adolescent Psychiatry—Modern Approaches, 3d ed. Oxford: Blackwell Scientific Publications, 1994, pp. 308–329.

2. Parry-Jones W: Psychiatric disorders of adolescence, in: Kendell RE, Zealley AK (eds.), Companion to Psychiatric Studies, 5th ed. Edinburgh, Scotland: Churchill-Livingstone, 1996, pp. 681–709.

3. American Psychiatric Association. Diagnostic and Statistical Manual of Mental Disorders, (DSM I). Washington, DC: American Psychiatric Association, 1952.

4. American Psychiatric Association. Diagnostic and Statistical Manual of Mental Disorders (DSM-II), 2d ed. Washington, DC: American Psychiatric Association 1968.

5. American Psychiatric Association. Diagnostic and Statistical Manual of Mental Disorders (DSM-III), 3d ed. Washington, DC: American Psychiatric Association 1980.

6. American Psychiatric Association. Diagnostic and Statistical Manual of Mental Disorders-revised (DSM-III-R), 3d ed. Washington, DC: American Psychiatric Association 1987.

7. American Psychiatric Association. Diagnostic and Statistical Manual of Mental Disorders (DSM-IV), 4th ed. Washington, DC: American Psychiatric Association 1994.

8. American Psychiatric Association. Diagnostic and Statistical Manual of Mental Disorders-text revised (DSM–IV-TR), 4th ed. Washington, DC: American Psychiatric Association, 2000.

9. World Health Organization. Mental Disorders: Glossary and Guides to their Classification in accordance with the 9th revision of the International Classification of diseases. WHO, Geneva, 1978.

10. World Health Organization. The ICD 10 Classification of Mental and Behavioral Disorders: Clinical Descriptions and Diagnostic Guidelines. WHO, Geneva, 1992.

11. Maugham B, Rowe R, Messer J, et al. J Child Psychol Psychiatry 2004;45:3.

12. Lahey BB, Waldman ID, McBurnett K: Annotation: The development of antisocial behavior: An integrative causal model. J Child Psychol Psychiatry 1999; 40:669–682.

13. Rowe R, Maughan BB, Pickles A, et al.: The relationship between DSM–IV oppositional defiant disorders and conduct disorders: Findings from the Great Smoky Mountain study. J Child Psychol Psychiatry 2002;43:365–373.

15. Taylor J, McGue M, Iacono WG: Sex difference, assertive mating and cultural transmission affects on adolescence delinquency: A twin family study. J Child Psychol Psychiatry 2000;41(4):433–440.

16. Raine A: Annotation: The role of prefrontal deficits, low autonomic arousal, and early health factors in the development of antisocial and aggressive behavior in children. J Child Psychol Psychiatry 2002;43(4): 417–434.

17. McBurnett K, Lahey BB, Rathauz PJ, et al.: Low salivary cortisol and persistent aggression in boys

referred for disruptive behavior. Arch J Psychiatry 2000;51:38–43.

18. Clark DB, Pollock N, Bukstein OG: Gender and co-morbid psychopathology in adolescents with alcohol dependence. J Am Acad Child Adolesc Psychiatry 1997;39(9):1195–1203.

19. Tomblin JB, Zhang X, Buck Walter P, et al.: The association of reading disability, behavioral disorders and language impairment amongst second grade children. J Child Psychol Psychiatry 2000;44(4):473–482.

20. Lewis DO, Yeager CA: Conduct disorders, in: Lewis M (ed.), Child and Adolescent Psychiatry. A Comprehensive Text Book, 3d Ed. New York, NY: Lippincott Williams & Williams, 2002.

21. Pajer KA: What happens to 'bad' girls? Am J Psychiatry 1998;155:862–870.

22. Barrichman L: Disruptive disorders, in: Greydanus DE, Patel DR, Pratt HD (eds.), PCNA, Vol. 50, no. 5, 2003, pp. 1004–1017.

23. Conner CK: Conner's Rating Scales Revised: Technical Manual. New York, NY: Multihealth Systems, 1997.

24. Achenbach TM: Manual for the Child Behavior Checklist 2-3 and 1992 Profile. Burlington, VT: University of Vermont, 1992.

26. Welner Z, Reich W, Herjanic B: Reliability, validity and parent -child agreement studies of the Diagnostic Interview for Children and Adolescents (DICA). J Am Acad Child Adolesc Psychiatry 1987;3(26):649–653.

27. Kazdin AE, Crowley M: Moderators of treatment outcome in cognitively based treatment of antisocial behavior. Cogn Ther 1997; R21:185–207.

28. Chamberlain P, Moore KA: Clinical model for parenting Juvenile offenders: A comparison of group care versus family care. Clin Child Psychol Psychiatry 1998; 3:375–386.

29. Stoolmiller M, Eddy JM, Reid JB: Detecting and describing preventive intervention effects in a Universal school based randomized trial targeting delinquent and violent behavior. J Consult Clin Psychol 2000;68:296–306.

30. Henggeler SW: Multisystemic therapy: Overview of clinical procedures, outcomes, and policy implications. Child Psychol Psychiatry Rev 1999;4:2–10.

31. Huey SJ Jr, Henggeler SW, Brondino MJ: Mechanisms of change in multisystemic therapy: Reducing delinquent behavior through therapist adherence and improved family and peer functioning. J Consult Clin Psychol 2000;68(3):451–467.

32. Findling RL, MacNamara NK, Branicky LA, et al.: A double blind pilot study of Risperidone in the treatment of conduct disorders. J Am Acad Child and Adolesc Psychiatry 2000;39:509–516.

33. Malone RP, Delaney MA, Leubbert JF, et al.: A double blind placebo controlled study of lithium in hospitalized aggressive children and adolescents with conduct disorder. Arch Gen Psychiatry 2000; 57:649–654.

36

MOOD DISORDERS IN ADOLESCENTS

Venus Paxton and Bennett L. Leventhal

INTRODUCTION

Mood disorders are among the most common medical conditions facing adolescents and presenting to the primary care clinician and mental health specialist. When properly diagnosed, these disorders can be very successfully treated, thus limiting significant disruption, disability, and premature death that may occur due to depression. Mood disorders come in many forms and can have a broad impact on youth leading to significant discomfort, genuine impairment in academic and social functioning, as well as increased medical morbidity and premature death related to suicide. Treatment of psychiatric disorders in adolescents can be complicated. Treatment requires a systematic approach that attends to the psychosocial influences from family, peers, school, and community factors that are omnipresent and play critical roles in adolescent functioning. Despite some controversy about treatment modalities, there are effective approaches that allow for early and effective interventions. This chapter presents an overview on mood disorders in adolescents.

HISTORICAL VIEW

Until relatively recently, it was a commonly held belief that children were not able to experience depression (Elliott and Smiga, 2003). The traditional psychoanalytic view was that the immature superego and personality structure of the child did not allow for any expression of depressive symptoms. Early researchers, such as Spitz (1946) and Bowlby (1960), did describe classical depressive symptoms; however, this work was largely in institutionalized children and was not felt to be generalizable. These children appeared depressed, reacted slowly to stimuli, had psychomotor retardation, and often cried; also, they had sleep and appetite difficulties. While this sort of psychoanalytic modeling was predominant, the notion of early-onset mood disorders was not foreign to all early psychiatrists. For example, Kraepelin (1921) reported that about 0.5% of manic patients seemed to have their first manic episode before the age of 10 years.

By the 1970s, there was a change in perspective on mood disorders. In 1977, Schulterbrandt and Raskin published *Depression in Childhood:*

Diagnosis, Treatment and Conceptual by Models; this work made it clear that depression was a serious condition that involved children and adolescents. A myriad of books and articles have concluded that depression criteria set for adults are generally accepted for the diagnosis of depression in adolescents, as long the youth's age and stage of development are considered (Chap. 1). Sadness and unhappiness, critical parts of the diagnosis of depression, are also part of the normal range of human emotions. Yet, there are critical differences in these sorts of experiences based on developmental level, language skills, and cognitive (not intellectual) capacity. These differences often lead to the necessity of seeking out signs and symptoms of depression in an age-appropriate manner; also, one should note that nonverbal and somatic signs and symptoms may predominate in these adolescents. Today, we understand mood disorders to be a developmental neurobehavioral syndrome of multiple etiologies that are often characterized as complex interactions among genetic, neurobiologic, and psychosocial components.

DIAGNOSIS

The two widely accepted classification systems of mood disorders are the DSM-IV (Diagnostic and Statistical Manual of Mental Disorders, 4th edition, American Psychiatric Association, 1994) and ICD-10 (World Health Organization, Geneva, Switzerland) with somewhat different diagnostic criteria for mood disorders in youth. In both systems, there are two major diagnostic categories for mood disorders: unipolar depressive disorders and bipolar disorders. Dysthymia, a third category is also allowed for children and adolescents. This discussion will be based on the American Psychiatric Association's DSM-IV classification system.

For *major depressive disorder*, the diagnostic criteria are virtually identical for children and adults (see American Psychiatric Association, 1994). One exception to the adult criteria is that depressive symptoms must be present for at least a 2-week period whereas for adolescents, an irritable mood lasting 2 weeks can be substituted for

depressed mood. Additionally, the weight change criteria are changed for youth to include the possibility of a failure to make *expected* weight gains in the place of weight loss in adults.

Bipolar disorder represents a more complex and controversial presentation of mood disorder that includes variations in the extremes of mood from severe depression to euphoria (American Psychiatric Association, 1994). The clinical presentation and differential diagnosis in youth and common comorbidity make this diagnosis more difficult. *Dysthymia* is a milder form of depression that is a more persistent state of dysphoria (see American Psychiatric Association, 1994). For this diagnosis, there is a modification of criteria so that the symptoms have to be present for only 1 year for adolescence, instead of 2 years required for adults. Additionally, coexisting psychiatric disorders are also common in adolescents, especially anxiety (Chap. 37) and behavior disorder, so combinations of diagnoses may be appropriate.

SUICIDE

Suicide is the third leading cause of death in adolescents, second only to accidents and homicides (Chap. 2). The death rate associated with suicide is estimated at 13/100,000. More than 90% of youths who complete suicide have an associated psychiatric illness, most commonly a mood disorder. Other risk factors include a previous attempt (25%), substance abuse (Chap. 34), chronic illness (Chap. 5), psychosis (Chap. 39), and family issues, such as a positive family history for suicide or abuse. Suicidal activities include both attempts and completed suicides, with considerable morbidity associated with the attempts. Females make more attempts than males by a ratio of approximately 4:1. The use of a firearm is the most common completed method for both sexes. Other common means of suicide attempts include overdose/self-poisoning, hanging, and suffocation.

Evaluating suicidal ideation and plans requires careful clinical examination. The clinician is never wrong to inquire about suicidal thoughts and plans; asking adolescents about suicidal thoughts and plans does not increase the likelihood of suicidal behavior and may actually decrease the risk of competed suicide. Therefore, detailed inquiry about patient safety is possible and recommended as a routine practice in the primary care office, especially given the significant morbidity and mortality of this behavior in adolescents.

EPIDEMIOLOGY

Epidemiologic studies report a 0.3% incidence rate of depression for preschoolers and 1%–2% for elementary age children (Anderson et al., 1987; Bird et al., 1988). Major depressive disorder tends to have a higher incidence in adolescents than in preschool children. Epidemiologic studies report a 4.7% incidence with a prevalence of 0.4%–8% of depression in adolescents. The lifetime prevalence has been reported to range from 15% to 20%. Data indicate that the sex ratio is equal in depressed children. However, a change begins around the age of 10 years when there is a gradual relative increase in rates of depression in females, so that the rates ultimately match rates in adult women. Less is known about the epidemiology of bipolar disorder in adolescents. Carlson and Kashani (1988) reported a prevalence of 0.6% in a community sample compared to 1% of adults. Some researches note an incidence of 3.4% for bipolar illness in a sample of adolescent inpatients. Methodological problems account for uncertainties and variability in rates found in the literature for children and adolescents (Geller and Luby, 1997).

Mood disorders that first appear in adolescents have a significant likelihood of being recurrent with multiple relapses. Compared to adults *without* early-onset mood disorders, adults *with* a history of childhood or adolescent mood disorder have a higher rate of adult mood disorder and anxiety disorders. Lewinsohn et al. (2000), using a community sample of formerly depressed adolescents, reported specific factors significantly related to the recurrence of major depressive disorder during early adulthood; these include multiple severe depressive episodes in adolescence, female gender, family history of mood disorder incidence, and the presence of personality disorder symptoms, especially borderline personality disorder. In contrast, adolescents with depression are less likely to have a recurrence if they had only a single episode of major depressive disorder, low levels of excessive emotional reliance, low or no family history of mood disorder, and low levels of personality disorder symptoms. Comorbidity plays a role in the recurrence risk of any psychiatric illness associated with mood disorders; the greatest comorbidity is with substance abuse disorders, anxiety disorders, and antisocial symptoms.

McCauley et al. (1993) have shown that, as in adults, more severe depressions are associated with a longer duration of the index episode, length of treatment, and female gender. Recurrences also occur sooner when there is a longer duration of the initial episode, higher socioeconomic status, and endogenicity. Some studies have shown that girls, in comparison to boys, reported higher levels of depressive symptoms, including depressed mood and lower self-esteem (Avison and Mcalpine, 1992; Allgood-Merten and Lewinsohn, 1990). On the other hand, boys may have greater reports of irritability. Adolescents with major depressive disorder are also at increased risk for developing bipolar disorder (Kovacs, 2001; McCauley et al., 1993).

ETIOLOGY/PATHOLOGY

There is no known etiology for mood disorders, though there are many theories (Table 36-1). It has long been suggested that neurotransmitter regulatory function plays a significant role in mood regulation and the pathophysiology of mood disorders. Serotonin, catecholamines, and acetylcholine are biogenic amines that have been implicated in

TABLE 36-1

ETIOLOGIC THEORIES OF MOOD DISORDERS

Biologic models
Psychoanalytical model
Cognitive-behavioral model
Learned helplessness model
Others

causal mechanisms for mood disorders. Drugs that deplete monoamines have been repeatedly shown to cause depression; also, antidepressant medications that target these neurotransmitters seem to be effective antidepressants. Neuroendocrine abnormalities have also been suggested, including abnormalities in cortisol, thyroid, and growth hormone regulation (Kutcher et al., 1988; Dahl et al., 1992).

Multiple studies have indicated significant genetic contribution in the etiology of mood disorders. Concordance rates are higher in monozygotic twins (~50%) in comparison to dizygotic twins (~25%) for depression. These results parallel those found in adult twin studies. Compared to rates in the general population, first-degree relatives of depressed adolescents have a significantly higher lifetime rate of mood disorders, ranging from 17% to 46%. Also, family studies, comparing control subjects to relatives of depressed subjects, report a two to three times increase in lifetime rates of mood disorders. In children of depressed parents, a lifetime risk for major depressive disorder has been found to range from 15% to 45%. Other risk factors include early-onset, recurrence, and both parents having depression.

There is a particularly strong suggestion of genetic influences for bipolar illness. Monozygotic twins have a concordance rate of 65% compared to 14% in dizygotic twins (Nurnberger and Gershon, 1982). Similar to depressive disorders, family studies report increased rates of bipolar illness among relatives of adolescents with bipolar illness. Early-onset bipolar illness is associated with higher rates of major depressive disorder, substance abuse, antisocial personality disorder, and attention-deficit/hyperactivity disorder (ADHD) (Chap. 38).

Psychosocial influences have been theorized in the etiology and pathology of mood disorders. The *psychoanalytical model* suggests that depression is aggression turned inward after the loss of an ambivalently loved object. Gabbard (1995) pointed out four key themes in the psychodynamic explanation of depression with loss being a central theme. However, there is little evidence of pathologic grief being associated with most depressions; Akiskal (1995) reported this in less than 10%–15% of children and 2%–5% of adults.

The loss itself may not be detrimental, but the lack of care given afterward can be. In studies by Brent et al. (1993), exposure to suicide was reported as a stressful event that was associated with a threefold increase in acute and major depressive illness in mothers, siblings, and friends of suicide victims. The risk of developing depression was found to be proportional to one's closeness to the victim and intensity of exposure. In the *cognitive-behavioral model*, depression is viewed as distorted, negative thoughts. The individual is said to have low self-esteem with negative thoughts about him/herself, his/her experiences, and his/her future—the so-called "cognitive triad."

Similar to cognitive theories of depression, the *learned helplessness model* (Seligman and Peterson, 1986) suggests that uncontrollable life events lead to helplessness in motivational, cognitive, and emotional reactions. Family interactions have also been implicated in the etiology of mood disorders, especially in families characterized as conflictual, rejecting, abusive, and with decreased expression of affect. There is also evidence that a child's own characteristics can elicit negative parental reactions that can lead to depression (Cook et al., 1991). This bidirectional influence can contribute to the risk of psychopathology in the child. Lewinsohn et al. (1994) reported multiple psychosocial influences associated with a community sample of 1508 adolescents. The actual mechanisms of contribution from these factors are not entirely clear, but it seems to increase one's vulnerability.

ASSESSMENT/CLINICAL PRESENTATION

In evaluating an adolescent for a mood disorder, it is essential that the clinician interview the adolescent and family members separately, as well as together. In order to evaluate youth successfully, one must also screen parents for psychopathology, as this contributes to the risk and clinical picture; additionally, information from teachers, peers, or direct observation, can be helpful. It should be noted that parents are often better at reporting behavior problems, whereas adolescents are better at reporting their internal mood states and experiences.

TABLE 36-2

STANDARDIZED RATING INSTRUMENTS
FOR MOOD DISORDERS

KSADS
DISC
Childhood Depression Rating Scale-revised (CDRS-R) (Poznanski et al., 1999)
Childhood Depression Inventory (CDI) (Kovacs et al., 1985)
Youth Mania Rating Scale (Fristad et al., 1992, 1995)
Child Behavior Checklist (CBCL) (Achenbach, 1992)
Child Symptom Inventory (CSI) (Gadow and Sprafkin, 1994)

TABLE 36-3

USUAL PRINCIPLE SYMPTOMS OF MOOD
DISORDERS

Depressed or irritable mood
Suicidal thoughts
Neurovegetative symptoms
Anhedonia
Decreased concentration
Feelings of hopelessness, worthlessness, or guilt
Suicidal ideations and plans

In addition to the direct clinical assessment, the use of standardized rating instruments (Table 36-2) can be helpful in evaluation and measures of progress. The KSADS (Chambers et al., 1985) is a semistructured, interviewer-based instrument that covers a broad spectrum of psychopathology. There is also an equally comprehensive diagnostic instrument that can be self-administered on a computer, the DISC (Diagnostic Interview Schedule for Children) (Shaffer et al., 2000). Other rating scales are listed in Table 36-2. These and other clinical rating scales are often used as a part of routine care as they can facilitate diagnosis, help determine severity of illness, and assist in monitoring responses to treatment.

The clinical presentation of mood disorders can have significant developmental differences. For adolescents, the individual's developmental level may not be the same as the chronologic age; this must be kept in mind in determining whether a symptom is clinically significant or not. The usual principle symptoms are listed in Table 36-3. In addition to traditional signs and symptoms, a number of other features may be associated with the mood disturbance; these include somatic complaints, psychomotor agitation, emotional arousal, phobias, separation anxiety, mood-congruent hallucinations, anxiety, substance abuse, and antisocial as well as aggressive behaviors (Kovacs et al., 1989; Carlson and Kashani, 1988; Birmaher et al., 1996; Weller and Weller, 1990).

In particular, adolescents who are depressed may present with overt behavior problems and not sadness or depressed mood. They may also show deviations from their otherwise typical involvement with their peer group; they may instead present with apathy, boredom, loneliness, or increasing social withdrawal. A decline in grades or even school failure may result from a lack of energy or concentration associated with an undetected depression. Twenty percent of adolescents with a mood disorder present with drug abuse. Similar to adults, males tend to report acting-out behaviors like drug abuse, running away, and theft in comparison to females.

Dysthymic disorder is a milder, less acute form of depression that can appear in adolescents. The average length of an early-onset episode of dysthymia is 4 years. It is associated with an increased risk for major depressive disorder (70%), bipolar disorder (13%), and substance abuse (15%) (Keller et al., 1988; Kovacs et al., 1994; Lewinsohn et al., 1991). Both boys and girls are equally represented with little differentiation in reference to age, socioeconomic status, parent's marital status, IQ, or school difficulties (Kovacs et al., 1994; Ferro et al., 1994).

One of the challenges with bipolar disorder is accurate diagnosis in adolescents. A broader phenotype includes adolescents who do not quite meet criteria for bipolar disorder, but still are impaired by symptoms of mood instability. This is a controversial topic with a growing discussion about whether bipolar symptoms in youth are dissimilar to those of adults. Mania in youth may include features listed in Table 36-4. Adolescents may have a

TABLE 36-4

FEATURES OF MANIA IN ADOLESCENTS

Irritability with aggressive temper outbursts rather than euphoria

Disordered sleep patterns

Impulsivity

Hyperactivity with goal-directed behavior (often associated with a high level of danger)

Disruptive behavior

Poor concentration

Mixed features

greater prolonged early course and are less responsive to treatment (McGlashan 1988; Strober et al., 1995). A manic episode may not occur first; therefore, one must take a comprehensive history, particularly regarding the family history and previous episodes of depression. Also, manic symptoms may not be clinically obvious. They may be gradually developing or be confounded with ADHD, anxiety, or with psychotic or behavioral symptoms. Irritability, labile mood, insomnia, and grandiosity are more common than euphoria. Early-onset usually predicts a worse course of illness, and the rate of onset of bipolar illness is higher in early-onset depression (Carlson et al., 2000).

No specific laboratory tests exist for the diagnosis of depression or bipolar disorder. However, a complete physical examination and appropriate laboratory tests are recommended to rule out specific elements of the differential diagnosis, including encephalopathies and neuroendocrine disturbances. Electroencephalography, CT scanning, or MRI ought to be performed only if clinically indicated. While abnormalities have been reported in neuroimaging studies, these are not of clinical use at this time.

DIFFERENTIAL DIAGNOSIS/COMORBIDITY

Comorbidity is a great concern and, indeed, is the rule rather than exception. Multiple epidemiologic and clinical studies have shown that up to 40%–70%

of depressed children and adolescents have a comorbid psychiatric diagnosis. Dysthymic disorder, anxiety disorder (Chap. 37), disruptive behavior disorders (Chap. 35), and substance abuse disorders (Chap. 34) are the most frequently diagnosed comorbid conditions. Also, increasing rates of ADHD (Chap. 38) and enuresis or encopresis have been reported. Both physical abuse and sexual abuse have been associated with depressive symptoms (Chap. 23).

Due to atypical presentations of disruptive behavior in youth, externalizing disorders have been confused with bipolar disorder, particularly in relation to impulsivity, hyperactivity, distractibility, and emotional lability. Studies have shown that in bipolar patients, the rates of ADHD vary from 22% to 98% (Geller and Luby, 1997; West et al., 1995; Wozniak et al., 1995; Carlson, 1990). Anxiety disorders were found in about 33% of prepubertal bipolar patients and 12% of adolescent bipolar patients (Geller et al., 1995).

Medical illnesses can be associated with depressive or manic symptoms and must be considered in the differential diagnosis of acute onset illness. Depressive symptoms can result from a number of disorders (Table 36-5). Particularly, right-hemisphere disease and frontal lobe damage can result in anhedonia, apathy, and bradykinesia. Manic symptoms can also result from exposure to prescription drug use, especially antidepressants, steroids, or stimulants; cocaine or amphetamine intoxication must be

TABLE 36-5

MEDICAL DISORDERS LEADING TO MOOD DISORDERS

Endocrine disorders such as diabetes or hypothyroidism

Brain injury or mass

Seizure disorder

Metabolic abnormalities

Infections

Multiple sclerosis

Malignancy

Acquired immunodeficiency syndrome (AIDS)

Migraine headaches

Medications (see text)

Others

considered when evaluating adolescents for mania. Less commonly, metabolic abnormalities, systemic infections, hyperthyroidism, and porphyria may lead to manic symptoms.

TREATMENT

As soon as an affirmative diagnosis is made, it is important to initiate treatment as soon as possible, due to the significant morbidity and mortality associated with adolescent mood disorders. In general, treatments for adolescent mood disorders should take place in the context of a biopsychosocial approach (Table 36-6). This approach mandates consideration of both biologic and environmental interventions. Biologic interventions are largely focused on psychotropic medications; however, the use of endocrinologic agents, electroconvulsive therapy (ECT), and transcranial magnetic stimulation (TMS) should not be ruled out. Environmental interventions could include one or more types of individual and group psychotherapy as well as interventions directed at school or work, social skills, behavioral functioning, and comorbidity.

The initial approach to treatment, to some extent, depends on the severity of presenting symptoms, comorbidity, prior history, and motivation for treatment. If the depression is mild, an initial approach can be supportive to alleviate stress. However, in moderate-to-severe depression, targeting symptoms with psychotherapy and medication may limit the severity of the episode. In some cases of severe depression, hospitalization may be indicated. This is especially the case when there are pronounced suicidal ideations or intentions and/or the presence of psychosis.

In general, there are three phases of treatment of mood disorders in adolescents: acute, continuation, and maintenance. The *acute phase* lasts about 6–12 weeks and treatment goals are to obtain a significant reduction in symptoms for at least 2 weeks. The *continuation phase* is an attempt to arrive at a full remission or at least 2–8 weeks of no or mild symptoms. The *maintenance* phase, often 4–12 months since initiation of treatment, is focused on relapse prevention. For individuals with recurrent episodes, the maintenance phase may last for years or even a lifetime. Despite the dearth of data, it is important for the clinician to begin treatment by attempting to educate the patient and family about the diagnosis, the target symptoms, available treatments, and expected results. This not only facilitates treatment planning but also compliance.

PHARMACOTHERAPY

Much has been written about the lack of randomized-controlled studies for the use of psychotropic medication (Table 36-7) for the treatment of children and adolescents with mood disorders. Even when studies exist, sample sizes are generally small, follow-up duration is limited to the acute phase of illness, and prevention of relapse is undetermined. A vexing problem for clinicians is the dearth of controlled trials that are conducted in adolescents, have ample size, and address the developmental challenges unique to this age group. The severity of the morbidity and mortality in teenagers is significant and provides compelling data to support interventions even with moderate treatment effect sizes.

For now, *selective serotonin reuptake inhibitors* (SSRIs) are the first-line pharmacologic treatment for major depression. Although *tricyclic antidepressants* were once considered first-line treatment, SSRIs appear to be much safer and at least as

T A B L E   3 6 - 6

TREATMENT OPTIONS FOR ADOLESCENTS WITH MOOD DISORDERS

Biological interventions
Psychotropic medications
Endocrinologic agents
Electroconvulsive therapy
Transcranial magnetic stimulation

Environmental interventions
Family therapy
Individual psychotherapy
Group psychotherapy
Others (see text)

TABLE 36-7

PSYCHOTROPIC AGENTS FOR MOOD DISORDERS (WITH DAILY DOSAGE RANGES)

Tricyclic antidepressants (not to exceed 3.5 mg/kg/day)
Imipramine (Tofranil) (50–200 mg/day)
Desipramine (Norpramin) (50–200 mg/day)
Nortriptyline (Pamelor) (20–100 mg/day)
Amitriptyline (Elavil) (50–200 mg/day)
Selective serotonin reuptake inhibitors
Fluoxetine (Prozac) (5–60 mg/day)
Fluvoxamine (Luvox) (50–200 mg/day)
Paroxetine (Paxil) (10–30 mg/day)*
Sertraline (Zoloft) (25–150 mg/day)
Citalopram (Celexa) (20–40 mg/day)
Escitalopram (Lexapro) (10–20 mg/day)
Other antidepressants
Bupropion (Wellbutrin) (75–400 mg/day)
Venlafaxine (Effexor) (50–200 mg/day)
Trazodone (Deseryl) (50–600 mg/day)
Mirtazapine (Remeron) (15–60 mg/day)

*In June, 2003, the Food and Drug Administration advised against the use of paroxetine in children and adolescents because of concerns it sometimes might increase the risk of suicidal ideation.
Source: Elliott DR, Smiga S: Depression in the child and adolescent. *Pediatr Clin North Am* 2003;50:1101.

effective. The SSRIs have relatively long half-lives, making once a day dosing generally possible (Chap. 37). Even though SSRIs do not appear to have a dose-dependent relationship with regard to therapeutic response, it seems clear that increasing dose is associated with an increase in side effects (Table 36-8). A potential link between antidepressants and risk of suicide is under study (Jick et al., 2004; Wessely and Kerwin, 2004; Whittington et al., 2004) and has resulted is the Federal Drug Administration (FDA) issuing a black box warning in 2004 for SSRIs regarding this potential. There clearly appears to be discontinuation syndromes associated with acute withdrawal from SSRIs; therefore, a tapering discontinuation schedule, especially with short half-life compounds, is advisable (Chap. 37).

TABLE 36-8

SSRI SIDE EFFECTS

Suicidality (FDA black box warning)
Nausea
Diarrhea
Constipation
Weight gain
Dyspepsia
Anorexia
Xerostomia
Decreased libido
Impotence
Anorgasmia
Ejaculation difficulties
Headache
Insomnia
Anxiety or nervousness
Somnolence
Amotivation syndrome
Tremor
Dizziness
Precipitate hypomania or mania (10% vs. 0.5–5% in adults)
Discontinuation syndrome
Aggressiveness
Hyperkinesis
Urinary incontinence
Epistaxis; purpura
Sinusitis
Akathisia (motor restlessness)
Especially in combination with neuroleptics
Linked to suicidality
Gastrointestinal bleeding (due to platelet function inhibition)
Hyponatremia
Growth attenuation
Discontinuation syndrome
Agitation, anxiety, anorexia, confusion, diarrhea, headache, sweating, tremor, emesis, flu-shock-like
Serotonin syndrome due to drug interactions
Isoniazid
Tramadol
St. Johns' Wart
Dextromethorphan

There are a very limited number of double-blind, placebo-controlled studies on the efficacy and safety of SSRIs in children and adolescents. The first study, reported by Emslie et al. (1997), found fluoxetine to be superior to placebo in the acute-phase treatment for both children and adolescents with major depressive disorder. At the completion of the study, 56% of patients treated with fluoxetine versus 33% given placebo were rated "much" or "very much" improved. Although a significant response was reported, many subjects only partially improved and did not achieve remission. This suggests that a higher dose of fluoxetine or longer treatment may have been helpful.

In another double-blind, placebo-controlled study, Keller et al. (2001) examined the efficacy of the SSRI, paroxetine (Paxil), as compared with the tricyclic antidepressant, imipramine (Tofranil and others), in 275 depressed adolescents. An 8-week, randomized, multicenter, parallel-design comparison of paroxetine and placebo to imipramine and placebo found that paroxetine was reported to be significantly more effective than placebo for depressed mood; also, the response to imipramine was not significantly different from placebo. Ambrosini et al. (1999) reported that SSRIs have a response rate of between 70% and 90% in open trials. Also, SSRIs were generally well tolerated.

Antidepressants that have a variety of mechanisms of actions are available for use in adults; however, few have been used in studies in youth. Current medications with limited, open-label studies include venlafaxine (Effexor), bupropion (Wellbutrin), and trazodone (Desyrel). The tricyclic antidepressants are probably no longer indicated for use in the treatment of depression in adolescents. This largely follows from side effects and safety factors, but there is also a general lack of scientific support for their efficacy in youth (Hazell et al., 1995; Ambrosini et al., 1993).

While SSRIs are generally effective in the treatment of depression, there are cases of treatment-resistant depression. In these cases, the first step is to clarify the patient's diagnosis and comorbidities. Secondly, one has to assess the level of compliance with treatment. If indications are that the diagnosis is correct and the compliance has been good, then one should optimize the current antidepressant dosage before switching to another medication. Pharmacologic treatment trials should occur for at least 6 weeks and, preferably, up to 10–12 weeks in partial responders. If medication changes do not prove to be effective, then augmentation strategies or combinations of psychopharmacologic agents should be considered. Adding lithium, 1-triiodothyronine (T3) at 25–50 µg/day, a stimulant medication, or another antidepressant has been show to be effective in adults; however, studies in children and adolescents in this regard are not available. When there is profound treatment failure and persistence of severe depressive symptoms, the use of ECT may be considered. However, there are no controlled studies in adolescents.

PSYCHOTHERAPY

For moderate-to-severe depressions, some form of psychosocial intervention should accompany medication management. There are five general types of psychosocial therapies for depression in adolescent, as listed in Table 36-9; these therapies can be used alone or in conjunction with each other, depending on the presenting problem and needs of the patient and family. Cognitive-behavior therapy (CBT) has been the subject of the most rigorous empirical study and the meta-analysis by Reinecke et al. (1998) was able to demonstrate a strong case for the use of CBT to treat adolescent depression. Clinical trials of interpersonal psychotherapy (IPT) suggest that the efficacy of IPT is equivalent to CBT; however, the complete absence of proper

TABLE 36-9

TYPES OF PSYCHOSOCIAL THERAPIES FOR DEPRESSION IN ADOLESCENTS

Cognitive-behavior therapy
Psychodynamic psychotherapy
Interpersonal psychotherapy
Group psychotherapy
Family therapy

controlled trials makes it difficult to assess the efficacy of psychodynamic psychotherapy, group therapy, and family therapy.

The Treatment of Adolescent Depression Study (TADS) was a multicenter, randomized control trial with 439 adolescents; it compared fluoxetine, CBT in combination, and alone against placebo, and provides the soundest evidence in support of successful treatment of depression in adolescents (Martin et al., 2003; Weiner annd Dulcan, 2004). Fluoxetine with CBT (71% improved) and fluoxetine (60.6%) or CBT (43.2%) alone were significantly superior to placebo (34.8%). Suicidal ideations were noted in 29% of the sample at baseline and improved steadily throughout the course of treatment with the eventual result of seven suicide attempts (1.6%) and no completed suicides.

BIPOLAR DISORDER

There has been a growing interest and much controversy concerning the diagnosis and treatment of bipolar illness in adolescents. As with major depressive disorder, pharmacologic treatments for bipolar disorder are largely extrapolated from studies done in adults and through anecdotal reports. Few placebo-controlled studies of adequate size and control are reported for bipolar illness in children and adolescents, thus making conclusions about the role of medications in the treatment of mania difficult to reach at this time.

In addition to the use of antidepressants, three basic medications have been used to treat bipolar disorder: lithium, mood stabilizers, and neuroleptics. Limited double-blind, randomized, placebo-controlled prospective studies and many case reports confirm the efficacy of lithium use in adolescents with bipolar illness (Geller et al., 1998; Keck et al., 2000; Kowatch et al., 2000). Careful monitoring of blood levels and side effects is essential as part of treatment (Silva et al., 1992; Geller and Fetner, 1989).

Similar to adults, anticonvulsants are more effective in mixed-states and rapid-cycling bipolar illness. The most common anticonvulsants used are valproic acid (Depakote and others) and carbamazepine (Tegretol) (Chap. 13). Both have been shown to be effective in youths (Donovan et al., 1997; Delito et al., 1998; Post et al., 1996; Solomon et al., 1996). Since these compounds have both mild and potentially lethal side effects, they are very carefully used in adolescents. Carbamazepine is typically used at a level of 6–12 µg/mL, while valproate is at levels of 80–110 µg/mL. Other anticonvulsants (lamotrigine [Lamictal], gabapentin [Neurontin], and topiramate [Topamax]) apparently have mood stabilizing properties as well, but have thus far not been the focus of adequate trials.

Antipsychotics have been FDA approved for acute mania in adults, but no controlled studies have been done for adolescents with mania. However, these medications, in particular atypical neuroleptics (risperidone [Risperdal], olanzepine [Zyprexa], aripiperazole [Abilify], ziprasadone [Geodon], quetiapine [Seroquel], are in common clinical use (Chap. 39).

COURSE/PROGNOSIS

The dearth of population-based trials and extensive follow-up studies make it very difficult to determine the actual course and outcome of mood disorders in adolescents. Studies have shown that youth with two or more depressive episodes seem to have poorer functioning than those with nonrecurrent episodes (Rao et al., 1995; Warner et al., 1995). In a large follow-up study of a clinically referred population (Kovacs et al., 1989, 1994), 26% of adolescents relapsed in a year, and 40% within 2 years of the initial depressive episode; by 5 years, two-thirds had a subsequent episode. Strober et al. (1993) reported recovery for adolescent inpatients to be 90% by 2 years. In other reports, a more protracted course seems to be associated with earlier onset (Lewinsohn et al., 1994; McCauley et al., 1993). Factors that have been associated with poorer prognosis include female sex, comorbid conditions (ADHD, conduct, or anxiety disorders), and exposure to negative events.

SUMMARY

Mood disorders are among the most common disorders to be experienced by adolescents; also, they are highly associated with significant morbidity and mortality in adolescents, including school and social failure as well as suicidality. While the diagnosis and treatment of psychiatric illness in adolescents can be complicated, safe and effective treatments are available. All treatments begin with a careful diagnostic assessment followed by thoughtful patient and family education. The use of psychotropic medications, including the SSRIs, atypical neuroleptics, and mood stabilizers, can be effective. Now, there is also growing evidence of the use of at least some forms of psychotherapy that, in combination with medications, can lead to improvement rates well in excess of 70% for adolescent patients.

The real limits to treatment and outcome rest in the failure to diagnose and adequately treat these disorders. Unfortunately, these limits to management are aggravated by a healthcare system that has systematic biases by insurance plans and practitioners, as well as community-prejudices against adolescent patients and their families in which psychiatric illness is present. Science will continue to lead to safer and more effective treatments, but changes in personal and community beliefs as public policy will be necessary to assure that all of our youth have access to proper diagnostic and treatment services for mood disorders and other psychiatric illnesses.

Bibliography

Achenbach TM: *Manual for the Child Behavior Checklist/2-3 and 1992 Profile*. Burlington, VT: University of Vermont, 1992.

Akiskal HS: Mood disorders: Introduction and overview, in: Kaplan HI, Sadock BJ (eds.), *Comprehensive Textbook of Psychiatry*, 4th ed. Baltimore, MD: Williams & Wilkins, 1995, pp. 1067–1069.

Allgood-Merten B, Lewinsohn PM. Hops H: Sex differences and adolescent depression. *J Abnormal Psychol* 1990;99:55–63.

Ambrosini PJ, Bianchi MD, Rabinovich H, et al.: Antidepressant treatments in children and adolescents, I: Affective disorders. *J Am Acad Child Adolesc Psychiatry* 1993;32:1–6.

Ambrosini PJ, Wagner KD, Biederman J, et al.: Multicenter open-label sertraline study in adolescent outpatients with major depression. *J Am Acad Child Adolesc Psychiatry* 1999;38:566–572.

American Psychiatric Association. *Diagnostic and Statistical Manual of Mental Disorders*, 4th ed. Washington, DC, 1994.

American Psychiatric Association. *Diagnostic and Statistical Manual of Mental Disorders*, 4th ed. Text Revision (DSM-IV-TR). Washington, DC, 2003.

Anderson JC, Williams S, McGee R, et al.: DSM-III disorders in preadolescent children: Prevalence in a large sample from the general population. *Arch Gen Psychiatry* 1987;44:69–76.

Avison WR, Mcalpine DD: Gender differences in symptoms of depression among adolescents. *J Health Soc Behav* 1992;33:77–96.

Bird HR, Canino G, Rubio-Stipec M, et al.: Estimates of the prevalence of childhood maladjustment to a community survey in Puerto Rico: The use of combined measures. *Arch Gen Psychiatry* 1988;45:1120–1126.

Birmaher B, Ryan ND, Williamson DE, et al.: Childhood and adolescent depression: A review of the past 10 years. Part II. *J Am Acad Child Adolesc Psychiatry* 1996;35:1575–1583.

Bowlby J: Grief and mourning in infancy and early childhood. *Psychoanal Study Child* 1960;15:9–52.

Brent DA, Perper JA, Moritz G, et al.: Psychiatric risk factors for adolescent suicide: A case-control study. *J Am Acad Child Adolesc Psychiatry* 1993;32: 521–529.

Burns JJ, Cottrell L, Perkins K, et al.: Depressive symptoms and health risk among rural adolescents. *Pediatrics* 2004;113:1313–1320.

Carlson GA: Child and adolescent mania-diagnostic considerations. *J Child Psychol Psychiatry* 1990;31: 331–341.

Carlson GA, Kashani JH: Manic symptoms in a non-referred adolescent population. *J Affect Disord* 1988;15:219–226.

Carlson GA, Bromet EJ, Sievers S: Phenomenology and outcome of subjects with early and adult-onset psychotic mania. *Am J Psychiatry* 2000;157:213–219.

Chambers WJ, Puig-Antich J, Hirsch M, et al.: The assessment of affective disorders in children and adolescents by semistructured interview. *Arch Gen Psychiatry* 1985;42:696–702.

Cook WL, Kenny DA, Goldstein MJ: Parental affective style risk and the family system: A social relations model analysis. *J Abnorm Psychol* 1991;100: 492–501.

Dahl RE, Ryan ND, Williamson DE, et al.: Regulation of sleep and growth hormone in adolescent depression. *J Am Acad Child Adolesc Psychiatry* 1992;31: 615–621.

Delito JA, Levitan J, Damore J, et al.: Naturalistic experience with the use of divalproex sodium on an inpatient unit for adolescent psychiatric patients. *Acta Psychiatric Scand* 1998;97:236–240.

Donovan SJ, Susser ES, Nunes EV, et al.: Divalproex treatment of disruptive adolescents: A report of 10 cases. *J Clin Psychiatry* 1997;58:12–15.

Elliott GR, Smiga S: Depression in the child and adolescent. *Pediatr Clin North Am* 2003;50:1093–1106.

Emslie GJ, Rush AJ, Weinberg WA, et al.: A double-blind, randomized, placebo-controlled trial of fluoxetine in children and adolescents with depression. *Arch Gen Psychiatry* 1997;54:1031–1037.

Ferro T, Carlson GA, Grayson P, et al.: Depressive disorders: Distinctions in children. *J Am Acad Child Adolesc Psychiatry* 1994;33:664–670.

Fristad MA, Weller EB, Weller RA: The Mania Rating Scale: Can it be used in children? A preliminary report. *J Am Acad Child Adolesc Psychiatry* 1992;31:252-257.

Fristad MA, Weller RA, Weller EB: The Mania Rating Scale: Further reliability and validity studies with children. *Ann Clin Psychiatry* 1995;7:127–132.

Gabbard GO: Mood disorders: Psychodynamic etiology, in: Kaplan HI, Saddock BJ (eds.), *Comprehensive Textbook of Psychiatry*, 6th ed. Baltimore, MD: Williams & Wilkins, 1995, pp. 1116–1123.

Gadow KD, Sprafkin J: *Child Symptom Inventory*. Stony Brook, NY: Checkmate Plus, 1994.

Geller B, Sun K, Zimerman B, et al: Complex and rapid-cycling in bipolar children and adolescents: A preliminary study. *J Affect Dis* 1995;34:259–268.

Geller B, Cooper TB, Sun, K, et al.: Double-blind and placebo-controlled study of lithium for adolescent bipolar disorders with secondary substance abuse dependency. *J Am Acad Child Adolesc Psychiatry* 1998;37:171–178.

Geller B, Fetner HH: Children's 24-hour serum lithium level after a single dose predicts initial steady-state plasma level (letter). *J Clin Psychopharmacol* 1989;9:155.

Geller B, Luby J: Child and adolescent bipolar disorder: A review of the past 10 years. *J Am Acad Child Adolesc Psychiatry* 1997;36:1168–1176.

Gould MS, Marrocco FA, Kleinman M, et al: Evaluating iatrogenic risk of youth suicide screening programs: A randomized controlled trial. *JAMA* 2005;293:1635–1643.

Hazell P, O'Connell D, Healthcote D, et al.: Efficacy of tricyclic drugs in treating child and adolescent bipolar depression: A meta-analysis. *BMJ* 1995;310:897–901.

Homicide and suicide rates—national violent death reporting system, 2003. *MMWR* 2005;54:377–380.

Jick H, Kaye JA, Jick SS: Antidepressants and the risk of suicide behaviors. *JAMA* 2004;292:338–343.

Keck, PE Jr, Mendlwicz J, Calabrese JR, et al.: A review of randomized, controlled clinical trials in acute mania. *J Affect Disord* 2000;59:S31–S39.

Keller MB, Beardslee W, Lavori PW, et al.: Course of major depression in non-referred adolescents: A retrospective study. *J Affect Disord* 1988;15:235–243.

Keller MB, Ryan ND, Strober M, et al.: Efficacy of paroxetine in the treatment of adolescent major depression: A randomized, controlled trial. *J Am Acad Child Adolesc Psychiatry* 2001;40:762–772.

Kovacs M: The children's depression inventory (CDI). *Psychopharm Bull* 1985;21:995–998.

Kovacs M: Gender and the course of major depressive disorder through adolescence in clinically referred youngsters. *J Am Acad Child Adolesc Psychiatry* 2001;40:1079–1085.

Kovacs M, Gatsonis C, Paulauskas SI, et al.: Depressive disorders in childhood, IV: A longitudinal study of comorbidity with and risk for anxiety disorders. *Arch Gen Psychiatry* 1989;46:776–782.

Kovacs M, Akiskal HS, Gatsonis C, et al.: Childhood-onset dysthymic disorder. Clinical features and prospective naturalistic outcome. *Arch Gen Psychiatry* 1994;51:365–374.

Kowatch RA, Suppes T, Carmody TJ, et al.: Effect size of lithium, divalproex sodium, and carbamazepine in children and adolescents with bipolar disorder. *J Am Acad Child Adolesc Psychiatry* 2000;39:713–720.

Kraepelin E: Manic-Depressive Insanity and Paranoia. Edinburgh, Scotland: Churchill-Livingstone, 1921.

Kutcher SP, Williamson P, Silverberg J, et al.: Nocturnal growth hormone secretion in depressed older adolescents. *J Am Acad Child Adolesc Psychiatry* 1988;27: 751–754.

Lewinsohn PM, Clarke GN, Seeley JR, et al.: Major depression in community adolescents: age at onset, episodic duration, and time to recurrence. *J Am Acad Child Adolesc Psychiatry* 1994;33:809–818.

Lewinsohn PM, Rohde P, Seeley JR, et al.: Comorbidity of unipolar depression, I: Major depression with dysthymia. *J Abnorm Psychol* 1991;100:205–213.

Lewinsohn PM, Roberts RE, Seeley JR, et al.: Adolescent psychopathology, II: Psychosocial risk factors for depression. *J Abnorm Psychol* 1994;103:302–315.

Lewinsohn PM, Rohde P, Seeley JR, et al.: Natural course of adolescent major depressive disorder in a community sample: Predictors of recurrence in young adults. *Am J Psychiatry* 2000;157:1584–1591.

McCauley E, Myers K, Mitchell J, et al.: Depression in young people: Initial presentation and clinical course. *J Am Acad Child Adolesc Psychiatry* 1993;32: 714–722.

McGlashan TH: Adolescent versus adult onset mania. *Am J Psychiatry* 1988;145:221–223.

Martin A, Scahill L, Charney D, Leckman J: *Pediatric Psychopharmacology: Principles and Practice.* NYC: Oxford University Press, 2003, p. 816.

Nurnberger JI, Gershon E: Genetics, in: Pakel ES (ed.), *Handbook of Effective Disorders.* Edinburgh, Scotland: Churchill-Livingston, 1982, pp. 126–145.

Post RM, Ketter TA, Denicoff K, et al.: The place of anticonvulsant therapy in bipolar illness. *Psychopharmacology* 1996;128:115–129.

Poznansky E, Mokros HB: Children's Depression Rating Scale-Revised. Los Angeles: Western Psychological Services, 1999.

Rao U, Ryan ND, Birmaher B, et al.: Unipolar depression in adolescents: Clinical outcome in adulthood. *J Am Acad Child Adolesc Psychiatry* 1995;34: 566–578.

Reinecke MA, Ryan ND, Dubois DL: Cognitive–behavioral therapy of depression and depressive symptoms during adolescence: A review and meta-analysis. *J Am Acad Child Adolesc Psychiatry* 1998; 37:26–34.

Schatzberg AF, Nemeroff CB: *The American Psychiatric Publishing Textbook of Psychopharmacology,* 3d ed. Washington, DC: American Psychiatric Publishing, 2004, p. 1248.

Seligman ME, Peterson C: A learned helplessness perspective on child depression: Theory and research, in: Rutter M, Izard CE, Read PB (eds.), *Depression in Young People.* New York: Guilford, 1986, pp. 223–249.

Shaffer D, Lucas C, Fisher P. *The Computerized Diagnostic Interview Schedule for Children.* New York, NY: The DISC Development Group, Columbia University, 2000, p. 10032.

Silva RR, Campbell M, Golden RR, et al.: Side effects associated with lithium and placebo administration in aggressive children. *Psychopharmacol Bull* 1992;28: 319–326.

Solomon DA, Keitner GI, Ryan CE, et al.: Polypharmacy in bipolar I disorder. *Psychopharmacol Bull* 1996;32: 579–587.

Spady DW, Schopflocher DP, Svenson LW et al: Medical and psychiatric comorbidity and health care among children 6 to 17 years of age. *Arch Pediatr Adolesc Med* 2005;159:231–237.

Spitz R: Anaclitic depression. *Psychoanal Study Child* 1946;2:113–117.

Strober M, Lampert C, Schmidt S, et al.: The course of major depressive disorder in adolescents, I: Recovery and risk of manic switching in a follow-up of psychotic and nonpsychotic subtypes. *J Am Acad Child Adolesc Psychiatry* 1993;32:34–42.

Strober M, Schmidt-Lackner S, Freeman R, et al.: Recovery and relapse in adolescents with bipolar affective illness: A five-year naturalistic, prospective follow-up. *J Am Acad Child Adolesc Psychiatry* 1995;34:724–731.

Warner V, Mufson L, Weissman MM: Offspring at high and low risk for depression and anxiety: mechanisms of psychiatric disorder. *J Am Acad Child Adolesc Psychiatry* 1995;34:786–797.

Weiner JM, Dulcan MK (eds.): *The American Psychiatric Publishing Textbook of Child and Adolescent Psychiatry,* 3d ed. Washington, DC: American Psychiatric Publishing, 2004, p. 1114.

Weller EB, Weller RA: Depressive disorders in children and adolescents, in: Garfinkel BD (ed.), *Psychiatric Disorders in Children and Adolescents.* Philadelphia, PA: W.B. Saunders, 1990, pp. 3–20.

Wessely S, Kerwin R: Suicide risk and the SSRIs. *JAMA* 2004;292:379–381.

West SA, McElroy SL, Strakowski SM, et al.: Attention deficit hyperactivity disorder in adolescent mania. *Am J Psychiatry* 1995;152:271–273.

Whittington J, Kendall T, Fonagy P, et al.: Selective serotonin reuptake inhibitors in childhood depression: Systemic review of published versus unpublished data. *Lancet* 2004;363:1341–1345.

Wozniak J, Biederman J, Kiely K, et al.: Mania-like symptoms suggestive of childhood-onset bipolar disorder in clinically referred children. *J Am Acad Child Adolesc Psychiatry* 1995;34:867–876.

37

ANXIETY DISORDERS IN THE ADOLESCENT

Leah K. Andrews and John Scott Werry

I worry about everything . . . when I get up in the morning I worry about what I will wear. Then I worry about whether my friend will remember that she is walking with me, and if she will be on time, and if I will have to stand and wait for her and if people will think I'm a loser because I am alone standing waiting for someone and my clothes aren't right, and I must be a loser if they haven't turned up . . . and I haven't even told you about how I worry about my mum do you think she is drinking again? and about my schoolwork—have we got time for that?"

> "Kerry" aged 13 years, in treatment
> for generalized anxiety disorder.

OUTLINE

Anxiety disorders are characterized by severe anxiety sufficient to cause significant disability in function and/or subjective well-being; they occur in about 5% of adolescents, especially females and increase in frequency with age. They probably are most often due to an interaction between genetic/temperamental vulnerability and psychosocial stress, though physical disorders and medications can contribute. There are seven different types which are defined, although more than one can co-occur, as can other

psychiatric disorders. They can be mistaken for physical disorders and be over-investigated by clinicians. Treatment varies from commonsense advice to specialist procedures, such as cognitive behavior therapy (CBT). Medication, primarily selective serotonin reuptake inhibitor (SSRI) antidepressants, has a secondary role to play in some cases and should be reserved for the most severe cases; specialist advice and assistance is recommended.

INTRODUCTION

Anxiety is a subjective feeling of unease akin to fear, often accompanied by physical symptoms of arousal. It is a normal experience, necessary to performance, motivation, and development which can be expressed *internally* with thoughts of fear or apprehension, or *externally* with a broad range of behaviors and somatic symptoms. Normal anxiety promotes a protective response to threat and is therefore adaptive. For anxiety to meet the criteria as a disorder as in the American Psychiatric Association's *Diagnostic and Statistical Manual of Mental Disorders (DSM-IV)*,[2] there must be clear and significant impairment of social, educational, occupational, or developmental functioning directly due to the symptoms. Inaccurate media reports often try to dismiss DSM-IV as pathologizing normal temperamental variations by ignoring this vital criterion.

Anxiety disorders are common, and adolescence is the time when their incidence, particularly of "adult-style" anxiety disorders, really begins; rates increase with age and with female gender. Around 20% of adolescents will have some symptoms of anxiety, but only 5% of 13–15-year olds will have anxiety symptoms which are excessive or disabling.[1] Separation anxiety and selective mutism are more common in younger children; however, in adolescence, the incidence of panic disorder, generalized anxiety disorder (GAD), and social phobia become predominant.[1]

Anxiety disorders are under-diagnosed, for a range of reasons. There is generally a poor association between parents' and youth's report of all mental health symptoms[3]; also, adults can be dismissive of adolescents' complaints, regarding them as "teenage stuff." In anxiety disorders the young person's own account of symptoms is paramount. This is not to dismiss adult reports which are especially helpful to describe change in function and the degree of resulting disability; however, relying on them alone can both miss the diagnosis and underestimate the degree of internal distress being experienced by the young person. Second, anxiety disorders are often comorbid and therefore obscured by other conditions much more annoying to adults.

Comorbidity is a major issue to consider, especially in patients seen in mental health clinics. Anxiety is strikingly associated with depression in adolescents (30%–50% of cases) and linked to suicide in youth (Chap. 36).[4] Anxiety disorders are also frequently (14%)[5] comorbid with another anxiety disorder. Twenty percent of adolescents with externalizing disorders such as conduct and attention-deficit/hyperactivity disorder (ADHD) also have an anxiety disorder (Chaps. 35 and 38).[6] Anxiety disorders are also common in other psychiatric disorders, for example, eating disorders[7] and bipolar affective disorder (Chaps. 30 and 36).[8] Anxiety symptoms and disorders are common in adolescents presenting with unexplained physical complaints[9,10] and in chronic illness[11–17] and are often poorly identified. There are significant associations with other problems—substance abuse

problems (Chap. 34),[18] cigarette smoking,[19] childhood sexual and physical abuse (Chap. 23),[20] incarceration (especially panic),[21] and lower levels of educational achievement[22] due to school dropout.

Anxiety is commonly regarded as a reaction to environmental stressors, but often the seed seems to fall on fertile soil, and something that stresses one young person may leave another unaffected. Many researchers have noted a strong association between anxiety disorders in young people and in first-degree relatives[23] with odds ratios from 4 to 6[24] and heritability calculations of 0.43 for panic disorder and 0.32 for GAD. This anxiety in relatives not only suggests that the etiology of anxiety disorders is complicated, but compounds the difficulty of managing the adolescent.

ANXIETY DISORDERS AFFECTING ADOLESCENTS: DESCRIPTIONS AND DIAGNOSES

Teenagers may experience a range of anxiety disorders that are now reviewed (Table 37-1).

Panic Attacks/Panic Disorder

Panic attacks are discreet episodes of intense fear or distress, usually developing suddenly and lasting about 10 minutes. DSM-IV requires the presence

TABLE 37-1

ANXIETY DISORDERS AFFECTING ADOLESCENTS

Panic attacks/panic disorder (with and without agoraphobia)
Specific phobia
Social phobia
Separation anxiety
Obsessive-compulsive disorder
Post-traumatic stress disorder
Generalized anxiety disorder
Anxiety disorder due to a medical condition
Substance-induced anxiety disorder

of at least four of the following: palpitations, sweating, trembling, sensations of shortness of breath, feelings of choking, chest pain, nausea or abdominal distress, feeling dizzy or faint, feelings of unreality or detachment, numbness or tingling sensation, chills or hot flushes. Further criteria are fears of dying, vomiting, or loss of control.[2]

Many young people experience panic attacks without having panic disorder. Community rates of panic attacks in adolescents are 17% for a full-blown panic attack and 36% for some symptoms without the full picture.[25] However, only 7% reported that panic attacks interfered with their daily lives, i.e., met the criteria for a panic disorder. Panic attacks may occur in any anxiety disorder, but are particularly seen in social phobia, obsessive-compulsive disorder (OCD), GADs, and specific phobias.[26] Panic can also be induced by a wide range of medical conditions, e.g., hyperthyroidism, pheochromocytoma, complex seizures, cardiac conditions, and medications (both licit and illicit), including cocaine, amphetamines, caffeine, or withdrawal from depressants such as alcohol.

> "Georgia", a 12 year old girl whose parents had recently separated, presented with marked physical anxiety symptoms, particularly hyperventilation and rapid heart beat. She started Cognitive-behavior therapy but did not improve and a physical review detected an abdominal mass, which was a pheochromocytoma. Surgical removal of the mass alleviated all symptoms. Diagnosis was Anxiety due to a general medical condition, now resolved.

Few adolescents recognize panic attacks as psychologic problems, instead seeing themselves as about to die or seriously ill. Thus, the doctor's role in identifying them is central. Clinicians can inadvertently contribute to iatrogenic ill-effects by medical over-investigation without a good, supportive history. Failure to recognize panic attacks can also lead to secondary chronic avoidance, such as agoraphobia and social isolation.

Specific Phobias

These are fears of specific objects, such as insects, animals, heights, flying, blood, and needles all of which are common in normal youth: to constitute phobic disorder, the fears need to be developmentally excessive, out of keeping with the situation, and cause impairment of functioning. Adolescents with specific phobic disorders also commonly experience panic attacks when confronted with the feared situation, and many have other anxiety disorders in addition to the phobia. Phobias are common, for example in a birth cohort of New Zealand 15 years old 3.6% had a specific phobic disorder.[27] Similar rates have been found in other community samples.

> "Jessica", 14, was seen by her pediatrician because of acne. During the interview she confided that she had "arachnophobia" with concerns about being bitten by a poisonous spider since a nest of these had been found at the school. She continued to attend school regularly and her grades and social activities were fine. Jessica's self-diagnosis seemed inaccurate and she was reassured that concerns about poisonous creatures are not necessarily abnormal.

Social Phobias

Social phobia is a relatively common disorder (lifetime prevalence 7.3% in a study of 3000 14–24-year olds[28]), has a peak incidence at age 16 years, and is more common in females. Young people with social phobia experience intense distress, sometimes with panic attacks or other acute anxiety symptoms in social situations and generally avoid these. Shyness alone is not sufficient for a social phobia diagnosis: as in all disorders, there must be a major impact on the adolescent's occupational or academic functioning and socialization.

Those with social phobia often "freeze" in social situations, hide from sight, may become electively mute, shrink from contact with others, but may also show secondary aggressive or difficult behavior. Although most adolescents will recognize that their fears of social situations are excessive, not all will be able to verbalize this and the observations of parents or teachers are needed. Unlike those with autistic spectrum disorder, young people with social phobia do make good intimate social relationships with known and familiar people.

"James", 14, had not attended school for a year. He had many episodes of abdominal pain, which he rated "10 out of 10" in severity. Extensive gastroenterology work-up had not found any disorder. James was observed to be restless, anxious, and sweaty when getting ready for school and teachers said that he appeared frightened to speak; however, he denied any worries or concerns except for his pain. James was diagnosed with Social Phobia and treated with fluoxetine (20 mg daily) but wouldn't take part in any Cognitive Behavior Therapy approaches. He began a home-schooling program and continued to play in a youth orchestra.

Separation Anxiety Disorder

Childhood fears of separation from important figures are normal and usually peak in the preschool years. However, some children have ongoing severe fears of separation from others which interfere with their schooling and relationships. Although separation anxiety disorder (SAD) is more common in preadolescents, it can continue into the teenage years. Anxiety about separation may range from mild to extreme and may involve fears of death or injury to important figures, fears of being alone, and refusal to sleep alone. Somatic symptoms such as abdominal pain or headache are highly associated with SAD.[29] Adolescents are usually brought to treatment because of school refusal, somatic symptoms, or panic attacks. There is some evidence that SAD may predispose to panic attacks in adulthood.[30] However, school refusal starting in adolescence is more likely due to social phobia not SAD. It is usually easy to differentiate this because the adolescent with social phobia is often happy to be alone at home, whereas one with SAD cannot separate from the primary caregiver.

Generalized Anxiety Disorder

As the name suggests, young people with GAD are fearful of almost everything; they are life's worriers. Multiple physical and psychologic symptoms are common. Common areas of concern are competence at school or in recreation, concerns about lateness, about world-wide events such as war, and

about health-related matters. The diagnosis cannot be made without at least one physical symptom (i.e., physical restlessness, feeling *keyed up*, difficulty concentrating, irritability, muscle tension, or sleep disturbance) in addition to psychologic ones.

Obsessive-Compulsive Disorder

Young people with OCD have recurrent obsessions (intrusive, repetitive thoughts) or compulsions (repetitive behaviors) severe enough to interfere with functioning. Around 2%–3% of late adolescents meet OCD criteria at some point in their lives, with around 50% of cases starting prior to age 15.[31] Young people often recognize their symptoms are "silly" and hide them due to embarrassment. Common symptoms include excessive concerns about family safety, contamination, sexual matters, and bodily preoccupations; compulsions include excessive washing, checking, counting, ordering, and touching.[32]

When news reports of avian influenza became prominent, "Jay", 14 years, stopped attending school and told his mother that his classmates had "AIDS or something." He had been washing his hands excessively and opening doors with his elbows for about a year. He told the interviewer that "birds fly everywhere and bacteria are everywhere" and that he had to stay home to keep safe. After an inpatient admission, treatment with fluoxetine (40 mg) and a behavioral program with a focus on response-prevention and anxiety management, he returned to school.

Posttraumatic Stress Disorder and Acute Stress Disorder

Posttraumatic stress disorder (PTSD) and acute stress disorder (ASD) develop in response to an extreme traumatic event or series of events. ASD is thought to be more self-limiting, although there has been little research in the field and there is a lack of clarity between the two diagnoses.[33] ASD symptoms are often dissociative in nature (e.g., feelings of being in a daze), last between days to weeks, and occur soon after the precipitating event. Up to 80% of children and adolescents show at least one ASD symptom after a traffic accident and a third have the full diagnosis.[34]

PTSD is characterized by increased arousal (such as problems with sleep, difficulty concentrating, hypervigilance, exaggerated startle response) and symptoms related to reexperiencing or avoiding the trauma (e.g., recurrent images or thoughts of the event, distressing dreams, feelings of reliving the event, avoidance of stimuli related to the event). Both PTSD and ASD require clinically significant impairment in function. PTSD symptoms can be quite variable and there is comorbidity with other disorders, especially depressive disorders (Chap. 36) and externalizing disorders such as ADHD (Chap. 38) is common.[35] A common error is to diagnose PTSD or ASD from the history of a severe trauma alone, without the presence of core symptoms and disability.

ASSESSMENT OF ADOLESCENTS WITH ANXIETY

Anxiety disorders should be considered in young people who have recurrent, difficult to explain symptoms, multiple visits without clear diagnosis, and in any young person who reports worries or fears. Some symptoms such as recurrent headache or abdominal pain are highly associated with anxiety disorders, as are many chronic illnesses. Anxiety is not a diagnosis of exclusion by doing multiple physical tests but must be actively enquired about and considered.

For diagnosis of anxiety disorders, a history of symptoms and their relation to various stresses or stimuli is needed. A HEADSS[36] assessment (Chap. 2) can be helpful in finding out more about the young person's life and challenges, and can alert the clinician to any likely issues for further assessment and treatment. Abuse needs to be specifically enquired for and considered by the examiner. Basic questions such as "Is there anything that worries you?" can also be asked. If the response to this question is positive, specific information should be elicited; this particularly includes inquiry about the form, nature, severity, frequency, and situation in which the symptoms are experienced. Comorbidities, especially depression and a family history of anxiety disorders, should also be queried.

If the young person is presenting with anxiety symptoms, a careful history and physical examination will still be required, since some physical symptoms of anxiety are also found in medical disorders, such as thyrotoxicosis; there is also an association with medications, such as steroids, sympathomimetics, and some alternative medicines including St. John's Wort. Enquiry should be made into the use of caffeine, and any drug, licit or illicit. Significant anxiety symptoms can occur both in association with *active* use of substances such as marijuana or amphetamine-type drugs, as well as *abstinence* from regular use of drugs.

There are many assessment instruments for anxiety disorders in adolescents, although not all are suitable for a primary care setting. These include the Multi-Dimensional Anxiety Scale for Children (MASC),[37] the Screen for Child Anxiety-related Emotional Disorders (SCARED),[38] and the Pediatric Anxiety Rating Scale (PARS).[39] Where OCD is suspected the children's Yale-Brown Obsessive-Compulsive Scale (YBOCS)[40] may be used.

TREATMENT

Treatment for anxiety disorders ranges from the simplest to the most intensive, depending on severity, duration, and associated effects on functioning (Table 37-2). Mild anxiety disorders in

TABLE 37-2

TREATMENT OF ANXIETY DISORDERS

Explanation, support, and building a collaborative relationship

Practical issues (sleep, eating, exercise), record-keeping

Specific strategies for reducing avoidance, usually related to school attendance and socialization

Development of coping strategies (relaxation, distraction)

Psychologic treatments (CBT)

Medications (SSRIs and others)

well-functioning adolescents may improve with good explanation alone, while severe disorders can lead to lifelong disability. More severe disorders are likely to require combination treatments and are unlikely to be suited to full management in primary care settings. Clinicians who do not have the time or skills to take good histories or use medication as first line of intervention should refer youth to mental health specialists for proper evaluation and treatment.

Explanation of Anxiety Symptoms

All treatments should start with a careful explanation of the nature and form of anxiety, since knowledge about the wide range of physical and psychologic symptoms occurring in anxiety disorders is frequently lacking even in families with high levels of education. Stigma in the area of mental health can also result in families and doctors being more willing to consider a physical diagnosis than a psychologic one. Explanations of anxiety are more likely to be acceptable to patients and families if the doctor matter-of-factly emphasizes the lack of separation between physical and psychologic symptoms and uses terms such as "physical and psychologic stress symptoms." Adolescents can be extremely sensitive to any implication that their symptoms are "in the mind," and therefore openly refuting this issue aids engagement. Some specific terms and phrases are often useful, such as "Pain from anxiety hurts just as much as pain from any other cause."

Practical Issues

It is common for the clinician to identify practical issues which are perpetuating or even causing anxiety symptoms, e.g., the use of caffeinated drinks or ongoing consumption of anxiety-inducing drugs. Sleep, diet, and exercise may all need to be specifically addressed. Many young people with anxiety symptoms affecting sleep initiation also have poor sleep hygiene (Chap. 14); they may stay up watching TV or playing computer games (often in bed!) and sleep late. Advice about structure and routine may be helpful in getting back into usual activities.

Young people can be advised that there is some evidence that moderate exercise helps mental

health symptoms[41] and encouraged to pursue this if they are inactive. The role of smoking and substance use in anxiety should be discussed with the aim of reducing or quitting. Since anxiety symptoms occur in a range of settings, contact with parents, schools, sporting, or religious groups can sometimes be very helpful in maintaining or resuming schooling, social, and other relationships. Anxious adolescents may need medical recommendations to access specific educational programs.

Coping Strategies

Coping strategies of a general kind should be reviewed; for example, many teenagers distract themselves from anxious thoughts and stimuli with music, social activities, or reading. Counting or visualizing a positive scene can be used. Specific training in self-distraction is part of CBT and other behavioral programs; relaxation exercises may also be helpful. Since adolescents sometimes lack the patience for more formal relaxation methods such as applied relaxation,[42] it can be helpful to teach them fast and unobtrusive methods, such as breathing techniques or brief isometric exercises.[43]

Reduction of Avoidance

Much of the disability from anxiety in young people arises from the secondary consequences of the disorder, as for example, avoidance of school or social situations in social phobia. Systematic and graduated reduction of avoidance is therefore a key strategy in any treatment program. Families often help their child avoid the anxiety-provoking situations out of a sense of compassion. If the role of avoidance in maintaining symptoms is explained, and firm but sympathetic directions are given, well-motivated patients and their families may be able to develop and carry out their own realistic graded behavioral program. An example of a graded exposure plan is shown in Table 37-3.

Record-Keeping

Young people with anxiety disorders can be helped to understand their symptoms and precipitating

TABLE 37-3

EXAMPLE OF A DESENSITIZATION PROGRAMME FOR RETURNING TO SCHOOL FOR MILD SCHOOL AVOIDANCE ASSOCIATED WITH SOCIAL PHOBIA

Get up in morning in time for school, dress in school clothes, gather school books, and lunch. Plan strategies for coping with anxiety symptoms. In all cases remain in the setting until symptoms subside if possible: if this is not possible, move one step down only.

Drive in vicinity of school while in session.

Stop outside school while in session.

Stop near school after hours, walk around grounds.

Attend school out of hours, walk around classrooms, and stay seated in one.

Attend least-feared school class with withdrawal to library at other times, half-time attendance.

Attend two classes, withdrawal at other times, and so forth.

Resume normal full-time school attendance.

stimuli if these are unclear by simple record-keeping. This is also invaluable for determining the effectiveness of medications and is a key strategy in CBT. A notebook or personal organizer with columns in which the teenager records two or three typical symptoms rated on a 5-point scale may be sufficient for monitoring therapy, although more specific record-keeping is required for most psychologic therapies.

Psychologic Treatments

CBT is the preferred mode of treatment for most anxiety disorders that do not respond to the simple measures noted above and there are reports of its use with all the common anxiety diagnoses in young people.[44] It is, however, a specialist treatment, which typically employs a four-part model to engage children in managing their anxiety. For example, Kendall's group use the acronym "FEAR" which covers Feeling frightened, Expecting bad things to happen, Attitudes and Actions that help, and Results and Rewards[45] in their C.A.T. Project programmes for anxious adolescents

CBT treatments are usually around 12 sessions in duration and depend on an active, collaborative approach. They require the ability to think about practical, concrete issues rather than abstract ones, which makes CBT suited to use with both younger and older adolescents. Primary care physicians are unlikely to be able to provide CBT, but they can easily use CBT concepts (which typically link thinking, feelings, and behaviors) when discussing anxiety and its treatment. There are a number of books and on-line resources which can help in this regard.[46] In addition to CBT, exposure and response-prevention have shown benefit for anxiety disorders in mixed groups of children and adolescents. In a review of the field, Ollendick and King[47] found that modeling and desensitization are probably useful for anxiety disorders.

Medications

Medication should be regarded as a specialist area undertaken only on the advice or under the aegis of an adolescent psychiatrist or pediatrician with proper advanced training. This is because accurate diagnosis and an intimate knowledge of effects and side effects are essential for prescribing in this area. With one or two exceptions medications should be the second line of treatment, used only in conjunction with or after CBT. Except in OCD, good evidence for their efficacy in adolescents is lacking. Since anxiety disorders tend to be persistent,[48] symptoms may return when medications are stopped. Further, some symptoms of anxiety, such as avoidant behavior, are not especially responsive to pharmacologic intervention. This means that psychosocial strategies are an important part of overall treatment.

However, medications can be considered where anxiety is severe and disabling,[49] although clinicians must be mindful of the recent challenges and warnings regarding the efficacy and safety of SSRIs in children and adolescents (Chap. 36).[50] At this time fluoxetine, sertraline, and fluvoxamine are FDA-approved for use in adolescents for the treatment of OCD.[51,52] Strangely, no warnings exist for other medications such as tricyclic antidepressants (TCAs) which generally have more adverse events including cardiotoxicity.

Selective Serotonin Reuptake Inhibitors

SSRIs (fluoxetine, paroxetine, citalopram, sertraline, venlafaxine, and fluvoxamine) are the most commonly prescribed medications for the treatment of anxiety disorders; they have been shown to be moderately effective in adults for panic disorder, social phobia, generalized anxiety, and OCD.[53]

Most evidence for SSRIs in youth is for OCD, where controlled trials and an open trial for citalopram[54] have shown efficacy for fluoxetine,[55] sertraline,[56] fluvoxamine,[57] and paroxetine.[58] A recent meta-analysis of OCD trials involving more than 1000 children and adolescents suggested that these four SSRIs are of equivalent efficacy in this disorder[59]although all SSRIs were slightly less effective than the tricyclic clomipramine.

Most studies are for relatively short duration, between 8 and 12 weeks, although usual recommendations on duration of treatment are for longer. Social phobia has been treated in adolescents with paroxetine and fluvoxamine, with some evidence of efficacy[60,61]; separation anxiety has been treated with fluvoxamine.[61] There are also positive controlled trials of venlafaxine (reviewed by Weller et al.[62]) and fluvoxamine[61] for GAD in adolescents. The numbers involved in theses studies remain quite small and not sufficiently robust for government approval. There are no controlled trials of SSRI use in specific phobias, PTSD, or selective mutism.

All the SSRIs may induce headache, nausea, and sedation. Reduced appetite and alterations in sleep state (both insomnia and drowsiness) are common. Activation may also occur with subjective (and in more severe cases, objective) restlessness and agitation; even mania may occur.[63] This activation is thought to sometimes cause an increase in suicidal behavior (though interestingly, increased SSRI use has been correlated with a marked decline in suicide rates in many countries!); thus, clinicians should warn patients about SSRIs and advise reduction or cessation of the drug if suicidal ideation arises after starting this drug. Some may become apathetic and listless taking SSRIs.[64] A recent chart review study[65] found a 20% rate of psychiatric adverse effects, most appearing later in treatment (median 91 days).

A severe effect of SSRIs is the *serotonin syndrome*, which includes changes in mental state, agitation, myoclonus, sweating, tremor, and sometimes fever. This may require urgent supportive and medical treatment with antiserotonin agents such as cyproheptadine. There have been reports of serotonin syndrome in adolescents and it is thought to occur more readily at higher dosages[63] and with concomitant use of serotonergic drugs or those that interfere with cytochrome P450 enzymes. Patients may also experience serotonin withdrawal states, especially when agents with shorter half-lives are used or doses are missed. Symptoms include dizziness, problems with balance, nausea, chills, changes in sleep, and increased levels of anxiety.[66] They usually resolve over a day or two but can be frightening, especially since young people with anxiety often have increased concern about physical symptoms.

Conversely, SSRIs are generally safe in overdose, an issue of importance in treating adolescents. Most cases of single-agent SSRI overdoses will resolve with gastric lavage and supportive care. All SSRIs are metabolized in the liver and inhibit the cytochrome P450 system to varying degrees, which raises the potential for interactions with a wide range of drugs. The inhibition of metabolism of contemporaneously administered TCAs and some antipsychotics leading to toxicity has been reported.[63]

SSRI dosages for young people vary widely; Table 37-4 outlines common doses. When prescribing SSRIs for adolescents with anxiety, it is good

TABLE 37-4

USUAL MEDICATION DOSES FOR ANXIETY IN ADOLESCENTS

	Usual Dosage
Fluoxetine	10–60 mg
Paroxetine	10–40 mg
Fluvoxamine	25–250 mg
Sertraline	25–150 mg
Citalopram	10–40 mg
Venlafaxine	37.5–150 mg, divided
Imipramine	25–150 mg
Clomipramine	25–200 mg (OCD)

practice to use low doses, to increase slowly (since improvement can take 4–6 weeks), and to monitor closely for side effects. It is also important to understand the wide variability in half-lives of these drugs and their propensity for interactions. Healthy adolescents are efficient metabolizers of SSRIs and may need higher doses for weight compared to adults. There is no evidence that any one SSRI is more effective than any other. SSRI treatment duration for adolescents with anxiety disorders is not established.[67] When the drugs are withdrawn, this should be slow, with tapering over several weeks if possible. Discussion of these issues with patients and their families may help prevent abrupt discontinuation of medications.

Tricyclic Antidepressants and Anxiolytics

TCAs have a long history of use for anxiety disorders in adults and have been used to some extent with adolescents (especially clomipramine and imipramine); however, study in youth has been limited[68] and SSRIs are now more popular. Because of greater toxicity, including cardiotoxicity, TCAs are ordinarily reserved for severe cases (e.g., OCD) which have not responded to SSRIs or where SSRIs cause unacceptable side effects. ECG monitoring is recommended for those on TCAs.[4] Because anxiety disorders are typically chronic or recurring, *benzodiazepines* are not recommended for other than acute and very time limited use in adolescents as they carry the risk in this vulnerable group of abuse and dependence. Further, evidence of their efficacy is lacking. *Buspirone*, an atypical anxiolytic, has sometimes been used; however, despite initial promise, it seems to have failed to attract good studies of safety and efficacy.[68] No other medications have been shown to have any place in the management of anxiety disorders in adolescents.

CONCLUSION

In conclusion, anxiety disorders are common in adolescents, carry significant risk for ongoing morbidity, and require informed as well as thoughtful treatment. Psychoeducation, behavioral treatments, and CBT are important interventions. SSRIs show some promise but should not be the only line of treatment. Primary care clinicians play a central role in the recognition, assessment, and management of adolescents with anxiety disorders.

Bibliography

1. Ford T, Goodman R, Meltzer H. The British child and adolescent mental health survey 1999: The prevalence of DSM-IV disorders. *J Am Acad Child Adolesc Psychiatry* 2003;42(10):1203–1211.
2. American Psychiatric Association. *Diagnostic and Statistical Manual of Mental Disorders*, 4th ed. Washington, DC: American Psychiatric Association, 1994.
3. Grills A, Ollendick T. Issues in parent-child agreement: The case of structured diagnostic interviews. [Review] [89 refs]. *Clin Child Fam Psychol Rev* 2002;5(1):57–83.
4. Varley CK, Smith CJ. Anxiety disorders in the child and teen. *Pediatr Clin North Am* 2003;50(5):1107–1138.
5. McGee RF, Feehan M, Williams S, Partridge F, Silva PA, Kelly J. DSM-III disorders from age 11 to age 15 years. *J Am Acad Child Adolesc Psychiatry* 1992;31:50–59.
6. Last C, Perrin S, Hersen M. DSM-III-R anxiety disorders in children. *J Am Acad Child Adolesc Psychiatry* 1992;31:1070–1076.
7. Jordan J, Joyce P, Carter F, et al. Anxiety and psychoactive substance use disorder comorbidity in anorexia nervosa or depression. *Int J Eat Disord* 2003;34(2):211–219.
8. Birmaher B, Kennah A, Brent D, Ehmann M, Bridge J, Axelson D. Is bipolar disorder specifically associated with panic disorder in youths? *J Clin Psychiatry* 2002;63(5):414–419.
9. Dorn L, Campo J, Thato S, et al. Psychological comorbidity and stress reactivity in children and adolescents with recurrent abdominal pain and anxiety disorders. *J Am Acad Child Adolesc Psychiatry* 2003;42(1):66–75.
10. Egger HL, Angold A, Costello EJ. Headaches and psychopathology in children and adolescents. *J Am Acad Child Adolesc Psychiatry* 1998;37:951–958.
11. Dantzer C, Swendsen J, Maurice-Tison S, Salamon R. Anxiety and depression in juvenile

diabetes: A critical review. *Clin Psychol Rev* 2003; 23(6):787–800.

12. Goodwin RD. Asthma and anxiety disorders. *Adv Psychosom Med* 2003;24:51–71.

13. Williams J, Steel C, Sharp G, et al. Anxiety in children with epilepsy. *Epilepsy Behav* 2003;4(6): 729–732.

14. Hobbie W, Stuber M, Meeske K, et al. Symptoms of posttraumatic stress in young adult survivors of childhood cancer. *J Clin Oncol* 2000;18(24): 4060–4066.

15. Koot H, Bouman N. Potential uses for quality-of-life measures in childhood inflammatory bowel disease. *J Pediatr Gastroenterol Nutr* 1999;28(4):556–561.

16. Garralda ME, Rangel L. Annotation: Chronic fatigue syndrome in children and adolescents. *J Child Psychol Psychiatry Allied Disciplines* 2002;43(2): 169–176.

17. Albrecht S, Naugle A. Psychological assessment and treatment of somatization: Adolescents with medically unexplained neurologic symptoms. *Adolesc Med* 2002;13(3):625–641.

18. Zimmermann P, Wittchen H, Hofler M, Pfister H, Kessler R, Lieb R. Primary anxiety disorders and the development of subsequent alcohol use disorders: A 4-year community study of adolescents and young adults. *Psychol Med* 2003;33(7):1211–1222.

19. Johnson JG, Cohen P, Pine DS, Klein DF, Kasen S, Brook JS. Association between cigarette smoking and anxiety disorders during adolescence and early adulthood [see comment]. *JAMA* 2000;284(18): 2348–2351.

20. Levitan RD, Rector NA, Sheldon T, Goering P. Childhood adversities associated with major depression and/or anxiety disorders in a community sample of Ontario: Issues of co-morbidity and specificity. *Depress Anxiety* 2003;17(1):34–42.

21. Domalanta DD, Risser WL, Roberts RE, Risser JM. Prevalence of depression and other psychiatric disorders among incarcerated youths. *J Am Acad Child Adolesc Psychiatry* 2003;42(4):477–484.

22. Van Ameringen M, Mancini C, Farvolden P. The impact of anxiety disorders on educational achievement. *J Anxiety Disord* 2003;17(5):561–571.

23. Pine DS. Pathophysiology of childhood anxiety disorders. [Review] [80 refs]. *Biol Psychiatry* 1999;46(11):1555–1566.

24. Hettema JM, Neale MC, Kendler KS. A review and meta-analysis of the genetic epidemiology of anxiety disorders. *Am J Psychiatry* 2001;158:1568–1578.

25. King NJ, Gallone E, Tonge BJ, Ollendick TH. Self-reports of panic attacks and manifest anxiety in adolescents. *Behav Res Therap* 1993;31:111–116.

26. Mattis SG, Ollendick TH. *Panic Disorder and Anxiety in Adolescence.* Victoria, Australia: ACER Press, 2004.

27. McGee R, Feehan M, Williams S, Partridge F, Silva P, Kelly J. DSM III disorders in a large sample of adolescents. *J Am Acad Child Adolesc Psychiatry* 1990;29:611–619.

28. Wittchen HU, Fehm L. Epidemiology and natural course of social fears and social phobia. *Acta Pschiatr Scand* 2003;108(Suppl 417):4–18.

29. Last CG. Somatic complaints in anxiety disordered children. *J Anxiety Disorders* 1991;5:125–138.

30. Manicavasagar V, Silove D, Curtis J, Wagner R. Continuities of separation anxiety from early life into adulthood. *J Anxiety Disorders* 2000;14(1): 1–18.

31. Zohar AH. The epidemiology of obsessive-compulsive disorder in children and adolescents. *Child Adolesc Psychiatr Clin North Am* 1999;8(3): 445–460.

32. Rapoport JL, Inoff-Germain G. Practitioner review: Treatment of obsessive-compulsive disorder in children and adolescents. *J Child Psychol Psychiatry Allied Disciplines* 2000;41(4):419–431.

33. March JS. Acute stress disorder in youth: A multivariate prediction model. [Review] [55 refs]. *Biol Psychiatry* 2003;53(9):809–816.

34. Winston FK, Kassam-Adams N, Vivarelli-O'Neill C, Ford J, Newman E, Baxt C. Acute stress disorder symptoms in children and their parents after pediatric traffic injury. *Pediatrics* 2002;109:e90.

35. Donnelly CL, Amaya-Jackson L. Post-traumatic stress disorder in children and adolescents. *Pediatr Drugs* 2002;4(3):159–170.

36. Goldenring J, Cohen E. Getting into adolescent heads. *Contemp Pediatr* 1988;5:75–90.

37. March JS, Parker J, Sullivan K. The multi-dimensional anxiety scale for children (MASC): Factor structure, reliability and validity. *J Am Acad Child Adolesc Psychiatry* 1997;36:844–852.

38. Birmaher B. *Screen for Child Anxiety Related Emotional Disorders (SCARED).* Pittsburgh: Division of Child Psychiatry, Western Psychiatric Clinic and Institute, 1999.

39. The Research Units on Pediatric Psychopharmacology Study Group. The pediatric anxiety rating scale (PARS). *J Am Acad Child Adolesc Psychiatry* 2002; 41(9):1061–1069.

40. Scahill L, Riddle MA, McSwiggin-Hardin M. Children's Yale-Brown obsessive-compulsive scale (CY-BOCS). *J Am Acad Child Adolesc Psychiatry* 1997;36:844–852.

41. Calfas K, Taylor W. Effects of physical exercise on psychological variables in adolescents. *Pediatr Exerc Sci* 1994;6:406–423.

42. Ost LG. Applied relaxation: Description of a coping technique and review of controlled studies. *Behav Res Therap* 1987;25(5):397–409.

43. Giarrantino L. *Clinical Skills for Treating Traumatised Adolescents.* Sydney, Australia: Talomin Books, 2004.

44. Foa E, Keane T, Friedman M. Introduction. In: Friedman M (ed.), *Effective Treatments for PTSD. Practice Guidelines from the International Study for Traumatic Stress Studies.* New York: The Guilford Press, 2000, pp. 1–17.

45. Kendall PC, Choudhary M, Hudson J, Webb A. *The C.A.T. Project Manual for the Cognitive-Behavioral Treatment of Anxious Adolescents.* Ardmore, PA: Workbook Publishing, 2002.

46. Stallard P. *Think Good—Feel Good.* Chichester, UK: John Wiley & Sons, 2002.

47. Ollendick TH, King NJ. Empirically supported treatments for children with phobic and anxiety disorders: Current status. *J Clin Child Psychol* 1998;27(2):156–167.

48. Keller M, Lavori P, Wunder J, Beardslee W, Schwartz C, Roth J. Chronic course of anxiety disorders in children and adolescents. *J Am Acad Child Adolesc Psychiatry* 1992;31:1110–1119.

49. American Academy of Child and Adolescent Psychiatry. Practice Parameters for the assessment and treatment of children and adolescents with anxiety disorders. *J Am Acad Child Adolesc Psychiatry* 1997;36(Suppl 10):69S–84S.

50. Jureidini JN, Doecke CJ, Mansfield PR, Menkes DB, Tonkin AL. Efficacy and safety of antidepressants for children and adolescents. *Br Med J* 2004;328(3):879–888.

51. Committee on Safety of Medicines. Selective Serotonin Reuptake Inhibitors (SSRIs): Overview of regulatory status and CSM advice relating to major depressive disorder (MDD) in children and adolescents including a summary of available safety and efficacy data. Available at: *http://www.mca.gov.uk/aboutagency/regframework/csm/csmhome.htm.* Accessed 14/6/04.

52. Federal Drug Administration. Public Health Advisory: Worsening depression and suicidality in patients being treated with antidepressant medications. Available at: *http://www.fda.gov/cder/drug/antidepressants/AntidepressanstPHA.htm.* Accessed 14/6/04.

53. Roy-Byrne PP, Cowley DS. Pharmacological treatments for panic disorder, generalized anxiety disorder, specific phobia and social anxiety disorder. In: Groman JM (ed.), *A Guide to Treatments that Work,* 2d. New York: Oxford University Press, 2002, pp. 337–365.

54. Thomsen PH, Ebbesen C, Persson C. Long-term experience with citalopram in the treatment of adolescent OCD. *J Am Acad Child Adolesc Psychiatry* 2001;40(8):895–902.

55. Riddle MA, Scahill L, King RA, et al. Double-blind, crossover trial of fluoxetine and placebo in children and adolescents with obsessive-compulsive disorder. *J Am Acad Child Adolesc Psychiatry* 1992;31(6):1062–1069.

56. Cook EH, Wagner KD, March JS, et al. Long-term sertraline treatment of children and adolescents with obsessive-compulsive disorder. *J Am Acad Child Adolesc Psychiatry* 2001;40(10):1175–1181.

57. Riddle MA, Reeve EA, Yaryura-Tobias JA, et al. Fluvoxamine for children and adolescents with obsessive-compulsive disorder: A randomized, controlled, multicenter trial. *J Am Acad Child Adolesc Psychiatry* 2001;40(2):222–229.

58. Geller D, Wagner K, Emslie G, et al. *Efficacy of Paroxetine in Pediatric OCD: Results of a Multicenter Study.* Annual Meeting New Research Program and Abstracts. Washington, DC: American Psychiatric Association, 2002, p. 39.

59. Geller DA, Biederman J, Stewart SE, et al. Which SSRI? A meta-analysis of pharmacotherapy trials in pediatric obsessive-compulsive disorder. *Am J Psychiatry* 2003;160(11):1919–1928.

60. Van Ameringen M, Mancini C, Farvolden P, Oakman J. Pharmacotherapy for social phobia: What works, what might work and what does not work at all. *CNS Spectr* 1999;4:61–68.

61. Research Units on Pediatric Psychopharmacology Study Group. Fluvoxamine for the treatment of anxiety disorders in children and adolescents. *N Engl J Med* 2001;344(17):1279–1285.

62. Weller EB, Weller RA, Davis GP. Use of venlafaxine in children and adolescents: A review of current literature. *Depress Anxiety* 2000;12(Suppl 1):85–89.

63. Leonard HL, March J, Rickler KC, Allen AJ. Pharmacology of the selective serotonin reuptake inhibitors in children and adolescents. *J Am Acad Child Adolesc Psychiatry* 1997;36(6):725–736.

64. Garland EJ, Baerg EA. Amotivational syndrome associated with selective serotonin reuptake inhibitors in children and adolescents. *J Child Adolesc Psychopharmacol* 2001;11(2):181–186.

65. Wilnes TE, Biederman J, Kwon A, et al. A systematic chart review of the nature of psychiatric adverse events in children and adolescents treated with selective serotonin reuptake inhibitors. *J Child Adolesc Psychopharmacol* 2003;13(2): 143–152.

66. Zajecka J, Tracy KA, Mitchell S. Discontinuation symptoms after treatment with selective serotonin reuptake inhibitors: A literature review. *J Clin Psychiatry* 1997;58:291–297.

67. Yorbik O, Birmhauer B. Pharmacological treatment of anxiety disorders in children and adolescents. *Bull Clin Psychopharmacol* 2003;13:133–141.

68. McClellan JM, Werry JS. Evidence based treatments in child and adolescent psychiatry: An inventory. *J Am Acad Child Adolesc Psychiatry* 2003;42: 1388–1400.

38

ATTENTION-DEFICIT/ HYPERACTIVITY DISORDER IN ADOLESCENTS

Donald E. Greydanus and Helen D. Pratt

INTRODUCTION

Attention-deficit/hyperactivity disorder (ADHD) is the most commonly diagnosed disorder of childhood (3%–9% of school-age youth) and occurs three times more often in boys than in girls. ADHD is a chronic disorder that refers to a family of related neurobiologic and behavioral symptoms that interfere with an individual's capacity to function in developmentally appropriate ways. The primary areas of difficultly include the adolescent's inability to attend to tasks (inattention), regulate activity levels (hyperactivity), inhibit behavior (impulsivity) (American Psychiatric Association). The severity of these symptoms can have an impact on the adolescent's functioning that ranges from minimal to severe. The factors governing that impact involve (a) *individual factors* (intelligence and temperament), (b) *family factors* (tolerance, support, attachment, resources [parents' support systems], and temperament), (c) *peer relationships* (supportive, nurturing, accepting and intimate friendships and acceptance by acquaintances), and (d) *environmental resources* (access to health care, academic supports, tutoring, supportive teachers, and so on).

Youth who have high intellectual functioning, strong family supports, good friends, are accepted by their peers, and nurtured by their teachers can often manage their mild-to-moderate symptoms and have a very good prognosis. Youth who have low average to borderline intellectual functioning, minimal family supports, few friends, are not accepted by their peers or nurtured by their teachers, or have one or more comorbid psychiatric disorders, may suffer more severely from their disorder. Deficits in attention, self-regulation, and self-control can have a serious impact on learning, social skills development, and psychologic and emotional adjustment. An individual's ability to learn is in part strongly influenced by the ability to sustain attention long enough to recognize and discriminate between relevant and irrelevant aspects of the environment. Youth who cannot regulate or control their actions may also be so engaged in extraneous activities that they may miss important opportunities to mature socially, emotionally, and intellectually. The outcome can result in learning, behavior, and/or emotional problems. Therefore, it is essential that youth with ADHD receive adequate evaluation and treatment.

Diagnosis

A number of publications address details of diagnosis and evaluation of ADHD (Barkley, 1998; NIMH, 2001; Reif, 2003; Stein, 2004). Table 38-1 compares diagnostic criteria from The International Classification of Diseases, 10th ed. (ICD-10) World Health Organization (1993) and Diagnostic and Statistical Manual of Mental Disorders (DSM-IV-TR), 4th ed., Text Revision (American Psychiatric Association, 2000), The Classification of Child and Adolescent Mental Diagnoses in Primary Care: Diagnostic and Statistical Manual for Primary Care (DSM-PC): Child and Adolescent Version (Wolraich and Felice, 1996).

The DSM-IV-TR provides the most detailed list of the symptoms by classification with diagnostic codes and criteria for labeling a disorder. The ICD-10 is often used by insurance companies and provides more flexibility in diagnosing and labels ADHD as attention-deficit/hyperkinetic disorder. The DSM-PC is used in primary care settings and employs a developmental approach to diagnosing and differentiates among variations (slightly abnormal), problems, and disorders. Each of the classification systems provides information on differential diagnosis. The DSM-IV-TR is the foundation for the DSM-PC and therefore differential diagnosis, comorbidity, and criteria for diagnosis of disorders are virtually identical.

Differential Diagnosis

Problems with attention, self-regulation, and self-control can be caused by other factors and are also symptoms listed as part of the criteria for other disorders (Table 38-2). It is important that the clinician carefully assess the severity of the symptoms to be sure they are not due to other psychiatric disorders or medical factors. Adolescents can be diagnosed with more than one psychiatric disorder (e.g., mental retardation, pervasive developmental disorder, anxiety disorders, and mood disorders)

but the symptoms of inattention, inhibition, and/or hyperactivity must exceed the criteria necessary to diagnose another psychiatric disorder.

Comorbid Conditions

Adolescents who experience deficits in attention, self-regulation, and inhibition may also have a variety of comorbid disorders. Psychiatric disorders are estimated to be present in up to 44% of youth diagnosed with ADHD; 32% have at least two disorders and 11% are diagnosed with three or more (Barkley, 1998). Although the disorders listed above can be the soul cause of the primary symptoms of ADHD, disorders such as anxiety and depression can coexist with ADHD. Other developmental disorders that may be present are: reading disorders, mathematic disorders, disorders of written expression, developmental coordination disorders, communication disorders, and Tourette syndrome (TS). Youth with ADHD may also have mental retardation but symptoms must exceed those that are caused by the retardation.

EVALUATION

The diagnosis of ADHD should include assessments of the adolescents functioning at home, school, work (if applicable) and should include information on peer relationships, family psychopathology, family conflict history, and any information on the adolescent's trauma history. Behavioral, neurologic, psychosocial, and psychologic tests can measure all aspects of ADHD but are not definitive. The data derived from those instruments must be used in conjunction with appropriate assessment data and then interpreted by a trained clinician. Test instruments and check lists can be used that allow the clinician to gather much of this information in an efficient manner. Data from the adolescent, parents or care providers, and teachers should include the presenting symptoms, differential diagnosis, possible comorbid conditions, as well as medical, developmental, school, psychosocial, and family histories. Understanding why the family is seeking help at this point will also provide clues regarding current stressors in the lives of the family.

TABLE 38-1
CRITERIA AND DIAGNOSTIC CODES FOR ATTENTION-DEFICIT/HYPERACTIVITY DISORDER (ADHD)

DSM-IV and DSM-PC

Criterion A: Six or more of the following symptoms from either section 1 (inattention) or section 2 (hyperactivity-impulsivity that have persisted for at least 6 months. Those behaviors must occur at an intensity that is maladaptive and inconsistent with the individual's developmental level:
1. Symptoms of inattention
    a. Often fails to pay close attention to details or makes careless mistakes on school work, work or other activities.
    b. Often has difficulty sustaining attention in tasks or play activities
    c. Often does not seem to listen when spoken to directly.
    d. Often does not follow through on instructions and fails to finish school work, chores, or duties in the workplace (not due to oppositional behavior or failure to understand instructions).
    e. Often has difficulty organizing tasks and activities.
    f. Often avoids, dislikes, or is reluctant to engage in tasks that require sustained mental efforts (such as schoolwork or homework).
    g. Often loses things necessary for tasks or activities (e.g., toys, school assignments, pencils, books, or tools).
    h. Is often easily distracted by extraneous stimuli.
    i. Is often forgetful in daily activities.
2. Symptoms of hyperactivity-impulsivity
    Hyperactivity
    a. Often fidgets with hands or feet or squirms in seat.
    b. Often leaves seat in classroom or in other situations in which remaining seated is expected.
    c. Often runs about or climbs excessively in situations in which it is inappropriate (in adolescents or adults, may be limited to subjective feelings of restlessness).
    d. Often has difficulty playing or engaging in leisure activities quietly.
    e. Is often "on the go" or often acts as if "driven by a motor."
    f. Often talks excessively.
    Impulsivity
    g. Often blurts out answers before questions have been completed.
    h. Often has difficulty awaiting turn.
    i. Often interrupts or intrudes on others (e.g., butts into conversations or games).
Criterion B: Some hyperactive-impulsive or inattentive symptoms that caused impairment were present before age 7 years.
Criterion C: Some impairment from the symptoms is present in two or more settings (e.g., at school [or work] and at home).
Criterion D: There must be clear evidence of clinically significant impairment in social, academic, or occupational functioning.
Criterion E: (differential diagnosis): The symptoms do no occur exclusively during the course of a pervasive developmental disorder, schizophrenia, or other psychotic disorder and are not better accounted for by another mental disorder (e.g., mood disorder, anxiety disorder, dissociative disorder, personality or autistic disorder, posttraumatic stress disorder, separation anxiety disorder, social phobias, dysthymic disorder, avoidant personality disorder, substance abuse (cocaine phencyclidine, stimulants) and mental retardation unless symptoms are in excess of those associated with MR.

(Continued)

T A B L E   3 8 - 1

CRITERIA AND DIAGNOSTIC CODES FOR ATTENTION-DEFICIT/HYPERACTIVITY
DISORDER (ADHD) (*CONTINUED*)

DSM-IV-TR Diagnostic Codes (Must Meet Criteria for 6 Months)	*ICD-9 CM Diagnostic Codes*	*DSM-PC Diagnostic Codes (Must Meet Criteria for 6 Months)*
314.01 Attention-deficit/ hyperactivity disorder, combined type: meets criteria A1 and A2.	314 Hyperkinetic syndrome of childhood Excludes: hyperkinesis as a symptom of underlying disorder—code the underlying disorder	Impulsive/hyperactive or inattentive behaviors Developmental variation
314.00 Attention-deficit/ hyperactivity disorder, predominately inattentive type: meets criterion A1 but not criterion A2.	314.0 Attention-deficit disorder Adult Child	V65.49 Hyperactive/impulsive variation During adolescence activity may be high in play situations and impulsive behavior may normally occur, especially in peer pressure situations. Does not impair function.
314.01 Attention-deficit/ hyperactivity disorder, predominately hyperactive type: meets criterion A2 but does not meet criterion A1.	314 00 Without mention of hyperactivity Predominately inattentive type	Developmental problem
314.9 Attention-deficit/ hyperactivity disorder, not otherwise specified (individuals who exhibit prominent symptoms of ADHD, inattentive type or hyperactivity-impulsivity but do not meet criteria are given this diagnosis (e.g., those whose symptoms are not present prior to age 7 years or those who present with symptoms of inattention but do not meet full criteria and have a behavioral pattern marked by sluggishness, daydreaming, and hypoactivity).	314.01 With hyperactivity Combined type Overactivity NOS Predominately hyperactive/ impulsive type Simple disturbance of attention with overactivity	V40.3 Hyperactive/impulsive behavior problem Behaviors are intense enough to begin to disrupt relationships with others or impede the acquisition of age-appropriate skills. But not intense enough to meet criteria for ADHD, a mood disorder or symptoms of anxiety. Rule out sexual abuse, physical abuse, chronic stress. Adolescents may engage in lots of fooling around behaviors that begins to annoy others and fidgets in class or while watching television. Likely to be accompanied by other behaviors such as negative emotional behaviors or aggressive/oppositional behaviors.
	314.1 Hyperkinesis with developmental delay Use additional code to identify any associated neurologic disorder	
	314.2 Hyperkinetic conduct disorder Hyperkinetic conduct disorder without developmental delay excludes hyperkinesis with significant delays in specific skills (314.1)	
	314.8 Other specified manifestations of hyperkinetic syndrome	314.01 Attention-deficit/hyperactivity disorder: predominately hyperactive-impulsive type (same as DSM-IV-TR)
	314.9 Unspecified hyperkinetic syndrome Hyperkinetic reaction of childhood or adolescence NOS Hyperkinetic syndrome NOS	

TABLE 38-1

CRITERIA AND DIAGNOSTIC CODES FOR ATTENTION-DEFICIT/HYPERACTIVITY DISORDER (ADHD) (*CONTINUED*)

DSM-IV-TR Diagnostic Codes (Must Meet Criteria for 6 Months)	*ICD-9 CM Diagnostic Codes*	*DSM-PC Diagnostic Codes (Must Meet Criteria for 6 Months)*
		314.01 Attention-deficit/ hyperactivity disorder: combined type (same as DSM-IV-TR)
		314.9 Attention-deficit/ hyperactivity disorder: NOS (same as DSM-IV-TR)
		V40.3 Inattention problem (does not meet criteria for diagnosis of ADHD, predominately inattentive type)
		314.00 Attention-deficit/ hyperactivity disorder predominately inattentive type

Source: Reprinted with Permission from: American Psychiatric Association. *Diagnostic and Statistical Manual of Mental Disorders*, 4th ed., Text Revision. Washington, DC: Author, 2000, pp. 85–93.

Source: Reprinted with Permission from: Wolraich ML, Felice ME, Drotar D. *Impulsive/Hyperactive or Inattentive Behaviors the Classification of Child and Adolescent Mental Diagnosis in Primary Care: Diagnostic and Statistical Manual for Primary Care (DSM-PC) Child and Adolescent Version.* Elk Grove, IL: American Academy of Pediatrics, pp. 91–110.

Source: Reprinted with Permission from: *Practice Management Information Corporation: International Classification of Diseases, 9th revision: Clinical Modifications*, 6th ed. Los Angeles, CA: Author, pp. 223–224.

In addition to screening for ADHD symptoms, it is essential that the adolescent be screened for psychosis, mood disorders, anxiety, and trauma.

A note of caution when diagnosing an adolescent with ADHD: Assigning a label of ADHD is a serious diagnosis that can result in adverse consequences for youth when they reach adulthood. Clinicians should be aware that there are some careers that may be off limits to even the most accomplished youth who have the mention of ADHD in their medical files. For example, very gifted individuals who have been diagnosed with ADHD during early childhood and taken medication to treat the disorder, then "outgrow" the symptoms and do not take medications during adolescence, can be denied acceptance into high-level military careers or any other career where deficits in attention and impulsivity are considered as undesirable characteristics. Very few clinicians envision this type of negative outcome for their

patients, especially when their interventions are meant to improve the health care and quality of life for their patients.

Educational evaluation issues: Educational systems are required by federal mandates to provide academic or psychologic evaluation for adolescents who are suspected of having a disability that impairs academic functioning. That impairment must be significant, which means the adolescent is two to three grade levels below their age appropriate peers in academic functioning. The individuals with Disabilities Act (IDEA) guarantees appropriate services and a public education to children with disabilities from ages 3 to 21. IDEA specifically lists ADHD as a qualifying condition for special education services. If the school assessment is inadequate or inappropriate, parents may request that an independent evaluation be conducted with an outside expert, at the school's expense. Adolescents who have multiple comorbid

TABLE 38-2

DIFFERENTIAL DIAGNOSIS: OTHER DISORDERS THAT CAN CAUSE INATTENTION, HYPERACTIVITY, IMPULSIVITY

	Inattention	Impulsivity	Hyperactivity
Mental retardation unless symptoms are in excess of those associated with MR	X	X	X
Pervasive developmental disorder: Autism	X	X	X
Anxiety disorders: Generalized anxiety disorder, separation anxiety	X	X	X
Mood disorders: Depression [both manic and hypomanic episode of depression], dysthymic disorder; bipolar disorder; cyclothymic disorder	X	X	X
Psychotic disorders: Schizophrenia or other dissociative disorder	X	X	X
Personality disorders: Avoidant personality disorder	X	X	X
Substance abuse: Cocaine, phencyclidine, stimulants	X	X	X
Impulse-control disorders			X
Behavioral disorders Oppositional defiant disorder Conduct disorder	X	X	X

disorders may qualify for special education services within the public schools, under the category of "Other Health Impaired." Clinicians can encourage parents to request an Individualized Education Program (IEP).

PSYCHOLOGIC MANAGEMENT

The literature on treating ADHD describes a wide variety of psychologic treatments used to treat the symptoms and problems associated with youth diagnosed with ADHD: psychotherapy, cognitive-behavior therapy (CBT), behavior therapy (BT), and psychosocial interventions (which may include support groups, and parent and educator skills, biofeedback, peer mediation to resolve interpersonal conflict, compliance training, self-management training, and social skills training). Little empirical evidence exists for most therapies except for CBT (National Institutes of Mental Health [NIMH], 2000, 2001). Most adolescents diagnosed with ADHD are treated

with prescription medications alone. Many youth would benefit from a combination of pharmacologic and psychosocial interventions. Some researchers argue that stimulant therapies have serious limitations of short treatment duration: (a) positive changes occur in only a few functional problem domains; (b) some youth suffer physiologic side effects; (c) not all adolescents can be given these medications; (d) finally, not all who take stimulant medications improve (Cunningham, 1998; Whalen and Henker, 1991).

PSYCHOPHARMACOLOGY OF ADHD

Over 60 years of research has revealed there are various medications that can improve the concentration ability of an adolescent with ADHD, probably related to pharmacologic effects on the noradrenergic and/or dopaminergic systems of the central nervous system. Their beneficial medications are reviewed in Table 38-3 and include *stimulants, antidepressants,*

TABLE 38-3

MEDICATIONS USED IN ATTENTION DISORDERS

Medication	Daily Dose Schedule (mg/kg)	Common Untoward Effects
Stimulants		
MPH	0.3–2.0 (10–80 mg/day) in 2–4 divided doses	Insomnia, decreased appetite, abdominal pain, headache, depression, loss of weight, rebound symptoms, decreased velocity vs. growth delay; see text
Magnesium pemoline	0.5–3.0 (37.5–131.25 mg/day) in 1–2 divided doses	Same as MPH + possible liver toxicity (FDA "black box" warning)
Dextroamphetamine	0.1–1.5 (5–80 mg/day) in 2–4 divided doses	Same as MPH but more depression
Antidepressants		
TCAs	1–5	Anticholinergic effects, others. See text
Imipramine, Desipramine	1–5	
Nortriptyline	0.5–3	
Bupropion	3–6 (50–300 mg/day) in 2–3 divided doses	Insomnia, irritability, drug-induced seizures (with doses >6 mg/kg): contraindicated in bulimic patients
Alpha$_2$-agonists		
Clonidine	3–10 µg/kg (0.05–0.4 mg/day) in 2–4 divided doses	Sedation (very frequent), depression, dry mouth, rebound hypertension, hypotension (rare), confusion (with high doses), localized irritation with transdermal preparation
Guanfacine	15–43 µg/kg (0.5–4.0 mg/day) in 1–2 divided doses	Same as clonidine but much less sedation, less hypotension
Norepinephrine reuptake inhibitors		
Atomoxetine	0.5–1.4 mg/kg/day in 1–2 divided doses	Decreased appetite, dyspepsia, dizziness, fatigue, sedation, nausea emesis, mood swings, growth delay

Source: Modified with permission from: Greydanus DE, Sloane M, Rappley M: Psychopharmacology of ADHD in adolescents. *Adolesc Med* 2002;13:600.

alpha$_2$ agonists, and *norepinephrine reuptake inhibitors*. Important principles of psychopharmacology to consider in this regard are provided in Table 38-4.

Stimulation Medication

Since the 1937 publication of Bradley revealing the positive effects of benzedrine on children with ADHD, several hundred research trials (randomized-controlled studies) have been conducted showing the beneficial effects of stimulant medications in 75%–95% of children, adolescents, and adults with ADD/ADHD (Table 38-5). The most comprehensive study looked at methylphenidate (MPH) and was conducted by the National Institute of Mental Health (NIHM) and was called the NIMH Collaborative Multisite Multimodal Treatment Study of Children

TABLE 38-4
PRINCIPLES OF PSYCHOPHARMACOLOGIC MANAGEMENT FOR ADHD

1. Educate the patient and parents ("family") about purpose of these medications; clarify the goals of medications (improving concentration, decreasing impulsivity, others). The clinician should avoid focusing only on medication in the clinical encounter. This implies to families that medication use alone should be the remedy to all problems. It further implies that when things are not going well, the problem must be with the choice or dose of medication. This shifts responsibility for problems completely to the clinician who must then urgently find the right medication.

2. Be sure the patient and parents understand that medications are not curative.

3. Correct any "myths" about medication the family may have. For example, medication will not correct family problems (i.e., alcoholism in a parent, contentious custody battles).

4. Wait for the patient/family to approve of a trial medication period before embarking on medication management. Do not force medication on a child or adolescent.

5. Educate the patient/family about potential side effects of medications and how you will deal with them; follow these patients on a regular basis to monitor efficacy and adverse effects.

6. Provide a thorough evaluation of the patient and family to determine possible comorbidities that may benefit from other medications.

7. Be supportive of other management tools (i.e., psychoeducation strategies, behavioral therapy).

8. Begin with a low dose and increase slowly until identified target symptoms are sufficiently improved; stop the medication(s) if side effects are unacceptable or upper medication levels are reached without amelioration of target symptoms.

9. Specific medications and doses may vary from patient to patient and are identified by careful trial and error. Medication(s) that are helpful may change as the child emerges to adolescence and adulthood.

10. Adolescents may require a medication dose higher than needed for adults because of increased renal clearance of drugs, lower body fat percentage, increased liver metabolism, or idiosyncratic medication metabolism.

11. Strive to achieve complete syndrome remission if feasible (rather than settling for symptom improvement).

12. Share responsibility explicitly by clearly stating what issues the family must work on, the school must work on, the child or adolescent must work on, and the physician must work on.

Source: Modified with permission from: Greydanus DE, Pratt HD, Sloane M, Rappley M: Attention-deficit/hyperactivity disorder in children and adolescents: Interventions for a complex costly clinical conundrum. *Pediatr Clin North Am* 2003;50:1061–1062.

with Attention-Deficit/Hyperactivity Disorder (abbreviated as the *MTA* study). The MTA study looked at nearly 600 children aged 7–9 and noted the effectiveness of MPH. Today, at least 6% of children aged 5–15 in the United States are placed on a psychostimulant medication.

Methylphenidate

MPH is the most commonly prescribed psychostimulant that has been used for over four decades to treat patients with ADD/ADHD. It is a schedule II medication that selectively binds the presynaptic dopamine transporter in striatal and prefrontal areas of the central nervous system, leading to an increase in extracellular dopamine. MPH also affects the norepinephrine system with resultant blockade of the norepinephrine transporter. The most common form of MPH has been Ritalin, though other forms have been developed over the past 15 years and are now available (Table 38-6). MPH is taken orally and crosses the blood-brain barrier leading to pharmacologic effects in 30–45 minutes that typically peak in 1–2 hours and wan over 3–5 hours. The half-life of MPH (Ritalin) is 2–4 hours and thus, another dose of this mediation is provided if beneficial stimulant effects are desired or needed.

TABLE 38-5

POTENTIAL BENEFITS OF STIMULANT MEDICATIONS

Enhanced concentration

Reduced hyperarousal

Reduced impulsivity

Reduced motor restlessness (i.e., decreased gross/fine motor movement, less finger tapping)

Improved homework completion

Improved school and/or work performance

Less aggressive and antisocial behavior

Source: Modified with permission from: Greydanus DE, Pratt HD, Sloane M, Rappley M: Attention-deficit/hyperactivity disorder in children and adolescents: Interventions for a complex costly clinical conundrum. *Pediatr Clin North Am* 2003;50:1062.

The adolescent with ADD/ADHD is often provided with a dose of MPH at breakfast, and this is repeated at noon and late afternoon if needed. Start with a low dose (as 2.5–5 mg) and slowly increase in 2.5–5 mg doses to find the best doses for the individual youth. The dosage range is 0.3–2.0 mg/kg/day; a single dose of over 20 mg or daily doses over 60–80 mg are not recommended. There is no correlation between the weight of the adolescent and the MPH efficacy; also, plasma levels of MPH do not correlate with medication efficacy. The best dose for each patient with ADD/ADHD must be carefully titrated. Various methods are used to verify the effectiveness of the medication, including patient/family interview, report cards, parent ratings, and/or teacher ratings. Reasons for the failure of MPH to be effective in a patient are listed in Table 38-7.

Stimulant Side Effects

Table 38-8 lists stimulant medication side effects, some of which may be minimized if the medication is started at a low dose and slowly titrated upward; some of these adverse events wan over time. Contraindications to stimulant medications include overt sensitivity to these medications, psychosis, hyperthyroidism, drug dependence, uncontrolled hypertension, symptomatic cardiovascular disease, and glaucoma; also, stimulants should not be used

TABLE 38-6

AVAILABLE METHYLPHENIDATE MEDICATIONS

Ritalin (MPH immediate-release; 5, 10, 20 mg tablets) (Novartis)

Ritalin-SR (20 mg MPH tablet, sustained-release) (Novartis)

Generic MPH (both immediate-release and sustained-release; tablet options same as Ritalin) (Geneva)

Ritalin LA (Ritalin developed for 8–9 h duration; 20, 30, 40 mg capsules) (Novartis)

Metadate ER (sustained-release [8 h] MPH; 20 mg tablets) (Celltech)

Methylin ER (sustained-release [8 h] MPH; 10, 20 mg tablets) (Mallinckrodt)

Concerta (MPH HCl: extended-release tablets: 18, 36, 54 mg; up to 12 h MPH duration) (Alza-McNeil)

Metadate CD (MPH HCl: extended-release 20 mg capsules; 8–9 h of MPH duration) (Celltech)

Focalin (dexmethylphenidate [purified D-methylphenidate] to last 4–6 h at half the usual dose; 2.5, 5, 10 mg tablets) (Novartis)

MethyPatch (once a day MPH patch) (Noven)

Source: Modified with permission from: Greydanus DE, Pratt HD, Sloane M, Rappley M: Attention-deficit/hyperactivity disorder in children and adolescents: Interventions for a complex costly clinical conundrum. *Pediatr Clin North Am* 2003;50:1063.

TABLE 38-7

REASONS FOR FAILURE OF METHYLPHENIDATE

Inaccurate diagnosis

Comorbid disorders that overshadow the ADHD

Medication doses that are too high or not high enough

Medication is diverted to others in or outside the family

Intolerable medication side effects

Medication is used as a drug of abuse for its euphoric effects

Patient and/or family not accepting of medication

Patient does not respond to MPH but does to other stimulants or alternative medications

Patient does not respond to medications of any kind

Source: Modified with permission from: Greydanus DE, Sloane M, Rappley M: Psychopharmacology of ADHD in adolescents. *Adolesc Med* 2002;13:604.

TABLE 38-8

POTENTIAL SIDE EFFECTS OF METHYLPHENIDATE

Headache*
Abdominal pain*
Jitteriness*
Dizziness
Anorexia*
Insomnia (delayed onset of sleep)*
Social withdrawal*
Weight loss (due to decreased appetite)*
Moodiness (irritability)
Nausea
Dry mouth
Constipation
Increase in heart rate, blood pressure, and palpitations
"Unmasking" of Tourette syndrome (TS)
Appearance of being "dazed or drugged"; perseveration and withdrawal
Rebound phenomenon
Increased hyperactivity
Appearance of psychosis or psychotic features
Personality change
Tolerance
Skin rash (rare)

*Commonly seen adverse effects.
Source: Modified with permission from: Greydanus DE, Sloane M, Rappley M: Psychopharmacology of ADHD in adolescents. *Adolesc Med* 2002;13:607.

with monoamine oxidase inhibitors, since a hypertensive crisis may develop. Combining stimulants with a tricyclic antidepressant (TCA) should be done cautiously, since rare sudden death from cardiac arrhythmia has been reported. MPH can interact with the metabolism of some anticonvulsants (such as phenobarbital, phenytoin, and ethosuximide). Combining antihistamines with stimulants may reduce stimulant efficacy.

Heart rate and blood pressure often increase to a mild extent when stimulant medication is started and is not of concern if the cardiovascular system is not compromised. Headaches may develop, either in relation to peaking plasma levels of MPH or to withdrawal of the medication. A different stimulant

may improve the headache pattern. Dizziness may develop on stimulants and be worsened with short-acting versus long-acting medication; evaluate for dehydration or blood pressure alterations if dizziness develops. Nausea or abdominal pain that develops on these medications may be improved if the MPH is taken with food or liquids. Table 38-9 suggests measures to consider if stimulant-associated appetite suppression arises. Weight loss and nutrition-deficient growth delay have been reported, though ultimate height potential is not limited. Some youth with ADHD have constitutional delay of growth and adolescence and careful assessment of growth is necessary if any questions about growth are raised.

Tolerance has been described in some patients who are on high doses of stimulants. It does not indicate that addiction has occurred and management includes trying another stimulant or using the same stimulant at a lower dose after a period of being off the medication. Youth who develop recurrent tolerance to various medications may be helped by changing the stimulant on a frequent

TABLE 38-9

MANAGEMENT OF ANOREXIA AND WEIGHT LOSS DUE TO STIMULANTS

Encourage meal intake when stimulant effects wear off, as in the evening
Provide higher-caloric foods (i.e., milk shakes, homogenized milk [vs. nonfat], food supplements)
Encourage a number of small meals vs. a large meal for some
Have the child or adolescent take the medication after a meal
Do not force meals
Be sure the child or adolescent is not using the stimulant to lose weight
Take the patient off stimulants as possible (as on weekends, summers, and others)
Try another stimulant or anti-ADD medication
Stop the stimulants if necessary

Source: Modified with permission from: Greydanus DE, Pratt HD, Sloane M, Rappley M: Attention-deficit/hyperactivity disorder in children and adolescents: Interventions for a complex costly clinical conundrum. *Pediatr Clin North Am* 2003;50:1070.

basis, as every 3 months. *Rebound* refers to the occurrence of worsening ADHD symptoms (including irritability and rage attacks) as the medication is wearing down; it may be seen in the late morning or late afternoon as a short-acting stimulant is wearing off or late afternoon if a morning dose of a long-acting stimulant is waning. Late afternoon rebound may improve by prescribing a longer-acting medication, reducing intervals between doses, or reducing late day doses. It may be difficult to manage early evening rebound since stimulant effect still present in the evening often interferes with sleep; other anti-ADD medications that cause sedation may be helpful in this regard, such as TCA, bupropion, or an alpha$_2$ agonist. Other medications that have been added to help sleep dysfunction include melatonin (3–6 mg before bedtime), trazodone (25–50 mg before sleep), or mirtazapine (Remeron, 7.5–15 mg before sleep). A careful search for other factors causing sleep dysfunction is also important.

ADHD is noted in 50%–75% of adolescents with TS and the TS may be noted in some cases after starting stimulant medication. The presence of tics is a relative, not absolute contraindication to using stimulant medication for ADHD. Antitic medication (as pimozide, haloperidol, or risperidone) may be given along with the stimulant medication, if beneficial effects are noted with the stimulant. If stimulants worsen the tic disorder, other anti-ADD medications may be tried that usually do not worsen the tic condition; these medications include TCAs, α_2 agonists (as clonidine or guanfacine), selegiline (monoamine oxidase B inhibitor), and atomoxetine. Bupropion may also improve the ADD symptoms and sometimes will worsen the tic condition.

Some youth on stimulant medication may develop self-manipulative behavior, including nail biting, skin cutting or pulling, and hair pulling. A change of stimulant medication or dosage may correct this condition. Some youth placed on too high a stimulant dose become very quiet, and withdrawn while perseverating about different issues; a reduction in stimulant dosage may be helpful. High stimulant doses may also induce compulsive behaviors and in rare conditions, movement disorders.

Though MPH can be abused to cause euphoria, there is no evidence that adolescents with ADHD who benefit from MPH are at increased risk to develop drug addiction with MPH or other drugs. The risk for abuse of amphetamines is well-known. Stimulant medications should be monitored closely by the clinician prescribing it, and this includes observing that the medication is not diverted to family members or peers of the adolescent. Some youth on stimulant medication develop depression or anxiety, and a careful assessment is necessary to identify if there is a comorbid depressive or anxiety state that is present or if these symptoms represent an adverse effect of the stimulant on this particular youth. More depressive symptoms are reported with amphetamine than MPH. Also, patients with latent bipolar affective disorder may develop acute mania while on stimulant mediation. In rare cases, youth on stimulant medication have developed overt psychosis.

MPH Preparations

Ritalin and Ritalin-SR have been the most popular brands of MPH until the past decade. Many patients do not like the need to take Ritalin (or its generic equivalent) two to four times a day if sustained effect is needed. Ritalin-SR is a sustained-release (SR) product that is only produced as a 20 mg formulation and may deliver an equivalent of 7 mg of MPH for several hours; it has a generic equivalent and may be combined with the short-acting version. Because of the limited formulations of Ritalin-SR and the erratic absorption noted in half or more of users, many other longer-acting MPH products have been developed over the past decade (Table 38-6). There are limited scientific data at this time to help the clinician and patient decide what is the best stimulant or combination of medications for a specific patient. Trial and error along with individual clinician preference is the current process. Table 38-10 compares the duration of action of various MPH products. If the adolescent has trouble swallowing pills, the long-acting products with a bead mechanism are helpful, since these products can be opened and the beads added to

TABLE 38-10

STIMULANTS: DURATION OF ACTION

Short-acting (3–6 h)
Ritalin
Methylin
Dexadrine
Dextrostat
Focalin
Intermediate-acting (6–8 h)
Ritalin-SR
Methylin ER
Adderall
Metadate ER
Once-daily (8 + h)
Dexedrine Spansules
Concerta
Adderall XR
Metadate CD
Ritalin LA
Focalin LA

Source: Modified with permission from: Greydanus DE, Pratt HD, Sloane M, Rappley M: Attention-deficit/hyperactivity disorder in children and adolescents: Interventions for a complex costly clinical conundrum. *Pediatr Clin North Am* 2003;50:1065.

food; these drugs include Ritalin LA, Metadate CD, Dexedrine Spansule, and Adderall XR. These newer products are now reviewed.

Newer MPH Formulations

Concerta uses a trilayer core covered by a membrane that is semipermeable allowing gradual MPH release via a hole on one end that is laser-drilled. Approximately 22% of MPH is in the overcoat and after swallowing, a plasma MPH peak is produced in 1–2 hours. This OROS mechanism is an osmotic time-released process allowing the extended-release MPH tablet to last 10–16 hours and produce an ascending MPH profile. The capsule is nearly impossible to alter and use as a drug of abuse. The 18 mg capsule gives 4 mg of immediate-release (IR) MPH while the 36 mg capsule allows 8 mg of IR MPH and the 54 mg capsule gives 12 mg of IR MPH. When switching from IR MPH to Concerta, one can use this general guideline: if the youth is

taking 5 mg IR MPH, start with an 18 mg Concerta capsule; if on 10 mg of IR MPH two or three times daily, use a 36 mg capsule; finally, if on 15 mg IR MPH two or three times a day, use a 54 mg capsule.

Ritalin LA is an MPH capsule (20, 30, 40 mg) with similar amounts of IR and SR beads that allows up to 8 hours of MPH efficacy based on the release of two doses 4 hours apart. Start with the 20 mg capsule and slowly advanced as necessary and as tolerated up to 60 mg/day. *Methylin* is produced as 5, 10, and 20 mg regular acting MPH tablets; *Methylin ER* is an extended-release MPH tablet (10 and 20 mg) that can provide MPH up to 8 hours. *Metadate CD* is a long-acting MPH, 20 mg capsule made of coated beads; 30% of the MPH is released immediately and the remaining MPH is released over the next 6–10 hours. The adolescent begins with the 20 mg capsule and gradually increases, up to 60 mg/day. A dose of 20 mg IR MPH twice a day is similar to taking 40 mg of *Metadate CD* a day. *Focalin* (dexmethylphenidate HCl—2.5, 5, and 10 mg tablets) is the D-threo-enantiomer of racemic MPH; this MPH form may be more pharmacologically active than the L-threo-enantiomer, possibly with less side effects; half the regular MPH dose is used for an effect of 4–6 hours a longer-acting version is Focalin LA. *MethyPatch (MTS)* is a patch with MPH that is absorbed through the skin; as with any patch, erythema around the patch site may develop.

AMPHETAMINE PRODUCTS

Dextroamphetamine (Dexedrine; Dextrostat) is an alternative to MPH, lasts 3–6 hours (average of 5 hours), and is useful for those who do not respond to MPH or cannot tolerate MPH. Side effects of amphetamine are the same as MPH and the mechanisms of action are reviewed in Table 38-11. Available amphetamine products are listed in Table 38-12. The action of amphetamine is a bit longer than IR MPH and may allow a smoother transition from one dose to the other. It may be more likely to induce depression than MPH. Both MPH and amphetamines are closely regulated, though amphetamine may be more difficult to obtain, due to its well-known abuse potential.

TABLE 38-11

AMPHETAMINE MECHANISM OF ACTION

Selectively binds to the dopamine transporter (increasing extracellular synaptic dopamine)

Leads to the direct release of dopamine into the synapse through several mechanisms

Norepinephrine reuptake inhibition

Weak effects on the serotonin system

Dextroamphetamine is taken one to three times daily and is found as 5 mg (Dexedrine; Dextrostat) and 10 mg scored tablets (Dextrostat); a generic version is also available. Gradual titration is recommended with a dosage range of 0.15–0.5 mg/kg/day—up to 40–50 mg daily. Dexedrine Spansule (5, 10, and 15 mg capsules) is given once daily and produces an IR as well as an effect up to 8–10 hours; its release of medication is more gradual and longer than noted with the IR of MPH in Ritalin-SR. Short- and long-acting amphetamines can be given together and the maximum dose of the long-acting form is 30 mg two or three times daily. Amphetamine and MPH products should not be combined and any long-acting stimulant may lead to evening sleep dysfunction as well as evening anorexia.

TABLE 38-12

AVAILABLE AMPHETAMINE STIMULANT MEDICATIONS

Dexedrine (dextroamphetamine tablets; short-acting) (GlaxoSmithKline)

Dexedrine Spansule (long-acting dextroamphetamine) (GlaxoSmithKline)

Dextroamphetamine generic (Barr)

Dextrostat (dextroamphetamine) (Shire US)

Adderall (mixed-salts amphetamine with extended-release) (Shire US)

Adderall XR (mixed-salts amphetamine with extended-release) (Shire US)

Desoxyn (methamphetamine) (Abbott)

Source: Modified with permission from: Greydanus DE, Pratt HD, Sloane M, Rappley M: Attention-deficit/hyperactivity disorder in children and adolescents: Interventions for a complex costly clinical conundrum. *Pediatr Clin North Am* 2003;50:1075.

Methamphetamine (Desoxyn [5 mg tablets]) is a potent stimulant that lasts for about 4 hours, is often difficult to find, and has the greatest addiction potential of all the stimulants. Adderall is a mixed-salts amphetamine (75% of the D-isomer and 25% of the L-isomer) with a side effect profile similar to dextroamphetamine. It is composed of 25% dextro (D)-amphetamine saccharate, 25% D-L-amphetamine aspartate, 25% D-amphetamine sulfate, and 25% D-L-amphetamine sulfate. Various dosage scored tablets are available: 5, 7.5, 10, 12.5, 15, 20, and 30 mg. It is a longer-acting stimulant with effects up to 8–10 hours that is given once in the morning, twice a day, and sometimes three times a day. Adderall XR is available as 5, 10, 15, 20, 25, and 30 mg capsule that gives a pulsed amphetamine salts release with effects up to 12 hours. There is a biphasic release of short-acting and extended-release stimulant action.

Pemoline

Pemoline (Cylert) is a schedule III, non-MPH, and nonamphetamine stimulant provided as magnesium pemoline in 18.75, 37.5, and 75 mg tablets; a 37.5 mg chewable tablet has also been available. It is taken once daily with a dosage range of 0.5–3.0 mg/kg/day—maximum of 112.5–131.25 mg/day. Chemical hepatitis develops in 3% after several months of use and a rare incidence of irreversible liver failure noted with pemoline use has resulted in this medication receiving an FDA "black box" warning. Patients and families must be informed of this possibility and careful patient monitoring is necessary, including baseline and periodic blood counts along with biweekly liver function tests. Parents must be given written informed consent acknowledging the potential risk of liver failure and death for anyone on pemoline. An infrequent movement disorder has been associated with this medication as well. It is now listed as an alternative stimulant for patients with ADD/ADHD.

NONSTIMULANT MEDICATIONS

Clonidine

Clonidine (Catapres) is a presynaptic, central-acting alpha$_2$-adrenergic agonist that is available as a pill and as a patch in 0.1, 0.2, and 0.3 mg dosages. Its benefit for patients with ADHD may lie in its sedative properties, improving the sleep-dysfunction properties of MPH (Table 38-13). Clonidine is given two to four times a day or at bedtime; it is begun at 0.1 mg once or twice a day; daily dosage range is 0.05–0.4 mg/day. Slow titration is recommended to reduce the incidence of adverse effects (Table 38-14) and it may take several weeks to months for full beneficial effects to be noted. Rebound hypertension may develop if the medication is not tapered slowly when getting the patient off clonidine. If a patch is used, begin with a 0.1 mg dose and titrate upward, slowly, as necessary; the patch is effective for 3–7 days.

Beginning with a low dose and slow titration may reduce the sedative effects of clonidine. A baseline blood pressure, pulse, and blood glucose should be taken, and then repeated periodically, sometimes when changing doses. A baseline electrocardiogram (ECG) is recommended and repeated every 6 months that the patient is on clonidine. It is not recommended in those with only attentional dysfunction, since its sedative properties may impair neuropsychologic function. Tolerance is noted and activation of hepatic enzymes may lead to an increase in dose after several months. There have been a few deaths of patients taking both MPH and clonidine. The clonidine patch may improve or prevent sedation side effects and rebound blood pressure problems. Dermatitis, as with any such patch, may occur.

Guanfacine

Guanfacine (Tenex) is an alpha$_{2A}$-adrenergic agonist related to clonidine, and also without proven benefit for concentration deficits of ADHD.

TABLE 38-13

USES OF CLONIDINE

Alternative or adjunctive medication to MPH
Treatment of TS (Tourette Syndrome)
Treatment of posttraumatic stress disorder
Treat severe aggressiveness seen with conduct disorder or oppositional defiant disorder

TABLE 38-14

SIDE EFFECTS OF CLONIDINE

Sedation (50%)
Dry mouth
Headache
Attention impairment
Decreased glucose tolerance
Depression
Dermatitis (from the patch)
Dizziness
Dysphoria
Fatigue
Inconsistent effects
Irritability
Itchy eyes
Postural hypotension
Potentiation of neuroleptic anticholinergic side effects
Rebound phenomenon
Tolerance
Weight gain
Withdrawal effects (rebound tachycardia and severe hypertension from sudden clonidine cessation)
Worsening of preexisting cardiac arrhythmias

Source: Modified with permission from: Greydanus DE, Sloane M, Rappley M: Psychopharmacology of ADHD in adolescents. *Adolesc Med* 2002;13:615.

In contrast to clonidine, guanfacine may produce less sedation as well as less hypotension along with an increased duration of action. Side effects are otherwise similar to clonidine, though more headaches and agitation may be noted. Guanfacine is available as 1 and 2 mg tablets and prescribed in a daily dosage range from 0.5 to 4.0 mg.

ANTIDEPRESSANTS

Tricyclic Antidepressants

Research does support the beneficial effect of TCA (Table 38-15) for ADHD and it is often used as alternative medication for ADHD if stimulants are not effective or not tolerated. Mechanism of action includes blockage of norepinephrine and serotonin reuptake and down regulation of beta-adrenergic

TABLE 38-15

TRICYCLIC ANTIDEPRESSANTS DOSAGE RANGE

Imipramine (Tofranil, others) 50–200 mg/day

Desipramine (Norpramin, Desipramine)
  50–200 mg/day

Amitriptyline (Elavil) 50–200 mg/day

Nortriptyline (Pamelor) 20–100 mg/day

receptors. Uses of TCAs are listed in Table 38-16, though the only FDA-approved uses in pediatrics are for enuresis (imipramine) and obsessive-compulsive disorder (clomipramine). Start imipramine at a low dose (0.5 mg/kg/day—25 or 50 mg/day) and raise slowly up to 2.5–5.0 mg/kg/day for the best dose with least adverse effects. The desipramine dose is 1–5 mg/kg/day and daily ranges of imipramine and desipramine are 50–200 mg for adults; the daily range for nortriptyline is 50–150 mg or 0.5–3.0 mg/kg/day.

TCA side effects are listed in Table 38-17, many of which are anticholinergic. Careful monitoring of the adolescent taking TCA is important, including monitoring of the vital signs, complete blood count, serum TCA levels, and ECG; management protocols are available (Varley, 2001). TCAs lead to less rebound than stimulants, but tolerance does develop. Plasma levels and efficacy of the medication do not correlate. Imipramine has a more sedative effect than desipramine or nortriptyline and can be severe. Tremor may be improved by

TABLE 38-16

USES OF TRICYCLIC ANTIDEPRESSANT

ADHD

Depression

Anxiety disorders (as panic disorder or obsessive
  compulsive disorder)

Insomnia

Tourette syndrome

Enuresis

Migraine headaches

Aggression

TABLE 38-17

TRICYCLIC ANTIDEPRESSANT SIDE EFFECTS

Blood dyscrasias

Blurred vision (including cycloplegia and mydriasis)

Cholestatic jaundice

Confusion

Constipation

Delirium (in high doses)

Dizziness

Drowsiness and sedation

Drug interactions (as with SSRIs)

Dry mouth (with decreased salivary flow and
  increased tooth decay)

ECG changes (sinus tachycardia, AV blocks,
  increased QRS interval, increased QTc interval)

Exercise-induced tachycardia

Hypotension

Increase in heart rate (10–15 bpm) and blood
  pressure (up to 8–10 mmHg)

Lowered seizure threshold

Peripheral neuropathy

Priapism

Respiratory failure and death from an overdose

Skin rash

Sudden death

Tachycardia

Tremor

Urinary retention

Weight gain

Source: Modified with permission from: Greydanus DE, Pratt HD, Sloane M, Rappley M: Attention-deficit/hyperactivity disorder in children and adolescents: Interventions for a complex costly clinical conundrum. *Pediatr Clin North Am* 2003;50:1079.

carefully lowering the TCA dose or adding propranolol (10–40 mg daily), though this may induce depression in some. TCA-induced agitation may improve by lowering the dose or adding a benzodiazepine. Toxic TCA levels may arise if TCAs and SSRIs are combined; TCA serum levels may also increase if MPH is added. Mixing TCAs and alcohol may cause respiratory depression and death. TCA may induce mania in a patient with latent bipolar disorder or psychosis in someone with latent schizophrenia. Discontinuation may develop if TCAs are stopped too soon; symptoms include nausea, emesis, fatigue, or worsening behavior. Rare cases of sudden death are reported, mainly with desipramine.

Bupropion

Bupropion (Wellbutrin) (Table 38-18) uses noradrenergic/dopaminergic effects to improve attention span, reduce irritability, and improve depression if present. In an alternate formulation, bupropion (Zyban) is used to blunt nicotine addiction in some tobacco abusers seeking to stop smoking. Bupropion is FDA-approved for use in adults with depression, but not in adolescents with depression or ADHD. Bupropion is available as 75 and 100 mg tablets and its dosage range is 50–300 mg/day (3.0–6.0 mg/kg). It is also seen in a sustained-release form, Wellbutrin-SR (100 and 150 mg) that is prescribed as 100–150 mg twice daily. Wellbutrin XL is a once-a-day bupropion product (150 mg, 300 mg).

Bupropion side effects are listed in Table 38-18 and include seizures—0.1% under 300 mg/day and 0.4% with doses over 300 mg/day. Seizure thresholds are reduced and bupropion is contraindicated in patients with seizure disorders and with eating disorders, such as bulimia nervosa. The risks for a seizure can also be reduced by not taking doses less than 8 hours apart, slow titration of the drug, using the SR formulation, and not using high doses of the regular formulation. Bupropion does not induce cardiac conduction delays and drug-to-drug interactions are minimal.

Atomoxetine

Atomoxetine (Strattera) is a nonstimulant medication that is FDA-approved for children (6 years and up), adolescents, and adults. Its beneficial effects on ADHD are related to a blockade of presynaptic norepinephrine transporter in the prefrontal cortex. Atomoxetine is available as 10-, 18-, 25-, 40-, and 60-mg capsules and side effects are listed in Table 38-19. A starting dose is 0.5 mg/kg/day, leading to a maximum dose of 1.0–1.4 mg/kg/day—up to 100 mg daily over a twice daily or once daily regimen. It serves as an alternative anti-ADHD drug, used for those not wishing to take a stimulant, not wishing to take a controlled drug, or those who do not respond to stimulants (Med Lett 2004; Staufer, 2005). Drug-to-drug interactions include those that are metabolized by cytochrome P450 2D6, including SSRIs. However, atomoxetine has low affinity for a number of receptors, including histaminic, serotonergic, cholinergic, alpha$_1$-adrenergic, and alpha$_2$-adrenergic. There is no increase in tics, cardiovascular complications, drug addiction, or drug diversion.

Miscellaneous

Venlafaxine (Effexor) is an atypical antidepressant that is produced in 25, 50, 75, and 100 mg tablets; it is also found as extended-release capsules (Effexor XR—37.5, 75, and 150 mg). It inhibits serotonin and norepinephrine reuptake and is FDA-approved for adults with depression and generalized

TABLE 38-18

BUPROPION SIDE EFFECTS

Anorexia
Agitation
Nausea
Restlessness
Drowsiness
Headache
Tics (exacerbation)
Seizures (0.1% under 300 mg/day and 0.4% over 300 mg/day)

TABLE 38-19

ATOMOXETINE SIDE EFFECTS

Anorexia
Nausea
Emesis
Sedation
Fatigue
Dizziness
Mood swings
Dyspepsia
Growth delay

TABLE 38-20

NON-RESEARCH-SUPPORTED ADHD TREATMENT OPTIONS

Antiyeast medications
Chiropractic manipulation
Dietary manipulation
Electroencephalographic-biofeedback training
Herbal treatments
Megavitamin therapy
Sensory integrative training
"Herbal" products
Acetyl carnitine
DMAE (dimethylaminoethanol [Deaner])
Ginkgo
Phosphatidylserine (CNS phospholipid)
Essential fatty acids (gamma-linolenic acid, docosahexaenoic acid)

anxiety disorder. Its role in ADHD is under research, especially if anxiety is also present. Side effects (as dizziness, anorexia, sedation, and nausea) may be reduced by beginning with a low dose and slowing titrating a larger dose. There is also research on the antinarcolepsy drug, *Modafinil* (Provigil), to see if its reticular activating effects will benefit patients with ADHD. A number of central nervous system nicotinic cholinergic agonist agents are under active study as well for possible benefit in the management of ADHD. Table 38-20 lists a number of treatment options that have been used, but without research support for any benefit in ADHD patients.

Bibliography

American Psychiatric Association. *Diagnostic and Statistical Manual of Mental Disorders*, 4th ed., Text Revision. Washington, DC: Author, 2000, pp. 85–93.

Atomoxetine: Strattera revisited. *Med Lett* 2004;46:65.

Barkley RA: Attention-deficit/hyperactivity disorder. *Sci Am* 1998a;66–71.

Barkley RA (ed.).: *Attention Deficit Hyperactivity Disorder: A Handbook for Diagnosis*, 2d ed. New York: Guilford Press, 1998b.

Bradley C: The behavior of children receiving benzedrine. *Am J Psychiatry* 1937;94:577–585.

Clarke SD: ADHD in adolescence. *J Adolesc Health* 2000;27:77–78.

Cunningham CF: A large-group, community-based, family systems approach to parent training. In: Barkley RA (ed.), *Attention Deficit Hyperactivity Disorder: A Handbook for Diagnosis*, 2d ed. New York: Guilford Press, 1998.

Greydanus DE, Sloane MA, Rappley MD: Psychopharmacology of ADHD in adolescents. *Adolesc Med* 2002;13:599–624.

Greydanus DE, Pratt HD, Sloane MA, et al.: Attention-deficit/hyperactivity disorder in Children and adolescents: Interventions for a complex costly clinical conundrum. *Pediatr Clin North Am* 2003;50: 1049–1092.

Greydanus DE: Psychopharmacology of ADHD in adolescents: Quo vadis? *Psychiatr Times* 2003;20: 5–9.

Greydanus DE, Patel DR: The adolescent and substance abuse: Current concepts. *Curr Probl Pediatr Adolesc Health Care* 2005;35(3):78–98.

Jensen PS, Hinshaw SP, Swanson JM, Greenhill LL, Conners CK, et al.: Findings from the NIMH Multimodal Treatment Study of ADHD (MTA): Implications and applications for primary care providers. *J Dev Behav Pediatr* 2001;22:60–73.

National Institute of Mental Health (NIMH): *Attention Deficit Hyperactivity Disorder*. NIMH, NIH Publication No. 01-4589, 2001. Available at: *http://www.nimh.nih.gov/publicat/helpchild.cfm*.

National Institute of Mental Health: *NIMH Research on Treatment for Attention Deficit Hyperactivity Disorder (ADHD): The Multimodal Treatment Study—Questions and Answers*. Washington, DC: NIMH, 2000. Available at: *http://www.nimh.nih.gov/events/mtaqa.cfm*

National Institute of Health (NIH): *Diagnosis and Treatment of Attention Deficit Hyperactivity Disorder*. NIH Consensus Statement Online 1998:Nov 16–18; [cited year, month, day]; 16(2): 1–37.

Pliszka SR, Greenhill LL, Crismon ML, et al.: The Texas children's medication algorithm project: report of the Texas consensus conference panel on medication treatment of childhood. attention-deficit/hyperactivity disorder. Part I. *J Am Acad Child Adolesc Psychiatry* 2001;39:908–919.

Pratt HD: Neurodevelopmental issues in the assessment and treatment of deficits in attention, cognition, and learning during adolescence. *Adolesc Med* 2002; 13(3):579–598.

Rappley MD: ADHD. *N Engl J Med* 2005;352: 165–173.

Reiff MI, Stein MT: ADHD evaluation and diagnosis: A practical approach to office practice. *Pediatr Clin North Am* 2003;50:1019–1048.

Schubiner H, Robin AL, Young J: Attention-deficit/hyperactivity disorder in adolescent males. *Adolesc Med* 2003;14:663–676.

Solanto MV, Arnsten AFT, Castellanos FX: The neuroscience of stimulant drug action in ADHD. In: Solanto MV, Arnsten AFT, Castellanos FX (eds.), *Stimulant Drugs and ADHD*. London: Oxford University Press, 2001, pp. 355–379.

Staufer WB, Greydanus DE: Attention-deficit/hyperactivity disorder psychopharmacology for college students. *Pediatr Clin North Am* 2005;52:71–84.

Stein MT: ADHD: The diagnostic process from different perspectives. *Dev Behav Pediatr* 2004;25: 53–57.

Swanson JM and MTA Cooperative Group: National Institute of Mental Health Multimodal Treatment Study of ADHD Follow-up: Changes in effectiveness and growth after the end of treatment. *Pediatrics* 2004;113:762–769.

Varley C: Sudden death of a child treated with imipramine. *J Child Adolesc Psychopharmacol* 2000; 10:321–325.

Varley CK: Sudden death related to selected tricyclic antidepressants in children: Epidemiology, mechanisms and clinical implications. *Paediatr Drugs* 2001;3: 613–627.

Wender EH: Managing stimulant medication for attention-deficit/hyperactivity disorder: An update. *Pediatr Rev* 2002;23:234–236.

Whalen CK, Henker B: Therapies for hyperactive children: Comparisons, combinations, and compromises. *J Consult Clin Psychol* 1991;59(1):126–137.

Wolraich ML, Felice ME: *The Classification of Child and Adolescent Mental Diagnoses in Primary Care: Diagnostic and Statistical Manual for Primary Care (DSM-PC): Child and Adolescent Version*. Elk Grove Village, IL: American Academy of Pediatrics, 1986, pp. 93–110.

Zito JM, Safer DJ, dosReis S, et al.: Psychotropic practice patterns for youth. A 10-year perspective. *Arch Pediatr Adolesc Med* 2003;157:17–25.

39

SCHIZOPHRENIA IN THE ADOLESCENT

Glenn Craig Davis

INTRODUCTION

Schizophrenia is a well-characterized psychiatric syndrome of unknown and probably heterogeneous etiology with a median age of onset between the ages of 15–24 years in males and 25–34 years in females. It affects between 0.5% and 1.5% of the population. This illness has a devastating effect on the lives of patients and their families, disrupting the normal progress of adolescent development, including the acquisition of learning, socialization, and cognitive skills. Schizophrenia ranks among the top 10 causes of disability worldwide. The course of the illness has both chronic continuous and episodic forms. Pharmacologic and psychosocial treatments aim to reduce the intensity and frequency of the syndrome's symptoms (e.g., hallucinations and delusions) as well as reduce social impairment associated with the illness. Much attention should be focused on patient education, development of good compliance as well as relapse prevention, and the early as well as effective management of relapse. Treatment may be less effective in ameliorating the underlying cognitive, perceptual, motor, and affective disturbances over time.

While the pharmacologic management of adolescents differs little from treatment in other decades of life, the consequences of inappropriate or delayed treatment have life-long effects. The importance of adhering to a high standard of treatment during adolescence lies in salutary effects of education on improving the adjustment of the patient to this illness and forging healthy doctor-patient relationships that have been shown to lead, in the long term, to better outcomes. This chapter focuses on the *psychopharmacologic* management of schizophrenia in adolescence.

Relevant Diagnostic Issues that Bear on Treatment

The diagnosis of schizophrenia requires that a patient has at least two of five clusters of symptoms for a significant portion of time during a 1-month period. These symptom clusters include (1) delusions, (2) hallucinations, (3) profoundly disorganized speech, (4) grossly disorganized or catatonic behavior, and (5) so-called "negative symptoms" that include features such as poverty of thought and speech as well as affective flattening (American Psychiatric Association, 2000).

While the diagnosis requires the presence of two symptom clusters for a month, continuous signs of the disturbance must persist for at least 6 months.

During this 6-month period, prodromal and residual symptoms may also be present. There must be social and/or occupational dysfunction for a significant portion of time since the onset of symptoms. Such dysfunction includes one or more disturbances of function that include work, interpersonal relationships, and self care. Particularly in childhood or adolescence, the clinician may observe failure to achieve expected levels of interpersonal, academic, and occupational achievement. There are additional and more complex rules (differential diagnostic points) that relate to excluding schizoaffective and other affective disorders that may often be associated with similar psychotic symptoms and functional impairments. Substance abuse (Chap. 34) and several general medical conditions may also present with similar symptom clusters and need to be ruled out (American Psychiatric Association, 2000).

Impact of Age of Onset or Schizophrenic Subtype in the Determination of Proper Treatment

Age of onset and schizophrenic subtype do predict treatment type and outcome in several ways. As a rule, childhood, latency, and occasionally early adolescent onset of symptoms are associated with poorer prognosis, chronic continuous course, more behavioral and speech disorganization, fewer hallucinations and delusions, and a poor response to antipsychotic medications. These patients with younger onset are more frequently diagnosed with disorganized, undifferentiated, or even catatonic subtypes of schizophrenia (American Psychiatric Association, 2000). Late adolescent or young adult onset is associated with better prognosis, an episodic course, fewer symptoms of disorganization (particularly interepisode), presence of hallucinations and delusions (particularly persecutory and grandiose), and, in general, a good response to antipsychotic drugs. These patients are more frequently diagnosed with the paranoid subtype of schizophrenia.

Schizophrenia, Childhood Onset

The childhood onset schizophrenic patient has peculiar behavior, including poor social development and

social relations; there are also expressions of other types of social impairment, including impaired school performance, odd speech and thought as well as less independence. Such a patient may have more typical psychotic symptoms, such as hallucinations and delusions, but such symptoms tend to be less associated with disturbances in arousal (agitation). If the psychotic symptoms are typical, a trial of an antipsychotic is appropriate (see below). If there is an absence of clear hallucinations or delusions, antipsychotic medications may be of little use, though an empirical trial of 4–8 weeks with attention to recovery of clearly identified target symptoms may still be appropriate.

Often the physician who cares for an adolescent patient with a history of childhood onset schizophrenia also inherits a history of treatment with antipsychotics. If, on taking a good history, the clinician determines that there has never been a clear response to treatment, it may be advisable to withdraw medications slowly and determine what management is necessary. Social therapies, parental support, occasional hospitalization, and regular follow-up by psychologists or social workers may be the major treatment approaches in such situations.

Schizophrenia, Adolescent Onset

The patient with adolescent onset schizophrenia generally presents with paranoid delusions, auditory hallucinations, and severe agitation. Antipsychotic medications should be introduced promptly after discussion with parents and patient about adverse effects and treatment expectations. Hospitalization, though dependent on disease severity, is often necessary. During the initial hospitalization period, a low-to-moderate dose of an antipsychotic medication should be initiated. Tables 39-1 and 39-2 show a list of commonly used antipsychotic drugs.

Antipsychotic Agents

There are many antipsychotic (often called neuroleptic) medications available for the treatment of the acute symptoms of schizophrenia and other psychotic disorders. The first class of drugs to be successfully used emerged in the 1950s—the phenothiazines (Table 39-1). Many phenothiazines came into use in

TABLE 39-1

CLASSES OF TYPICAL ANTIPSYCHOTIC MEDICATIONS

	Dose Range (mg/day)
Phenothiazines	
Chlorpromazine (Thorazine)	100–1000
Thioridazine (Mellaril)	100–800
Mesoridazine (Serentil)	50–400
Trifluoperazine (Stelazine)	5–60
Perphenazine (Trilafon)	8–64
Fluphenazine (Prolixin)	2–60
Loxapine (Loxitane)	20–160
Butyrophenones	
Haloperidol (Haldol)	2–30
Thioxanthenes	
Thiothixine (Navane)	2–120
Dihydroindolones	
Molindone (Moban)	20–200

the 1950s and 1960s; chlorpromazine (Thorazine) is still in use. Later entries to the market, such as fluphenazine, are more potent and became first-line treatment. The release of haloperidol (Haldol), a butyrophenone, provided a highly potent neuroleptic that is still in common use today; haloperidol is often used as the comparison drug in double-blind

TABLE 39-2

CLASSES OF A TYPICAL ANTIPSYCHOTIC MEDICATIONS

	Dose Range (mg/day)
Benzisoxazoles	
Risperidone (Risperdal)	2–6
Ziprasidone (Geodon)	40–160
Tricyclic benzodiazepines	
Clozapine (Clozaril)	300–900
Olanzapine (Zyprexa; Zydis)	5–10
Quetiapine (Seroquel)	300–700
Other	
Aripiprazole (Abilify)	15–30

clinical trials. Phenothiazine, butyrophenone, thioxanthene, dibenzoxazepine, and dihydroindolone neuroleptics all cause extrapyramidal side effects. These particular side effects are disturbing at the least, and disabling, at worst. They have been a major cause of noncompliance by patients over the years. The next set of compounds to emerge in the market have been so-called "atypical" antipsychotics including clozapine, olanzapine, risperidone, quetiapine, ziprasidone, and aripiprazole.

The "atypical" antipsychotics (Table 39-2) demonstrate a far lower propensity for extrapyramidal side effects. There is much debate about the relative effectiveness of the atypicals in contrast to earlier drugs. In general, most expert opinion leans toward the equal effectiveness of all antipsychotic drugs currently on the market for the positive symptoms of schizophrenia. Current debate centers on claims that the "atypicals" may be more effective in treating negative symptoms of schizophrenia. All antipsychotics have a broad range of side effects that must be understood and managed in the course of the treatment. Were it not for the differences in adverse effects and some evidence of greater improvement negative symptoms for the atypical antipsychotics, clinicians would need only a few of the many drugs currently available.

Discovery of Antipsychotics Emphasizing Atypicals

The phenothiazine antipsychotics were the first to be discovered in the 1950s and 1960s with other typical agents arriving in the 1960s and 1970s. The impact of their discovery on the management of psychotic illnesses was dramatic and the number of hospital beds occupied by psychotic patients dropped dramatically. Nevertheless, untreated negative symptoms, frequent relapse, and a disturbing pattern of adverse effects and noncompliance led to an aggressive search for additional compounds. The reasons for the transition from using typical to atypical antipsychotic medications as first-line treatment of schizophrenia has been their better adverse effect profile: less likelihood of extrapyramidal symptoms (EPS) (especially tardive dyskinesia), less likelihood of prolactin elevation, some evidence of improved effectiveness in negative symptoms of schizophrenia (for example, poverty of speech and social withdrawal), and some evidence of greater effectiveness in otherwise treatment-resistant adult cases.

In 1989, clozapine was introduced and provided another tool in the management of treatment-resistant cases or in the management of patients who are exquisitely sensitive to the extrapyramidal consequences of the use of typicals. However, it became clear that agranulocytosis occurred in a number of cases (1–2% risk) and that close monitoring is required to manage patients on clozapine. Other side effects included weight gain (true for most antipsychotics), seizures, hypersalivation, tachycardia, and dizziness.

Risperidone was introduced shortly thereafter in 1994. In children and adolescents, there has been some success in treating developmentally disabled populations where it may help with agitation, aggression, and psychotic symptoms. Olanzapine, quetiapine, ziprasidone and most recently, aripiprazole have been introduced as additional atypical antipsychotics. For most of these compounds, one should use about half the adult dosage range (e.g., olanzapine 2.5–5 mg/day for teens). Weight gain tends to accompany each of these agents. One should consult the package insert or papers cited in the references for detailed dosing recommendations. The side effects of these medications are discussed later in the chapter.

Treatment of Acute Psychotic Symptoms

On the whole, current treatment guidelines recommend using atypical antipsychotics (with the exception of clozapine the adverse effects of which profile includes agranulocytosis) as the first-line treatment in patients newly diagnosed with schizophrenia.

Determining When and Whether the Patient is Improving

The acute symptoms of schizophrenia (target symptoms) that are likely to respond to antipsychotic treatment fall into the following categories:

arousal, affect, thought disorder, psychomotor activity, and social adjustment. Thought disorder symptoms fall into two groups: *content disorders* (such as hallucinations and delusions) and *formal thought disturbances* (such as loose associations, tangential thinking, and poverty of thought). Arousal symptoms (e.g., agitation) are among the first symptoms to respond to drug therapy, taking anywhere from 1 to 3 days at appropriate dosages. The profound sedating effects of neuroleptics may be confused with specific effects on arousal and may be seen within a few hours. Psychomotor agitation is reduced initially as well. Affective symptoms accompanying the arousal improve promptly, but affect associated with the paranoid ideas may take some time to improve; days to a few weeks may be necessary for substantial improvement. Hallucinations may appear to respond quickly; however, a significant reduction in hallucinations may take days to weeks. Thought content, persecutory delusions for example, may take a substantial period of time to improve while social impairment recovers last.

Medication Management—Increasing Dose

Since response takes days to weeks, initial dosing is focused on reducing arousal and affect to manageable levels; manageable levels depend on the setting, whether locked ward, open medical ward, home, or half-way house. It is common to use more than is necessary to treat the psychosis in order to reduce combativeness as well as high levels of arousal and agitation. Consideration for reducing dose should take place if sedation is significant over the first days.

Dosages for Antipsychotic Drugs

Since there is a lag in the response of psychotic symptoms to treatment, patience is a virtue. Symptoms, particularly cognitive symptoms and delusional content (e.g., thinking that the FBI is after one), may improve several weeks to a month after treatment with an appropriate dose. Initial treatment as mentioned earlier is targeted to control agitation, arousal, and motor hyperactivity. Decision to reduce the dose may be made if target symptoms come into control, excessive sedation occurs or feelings of "mental constraint" arise; on the other hand, continued affective, cognitive, and disorganized behavior lead to increases in antipsychotic dosage over a period of weeks.

Factors that Impact Length of Hospital Stay

If the adolescent is hospitalized for psychotic symptoms, continued hospitalization is generally supported until behavior comes under moderate control. The patient should demonstrate significant improvement in psychotic behavior and improved organizational capabilities. To be discharged, the patient must be seen as being able to be managed and expected to demonstrate continued improvement in a partial hospital program, or a day program; in less resourced or more remote areas of the country, these youth must be manageable at home. In this age and because of constraints placed on length of stay, schizophrenic patients are often discharged with residual psychotic symptoms. Nevertheless, one should aggressively discuss with third parties the dangers of discharging patients with significant residual psychotic symptoms with little insight or willingness to continue therapy. It is, of course, important for the schizophrenic adolescent to have a tightly supervised home milieu where discharge occurs before significant remission of psychotic symptoms develops.

Factors that Impact Duration of Antipsychotic Treatment

Patients experiencing their first psychotic episode should be maintained on antipsychotic medications for a minimum of 6–12 months; most psychiatrists would lean toward 12 months from the point of maximum improvement. There are a number of extremely well conducted discontinuation studies that demonstrate a significantly increased relapse rate in the year following treatment in patients randomized to placebo. The decision whether to continue antipsychotic medication is dependent on a number of factors; these include diagnostic confidence, duration and severity of symptoms, rate of response, and compliance with treatment. Since the disorder, even in its "good prognosis" form, is associated with many episodes, treatment tends to be continuous. This is particularly true in patients who have long and frequent psychotic episodes of significant severity.

Common Adverse Effects of Antipsychotic Medications

It is important for clinicians to use only those medications that are well-known by the prescriber. Physicians should consult textbooks, reliable internet sites, journal articles, or the package inserts to determine the most frequent side effects of the particular antipsychotic medication that they select. In general, adverse effects may be classed as *anticholinergic* (e.g., dry mouth, difficulty urinating, blurred vision), *alpha-adrenergic* (e.g., orthostatic hypertension, impotence), *dopaminergic* (e.g., extrapyramidal movement disorders, galactorrhea, amenorrhea, other dyskinesias and weight gain), and *antihistaminic*.

There are a number of rare but serious consequences, including agranulocytosis (clozapine, as noted, is the most common offender), and sometimes irreversible movement disorders, such as tardive dyskinesia, and neuroleptic malignant syndrome. Stigmatizing effects, such as movement disorders, cause noncompliance, and noncompliance often leads to recurrence of psychotic symptoms and rehospitalization. There are also a wide variety of adverse effects beyond those described and include (but are not limited to) weight gain, glucose metabolism effects, seizures, and adverse cardiac events. The wide range of medication-induced adverse effects is particularly concerning to patients and clinicians alike.

It is beyond the scope of this chapter to provide detailed, individualized drug profiles; however, *selective* comments on side effects of atypicals are presented. Adverse effects of risperidone include weight gain that can be profound, sedation, and hyperprolactinemia. Olanzapine can induce weight gain (that can be substantial), lipidopathies, type 2 diabetes mellitus, and constipation; it has a low incidence of inducing prolactin changes and has a low EPS profile. Moderate weight gain and sedation are reported adverse events of quetiapine (introduced in 1997), but there appears to be little EPS; cataracts are noted in animal studies and in a case report, prompting some to suggest obtaining baseline and intermittent slit lamp examinations. Ziprasidone was released in 2001 and may induce only minimal weight gain; ECG may show an increased QTc interval, and it should not be combined with drugs that prolong the QTc interval; also, it should be avoided in those with QT syndrome or cardiac arrhythmias.

The Role of Serum or Plasma Levels of Antipsychotics Treatment

While very high serum/plasma levels are associated with adverse effects, there are no reliable dose-response relationships, thus, blood levels have failed to be useful in the management of schizophrenia.

The Role of Other Medications in Treatment

Often heavy doses of anxiolytic or sedative hypnotics are used concomitantly in patients with schizophrenia. Such medications do not appear to have specific effects on the symptoms of schizophrenia, but may be useful in the acute management of the psychotic presentation. Also, patients may be anxious in the remitted state and therefore, may benefit from an anxiolytic (Chap. 37). Benzodiazepines continue to be the anxiolytics of choice in this situation.

There are no other medications that are considered specific for the symptoms of schizophrenia, although many have been tried. Much work has been done to determine whether antidepressants may be of help (Chaps. 36 and 37). They are not indicated unless it can be demonstrated that the patient meets criteria for depression when the psychotic symptoms have remitted.

CONCLUSION

Studies of atypical antipsychotic use in the pediatric age range are quite limited. There have been some studies of the use of atypicals in tic disorders, pervasive developmental disorders, disruptive behavioral disorders, mood disorders (with psychotic features), mania, self-injurious behavior, and hyperactivity. It is important to note that the Federal Drug Administration (FDA) has only approved typical antipsychotic drugs for pediatric use; this is because of the limited research that has been conducted thus far on children and adolescents. When prescribing atypical antipsychotic drugs for pediatric patients because of their better therapeutic and adverse symptom profile, it is important to recognize the additional risks of using medications prior to FDA approval, or anticipated approval. Finally, it is always preferable for the primary care clinician to refer an adolescent schizophrenic patient, when possible. Pharmacotherapy forms just one arm of a comprehensive treatment plan. There are a variety of psychotherapeutic, psychosocial, psychoeducational, and rehabilitative approaches that enhance the overall management, promote adjustment, and integrate adolescents with schizophrenia into more normal social relationships. Families often become lifelong partners with the physician to maintain their child (eventually, adult child) at the highest levels of social and vocational functioning that are possible.

Bibliography

American Psychiatric Association: Practice guidelines for the treatment of patients with schizophrenia. *Am J Psychiatry* 1997;154(Suppl):1.

American Psychiatric Association: *Diagnostic and Statistical Manual of Mental Disorders*, 4th ed. *Text Revision, DRM-IV-TR*. Washington, DC: American Psychiatric Association, "Schizophrenia and other Psychotic Disorders, pp. 297–337, 2000.

Bryden KE, Carrey NJ, Kutcher SP: Update and recommendations for the use of antipsychotics in early-onset psychoses. *J Child Adolesc Psychopharmacol* 2001;11:113–130.

Buck ML: Using the atypical antipsychotic agents in children and adolescents. *Pediatr Pharmacother* 2001;7:1.

Carpenter WT Jr, Buchanan RW: Schizophrenia. *N Engl J Med* 1994;330:681–690.

Citrome L, Volavka J: The promise of atypical antipsychotics. *Postgrad Med* 2004;116:49–63.

Cooper WO, Hickson GB, Fuchs C, et al.: New users of antipsychotic medications among children enrolled in TennCare. *Arch Pediatr Adolesc Med* 2004;158:753–759.

Findling RL, McNamara NK, Youngstrom EA, et al.: A prospective, open-label trial of olanzapine in adolescents with schizophrenia. *J Am Acad Child Adolesc Psychiatry* 2003;42:170–175.

Freedman R: Schizophrenia. *N Engl J Med* 2003;349: 1838–1849.

Gerber DJ, Tonegawa S: Psychotomimetic effects of drugs: A common pathway to schizophrenia? *N Engl J Med* 2004;350:1047–1048.

Goff DC: A 23-year old man with schizophrenia. *JAMA* 2002;287:3249–3257.

Martin A, Scahill L, Charney DS, Leckman JF (eds.): *Pediatric Psychopharmacology. Principles and Practice.* New York: Oxford University Press, p. 791, 2003.

McClellan J, Werry J: Work Group on Quality Issues. Practice parameters for the assessment and treatment of children and adolescents with schizophrenia. American Academy of Child and Adolescent Psychiatry. *J Am Acad Child Adolesc Psychiatry* 2001;40(Suppl 7):S4–S23.

McConville BJ, Arvanitis LA, Thyrum PT, et al.: Pharmacokinetics, tolerability and clinical effectiveness of quetiapine fumarate: An open-label trial in adolescents with psychotic disorders. *J Clin Psychiatry* 2000;61:252–260.

McCracken JT, McGough J, Shah B, et al.: Risperidone in children with autism and serious behavior problems. *N Engl J Med* 2002;347:314–321.

McDougle CJ, Kem DL, Posey DJ: Case series: use of ziprasidone for maladaptive symptoms in youths with autism. *J Am Acad Child Adolesc Psychiatry* 2002; 41:921–927.

Meighen KG, Shelton HM, McDougle CJ: Ziprasidone treatment of two adolescents with psychosis. *J Child Adolesc Psychopharmacol* 2004;14:139–144.

Olanzapine/fluoxetine for bipolar depression. *Med Lett* 2004;46:23–24.

Remschmidt H, Henninghausen K, Clement HW, et al.: Atypical neuroleptics in child and adolescent psychiatry. *Eur Child Adolesc Psychiatr* 2000;9 (Suppl 1):9–19.

Research Units on Pediatric Psychopharmacology Autism Network. Risperidone in children with autism and serious behavioral problems. *N Engl J Med* 2002;347:314–321.

Riddle MA, Kastelic DA, Frosch E: Pediatric psychopharmacology. *J Child Psychol Psychiatry* 2001;42:73–90.

Schatzberg AF, Nemeroff CB: *The American Psychiatric Publishing Textbook of Psychopharmacology*, 3d ed. Washington, DC: American Psychiatric Publishing, p. 1248, 2004.

Sikich, Hamer RM, Sheitman BB, Lieberman JA: A pilot study of risperidone, olanzapine, and haloperidol in psychotic youth: a double-blind, randomized, 8-week trial. *Neuropsychopharmacol* 2004;29(1): 133–145.

Stigler KA, Potenza MM, McDougle CJ: Tolerability profile of atypical antipsychotics in children and adolescents. *Paediatr Drugs* 2001;3:927–942.

Turetz M, Mozes T, Toren P, et al.: An open trial of clozapine in neuroleptic resistant childhood-onset schizophrenia. *Br J Psychiatry* 1997;170: 507–510.

Weiner JM, Dulcan MK (eds.): *The American Psychiatric Publishing Textbook of Child and Adolescent Psychiatry*, 3d ed. Washington, DC: American Psychiatric Publishing, p. 1114, 2004.

World Health Organization: *The World Health Report 2001—Mental Health: New Understanding, New Hope.* Geneva: World Health Organization, 2001.

Wyatt RJ, Damiani LM, Henter ID: First-episode schizophrenia. Early intervention and medication discontinuation in the context of course and treatment. *Br J Psychiatry* 1998;172(Suppl 33):77.

INDEX

Page numbers followed by italic *f* or *t* denote figures or tables, respectively.

Orthostatic hypotension, 270–271
Orthostatic proteinuria, 335–336
OSA. *See* Obstructive sleep apnea
Osgood-Schlatter disease, 689
Osmotic diarrhea, 162. *See also* Diarrhea
Osteoblastoma, 193
Osteochondritis, 450–451
Osteochondritis dissecans, 189–190, 189*t*
Osteogenesis imperfecta, 473
Osteoid osteoma, 192–193, 193*t*
Osteolysis, atraumatic, 682–683
Osteomalacia, 227
Osteomyelitis
  hematogenous, 448–451
  nonhematogenous, 450–453
  vertebral, 186
Osteopenia
  in anorexia nervosa, 643, 646
  in cystic fibrosis, 118–119
  evaluation and screening, 227
  treatment, 228, 646
Osteoporosis
  alcohol consumption and, 619
  anorexia nervosa and, 643
  calcium intake and, 616, 619, 620
  in cystic fibrosis, 118–119
  pathophysiology, 227
  risk factors, 227
  screening, 227
  treatment, 228
Osteotomy, 216
Otitis externa, 87–88, 88*t*
Otitis media, 89–90, 89*t*
Otorrhea, 90
Ovarian fibroma, 611
Ovarian tumors
  benign, 611, 614
  malignant, 549, 610*t*, 611–613
Overuse injuries
  elbow, 683–684, 683*t*
  knee, 687–689, 687*t*, 688*t*
  pathophysiology, 678–679, 679*t*
  shoulder, 681–683, 682*t*
  treatment, 679
  wrist, 684–685
Oxaprozin, 213*t*
Oxcarbazepine, 246*t*
Oxybutynin, 357, 357*t*
Oxycodone
  abuse, 711
  dosage and half-life, 72*t*

P

Pain management
  in end-of-life care, 71, 72*t*, 73*t*
  in sickle cell disease, 389
Palilalia, 276
PAN. *See* Polyarteritis nodosa
Pancreas, artificial, 314
Pancreatitis, 172–173
Panic attacks/panic disorder, 740–741
PAP devices. *See* Positive airway pressure (PAP)
  devices
Papilledema, 263–265, 264*t*
Parasomnias, 287–288
Parathyroid hormone, for osteoporosis, 228
Parenting, adolescent, 568–569
Parotid hypertrophy, in bulimia nervosa, 640
Partner violence, 486
Patellar dislocation, 687
Patent ductus arteriosus (PDA), 142
PCN. *See* Percutaneous nephrolithopaxy
PCP. *See* Phencyclidine
PDA. *See* Patent ductus arteriosus
Pectus carinatum, 106–107, 106*f*
Pectus excavatum, 106, 106*f*
Pediatric oncologists, 400–401
Pediculosis, 430–431, 541
Pediculus humanus capitis, 430
Pediculus humanus humanus, 430
Pelvic congestion syndrome, 596–597
Pelvic examination
  for oral contraceptive prescription, 550
  for sexually transmitted infection detection, 518
Pelvic inflammatory disease (PID)
  clinical manifestations, 525–526
  complications and sequelae, 223
  diagnostic tests, 525–526, 525*t*
  epidemiology, 525
  etiology, 525
  follow-up, 523*t*
  oral contraceptives and, 549
  partner referral, 523*t*
  treatment, 526–527, 526*t*
Pemoline, 763
Penis, 367–368
Peptic ulcer disease, 159, 160*t*
Percutaneous nephrolithopaxy (PCN), 354
Periappendicitis, 520
Pericarditis, 151–152
Pericardium, as source of chest pain, 132
Perihepatitis, 520, 524
Perimolysis, 101